HUMAN PHYSIOLOGY AND MECHANISMS OF DISEASE

FOURTH EDITION

ARTHUR C. GUYTON, M.D.

Chairman and Professor
Department of Physiology and Biophysics
University of Mississippi, School of Medicine

1987
W. B. SAUNDERS COMPANY
Philadelphia London Toronto Mexico City
Rio de Janeiro Sydney Tokyo Hong Kong

W. B. Saunders Company: West Washington Square
Philadelphia, PA   19105

Library of Congress Cataloging-in-Publication Data

Guyton, Arthur C.

Human physiology and mechanisms of disease.

Includes bibliographies and index.

1. Human physiology.   2. Physiology, Pathological.
I. Title.

QP34.5.G87 1987   612   86–15530

ISBN 0–7216–2114–7

Editors: W. B. Saunders Staff

Developmental Editor: Kitty McCullough

Designer: Karen O'Keefe

Production Manager: Carolyn Naylor

Manuscript Editor: Lorraine Zawodny

Cover Illustrator: Philip Ashley

Illustration Coordinator: Peg Shaw

Indexer: Ann Cassar

Listed here are the latest translated editions of this book together with
the language of the translation and the publisher.

Bahasa Malaysia (3rd Edition)—Universiti Sains Malaysia, Minden, Malaysia

Greek (3rd Edition)—C. G. Listsas, Athens, Greece

Portuguese (2nd Edition)—DISCO CBS Industria e Comercio Ltd., Rio de Janeiro, Brazil

Spanish (2nd Edition)—Nueva Editorial Interamericana, S.A.

Human Physiology and Mechanisms of Disease   ISBN   0-7216-2114-7

Last digit is the print number: 9   8   7   6   5   4   3   2   1

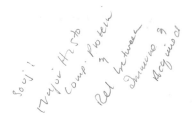

Preface

This textbook, entitled *HUMAN PHYSIOLOGY AND MECHANISMS OF DISEASE*, is written for those college and professional students, both medical and nonmedical, who cannot afford the time to study one of the more formidable books and yet require more than an elementary introduction to the physiology of the human body. In general, the types of material presented are twofold: first, the basic fundamental principles of life itself, beginning with the biology of cellular function as based on well-known physical, chemical, and molecular laws and, second, the important concepts and principles of physiology that are necessary for understanding the overall, integrated functions of the human body.

This is the fourth edition of this text. The changes that have been made from the third edition are mainly a shift in emphasis toward more fundamental molecular mechanisms of physiology. The principal reason for this shift is that this is the area of greatest advance in physiology. Fortunately, this new knowledge also simplifies many of the explanations for which only speculation could previously be used.

A continuing effort has also been made to use feedback from students to modify the portions of the text that the students find difficult. Special examples occur in Chapters 4 and 5, wherein the descriptions of membrane transport, membrane potentials, and action potentials have been reworked to give even more basic discussions yet greatly simplified exposition of the phenomena.

I hope that this text can convey to the student that our bodies are among the most complex and beautiful of all functional mechanisms. I hope that he or she will understand that each individual living cell carries within its nucleus all the genetic information required to create an entire human being and yet that this same genetic pool includes a myriad of intracellular control systems that regulate literally thousands of chemical reactions within each cell. Also, I hope that all students will begin to realize, as a special example, that the human brain is a computer having capabilities and functions that all the electronic computers in the world cannot at present achieve. I could go on detailing the miracles of the human body. That, indeed, is the purpose of this entire text, and the success of the book will be measured by the degree of excitement that it leaves with the student as a motive for further study in the field of physiology or for a lifetime of physiological thinking.

A small but important portion of this text presents not only knowledge that has come from basic experiments in animals but also knowledge that has come from human experiments, especially unplanned experiments caused by disease. For instance, a major share of our knowledge of the regulation of blood glucose and of the mechanisms of carbohydrate metabolism has come from study of diabetes mellitus, a disease that alters these physiological functions profoundly and that is widespread among the human population. Likewise, literally thousands of human "experiments" proceed each day in the fields of high blood pressure, congestive heart failure, gastrointestinal disturbances, respiratory diseases, and so forth. The physiology of each of these abnormalities is discussed briefly, partly because study of the diseases themselves can be enlightening but even more, because they give important insights into basic physiological concepts.

Finally, I would like to thank many others who have contributed to the development of this text. For the figures in the text I am especially indebted to Ms. Tomiko Mita, and for excellent secretarial services I owe my gratitude to Mrs. Ivadelle Osberg Heidke and Ms. Gwendolyn Robbins. I also extend my appreciation to the staff of the W. B. Saunders Company for its continued excellence in all publication matters, with appreciation especially to Mr. Dana Dreibelbis, Editor; Karen O'Keefe, Designer; Carolyn Naylor, Production Manager; Lorraine Zawodny, Manuscript Editor; and Peg Shaw, Illustration Coordinator, whose editorial and technical help have been invaluable.

ARTHUR C. GUYTON, M.D.

Contents

I Introduction to Physiology: The Cell and General Physiology **1**

1 Functional Organization of the Human Body and Control of the
  Internal Environment 2

2 The Cell and Its Function 8

3 Genetic Control of Cell Function—Protein Synthesis and Cell
  Reproduction 20

4 Transport Through the Cell Membrane 32

II Nerve and Muscle **43**

5 Membrane Potentials, Action Potentials, Excitation, and
  Rhythmicity 44

6 Contraction of Skeletal Muscle 57

7 Neuromuscular Transmission; Function of Smooth Muscle 69

III The Heart **79**

8 Heart Muscle; the Heart as a Pump 80

9 Rhythmic Excitation of the Heart 90

10 The Electrocardiogram 98

IV The Circulation **109**

11 Physics of Blood, Blood Flow, and Pressure: Hemodynamics 110

12 The Systemic and Pulmonary Circulation 118

13 Local Control of Blood Flow by the Tissues; Nervous and
Humoral Regulation 129

14 Nervous Reflex and Hormonal Mechanisms for Short-Term
Arterial Pressure Control 139

15 Long-Term Regulation of Mean Arterial Pressure;
Hypertension 147

16 Cardiac Output and Circulatory Shock 156

17 Coronary Blood Flow; Cardiac Failure; Heart Sounds; Valvular
and Congenital Heart Defects 169

18 Muscle Blood Flow During Exercise; Cerebral, Splanchnic, and
Skin Blood Flows 183

V **Blood Cells, Immunity, and Blood Clotting** **193**

19 Red Blood Cells, White Blood Cells, and Resistance of the
Body to Infection 194

20 Immunity, Allergy, Blood Groups, Transfusion, and
Transplantation 206

21 Hemostasis and Blood Coagulation 218

VI **The Body Fluids and the Kidneys** **227**

22 Capillary Dynamics; Exchange of Fluid Between the Blood and
Interstitial Fluid 228

23 The Lymphatic System, Interstitial Fluid Dynamics, Edema, the
Pulmonary Fluid, and the Special Fluid Systems 237

24 Formation of Urine by the Kidneys 247

25 Regulation of Blood Fluids and Their Constituents by the
Kidneys and the Thirst Mechanism 266

26 Regulation of Acid-Base Balance; Renal Disease; Micturition 279

VII **Respiration** **293**

27 Pulmonary Ventilation and Physical Principles of Gaseous
Exchange 294

28 Transport of Oxygen and Carbon Dioxide Between the Alveoli
and the Tissue Cells 305

29 Regulation of Respiration and Respiratory Insufficiency 318

VIII   Aviation, Space, and Deep Sea Diving Physiology 331

30   Aviation, Space, and Deep Sea Diving Physiology 332

IX   The Central Nervous System 343

31   Organization of the Nervous System; Basic Functions of
Synapses and Neuronal Circuits 344

32   Sensory Receptors and Mechanoreceptive Somatic Sensations 363

33   Somatic Sensations: Pain, Visceral Pain, Headache, and
Thermal Sensations 377

34   The Spinal Cord and Brain Stem Reflexes and Function of the
Vestibular Apparatus 386

35   Motor Control by the Motor Cortex, the Basal Ganglia, and
the Cerebellum 400

36   The Cerebral Cortex and Intellectual Functions of the Brain 415

37   Activation of the Brain; Wakefulness and Sleep; Behavioral
Functions of the Brain 425

38   The Autonomic Nervous System; the Adrenal Medulla 439

X   The Special Senses 447

39   The Eye: I. Optics of Vision and Function of the Retina 448

40   The Eye: II. Neurophysiology of Vision 462

41   The Sense of Hearing and the Chemical Senses of Taste and
Smell 472

XI   The Gastrointestinal Tract 485

42   Movement of Food Through the Alimentary Tract 486

43   Secretory Functions of the Alimentary Tract 497

44   Digestion and Absorption in the Gastrointestinal Tract;
Gastrointestinal Disorders 510

XII   Metabolism and Temperature Regulation 521

45   Metabolism of Carbohydrates and Formation of Adenosine
Triphosphate 522

46 Lipid and Protein Metabolism 531

47 Energetics, Metabolic Rate, and Regulation of Body Temperature 542

48 Dietary Balances, Regulation of Feeding, Obesity, and Vitamins 553

XIII Endocrinology and Reproduction 563

49 Introduction to Endocrinology; the Pituitary Hormones 564

50 The Thyroid Metabolic Hormones 576

51 The Adrenocortical Hormones 585

52 Insulin, Glucagon, and Diabetes Mellitus 595

53 Parathyroid Hormone, Calcitonin, Calcium and Phosphate Metabolism, Vitamin D, Bone, and Teeth 605

54 Reproductive Functions of the Male, the Male Sex Hormones, and the Pineal Gland 619

55 Prepregnancy Reproductive Functions in the Female and the Female Hormones 629

56 Pregnancy, Lactation, and Fetal and Neonatal Physiology 640

XIV Sports Physiology 655

57 Sports Physiology 656

Index 669

I

INTRODUCTION TO PHYSIOLOGY: THE CELL AND GENERAL PHYSIOLOGY

1 ■ Functional Organization of the Human Body and Control of the Internal Environment

2 ■ The Cell and Its Function

3 ■ Genetic Control of Cell Function—Protein Synthesis and Cell Reproduction

4 ■ Transport Through the Cell Membrane

1

Functional Organization of the Human Body and Control of the Internal Environment

CELLS AS THE LIVING UNITS OF THE
  BODY
THE EXTRACELLULAR FLUID—THE
  INTERNAL ENVIRONMENT
HOMEOSTATIC MECHANISMS OF THE
  MAJOR FUNCTIONAL SYSTEMS
  HOMEOSTASIS
  *THE EXTRACELLULAR FLUID
    TRANSPORT SYSTEM—THE
    CIRCULATORY SYSTEM*

*ORIGIN OF NUTRIENTS IN THE
  EXTRACELLULAR FLUID*
*REMOVAL OF METABOLIC END-
  PRODUCTS*
*REGULATION OF BODY FUNCTIONS
REPRODUCTION*
THE CONTROL SYSTEMS OF THE BODY
  *EXAMPLES OF CONTROL
    MECHANISMS*
AUTOMATICITY OF THE BODY

In human physiology we attempt to explain the specific characteristics and mechanisms of the human body that make it a living being. The very fact that we remain alive is almost beyond our own control, for hunger makes us seek food and fear makes us seek refuge. Sensations of cold make us provide warmth, and other forces cause us to seek fellowship and to reproduce. Thus, the human being is actually an automaton, and the fact that we are sensing, feeling, and knowledgeable beings is part of this automatic sequence of life; these special attributes allow us to exist under widely varying conditions that otherwise would make life impossible.

CELLS AS THE LIVING UNITS OF THE BODY

The basic living unit of the body is the cell, and each organ is an aggregate of many different cells held together by intercellular supporting structures. Each type of cell is specially adapted to perform one or a few particular functions. For instance, the red blood cells, 25 trillion in all, transport oxygen from the lungs to the tissues. Though this type of cell is

perhaps the most abundant, there are approximately another 50 trillion cells. The entire body, then, contains about 75 trillion cells.

Though the many cells of the body often differ markedly from each other, all of them have certain basic characteristics that are alike. For instance, in all cells oxygen combines with carbohydrate, fat, or protein to release the energy required for cell function. Furthermore, the general mechanisms for changing nutrients into energy are basically the same in all cells, and all the cells also deliver the end-products of their chemical reactions into the surrounding fluids.

Most cells of the body also have the ability to reproduce, and whenever cells of a particular type are destroyed from one cause or another, the remaining cells of this type usually divide again and again until the appropriate number is replenished.

THE EXTRACELLULAR FLUID— THE INTERNAL ENVIRONMENT

About 56 per cent of the adult human body is fluid. Though most of this fluid is inside the cells and is called *intracellular fluid,* about one third is in the spaces outside the cells and is called *extracellular fluid.* This extracellular fluid is in constant motion throughout the body. It is rapidly transported by the blood circulation and then mixed between the blood and the tissue fluids by diffusion through the capillary walls. In the extracellular fluid are the ions and nutrients needed for maintenance of cellular life. Therefore, all cells live in essentially the same environment, that is, the extracellular fluid. For this reason the extracellular fluid is called the *internal environment* of the body, or the *milieu intérieur,* a term introduced a hundred years ago by the great 19th century French physiologist Claude Bernard.

Cells are capable of living, growing, and providing their special functions so long as the proper concentrations of oxygen, glucose, the different ions, amino acids, and fatty substances are available in this internal environment.

Differences Between Extracellular and Intracellular Fluids. The extracellular fluid contains large amounts of sodium, chloride, and bicarbonate ions, plus nutrients for the cells, such as oxygen, glucose, fatty acids, and amino acids. It also contains carbon dioxide that is being transported from the cells to the lungs to be excreted and other cellular products that are being transported to the kidneys for excretion.

The intracellular fluid differs significantly from the extracellular fluid; particularly, it contains large amounts of potassium, magnesium, and phosphate ions instead of the sodium and chloride ions found in the extracellular fluid. Special mechanisms for transporting ions through the cell membranes maintain these differences. These mechanisms will be discussed in Chapter 4.

HOMEOSTATIC MECHANISMS OF THE MAJOR FUNCTIONAL SYSTEMS

HOMEOSTASIS

The term *homeostasis* is used by physiologists to mean *maintenance of static,* or *constant, conditions in the internal environment.* Essentially all the organs and tissues of the body perform functions that help to maintain these constant conditions. For instance, the lungs provide oxygen to the extracellular fluid to replenish continually the oxygen that is being used by the cells; the kidneys maintain constant ion concentrations; and the gastrointestinal system provides nutrients. A large segment of this text is concerned with the manner in which each organ or tissue contributes to homeostasis. To begin this discussion, the different functional systems of the body and their homeostatic mechanisms will be outlined briefly.

THE EXTRACELLULAR FLUID TRANSPORT SYSTEM— THE CIRCULATORY SYSTEM

Extracellular fluid is transported through all parts of the body in two different stages. The first stage

entails movement of blood around and around the circulatory system, and the second, movement of fluid between the blood capillaries and the cells. Figure 1–1 illustrates the overall circulation of blood, showing that the heart is actually two separate pumps, one of which propels blood through the lungs and the other through the systemic circulation. All the blood in the circulation traverses the entire circuit of the circulation an average of once each minute at rest and as many as six times each minute when a person becomes extremely active.

As blood passes through the capillaries, continual fluid exchange occurs between the plasma portion of the blood and the interstitial fluid that fills the spaces between the cells—the intercellular spaces. This process is illustrated in Figure 1–2. Note that the capillaries are porous so that large amounts of fluid and its dissolved constituents can *diffuse* back and forth between the blood and the tissue spaces, as illustrated by the arrows. This process of diffusion is caused by kinetic motion of the molecules in both the plasma and the interstitial fluid. That is, the fluid and dissolved molecules are continually moving and bouncing in all directions within the fluid itself and also through the pores as well as through the tissue spaces. Almost no cell is located more than 25 to 50 microns from a capillary, which insures diffusion of almost any substance from the capillary to the cell within a few seconds. Thus, the extracellular fluid everywhere in the body, both that of the plasma and that in interstitial spaces, is continually being mixed, thereby maintaining almost complete homogeneity.

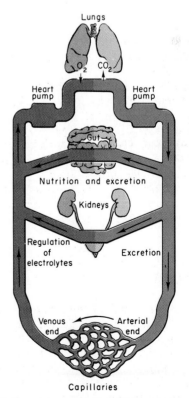

Figure 1–1. General organization of the circulatory system.

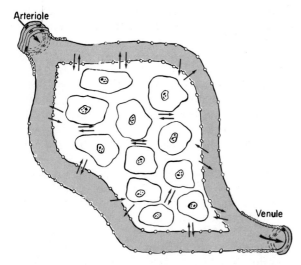

Figure 1–2. Diffusion of fluids through the capillary walls and through the interstitial spaces.

ORIGIN OF NUTRIENTS IN THE EXTRACELLULAR FLUID

The Respiratory System. Figure 1–1 shows that each time the blood passes through the body it also flows through the lungs. The blood picks up oxygen in the alveoli, thus acquiring the oxygen needed by the cells. The membrane between the alveoli and the lumen of the pulmonary capillaries is only 0.4 to 2.0 microns in thickness, and oxygen diffuses through this membrane into the blood in exactly the same manner that water and the ions diffuse through the tissue capillaries.

The Gastrointestinal Tract. A large portion of the blood pumped by the heart also passes through the walls of the gastrointestinal organs. Here different dissolved nutrients, including carbohydrates, fatty acids, amino acids, and others, are absorbed into the extracellular fluid.

The Liver and Other Organs That Perform Primarily Metabolic Functions. Not all substances absorbed from the gastrointestinal tract can be used in their absorbed form by the cells. The liver changes the chemical compositions of many of these to more usable forms, and other tissues of the body—the fat cells, the gastrointestinal mucosa, the kidneys, and the endocrine glands—help to modify the absorbed substances or store them until they are needed at a later time.

Musculoskeletal System. Sometimes the question is asked: How does the musculoskeletal system fit into the homeostatic functions of the body? The answer to this is obvious and simple: Were it not for this system, the body could not move to the appropriate place at the appropriate time to obtain the foods required for nutrition. The musculoskeletal system also provides motility for protection against adverse surroundings, without which the entire body, and along with it all the homeostatic mechanisms, could be destroyed instantly.

REMOVAL OF METABOLIC END-PRODUCTS

Removal of Carbon Dioxide by the Lungs. At the same time that blood picks up oxygen in the lungs, carbon dioxide is released from the blood into the alveoli, and the movement of air into and out of the alveoli during breathing carries the carbon dioxide to the atmosphere. Carbon dioxide is the most abundant of all the end-products of metabolism.

The Kidneys. Passage of the blood through the kidneys removes most substances from the plasma that are not needed by the cells. These substances include especially different end-products of cellular metabolism as well as excesses of ions and water that might have accumulated in the extracellular fluid. The kidneys perform their function by, first, filtering large quantities of plasma through the glomeruli into the kidney tubules and then reabsorbing into the blood those substances needed by the body such as glucose, amino acids, appropriate amounts of water, and many of the ions. However, the substances not needed by the body, for instance, the metabolic end-products such as urea, are not reabsorbed at all or only poorly so; instead, they pass on through the renal tubules into the urine.

REGULATION OF BODY FUNCTIONS

The Nervous System. The nervous system is composed of three major parts: the *sensory portion,* the *central nervous system* (or *integrative portion*), and the *motor portion.* Sensory receptors detect the state of the body or the state of the surroundings. For instance, receptors present everywhere in the skin apprise one every time an object touches the skin. The eyes are sensory organs that give one a visual image of the surrounding area.

The central nervous system is composed of the brain and spinal cord. The brain can store information, generate thoughts, create ambition, and determine reactions the body performs in response to the sensations. Appropriate signals are then transmitted to the muscles, glands, and other organs through the motor portion of the nervous system to carry out the person's desires.

A large segment of the nervous system is called the *autonomic system.* It operates at a subconscious level and controls many functions of the internal organs, including the action of the heart, the movements of the gastrointestinal tract, and the secretion by different glands.

The Hormonal System of Regulation. Located in the body are eight major endocrine glands that secrete special chemical substances, the *hormones,* that are transported in the extracellular fluid to all parts of the body to help regulate cellular function. For instance, thyroid hormone increases the rates of most chemical reactions in all cells. In this way thyroid hormone helps to set the tempo of bodily activity. Likewise, insulin controls glucose metabolism; adrenocortical hormones control ion and protein metabolism; and parathormone controls bone metabolism.

Thus, the hormones are a system of regulation that complements the nervous system. The nervous system, in general, regulates mainly muscular and secretory activities of the body, whereas the hormonal system regulates mainly the metabolic functions.

REPRODUCTION

Reproduction sometimes is not considered to be a homeostatic function. But it does help to maintain static conditions by generating new beings to take the place of ones that are dying. This perhaps sounds like a farfetched usage of the term homeostasis, but it does illustrate that, in the final analysis, essentially all structures of the body are so organized that they help maintain the automaticity and the continuity of life.

THE CONTROL SYSTEMS OF THE BODY

The human body has literally thousands of control systems in it. The most intricate of all these are the genetic control systems that operate within all cells to control intracellular function, and also to control all life processes, a subject that will be discussed in detail in Chapter 3. Many other control systems operate within the organs to control functions of individual parts of the organs; others operate throughout the entire body to control the interrelationships between the organs. For instance, the respiratory system, operating in association with the nervous system, regulates the concentration of carbon dioxide in the extracellular fluid. The liver and the pancreas regulate the concentration of glucose in the extracellular fluid. And the kidneys regulate the concentrations of hydrogen, sodium, potassium, phosphate, and other ions in the extracellular fluid.

EXAMPLES OF CONTROL MECHANISMS

Regulation of Oxygen and Carbon Dioxide Concentrations in the Extracellular Fluid. Since oxygen is one of the major substances required for chemical reactions in the cells, it is fortunate that the body has a special control mechanism to maintain an almost exact and constant oxygen concentration in the extracellular fluid. This mechanism depends principally on the chemical characteristics of *hemoglobin,* which is present in all the red blood cells. Hemoglobin combines with oxygen as the blood passes through the lungs. Then, as the blood passes through the tissue capillaries, the hemoglobin will not release oxygen into the tissue fluid if too much oxygen is already there, but if the oxygen concentration is too little, sufficient oxygen will be released to re-establish an adequate tissue oxygen concentration. Thus, the regulation of oxygen concentration in the tissues is vested principally in the chemical characteristics of hemoglobin itself. This regulation is called the *oxygen-buffering function of hemoglobin.*

Carbon dioxide concentration in the extracellular fluid is regulated in quite a different way. Carbon dioxide is one of the major end-products of the oxidative reactions in cells. If all the carbon dioxide formed in the cells should continue to accumulate in the tissue fluids, the mass action of the carbon dioxide itself would soon halt all the energy-giving reactions of the cells. Fortunately, a high carbon dioxide concentration *excites the respiratory center,* located in the basal regions of the brain, causing the person to breathe rapidly and deeply. This increases the expiration of carbon dioxide and therefore increases its removal from the blood and extracellular fluid, and the process continues until the concentration returns to normal.

Regulation of Arterial Pressure. Several different systems contribute to the regulation of arterial pressure. One of these, the *baroreceptor system,* is a very simple and excellent example of a control mechanism. In the walls of most of the great arteries of the upper body, especially in the bifurcation region of the carotids and the arch of the aorta, are many nerve receptors, called *baroreceptors,* which are stimulated by stretch of the arterial wall. When the arterial pressure becomes great, these baroreceptors are stimulated excessively, and nerve signals are transmitted to the medulla of the brain. Here the signals inhibit the *vasomotor center,* which in turn decreases nerve signals transmitted through the sympathetic nervous system to the heart and blood vessels. Lack of these signals causes diminished pumping activity by the heart and increased ease of blood flow through the peripheral vessels, both of which lower the arterial pressure back toward normal. Conversely, a fall in arterial pressure relaxes the stretch receptors, allowing the vasomotor center to become more active than usual and thereby causing the arterial pressure to rise back toward normal.

Negative Feedback Nature of Control Systems

Most of the control systems of the body act by a process of *negative feedback,* which can be explained best by analyzing the baroreceptor pressure-regulating mechanism that was just discussed. In this mechanism, it is clear that a high pressure causes a series of reactions that promote a lowered pressure, or a low pressure causes a series of reactions that promote an elevated pressure. In both instances these effects are opposite to, or *negative* to, the initiating stimulus, hence the term "negative feedback."

Essentially all other control mechanisms of the body also operate by the process of negative feedback. For instance, if the oxygen concentration in the body fluids falls too low, the mechanisms for controlling oxygen automatically return the oxygen back to a higher level. Thus, the effect is *negative* to the initiating stimulus. Likewise, elevated carbon dioxide concentration in the body fluids causes increased respiration, which then removes the excess carbon dioxide. Again, the response is negative to the stimulus. Essentially all of the endocrine control systems also operate in this manner. For instance, when the concentration of potassium falls too low in the extracellular fluid, the adrenal glands decrease their secretion of the hormone aldosterone, and lack of this hormone decreases the rate of potassium excretion by the kidneys into the urine. Therefore, potassium accumulates in the extracellular fluid until its concentration returns to normal. This is still another example of negative feedback.

Thus, in general, if some factor becomes excessive or too little, a control system initiates *negative feedback*, which consists of a series of changes that returns the factor toward a certain mean value, thus maintaining homeostasis.

Amplification, or Gain, of a Control System. The degree of effectiveness with which a control system maintains constant conditions is called the *amplification,* or *gain,* of the system.

For instance, let us assume that a large volume of blood is suddenly transfused into a person and that this immediately raises the arterial pressure from a normal value of 100 mm Hg up to 160 mm Hg. However, within 15 to 30 seconds the baroreceptor control mechanism becomes fully operative, and the arterial pressure is reduced back to 120 mm Hg. Thus, the pressure is corrected 40 mm Hg, while the final abnormality is only 20 mm Hg instead of the 60 mm Hg that would have occurred without the control system. The gain of the mechanism is calculated by the following equation:

$$\text{Gain} = \frac{\text{Amount of correction of abnormality}}{\text{Amount of abnormality still remaining}}$$

In the above example the correction is −40 mm Hg, and the amount of abnormality still remaining is 20 mm Hg; therefore, the gain of the baroreceptor system for control of arterial pressure is approximately −2.

The gains of different control systems of the body vary markedly, with gains as low as −1 to −2 for control of arterial pressure by a hormone called renin, which is released from the kidney, and as high as −30 for control of body temperature in the face of changing atmospheric temperature. In other words, the pressure-controlling ability of the renin mechanism is only moderate, while the temperature-controlling ability of the temperature feedback system is very great.

AUTOMATICITY OF THE BODY

The purpose of this chapter has been to point out, first, the overall organization of the body and, second, the means by which the different parts of the body operate in harmony. To summarize, the body is actually a *social order of about 75 trillion cells* organized into different functional structures, some of which are called *organs*. Each functional structure provides its share in the maintenance of homeostatic conditions in the extracellular fluid, which is often called the *internal environment*. As long as normal conditions are maintained in this internal environment, the cells of the body will continue to live and function properly. Thus, each cell benefits from homeostasis, and each in turn contributes its share toward the maintenance of homeostasis. This reciprocal interplay provides continuous automaticity of the body until one or more functional systems lose their ability to contribute their share of function. When this happens, all the cells of the body suffer. Extreme dysfunction leads to death, while moderate dysfunction leads to sickness.

QUESTIONS

1. Approximately how many cells are there in the body?
2. Explain what is meant by the "internal environment."
3. Explain the differences between the extracellular and intracellular fluids.
4. What is the meaning of the word *homeostasis*?
5. What role does the circulatory system play in homeostasis?
6. Explain what is meant by diffusion.
7. What is the role of the kidneys in homeostasis?
8. What are the three major portions of the nervous system?
9. Explain the importance of *negative feedback* as the basis for most control mechanisms.
10. If the arterial blood pressure suddenly becomes 80 mm Hg too high, but one of the pressure-controlling mechanisms then returns the pressure to a level that is only 10 mm Hg too high, what is the gain of that control mechanism?

References

Adolph, E. F.: Origins of Physiological Regulations. New York, Academic Press, 1968.

Adolph, E. F.: Physiological integrations in action. The Physiologist 25:(Suppl.) 1, 1982.

Bernard, C.: Lectures on the Phenomena of Life Common to Animals and Plants. Springfield, Ill., Charles C. Thomas, 1974.

Borow, M.: Fundamentals of Homeostasis: A Clinical Approach to Fluid

Electrolyte Acid-Base Energy Metabolism in Health and Disease. Flushing, N.Y., Medical Examination Publishing Co., 1977.

Bryant, P. J., and Simpson, P.: Intrinsic and extrinsic control of growth in developing organs. Q Rev Biol 59:387, 1984.

Cannon, W. B.: The Wisdom of the Body. New York, W. W. Norton & Co., 1932.

Frisancho, A. R.: Human Adaptation. St. Louis, C. V. Mosby Co., 1979.

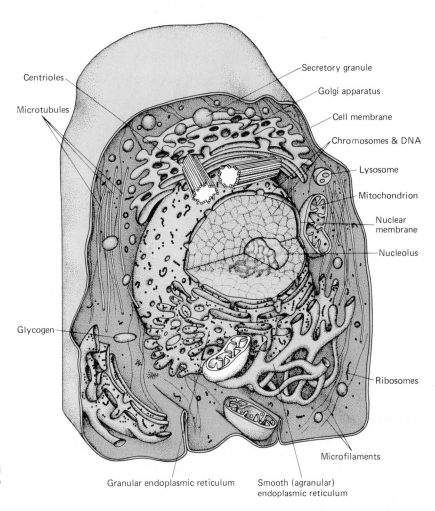

Figure 2–2. Reconstruction of a typical cell, showing the internal organelles in the cytoplasm and in the nucleus.

the other hand, often penetrate all the way through the membrane, thus interrupting the continuity of the lipid barrier and therefore providing pathways for passage of specific substances through the membrane. Also, many of the membrane proteins are enzymes that catalyze a multitude of different chemical reactions which will be the subjects of many discussions in this and future chapters.

The Cell Membrane

The Lipid Barrier of the Cell Membrane. Figure 2–3 illustrates the cell membrane. Its basic structure is a *lipid bilayer,* which is a thin film of lipids only 2 molecules thick that is continuous over the entire cell surface. Interspersed in this lipid film are large globular protein molecules.

The lipid bilayer is composed almost entirely of phospholipids and cholesterol. One part of each phospholipid or cholesterol molecule is *hydrophilic,* that is, soluble in water, whereas the other part is *hydrophobic,* that is, soluble only in fats. The phosphate radical of the phospholipid is hydrophilic, and the fatty acid radicals are fat-soluble. The cholesterol has a hydroxyl radical that is water soluble and a steroid nucleus that is fat soluble. Because the hydrophobic

portions of both these molecules are repelled by water but are mutually attracted to each other, they have a natural tendency to line up to form a membrane two molecules thick, as illustrated in Figure 2–3, so that the fatty portions occupy the center of the membrane and the hydrophilic portions project to the two surfaces in contact with the surrounding water.

The membrane lipid bilayer is a major impermeable barrier to the usual water-soluble substances such as ions, glucose, urea, and others. On the other hand, fat-soluble substances such as oxygen and alcohols can penetrate this portion of the membrane with ease.

A special feature of the lipid bilayer is that it is a *fluid* and not a solid. Therefore, portions of the membrane can literally flow from one point to another in the membrane. Proteins or other substances dissolved in or floating in the lipid bilayer tend to diffuse to all areas of the cell membrane.

The Cell Membrane Proteins. Figure 2–3 illustrates globular masses floating in the lipid bilayer. These are membrane proteins, most of which are *glycoproteins.* Two types of proteins occur: the *integral proteins* that protrude all the way through the membrane and the *peripheral proteins* that are attached only to the surface of the membrane and do not penetrate.

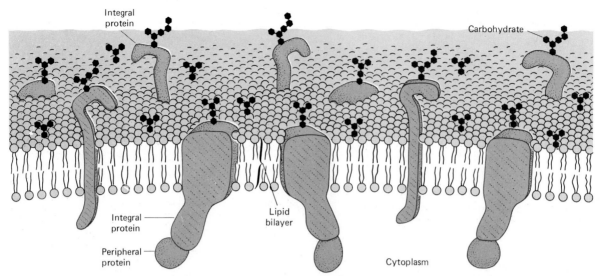

Figure 2–3. Structure of the cell membrane, showing that it is composed mainly from a lipid bilayer but with large numbers of protein molecules protruding through the layer. Also, carbohydrate moieties are attached to the protein molecules on the outside of the membrane and additional protein molecules on the inside. (From Lodish and Rothman: *Sci. Am.,* 240:48, 1979. ©1979 by Scientific American, Inc. All rights reserved.)

The integral proteins provide structural *channels* (or *pores*) through which water-soluble substances, especially the ions, can diffuse between the extracellular and intracellular fluid. However, these proteins have selective properties that cause preferential diffusion of some substances more than others. Some of them also act as *carrier proteins* for transporting substances that are too large to diffuse through the channels.

The peripheral proteins occur either entirely or almost entirely on the inside of the membrane, and they are normally attached to one of the integral proteins. These peripheral proteins function almost entirely as *enzymes*.

The Membrane Carbohydrates—The Cell Glyco-calyx. The membrane carbohydrates occur almost invariably in combination with proteins and lipids in the form of *glycoproteins* and *glycolipids*. In fact, most of the integral proteins are glycoproteins, and about one tenth of the lipid molecules are glycolipids. The "glyco-" portions of these molecules almost invariably protrude to the outside of the cell, dangling outward from the cell surface. Many other carbohydrate compounds, called *proteoglycans*, which are mainly carbohydrate substances bound together by small protein cores, are often loosely attached to the outer surface of the cell as well. Thus, the entire surface of the cell often has a loose carbohydrate coat called the *glycocalyx*.

These carbohydrate moieties attached to the outer surface of the cell have several important functions: (a) Many of them are negatively charged, which gives most cells an overall negative surface charge that repels other negative objects. (b) The glycocalyx of some cells attaches to the glycocalyx of other cells, thus attaching the cells to each other as well. (c) Some carbohydrates act as receptor substances for binding hormones like insulin that stimulate specific types of activity in the cells. (d) And some enter into immune reactions, as we shall discuss in Chapter 20.

THE CYTOPLASM AND ITS ORGANELLES

The cytoplasm is the fluid compartment between the cell membrane and the nuclear membrane. It is filled with both minute and large dispersed particles as well as organelles ranging in size from a few nanometers to many microns. The clear fluid portion of the cytoplasm in which the particles are dispersed is called *cytosol;* this contains mainly dissolved proteins, electrolytes, glucose, and small quantities of phospholipids, cholesterol, and esterified fatty acids.

Among the large dispersed particles in the cytoplasm are *neutral fat globules, glycogen granules, ribosomes, secretory granules,* and four especially important organelles—the *endoplasmic reticulum,* the *Golgi apparatus,* the *mitochondria,* and the *lysosomes.*

The Endoplasmic Reticulum

Figure 2–2 illustrates in the cytoplasm a network of tubular and flat vesicular structures called the *endoplasmic reticulum.* The tubules and vesicles all interconnect with each other in the manner illustrated in Figure 2–4. Also, their walls are constructed of lipid bilayer membranes containing large amounts of proteins, similar to the cell membrane. The total surface area of this structure in some cells—the liver cells, for instance—can be as much as 30 to 40 times as great as the cell membrane area.

The detailed structure of a small portion of endoplasmic reticulum is illustrated in Figure 2–4. The space inside the tubules and vesicles is filled with *endoplasmic matrix,* a fluid medium that is different from the fluid outside the endoplasmic reticulum.

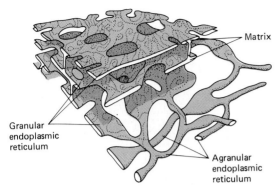

Figure 2-4. Structure of the endoplasmic reticulum. (Modified from De Robertis, Saez, and De Robertis: Cell Biology. 6th ed. Philadelphia, W. B. Saunders Company, 1975.)

Substances formed in different parts of the cell enter the space of the endoplasmic reticulum and are then conducted to other parts of the cell. Also, the vast surface area of the reticulum, as well as the many enzyme systems along the surfaces of its membranes, provides the machinery for a major share of the metabolic functions of the cell.

Ribosomes and the Granular Endoplasmic Reticulum. Attached to the outer surfaces of many parts of the endoplasmic reticulum are large numbers of small granular particles called *ribosomes* that function in the synthesis of proteins, as we shall discuss more fully later in this and the following chapter. Where these are present, the reticulum is frequently called the *granular endoplasmic reticulum.*

The Agranular Endoplasmic Reticulum. Part of the endoplasmic reticulum has no attached ribosomes. This part is called the *agranular,* or *smooth, endoplasmic reticulum.* The agranular reticulum functions in the synthesis of lipid substances and in many other enzymatic processes of the cell.

Golgi Apparatus

The Golgi apparatus, illustrated in Figure 2–5, is closely related to the endoplasmic reticulum. It has membranes similar to those of the agranular endo-

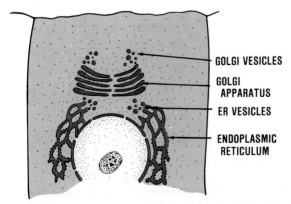

Figure 2-5. A typical Golgi apparatus and its relationship to the endoplasmic reticulum and the nucleus.

plasmic reticulum. It is usually composed of four or more stacked layers of thin, flat vesicles lying near the nucleus. This apparatus is very prominent in secretory cells; in these it is located on the side of the cell from which the secretory substances will be extruded.

The Golgi apparatus also functions in association with the endoplasmic reticulum. As illustrated in Figure 2–5, small "transport vesicles" continually pinch off from the endoplasmic reticulum and shortly thereafter fuse with the Golgi apparatus. In this way substances are transported from the endoplasmic reticulum to the Golgi apparatus. The transported substances are then processed in the Golgi apparatus to form *lysosomes, secretory vesicles,* or other cytoplasmic components to be discussed later in the chapter.

The Lysosomes

The lysosomes, which are formed by the Golgi apparatus, provide an intracellular digestive system that allows the cell to digest and thereby remove unwanted substances, such as bacteria. The lysosome, illustrated in Figure 2–2, is quite different from one cell to another, but it is usually 250 to 750 nanometers in diameter. It is surrounded by a typical lipid bilayer membrane and is filled with large numbers of small granules 5 to 8 nanometers in diameter, which are protein aggregates of digestive enzymes. Proteins are digested to form amino acids, and the different carbohydrates are digested mainly to form glucose. More than 40 different *acid hydrolases* (digestive enzymes) have been found in lysosomes, and the principal substances that they digest are proteins, nucleic acids, mucopolysaccharides, lipids, and glycogen.

Ordinarily, the membrane surrounding the lysosome prevents the enclosed hydrolytic enzymes from coming in contact with other substances in the cell. However, many different conditions of the cell will break the membranes of some of the lysosomes, allowing release of the enzymes. These enzymes then split the organic substances with which they come in contact into small, highly diffusible substances, such as amino acids and glucose. Some of the more specific functions of lysosomes are discussed later in the chapter.

The Mitochondria

Dispersed widely in the cytoplasm, as illustrated in Figure 2–2, are large numbers of mitochondria, which are called the "powerhouses" of the cell. Without them the cells would be unable to extract significant amounts of energy from the nutrients and oxygen, and as a consequence essentially all cellular functions would cease. The number of mitochondria per cell varies from less than a hundred up to as many as several thousand, depending upon the amount of energy required by each cell.

The basic structure of the mitochondrion is illustrated in Figure 2–6, which shows it to be composed

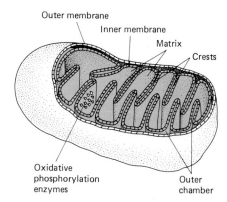

Figure 2–6. Structure of a mitochondrion. (Modified from De Robertis, Saez, and De Robertis: Cell Biology. 6th ed. Philadelphia, W. B. Saunders Company, 1975.)

mainly of two lipid bilayer-protein membranes: an *outer membrane* and an *inner membrane*. Many infoldings of the inner membrane form *shelves* onto which oxidative enzymes are attached. In addition, the inner cavity of the mitochondrion is filled with a gel *matrix* containing large quantities of dissolved enzymes that are also necessary for extracting energy from nutrients. The liberated energy is used to synthesize a high-energy substance called *adenosine triphosphate (ATP)*. ATP is then transported out of the mitochondrion, and it diffuses throughout the cell to release its energy wherever it is needed for performing cellular functions. The details of ATP formation by the mitochondrion are given in Chapter 45; however, some of the important functions of ATP in the cell are introduced later in this chapter.

Other Cytoplasmic Structures and Organelles

Throughout this text we learn that there are literally hundreds of different types of cells, and each of these has special unique structures. For instance, some of the cells are rigid. This is usually achieved by the presence in the cytoplasmic compartment of large numbers of filamentous or tubular structures composed of fibrillar proteins. Also, some of the tubular structures, called *microtubules,* can actually transport substances from one part of a cell to another, thus providing an intracellular circulatory system. Also, it is structures composed of microtubules that form the rigid structures of (a) cilia that protrude from certain cell surfaces and move fluids along the surfaces, (b) the tail of the sperm that beats rhythmically and propels the sperm through the genital tract of the female, and (c) the mitotic apparatus that plays an essential role in cell division.

Fibrillar proteins also form the contractile apparatus of muscle cells, which we shall discuss in great detail in Chapter 6.

Finally, one of the important functions of many cells is to secrete special substances. All such substances are formed by the endoplasmic reticulum–Golgi apparatus system and are released from the Golgi apparatus into the cytoplasm inside storage vesicles called *secretory vesicles* or *secretory granules.* Then, at a later time, these are expelled through the cell membrane, as we shall discuss later in this chapter.

THE NUCLEUS

The nucleus, illustrated in Figure 2–7, is the control center of the cell. It controls both the chemical reactions that occur in the cell and reproduction of the cell. Briefly, the nucleus contains large quantities of *deoxyribonucleic acid,* which we have called *genes* for many years. The genes determine the characteristics of the protein structures and enzymes of the cytoplasm, and in this way control cytoplasmic activities. These activities of the nucleus are considered in detail in the following chapter.

The appearance of the nucleus under the microscope does not give much of a clue to the mechanisms by which it performs its control functions. Figure 2–7 illustrates the light microscopic appearance of the interphase nucleus (period between mitoses), showing darkly staining *chromatin material* throughout the *nucleoplasm.* During mitosis, the chromatin material becomes readily identifiable as part of the highly structured *chromosomes,* which can then be seen easily with the light microscope.

The Nuclear Envelope

The nuclear envelope is frequently called the *nuclear membrane.* However, it is actually two separate membranes, one inside the other. The outer membrane is continuous with the endoplasmic reticulum, and the space between the two nuclear membranes is also continuous with the compartment inside the endoplasmic reticulum.

The nuclear envelope is penetrated by several thousand very large *nuclear pores,* large enough to allow protein molecules as large as 44,000 molecular weight to pass through with relative ease and proteins with molecular weight less than 15,000 to pass extremely rapidly. It is through these pores that the large RNA molecules formed in the nucleus pass into the cyto-

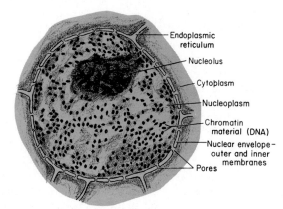

Figure 2–7. Structure of the nucleus.

plasm, where they control protein synthesis. We shall discuss this important function in the following chapter.

Nucleoli

The nuclei of many cells contain one or more lightly staining structures called *nucleoli*. The nucleolus contains large amounts of *ribonucleic acid* and proteins of the types found in ribosomes. The nucleolus becomes considerably enlarged when a cell is actively synthesizing proteins. The genes of several of the chromosome pairs synthesize the ribonucleic acid and then store it in the nucleolus, forming granular "subunits" of ribosomes. These in turn are transported through the nuclear membrane pores into the cytoplasm where they assemble together to form the "mature" ribosomes that play an essential role for the formation of proteins.

FUNCTIONAL SYSTEMS OF THE CELL

In the remainder of this chapter we will discuss several representative functional systems of the cell that make it a living organism.

INGESTION BY THE CELL—ENDOCYTOSIS

If a cell is to live and grow, it must obtain nutrients from the surrounding fluids. Substances can pass through a cell membrane in three separate ways: (1) by *diffusion* through the pores in the membrane or through the membrane matrix itself; (2) by *active transport* through the membrane, a mechanism in which enzyme systems and special carrier proteins transport the substances through the membrane; and (3) by *endocytosis,* a mechanism by which the membrane actually engulfs particulate matter or extracellular fluid and its contents. The important subject of transport of substances by diffusion and active transport, the means by which most nutrients and other substances enter the cell, will be considered in detail in Chapter 4. Endocytosis is a specialized cellular function that merits mention here.

Endocytosis begins by the formation of small vesicles at the cell membrane; these vesicles then pinch off to the interior of the cell and float freely in the cytoplasm. The two principal forms of endocytosis are called *pinocytosis* and *phagocytosis*. Pinocytosis means the formation of extremely small vesicles containing extracellular fluid. Phagocytosis means ingestion of large particles, such as bacteria, cells, or portions of degenerating tissue.

Pinocytosis. Pinocytosis occurs continually at the cell membranes of most cells, but especially rapidly in some cells. For instance, it occurs so rapidly in certain white blood cells that about 3 per cent of the total membrane is engulfed in the form of vesicles each minute. Even so, the pinocytic vesicles are so small, usually only 100 to 200 nanometers in diameter,

that most of their characteristics can be discerned only with the electron microscope.

Pinocytosis is the only means by which some very large macromolecules, such as most protein molecules, can enter cells. In fact, the rate at which pinocytic vesicles form usually is enhanced when such macromolecules attach to the cell membrane.

Figure 2–8 illustrates the successive steps of pinocytosis, showing three molecules of protein attaching to the membrane. These molecules usually attach to *receptors* in the membrane that are specific for the types of proteins that are to be absorbed, and these receptors generally are concentrated in small pits in the cell membrane, called *coated pits*. The inside surfaces of these pits, in turn, are coated with a dense material containing contractile filaments. Once the protein molecules have bound with the receptors, the surface properties of the membrane change in such a way that the entire pit invaginates inward and its borders close over the attached proteins, as well as over a small amount of extracellular fluid. Immediately thereafter, the invaginated portion of the membrane breaks away from the surface of the cell, forming a *pinocytic vesicle.*

Phagocytosis. Phagocytosis occurs in much the same way as pinocytosis, except that it involves large particles such as bacteria or dead tissues rather than macromolecules. Only certain cells have the capability of phagocytosis, most notably the tissue macrophages and some of the white blood cells. A postulated cause of phagocytosis is the presence of positive electrical charges on the surfaces of the phagocytized particles. Most normal particles in the extracellular fluid are negatively charged, the same as the outsides of the macrophages and white blood cells. Therefore, these particles are repelled from the cell surfaces. On the other hand, damaged tissues and bacteria that have been attacked by antibodies (a process called *opsonization,* which is discussed in Chapters 19 and 20) often acquire positive charges or other surface properties that allow them to be phagocytized.

Phagocytosis occurs in the following steps: First,

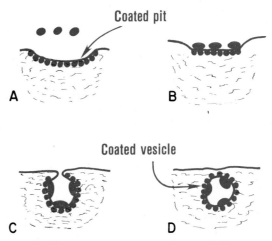

Figure 2–8. Mechanism of pinocytosis.

the cell membrane attaches to the surface of the object. Second, the edges of the membrane around the point of attachment suddenly evaginate outward and completely engulf the object within a fraction of a second. Third, the membrane contracts and pulls the object to the interior. And, fourth, the phagocytic vesicle pinches off to the interior of the cell in the same way that pinocytic vesicles are formed.

DIGESTION OF FOREIGN SUBSTANCES IN THE CELL—FUNCTION OF THE LYSOSOMES

Almost immediately after a pinocytic or phagocytic vesicle appears inside a cell, one or more lysosomes become attached to the vesicle and empty their digestive enzymes into the vesicle, as illustrated in Figure 2–9. Thus, a *digestive vesicle* is formed in which the hydrolases begin digesting the proteins, glycogen, nucleic acids, mucopolysaccharides, and other substances in the vesicle. The products of digestion are small molecules of amino acids, glucose, phosphates, and so forth that can then diffuse through the membrane of the vesicle into the cytoplasm. What is left of the digestive vesicle, called the *residual body,* represents the undigestible substances. In most instances this is finally excreted through the cell membrane by a process called *exocytosis,* which is essentially the opposite of endocytosis.

Thus, the lysosomes may be called the *digestive organs* of the cells.

The lysosomes also contain bactericidal agents that can kill phagocytized bacteria before they can cause cellular damage. These agents include *lysozyme* that dissolves the bacterial cell membrane, *lysoferrin* that binds iron and other metals that are essential for bacterial growth, and acid at a pH of about 5.0 that activates the digestive enzymes and at the same time inactivates some of the bacterial metabolic systems.

SYNTHESIS AND FORMATION OF CELLULAR STRUCTURES BY THE ENDOPLASMIC RETICULUM AND THE GOLGI APPARATUS

The extensiveness of the endoplasmic reticulum and the Golgi apparatus, especially in secretory cells, has already been emphasized. These two structures are made primarily of lipid bilayer membranes, and their walls are literally loaded with protein enzymes that catalyze the synthesis of many of the substances required by the cell.

In general, most synthesis begins in the endoplasmic reticulum; then the products formed in the endoplasmic reticulum are passed on to the Golgi apparatus where they are further processed prior to release into the cell. But, first, let us note the specific products that are synthesized in the specific portions of the endoplasmic reticulum and the Golgi apparatus.

Formation of Proteins by the Granular Endoplasmic Reticulum. The granular endoplasmic reticulum is characterized by the presence of large num-

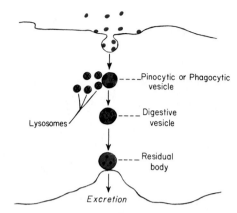

Figure 2–9. Digestion of substances in pinocytic vesicles by enzymes derived from lysosomes.

bers of ribosomes attached to the outer surfaces of the reticulum membrane. As we shall discuss in the following chapter, protein molecules are synthesized within the structures of the ribosomes. The ribosomes extrude many of the synthesized protein molecules through the endoplasmic reticulum wall into the endoplasmic matrix.

Almost as rapidly as the protein molecules enter the endoplasmic matrix, enzymes in the endoplasmic reticulum wall cause rapid changes in these molecules. First, almost all of them are immediately glycosylated, that is, conjugated with carbohydrates, to form *glycoproteins.* Therefore, essentially all the endoplasmic proteins are glycoproteins, in contrast to the proteins that are formed by the ribosomes floating freely in the cytosol which mainly form free proteins. Second, the proteins are cross-linked and folded to form more compact molecules.

Synthesis of Lipids by the Endoplasmic Reticulum, Especially by the Smooth Endoplasmic Reticulum. The endoplasmic reticulum also synthesizes lipids, especially phospholipids and cholesterol. These are rapidly incorporated into the lipid bilayer of the endoplasmic reticulum itself, thus causing the endoplasmic reticulum to grow continually. This occurs mainly in the smooth portion of the endoplasmic reticulum.

To keep the endoplasmic reticulum from growing beyond the limits of the cell, however, small vesicles called *endoplasmic reticulum vesicles,* or *transport vesicles,* continually break away from the smooth reticulum; we shall see later that most of these vesicles migrate rapidly to the Golgi apparatus.

Synthetic Functions of the Golgi Apparatus. Though the major function of the Golgi apparatus is to process substances already formed in the endoplasmic reticulum, it also has the capability of synthesizing certain carbohydrates that cannot be formed in the endoplasmic reticulum. It especially causes the formation of very large saccharide polymers bound with only small amounts of protein; the most important of these are hyaluronic acid and chondroitin sulfate. A few of the many functions of hyaluronic acid and chondroitin sulfate in the body are: (1) They

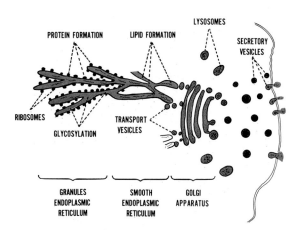

Figure 2–10. Formation of proteins, lipids, and cellular vesicles by the endoplasmic reticulum and Golgi apparatus.

are the major components of proteoglycans secreted in mucus and other glandular secretions. (2) They are the major components of the ground substance in the interstitial spaces, acting as a filler between the cells. (3) They are principal components of the organic matrix in both cartilage and bone.

Processing of Endoplasmic Secretions by the Golgi Apparatus—Formation of Intracellular Vesicles. Figure 2–10 summarizes the major functions of the endoplasmic reticulum and Golgi apparatus. As substances are formed in the endoplasmic reticulum, especially the proteins, they are transported through the tubules toward the portions of the smooth endoplasmic reticulum that lie nearest the Golgi apparatus. At this point small "transport" vesicles of smooth endoplasmic reticulum continually break away and diffuse to the innermost layers of the Golgi apparatus. Inside these transport vesicles are the synthesized proteins and other products. These vesicles instantly fuse with the Golgi apparatus and empty their contained substances into the vesicular spaces of the Golgi apparatus. Here, additional carbohydrate moieties are added to the secretions. Also, a most important function of the Golgi apparatus is to compact the endoplasmic reticular secretions into highly concentrated packets. As the secretions pass toward the outermost layers of the Golgi apparatus, the compaction and processing proceed; finally, at the outer layer both small and large vesicles continually break away from the Golgi apparatus, carrying with them the compacted secretory substances.

To give one an idea of the timing of these processes, when a glandular cell is stimulated to produce proteins, newly formed protein molecules can be detected in the granular endoplasmic reticulum within 3 to 5 minutes. Within 20 minutes the newly formed proteins are present in the Golgi apparatus, and within 1 to 2 hours they are secreted from the surface of the cell.

Types of Vesicles Formed by the Golgi Apparatus—Secretory Vesicles and Lysosomes. In a highly secretory cell, the vesicles that are formed by the Golgi apparatus are mainly *secretory vesicles,* containing especially the protein substances that are to be secreted through the surface of the cell. These vesicles diffuse to the cell membrane, then fuse with it and empty their substances to the exterior by a mechanism called *exocytosis,* which is essentially the opposite of endocytosis. Exocytosis, in most cases, is stimulated by entry of calcium ions into the cell; the calcium ions interact with the vesicular membrane, in some way not yet understood, to cause its fusion with the cell membrane.

On the other hand, some of the vesicles are destined for intracellular use. For instance, specialized portions of the Golgi apparatus form the *lysosomes* that have already been discussed. And another type of vesicle formed in the same way is *peroxisomes* that in turn form peroxides used in the cell to cause strong oxidizing chemical reactions.

Use of Intracellular Vesicles to Replenish Cellular Membranes. Many of the vesicles finally fuse with the cell membrane or with the membranes of other intracellular structures such as the mitochondria and even the endoplasmic reticulum itself. This obviously increases the expanse of these membranes and thereby replenishes them as they themselves are destroyed. For instance, the cell membrane loses much of its substance every time it forms a phagocytic or pinocytic vesicle, and it is vesicles from the Golgi apparatus that continually replenish the cell membrane.

Thus, in summary, the membranous system of the endoplasmic reticulum and the Golgi apparatus represents a highly metabolic organ capable of forming both new cellular structures and secretory substances to be extruded from the cell.

EXTRACTION OF ENERGY FROM NUTRIENTS—FUNCTION OF THE MITOCHONDRIA

The principal substances from which cells extract energy are oxygen and one or more of the foodstuffs—carbohydrates, fats, and proteins. In the human body essentially all carbohydrates are converted into *glucose* before they reach the cell, the proteins are converted into *amino acids,* and the fats are converted into *fatty acids.* Figure 2–11 shows oxygen and the foodstuffs—glucose, fatty acids, and amino acids—all entering the cell. Inside the cell, the foodstuffs react chemically with the oxygen under the influence of various enzymes that control their rates of reactions and channel the energy that is released in the proper direction.

Almost all these oxidative reactions occur inside the mitochondria, and the energy that is released is used to form adenosine triphosphate. Then, the adenosine triphosphate, not the original foodstuffs themselves, is used throughout the cell to energize almost all the intracellular metabolic reactions. Thus, the adenosine triphosphate is an intracellular storehouse of energy.

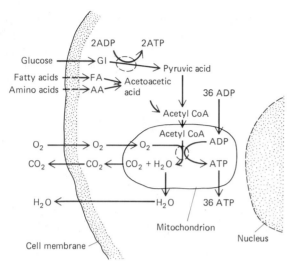

Figure 2–11. Formation of adenosine triphosphate in the cell, showing that most of the ATP is formed in the mitochondria.

Functional Characteristics of Adenosine Triphosphate (ATP). The formula for adenosine triphosphate, generally called simply ATP, is as follows:

ATP is a nucleotide composed of the nitrogenous base *adenine*, the pentose sugar *ribose,* and three *phosphate radicals.* The last two phosphate radicals are connected with the remainder of the molecule by so-called *high-energy phosphate bonds,* which are represented by the symbol ~. Each of these bonds contains about 12,000 calories of energy per mole of ATP under the physical conditions of the body (7,300 calories under standard conditions). This is much greater than the energy stored in the average chemical bond of other organic compounds, thus giving rise to the term *high-energy bond.* Furthermore, the high-energy phosphate bond is very labile so that it can be split instantly on demand whenever energy is required to promote other cellular reactions.

When ATP releases its energy, a phosphoric acid radical is split away, and *adenosine diphosphate (ADP)* is formed. Then, energy derived from the

oxidation of nutrients in the mitochondria causes the ADP and phosphoric acid to recombine to form new ATP, the entire process continuing over and over again. For these reasons, ATP has been called the *energy currency* of the cell, for it can be spent and remade again and again.

Formation of ATP in the Mitochondria. Inside the mitochondria the cellular nutrients—the carbohydrates, the fatty acids, and the amino acids—are split into their two most important component parts, hydrogen atoms and carbon dioxide. The carbon dioxide, in turn, diffuses out of the mitochondria and eventually out of the cell. The hydrogen atoms, on the other hand, combine with carrier substances and are carried to the surfaces of the shelves that protrude into the mitochondrial cavity as shown in Figure 2–6. Attached to these shelves are the so-called *oxidative enzymes* as well also protruding molecules of *ATP synthetase,* the enzyme that catalyzes the conversion of ADP to ATP. The oxidative enzymes, by a series of sequential reactions, cause the hydrogen atoms to combine with oxygen. The enzymes are arranged on the surfaces of the shelves in such a way that the products of one chemical reaction are immediately relayed to the next enzyme, then to the next, and so on until the complete sequence of reactions has taken place. During the course of these reactions, the energy released from the combination of hydrogen with oxygen is used to activate the ATP synthetase and drive the reaction to manufacture tremendous quantities of ATP from ADP. The ATP is then transported out of the mitochondrion into all parts of the cytoplasm and nucleoplasm where its energy is used to energize the functions of the cell.

The details of ATP formation and many of its metabolic functions in the body will be presented in Chapters 45 through 47.

Uses of ATP for Cellular Function. ATP is used to promote three major categories of cellular functions: (1) *membrane transport,* (2) *synthesis of chemical compounds* throughout the cell, and (3) *mechanical work.* These three different uses of ATP are illustrated in Figure 2–12: (a) to supply energy for the transport of sodium through the cell membrane, (b) to promote protein synthesis by the ribosomes, and (c) to supply the energy needed during muscle contraction.

In addition to membrane transport of sodium, energy from ATP is required in all cells for transport of potassium ions and, in certain cells, calcium ions, phosphate ions, chloride ions, urate ions, hydrogen ions, and many other special substances. Membrane transport is so important to cellular function that some cells, the renal tubular cells for instance, utilize as much as 80 per cent of the ATP formed in the cells for this purpose alone.

In addition to synthesizing proteins, cells also synthesize phospholipids, cholesterol, purines, pyrimidines, and a great host of other substances. Synthesis of almost any chemical compound requires energy. For instance, a single protein molecule might be

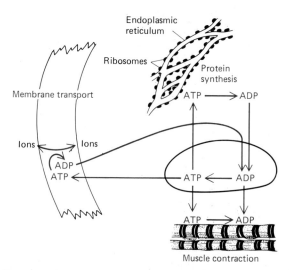

Figure 2–12. use of adenosine triphosphate to provide energy for three major cellular functions: (1) membrane transport, (2) protein synthesis, and (3) muscle contraction.

composed of as many as several thousand amino acids attached to each other by peptide linkages; the formation of each of these linkages requires the breakdown of four high-energy bonds; thus many thousand ATP molecules must release their energy as each protein molecule is formed. Indeed, some cells utilize as much as 75 per cent of all the ATP formed in the cell simply to synthesize new chemical compounds; this is particularly true during the growth phase of cells.

The final major use of ATP is to supply energy for special cells to perform mechanical work. We shall see in Chapter 6 that each contraction of a muscle fiber requires expenditure of tremendous quantities of ATP. Other cells perform mechanical work in two additional ways, by *ciliary motion* and *ameboid motion*, both of which will be described later in this chapter. The source of energy for all these types of mechanical work is ATP.

In summary, therefore, ATP is always available to release its energy rapidly and almost explosively wherever in the cell it is needed. To replace the ATP used by the cell, other much slower chemical reactions break down carbohydrates, fats, and proteins and use the energy derived from these to form new ATP. About 95 per cent of this ATP is formed in the mitochondria, which accounts for the name given to the mitochondria, the "powerhouses" of the cell.

AMEBOID LOCOMOTION OF CELLS

By far the most important type of cell movement that occurs in the body is that of the specialized muscle cells in skeletal, cardiac, and smooth muscle, which comprise almost 50 per cent of the entire body mass. The specialized functions of these cells will be discussed in Chapters 6 through 8. However, two other types of movement occur in other cells, *ameboid locomotion* and *ciliary movement*.

Ameboid Locomotion. Ameboid locomotion means movement of an entire cell in relation to its surroundings, such as the movement of white blood cells through tissues. However, it has received its name from the fact that amebae move in this manner and have provided the best tool for studying the phenomenon. Typically, ameboid locomotion begins with protrusion of a *pseudopodium* from one end of the cell. The pseudopodium projects far out, away from the cell body, and then the remainder of the cell moves toward the pseudopodium. Figure 2–13 illustrates this process, showing an elongated cell the right-hand end of which is a protruding pseudopodium. The membrane of this end of the cell is continually moving forward, and the membrane at the left-hand end of the cell is continually following along as the cell moves.

It is believed that ameboid locomotion is caused in the following way: The outer portion of the cytoplasm is in a *gel* state and is called the *ectoplasm,* whereas the central portion of the cytoplasm is in a *sol* state and is called *endoplasm.* In the gel are numerous microfilaments composed of *actin*, and also present are many *myosin molecules* that can interact with the actin filaments to cause contraction, the same as occurs in muscle. These filaments contract in the presence of ATP and calcium ions, and normally there is a continual tendency for the ectoplasm to contract. However, in response to an external chemical or physical stimulus the ectoplasm at one end of the cell becomes thin, causing a pseudopodium to bulge outward in the direction of the "chemotactic" source. Thus, the pseudopodium moves forward. At the same time, the ectoplasm at the opposite end of the cell contracts, which pushes the endoplasm into the pseudopodium and causes it to extend even further. Also, the membrane of the pseudopodium often becomes attached to some of the surrounding tissue elements so that when the ectoplasm in the remainder of the cell contracts, this literally pulls the main body of the cell toward the pseudopodium.

Types of Cells That Exhibit Ameboid Locomotion. The most common cells exhibiting ameboid locomotion in the human body are the *white blood cells* moving out of the blood into the tissues in the form of *tissue macrophages* and *microphages*. However,

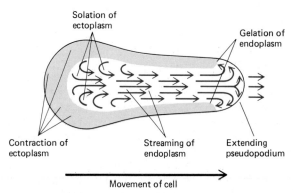

Figure 2–13. Ameboid motion by a cell.

many other types of cells can move by ameboid locomotion under certain circumstances. For instance, fibroblasts will move into any damaged area to help repair the damage, and even some of the germinal cells of the skin, though ordinarily completely sessile cells, will move toward a cut area to repair the rent. Finally, cell locomotion is especially important in the development of the fetus, for embryonic cells often migrate long distances from the primordial sites of origin to new areas during the development of special structures.

Control of Ameboid Locomotion—Chemotaxis. The most important factor that initiates ameboid locomotion is the appearance of certain chemical substances in the tissues. This phenomenon is called *chemotaxis*, and the chemical substance that causes it to occur is called a *chemotactic substance*. The chemotactic substance causes pseudopodia to form by altering the cell membrane on the side where the chemotactic substance contacts the cell; it does this by changing the permeability of the membrane, changing its electrical potential, or changing some other characteristic.

CILIA AND CILIARY MOVEMENTS

A second type of cellular motion, *ciliary movement,* is a whiplike movement of cilia on the surface of cells. This occurs in only two places in the human body: on the inside surfaces of the respiratory airways and on the inside surfaces of the uterine tubes (fallopian tubes) of the reproductive tract. In the nasal cavity and lower respiratory airways, the whiplike motion of the cilia causes a layer of mucus to move at a rate of about 1 cm/min toward the pharynx, in this way continually clearing these passageways of the mucus and any particles that have become entrapped in the mucus. In the uterine tubes, the cilia cause slow movement of fluid from the ostium of the uterine tube toward the uterine cavity; it is this movement of fluid that transports the ovum from the ovary to the uterus.

As illustrated in Figure 2–14, a cilium has the appearance of a sharp-pointed curved hair that projects 3 to 4 microns from the surface of the cell. Many cilia project from each single cell—for instance, there are as many as 200 cilia on the surface of each epithelial cell in the respiratory tract. The cilium is covered by an outcropping of the cell membrane, and it is supported by 11 microtubules, 9 double tubules located around the periphery of the cilium and 2 single tubules down the center, as shown in the cross-section illustrated in the figure.

The *flagellum of a sperm* is also similar to a cilium; in fact, it has much the same type of structure and same type of contractile mechanism. However, it is much longer and moves in quasisinusoidal waves instead of with whiplike movements.

In the inset of Figure 2–14 movement of the cilium is illustrated. The cilium moves forward with a sudden rapid stroke, 10 to 20 times per second, bending

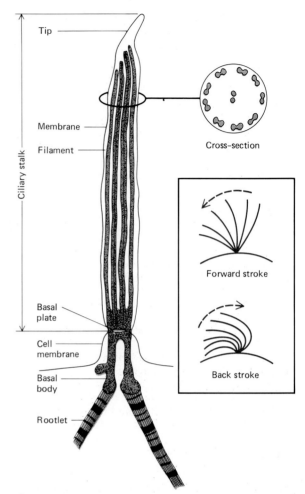

Figure 2–14. Structure and function of the cilium. (Modified from Satir: *Sci. Am., 204*:108, 1961. © 1961 by Scientific American, Inc. All rights reserved.)

sharply where it projects from the surface of the cell. Then it moves backward very slowly in a relaxed whiplike manner. The rapid forward movement pushes the fluid lying adjacent to the cell in the direction that the cilium moves, then the slow relaxed movement in the other direction has almost no effect on the fluid. As a result, fluid is continually propelled in the direction of the forward stroke. Since most ciliated cells have large numbers of cilia on their surfaces, and since all the cilia are oriented in the same direction, this is a very effective means for moving fluids from one part of the surface to another.

Mechanism of Ciliary Movement. Though all aspects of ciliary movement are not yet clear, we do know the following: First, the nine double tubules and the two single tubules are all linked to each other by a complex of protein cross-linkages; this total complex of tubules and cross-linkages is called the *axoneme.* Second, even after removal of the membrane and destruction of other elements of the cilium besides the axoneme, the cilium can still beat under appropriate conditions. Third, there are two necessary conditions for continued beating of the axoneme: (1) the presence of ATP and (2) appropriate ionic conditions, including, especially, appropriate concentrations of magnesium and calcium. Fourth, the tubules on the front edge of the bending cilium slide outward toward the tip of the cilium while the tubules on the back edge of the bending cilium remain in place. Fifth, three protein arms, composed of the protein *dynein* that has ATPase activity, project from each set of peripheral tubules toward the next set.

Given this basic information, it has been postulated that the release of energy from ATP in contact with the ATPase dynein arms causes the arms to "crawl"

along the surface of the adjacent pair of tubules. If the front tubules crawl outward while the back tubules remain stationary, this obviously will cause bending.

The way in which cilia contraction is controlled is not yet understood. However, the cilia of some genetically abnormal cells do not have the two central single tubules, and these cilia fail to beat at all. Therefore, it is presumed that some signal, perhaps an electrochemical signal, is transmitted along these two tubules to activate the ATPase activity of the dynein arms.

QUESTIONS

1. Name the membranous structures of the cell.
2. Discuss the chemical and physical characteristics of the cell membrane.
3. What are the roles of cell membrane proteins and carbohydrates?
4. Describe the endoplasmic reticulum and its synthesis functions.
5. How does the role of the Golgi apparatus differ from that of the endoplasmic reticulum?
6. How are the lysosomes formed, and what are the principal constituents of the lysosomes?
7. What is the structure of the mitochondria, and what is the special significance of the enzymes located in the mitochondrial shelves?
8. What are the characteristics of the nuclear pores?
9. Explain the mechanisms of pinocytosis and phagocytosis?

10. Describe the digestive vesicle and the events that take place in it.
11. Trace the synthesis of proteins by the granular endoplasmic reticulum, their transport to the Golgi apparatus, the formation of secretory vesicles, and final extrusion of secretory proteins through the cell surface.
12. What are some of the special substances and organelles formed by the Golgi apparatus?
13. Explain the special characteristics of the chemical substance adenosine triphosphate that allow it to function as "energy currency" in a cell.
14. Explain briefly the role of the mitochondrion in the formation of ATP.
15. What are the uses of ATP in the cell?
16. Describe ameboid and ciliary motions and their mechanisms.

References

Agard, D. A.: Optical sectioning microscopy: Cellular architecture in three dimensions. Ann Rev Biophys Bioeng 13:191, 1984.

Almers, W., and Stirling, C.: Distribution of transport proteins over animal cell membranes. J Membr Biol 77:169, 1984.

Baker, P. F., and Knight, D. E.: Chemiosmotic hypotheses of exocytosis: A critique. Biosci Rep 4:285, 1984.

Busch, H., ed.: The Cell Nucleus. Nuclear Particles. New York, Academic Press, 1981.

de Brabander, M., et. al., eds.: Cell Movement and Neoplasia. New York, Pergamon Press, 1980.

DeDuve, C.: A Guided Tour of the Living Cell. New York, W. H. Freeman, 1985.

Fawcett, D. W.: The Cell. Philadelphia, W. B. Saunders Co., 1966.

Hammersen, F.: Histology: A Color Atlas of Cytology, Histology, and Microscopic Anatomy. Baltimore, Urban & Schwarzenberg, 1980.

Macnab, R. M., and Aizawa, S.-I.: Bacterial motility and the bacterial flagellar motor. Annu Rev Biophys Bioeng 13:51, 1984.

McCloskey, M., and Poo, M. M.: Protein diffusion in cell membranes: Some biological implications. Int Rev Cytol 87:19, 1984.

Tseng, H.: Atlas of Ultrastructure. New York, Appleton-Century-Crofts, 1980.

Wall, D. A., and Maack, T.: Endocytic uptake, transport, and catabolism of proteins by epithelial cells. Am J Physiol 248:C12, 1985.

Wheatley, D. N.: Mini-review. On the possible importance of an intracellular circulation. Life Sci 36:299, 1985.

Willingham, M. C., and Pastan, I.: Endocytosis and exocytosis: Current concepts of vesicle traffic in animal cells. Int Rev Cytol 92:51, 1984.

3

Genetic Control of Cell Function— Protein Synthesis and Cell Reproduction

THE GENES
THE GENETIC CODE
FORMATION OF RIBONUCLEIC ACID (RNA)—THE PROCESS OF TRANSCRIPTION
MESSENGER RNA—THE CODONS
TRANSFER RNA—THE ANTICODONS
RIBOSOMAL RNA
FORMATION OF PROTEINS ON THE RIBOSOMES—THE PROCESS OF TRANSLATION
SYNTHESIS OF OTHER SUBSTANCES IN THE CELL

CONTROL OF GENETIC FUNCTION AND BIOCHEMICAL ACTIVITY IN CELLS
GENETIC REGULATION
CONTROL OF ENZYME ACTIVITY
CELL REPRODUCTION
REPLICATION OF THE DNA
THE CHROMOSOMES
MITOSIS
CONTROL OF CELL GROWTH
CANCER

Almost everyone knows that the genes control heredity from parents to children, but most persons do not realize that the same genes control the reproduction of and day-by-day function of all cells. The genes control cell function by determining what substances will be synthesized within the cell—what structures, what enzymes, what chemicals.

Figure 3–1 illustrates the general schema of genetic control. Each gene, which is a nucleic acid called *deoxyribonucleic acid (DNA)*, automatically controls the formation of another nucleic acid, *ribonucleic acid (RNA)*, which spreads throughout the cell and controls the formation of a specific protein. Some proteins are *structural proteins* which, in association with various lipids, form the structures of the various organelles that were discussed in the preceding chapter. But by far the majority of the proteins are *enzymes* that catalyze the different chemical reactions in the cells. For instance, enzymes promote all the oxidative reactions that supply energy to the cell, and they promote the synthesis of various chemicals such as lipids, glycogen, adenosine triphosphate, and so on.

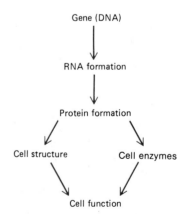

Figure 3–1. General schema by which the genes control cell function.

THE GENES

The genes are contained, large numbers of them attached end on end, in long, double-stranded, helical molecules of *deoxyribonucleic acid (DNA)* having

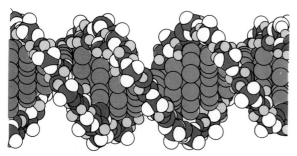

Figure 3–2. The helical, double-stranded structure of the gene. The outside strands are composed of phosphoric acid and the sugar deoxyribose. The internal molecules connecting the two strands of the helix are purine and pyrimidine bases; these determine the "code" of the gene.

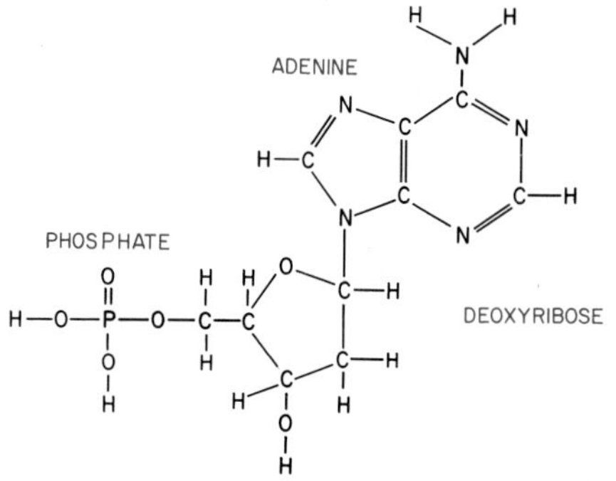

molecular weights measured in the billions. A very short segment of such a molecule is illustrated in Figure 3–2. This molecule is composed of several simple chemical compounds arranged in a regular pattern explained in the following few paragraphs.

The Basic Building Blocks of DNA. Figure 3–3 illustrates the basic chemical compounds involved in the formation of DNA. These include (1) *phosphoric acid,* (2) a sugar called *deoxyribose,* and (3) four nitrogenous *bases* (two purines, *adenine* and *guanine,* and two pyrimidines, *thymine* and *cytosine*). The phosphoric acid and deoxyribose form the two helical strands of the DNA molecule, and the bases lie between the strands and connect them together.

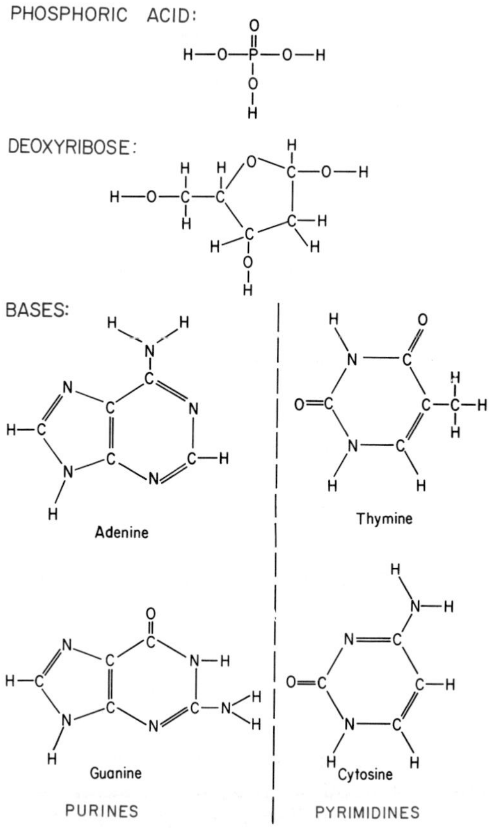

Figure 3–4. Deoxyadenylic acid, one of the nucleotides that make up DNA.

The Nucleotides. The first stage in the formation of DNA is the combination of one molecule of phosphoric acid, one molecule of deoxyribose, and one of the four bases to form a nucleotide. Four separate nucleotides are thus formed, one for each of the four bases: *deoxyadenylic, deoxythymidylic, deoxyguanylic,* and *deoxycytidylic* acids. Figure 3–4 illustrates the chemical structure of adenylic acid, and Figure 3–5 illustrates simple symbols for all the four basic nucleotides that form DNA.

Organization of the Nucleotides to Form DNA. Figure 3–6 illustrates the manner in which multiple numbers of nucleotides are bound together to form DNA. Note that these are combined in such a way that phosphoric acid and deoxyribose alternate with each other in the two separate strands, and these strands are held together by loose bonds between the purine and pyrimidine bases. But note carefully that

(1) the purine base *adenine* always bonds with the pyrimidine base *thymine;* and

(2) the purine base *guanine* always bonds with the pyrimidine base *cytosine.*

Thus, in Figure 3–6 the sequence of complementary pairs of bases is CG, CG, GC, TA, CG, TA, GC, AT, and AT. However, the bases are bound together by very loose *hydrogen bonding,* represented in the figure by dashed lines. Because of the looseness of these bonds, the two strands can pull apart with ease, and they do so many times during the course of their function in the cell.

Figure 3–3. The basic building blocks of DNA.

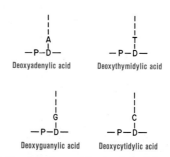

Figure 3–5. Combinations of the basic building blocks of DNA to form nucleotides. (*P,* phosphoric acid; *D,* deoxyribose.) The four nucleotide bases are *A,* adenine; *T,* thymine; *G,* guanine; and *C,* cytosine. These four different types of nucleotides make up DNA.

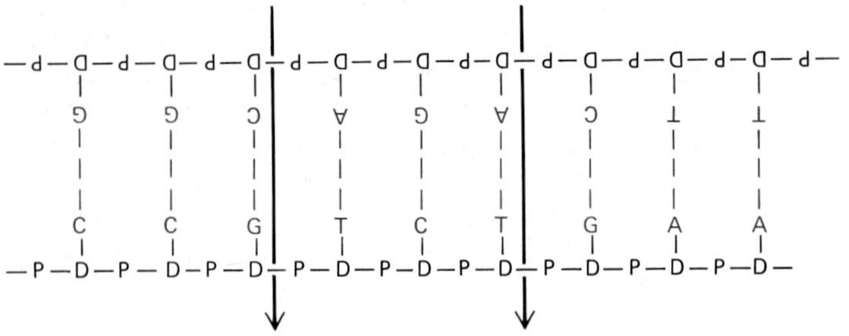

—d—◖—d—◖—d—◖—d—◖—d—◖—d—◖—d—◖—d—◖—d—◖—d—
     | | | | | | | | |
    G   G   C   A   G   A   C   T   T
    C   C   G   T   C   T   G   A   A
—P—D—P—D—P—D—P—D—P—D—P—D—P—D—P—D—P—D—

Figure 3–6. Arrangement of deoxyribose nucleotides in DNA.

Now, to put the DNA of Figure 3–6 into its proper physical perspective, one needs merely to pick up the two ends and twist them into a helix. Ten pairs of nucleotides are present in each full turn of the helix in the DNA molecule, as was illustrated in Figure 3–2.

THE GENETIC CODE

The importance of DNA lies in its ability to control the formation of other substances in the cell. It does this by means of the so-called *genetic code.* When the two strands of a DNA molecule are split apart, this exposes the purine and pyrimidine bases projecting to the side of each strand. It is these projecting bases that form the code.

Research studies in the past few years have demonstrated that the genetic code consists of successive "triplets" of bases—that is, each three successive bases are a code word. And the successive triplets control the sequence of amino acids in a protein molecule that is to be synthesized in the cell. Note in Figure 3–6 that each of the two strands of the DNA molecule carries its own genetic code. For instance, the top strand, reading from left to right, has the genetic code GGC, AGA, CTT, the triplets being separated from each other by the arrows. As we follow this genetic code through Figures 3–7 and 3–8, we shall see that these three respective triplets are responsible for placement of the three amino acids, *proline, serine,* and *glutamic acid,* in a molecule of protein. Furthermore, these three amino acids will be lined up in the protein molecule in exactly the same sequence that the genetic code is lined up in this strand of DNA.

FORMATION OF RIBONUCLEIC ACID (RNA)—THE PROCESS OF TRANSCRIPTION

Since almost all DNA is located in the nucleus of the cell and yet most of the functions of the cell are carried out in the cytoplasm, some means must be available for the genes of the nucleus to control the chemical reactions of the cytoplasm. This is achieved through the intermediary of another type of nucleic acid, *ribonucleic acid (RNA),* the formation of which is controlled by the DNA of the nucleus; in this process the code is transferred to the RNA, which is called *transcription.* The RNA is then transported from the nucleus into the cytoplasmic cavity where it controls protein synthesis.

Synthesis of RNA

During synthesis of RNA, the two strands of the DNA molecule separate temporarily; one of these strands is then used as a template for synthesis of the RNA molecules. The code triplets in the DNA cause the formation of *complementary* code triplets (called *codons*) in the RNA; these codons in turn will control the sequence of amino acids in a protein to be synthesized later in the cytoplasm. When one strand of DNA is used in this manner to cause the formation of RNA, the opposite strand remains inactive. Each DNA helix is such a large molecule that it carries the code for more than 1000 genes.

The Basic Building Blocks of RNA. The basic building blocks of RNA are almost the same as those of DNA except for two differences. First, the sugar

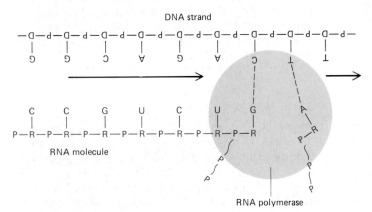

DNA strand

RNA molecule

Figure 3–7. Combination of ribose nucleotides with a strand of DNA to form a molecule of ribonucleic acid (RNA) that carries the DNA code from the gene to the cytoplasm. The RNA polymerase moves along the DNA strand and builds the RNA molecule.

RNA polymerase

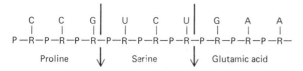

Figure 3–8. Portion of a ribonucleic acid molecule, showing three "code" words, CCG, UCU, and GAA, which represent the three amino acids *proline, serine,* and *glutamic acid.*

deoxyribose is not used in the formation of RNA. In its place is another sugar of very slightly different composition, *ribose.* Second, thymine is replaced by another pyrimidine, *uracil.*

Formation of RNA Nucleotides. The basic building blocks of RNA first form nucleotides exactly as described above for the synthesis of DNA. Here again, four separate nucleotides are used in the formation of RNA. These nucleotides contain the bases *adenine, guanine, cytosine,* and *uracil.* Note that these are the same as the bases in DNA except for one of them; the uracil replaces the thymine in DNA.

Assembly of the RNA Molecule from Nucleotides Using the DNA Strand as a Template—The Process of Transcription. Assembly of the RNA molecule is accomplished in the manner illustrated in Figure 3–7 under the influence of the enzyme *RNA polymerase.* This is a very large enzyme that has many functional properties necessary for the formation of the RNA molecule. These are:

(1) In the DNA strand immediately ahead of the initial gene is a sequence of nucleotides called the *promoter.* The RNA polymerase has an appropriate complementary structure that recognizes this promoter and becomes attached to it. This is the essential step in initiating the formation of the RNA molecule.

(2) Then the polymerase moves along the DNA strand, temporarily unwinding and separating the two DNA strands at each stage of its movement. As it moves along, it forms the RNA molecule by the following steps:

(3) First, it causes hydrogen bonds between the bases of the DNA strand and the bases of appropriate RNA nucleotides in the nucleoplasm.

(4) Then, one at a time, the RNA polymerase breaks two of the three phosphate radicals away from each of these RNA nucleotides, liberating large amounts of energy from the broken high energy phosphate bonds; this energy is used to cause covalent linkage of the remaining phosphate on the nucleotide with the ribose on the end of the growing RNA molecule.

(5) When the RNA polymerase reaches the end of the gene or sequence of genes, it encounters a new sequence of DNA nucleotides called the *chain-terminating sequence;* this causes the polymerase to break away from the DNA strand. Then the polymerase can attach somewhere else to be used again and again for forming new RNA molecules.

(6) As the new RNA strand is formed, its hydrogen bonds with the DNA template break away. In this way, the RNA molecule is released into the nucleoplasm.

It should be remembered that there are four different types of DNA bases and also four different types of RNA nucleotide bases. Furthermore, these always combine with each other in specific combinations. Therefore, the code that is present in the DNA strand is transmitted in *complementary* form to the RNA molecule. The ribose nucleotide bases always combine with the deoxyribose bases in the following combinations:

DNA base	RNA base
guanine	cytosine
cytosine	guanine
adenine	uracil
thymine	adenine

There are three separate types of RNA, each of which plays an independent and entirely different role in protein formation. These are

(1) *messenger RNA,* which carries the genetic code to the cytoplasm for controlling the formation of the proteins;

(2) *transfer RNA,* which transports activated amino acids to the ribosomes to be used in assembling the protein molecules; and

(3) *ribosomal RNA,* which, along with almost 100 proteins, forms the *ribosomes,* the physical and chemical structures on which protein molecules are actually assembled.

MESSENGER RNA—THE CODONS

Messenger RNA molecules are long strands that are suspended in the cytoplasm. These molecules are usually composed of several hundred to several thousand nucleotides in unpaired strands, and they contain *codons* that are exactly complementary to the code triplets of the genes. Figure 3–8 illustrates a small segment of a molecule of messenger RNA. Its codons are CCG, UCU, and GAA. These are the codons for the amino acids proline, serine, and glutamic acid. The transcription of these codons from the DNA molecule was demonstrated in Figure 3–7.

RNA Codons. Table 3–1 gives the RNA codons for the 20 common amino acids found in protein molecules. Note that most of the amino acids are represented by more than one codon; also, one codon represents the signal "start manufacturing a protein molecule" and three codons represent "stop manufacturing a protein molecule." In Table 3–1, these two types of codons are designated CI for "chain-initiating" and CT for "chain-terminating."

TRANSFER RNA—THE ANTICODONS

Another type of RNA that plays a prominent role in protein synthesis is called *transfer RNA* because it transfers amino acid molecules to protein molecules as the protein is synthesized. There are basically 20 types of transfer RNA, each type combining specifically with only one of the 20 amino acids that are to be incorporated into proteins. The transfer RNA then

Table 3–1. RNA CODONS FOR THE DIFFERENT AMINO
ACIDS AND FOR START AND STOP

Amino Acid	RNA Codons					
Alanine	GCU	GCC	GCA	GCG		
Arginine	CGU	CGC	CGA	CGG	AGA	AGG
Asparagine	AAU	AAC				
Aspartic acid	GAU	GAC				
Cysteine	UGU	UGC				
Glutamic acid	GAA	GAG				
Glutamine	CAA	CAG				
Glycine	GGU	GGC	GGA	GGG		
Histidine	CAU	CAC				
Isoleucine	AUU	AUC	AUA			
Leucine	CUU	CUC	CUA	CUG	UUA	UUG
Lysine	AAA	AAG				
Methionine	AUG					
Phenylalanine	UUU	UUC				
Proline	CCU	CCC	CCA	CCG		
Serine	UCU	UCC	UCA	UCG	AGC	AGU
Threonine	ACU	ACC	ACA	ACG		
Tryptophan	UGG					
Tyrosine	UAU	UAC				
Valine	GUU	GUC	GUA	GUG		
Start (CI)	AUG					
Stop (CT)	UAA	UAG	UGA			

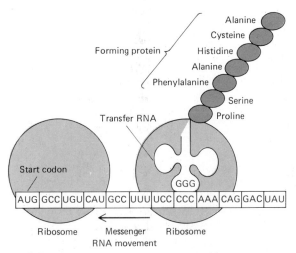

Figure 3–9. Mechanism by which a protein molecule is formed in ribosomes in association with messenger RNA and transfer RNA.

acts as a *carrier* to transport its specific type of amino acid to the ribosomes where protein molecules are formed. In the ribosomes, each specific type of transfer RNA recognizes a particular codon on the messenger RNA, as is described below, and thereby delivers the appropriate amino acid to the appropriate place in the chain of the newly forming protein molecule.

Transfer RNA, containing only about 80 nucleotides, is a relatively small molecule in comparison with messenger RNA. It is a folded chain of nucleotides with a cloverleaf appearance similar to that illustrated in Figure 3–9. At one end of the molecule is always an adenylic acid; it is to this that the transported amino acid attaches.

Since the function of transfer RNA is to cause attachment of a specific amino acid to a forming protein chain, it is essential that each type of transfer RNA also have specificity for a particular codon in the messenger RNA. The specific code in the transfer RNA that allows it to recognize a specific codon is again a triplet of nucleotide bases and is called an *anticodon*. This is located approximately in the middle of the transfer RNA molecule (at the bottom of the cloverleaf configuration illustrated in Figure 3–9). During formation of a protein molecule, the anticodon bases combine loosely by hydrogen bonding with the codon bases of the messenger RNA. In this way the respective amino acids are lined up one after another along the messenger RNA chain, thus establishing the appropriate sequence of amino acids in the protein molecule.

RIBOSOMAL RNA

The third type of RNA in the cell is ribosomal RNA; it constitutes about 60 per cent of the ribo-

some. The remainder of the ribosome is protein, containing almost 100 different types of proteins that are both structural proteins and enzymes needed in the manufacture of protein molecules.

The ribosome is the physical and chemical structure in the cytoplasm on which protein molecules are actually synthesized. However, it always functions in association with both the other types of RNA as well: transfer RNA transports amino acids to the ribosomes for incorporation into the developing protein molecules, while messenger RNA provides the information necessary for sequencing the amino acids in proper order for each specific type of protein to be manufactured.

Formation of Ribosomes in the Nucleolus. When the ribosomal RNA first forms in the nucleus, it collects in the *nucleolus*, a specialized structure lying adjacent to the chromosomes. Here the ribosomal RNA is specially processed and combined with "ribosomal proteins" to form granular condensation products that are primordial subunits of the ribosomes. These subunits are then released from the nucleolus and transported through the large pores of the nuclear envelope to almost all parts of the cytoplasm. Only after the subunits enter the cytoplasm are they assembled to form mature, functional ribosomes. Therefore, proteins are *not* formed in the nucleus because the nucleus does not contain mature ribosomes.

FORMATION OF PROTEINS ON THE RIBOSOMES—THE PROCESS OF TRANSLATION

When a molecule of messenger RNA comes in contact with a ribosome, it travels through the ribosome, and, as illustrated in Figure 3–9, this causes a protein molecule to be formed—a process called *translation*. Thus, the ribosome reads the code of the messenger RNA in much the same way that a tape is "read" as it passes through the playback head of a tape recorder. Then, when a "stop" (or "chain-terminating") codon slips past the ribosome, the end of the protein molecule is signaled, and the protein is freed into the cytoplasm.

Attachment of Ribosomes to the Endoplasmic Reticulum. In the previous chapter it was noted that many of the ribosomes become attached to the endoplasmic reticulum. This does not occur until the ribosomes begin to form the protein molecules. However, the initial ends of certain types of protein molecules, as they are being synthesized, immediately attach themselves to specific receptor sites on the endoplasmic reticulum, which causes these molecules then to penetrate the reticulum wall and enter the endoplasmic reticulum matrix. Because this occurs while the protein molecule is still being formed by the ribosome, this pulls the ribosome against the endoplasmic reticulum, thereby giving the "granular" appearance to the reticulum. The reason these proteins attach to the endoplasmic reticulum is that they have a special sequence of amino acids on their initial ends with specific binding affinity for the receptors on the reticulum. These initial amino acids are then removed as the protein enters the reticulum matrix and are replaced by saccharide moieties, giving rise to the typical glycosylated proteins that are processed in the endoplasmic reticulum.

Figure 3–10 shows the functional relationship of messenger RNA to the ribosomes and also the manner in which the ribosomes attach to the membrane of the endoplasmic reticulum. Note the process of translation occurring in several ribosomes at the same time in response to the same strand of messenger RNA. And note also the newly forming polypeptide chains passing through the endoplasmic reticulum membrane into the endoplasmic matrix.

Yet, it should be noted that, except in glandular cells that form large amounts of protein-containing secretory vesicles, most proteins formed on the ribosomes are released directly into the cytosol rather than into the endoplasmic reticulum and are not of the glycosylated variety. These are the enzymes and structural proteins of the cytosol.

Peptide Linkage. The successive amino acids in the protein chain combine with each other according to the following typical reaction:

$$\underset{R-C}{\overset{NH_2}{|}} \quad \underset{C}{\overset{O}{\|}} \quad OH \; + \; H \; - \underset{R-C}{\overset{H}{|}} \underset{C}{\overset{R}{|}} - COOH \;\rightarrow$$

$$\underset{R-C}{\overset{NH_2}{|}} \quad \underset{C}{\overset{O}{\|}} \quad \underset{N}{\overset{H}{|}} \quad \underset{C}{\overset{R}{|}} - COOH + H_2O$$

In this chemical reaction, a hydroxyl radical is removed from the COOH portion of one amino acid while a hydrogen of the NH_2 portion of the other amino acid is removed. These combine to form water, and the two reactive sites left on the two successive amino acids combine, resulting in a single molecule. This process is called *peptide linkage.*

For each peptide linkage formed during the manufacture of a protein molecule in the ribosome, a very large amount of energy is consumed, requiring the breakdown of four molecules of ATP. Thus, protein synthesis is one of the most energy-consuming of all the life processes of the cell.

SYNTHESIS OF OTHER SUBSTANCES IN THE CELL

Many thousand protein enzymes formed in the manner just described control essentially all the other chemical reactions that take place in cells. These enzymes promote synthesis of lipids, glycogen, purines, pyrimidines, and hundreds of other substances. We will discuss many of these synthetic processes in relation to carbohydrate, lipid, and protein metabolism in Chapters 45 and 46. It is by means of all these different substances that the many functions of the cells are performed.

CONTROL OF GENETIC FUNCTION AND BIOCHEMICAL ACTIVITY IN CELLS

There are basically two different methods by which the biochemical activities in the cell are controlled. One of these is called *genetic regulation,* in which the activities of the genes themselves are controlled, and

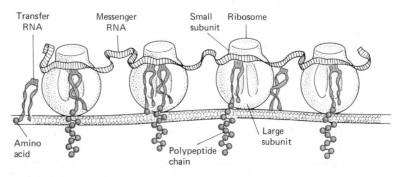

Figure 3–10. An artist's concept of the physical structure of the ribosomes as well as their functional relationship to messenger RNA, transfer RNA, and the endoplasmic reticulum during the formation of protein molecules. (From Bloom and Fawcett: A Textbook of Histology. 10th ed. Philadelphia, W. B. Saunders Company, 1975.)

the other *enzyme regulation,* in which the activity rates of the enzymes within the cell are controlled.

Strange as it may seem, every nucleated cell of the body contains the same set of genes as those originally present in the fertilized ovum from which the body was formed. Therefore, the vast differences in the different types of cells result not from different types of genes in the cells but instead from repression or activation of different genes in different cells. This effect is called *differentiation* of the cells. The respective genes are repressed or activated by special intracellular genetic control mechanisms that allow expression of different functional characteristics in separate types of "differentiated" cells, some providing muscle activity, others glandular secretion, and still others the many other bodily functions.

GENETIC REGULATION

The Operon and Its Control of Biochemical Synthesis—Function of the Promoter. The synthesis of a cellular biochemical product usually requires a series of reactions, and each of these reactions is catalyzed by a special protein enzyme. This process has been studied very thoroughly in bacteria, especially in the colon bacillus, but the same principles apply in different mechanistic ways to nucleated cells as well. In the colon bacillus, formation of all the enzymes needed for the synthetic process is often controlled by a sequence of genes located in series one after the other on the same chromosomal DNA strand. This area of the DNA strand is called an *operon,* and the genes responsible for forming the respective enzymes are called the *structural genes.* In Figure 3–11, three respective structural genes are illustrated in an operon, and it is shown that they control the formation of three respective enzymes utilized in a particular biochemical synthetic process.

Now note in the figure the segment on the DNA strand called the *promoter.* This is a series of nucleotides that has specific affinity for RNA polymerase, as already discussed. The polymerase must bind with this promoter before it can begin traveling along the DNA strand to synthesize RNA. Therefore, the promoter is the essential element in activating the operon.

Control of the Operon by a Repressor Protein— The Repressor Operator. Also note an additional band of nucleotides lying in the middle of the promoter. This area is called a *repressor operator* because a regulatory protein can bind here and prevent attachment of RNA polymerase to the promoter, thereby blocking transcription of the genes. Such a regulatory protein is called a *repressor protein.* However, each regulatory repressor protein generally exists in two different physical forms, one that can bind with the operator and repress transcription and the other that does not bind. That is, one of its forms might be a straight protein molecule and the other the same molecule bent at an angle in the middle. Only one of these forms can repress the operator. In

turn, various nonprotein substances in the cell, such as some of the cell metabolites, can bind with the repressor protein to change its physical state. A substance that causes it to change so that it will bind with the operator and stop transcription is called a *repressor substance* or *inhibitor substance.* On the other hand, a substance that changes the repressor protein so that it will break its bond with the operator is called an *activator substance* or *inducer substance* because it activates, or induces, the transcription process by removing the repressor protein.

To illustrate the control of gene transcription by a repressor protein, let us give an example. The saccharide lactose usually is not available to cells as a food substrate. Therefore, the cells normally will not synthesize the required enzymes for metabolic breakdown of lactose. However, when lactose does become available, it induces a physical change in a repressor protein, causing it to break away from a repressor operator on the operon that transcribes for the necessary metabolic enzymes. Therefore the operon becomes derepressed, and within a few hours the appropriate enzymes are present in the cell to cause breakdown of the lactose. Then, as the lactose begins to disappear from within the cell, the rate of synthesis of the enzymes also decreases back to that level required only for the amount of lactose that is available. Thus one can see the logic of having such regulatory systems in the cell.

Control of the Operon by an Activator Protein— The Activator Operator. Now note in Figure 3–11 another operator, called the *activator operator,* that lies adjacent to but ahead of the promoter. When a regulatory protein binds to this operator, it helps to attract the RNA polymerase to the promoter, in this way activating the operon. Therefore, a regulatory protein of this type is called an *activator protein.* The operon can be activated or inhibited through the activator operator in ways exactly opposite to the control of the repressor operator.

Negative Feedback Control of the Operon. Finally, note in Figure 3–11 that the presence of a critical amount of a synthesized product in the cell can cause

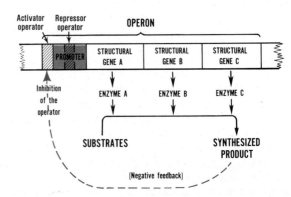

Figure 3–11. Function of the operon in controlling biosynthesis. Note that the synthesized product exerts a negative feedback to inhibit function of the operon, in this way automatically controlling the concentration of the product itself.

negative feedback inhibition of the operon that is responsible for its synthesis. It can do this either by causing a regulatory repressor protein to bind at the repressor operator or a regulatory activator protein to break its bond with the activator operator. In either case, the operon becomes inhibited. Therefore, once the required synthesized product has become abundant enough, the operon becomes dormant. On the other hand, when the synthesized product becomes degraded in the cell and its concentration falls, the operon once again becomes active. In this way, the concentration of the product is automatically controlled.

Other Mechanisms for Control of Transcription by the Operon. Variations in the basic mechanism for control of the operon have been discovered with rapidity in the last few years. Without giving details, let us mention two of these:

(1) An operon is frequently controlled by a *regulatory gene* located elsewhere in the genetic complex of the nucleus. That is, the regulatory gene causes the formation of a *regulatory protein* that in turn acts either as an activator or a repressor substance to control the operon.

(2) Occasionally, many different operons are controlled at the same time by the same regulatory protein. And in some instances, the same regulatory protein functions as an activator for one operon and as a repressor for another operon. When multiple operons are controlled simultaneously in this manner, all the operons that function together are called a *regulon.*

Because there are as many as 30,000 to 100,000 different genes in each cell, the large number of different ways in which genetic activity can be controlled is not surprising. Through these control mechanisms, especially through negative feedback controls, the cell is able to maintain appropriate concentrations of its necessary functional biochemicals. The genetic control systems are especially important for controlling the intracellular concentrations of amino acids, amino acid derivatives, and many if not most of the intermediate substrates of carbohydrate, lipid, and protein metabolism.

CONTROL OF ENZYME ACTIVITY

In the same way that inhibitors and activators can affect the genetic regulatory system, so also can the enzymes themselves be directly controlled by other inhibitors or activators. This, therefore, represents a second category of mechanisms by which cellular biochemical functions can be controlled.

Enzyme Inhibition. A great many of the chemical substances formed in the cell have a direct feedback effect in inhibiting the respective enzyme systems that synthesize them. Almost always the synthesized product acts on the first enzyme in a sequence, rather than on the subsequent enzymes, usually binding directly with the enzyme and causing a physical change that inactivates it.

This process of enzyme inhibition is another example of negative feedback control; it is responsible for controlling the intracellular concentrations of some of the amino acids that are not controlled by the genetic mechanism as well as the concentrations of the purines, the pyrimidines, vitamins, and many other substances.

Enzyme Activation. Enzymes that are either normally inactive or that have been inactivated by some inhibitor substance often can be activated. An example of this occurs when most of the adenosine triphosphate has been depleted in a cell. One of the products of the ATP breakdown, cyclic AMP, immediately activates the glycogen-splitting enzyme phosphorylase, liberating glucose molecules that are rapidly used for replenishment of the ATP stores. Thus, in this case the cyclic AMP acts as an enzyme activator and thereby helps control intracellular ATP concentration.

In summary, there are two principal methods by which the cells control proper proportions and proper quantities of different cellular constituents: (1) the mechanism of genetic regulation, and (2) the mechanism of enzyme regulation. The genes can be either activated or inhibited, and, likewise, the enzyme systems can be either activated or inhibited. Most often, these regulatory mechanisms function as feedback control systems that continually monitor the cell's biochemical composition and make corrections as needed. But, on occasion, substances from outside the cell (especially some of the hormones that will be discussed later in this text) also control the intracellular biochemical reactions by activating or inhibiting one or more of the intracellular control systems.

CELL REPRODUCTION

Cell reproduction is another example of the pervading, ubiquitous role that the DNA-genetic system plays in all life processes. It is the genes and their regulatory mechanisms that determine the growth characteristics of the cells and also when or whether these cells will divide to form new cells. In this way, this all-important genetic system controls each stage in the development of the human being from the single-cell fertilized ovum to the whole functioning body. Thus, if there is any central theme to life it is the DNA-genetic system.

The Life Cycle of the Cell. The life cycle of a cell is the period of time from reproduction to reproduction. When cells are reproducing as rapidly as they can, this life cycle lasts for 10 to 30 hours. It is terminated by a series of distinct physical events called *mitosis* that cause division of the cell into two new daughter cells. The events of mitosis are illustrated in Figure 3–12 and will be described later. The actual stage of mitosis, however, lasts for only about 30 minutes, so that more than 95 per cent of the life cycle is represented by the interval between mitosis, called *interphase.* In fact, except in special conditions

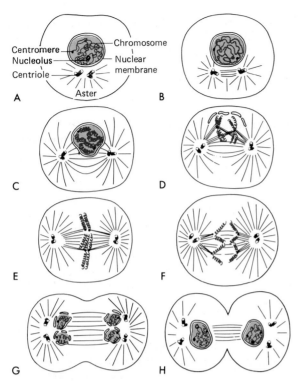

Figure 3–12. Stages in the reproduction of the cell. *A, B,* and *C,* prophase; *D,* prometaphase; *E,* metaphase; *F,* anaphase; *G* and *H,* telophase. (Redrawn from Mazia: *Sci. Am., 205:*102, 1961. © by Scientific American, Inc. All rights reserved.)

of rapid cellular reproduction, inhibitory controls almost always slow or stop the uninhibited life cycle of the cell. Therefore, different cells of the body have life cycle periods that vary from as little as 10 hours for stimulated bone marrow cells to an entire lifetime of the human body for nerve and striated muscle cells.

Immediately after new daughter cells are formed, they are still small, but they enter an initial period of rapid growth consisting of rapid formation of RNA, extensive protein synthesis, and accumulation of increased quantities of nucleoplasm and cytoplasm. During rapid cell reproduction, this period lasts for 20 to 40 per cent of the total life cycle.

REPLICATION OF THE DNA

As is true of almost all other important events in the cell, reproduction begins in the nucleus itself. The first step is *replication (duplication) of all DNA in the chromosomes.* Only after this has occurred can mitosis take place.

The DNA begins to be duplicated some 5 to 10 hours before mitosis, and this is completed in 4 to 8 hours. The DNA is duplicated only once, so that the net result is two exact *replicates* of all DNA. These replicates, in turn, become the DNA in the two new daughter cells that will be formed at mitosis. Following replication of the DNA there is another period of 1 to 2 hours before mitosis begins abruptly. However, even during this period, preliminary changes

are already beginning to take place that will lead to the mitotic process.

Chemical and Physical Events of DNA Replication. DNA is replicated in much the same way that RNA is transcribed by DNA except for a few important differences:

(1) Both strands of the DNA are replicated, not simply one of them.

(2) Both entire strands of the DNA helix are replicated from end to end rather than small portions of them as occurs in the transcription of RNA by the genes. The two DNA strands of each chromosome contain more than 1000 genes.

(3) The principal enzyme for replicating DNA is *DNA polymerase* rather than RNA polymerase. It lines up the DNA nucleotides in the appropriate order while the enzyme *DNA ligase* causes attachment of the successive nucleotides to each other, utilizing high energy phosphate bonds to energize these attachments.

(4) Each newly formed strand of DNA remains attached to the original DNA strand that is used as its template. Therefore, two new DNA helixes are formed that are exact duplicates of each other and that are still coiled together.

DNA Repair and DNA "Proofreading." During the few hours between DNA replication and the beginning of mitosis, there is a period of very active repair and "proofreading" of the DNA strands. That is, wherever inappropriate DNA nucleotides have been matched up with the nucleotides of the original template strand, special enzymes cut out the defective areas and replace these with the appropriate complementary nucleotides. This is achieved by the same DNA polymerase and DNA ligase that are used in the process of replication. This repair process is referred to as *DNA proofreading.*

Because of repair and proofreading, the transcription process almost never makes a mistake. But when a mistake is made, this is called a *mutation;* it in turn will cause the formation of some abnormal protein in the cell, often leading to abnormal cellular function and sometimes even to death. Yet, because of the precision of the transcription process, it has been calculated that each human gene mutates only about once in every 200,000 years of human life. Nevertheless, when one realizes that there are 30,000 to 100,000 genes in the human genome and that the period from one generation to another is about 30 years, one would still expect as many as three to ten mutations in the passage of the genome from parent to child. Fortunately, though, each human genome is represented by two separate sets of chromosomes with almost identical genes so that one functional gene almost always is still available to the child despite a mutation.

THE CHROMOSOMES

The DNA helixes of the nucleus are packaged in the chromosomes. The human cell contains 46 chromosomes arranged in 23 pairs. Most of the genes in the two chromosomes of each pair are identical or almost identical with each other, so that it is usually stated that the different genes also exist in pairs, though occasionally this is not the case.

Aside from the DNA in the chromosome there is also a large amount of protein, composed mainly of many small molecules of electropositively charged *histones*. The histones are organized into vast numbers of small, bobbin-like cores. Successive segments of each DNA helix are coiled sequentially around one core after another. Then the successive cores are packed one on top of the other, thus allowing the tremendously long DNA molecule, having a linear length of 6 cm and a molecular weight of about 60 billion, to be packaged in a coiled and folded arrangement that is only a few microns in length.

The histone cores of the chromosome probably also play an important role in the regulation of DNA activity, because as long as the DNA is packaged tightly it cannot function as a template either for the formation of RNA or for replication of new DNA. Furthermore, some of the regulatory proteins have been shown to decondense the histone packaging of the DNA and to allow large segments at a time to form RNA. Thus, this is still a higher order of regulation than the types of regulation discussed earlier, and it functions especially in nucleated cells.

MITOSIS

The actual process by which the cell splits into two new cells is called *mitosis*. Once the genes have been duplicated and each chromosome has split to form two daughter chromosomes, called *chromatids*, mitosis follows automatically within an hour or two.

The Mitotic Apparatus. One of the first events of mitosis takes place in the cytoplasm. As illustrated in Figure 3–12, two pairs of centrioles lie close to each other near one pole of the nucleus. Each centriole is a small cylindrical body about 0.4 micron long and about 0.15 micron in diameter, consisting mainly of nine parallel, tubule-like structures arranged around the inner wall of the cylinder. The two centrioles of each pair lie at right angles to each other.

Shortly before mitosis is to take place, the two pairs of centrioles begin to move apart from each other. This is caused by the growth of protein microtubules between the respective pairs that actually pushes them apart. At the same time, other microtubules grow radially away from each of the centriole pairs, forming a spiny star, called the *aster*, in each end of the cell. Some of the spines penetrate the nucleus and will play a role in separating the two sets of chromatids during mitosis. The complex of microtubules connecting the two centriole pairs is called the *spindle*, and the entire set of microtubules plus the two pairs of centrioles is called the *mitotic apparatus*.

Prophase. The first stage of mitosis, called *prophase*, is shown in Figure 3–12A, B, and C. While the spindle is forming, the chromosomes of the nucleus, which in interphase consist of loosely coiled strands, become condensed into well-defined chromosomes.

Prometaphase. During this stage (Fig. 3–12D), the nuclear envelope fragments. At the same time, a new set of microtubules begins to extend outward from a small condensed portion of each chromatid called the *kinetochore*. These new microtubules, in turn, either become attached to or interact with the microtubules from the two asters of the mitotic apparatus, with one chromatid connecting to one of the asters and the other chromatid connecting to the opposite aster.

Metaphase. During metaphase (Fig. 3–12E), the two asters of the mitotic apparatus are pushed farther apart by additional growth of the mitotic spindle. Simultaneously the chromatids are pulled tightly by the attached microtubules to the very center of the cell, lining up to form the *equatorial plate* of the mitotic spindle.

Anaphase. During this phase (Fig. 3–12F), the two chromatids of each chromosome are pulled apart. Exactly how the microtubular system causes this is not known, except that it is known that the microtubules contain *actin*, which is one of the contractile proteins of muscle. Therefore, it has been presumed that the microtubules might contract or that the chromosomal tubules might in some way interact with the microtubules of the aster to cause the pulling force. Regardless of the mechanism, all 46 pairs of chromatids are separated, forming two separate sets of 46 *daughter chromosomes*. One of these sets is pulled toward one mitotic aster and the other toward the other aster at the two respective poles of the dividing cell.

Telophase. In telophase (Fig. 3–12G and H), the two sets of daughter chromosomes are now pulled completely apart. Then the mitotic apparatus dissolutes and a new nuclear membrane develops around each set of chromosomes, this membrane being formed from portions of the endoplasmic reticulum that are already present in the cytoplasm. Shortly thereafter, the cell pinches in two midway between the two nuclei, for reasons mainly unexplained at present, except: (1) It is the two asters that initiate the cell division, each of the two daughter cells being composed of the portion of the cell occupied by a dissoluting aster. And (2) a contractile ring of *microfilaments* composed of *actin* and probably *myosin*, the two contractile proteins of muscle, develops at the juncture of the newly developing cells and pinches them off from each other.

CONTROL OF CELL GROWTH

In the normal human body, regulation of cell growth and reproduction is mainly a mystery. We know that certain cells grow and reproduce all the time, such as the blood-forming cells of the bone marrow, the germinal layers of the skin, and the epithelium of the gut. However, many other cells, such as smooth muscle cells, do not reproduce for many years. And a few cells, such as the neurons and striated muscle cells, usually do not reproduce during the entire life of the person.

If there is an insufficiency of certain types of cells in the body, these will grow and reproduce very rapidly until appropriate numbers of them are again available. For instance, seven-eighths of the liver can be removed surgically, and the cells of the remaining one-eighth will grow and divide until the liver mass returns almost to normal. The same effect occurs for almost all glandular cells, for cells of the bone marrow, the subcutaneous tissue, the intestinal epithelium, and almost any other tissue except highly differentiated cells, such as nerve and muscle cells.

We know very little about the mechanisms that maintain proper numbers of the different types of cells in the body. However, growth is often controlled by *growth factors* that come from other parts of the body. Some of these circulate in the blood, but others originate in adjacent tissues. For instance, the epithelial cells of some glands, such as the pancreas, will fail to grow without a growth factor from the sublying connective tissue of the gland. Also, cells grown in tissue culture often will stop growing when minute amounts of their own secretions are allowed to collect in the culture medium. This, too, could provide a means for feedback control of growth.

CANCER

Cancer is caused in all or almost all instances by *mutation* of cellular genes that control cell growth and cell mitosis. The mutated genes are called *oncogenes*. Usually two or more different oncogenes must occur in a cell before the cell will become cancerous.

Only a minute fraction of the cells that mutate in the body ever lead to cancer. There are several reasons for this: First, most mutated cells have less survival capability than normal cells and therefore simply die. Second, those cells that are potentially cancerous are usually destroyed by the body's immune system before they grow into a cancer. This occurs in the following way: Most mutated cells form abnormal proteins within their cell bodies because of their altered genes, and these proteins then stimulate the body's immune system, causing it to form antibodies against the cancerous cells, in this way destroying them. Indeed, it is believed that all of us are continually forming cells that are potentially cancerous but that our immune system acts as a scavenger that nips these abnormal cells in the bud before they can become established. In support of this is the fact that in persons whose immune systems have been suppressed, such as those who are taking immuno-

suppressant drugs following transplantation of a kidney or a heart, the probability of developing a cancer is multiplied severalfold.

But what is it that causes the mutations themselves? When one realizes that many trillions of new cells are formed each year in the human being, this question should probably better be asked in the following form: Why is it that we do not develop literally millions or billions of mutant cancerous cells? The answer is the incredible precision with which DNA chromosomal strands are replicated in each cell before mitosis takes place and also because the "proofreading" process cuts and repairs any abnormal DNA strand before the mitotic process is allowed to proceed.

Thus, chance alone is all that is required for mutations to take place, so we may suppose that a very large number of cancers are merely the result of an unlucky occurrence.

Yet, the probability of mutations can be increased manyfold when a person is exposed to certain chemical, physical, or biological factors. Some of these are the following:

(1) *Ionizing radiation* such as x-rays, gamma rays, and particle radiations from radioactive substances, and even ultraviolet light.

(2) *Chemical substances* of certain types, called *carcinogens*, also have a high propensity for causing mutations. The carcinogens that cause by far the greatest number of deaths in our present-day society are those in cigarette smoke. These cause about one quarter of all cancer deaths.

(3) *Physical irritants* can also lead to cancer, such as continued abrasion of the linings of the intestinal tract by some types of food.

(4) In many families there is a strong *hereditary tendency to cancer*.

Invasive Characteristic of the Cancer Cell. The two major differences between the cancer cell and the normal cell are: (1) The cancer cell does not respect usual cellular growth limits; the reason for this is that the cells presumably do not require the growth factors that are necessary to cause growth of normal cells. (2) Cancer cells are far less adhesive to each other than are normal cells. Therefore, they have a tendency to wander through the tissues, to enter the blood stream, and to be transported all through the body where they form nidi for numerous new cancerous growths.

Why Do Cancer Cells Kill? The answer to this is very simple: Cancer tissue competes with normal tissues for nutrients. Because cancer cells continue to proliferate indefinitely, their number multiplying day by day, one can readily understand that the cancer cells will soon demand essentially all the nutrition available to the body. As a result the normal tissues gradually suffer nutritive death.

QUESTIONS

1. What is a gene?
2. Give the overall schema by which genes control cellular function and reproduction.
3. What are the building blocks of DNA?
4. Explain the genetic code and how it is transferred from DNA to RNA and then to the formation of proteins.
5. What are the different types of RNA, and what are their specific functions?
6. How do the building blocks of RNA differ from those of DNA?
7. What is meant by the anticodons of transfer RNA and how do they function in relation to the codons of messenger RNA?
8. Explain the role of ribosomes in the formation of protein.
9. What is the role of peptide linkages in the formation of proteins, and how much energy is expended in the formation of each peptide linkage?
10. Explain the genetic regulation mechanism for regulating synthetic functions in a cell.
11. What is meant by an "operon"?
12. How do repressor substances and activator substances function in the regulation of cell activity?
13. Explain the difference between genetic regulation and enzyme regulation.
14. During cell reproduction, how is the replication of DNA different from the transcription process for the formation of RNA?
15. Explain the mechanism of DNA "proofreading."
16. Explain the formation of the mitotic apparatus as well as its functions during mitosis.
17. Describe the stages of mitosis.
18. What are some of the factors that control cell growth?
19. How do cancer cells differ from normal cells, and what prevents the formation of literally thousands of cancers in all persons?

References

Antoniades, H. N., and Owen, A. J.: Growth factors and regulation of cell growth. Annu Rev Med 33:445, 1982.

Bajaj, M., and Blundell, T.: Evolution and the tertiary structure of proteins. Annu Rev Biophys Bioeng 13:453, 1984.

Beers, R. F., ed.: Cell Fusion. Gene Transfer and Transformation. New York, Raven Press, 1984.

Bownes, M.: Differentiation of Cells. New York, Methuen, Inc., 1985.

Busch, H., ed.: The Cell Nucleus. Nuclear Particles. New York, Academic Press, 1981.

DeRecondo, A. M., ed.: New Approaches in Eukaryotic DNA Replication. New York, Plenum Publishing Corp., 1983.

Hall, A.: Oncogenes—implications for human cancer: A review. J R Soc Med 77:410, 1984.

Hunt, T., ed.: DNA Makes RNA Makes Protein. New York, Elsevier Science Publishing Co., 1983.

Kucherlapati, R., and Skoultchi, A. I.: Introduction of purified genes into mammalian cells. CRC Crit Rev Biochem 16:349, 1984.

Kulaev, J. S., ed.: Environmental Regulation of Microbial Metabolism. New York, Academic Press, 1985.

Lerman, L. S., et al.: Sequence-determined DNA separations. Annu Rev Biophys Bioeng 13:399, 1984.

Nomura, M., et al.: Regulation of the synthesis of ribosomes and ribosomal components. Annu Rev Biochem 53:75, 1984.

Pabo, C. O., and Sauer, R. T.: Protein-DNA recognition. Annu Rev Biochem 53:293, 1984.

Raff, E. C.: Genetics of microtubule systems. J Cell Biol 99:1, 1984.

Rigler, R., and Wintermeyer, W.: Dynamics of tRNA. Annu Rev Biophys Bioeng 12:475, 1983.

Schimke, R. T.: Gene amplification in cultured animal cells. Cell 37:705, 1984.

Smith, H. S., et al.: The biology of breast cancer at the cellular level. Biochem Biophys Acta 738:103, 1984.

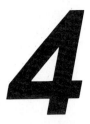

Transport Through the Cell Membrane

DIFFUSION
  DIFFUSION THROUGH THE CELL
    MEMBRANE
  NET DIFFUSION THROUGH THE
    PROTEIN CHANNELS OF THE CELL
    MEMBRANE AND FACTORS THAT
    AFFECT IT
  OSMOSIS ACROSS SELECTIVELY
    PERMEABLE MEMBRANES—NET
    DIFFUSION OF WATER

ACTIVE TRANSPORT
  BASIC MECHANISM OF ACTIVE
    TRANSPORT
  SECONDARY ACTIVE TRANSPORT:
    SODIUM COTRANSPORT OF
    GLUCOSE AND AMINO ACIDS

The fluid inside the cells of the body, called *intracellular fluid*, is very different from that outside the cells, called *extracellular fluid*. The extracellular fluid includes both the *interstitial fluid* that circulates in the spaces between the cells and also the fluid of the *blood plasma* that mixes freely with the interstitial fluid through the capillary walls. It is the extracellular fluid that supplies the cells with nutrients and other substances needed for cellular function. But before the cell can utilize these substances, they must also be transported through the cell membrane.

Figure 4–1 gives the approximate compositions of both the extracellular and intracellular fluids. Note that the extracellular fluid contains large quantities of *sodium* but only small quantities of *potassium*. Exactly the opposite is true of the intracellular fluid. Also, the extracellular fluid contains large quantities of chloride, while the intracellular fluid contains very little. But the concentrations of phosphates, essentially all of which are organic metabolic intermediates, and proteins in the intracellular fluid are considerably greater than in the extracellular fluid. These differences between the components of the intracellular and extracellular fluids are extremely important to the life of the cell. It is the purpose of this chapter to explain how these differences are brought about by the transport mechanisms in the cell membrane.

The Lipid Barrier and the Transport Proteins of the Cell Membrane

The structure of the cell membrane was discussed in Chapter 2 and shown in Figure 2–3. Basically, it consists of a *lipid bilayer* with large numbers of protein molecules floating in the lipid, many if not most of them penetrating all the way through, as illustrated in Figure 4–2.

	Extracellular fluid	Intracellular fluid
Na$^+$	142 mEq/L	10 mEq/L
K$^+$	4 mEq/L	140 mEq/L
Ca^{++}	5 mEq/L	<1 mEq/L
Mg^{++}	3 mEq/L	58 mEq/L
Cl$^-$	103 mEq/L	4 mEq/L
HCO$_3^-$	28 mEq/L	10 mEq/L
Phosphates	4 mEq/L	75 mEq/L
SO$_4^{--}$	1 mEq/L	2 mEq/L
Glucose	90 mg %	0 to 20 mg %
Amino acids	30 mg %	200 mg % ?
Cholesterol Phospholipids Neutral fat	0.5 g %	2 to 95 g %
Po$_2$	35 mm Hg	20 mm Hg ?
Pco$_2$	46 mm Hg	50 mm Hg ?
pH	7.4	7.0
Proteins	2 g % (5 mEq/L)	16 g % (40 mEq/L)

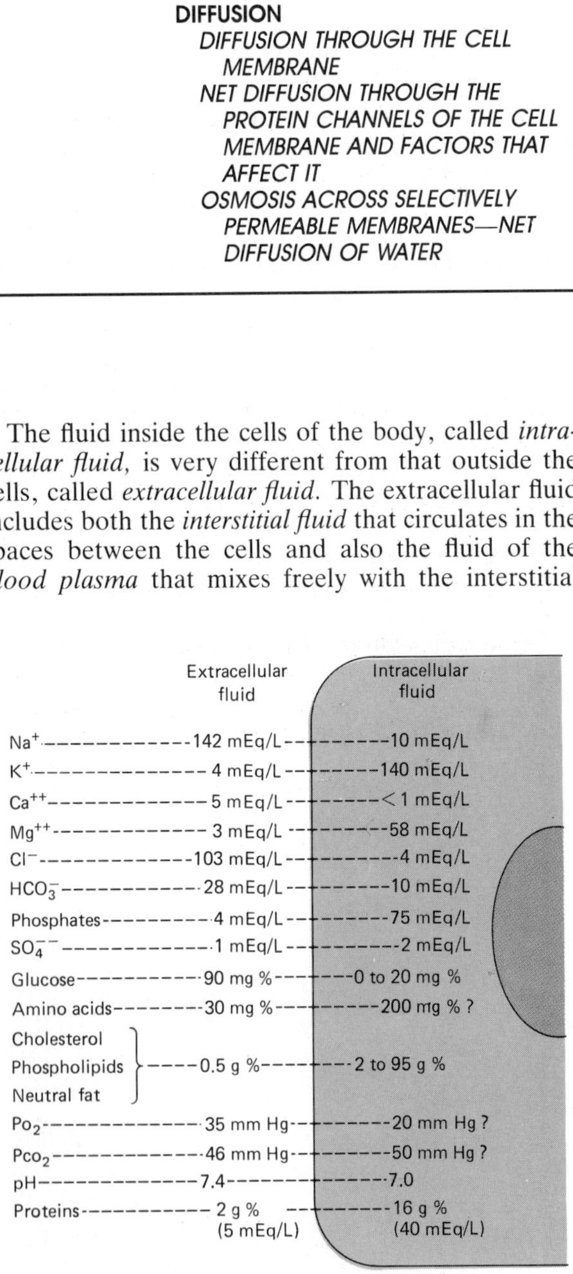

Figure 4–1. Chemical compositions of extracellular and intracellular fluids.

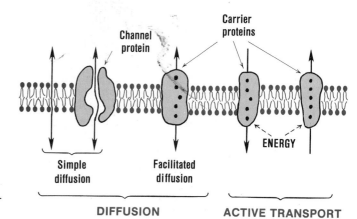

Figure 4–2. Transport pathways through the cell membrane and the basic mechanisms of transport.

The lipid bilayer is not miscible with either the extracellular or the intracellular fluid. Therefore, it constitutes a barrier for the movement of most water-soluble substances between the extracellular and intracellular fluid compartments. However, as illustrated by the left-hand arrow of Figure 4–2, a few substances can penetrate this bilayer and can either enter the cell or leave it, passing directly through the lipid substance itself.

The protein molecules, on the other hand, have entirely different transport properties. Their molecular structures interrupt the continuity of the lipid bilayer and therefore constitute an alternate pathway through the cell membrane. Most of these proteins, therefore, are *transport proteins*. Different transport proteins function differently. Some have watery spaces all the way through the molecule and allow free movement of certain ions or molecules; these are called *channel proteins*. Others, called *carrier proteins*, bind with substances that are to be transported, and conformational changes in the protein molecules then move the substances through the interstices of the molecules to the other side of the membrane. Both the channel proteins and the carrier proteins are highly selective in the type or types of molecules or ions that are allowed to cross the membrane.

Diffusion Versus Active Transport. Transport through the cell membrane, either directly through the lipid bilayer or through the proteins, occurs by one of two basic processes, *diffusion* (which is also called "passive transport") or *active transport*. Though there are many different variations of these two basic mechanisms, diffusion means random molecular movement of substances either through openings in the membrane or in combination with a carrier protein caused by the normal kinetic motion of matter. By contrast, active transport means movement of ions or other substances across the membrane in combination with a carrier protein but additionally capable of moving *against an energy gradient*, such as from a low concentration state to a high concentration state, a process that requires chemical energy to cause the movement. Let us explain in more detail the basic physics and physical chemistry of these two separate processes.

DIFFUSION

All molecules and ions in the body fluids, including both water molecules and dissolved substances, are in constant motion, each particle moving its own separate way. Motion of these particles is what physicists call heat—the greater the motion, the higher the temperature—and motion never ceases under any conditions except at absolute zero temperature. When a moving molecule, A, approaches a stationary molecule, B, the electrostatic and internuclear forces of molecule A repel molecule B, adding some of the energy of motion to molecule B. Consequently, molecule B gains kinetic energy of motion while molecule A slows down, losing some of its kinetic energy. Thus, as shown in Figure 4–3, a single molecule in solution bounces among the other molecules first in one direction, then another, then another, and so forth, bouncing randomly billions of times each second.

This continual movement of molecules among each other in liquids, or in gases, is called *diffusion*. Ions diffuse in exactly the same manner as whole molecules, and even suspended colloid particles diffuse in a similar manner, except that they diffuse far less rapidly than molecular substances because of their very large sizes.

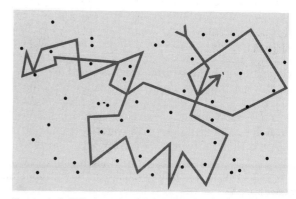

Figure 4–3. Diffusion of a fluid molecule during a billionth of a second.

DIFFUSION THROUGH THE CELL MEMBRANE

Simple Diffusion

Diffusion through the cell membrane is divided into two separate subprocesses called *simple diffusion* and *facilitated diffusion*. Simple diffusion means the molecular kinetic movement of molecules or ions through a membrane opening without the necessity of binding with carrier proteins in the membrane. The rate of diffusion is determined by the amount of substance available, by the velocity of kinetic motion, and by the number of openings in the cell membrane through which the molecules or ions can move. On the other hand, facilitated diffusion requires the interaction of the molecules or ions with a carrier protein that aids its passage through the membrane, probably by binding chemically with it and shuttling it through the membrane in this form.

Simple diffusion can occur through the cell membrane by two pathways: through the interstices of the lipid bilayer and through watery channels in some of the transport proteins, as illustrated to the left in Figure 4–2.

Diffusion Through the Lipid Bilayer

Diffusion of Lipid-Soluble Substances. One of the most important factors that determines how rapidly a substance will move through the lipid bilayer is the lipid solubility of the substance. For instance, the lipid solubilities of oxygen, nitrogen, and alcohols are very high, so that all these can dissolve directly in the lipid bilayer and diffuse through the cell membrane in exactly the same manner that diffusion occurs in a watery solution. For obvious reasons, the rate of diffusion of these substances through the membrane is directly proportional to their lipid solubility. Note especially that tremendous quantities of oxygen can be transported in this way; therefore, oxygen is delivered to the interior of the cell almost as though the cell membrane did not exist.

Transport of Water and Other Lipid-Insoluble Molecules. Even though water is highly insoluble in the membrane lipids, nevertheless it penetrates the cell membrane very readily, most of it passing directly through the lipid bilayer and still more passing through protein channels as well. The rapidity with which water molecules can penetrate the cell membrane is astounding. As an example, the total amount of water that diffuses in each direction through the red cell membrane during each second is approximately 100 times as great as the volume of the red cell itself.

The reason for the extreme diffusion of water through the lipid bilayer is still not certain, but it is believed that the water molecules are small enough and their kinetic energy great enough that they can simply penetrate like bullets through the lipid portion of the membrane before the "hydrophobic" character of the lipids can stop them.

Failure of Ions to Diffuse Through the Lipid Bilayer. Even though water and other very small uncharged molecules diffuse easily through the lipid bilayer, ions—even small ions such as hydrogen ions, sodium ions, potassium ions, and so forth—penetrate the lipid bilayer about one million times less rapidly than does water. Therefore, any significant transport of these through the cell membrane must occur through channels in the proteins, as we shall discuss shortly.

The reason for the impenetrability of the lipid bilayer to ions is the electrical charge of the ions; this impedes ionic movement in two separate ways: (1) The electrical charge of these ions causes multiple molecules of water to become bonded to the ions, forming so-called *hydrated ions*. This greatly increases the sizes of ions, which alone impedes penetration of the lipid bilayer. (2) Even more important, the electrical charge of the ion also interacts with the charges of the lipid bilayer in such a way that the ion is instantaneously repulsed.

To summarize, Table 4–1 gives the relative permeabilities of the lipid bilayer to a number of different molecules or ions of different diameters. Note especially the *extremely poor permeance of the ions* because of their electrical charges and the *poor permeance of glucose* because of its molecular diameter. But note also that glycerol penetrates the membrane almost as easily as urea even though its diameter is almost twice as great. The reason for this is a slight degree of lipid solubility.

Diffusion Through Protein Channels and "Gating" of These Channels

The protein channels are believed to be watery pathways through the interstices of the protein molecules. Therefore, substances can diffuse directly through these channels from one side of the membrane to the other. However, the protein channels are distinguished by two important characteristics: (1) They are often selectively permeable to certain substances. (2) Many of the channels can be opened or closed by *gates*.

Selective Permeability of Different Protein Channels. Most, but not all, protein channels are highly selective for the transport of one or more specific ions or molecules. This results from the characteristics

Table 4–1. RELATIVE PERMEABILITY OF THE CELL MEMBRANE LIPID BILAYER TO MOLECULES OF DIFFERENT SIZES

Substance	Diameter (nm)	Relative Permeability
Water molecule	0.3	1.0
Urea molecule	0.36	0.0006
Hydrated chloride ion	0.386	0.00000001
Hydrated potassium ion	0.396	0.0000000006
Hydrated sodium ion	0.512	0.0000000002
Glycerol	0.62	0.0006
Glucose	0.86	0.000009

of the channel itself, such as its diameter, its shape, and the nature of the electrical charges along its surfaces. To give an example, one of the most important of the protein channels, the so-called *sodium channel,* is only 0.3 by 0.5 nm in size, but more importantly the inner surfaces of these channels are *strongly negatively charged,* as illustrated by the negative signs in the top panel of Figure 4–4. These strong negative charges pull the sodium ions more than they pull other physiologically important ions into the channels, because the ratio of pulling force to ionic diameter is far greater for sodium than for the others. Once in the channel, the sodium ion then diffuses in either direction according to the usual laws of diffusion. Thus, the sodium channel is specifically selective for the passage of sodium ions.

On the other hand, another set of protein channels is selective for potassium transport, illustrated in the lower panel of Figure 4–4. These channels are slightly smaller than the sodium channels, only 0.3 by 0.3 nm, but *they are not negatively charged.* Therefore, no strong attractive force is pulling ions into the channels. On the other hand, the hydrated form of the potassium ion is considerably smaller than the hydrated form of sodium because the sodium ion has one whole orbital set of electrons less than the potassium ion, which allows the sodium nucleus to attract far more water molecules than can the potassium. Therefore, the smaller hydrated potassium ions can pass easily through this channel whereas sodium ions are mainly rejected, thus once again providing selective permeability for a specific ion.

Gating of Protein Channels. Gating of protein channels means simply the opening or closing of the

channels. This provides a means for controlling the permeability of the channels. This is illustrated in the upper and lower panels of Figure 4–4 for both the sodium and the potassium ion. It is believed that the gates are actual gate-like extensions of the transport protein molecule, which can close over the opening of the channel or can be lifted away from the opening by a physical change in the shape of the protein molecule itself.

The opening and closing of gates are controlled by at least two principal ways:

(1) *Voltage gating.* In this instance, the molecular conformation of the gate responds to the electrical potential across the cell membrane. This is the basic cause of action potentials in nerves that are responsible for nerve signals as we shall discuss in the following chapter.

(2) *Ligand gating.* Some protein channel gates are opened by the binding of another molecule with the protein, this also causing a physical change in the protein molecule that opens or closes the gate. This is called *ligand gating,* and the substance that binds is the *ligand.* One of the most important instances of ligand gating is the effect of acetylcholine on the so-called *acetylcholine channel.* This opens the gate of this channel, providing a pore about 0.65 nm in diameter that allows all molecules and positive ions smaller than this diameter to pass through. This gate is exceedingly important in the transmission of signals from one nerve cell to another (Chapter 31) and from nerve cells to muscle cells (Chapter 7).

Figure 4–5 illustrates an especially interesting characteristic of voltage-gated channels. This figure shows two recordings of electrical current flowing through a sodium channel when there was an approximate 25 millivolt potential gradient across the pore. Note that the pore conducts current either all or none. That is, the gate of the pore snaps open and then snaps closed, each snapping event occurring within a few

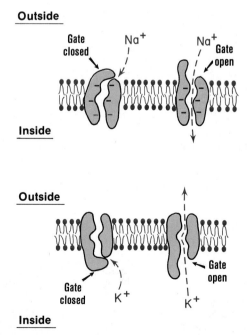

Figure 4–4. Transport of sodium and potassium ions through protein channels. Also shown are conformational changes of the channel protein molecules that open or close the "gates" guarding the channels.

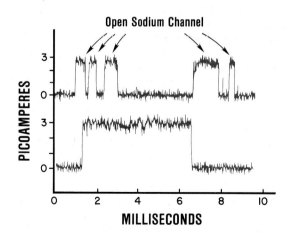

Figure 4–5. Record of current flow through a single voltage-gated sodium pore, demonstrating the all-or-none principle for opening the pore. (This type of record is obtained using a "patchclamp," which is a minute pipette, the tip of which abuts tightly against a small area of the cell membrane and allows current flow to be measured through individual pores.)

millionths of a second. This illustrates the rapidity with which the conformational changes can occur in the shape of the protein molecular gates. The figure also shows in the lower recording another important characteristic: at one voltage potential the pore may remain closed all the time or almost all the time, whereas at another voltage level it may remain open either all or most of the time. However, at in-between voltages, the pores tend to snap open and closed as illustrated in the upper recording, giving an average current flow somewhere between the minimum and the maximum.

Facilitated Diffusion

Facilitated diffusion is also called *carrier-mediated diffusion,* because a substance transported in this manner usually cannot pass through the membrane without a specific carrier protein helping it. That is, the carrier *facilitates* the diffusion of the substance to the other side.

Facilitated diffusion differs from simple diffusion through an open channel in the following very important way: whereas the rate of diffusion through an open channel increases proportionately with the concentration of the diffusing substance, in facilitated diffusion the rate of diffusion approaches a maximum as the concentration of the substance increases.

What is it that limits the rate of facilitated diffusion? A probable answer is that each time a molecule is transported by facilitated diffusion the molecule must first bind with a carrier protein and then be shuttled through the membrane by the carrier. Therefore, the rate of facilitated diffusion reaches a maximum when all the carrier proteins are functioning as rapidly as they can.

Among the most important substances that cross cell membranes by facilitated diffusion are *glucose* and the *amino acids.* Insulin can increase the rate of facilitated diffusion of glucose as much as 10- to 20-fold. This is the principal mechanism by which insulin controls glucose utilization in the body, as we shall discuss in Chapter 52.

NET DIFFUSION THROUGH THE PROTEIN CHANNELS OF THE CELL MEMBRANE AND FACTORS THAT AFFECT IT

By now it is evident that many different substances can diffuse either through the lipid bilayer of the cell membrane or through protein channels. However, please understand clearly that substances that diffuse in one direction can also diffuse in the opposite direction. Usually, what is important to the cell is not the total substance diffusing in both directions but the difference between these two, which is the *net rate of diffusion*; this is the difference between the rate of diffusion in one direction and that in the other direction. Some of the factors that affect this net diffusion are:

The Permeability of the Membrane. The permea- bility of a membrane is defined as the rate of transport through a unit area of membrane for a given concentration difference. Among the factors that affect the total permeability of the membrane protein channels are (a) the *number* of channels through which the substance can diffuse, (b) the degree of impediment to movement through each channel—that is, the *resistance* of the channel, (c) the *molecular weight* of the diffusing substance, and (d) the *temperature.* The effect of each of these on the permeability is obvious, with the possible exception of temperature and molecular weight.

A higher temperature increases the permeability because the thermal motion of all the molecules and ions in a solution increases directly with the temperature, thus more diffusion through the channels.

The molecular weight affects diffusion of molecules and ions mainly because the velocity of kinetic motion in a solution is inversely proportional to the square root of the molecular weight. Therefore, in general, the permeability of the membrane is also approximately inversely proportional to the square root of the molecular weight.

The following formula gives the approximate effect of all the above factors together on the permeability of the membrane for diffusion of any given substance:

$$\text{Permeability} = \frac{\begin{array}{c}\text{Number of channels per unit area}\\ \times \text{ temperature}\end{array}}{\begin{array}{c}\text{Resistance of each channel}\\ \times \text{ square root of molecular weight}\end{array}}$$

Effect of a Concentration Difference. Figure 4–6A illustrates a membrane with a substance in high concentration on the outside and low concentration on the inside. The rate at which the substance diffuses *inward* is proportional to the concentration of molecules on the outside, for this concentration determines how many of the molecules strike the outside of the channels each second. On the other hand, the rate at which the molecules diffuse *outward* is proportional to their concentration *inside* the membrane. Obviously, therefore, the rate of net diffusion into the cell is proportional to the concentration on the outside *minus* the concentration on the inside or

$$\text{Net diffusion} \propto P (C_o - C_i)$$

in which C_o is the concentration on the outside, C_i is the concentration on the inside, and P is the permeability of the membrane for the substance.

Effect of an Electrical Potential Difference. If an electrical potential is applied across the membrane as shown in Figure 4–6B, because of their electrical charges ions will move through the membrane even though no concentration difference exists to cause their movement. Thus, to the left in the figure, the concentrations of negative ions are exactly the same on both sides of the membrane, but a positive charge has been applied to the right side of the membrane and a negative charge to the left, creating an electrical

A.

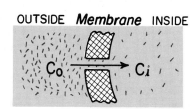

OUTSIDE *Membrane* INSIDE

$$C_o \longrightarrow C_i$$

B.

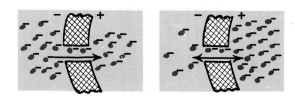

C.

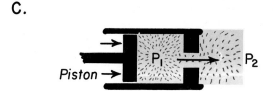

Piston → P_1 P_2

Figure 4–6. Effect of (*A*) concentration difference, (*B*) electrical difference, and (*C*) pressure difference on net diffusion of molecules and ions through a cell membrane.

gradient across the membrane. The positive charge attracts the negative ions while the negative charge repels them. Therefore, net diffusion occurs from left to right. After much time large quantities of negative ions will have moved to the right (if we neglect, for the time being, the disturbing effects of the positive ions of the solution), creating the condition illustrated on the right in Figure 4–6B, in which a concentration difference of the same ions has developed in the direction opposite to the electrical potential difference. Obviously, the concentration difference is now tending to move the ions to the left, while the electrical difference is tending to move them to the right. When the concentration difference rises high enough, the two effects will exactly balance each other. At normal body temperature (37°C), the electrical difference that will exactly balance a given concentration difference of *univalent* ions, such as Na$^+$, K$^+$, or Cl$^-$, can be determined from the following formula called the *Nernst equation:*

$$\text{EMF (in millivolts)} = \pm 61 \log \frac{C_1}{C_2}$$

in which EMF is the electromotive force (voltage) between side 1 and side 2 of the membrane, C_1 is the concentration on side 1, and C_2 is the concentration on side 2. The polarity of the voltage on side 1 in the above equation is + for negative ions and − for

positive ions. This relationship is extremely important in understanding the transmission of nerve impulses, for which reason it is discussed in even greater detail in the following chapter.

Effect of a Pressure Difference. At times considerable pressure difference develops between the two sides of a membrane. This occurs, for instance, at the capillary membrane, which has a pressure approximately 23 mm Hg greater inside the capillary than outside. Pressure actually means the sum of all the forces of the different molecules striking a unit surface area at a given instant. Therefore, when the pressure is higher on one side of a membrane than the other, this means that the sum of all the forces of the molecules striking the channels on that side of the membrane is greater than on the other side. This can result either from greater numbers of molecules striking the membrane per second or from greater kinetic energy of the average molecule striking the membrane. In either event, increased amounts of energy are available to cause net movement of molecules from the high pressure side toward the low pressure side. This effect is illustrated in Figure 4–6C, which shows a piston developing high pressure on one side of a cell membrane, thereby causing net diffusion through the membrane to the other side.

OSMOSIS ACROSS SELECTIVELY PERMEABLE MEMBRANES—NET DIFFUSION OF WATER

By far the most abundant substance to diffuse through the cell membrane is water. It should be recalled again that enough water ordinarily diffuses in each direction through the red cell membrane per second to equal about *100 times the volume of the cell itself.* Yet, *normally*, the amount that diffuses in the two directions is so precisely balanced that not even the slightest *net* movement of water occurs. Therefore, the volume of the cell remains constant. However, under certain conditions, a *concentration difference for water* can develop across a membrane, just as concentration differences for other substances can also occur. When this happens, net movement of water does occur across the cell membrane, causing the cell either to swell or to shrink, depending on the direction of the net movement. This process of net movement of water caused by a concentration difference of water is called *osmosis.*

To give an example of osmosis, let us assume the conditions shown in Figure 4–7, with pure water on one side of the cell membrane and a solution of sodium chloride on the other side. Referring back to Table 4–1, we see that water molecules pass through the cell membrane with extreme ease while sodium and chloride ions pass through only with extreme difficulty. Therefore, sodium chloride solution is actually a mixture of permeant water molecules and nonpermeant sodium and chloride ions, and the membrane is said to be *selectively permeable* (or sometimes "semipermeable"), i.e., permeable to water but not to sodium and chloride ions. Yet, the presence of the

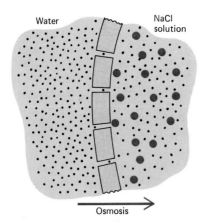

Figure 4–7. Osmosis at a cell membrane when a sodium chloride solution is placed on one side of the membrane and water on the other side.

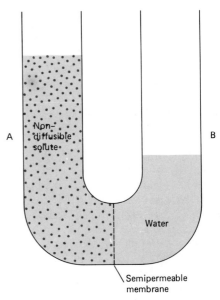

Figure 4–8. Demonstration of osmotic pressure on the two sides of a semipermeable membrane.

sodium and chloride has reduced the concentration of water molecules to less than that of pure water. As a result, in the example of Figure 4–7, more water molecules strike the channels on the left side where there is pure water than on the right side where the water concentration has been reduced. Thus, net movement of water occurs from left to right—that is, osmosis occurs from the pure water into the NaCl solution.

Osmotic Pressure

If in Figure 4–7 pressure were applied to the sodium chloride solution, osmosis of water into this solution could be slowed or even stopped. The amount of pressure required to stop osmosis completely is called the *osmotic pressure* of the sodium chloride solution.

The principle of a pressure difference opposing osmosis is illustrated in Figure 4–8, which shows a selectively permeable membrane separating two columns of fluid, one containing water and the other containing a solution of water and some solute that will not penetrate the membrane. Osmosis of water from chamber B into chamber A causes the levels of the fluid columns to become farther and farther apart, until eventually a pressure difference is developed that is great enough to oppose the osmotic effect. The pressure difference across the membrane at this point is the osmotic pressure of the solution containing the nondiffusible solute.

Importance of Numbers of Osmotic Particles (or of Molar Concentration) in Determining Osmotic Pressure. The osmotic pressure exerted by particles in a solution, whether they be molecules or ions, is determined by the *numbers* of particles per unit volume of fluid and not the mass of the particles. The reason for this is that each particle in a solution, regardless of its mass, exerts, on the average, the same amount of pressure against the membrane. That is, all particles are bouncing among each other with, on the average, equal energy because the large molecules move very slowly, whereas the small molecules move very rapidly. Consequently, the factor that determines the osmotic pressure of a solution is the concentration of the solution in terms of numbers of particles (which is the same as its *molar concentration* if it is a nondissociated molecule) and not in terms of mass of the solute.

Osmolality—The Osmole. Since the amount of osmotic pressure exerted by a solute is proportional to the concentration of the solute in numbers of molecules or ions, expressing the solute concentration in terms of mass is of no value in determining osmotic pressure. To express the concentration in terms of numbers of particles, the unit called the *osmole* is used in place of grams.

One osmole is the number of particles (molecules) in 1 gram molecular weight of undissociated solute. Thus, 180 grams of glucose, which is one gram molecular weight of glucose, is equal to 1 osmole of glucose, because glucose does not dissociate. On the other hand, if the solute dissociates into two ions, 1 gram molecular weight of the solute equals 2 osmoles, because the number of osmotically active particles is now twice as great as is the case in the undissociated solute. Therefore, 1 gram molecular weight of sodium chloride, 58.5 grams, is equal to 2 osmoles.

ACTIVE TRANSPORT

Often only a minute concentration of a substance is present in the extracellular fluid, and yet a large concentration of the substance is required in the intracellular fluid. For instance, this is true of potassium ions. Conversely, other substances frequently enter cells and must be removed even though their concentrations inside are far less than outside. This is true of sodium ions.

From the discussion thus far it is evident that *no substances can diffuse against an electrochemical gra-*

dient, which is the sum of all the diffusion forces acting at the membrane—the forces caused by concentration difference, electrical difference, and pressure difference. That is, it is often said that substances cannot diffuse "uphill." To cause movement of a substance uphill, energy must be imparted to the substance. This is analogous to the compression of air by a pump. Compression causes the concentration of the air molecules to increase, but to create this greater concentration, energy must be imparted to the air molecules by the piston of the pump as they are compressed. Likewise, as molecules are transported through a cell membrane from a dilute solution to a concentrated solution, energy must be imparted to the molecules to concentrate them. When a cell membrane moves molecules uphill against a concentration gradient (or uphill against an electrical or pressure gradient) the process is called *active transport.*

Among the different substances that are actively transported through cell membranes are sodium ions, potassium ions, calcium ions, iron ions, hydrogen ions, chloride ions, iodide ions, urate ions, several different sugars, and the amino acids.

BASIC MECHANISM OF ACTIVE TRANSPORT

Active transport depends on transport of substances by *carrier proteins* that penetrate through the membrane, the same as is true for facilitated diffusion. However, in active transport, the carrier protein functions differently from the carrier in facilitated diffusion, because the carrier must now impart energy to the substance that is being transported to move it against the electrochemical gradient. The energy for this purpose is derived from ATP. Furthermore, the active transport carrier proteins have ATPase activity, which means that they can cleave ATP to form ADP or AMP with release of the energy from the high energy phosphate bonds. Unfortunately, though, the manner in which this energy is coupled to cause transport of the substance against the electrochemical gradient is not yet clear.

The Sodium-Potassium "Pump"

The most ubiquitous active transport mechanism in the body is the one that transports sodium ions out of cells to the exterior and at the same time pumps potassium ions from the outside to the inside; it is called the *sodium-potassium pump.* This pump is present in all cells of the body, and it is responsible for maintaining the sodium and potassium concentration differences across the cell membrane as well as for establishing a negative electrical potential inside the cells. Indeed, we shall see in the next chapter that this pump is the basis of nerve function to transmit signals throughout the nervous system.

Figure 4–9 illustrates the basic components of the Na^+-K^+ pump. The *carrier protein* is a complex of two separate globular proteins. This complex has

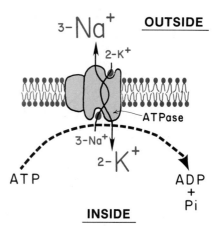

Figure 4–9. The postulated mechanism of the sodium-potassium pump.

three specific features that are important for function of the pump:

(1) It has three *receptor sites for binding sodium ions* on the portion of the protein that protrudes to the interior of the cell.

(2) It has two *receptor sites for potassium ions* on the outside.

(3) The inside portion of this carrier protein adjacent to or near the sodium binding sites has ATPase activity.

Now to put the pump into perspective: When three sodium ions bind on the inside of the carrier protein and two potassium ions on the outside, the ATPase function of the protein becomes activated. This then cleaves 1 molecule of ATP, splitting it to ADP and liberating a high energy phosphate bond of energy. This energy is then believed to cause a conformational change in the protein carrier molecule, extruding the three sodium ions to the outside and the two potassium ions to the inside.

Note also in Figure 4–9 that the concentration of sodium on the inside, as designated by the small size of the Na^+ symbol, is very slight, whereas the concentration of the sodium on the outside is very great. Conversely, the potassium ion concentration on the outside is very slight whereas its concentration on the inside is very great. Thus, both these ions are transported against very large energy gradients.

The Calcium Pump

Another very important pump is the calcium pump. Calcium ions are normally maintained at extremely low concentration in the intracellular fluid, at a concentration about 10,000 times less than that in the extracellular fluid. This is achieved by two calcium pumps: One is in the cell membrane and pumps calcium to the outside of the cell. The other pumps calcium ions into one or more of the internal vesicular organelles of the cell, such as into the sarcoplasmic reticulum of muscle cells and into the mitochondria in all cells. In both instances, the carrier protein responsible for pumping the calcium ions is an ATPase having the same capability to cleave ATP as the ATPase sodium-potassium carrier protein. The difference is that this protein has a binding site for calcium instead of sodium.

Saturation of Active Transport

Active transport "saturates" in exactly the same way that facilitated diffusion saturates. That is, at large concentrations, transport approaches a maximum, as is also true for facilitated diffusion. The saturation is caused by limitation of the rates at which the chemical reactions of binding, release, and carrier conformational changes can occur.

Energetics of Active Transport

The amount of energy required to transport a substance actively through a membrane (aside from energy lost as heat in the chemical reactions) is determined by the amount that the substance is concentrated during transport. Compared to the energy required to concentrate a substance tenfold, to concentrate it 100-fold requires twice as much energy, and to concentrate it 1000-fold requires three times as much. In other words, the energy required is proportional to the logarithm of the degree that the substance is concentrated, as expressed by the following formula:

$$\text{Energy (in calories per osmole)} = 1400 \log \frac{C_1}{C_2}$$

That is, in terms of calories, the amount of energy required to concentrate 1 osmole of substance tenfold is about 1400 calories. One can see that the energy expenditure for concentrating substances in cells or for removing substances from cells against a concentration gradient can be tremendous. Some cells, such as those lining the renal tubules, as well as many glandular cells perhaps expend as much as 90 per cent of their energy for this purpose alone.

SECONDARY ACTIVE TRANSPORT: SODIUM COTRANSPORT OF GLUCOSE AND AMINO ACIDS

Glucose and amino acids are transported into some cells against very large concentration gradients, even though the carrier protein for transport of these substances cannot cleave ATP to provide the required energy. Instead, the energy is provided by the concentration gradient of the sodium ions across the cell membrane. The mechanism of this is illustrated in Figure 4–10. Note that the carrier protein has two binding sites on its exterior side, one for sodium and one for glucose. But note also that the concentration of sodium is very high on the outside and very low on the inside. Therefore, sodium ions are always attempting to move down their energy gradient to the interior of the cell, causing continual stress on

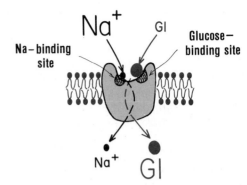

Figure 4–10. A postulated mechanism for sodium cotransport of glucose.

the carrier protein to let the sodium ions pass on through to the interior. However, another property of this carrier protein is that the conformational change of the protein molecule will not occur to allow the sodium to move to the interior unless a glucose molecule is also attached. But once both the sodium ion and the glucose molecule are attached, then the conformational change takes place and both the sodium and glucose are transported to the inside of the cell at the same time. Furthermore, this can occur even though the glucose must be transported "uphill" from a low concentration on the outside to a high concentration inside. That is, the energy gradient of the sodium ions literally pulls the glucose to the interior, thus utilizing energy from the sodium gradient to cause the uphill transport of the glucose. For obvious reasons, this type of transport has received both the names *secondary active transport* and *sodium-glucose cotransport.*

Sodium cotransport of the amino acids occurs in the same manner as for glucose except that it utilizes a different set of transport proteins. Five separate *amino acid transport proteins* have been identified, each of which is responsible for transporting one subset of amino acids with specific molecular characteristics.

Sodium cotransport of glucose and amino acids occurs especially in the epithelial cells of the intestinal tract and renal tubules to aid in the absorption of these substances into the blood, as we shall discuss in later chapters.

Sodium *countertransport* mechanisms also occur; these can cause transport in the *opposite direction* from the movement of the sodium. That is, a receptor site is present on the outside of the carrier protein for sodium but on the inside for the other substance, and movement of the sodium down its energy gradient to the inside of the cell causes the other substance to be transported to the exterior. Transport of this type has been observed in some cells for exchange of sodium and other ions, such as potassium or calcium, across the membrane.

It is clear that the ultimate source of the energy for sodium cotransport or countertransport is ATP, which drives the sodium-potassium pump to build up the necessary sodium concentration gradient.

QUESTIONS

1. What are the principal differences between the composition of extracellular fluid and that of intracellular fluid?
2. Describe the transport properties of the cell membrane lipid barrier. What substances penetrate this barrier with ease, and why?
3. Describe the characteristics of the transport proteins.
4. Explain the mechanism of diffusion. Also explain the difference between simple diffusion and facilitated diffusion.
5. What are some of the substances that are transported through the cell membrane by simple diffusion?
6. What are some of the substances transported through the cell membrane by facilitated diffusion? Why do both facilitated diffusion and active transport "saturate"—that is, why do each of these reach a maximum rate at which they can transport substances?
7. How do ions pass through the cell membrane? Explain what is meant by *gating* of protein transport channels. Also explain *voltage gating* and *ligand gating*.
8. Explain how each of the following factors affects net diffusion through the cell membrane: (a) permeability of the membrane, (b) concentration difference across the membrane, (c) electrical potential difference across the membrane, and (d) pressure difference across the membrane.
9. Give the Nernst equation. If the concentration of sodium ions is ten times as great inside a membrane as outside and only sodium ions can pass through the membrane, what is the electrical potential across the membrane?
10. Explain the mechanisms of osmosis and osmotic pressure.
11. Why is osmotic pressure determined by the molar concentration of a solution rather than by its mass concentration of the dissolved solute?
12. Give the numerical relationship between osmolality of a solution and its osmotic pressure.
13. In what way does active transport differ from facilitated diffusion?
14. Describe the mechanism of the sodium-potassium "pump."
15. What substances are transported by the mechanism of active transport in different cells of the body?
16. How much energy is required to concentrate one osmol of a substance 10-fold? To concentrate it 1000-fold?
17. Explain the mechanism of sodium cotransport. What important substances are normally transported by the mechanism of cotransport in many cells of the body?

References

Agnew, W. S.: Voltage-regulated sodium channel molecules. Annu Rev Physiol 46:517, 1984.

Almers, W., and Stirling, C.: Distribution of transport proteins over animal cell membranes. J Membr Biol 77:169, 1984.

Auerbach, A., and Sachs, F.: Patch clamp studies of single ionic channels. Annu Rev Biophys Bioeng 13:269, 1984.

Blachley, J. E., et al.: The harmful effects of ethanol on ion transport and cellular respiration. Am J Med Sci 289:22, 1985.

DiPolo, R., and Beauge, L.: The calcium pump and sodium-calcium exchange in squid axons. Annu Rev Physiol 45:313, 1983.

Ellis, D.: Na-Ca exchange in cardiac tissues. Adv Myocardiol 5:295, 1985.

Fettiplace, R., and Haydon, D. A.: Water permeability of lipid membranes. Physiol Rev 60:510, 1980.

Flatman, P. W.: Magnesium transport across cell membranes. J Membr Biol 80:1, 1984.

Gadsby, D. C.: The Na/K pump of cardiac cells. Annu Rev Biophys Bioeng 13:373, 1984.

Hess, G. P., et al.: Acetylcholine receptor-controlled ion translocation: Chemical kinetic investigations of the mechanism. Annu Rev Biophys Bioeng 12:443, 1983.

Ives, H. E., and Rector, F. C., Jr.: Proton transport and cell function. J Clin Invest 73:285, 1984.

Katz, A. M.: Basic cellular mechanisms of action of the calcium-channel blockers. Am J Cardiol 55:2B, 1985.

Latorre, R., and Alvarez, O.: Voltage-dependent channels in planar lipid bilayer membranes. Physiol Rev 61:77, 1981.

Macey, R. I.: Transport of water and urea in red blood cells. Am J Physiol 246:C195, 1984.

Malhotra, S. K.: The Plasma Membrane. New York, John Wiley & Sons, 1983.

Miller, C.: Integral membrane channels: Studies in model membranes. Physiol Rev 63:1209, 1983.

Naftalin, R. J.: The thermostatics and thermodynamics of cotransport. Biochem Biophys Acta 778:155, 1984.

Reuter, H.: Ion channels in cardiac cell membranes. Annu Rev Physiol 46:473, 1984.

Sakmann, B., and Neher, E.: Patch clamp techniques for studying ionic channels in excitable membranes. Annu Rev Physiol 46:455, 1984.

Schultz, S. G.: A cellular model for active sodium absorption by mammalian colon. Annu Rev Physiol 46:435, 1984.

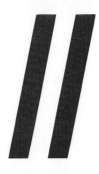

NERVE AND MUSCLE

5 ■ Membrane Potentials, Action Potentials, Excitation, and Rhythmicity

6 ■ Contraction of Skeletal Muscle

7 ■ Neuromuscular Transmission and Function of Smooth Muscle

5

Membrane Potentials, Action Potentials, Excitation, and Rhythmicity

BASIC PHYSICS OF MEMBRANE
  POTENTIALS
  *MEMBRANE POTENTIALS CAUSED BY
    DIFFUSION*
  *MEMBRANE POTENTIALS CAUSED BY
    ACTIVE TRANSPORT—THE
    SODIUM–POTASSIUM
    ELECTROGENIC "PUMP"*
  *MEASURING THE MEMBRANE
    POTENTIAL*
THE RESTING MEMBRANE POTENTIAL
  OF NERVES
  *ORIGIN OF NORMAL RESTING
    MEMBRANE POTENTIAL*
THE NERVE ACTION POTENTIAL
  *THE VOLTAGE–GATED SODIUM AND
    POTASSIUM CHANNELS*
  *SUMMARY OF EVENTS THAT CAUSE
    THE ACTION POTENTIAL*

*INITIATION OF THE ACTION
  POTENTIAL*
PROPAGATION OF THE ACTION
  POTENTIAL
RECHARGING THE FIBER MEMBRANE
  AFTER ACTION POTENTIALS—
  IMPORTANCE OF ENERGY
  METABOLISM
PLATEAU IN SOME ACTION POTENTIALS
RHYTHMICITY OF CERTAIN EXCITABLE
  TISSUES—REPETITIVE DISCHARGE
SPECIAL ASPECTS OF SIGNAL
  TRANSMISSION IN NERVE TRUNKS
  *VELOCITY OF CONDUCTION IN
    NERVE FIBERS*
EXCITATION—THE PROCESS OF
  ELICITING ACTION POTENTIAL
RECORDING MEMBRANE POTENTIALS
  AND ACTION POTENTIALS

Electrical potentials exist across the membranes of essentially all cells of the body, and some cells, such as nerve and muscle cells, are "excitable"—that is, capable of self-generation of electrochemical impulses at their membranes and employment of these impulses to transmit signals along the membranes. In still other types of cells, such as glandular cells, macrophages, and ciliated cells, changes in membrane potentials probably play significant roles in controlling other of the cell's functions.

BASIC PHYSICS OF MEMBRANE POTENTIALS

Before beginning this discussion, let us first recall that the fluids both inside and outside the cells are electrolytic solutions containing 150 to 160 mEq per liter of positive ions and the same concentration of negative ions. Generally, a very minute excess of negative ions (anions) accumulates immediately inside the cell membrane along its inner surface, as illustrated in Figures 5–1A and 5–2, and an equal number of positive ions (cations) accumulate immediately outside the membrane. The effect of this is the establishment of a *membrane potential* between the inside and outside of the cell.

The two basic means by which membrane potentials can develop are (1) diffusion of ions through the membrane as a result of ion concentration differences between the two sides of the membrane, thus creating an imbalance of negative and positive charges on the two sides of the membrane, and (2) active transport of ions through the membrane, thus also creating an imbalance of charges.

DIFFUSION POTENTIALS

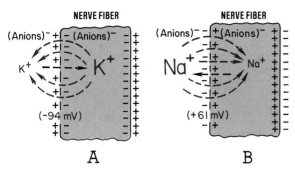

Figure 5–1. *A,* Establishment of a diffusion potential across a cell membrane, caused by potassium ions diffusing from inside the cell to the outside through a membrane that is selectively permeable only to potassium. *B,* Establishment of a diffusion potential when the membrane is permeable only to sodium ions. Note that the internal membrane potential is negative when potassium ions diffuse and positive when sodium ions diffuse because of opposite concentration gradients of these two ions.

MEMBRANE POTENTIALS CAUSED BY DIFFUSION

Figures 5–1A and B illustrate a nerve fiber when there is no active transport of either sodium or potassium. In Figure 5–1A the potassium concentration is very great inside the membrane while that outside is very low. Furthermore, the membrane is very permeable to the potassium ions but not to any other ions. Because of the large potassium concentration gradient from the inside toward the outside, there is a strong tendency for potassium ions to diffuse outward. As they do so, they carry positive charges to the outside, thus creating a state of electropositivity outside the membrane, and electronegativity on the inside because of the negative anions that remain behind. This potential difference across the membrane tends to repel the potassium ions in a backward direction from outside toward the inside. And within a millisecond or so the potential becomes great enough to block further diffusion of potassium ions to the exterior. The potential at this point is the

ELECTROGENIC POTENTIAL

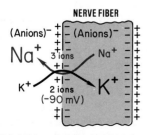

Figure 5–2. Establishment of a membrane potential as a result of sodium and potassium being pumped through the nerve membrane by the Na⁺–K⁺ electrogenic pump, with three soidum ions passing outward through the membrane for each two potassium ions passing inward.

Nernst potential for the potassium ions, as we shall discuss.

Figure 5–1B illustrates the same effect as that in Figure 5–1A but with a high concentration of sodium ions outside the membrane and a low sodium concentration inside. These ions are also positively charged. However, this time the membrane is highly permeable to the sodium ions and impermeable to all other ions; also, the excess of sodium ions diffuses to the inside, that is, in the opposite direction to the diffusion of potassium ions in Figure 5–1A. This diffusion creates a membrane potential now of opposite polarity, with negativity outside and positivity inside, and, again, the membrane potential rises high enough within milliseconds to block further net diffusion of the sodium ions to the inside, but this time the potential is called the *Nernst potential for the sodium ions.*

Thus, in both Figures 5–1A and B we see that a concentration difference of ions across a semipermeable membrane can, under appropriate conditions, cause the creation of a membrane potential. In later sections of this chapter, we shall see that many of the membrane potential changes observed during the course of nerve and muscle impulse transmission result from the occurrence of rapidly changing diffusion membrane potentials of this nature.

Relationship of the Diffusion Potential to the Concentration Difference—The Nernst Equation. When a concentration difference of a single type of ion across a membrane causes diffusion of ions through the membrane, thus creating a membrane potential, the magnitude of the potential *inside* the membrane versus the *outside* is determined by the ratio of the tendency for the ions to diffuse in one direction versus the other direction; for positive ions the following formula gives the quantitative value of the potential that develops:

$$\text{EMF (millivolts)} = -61 \log \frac{\text{Conc. inside}}{\text{Conc. outside}}$$

Thus, when the concentration of positive ions on the inside of a membrane is ten times that on the outside, the log of 10 is 1, and the potential difference calculates to be −61 millivolts. This equation is called the *Nernst equation,* and the developed potential is the *Nernst potential.*

Using the Nernst equation, let us now calculate the Nernst potential across the nerve membrane, first, when the membrane is permeable only to sodium ions and, second, when the membrane is permeable only to potassium ions:

The normal concentration of sodium ions inside the nerve membrane is approximately 14 mEq and outside approximately 142 mEq. Thus, the ratio of these two is 0.10, and the logarithm of 0.10 is −1.00. Multiplying this by −61 millivolts gives a Nernst potential for sodium of +61 millivolts inside the nerve fiber membrane.

The normal concentration of potassium ions inside the nerve fiber is approximately 140 mEq per liter and 4 mEq per liter on the outside. The ratio of these two is 35. The logarithm of 35 is 1.54; this times −61 millivolts equals a Nernst potential for potassium of −94 millivolts inside the membrane.

Therefore, if there were no pumping of ions through the nerve membrane and if the membrane were permeable only to sodium but not at all to other ions, the potential inside the nerve fiber would be +61 millivolts. Conversely, if the membrane were permeable to potassium but not permeable to any other ions, the membrane potential would be −94 millivolts. We shall see later in this discussion that under resting conditions the membrane potential averages about −90 millivolts, which is very near the −94 millivolts potassium Nernst potential. This is true because in the resting state the membrane is very permeable to potassium and only slightly permeable to sodium. On the other hand, when a nerve impulse is transmitted, the membrane, for a minute fraction of a second, becomes much more permeable to sodium than to potassium. Therefore, during this split second, the membrane potential rises to approximately +45 millivolts, which is much nearer the sodium Nernst potential than the potassium Nernst potential.

MEMBRANE POTENTIALS CAUSED BY ACTIVE TRANSPORT—THE SODIUM–POTASSIUM ELECTROGENIC "PUMP"

Figure 5–2 illustrates another method by which a membrane potential can develop—by active transport. It will be recalled from the discussions in the last chapter that the sodium-potassium pump pumps three sodium ions out of the cell for every two potassium ions pumped in. Thus, for each cycle of the pump the inside of the nerve fiber loses one positive charge. Because the membrane is almost totally impermeable to the negatively charged ions (anions) inside the cell, continuation of this process will lead to an excess of positive charges on the outside and an excess of negative charges inside, as illustrated in Figure 5–2. Thus, once again, the nerve membrane becomes negatively charged on the inside. And, because of the ability of the Na+-K+ pump to create such a membrane potential, it is called an *electrogenic pump*.

It was also clear from the discussions of the previous chapter that the Na+-K+ pump is responsible for establishing the normal sodium and potassium gradients across the cell membrane. That is, the continual pumping of sodium to the exterior leads to the normally greatly reduced sodium concentration inside the nerve fiber, whereas the pumping of the potassium ions to the interior helps establish the high concentration of potassium on the inside. We shall see later in the chapter that after many nerve impulses have been transmitted, the concentration gradients across the cell membrane of both sodium and potassium decrease because of diffusion of these ions through the membrane during the action potentials. But the Na+-K+ pump will soon re-establish the appropriate concentration gradients.

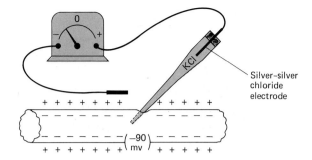

Figure 5–3. Measurement of the membrane potential of the nerve fiber using a microelectrode.

MEASURING THE MEMBRANE POTENTIAL

The method for measuring the membrane potential is simple in theory but often very difficult in practice because of the small sizes of many of the fibers. Figure 5–3 illustrates a small pipette filled with a very strong electrolyte solution (KCl) that is impaled through the cell membrane to the interior of the fiber. Then another electrode, called the "indifferent electrode," is placed in the interstitial fluids, and the potential difference between the inside and outside of the fiber is measured using an appropriate voltmeter. This is a highly sophisticated electronic apparatus that is capable of measuring very small voltages despite extremely high resistance to electrical flow through the tip of the micropipette, which has a diameter usually less than 1 micron and a resistance often as great as a billion ohms. For recording rapid *changes* in the membrane potential during the transmission of nerve impulses, the microelectrode is connected to an oscilloscope, as will be explained later in the chapter.

THE RESTING MEMBRANE POTENTIAL OF NERVES

The membrane potential of large nerve fibers when they are not transmitting nerve signals—that is, when in the so-called "resting" state—is about −90 millivolts (mv). This means that the potential *inside the fiber* is 90 mv more negative than the potential in the interstitial fluid on the outside of the fiber. In the next few paragraphs we will explain how this potential comes about, but before doing so we must describe the transport properties of the resting nerve membrane for sodium and potassium.

Active Transport of Sodium and Potassium Ions Through the Membrane—The Sodium-Potassium Pump. First, let us recall from the discussions of the previous chapter that all cell membranes of the body have a powerful sodium-potassium pump and that this continually pumps sodium to the outside of the fiber and potassium to the inside. Further, let us remember that this is an *electrogenic pump*, because more positive charges are pumped to the outside than to the inside, leaving a net deficit of positive ions on

OUTSIDE

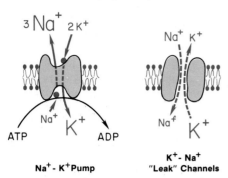

Figure 5–4. The functional characteristics of the Na⁺–K⁺ pump and also of the potassium-sodium "leak" channels.

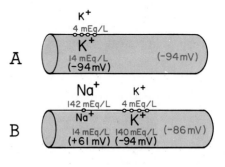

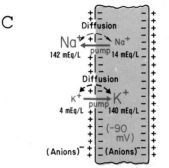

Figure 5–5. Establishment of resting membrane potentials in nerve fibers under three separate conditions: A, when the membrane potential is caused entirely by potassium diffusion alone; B, when the membrane potential is caused by diffusion of both sodium and potassium ions; and C, when the membrane potential is caused by diffusion of both sodium and potassium ions plus pumping of both these ions by the Na⁺–K⁺ pump.

the inside; this is the same as causing a negative charge inside the cell membrane.

This sodium-potassium pump causes the tremendous concentration gradients for sodium and potassium across the resting nerve membrane. These gradients are the following:

Na⁺ (outside):	142 mEq/L
Na⁺ (inside):	14 mEq/L
K⁺ (outside):	4 mEq/L
K⁺ (inside):	140 mEq/L

Leakage of Potassium and Sodium Through the Nerve Membrane. To the right in Figure 5–4 is illustrated a channel type of transport protein in the cell membrane through which potassium and sodium ions can leak. The channels through these proteins are called *potassium-sodium "leak" channels.* The emphasis is on the potassium because the channels are far more permeable to potassium than to sodium, normally about 100 times as permeable. This differential in permeability is exceedingly important in the establishment of the normal resting membrane potential.

ORIGIN OF NORMAL RESTING MEMBRANE POTENTIAL

Figure 5–5 illustrates the important factors in the establishment of the normal resting membrane potential of −90 mv. These are

Contribution of the Potassium Diffusion Potential. In Figure 5–5A, we make the assumption that the only movement of ions through the membrane is the diffusion of potassium ions, as illustrated by the open channel between the potassium inside the membrane and the outside. Because of the high ratio of potassium ions inside to the potassium ions outside, 35 to 1, the Nernst potential corresponding to this ratio is −94 mv. That is, the *diffusion potential* caused by the potassium would be −94 mv, as illustrated to the right inside the nerve fiber, if this were the only factor causing the resting nerve potential.

Contribution of Sodium Diffusion Through the Nerve Membrane. Figure 5–5B illustrates the addition of very slight permeability of the nerve membrane to sodium ions, thus also allowing minute diffusion of sodium ions through the K⁺-Na⁺ leak channels. The ratio of sodium ions from inside to outside the membrane is 0.1, and this gives a calculated Nernst potential for the inside of the membrane of +61 mv. But also shown in Figure 5–5B is the Nernst potential for potassium diffusion of −94 mv. However, because far more potassium ions leak through the channels than sodium ions, the potassium ions dominate the picture, and the actual diffusion potential is approximately −86 mv, as shown to the right in the figure, a value that is very close to the Nernst potential for potassium.

Contribution of the Na⁺-K⁺ Pump. Finally, in Figure 5–5C the additional contribution of the sodium-potassium pump is illustrated. The fact that more sodium ions are being pumped to the outside than potassium to the inside causes a continual loss of positive charges from inside the membrane, and this creates an additional small degree of negativity on the inside beyond that which can be accounted for by diffusion alone. Therefore, as illustrated in Figure 5–5C, the net membrane potential with all these factors operative at the same time is approximately −90 mv.

In summary, the diffusion potentials alone caused by potassium and sodium diffusion would give a membrane potential of approximately −86 mv, almost all of this being determined by the potassium diffusion. Then, an additional −4 mv is contributed to the membrane potential by the electrogenic Na⁺-K⁺ pump, giving a net resting membrane potential of −90 mv.

THE NERVE ACTION POTENTIAL

Nerve signals are transmitted by *action potentials,* which are rapid changes in the membrane potential. Each action potential begins with a sudden change from the normal resting negative potential to a positive membrane potential and then ends with an almost equally rapid change back again to the negative potential. To conduct a nerve signal, the action potential moves along the nerve fiber until it comes to the fiber's end. The upper panel of Figure 5–6 shows the electrical charge disturbances that occur at the membrane during the action potential, with transfer of positive charges to the interior of the fiber at its onset and return of positive charges to the exterior at its end. The lower panel illustrates graphically the successive changes in the membrane potential over a period of a few 10,000ths of a second, illustrating the explosive onset of the action potential and the almost equally rapid recovery.

The successive stages of the action potential are described by the following terms:

Resting Stage. This is the resting membrane potential before the action potential occurs. The membrane is said to be "polarized" during this stage because of the very large negative membrane potential that is present.

Depolarization Stage. At the onset of the action potential, the membrane suddenly becomes very permeable to sodium ions, allowing tremendous numbers of sodium ions to flow to the interior of the axon. The normal "polarized" state of −90 mv is lost, with the potential rising rapidly in the positive direction. This is called *depolarization.* In large nerve fibers, the membrane potential actually "overshoots" beyond the zero level and becomes slightly positive, but in some smaller fibers as well as many central nervous system neurons, the potential merely approaches the zero level and does not overshoot to the positive state.

Repolarization Stage. Within a few 10,000ths of a second after the membrane becomes highly permeable to sodium ions, the sodium channels close almost as rapidly as they had opened. Then, rapid diffusion of potassium ions to the exterior re-establishes the normal negative resting membrane potential. This is called *repolarization* of the membrane.

To explain more fully the factors that cause both the depolarization and repolarization processes, we need now to describe the special characteristics of yet two other types of transport channels through the nerve membrane: the voltage-gated sodium and potassium channels.

THE VOLTAGE–GATED SODIUM AND POTASSIUM CHANNELS

The principal actor in causing both depolarization and repolarization of the nerve membrane during the action potential is the *voltage-gated sodium channel.* However, the *voltage-gated potassium channel* also plays an important role in some nerve fibers for the rapid repolarization of the membrane. *These two voltage-gated channels are in addition to the Na⁺-K⁺ pump and also in addition to the Na⁺-K⁺ leak channels.*

The Voltage-Gated Sodium Channel— "Activation" and "Inactivation" of the Channel

The upper panel of Figure 5–7 illustrates the voltage-gated sodium channel in three separate states. This channel has two separate gates, one near the outside of the channel called the *activation gate* and another near the inside called the *inactivation gate.* To the left is shown the state of these two gates in the normal resting membrane when the membrane potential is −90 mv. In this state the activation gate is closed, which prevents any entry of sodium ions to the interior of the fiber through these sodium channels. On the other hand, the inactivation gate is open and does not at this time constitute any barrier to the movement of sodium ions.

Activation of the Sodium Channel. When the membrane potential becomes less negative than during the resting state, rising from −90 mv toward zero, it finally reaches a voltage, usually somewhere between −70 and −50 mv, that causes a sudden conformational change in the activation gate, flipping it to the open position. This is called the *activated state,* and

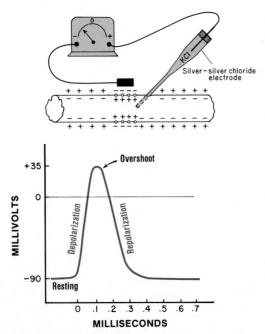

Figure 5–6. A typical action potential recorded by the method illustrated in the upper panel of the figure.

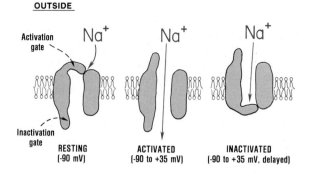

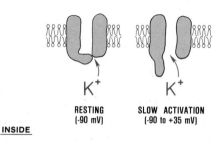

Figure 5–7. Characteristics of the voltage-gated sodium and potassium channels, showing both activation and inactivation of the sodium channels but activation of the potassium channels only when the membrane potential is changed from the normal resting negative value to a positive value.

during this state sodium ions can literally pour inward through the channel, increasing the sodium permeability of the membrane as much as 500- to 5000-fold.

Inactivation of the Sodium Channel. To the far right in the upper panel of Figure 5–7 is illustrated a final state of the sodium channel. The same increase in voltage that opens the activation gate also closes the inactivation gate. However, closure of the inactivation gate occurs a few 10,000ths of a second after the activation gate opens. That is, the conformational change that flips the inactivation gate to the closed state is a slower process. Therefore, after the sodium channel has remained open for a few 10,000ths of a second, it suddenly closes, and sodium ions can no longer pour to the inside of the membrane. At this point the membrane potential begins to recover back toward the resting membrane state, which is the repolarization process, caused principally by the leakage of potassium ions to the exterior through the leak channels.

A very important characteristic of the sodium channel inactivation process is that *the inactivation gate will not reopen again until the membrane potential returns either to or nearly to the original resting membrane potential level.* Therefore, it is not possible for the sodium channels to open again without the nerve fiber first repolarizing.

The Voltage-Gated Potassium Channels and Their Activation

The lower panel of Figure 5–7 illustrates the voltage-gated potassium channel in two separate states:

during the resting membrane state and during the action potential. During the resting state, the gate of the potassium channel is closed, as illustrated to the left in the figure, and potassium ions are prevented from passing to the exterior. When the membrane potential rises from −90 mv toward zero, this voltage change causes a slow conformational opening of the gate and allows increased potassium diffusion outward through the channel. However, because of the slowness of opening of these potassium channels, they open at the same time that the sodium channels are becoming inactivated and are closing. Thus, the decrease in sodium entry to the cell and simultaneous increase in potassium exit from the cell greatly speeds the repolarization process, leading within a few 10,000ths of a second to full recovery of the resting membrane potential.

SUMMARY OF EVENTS THAT CAUSE THE ACTION POTENTIAL

Figure 5–8 illustrates in summary form the sequential events that occur during the action potential.

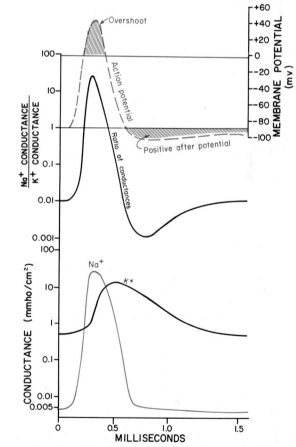

Figure 5–8. Changes in sodium and potassium conductances during the course of the action potential. Note that sodium conductance increases several thousandfold during the early stages of the action potential, whereas potassium conductance increases only about 30-fold during the latter stages of the action potential and for a short period thereafter. (Curves constructed from data in Hodgkin and Huxley papers but transposed from squid axon to apply to the membrane potentials of large mammalian nerve fibers).

These are:

At the bottom of the figure are shown the changes in membrane conductances for sodium and potassium ions. During the resting state, before the action potential begins, the conductance for potassium ions is shown to be already 50 to 100 times as great as the conductance for sodium ions. This is caused by much greater leakage of potassium ions through the leak channels than the leakage of sodium ions. However, at the onset of the action potential, the sodium channels instantaneously become activated and allow an up to 5000-fold increase in sodium conductance. Then the inactivation process almost as rapidly closes the sodium channels within another small fraction of a millisecond. The onset of the action potential also causes voltage gating of the potassium channels, causing them to begin opening a fraction of a millisecond after the sodium channels open.

In the middle portion of Figure 5–8 is shown the ratio of sodium conductance to potassium conductance at each instant during the action potential, and above this is shown the action potential itself. During the early portion of the action potential, this ratio increases more than a thousand-fold. Therefore, far more sodium ions now flow to the interior of the fiber than do potassium ions to the exterior. This is what causes the membrane potential to become positive. At this time the sodium channels become inactivated but at the same time the potassium channels open, and the ratio of conductance now shifts far in favor of high potassium conductance but low sodium conductance. This allows extremely rapid loss of potassium ions to the exterior while essentially no sodium ions flow to the interior. Consequently, the action potential quickly returns to its baseline level.

INITIATION OF THE ACTION POTENTIAL

Up to this point, we have explained the action potential itself but not what initiates the action potential. The answer to this is really quite simple:

First, as long as the membrane of the nerve fiber remains totally undisturbed, no action potential will occur. However, if any event at all causes enough initial rise in the membrane potential from -90 mv up toward the zero level, the rising voltage itself will affect the voltage-gated sodium channels, causing them to become activated (opened). This allows rapid inflow of sodium ions, which causes still further rise of the membrane potential, thus opening still more voltage-gated sodium channels and causing more streaming of sodium ions to the interior of the fiber. Thus, the process continues in a positive-feedback circle until all the voltage-gated sodium channels have become totally opened. But then within another fraction of a millisecond the rising membrane potential causes inactivation (closure) of the sodium channels, and the action potential soon terminates.

Threshold for Initiation of the Action Potential. An action potential will not occur until the initial rise in membrane potential is great enough to create the circle described in the last paragraph. Usually, a sudden rise in membrane potential of 15 to 30 mv is required. For instance, a sudden increase in the membrane potential in a large nerve fiber of from -90 mv up to about -65 mv will usually cause the explosive development of the action potential. This level of -65 mv is said to be the *threshold* for stimulation.

PROPAGATION OF THE ACTION POTENTIAL

In the preceding paragraphs we have discussed the action potential as it occurs at one spot on the membrane. However, an action potential elicited at any one point on an excitable membrane usually excites adjacent portions of the membrane, resulting in propagation of the action potential. The mechanism of this is illustrated in Figure 5–9. Figure 5–9A shows a normal resting nerve fiber, and Figure 5–9B shows a nerve fiber that has been excited in its midportion—that is, the midportion has suddenly developed increased permeability to sodium. The arrows illustrate a "local circuit" of current flow between the depolarized areas of the membrane and the adjacent resting membrane areas; that is, positive electrical charges flow inward through the depolarized membrane and also for several millimeters along the core of the axon. These positive charges increase the voltage for a distance of 1 to 3 mm inside large fibers to above the threshold voltage value for initiating an action potential. Therefore, the sodium channels in these new areas also activate, and, as illustrated in Figure 5–9C and D, the explosive action potential spreads. And these newly depolarized areas cause

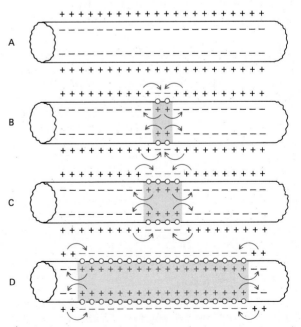

Figure 5–9. Propagation of action potentials in both directions along a conductive fiber.

local circuits of current flow still further along the membrane, causing progressively more and more depolarization. Thus, the depolarization process travels in both directions along the entire extent of the fiber. The transmission of the depolarization process along a nerve or muscle fiber is called a *nerve* or *muscle impulse.*

Direction of Propagation. It is now obvious that an excitable membrane has no single direction of propagation, but that the action potential can travel in both directions away from the stimulus—and even along all branches of a nerve fiber—until the entire membrane has become depolarized.

The All-or-Nothing Principle. It is equally obvious that, once an action potential has been elicited at any point on the membrane of a normal fiber, the depolarization process will travel over the entire membrane. This is called the all-or-nothing principle, and it applies to all *normal* excitable tissues. Occasionally, though, when the fiber is in an abnormal state the action potential will reach a point on the membrane at which it does not generate sufficient voltage to stimulate the adjacent area of the membrane. When this occurs the spread of depolarization will stop.

Propagation of Repolarization. The action potential normally lasts almost the same length of time at each point along a fiber. Therefore, repolarization normally occurs first at the point of original stimulus and then spreads progressively along the membrane, moving in the same direction that depolarization had previously spread but a few 10,000ths of a second later.

RECHARGING THE FIBER MEMBRANE AFTER ACTION POTENTIALS—IMPORTANCE OF ENERGY METABOLISM

Transmission of each impulse (action potential) along the nerve fiber reduces the concentration differences of sodium and potassium between the inside and outside of the membrane because of diffusion of sodium ions to the inside during depolarization and diffusion of potassium ions to the outside during repolarization. For a single action potential, this effect is so minute that it cannot even be measured. Indeed, 100,000 to 500,000 impulses can be transmitted by nerve fibers before the concentration differences have run down to the point that action potential conduction ceases. Yet, even so, with time it becomes necessary to re-establish the sodium and potassium membrane concentration differences. This is achieved by the action of the Na^+-K^+ pump in exactly the same way as that described earlier in the chapter for establishment of the original resting potential. That is, the sodium ions that, during the action potentials, have diffused to the interior of the cell and the potassium ions that have diffused to the exterior are returned to their original state by the sodium and potassium pump. Since this pump requires energy for

operation, this process of "recharging" the nerve fiber is an active metabolic one, utilizing energy derived from the adenosine triphosphate energy "currency" system of the cell.

A special feature of the sodium–potassium ATPase membrane pumping system is that its degree of activity is very strongly stimulated by excess sodium ions inside the cell membrane. In fact, the pumping activity increases approximately in proportion to the third power of the sodium concentration. That is, if the internal sodium concentration rises from 10 to 20 mEq per liter, the activity of the pump does not merely double but instead increases approximately eightfold. Therefore, it can easily be understood how the recharging process of the nerve fiber can rapidly be set into motion whenever the concentration differences of sodium and potassium across the membrane begin to "run down."

Heat Production by the Nerve Fiber. Figure 5–10 illustrates the relationship of heat production in a nerve fiber to the number of impulses transmitted by the fiber each second. The rate of heat production is a measure of the rate of metabolism in the nerve, because heat is always liberated as a product of the chemical reactions of energy metabolism. Note that the heat production increases markedly as the number of impulses per second increases. It is this increased use of energy that causes the "recharging" process.

PLATEAU IN SOME ACTION POTENTIALS

In some instances the excitable membrane does not repolarize immediately after depolarization, but, instead, the potential remains on a plateau near the peak of the spike sometimes for many milliseconds before repolarization begins. Such a plateau is illustrated in Figure 5–11, from which one can readily see that the plateau greatly prolongs the period of depolarization. This type of action potential occurs in the heart, where the plateau lasts for as long as three- to four-tenths of a second and causes contraction of the heart muscle during this entire period of time.

The cause of the action potential plateau is a

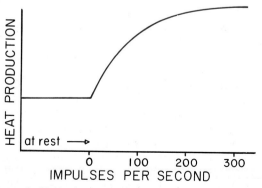

Figure 5–10. Heat production in a nerve fiber at rest and at progressively increasing rates of stimulation.

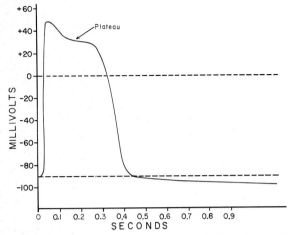

Figure 5-11. An action potential from a Purkinje fiber of the heart, showing a "plateau."

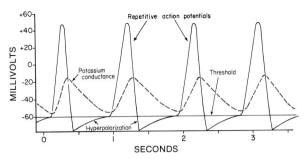

Figure 5-12. Rhythmic action potentials, and their relationship to potassium conductance and to the state of hyperpolarization.

combination of several different factors. First, in heart muscle, two separate types of channels enter into the depolarization process: (1) the usual voltage-activated sodium channels, called the *fast channels*, and (2) voltage-activated calcium-sodium channels, which are slow to be activated and also slow to be inactivated and therefore are called *slow channels*—these channels allow diffusion mainly of calcium ions but also of some sodium ions as well. Activation of the fast channels causes the spike portion of the action potential, whereas the slow but prolonged activation of the slow channels is mainly responsible for the plateau portion of this type of action potential.

RHYTHMICITY OF CERTAIN EXCITABLE TISSUES—REPETITIVE DISCHARGE

All excitable tissues can discharge repetitively if the threshold for stimulation is reduced low enough. For instance, even nerve fibers and skeletal muscle fibers, which normally are highly stable, discharge repetitively when they are placed in a solution containing the drug veratrine or when the calcium ion concentration falls below a critical value. Repetitive discharges, or rhythmicity, occur normally in the heart, in most smooth muscle, and also in many of the neurons of the central nervous system. It is these rhythmical discharges that cause the heart beat, that cause peristalsis, and that cause such neuronal events as the rhythmical control of breathing.

The Re-Excitation Process Necessary for Rhythmicity. For rhythmicity to occur, the membrane, even in its natural state, must already be permeable enough to sodium ions (or to calcium and sodium ions through the Ca^{++}-Na^+ slow channels) to allow automatic membrane depolarization. Thus, Figure 5-12 shows that the "resting" membrane potential is only -60 to -70 millivolts. This is not enough negative voltage to keep the sodium and calcium-sodium channels closed. That is, (a) sodium and calcium ions flow

inward and increase the membrane potential, (b) this further increases the membrane permeability, (c) still more ions flow inward, (d) the permeability increases more, and so forth, thus eliciting the regenerative process of sodium and calcium-sodium channel openings until an action potential is generated. Then, at the end of the action potential the membrane repolarizes. But shortly thereafter, the depolarization process begins again and a new action potential occurs spontaneously—this cycle continuing again and again and causing self-induced rhythmical excitation of the excitable tissue.

Yet, why does the next action potential not occur immediately after the membrane has become repolarized rather than delaying for nearly a second before the onset of the next action potential? The answer to this can be found by referring back to Figure 5-8, which shows that toward the end of the action potential, and continuing for a short period thereafter, the membrane becomes excessively permeable to potassium. This allows excessive outflow of potassium ions, which carries tremendous numbers of positive charges to the outside of the membrane and creates inside the fiber considerably more negativity than would otherwise occur. This is a state called *hyperpolarization*, which is illustrated in Figure 5-12. As long as this state exists, re-excitation will not occur; but gradually the excess potassium conductance (and the state of hyperpolarization) disappears, thereby allowing the membrane potential to rise once again until it reaches the *threshold* for excitation; then suddenly a new action potential results, the process occurring again and again.

SPECIAL ASPECTS OF SIGNAL TRANSMISSION IN NERVE TRUNKS

Myelinated and Unmyelinated Nerve Fibers. A typical nerve trunk is comprised of a few very large nerve fibers that occupy most of the cross-sectional area and many more small fibers lying between the large ones. The large fibers are *myelinated* and the small ones are *unmyelinated*. The average nerve trunk contains about twice as many unmyelinated fibers as myelinated fibers.

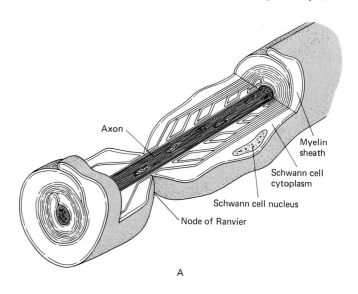

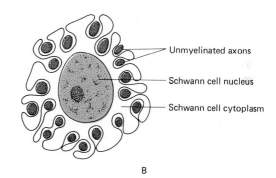

Figure 5–13. Function of the Schwann cell to insulate nerve fibers. *A,* The wrapping of a Schwann cell membrane around a large axon to form the myelin sheath of the myelinated nerve fiber. (Modified from Leeson and Leeson: Atlas of Histology. Philadelphia, W. B. Saunders Company, 1979.) *B,* Evagination of the membrane and cytoplasm of a Schwann cell around multiple unmyelinated nerve fibers.

Figure 5–13 illustrates a typical myelinated fiber. The central core of the fiber is the *axon,* and the membrane of the axon is the actual *conductive membrane.* The axon is filled in its center with *axoplasm,* which is a viscid intracellular fluid. Surrounding the axon is a *myelin sheath* that is often thicker than the axon itself, and about once every millimeter along the extent of the axon the myelin sheath is interrupted by a *node of Ranvier.*

The myelin sheath is deposited around the axon by Schwann cells in the following manner: The membrane of a Schwann cell first envelops the axon. Then the cell rotates around the axon many times, laying down multiple layers of cellular membrane containing the lipid substance *sphingomyelin.* This substance is an excellent insulator that prevents almost all flow of ions. In fact, it increases the resistance to ion flow through the membrane approximately 5000-fold. However, at the juncture between each two successive Schwann cells along the axon, a small, uninsulated area remains where ions can still flow with ease between the extracellular fluid and the axon. This area is the node of Ranvier.

Saltatory Conduction in Myelinated Fibers from Node to Node. Even though ions cannot flow significantly through the thick myelin sheaths of myelinated nerves, they flow with considerable ease through the nodes of Ranvier. Therefore, action potentials occur only at the nodes. Yet, the action potentials are conducted from node to node, as illustrated in Figure 5–14; this is called *saltatory conduction.* That is, electrical current flows through the surrounding extracellular fluids and also through the axoplasm from node to node, exciting successive nodes one after another. Thus, the nerve impulse jumps down the fiber, which is the origin of the term *saltatory.*

Saltatory conduction is of value for two reasons: First, by causing the depolarization process to jump long intervals along the axis of the nerve fiber, this mechanism increases the velocity of nerve transmission in myelinated fibers an average of five- to sev-

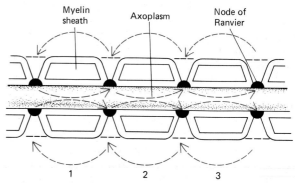

Figure 5–14. Saltatory conduction along a myelinated axon.

enfold. Second, saltatory conduction conserves energy for the axon, for only the nodes depolarize, allowing perhaps a hundred times smaller loss of ions than would otherwise be necessary and therefore requiring little extra metabolism for re-establishing the sodium and potassium concentration differences across the membrane after a series of nerve impulses.

VELOCITY OF CONDUCTION IN NERVE FIBERS

The velocity of conduction in nerve fibers varies from as little as 0.5 meter per second in very small unmyelinated fibers to as great as 100 meters per second (the length of a football field) in very large myelinated fibers. The velocity increases approximately with the fiber diameter.

EXCITATION—THE PROCESS OF ELICITING ACTION POTENTIAL

Chemical Stimulation. Basically, any factor that causes sodium ions to begin to diffuse inward through the membrane in sufficient numbers will set off the automatic, regenerative opening of the sodium channels that eventuates in the action potential. Thus, certain chemicals can stimulate a nerve fiber by increasing the membrane permeability. Such chemicals include acids, bases, almost any salt solution of very strong concentration, and, most importantly, the substance *acetylcholine.* Many nerve fibers, when stimulated, secrete acetylcholine at their endings where they synapse with other neurons or where they end on muscle fibers. The acetylcholine in turn stimulates the successive neuron or muscle fiber by opening pores in the membrane large enough for sodium ions to go through with ease. This is discussed in much greater detail in Chapter 7; it is one of the most important means by which nerve and muscle fibers are stimulated. Likewise, *norepinephrine* secreted by sympathetic nerve endings can stimulate cardiac muscle fibers and some smooth muscle fibers, and still other hormonal *transmitter substances* can stimulate neurons in the central nervous system.

Mechanical Stimulation. Crushing, pinching, or pricking a nerve fiber can cause a sudden surge of sodium influx and, for obvious reasons, can elicit an action potential. Even slight pressure on some specialized nerve endings can stimulate these; this will be discussed in Chapter 32 in relation to sensory perception.

Electrical Stimulation. An electrical current passed through a nerve from electrodes connected to a battery or some other electrical source causes excess flow of ions through the axonal membrane; this too can initiate an action potential and it is the usual means by which nerve fibers are excited when they are studied in the laboratory.

RECORDING MEMBRANE POTENTIALS AND ACTION POTENTIALS

The Cathode Ray Oscilloscope. Earlier in this chapter we noted that the potential changes at the membrane occur very rapidly throughout the course of an action potential. Indeed, most of the action potential complex of large nerve fibers takes place in less than $\frac{1}{1000}$ second. In some figures of this chapter an electrical meter has been shown recording these potential changes. However, it must be understood that any meter capable of recording them must be capable of responding extremely rapidly. For practical purposes the only type of meter that is capable of responding accurately to the very rapid membrane potential changes of most excitable fibers is the cathode ray oscilloscope.

Figure 5–15 illustrates the basic components of a cathode ray oscilloscope. The cathode ray tube itself is composed basically of an *electron gun* and a *fluorescent surface* against which electrons are fired. Where the electrons hit the surface, the fluorescent material glows. If the electron beam is moved across the surface, the spot of glowing light also moves and draws a fluorescent line on the screen.

In addition to the electron gun and fluorescent surface, the cathode ray tube is provided with two sets of plates: one set, called the *horizontal deflection plates,* is positioned on either side of the electron beam, and the other set, called the *vertical deflection plates,* is positioned above and below the beam. If a negative charge is applied to the left-hand plate and a positive charge to the right-hand plate, the electron beam will be repelled away from the left plate and attracted toward the right plate, thus bending the beam toward the right; this will cause the spot of light on the fluorescent surface of the cathode ray screen to move to the right. Likewise, positive and

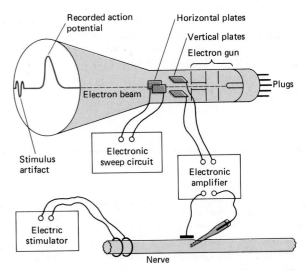

Figure 5–15. The cathode ray oscilloscope for recording transient action potentials.

negative charges can be applied to the vertical deflection plates to move the beam up or down.

Since electrons travel at extremely rapid velocity and since the plates of the cathode ray tube can be alternately charged positively or negatively within less than a millionth of a second, it is obvious that the spot of light on the face of the tube can also be moved to almost any position in less than a millionth of a second. For this reason, the cathode ray tube oscilloscope can be considered to be an inertialess meter capable of recording with extreme fidelity almost any change in membrane potential.

To use the cathode ray tube for recording action potentials, two electrical circuits must be employed. These are (1) an *electronic sweep circuit* that controls the voltages on the horizontal deflection plates and (2) an *electronic amplifier* that controls the voltages on the vertical deflection plates. The sweep circuit automatically causes the spot of light to begin at the left-hand side and move slowly toward the right. When the spot reaches the right side it jumps back immediately to the left-hand side and starts a new trace.

The electronic amplifier amplifies signals that come from the nerve. If a change in membrane potential occurs while the spot of light is moving across the screen, this change in potential will be amplified and will cause the spot to rise above or fall below the mean level of the trace, as illustrated in the figure. In other words, the sweep circuit provides the lateral movement of the electron beam while the amplifier provides the vertical movement in direct proportion to the changes in membrane potentials picked up by appropriate electrodes.

Figure 5–15 also shows an electric stimulator used to stimulate the nerve. When the nerve is stimulated, a small *stimulus artifact* usually appears on the oscilloscope screen prior to the action potential.

Recording the Action Potential. Throughout this chapter action potentials have been shown in different diagrams. To record these, an electrode such as that illustrated earlier in the chapter in Figure 5–3 must be inserted into the interior of the fiber. Then, as the action potential spreads down the fiber, the changes in the potential inside the fiber are recorded as illustrated earlier in the chapter in Figures 5–6, 5–8, 5–9, and 5–12.

QUESTIONS

1. What is meant by a membrane potential?
2. Explain how membrane potentials can be caused by diffusion of ions through a membrane.
3. Calculate the Nernst potentials for sodium and potassium for the normal nerve, using the concentration values given in the text.
4. Explain why the sodium-potassium pump is called an electrogenic pump.
5. Describe the method for measuring the membrane potential.
6. Why is the normal resting membrane potential nearly equal to the Nernst potential for potassium?
7. Explain the events that occur during the depolarization and repolarization stages of the action potential.
8. Describe the voltage-gated sodium and potassium channels. What is meant by *activation* of the sodium channel, and what is meant by *inactivation* of this channel?
9. Approximately how much does the sodium conductance increase during the early part of the action potential?
10. Explain how action potentials are initiated. What is meant by the *threshold* for initiation of the action potential?
11. Explain the means by which action potentials are propagated along the nerve fiber.
12. What is meant by the term *all-or-nothing principle?*
13. Why must a nerve fiber be recharged after nerve impulses have been transmitted? Approximately how many nerve impulses can be transmitted before the nerve fiber will "run down"?
14. What causes increased heat production in nerve fibers?
15. Explain what causes a plateau in some action potentials. In what tissues is one likely to find such action potentials?
16. Describe the re-excitation process that occurs in some tissues, such as the heart and some smooth-muscle organs, that causes repetitive discharge. What is the difference between a *myelinated* and an *unmyelinated* nerve fiber, and how does saltatory conduction occur in myelinated fibers?
17. Explain the different methods by which nerve fibers can be excited.
18. Describe the use of the oscilloscope for recording action potentials.

References

Agnew, W. S.: Voltage-regulated sodium channel molecules. Annu Rev Physiol 45:517, 1984.

Auerbach, A., and Sachs, F.: Patch clamp studies of single ionic channels. Annu Rev Biophys Bioeng 13:269, 1984.

Baker, P. F., et al.: The effects of changes in internal ionic concentrations on the electrical properties of perfused giant axons. J Physiol (Lond), 164:355, 1962.

Cole, K. S.: Electrodiffusion models for the membrane of squid giant axon. Physiol Rev 45:340, 1965.

Hille, B.: Gating in sodium channels of nerve. Annu Rev Physiol 38:139, 1976.

Hodgkin, A. L.: The Conduction of the Nervous Impulse. Springfield, Ill., Charles C Thomas, 1963.

Hodgkin, A. L., and Huxley, A. F.: Movement of sodium and potassium ions during nervous activity. Cold Spr Harb Symp Quant Biol 17:43, 1952.

Hodgkin, A. L., and Huxley, A. F.: Quantitative description of membrane current and its application to conduction and excitation in nerve. J Physiol (Lond), 117:500, 1952.

Katz, B.: Nerve, Muscle, and Synapse. New York, McGraw-Hill, 1968.

Kostyuk, P. G.: Intracellular perfusion of nerve cells and its effects on membrane currents. Physiol Rev 64:435, 1984.

Latorre, R., et al.: K$^+$ channels gated by voltage and ions. Annu Rev Physiol 46:485, 1984.

Malhotra, S. K.: The Plasma Membrane. New York, John Wiley & Sons, 1983.

Noble, D.: Applications of Hodgkin-Huxley equations to excitable tissues. Physiol Rev 46:1, 1966.

Rogart, R.: Sodium channels in nerve and muscle membrane. Annu Rev Physiol 43:711, 1981.

Snell, R. M., ed.: Transcellular Membrane Potentials and Ionic Fluxes. New York, Gordon Press Pubs., 1984.

Stefani, E., and Chiarandini, D. J.: Ionic channels in skeletal muscle. Annu Rev Physiol 44:357, 1982.

Vinores, S., and Guroff, G.: Nerve growth factor: Mechanism of action. Annu Rev Biophys Bioeng 9:223, 1980.

Windhager, E. E., and Taylor, A.: Regulatory role of intracellular calcium ions in epithelial Na transport. Annu Rev Physiol 45:519, 1983.

Wright, E. M.: Electrophysiology of plasma membrane vesicles. Am J Physiol 246:F363, 1984.

6
Contraction of Skeletal Muscle

PHYSIOLOGICAL ANATOMY OF
   SKELETAL MUSCLE
   THE SKELETAL MUSCLE FIBER
MOLECULAR MECHANISM OF MUSCLE
   CONTRACTION
   *MOLECULAR CHARACTERISTICS OF
      THE CONTRACTILE FILAMENTS*
   *DEGREE OF ACTIN AND MYOSIN
      FILAMENT OVERLAP—EFFECT ON
      TENSION DEVELOPED BY THE
      CONTRACTING MUSCLE*
INITIATION OF MUSCLE
   CONTRACTION: EXCITATION-
   CONTRACTION COUPLING

THE MUSCLE ACTION POTENTIAL
*RELEASE OF CALCIUM IONS BY THE
   SARCOPLASMIC RETICULUM*
EFFICIENCY OF MUSCLE
   CONTRACTION
CHARACTERISTICS OF A SINGLE
   MUSCLE TWITCH
MECHANICS OF SKELETAL MUSCLE
   CONTRACTION
   THE MOTOR UNIT
   *SUMMATION OF MUSCLE
      CONTRACTION*
MUSCLE FATIGUE
MUSCLE HYPERTROPHY
MUSCLE ATROPHY

Approximately 40 per cent of the body is skeletal muscle and almost another 10 per cent is smooth and cardiac muscle. Many of the same principles of contraction apply to all these different types of muscle, but in the present chapter the function of skeletal muscle is mainly considered; the specialized functions of smooth muscle will be discussed in the following chapter, and cardiac muscle in Chapter 8.

PHYSIOLOGICAL ANATOMY OF SKELETAL MUSCLE

THE SKELETAL MUSCLE FIBER

Figure 6–1 illustrates the organization of skeletal muscle, showing that all skeletal muscles are made of numerous fibers ranging between 10 and 80 microns in diameter. In most muscles the fibers extend the entire length of the muscle, and, except for about 2 per cent of the fibers, each is innervated by only one nerve ending, located near the middle of the fiber.

The Sarcolemma. The sarcolemma is the cell membrane of the muscle fiber. However, the sarcolemma consists of a true cell membrane, called the *plasma membrane,* and an outer coat consisting of a thin layer of polysaccharide material containing numerous thin collagen fibrillae. At the end of the muscle fiber, this surface layer of the sarcolemma fuses with a tendon fiber, and the tendon fibers in turn collect into bundles to form the muscle tendons and thence insert into the bones.

Myofibrils; Actin and Myosin Filaments. Each muscle fiber contains several hundred to several thousand *myofibrils,* which are illustrated by the many small open dots in the cross-sectional view of Figure 6–1C. Each myofibril (Figure 6–1D) in turn has, lying side-by-side, about 1500 *myosin filaments* and 3000 *actin filaments,* which are large polymerized protein molecules that are responsible for muscle contraction. These can be seen in longitudinal view in the electron micrograph of Figure 6–2. The thick filaments are *myosin* and the thin filaments are *actin.* Note that the myosin and actin filaments partially interdigitate and thus cause the myofibrils to have alternate light and dark bands. The light bands contain only actin filaments and are called *I bands* because they are mainly *isotropic* to polarized light. The dark bands contain the myosin filaments as well as the ends of the actin filaments where they overlap the myosin and are called *A bands* because they are *anisotropic* to polarized light. Note also the small projections from the

SKELETAL MUSCLE

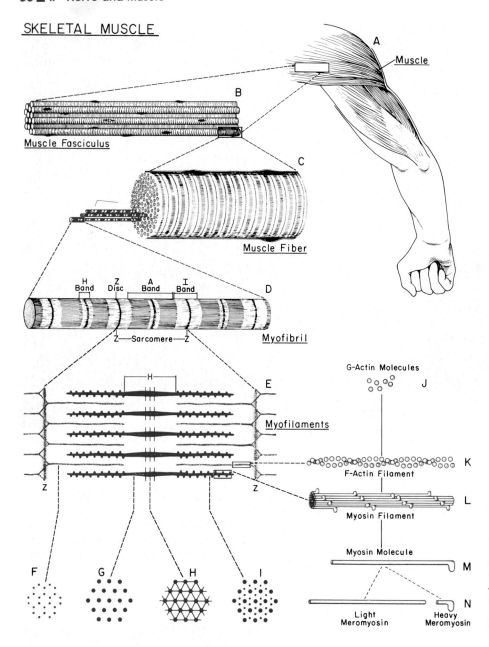

Figure 6–1. Organization of skeletal muscle, from the gross to the molecular level. F, G, H, and I are cross-sections at the levels indicated. (From Bloom and Fawcett: A Textbook of Histology. Philadelphia, W. B. Saunders Company, 1975. Drawn by Sylvia Colard Keene.)

sides of the myosin filaments. These are called *cross-bridges.* They protrude from the surfaces of the myosin filaments. It is interaction between these cross-bridges and the actin filaments that causes contraction.

Figure 6–1E shows that the actin filaments are attached to the so-called *Z disc,* and the filaments extend on either side of the Z disc to interdigitate with the myosin filaments. The Z disc also passes from myofibril to myofibril, attaching the myofibrils to each other all the way across the muscle fiber. Therefore, the entire muscle fiber has light and dark bands, as is also true of the individual myofibrils. These bands give skeletal and cardiac muscle their striated appearance.

The portion of a myofibril (or of the whole muscle fiber) that lies between two successive Z discs is called a *sarcomere.* When the muscle fiber is at its normal, fully stretched resting length, the length of the sarcomere is about 2.0 microns. At this length, the actin filaments completely overlap the myosin filaments and are just beginning to overlap each other. We shall see later that at this length the sarcomere is capable of generating its greatest force of contraction.

The Sarcoplasm. The myofibrils are suspended inside the muscle fiber in a matrix called *sarcoplasm,* which is composed of usual intracellular constituents. The sarcoplasm contains tremendous numbers of *mitochondria* that lie between and parallel to the myofi-

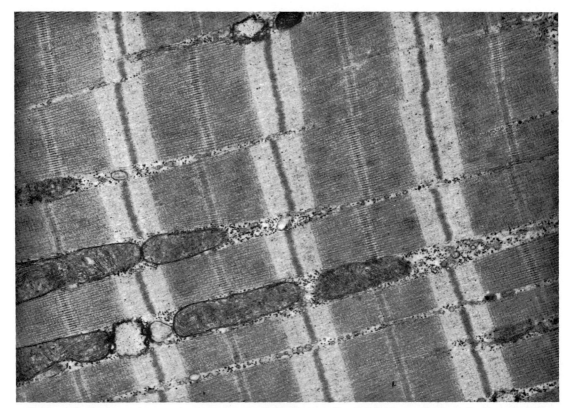

Figure 6–2. Electron micrograph of muscle myofibrils, showing the detailed organization of actin and myosin filaments. Note the mitochondria lying between the myofibrils. (From Fawcett: The Cell, 2d ed. Philadelphia, W. B. Saunders Company, 1981.)

brils, which is indicative of the great need of the contracting myofibrils for large amounts of ATP formed by the mitochondria.

The Sarcoplasmic Reticulum. Also in the sarcoplasm is an extensive endoplasmic reticulum, which in the muscle fiber is called the *sarcoplasmic reticu-* *lum.* This reticulum has a special organization that is extremely important in the control of muscle contraction, which will be discussed later in the chapter. The electron micrograph of Figure 6–3 illustrates the arrangement of this sarcoplasmic reticulum and shows how extensive it can be.

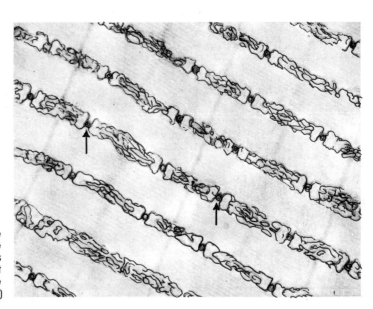

Figure 6–3. Sarcoplasmic reticulum surrounding the myofibril, showing the longitudinal system paralleling the myofibrils. Also shown in cross-section are the T tubules that lead to the exterior of the fiber membrane and that contain extracellular fluid (arrows). (From Fawcett: The Cell, 2d ed. Philadelphia, W. B. Saunders Company, 1981.)

MOLECULAR MECHANISM OF MUSCLE CONTRACTION

Sliding Mechanism of Contraction. Figure 6–4 illustrates the basic mechanism of muscle contraction. It shows the relaxed state of a sarcomere (above) and the contracted state (below). In the relaxed state, the ends of the actin filaments derived from two successive Z discs barely overlap each other while at the same time completely overlapping the myosin filaments. On the other hand, in the contracted state these actin filaments have been pulled inward among the myosin filaments so that they now overlap each other to a major extent. Also, the Z discs have been pulled by the actin filaments up to the end of the myosin filaments. Thus, muscle contraction occurs by a *sliding filament mechanism.*

But what causes the actin filaments to slide inward among the myosin filaments? Almost certainly, this is caused by mechanical, chemical, or electrostatic forces generated by the interaction of the cross-bridges of the myosin filaments with the actin filaments, as we shall discuss in the following sections.

Under resting conditions, the sliding forces between the actin and myosin filaments are inhibited, but when an action potential travels over the muscle fiber membrane, this causes the release of large quantities of calcium ions into the sarcoplasm surrounding the myofibrils. These calcium ions activate the forces between the filaments and contraction begins. But energy is also needed for the contractile process to proceed. This energy is derived from the high energy bonds of adenosine triphosphate (ATP), which is degraded to adenosine diphosphate (ADP) to give the energy required.

In the next few sections we will describe what is known about the details of the molecular processes of contraction. To begin this discussion, however, we must first characterize in detail the myosin and actin filaments.

MOLECULAR CHARACTERISTICS OF THE CONTRACTILE FILAMENTS

The Myosin Filament. The myosin filament is composed of multiple myosin molecules, each having a molecular weight of about 480,000. Figure 6–5A illustrates an individual molecule, and B illustrates the organization of the molecules to form a myosin filament, as well as its interaction with the ends of two actin filaments.

The *myosin molecule* is comprised of six polypeptide chains, two *heavy chains* each with a molecular weight of about 200,000 and four *light chains* with molecular weights of about 20,000 each. The two heavy chains coil around each other to form a double helix. However, one end of each of these chains is folded into a globular protein mass called the myosin *head.* Thus, there are two free heads lying side by side at one end of the double helix myosin molecule; the other nerve of the coiled helix is called the *tail.*

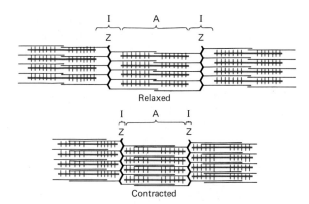

Figure 6–4. The relaxed and contracted states of a myofibril, showing sliding of the actin filaments (black) into the channels between the myosin filaments (red).

The four light chains are also parts of the myosin heads, two to each head. These light chains help control the function of the head during the process of muscle contraction.

The *myosin filament* is made up of about 200 individual myosin molecules. The central portion of one of these filaments is illustrated in Figure 6–5B, showing the tails of the myosin molecules bundled together to form the *body* of the filament, while many heads of the molecules hang outward to the sides of the body. Also, part of the helix portion of each myosin molecule extends to the side along with the head, thus providing an *arm* that extends the head outward from the body of the filament as shown in the figure. The protruding arms and heads together are called *cross-bridges,* and each of these is believed to be flexible at two points called *hinges,* one where the arm leaves the body of the myosin filament and the other where the two heads attach to the arm. The

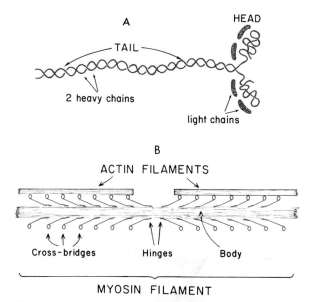

Figure 6–5. *A,* The myosin molecule. *B,* Combination of many myosin molecules to form a myosin filament. Also shown are the cross-bridges and the interaction between the heads of the cross-bridges and adjacent actin filaments.

hinged arms allow the heads to be extended either far outward from the body of the myosin filament or to be brought close to the body. The hinged heads are believed to participate in the actual contraction process.

The total length of the myosin filament is 1.6 microns. However, note that there are no cross-bridge heads in the very center of the myosin filament because the hinged arms extend toward both ends of the myosin filament away from the center; therefore, in the center there are only tails of the myosin molecules and no heads.

ATPase Activity of the Myosin Head. Another feature of the myosin head that is essential for muscle contraction is that it can function as an ATPase enzyme. As we shall see later, this property allows the head to cleave ATP and to use the energy derived from the ATP's high energy phosphate bond to energize the contraction process.

The Actin Filament. The actin filament is also complex. It is composed of three different components: *actin, tropomyosin,* and *troponin.*

The backbone of the actin filament is a double-stranded F-actin protein molecule, illustrated in Figure 6–6. The two strands are wound in a helix in the same manner as that in the myosin molecule.

Each strand of the double F-actin helix is composed of polymerized G-actin molecules, each having a molecular weight of 42,000. There are approximately 13 of these molecules in each revolution of each strand of helix. Attached to each one of the G-actin molecules is one molecule of ADP. It is believed that these ADP molecules are the active sites on the actin filaments with which the cross-bridges of the myosin filaments interact to cause muscle contraction.

Each actin filament is approximately 1 micron long. The bases of the actin filaments are inserted strongly into the Z discs, while their other ends protrude in both directions into the adjacent sarcomeres to lie in the spaces between the myosin molecules, as illustrated in Figure 6–4.

The Tropomyosin Strands. The actin filament also contains two additional protein strands that are polymers of *tropomyosin* molecules, each molecule having a molecular weight of 70,000 and extending a length of 40 nanometers. It is believed that each tropomyosin strand is loosely attached to an F-actin strand and that in the resting state it physically covers the active sites of the actin strands so that interaction cannot occur between the actin and myosin to cause contraction.

Troponin and Its Role in Muscle Contraction. Attached at multiple points along each tropomyosin molecule is a complex of three globular protein molecules called *troponin.* One of the globular proteins (troponin I) has a strong affinity for actin, another (troponin T) for tropomyosin, and a third (troponin C) for calcium ions. This complex is believed to attach the tropomyosin to the actin. The strong affinity of the troponin for calcium ions is believed to initiate the contraction process, as will be explained in the following section.

Interaction of Myosin and Actin Filaments to Cause Contraction

Inhibition of the Actin Filament by the Troponin-Tropomyosin Complex; Activation by Calcium Ions. A pure actin filament without the presence of the troponin-tropomyosin complex binds strongly with myosin molecules in the presence of ATP, which is normally abundant in the myofibril. But, if the troponin-tropomyosin complex is added to the actin filament, this binding does not take place. Therefore, it is believed that the active sites on the normal actin filament of the relaxed muscle are inhibited (or perhaps physically covered) by the troponin-tropomyosin complex. Consequently, they then cannot interact with the myosin filaments to cause contraction. Before contraction can take place the inhibitory effect of the troponin-tropomyosin complex must itself be inhibited.

Now, let us discuss the role of the calcium ions. In the presence of large amounts of calcium ions, the inhibitory effect of the troponin-tropomyosin on the actin filaments is itself inhibited. The mechanism of this is not known, but one suggestion is the following: When calcium ions combine with troponin C, the troponin complex supposedly undergoes a conformational change that in some way tugs on the tropomyosin protein strand and supposedly moves the tropomyosin strand deeper into the groove between the two actin strands. This "uncovers" the active sites of the actin, thus allowing contraction to proceed. Though this is a hypothetical mechanism, nevertheless it does emphasize that the normal relationship between the tropomyosin-troponin complex and actin is altered by calcium ions—a condition that leads to contraction.

Interaction Between the "Activated" Actin Filament and the Myosin Cross-Bridges—The "Walk-Along" Theory of Contraction. As soon as the actin filament becomes activated by the calcium ions, it is believed that the heads of the cross-bridges from the myosin filaments immediately become attracted to the active sites of the actin filament, and this causes contraction to occur. Though the precise manner by which this interaction between the cross-bridges and the actin causes contraction is still unknown, a suggested hypothesis for which considerable evidence exists is the *"walk-along" theory of contraction.*

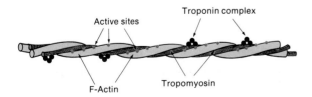

Figure 6–6. The actin filament, composed of two helical strands of F-actin and two tropomyosin strands that lie in the grooves between the actin strands. Attaching the tropomyosin to the actin are several troponin complexes.

Figure 6–7 illustrates the postulated walk-along mechanism for contraction. This figure shows the heads of two cross-bridges attaching to and disengaging from the active sites of an actin filament. It is postulated that when the head attaches to an active site this attachment simultaneously causes profound changes in the intramolecular forces in the head and arm of the cross-bridge. The new alignment of forces causes the head to tilt toward the arm and to drag the actin filament along with it. This tilt of the head of the cross-bridge is called the *power stroke*. Then, immediately after tilting, the head automatically breaks away from the active site and returns to its normal perpendicular direction. In this position it combines with an active site farther along the actin filament; then, a second tilt takes place to cause a new power stroke, and the actin filament moves another step. Thus, the heads of the cross-bridges bend back and forth and step by step walk along the actin filament, pulling it toward the center of the myosin filament.

Each one of the cross-bridges is believed to operate independently of all others, each attaching and pulling in a continuous but random cycle. Therefore, the greater the number of cross-bridges in contact with the actin filament at any given time, the greater, theoretically, is the force of contraction.

ATP as the Source of Energy for Contraction—Chemical Events in the Motion of the Myosin Heads. When a muscle contracts against a load, work is performed and energy is required. It is found that large amounts of ATP are cleaved to form ADP during the contraction process. Furthermore, the greater the amount of work performed by the muscle, the greater the amount of ATP that is cleaved. Though it is still not known exactly how ATP is used to provide the energy for contraction, the following is a sequence of events that has been suggested as the means by which this occurs:

1. Before contraction begins, the heads of the cross-bridges bind with ATP. The ATPase activity of the myosin head immediately cleaves the ATP but leaves the cleavage product ADP bound to the head. In this state, the conformation of the head is such that it extends perpendicularly toward the actin filament.

2. Next, when the inhibitory effect of the troponin-tropomyosin complex is itself inhibited by calcium ions, active sites on the actin filament are uncovered and the myosin heads bind with these, as illustrated in Figure 6–7.

3. The bond between the head of the cross-bridge and the active site of the actin filament causes a conformational change in the head, causing the head to tilt toward the arm of the cross-bridge. This provides the *power stroke* for pulling the actin filament. The energy that activates the power stroke is the energy already stored in the head at the time of cleavage of the ATP.

4. Once the head of the cross-bridge tilts, this allows release of the ADP and exposes a site on the head where a new molecule of ATP binds, and this binding in turn causes detachment of the head from the actin.

5. After the head has split away from the actin, the new molecule of ATP is also cleaved, and the energy again "cocks" the head back to its perpendicular position ready to begin a new power stroke cycle.

Thus, the process proceeds again and again until the actin filament pulls the Z membrane up against the ends of the myosin filaments or until the load on the muscle becomes too great for further pulling to occur.

DEGREE OF ACTIN AND MYOSIN FILAMENT OVERLAP—EFFECT ON TENSION DEVELOPED BY THE CONTRACTING MUSCLE

Figure 6–8 illustrates the effect of sarcomere length on the tension developed by a single, contracting, *isolated* muscle fiber. To the right are illustrated different degrees of overlap of the myosin and actin filaments at different sarcomere lengths. At point D on the diagram, the actin filament has been pulled all the way out to the end of the myosin filament with no overlap at all. At this point, the tension developed by the activated muscle is zero. Then, as the sarcomere shortens and the actin filament overlaps the myosin filament progressively more and more, the tension increases until the sarcomere length decreases

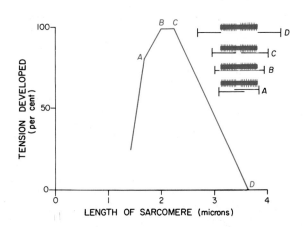

Figure 6–8. Length-tension diagram for a single sarcomere, illustrating maximum strength of contraction when the sarcomere is 2.0 to 2.2 microns in length. At the upper right are shown the relative positions of the actin and myosin filaments at different sarcomere lengths from point A to point D. (Modified from Gordon, Huxley, and Julian: *J. Physiol., 171*:28P, 1964.)

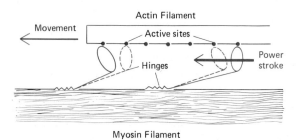

Figure 6–7. The "walk along" mechanism for contraction of the muscle.

to about 2.2 microns. At this point the actin filament has already overlapped all the cross-bridges of the myosin filament but has not yet reached the center of the myosin filament. Upon further shortening, the sarcomere maintains full tension until point B at a sarcomere length of approximately 2.0 microns. At this point the ends of the two actin filaments begin to overlap. As the sarcomere length falls from 2 microns down to about 1.65 microns, at point A, the strength of contraction decreases. It is at this point that the two Z discs of the sarcomere abut the ends of the myosin filaments. Then, as contraction proceeds to still shorter sarcomere lengths, the ends of the myosin filaments are actually crumpled, and as illustrated in Figure 6–8 the strength of contraction also decreases precipitously.

This diagram illustrates that maximum contraction occurs when there is maximum overlap between the actin filaments and the cross-bridges of the myosin filaments, and it supports the idea that the greater the number of cross-bridges pulling the actin filaments, the greater the strength of contraction.

INITIATION OF MUSCLE CONTRACTION: EXCITATION-CONTRACTION COUPLING

Initiation of contraction in skeletal muscle begins with action potentials in the muscle fibers. These elicit electrical currents that spread to the interior of the fiber where they cause release of calcium ions from the sarcoplasmic reticulum. It is the calcium ions that in turn initiate the chemical events of the contractile process. This overall process for controlling muscle contraction is called *excitation-contraction coupling.*

THE MUSCLE ACTION POTENTIAL

Almost everything discussed in Chapter 10 regarding initiation and conduction of action potentials in nerve fibers applies equally well to skeletal muscle fibers, except for quantitative differences. Some of the quantitative aspects of muscle potentials are the following:

1. Resting membrane potential: Approximately −90 millivolts in skeletal fibers—the same as in large myelinated nerve fibers.

2. Duration of action potential: 1 to 5 milliseconds in skeletal muscle—about five times as long as in large myelinated nerves.

3. Velocity of conduction: 3 to 5 meters per second—about 1/18 the velocity of conduction in the large myelinated nerve fibers that excite skeletal muscle.

Excitation of Skeletal Muscle Fibers by Nerves. In normal function of the body, skeletal muscle fibers are excited by large myelinated nerve fibers. These attach to the skeletal muscle fibers at the neuromuscular junction, which will be discussed in detail in the following chapter. Except for 2 per cent of the muscle fibers, there is only one neuromuscular junction to

each muscle fiber; this junction is located near the middle of the fiber. Therefore, the action potential spreads from the middle of the fiber toward its two ends. This dual direction of spreading from the center is important because it allows nearly coincident contraction of all sarcomeres of the muscles so that they can all contract together rather than separately.

Spread of the Action Potential to the Interior of the Muscle Fiber by Way of the Transverse Tubule System

The skeletal muscle fiber is so large that action potentials spreading along its surface membrane cause almost no current flow deep within the fiber. Yet, to cause contraction, these electrical currents must penetrate to the vicinity of all the separate myofibrils. This is achieved by transmission of the action potentials along very small *transverse tubules* (T tubules) that penetrate all the way through the muscle fiber from one side to the other. The T tubule action potentials in turn cause the sarcoplasmic reticulum to release calcium ions in the immediate vicinity of all the myofibrils, and these calcium ions in turn cause contraction. Now, let us describe this system in much greater detail.

The Transverse Tubule–Sarcoplasmic Reticulum System. Figure 6–9 illustrates a group of myofibrils surrounded by the transverse tubule–sarcoplasmic reticulum system. The transverse tubules are the very small tubules lying on top of the red-colored sarcoplasmic reticulum. They penetrate all the way from one side of the muscle fiber to the opposite side. Not shown in the figure is the branching of these tubules among themselves so that they form entire *planes* of T tubules interlacing among all the separate myofibrils. Also, it should be noted that where the T tubules originate from the cell membrane they are open to the exterior. Therefore, they communicate with the fluid surrounding the muscle fiber and contain extracellular fluid in their lumens. In other words, the T tubules are internal extensions of the cell membrane. Therefore, when an action potential spreads over a muscle fiber membrane, it spreads along the T tubules to the deep interior of the muscle fiber as well.

Figure 6–9 shows the extensiveness of the *sarcoplasmic reticulum* as well. This is composed of two major parts: (1) long *longitudinal tubules* that cover the surfaces of the myofibrils and terminate in (2) large chambers called *terminal cisternae* that abut the transverse tubules.

RELEASE OF CALCIUM IONS BY THE SARCOPLASMIC RETICULUM

One of the special features of the sarcoplasmic reticulum is that it contains calcium ions in very high concentration, and many of these ions are released when the adjacent T tubule is excited.

Figure 6–10 shows that the action potential of the T tubule causes current flow through the cisternae

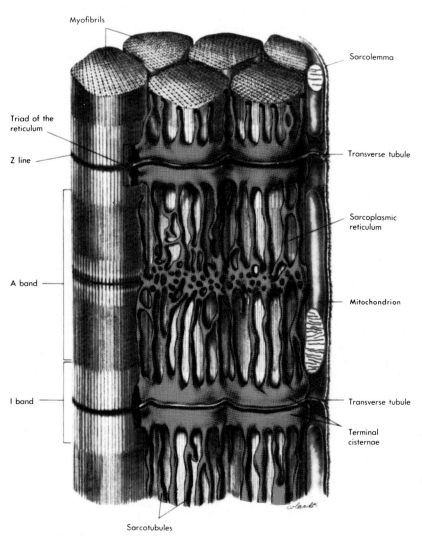

Myofibrils

Triad of the reticulum

Z line

A band

I band

Sarcotubules

Sarcolemma

Transverse tubule

Sarcoplasmic reticulum

Mitochondrion

Transverse tubule

Terminal cisternae

Figure 6–9. The transverse tubule-sarcoplasmic reticulum system. Note the *longitudinal tubules* that terminate in large *cisternae.* The cisternae in turn abut the transverse tubules. Note also that the transverse tubules communicate with the outside of the cell membrane. This illustration was drawn from frog muscle, which has one transverse tubule per sarcomere, located at the Z line. A similar arrangement is found in mammalian heart muscle, but mammalian skeletal muscle has two transverse tubules per sarcomere, located at the A-I junctions. (From Bloom and Fawcett: A Textbook of Histology. Philadelphia, W. B. Saunders Company, 1975. Modified after Peachey: *J. Cell Biol. 25:*209, 1965. Drawn by Sylvia Colard Keene.)

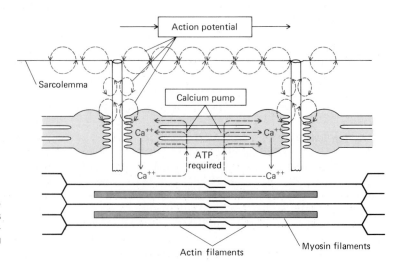

Action potential

Sarcolemma

Calcium pump

Ca^{++}

Ca^{++}

ATP required

Ca^{++}

Ca^{++}

Actin filaments

Myosin filaments

Figure 6–10. Excitation-contraction coupling in the muscle, showing an action potential that causes release of calcium ions from the sarcoplasmic reticulum and then reuptake of the calcium ions by a calcium pump.

where they abut the T tubule. The cisternae project *junctional feet* that surround the T tubule, presumably facilitating passage of electrical current from the T tubule into the cisternae. This current flow causes rapid release of calcium ions into the sarcoplasm from the cisternae and perhaps from the longitudinal tubules as well. Presumably this results from the opening of calcium channels similar to the opening of sodium channels at the onset of the action potential, though the actual mechanism is still unknown.

The calcium ions thus released from the sarcoplasmic reticulum diffuse to the adjacent myofibrils where they bind strongly with troponin C, as discussed in an earlier section, and this in turn elicits the muscle contraction, as has also been discussed.

The Calcium Pump for Removing Calcium Ions from the Sarcoplasmic Fluid. Once the calcium ions have been released from the cisternae and have diffused to the myofibrils, muscle contraction will then continue as long as the calcium ions remain in high concentration in the sarcoplasmic fluid. However, a continually active calcium pump located in the walls of the sarcoplasmic reticulum pumps calcium ions back out of the sarcoplasmic fluid and once again into the vesicular cavities of the reticulum. This pump can concentrate the calcium ions about 10,000-fold inside the sarcoplasmic reticulum. In addition, inside the reticulum is a protein called *calsequestrin* that can bind 40 times as much calcium as that in the ionic state, thus providing another 40-fold increase in the storage of calcium. Thus, this massive transfer of calcium in the sarcoplasmic reticulum causes almost total depletion of calcium ions in the fluid of the myofibrils. Therefore, except immediately after an action potential, the calcium ion concentration in the myofibrils is kept at an extremely low level.

The Excitatory "Pulse" of Calcium Ions. The normal "resting" concentration (less than 10^{-7} molar) of calcium ions in the cytosol that bathes the myofibrils is too little to elicit contraction. Therefore, in the resting state, the troponin-tropomyosin complex keeps the actin filaments inhibited and maintains a relaxed state of the muscle.

On the other hand, full excitation of the T tubule-sarcoplasmic reticulum system causes enough release of calcium ions to increase the concentration in the myofibrillar fluid to as high as 2×10^{-4} molar concentration, which is several times the level required to cause maximum muscle contraction (about 2×10^{-5} molar). Immediately thereafter, the calcium pump depletes the calcium ions again. The total duration of this calcium "pulse" in the usual skeletal muscle fiber lasts about $1/30$ of a second, though it may last several times as long as this in some skeletal muscle fibers and several times less in others (in heart muscle the pulse lasts for as long as 0.3 second because of the long duration of the cardiac action potential). It is during this calcium pulse that muscle contraction occurs. If the contraction is to continue without interruption for longer intervals, a series of such pulses must be initiated by a continuous series of repetitive action potentials, as will be discussed in more detail later in the chapter.

EFFICIENCY OF MUSCLE CONTRACTION

The efficiency of an engine or a motor is calculated as the percentage of energy input that is converted into muscle work instead of heat. The percentage of the input energy to a muscle (the chemical energy in the nutrients) that can be converted into muscle work is less than 20 to 25 per cent, the remainder becoming heat. The reason for this low efficiency is that about half of the energy in the foodstuffs is lost during the formation of ATP, and even then only 40 to 45 per cent of the energy in the ATP itself can later be converted into work. Also, maximum efficiency can be realized only when the muscle contracts at a moderate velocity. If the muscle contracts very slowly or without any movement at all, large amounts of *maintenance heat* are released during the process of contraction even though little or no work is being performed, thereby decreasing the efficiency. On the other hand, if contraction is too rapid, large proportions of the energy are used to overcome the viscous friction within the muscle itself, and this, too, reduces the efficiency of contraction. Ordinarily, maximum efficiency is developed when the velocity of contraction is about 30 per cent of maximum.

CHARACTERISTICS OF A SINGLE MUSCLE TWITCH

Many features of muscle contraction can be especially well demonstrated by eliciting single *muscle twitches*. This can be accomplished by instantaneously exciting the nerve to a muscle or by passing a short electrical stimulus through the muscle itself, giving rise to a single, sudden contraction lasting for a fraction of a second.

Isometric Versus Isotonic Contraction. Muscle contraction is said to be *isometric* when the muscle does not shorten during contraction and *isotonic* when it shortens while the tension on the muscle remains constant.

There are several basic differences between isometric and isotonic contractions. First, isometric contraction does not require much sliding of myofibrils among each other. Second, in isotonic contraction a load is moved, which involves the phenomena of inertia. That is, the weight or other type of object being moved must first be accelerated, and once a velocity has been attained the load has momentum that causes it to continue moving even after the contraction is over. Therefore, an isotonic contraction is likely to last considerably longer than an isometric contraction of the same muscle. Third, isotonic contraction entails the performance of external work.

Therefore, a greater amount of energy is used by the muscle.

Muscles can contract both isometrically and isotonically in the body, but most contractions are actually a mixture of the two. When standing, a person tenses the quadriceps muscles to tighten the knee joints and to keep the legs stiff. This is isometric contraction. On the other hand, when a person lifts a weight using the biceps, this is mainly an isotonic contraction. Finally, contractions of leg muscles during running are a mixture of isometric and isotonic contractions—isometric mainly to keep the limbs stiff when the legs hit the ground and isotonic mainly to move the limbs.

Characteristics of Isometric Twitches Recorded from Different Muscles. The body has many different sizes of skeletal muscles—from the very small stapedius muscle of only a few millimeters length and a millimeter or so in diameter up to the very large quadriceps muscle. Furthermore, the fibers may be as small as 10 microns in diameter or as large as 80 microns. And, finally, the energetics of muscle contraction vary considerably from one muscle to another. These different physical and chemical characteristics often manifest themselves in the form of different speeds of contraction: some muscles contract rapidly while others contract slowly.

Fast Versus Slow Muscle. Figure 6–11 illustrates isometric contractions of three different types of skeletal muscles: an ocular muscle, which has a duration of contraction of less than $1/100$ second; the gastrocnemius muscle, which has a duration of contraction of about $1/30$ second; and the soleus muscle, which has a duration of contraction of about $1/10$ second. It is interesting that these durations of contractions are adapted to the function of each of the respective muscles, for ocular movements must be extremely rapid to maintain fixation of the eyes upon specific objects, the gastrocnemius muscle must contract moderately rapidly to provide sufficient velocity of limb movement for running and jumping, while the soleus muscle is concerned principally with slow reactions for continual support of the body against gravity.

As we shall discuss more fully in Chapter 57 on sports physiology, every muscle of the body is composed of a mixture of so-called *fast* and *slow* muscle fibers, with still other fibers graduated between these two extremes. The muscles that react very rapidly usually are composed mainly of the fast fibers, which are much larger and contain a much more extensive sarcoplasmic reticulum than found in the slow fibers.

MECHANICS OF SKELETAL MUSCLE CONTRACTION

THE MOTOR UNIT

Each motor nerve fiber that leaves the spinal cord usually innervates many different muscle fibers, the number depending on the type of muscle. All the muscle fibers innervated by a single motor nerve fiber are called a *motor unit.* In general, small muscles that react rapidly and whose control is exact have few muscle fibers in each motor unit (as few as two to three in some of the laryngeal muscles) and have a large number of nerve fibers going to each muscle. On the other hand, the large muscles that do not require a very fine degree of control, such as the gastrocnemius muscle, may have several hundred muscle fibers in a motor unit. An average figure for all the muscles of the body can be considered to be about 150 muscle fibers to the motor unit.

SUMMATION OF MUSCLE CONTRACTION

Summation means the adding together of individual muscle twitches to make strong and concerted muscle movements. In general, summation occurs in two different ways: (1) by increasing the number of motor units contracting simultaneously, and (2) by increasing the rapidity of contraction of individual motor units. These are called, respectively, *multiple motor unit summation* and *wave summation* (or spatial summation and temporal summation).

Wave Summation and Tetanization. When a muscle is stimulated at progressively greater frequencies, its degree of contraction becomes progressively greater, which is *wave* summation. This is illustrated in Figure 6–12. Also, at the higher frequencies of stimulation the successive contractions fuse together and cannot be distinguished one from the other. This state is called *tetanization,* and the lowest frequency at which it occurs is called the *critical frequency.*

Tetanization results partly from the viscous properties of the muscle and partly from the nature of the contractile process itself. The muscle fibers are filled with sarcoplasm, which is a viscous fluid, and the fibers are encased in fasciae and muscle sheaths that have a viscous resistance to change in length. Therefore, these viscous factors play a role in causing the successive contractions to fuse with each other.

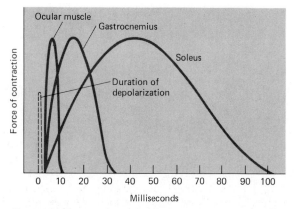

Figure 6–11. Duration of isometric contractions of different types of mammalian muscles, showing also a latent period between the action potential and muscle contraction.

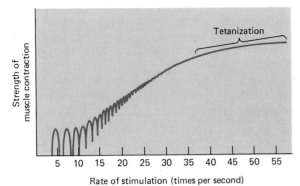

Figure 6–12. Wave summation and tetanization.

But in addition to the viscous property of muscle, the activation process itself lasts for a definite period of time, and successive pulsatile states of activation of the muscle fiber can occur so rapidly that they fuse into a long continual state of activation; that is, the level of free calcium ions in the myofibrils remains continuously above the level required for full activation of the contractile process, thus providing an uninterrupted stimulus for maintenance of contraction. Once the critical frequency for tetanization is reached, further increase in rate of stimulation increases the force of contraction only a few more per cent, as shown in Figure 6–12.

Maximum Strength of Contraction. The maximum strength of tetanic contraction of a muscle operating at a normal muscle length is about 3.5 kilograms per square centimeter of muscle, or 50 pounds per square inch. Since a quadriceps muscle can at times have as much as 16 square inches of muscle belly, as much as 800 pounds of tension may at times be applied to the patellar tendon. One can readily understand, therefore, how it is possible for muscles sometimes to pull their tendons out of the insertions in bones. This often occurs where the patellar tendon inserts in the tibia, and it occurs even more frequently where the Achilles tendon of the gastrocnemius muscle inserts at the heel.

MUSCLE FATIGUE

Prolonged and strong contraction of a muscle leads to the well-known state of muscle fatigue. Studies in athletes have shown that muscle fatigue increases in almost direct proportion to the rate of depletion of muscle glycogen. Therefore, most fatigue probably results simply from inability of the contractile and metabolic processes of the muscle fibers to continue supplying the same work output. However, experiments have also shown that transmission of the nerve signal through the neuromuscular junction can occasionally diminish following prolonged muscle activity, thus further diminishing muscle contraction.

Interruption of blood flow through a contracting muscle leads to almost complete muscle fatigue within

a minute or more because of the obvious loss of nutrient supply—especially loss of oxygen.

MUSCLE HYPERTROPHY

Forceful muscular activity causes the muscle size to increase, a phenomenon called hypertrophy. Most of the hypertrophy results from increase in the diameters of the fibers already present in the muscle, but the numbers of fibers can probably also increase to a very slight extent by splitting of fibers already present; this is called *hyperplasia*. As the diameters of the muscle fibers increase, the sarcoplasm increases, and the fibers gain in various nutrient and intermediary metabolic substances, such as adenosine triphosphate, phosphocreatine, glycogen, intracellular lipids, and even many additional mitochondria. It is likely that the myofibrils also increase in size and perhaps in numbers as well, but this has not been proved. Briefly, muscular hypertrophy increases both the motive power of the muscle and the nutrient mechanisms for maintaining increased motive power.

Weak muscular activity, even when sustained over long periods of time, does not result in significant hypertrophy. Instead, hypertrophy results mainly from *very* forceful muscle activity, though the activity might occur for only a few minutes each day. For this reason, strength can be developed in muscles much more rapidly when "resistive" or "isometric" exercise is used rather than simply prolonged mild exercise. Indeed, essentially no enlargement of the muscle fibers occurs unless the muscle contracts to at least 75 per cent of its maximum tension.

On the other hand, prolonged muscle activity does increase muscle endurance, causing increases in the oxidative enzymes, myoglobin, and even blood capillaries—all of which are essential to increased muscle metabolism.

MUSCLE ATROPHY

Muscle atrophy is the reverse of muscle hypertrophy; it results any time a muscle is not used or even when a muscle is used only for very weak contractions. Atrophy is particularly likely to occur when limbs are placed in casts, thereby preventing muscular contraction. As little as one month of disuse can sometimes decrease the muscle size to one-half normal.

Atrophy Caused by Muscle Denervation. When a muscle is denervated it immediately begins to atrophy, and the muscle continues to decrease in size for several years. If the muscle becomes reinnervated during the first three to four months, full function of the muscle usually returns, but after four months of denervation some of the muscle fibers usually will have degenerated. Reinnervation after two years rarely results in return of any function at all. Pathological studies show that the muscle fibers have by that time been replaced by fat and fibrous tissue.

Prevention of Muscle Atrophy by Electrical Stimulation. Strong electrical stimulation of denervated muscles, particularly when the resulting contractions occur against loads, will delay and in some instances prevent muscle atrophy despite denervation. This procedure is used to keep muscles alive until reinnervation can take place.

QUESTIONS

1. Describe the component parts of a skeletal muscle fiber, beginning with the fiber itself; then describe the nature of the myofibrils and the organization of myosin and actin filaments in the myofibrils.
2. How are the actin and myosin filaments organized within each sarcomere of the skeletal muscle fiber?
3. Describe the manner in which the sarcolemma attaches to the tendons.
4. Explain the manner in which the actin and myosin filaments interdigitate with each other to cause contraction.
5. How do multiple myosin molecules combine with each other to form the myosin filament?
6. Describe the cross-bridges of the myosin filaments and their component parts.
7. Describe the manner in which the actin molecules are combined together to form the actin filament.
8. Explain the relationship of tropomyosin and troponin to the actin filaments.
9. Explain the manner in which the myosin and actin filaments interact with each other to cause contraction by the "walk-along" mechanism.
10. Give the postulated steps for the mechanism by which ATP is used as an energy source to cause the power stroke of the myosin heads.
11. Explain why the strength of contraction of a skeletal muscle fiber is determined by the degree of overlap of the actin and myosin filaments. Also, what is the relationship between sarcomere length and strength of contraction?
12. Describe the organization of the sarcoplasmic reticulum in the skeletal muscle fiber, and also explain the relationship of the transverse tubules to this sarcoplasmic reticulum.
13. How does the muscle action potential travel to the interior of the skeletal muscle fiber?
14. Explain how the "pulse" of calcium ions in the sarcoplasm occurs and how the calcium ions disappear during each skeletal muscle twitch.
15. Explain the postulated mechanism by which calcium ions cause muscle contraction.
16. What is meant by efficiency of muscle contraction? Approximately how efficient is the contraction of most skeletal muscle?
17. Explain the difference between *isometric* and *isotonic* muscle contractions.
18. Explain how muscle contraction summates as a result of *multiple motor unit summation* and *wave summation*.
19. What is meant by *tetanization* during muscle contraction, and what causes this?
20. If a muscle has ten square centimeters of cross-sectional area, what will be its approximate maximal strength of contraction?
21. What factors can lead to muscle fatigue?
22. What type of muscle contraction leads to muscle hypertrophy, and what are the changes in the muscle itself?
23. What factors can lead to muscle atrophy? Following denervation, how long can a muscle fiber remain alive while awaiting a nerve fiber to reinnervate it?

References

American Physiological Society: Skeletal Muscle. Baltimore, Waverly Press, 1983.

Armstrong, R. B.: Mechanisms of exercise-induced delayed onset muscular soreness: A brief review. Med Sci Sports Exerc 16:529, 1984.

Burke, R. E.: Motor units: Anatomy, physiology, and functional organization. In Brooks, V. B., ed.: Handbook of Physiology. Sec. 1, Vol. 11. Bethesda, American Physiological Society, 1981, p. 345.

Freund, H.-J.: Motor unit and muscle activity in voluntary motor control. Physiol Rev 63:387, 1983.

Hasselbach, W., and Oetliker, H.: Energetics and electrogenicity of the sarcoplasmic reticulum calcium pump. Annu Rev Physiol 45:325, 1983.

Hockey, R.: Stress and Fatigue in Human Performance. New York, John Wiley & Sons, 1983.

Huxley, A. F., and Gordon, A. M.: Striation patterns in active and passive shortening of muscle. Nature (Lond.) 193:280, 1962.

Huxley, H. E., and Faruqi, A. R.: Time-resolved x-ray diffraction studies on vertebrate striated muscle. Annu Rev Biophys Bioeng 12:381, 1983.

Ikemoto, N.: Structure and function of the calcium pump protein of sarcoplasmic reticulum. Annu Rev Physiol 44:297, 1982.

Lamb, D. R.: Physiology of Exercises. Responses and Adaptations. New York, Macmillan Publishing Co., 1984.

Martonosi, A. N.: Mechanisms of Ca^{2+} release from sarcoplasmic reticulum of skeletal muscle. Physiol Rev 64:1240, 1984.

Morgan, D. L., and Proske, U.: Vertebrate slow muscle: Its structure, pattern of innervation, and mechanical properties. Physiol Rev 64:103, 1984.

Pollack, G. H.: The cross-bridge theory. Physiol Rev 63:1049, 1983.

Rash, J.: Neuromuscular Atlas. New York, Prager Publishers, 1984.

Schubert, D.: Developmental Biology of Cultured Nerve, Muscle and Glia. New York, John Wiley & Sons, 1984.

Stefani, E., and Chiarandini, D. J.: Ionic channels in skeletal muscle. Annu Rev Physiol 44:357, 1982.

Winegrad, S.: Regulation of cardiac contractile proteins. Correlations between physiology and biochemistry. Circ Res 55:565, 1984.

7

Neuromuscular Transmission; Function of Smooth Muscle

TRANSMISSION OF IMPULSES FROM
NERVES TO SKELETAL MUSCLE
FIBERS: THE NEUROMUSCULAR
JUNCTION
MYASTHENIA GRAVIS
CONTRACTION OF SMOOTH MUSCLE
TYPES OF SMOOTH MUSCLE
THE CONTRACTILE PROCESS IN
SMOOTH MUSCLE
MEMBRANE POTENTIALS AND
ACTION POTENTIALS IN SMOOTH
MUSCLE

EXCITATION–CONTRACTION
COUPLING—ROLE OF CALCIUM
IONS
NEUROMUSCULAR JUNCTIONS OF
SMOOTH MUSCLE
SMOOTH MUSCLE CONTRACTION
WITHOUT ACTION POTENTIALS—
EFFECT OF LOCAL TISSUE
FACTORS AND HORMONES
MECHANICAL CHARACTERISTICS OF
SMOOTH MUSCLE CONTRACTION

TRANSMISSION OF IMPULSES FROM NERVES TO SKELETAL MUSCLE FIBERS: THE NEUROMUSCULAR JUNCTION

The skeletal muscles are innervated by large, myelinated nerve fibers that originate in the large motor neurons of the anterior horns of the spinal cord. It was pointed out in the previous chapter that each nerve fiber normally branches many times and stimulates from three to several hundred skeletal muscle fibers. The nerve ending makes a junction, called the *neuromuscular junction*, with the muscle fiber approximately at the fiber's midpoint so that the action potential in the fiber travels in both directions. With the exception of about 2 per cent of the muscle fibers there is only one such junction per muscle fiber.

Physiologic Anatomy of the Neuromuscular Junction. Figure 7–1, Parts A and B, illustrates the neuromuscular junction. The nerve fiber branches at its end to form a complex of branching nerve *terminals* called the *end-plate,* which invaginates into the muscle fiber but lies entirely outside the muscle fiber plasma membrane. The entire structure is covered by one or more Schwann cells that insulate the end-plate from the surrounding fluids.

Figure 7–1C shows an electron micrographic sketch of the junction between one of the individual branching axon terminals and the muscle fiber. The invagination of the membrane is called the *synaptic gutter* or *synaptic trough*, and the space between the terminal and the fiber membrane is the *synaptic cleft.* The synaptic cleft is 20 to 30 nanometers wide and is filled with a thin layer of spongy reticular fibers through which diffuses extracellular fluid. At the bottom of the gutter are numerous smaller *folds* of the muscle membrane called *subneural clefts,* which greatly increase the surface area at which the synaptic transmitter can act. In the axon terminal are many mitochondria that supply energy mainly for synthesis of an excitatory transmitter, *acetylcholine* that, in turn, excites the muscle fiber. The acetylcholine is synthesized in the cytoplasm of the terminal but is rapidly absorbed into many small synaptic vesicles, approximately 300,000 of which are normally in the terminals of a single end-plate. Attached to the reticular fibers in the cleft are large quantities of the enzyme *acetylcholinesterase,* which is capable of destroying acetylcholine, a process to be explained in further detail.

Secretion of Acetylcholine by the Axon Terminals. When a nerve impulse reaches the neuromuscular

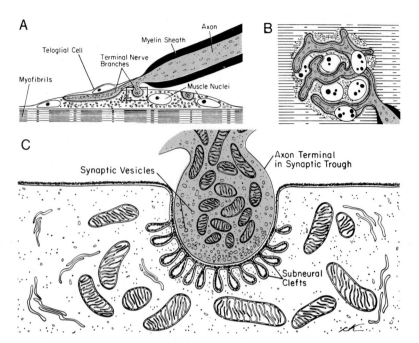

A

Teloglial Cell
Terminal Nerve
Branches
Myelin Sheath
Axon
Myofibrils
Muscle Nuclei

B

C

Synaptic Vesicles
Axon Terminal
in Synaptic Trough
Subneural
Clefts

Figure 7–1. Different views of the motor end-plate. A, Longitudinal section through the end-plate. B, Surface view of the end-plate. C, Electron micrographic appearance of the contact point between one of the axon terminals and the muscle fiber membrane, representing the rectangular area shown in A. (From Bloom and Fawcett, as modified from R. Couteaux: A Textbook of Histology. Philadelphia, W. B. Saunders Company, 1975.)

junction, about 300 vesicles of acetylcholine are released by the terminals into the synaptic clefts between the terminals and the muscle fiber membrane. The cause of this release is inflow of calcium ions from the extracellular fluid into the membranes of the terminals when the action potential depolarizes the membranes. The calcium ions cause the vesicles of acetylcholine to attach to and then rupture through the membrane.

Destruction of the Released Acetylcholine by Cholinesterase. Within approximately 1 millisecond after acetylcholine is released by the axon terminal, much of it has already diffused out of the synaptic gutter and no longer acts on the muscle fiber membrane, and virtually all the remainder is destroyed by the acetylcholinesterase in the cleft itself. The very short period of time that the acetylcholine remains in contact with the muscle fiber membrane—about 1 millisecond—is almost always sufficient to excite the muscle fiber, and yet the rapid removal of the acetylcholine prevents re-excitation after the muscle fiber has recovered from the first action potential.

Effect of Acetylcholine in Opening Acetylcholine-Gated Ion Channels. Even though the acetylcholine released into the cleft between the end-plate and the muscle membrane lasts for only a very small fraction of a second, during this time the permeability of the muscle membrane to positive ions in the cleft increases several thousandfold. This is because of the opening of *acetylcholine-gated ion channels*. On the external surface of each channel is a gate similar to that of the sodium channels discussed in Chapter 5. However, it is a *ligand-activated gate* rather than a voltage-activated gate, responding to acetylcholine as the ligand. The surface-protruding portion of this channel protein acts as a receptor for acetylcholine, and acetylcholine in turn causes a conformational change in the channel molecule to open the gate for about 1 millisecond.

The acetylcholine channels have a diameter of about 0.65 nanometers, which is large enough to allow all the important positive ions—Na^+, K^+, and Ca^{++}—to move easily through the channels. (Negative ions such as chloride ions do not pass through this channel because of strong negative charges in the wall of the channel.)

Yet, from a practical point of view only sodium ions flow through the channels, for the following reasons: First, the normal resting potential of the muscle fiber membrane is almost equal to the Nernst potential for potassium ions; therefore, opening the channels will not allow significant numbers of potassium ions to flow through the membrane—that is, the potassium concentration gradient is already approximately in equilibrium with the voltage gradient across the channels. On the other hand, both sodium and calcium ions have far greater concentrations outside the nerve fiber than inside, and their Nernst potentials are of opposite polarity to the resting membrane potential. Therefore, opening the acetylcholine channels allows both these ions to flow rapidly to the interior of the muscle fiber. However, the concentration of calcium ions in the extracellular fluid is less than one fiftieth the concentration of sodium ions, and their mobility is also less. Therefore, in essence, opening the acetylcholine channels allows very rapid influx of sodium ions to the interior of the fiber and little else. Nevertheless, even 1 millisecond influx of the sodium ions is still enough to excite an action potential in the muscle fiber.

The End-Plate Potential and Excitation of the Skeletal Muscle Fiber. The sudden insurgence of sodium ions into the muscle fiber when the acetylcholine channels open causes the membrane potential in the *local area of the end-plate* to increase in the positive direction as much as 50 to 75 millivolts, creating a *local potential* called the *end-plate potential*. If we recall from the previous chapter that a sudden increase in membrane potential of more than 15 to 30 millivolts is sufficient to initiate the positive feedback effect of sodium channel activation, one can understand that the end-plate potential created by the acetylcholine stimulation is normally far greater than the minimum required to initiate an action potential in the muscle fiber.

Drugs That Affect Transmission at the Neuromuscular Junction

Drugs That Stimulate the Muscle Fiber by Acetylcholine-Like Action. Many different compounds, including *methacholine, carbachol,* and *nicotine,* have the same effect on the muscle fiber as does acetylcholine. The difference between these drugs and acetylcholine is that they are not destroyed by cholinesterase or are destroyed very slowly, so that when once applied to the muscle fiber the action persists for many minutes to several hours. Moderate quantities of the above three drugs applied to a muscle fiber cause localized areas of depolarization, and every time the muscle fiber becomes repolarized elsewhere, these depolarized areas, by virtue of their leaking ions, cause new action potentials, thereby causing a state of spasm.

Drugs That Block Transmission at the Neuromuscular Junction. A group of drugs, known as the *curariform drugs,* can prevent passage of impulses from the end-plate into the muscle. Thus, D-*tubocurarine* affects the membrane, probably by competing with acetylcholine for the receptor sites of the membrane, so that the acetylcholine cannot increase the permeability of the acetylcholine channels sufficiently to initiate a depolarization wave.

Drugs That Stimulate the Neuromuscular Junction by Inactivating Acetylcholinesterase. Three particularly well-known drugs, *neostigmine, physostigmine,* and *diisopropyl fluorophosphate,* inactivate acetylcholinesterase so that the cholinesterase normally in the synapses will not hydrolyze the acetylcholine released at the end-plate. As a result, acetylcholine increases in quantity with successive nerve impulses so that extreme amounts of acetylcholine can accumulate and then repetitively stimulate the muscle fiber. This causes *muscular spasm* even when only a few nerve impulses reach the muscle; this can cause death due to laryngeal spasm, which smothers the person.

Diisopropyl fluorophosphate, which has military potential as a very powerful "nerve" gas, actually inactivates acetylcholinesterase for several weeks, which makes this a particularly lethal drug.

MYASTHENIA GRAVIS

The disease *myasthenia gravis,* which occurs in about one of every 20,000 persons, causes the person to become paralyzed because of inability of the neuromuscular junctions to transmit signals from the nerve fibers to the muscle fibers. Pathologically, the number of subneural clefts in the synaptic gutter is reduced and the synaptic cleft itself is widened as much as 50 per cent. Also, antibodies that attack the acetylcholine-gated transport proteins have been demonstrated in the bloods of these patients. Therefore, it is believed that myasthenia gravis is an autoimmune disease in which patients have developed antibodies against their own acetylcholine-activated ion channels.

Regardless of the cause, the end-plate potentials developed in the muscle fibers are too weak to stimulate the muscle fibers adequately. If the disease is intense enough, the patient dies of paralysis—in particular, of paralysis of the respiratory muscles. However, the disease can usually be ameliorated with several different drugs, as follows:

Treatment with Drugs. When a patient with myasthenia gravis is treated with a drug, such as neostigmine, that is capable of inactivating acetylcholinesterase, the acetylcholine secreted by the end-plate is not destroyed immediately. If a sequence of nerve impulses arrives at the end-plate, the quantity of acetylcholine present at the membrane increases progressively until finally the end-plate potential caused by the acetylcholine rises above threshold value for stimulating the muscle fiber. Thus, it is sometimes possible, by diminishing the quantity of acetylcholinesterase in the muscles of a patient with myasthenia gravis, to allow even the inadequate quantities of acetylcholine secreted at the end-plates to effect almost normal muscular activity.

CONTRACTION OF SMOOTH MUSCLE

In the previous chapter and thus far in the present chapter, the discussion has been concerned with skeletal muscle. We now turn to smooth muscle, which is composed of far smaller fibers—usually 2 to 5 microns in diameter and only 50 to 200 microns in length—in contrast to the skeletal muscle fibers that are as much as 20 times as large (in diameter) and thousands of times as long. Nevertheless, many of the principles of contraction apply to smooth muscle in the same way as to skeletal muscle. Most important, essentially the same chemical substances cause contraction in smooth muscle as in skeletal muscle, but the physical arrangement of smooth muscle fibers is entirely different, as we shall see.

TYPES OF SMOOTH MUSCLE

The smooth muscle of each organ is distinctive from that of most other organs in several different ways: physical dimensions, organization into bundles or sheets, response to different types of stimuli, characteristics of innervation, and function. Yet, for the sake of simplicity, smooth muscle can generally be divided into two major types, which are illustrated in Figure 7–2: *multiunit smooth muscle* and *visceral smooth muscle,* which is found in the walls of small blood vessels.

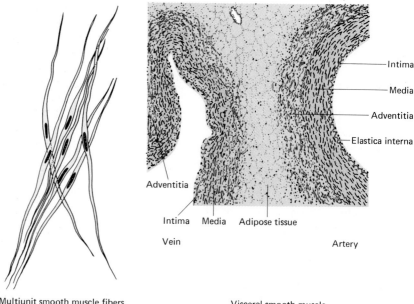

Figure 7–2. Visceral and multiunit smooth muscle fibers.

Multiunit smooth muscle fibers
A

Visceral smooth muscle
B

Multiunit Smooth Muscle. This type of smooth muscle is composed of discrete smooth muscle fibers. Each fiber operates entirely independently of the others and is often innervated by a single nerve ending, as occurs for skeletal muscle fibers.

The most important characteristic of multiunit smooth muscle fibers is that they usually contract only in response to nerve signals, the same as skeletal muscle fibers. This is in contrast to a major share of the control of visceral smooth muscle by non-nervous stimuli.

Some examples of multiunit smooth muscle are the smooth muscle fibers of the ciliary muscle of the eye, the iris of the eye, the nictitating membrane that covers the eyes in some lower animals, the piloerector muscles that cause erection of the hairs when stimulated by the sympathetic nervous system, and the smooth muscle of many of the larger blood vessels.

Visceral Smooth Muscle. Visceral smooth muscle fibers are usually arranged in sheets or bundles and the cell membranes contact each other at multiple points to form many *gap junctions* through which ions can flow freely from one cell to the next. Thus the fibers form a *functional syncytium* that usually contracts in large areas at once. This type of muscle is found in most of the organs of the body, especially in the walls of the gut, the bile ducts, the ureters, the uterus, and so forth.

When one portion of a visceral muscle tissue is stimulated, the action potential is conducted to the surrounding fibers by *direct electrical conduction* through the gap junctions. That is, the action potential generated in one area of the muscle electrically excites the adjacent fibers without secretion of any transmitter substance. Instead, electrical current flows through the gap junctions so easily that action potentials spread directly from one smooth muscle fiber to

the next almost as though cell membranes did not exist between the fibers.

THE CONTRACTILE PROCESS IN SMOOTH MUSCLE

The Chemical Basis for Smooth Muscle Contraction. Smooth muscle contains both *actin* and *myosin filaments,* having chemical characteristics similar to but not exactly the same as those of the actin and myosin filaments in skeletal muscle. Smooth muscle also contains *tropomyosin,* but it is doubtful whether troponin or a troponin-like substance exists in smooth muscle.

Chemical studies have shown that actin and myosin derived from smooth muscle interact with each other in the same way that this occurs for actin and myosin derived from skeletal muscle. Furthermore, the contractile process is activated by calcium ions, and ATP is degraded to ADP to provide the energy for contraction.

On the other hand, there are major differences between the physical organization of smooth muscle and that of skeletal muscle, as well as differences in other aspects of smooth muscle function, such as excitation-contraction coupling, control of the contractile process by calcium ions, duration of contraction, and amount of energy required for the contractile process.

The Physical Basis for Smooth Muscle Contraction. Smooth muscle does not have the same striated arrangement of the actin and myosin filaments as that found in skeletal muscle. Instead, recent special electron micrographic techniques suggest the physical organization illustrated in Figure 7–3. This shows large numbers of actin filaments attached to so-called *dense bodies.* Some of these bodies in turn are at-

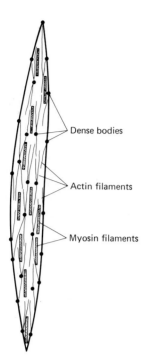

Figure 7–3. Arrangement of actin and myosin filaments in the smooth muscle cell. Note the attachment of the actin filaments to "dense bodies," some of which are themselves attached to the cell membrane.

tached to the cell membrane whereas others are located throughout the cell but are held in place by a scaffold of structural protein cross-attachments from one dense body to another. Interspersed among the actin filaments are a few thick filaments about 2.5 times the diameter of the thin actin filaments. These are assumed to be myosin filaments. However, there are only one twelfth to one fifteenth as many of these "myosin filaments" as actin filaments.

Despite the relative paucity of myosin filaments, it is assumed that they have sufficient cross-bridges to attract the many actin filaments and cause contraction by the sliding filament mechanism in essentially the same way that this occurs in skeletal muscle. And it is especially interesting to note that the maximum strength of contraction of smooth muscle is approximately equal to that of skeletal muscle, about 3 kg per square centimeter of cross-sectional area of the muscle.

Slowness of Contraction and Relaxation of Smooth Muscle. Though each smooth muscle tissue in the body has its own characteristics quite distinctive from the others, a typical smooth muscle tissue will begin to contract 50 to 100 milliseconds after it is excited, and will reach full contraction about half a second later. Then the contraction declines in another 1 to 2 seconds, giving a total contraction time of 1 to 3 seconds, which is about 30 times as long as the single-twitch contraction of skeletal muscle. However, smooth muscle contractions as short as 0.2 second and as long as 30 seconds also occur. This prolonged contraction seems to be caused by slowness of the

chemical reactions that cause the contraction. It has been calculated that the frequency of power strokes by the heads of the cross-bridges is only one tenth to one hundredth as rapid as in skeletal muscle.

Energy Required to Sustain Smooth Muscle Contraction. Measurements have shown that only one twentieth to one four-hundredth as much energy is required to sustain the same tension of contraction in smooth muscle as in skeletal muscle. This also is believed to result mainly from the very slow activity of the smooth muscle.

This economy of energy utilization by smooth muscle is exceedingly important to overall function of the body, because organs such as the intestines, the urinary bladder, the gallbladder, and other viscera must maintain moderate degrees of muscle contractile tone day in and day out.

MEMBRANE POTENTIALS AND ACTION POTENTIALS IN SMOOTH MUSCLE

Smooth muscle exhibits membrane potentials and action potentials similar to those that occur in skeletal muscle fibers. Furthermore, smooth muscle contraction can be elicited by depolarization of the membrane in the same way that contraction is initiated by depolarization of skeletal muscle fibers. However, there are both quantitative and qualitative differences in the membrane potentials and action potentials of smooth muscle that require special attention.

Membrane Potentials in Smooth Muscle. The quantitative value of the membrane potential of smooth muscle is variable from one type of smooth muscle to another, and it also depends on the momentary condition of the muscle. However, in the normal resting state, the membrane potential is usually about −50 to −60 millivolts, or about 30 millivolts less negative than in skeletal muscle.

Action Potentials in Visceral Smooth Muscle. Action potentials occur in visceral smooth muscle in the same way that they occur in skeletal muscle. However, action potentials probably do not normally occur in multiunit types of smooth muscle, as will be discussed in a subsequent section.

The action potentials of visceral smooth muscle occur in two different forms: (1) spike potentials and (2) action potentials with plateaus.

Spike Potentials. Typical spike action potentials, such as those seen in skeletal muscle, occur in most types of visceral smooth muscle. The duration of this type of action potential is 10 to 50 milliseconds, as illustrated in Figure 7–4A. Such action potentials can be elicited in many ways, such as by electrical stimulation, by the action of hormones on the smooth muscle, by the action of transmitter substances from nerve fibers, or as a result of spontaneous generation in the muscle fiber itself, as discussed below.

Action Potentials with Plateaus. Figure 7–5 illustrates an action potential with a plateau. The onset of this action potential is similar to that of the typical spike potential. However, instead of rapid repolari-

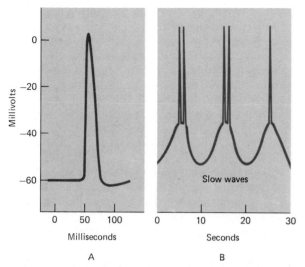

Figure 7–4. A, A typical smooth muscle action potential (spike potential) elicited by an external stimulus. B, A series of spike action potentials elicited by rhythmic, slow electrical waves occurring spontaneously in the smooth muscle wall of the intestine.

zation of the muscle fiber membrane, the repolarization is delayed for several hundred to several thousand milliseconds. The importance of the plateau is that it can account for the prolonged periods of contraction that occur in at least some types of smooth muscle. This type of action potential often occurs in the ureter, in the uterus under some conditions, and in some types of vascular smooth muscle.

Importance of Calcium Channels in Generating the Smooth Muscle Action Potential. The smooth muscle cell membrane has far more voltage-gated calcium channels than does skeletal muscle, but far fewer sodium channels. Therefore, sodium participates to a far less extent in the generation of the action potential in smooth muscle than in skeletal muscle. Instead, the flow of calcium ions to the interior of the fiber is mainly responsible for the action potential. This occurs in the same self-regenerative way as occurs for the sodium channels in nerve fibers and in skeletal muscle fibers. However, calcium channels open many times more slowly than do sodium channels. This accounts in large measure for the slow action potentials of smooth muscle fibers.

Slow Wave Potentials in Visceral Smooth Muscle and Spontaneous Generation of Action Potentials. Some smooth muscle is self-excitatory. That is, action potentials arise within the smooth muscle itself without an extrinsic stimulus. This is often associated with a basic *slow wave rhythm* of the membrane potential. A typical slow wave of this type is illustrated in Figure 7–4B. The slow wave itself is not an action potential. It is not a self-regenerative process that spreads progressively over the membranes of the muscle fibers. Instead, the slow waves are believed to be caused by waxing and waning of the pumping of sodium outward through the muscle fiber membrane; the membrane potential becomes more negative when sodium is pumped rapidly and less negative when the sodium pump becomes less active.

The slow waves themselves cannot cause muscle contraction, but when the potential of the slow wave rises above the level of approximately −35 millivolts (the approximate threshold for eliciting action potentials in most visceral smooth muscle), an action potential develops and spreads over the visceral smooth muscle mass, and then contraction does occur. Figure 7–4B illustrates this effect, showing that at each peak of the slow wave, one or more action potentials occur. This can obviously promote a series of rhythmical contractions of the smooth muscle mass. Therefore, the slow waves are frequently called *pacemaker waves.* This type of activity is especially prominent in some tubular types of smooth muscle masses, such as in the gut.

Depolarization of Multiunit Smooth Muscle Without Action Potentials. The smooth muscle fibers of multiunit smooth muscle normally contract mainly in response to nerve stimuli. The nerve endings secrete acetylcholine in the case of some multiunit smooth muscles and norepinephrine in the case of others. In both instances, these transmitter substances cause depolarization of the smooth muscle membrane, and this response in turn elicits the contraction. However, action potentials most often do not develop. The reason for this is that the fibers are too small to generate an action potential. (When action potentials are elicited in visceral smooth muscle, as many as 30 to 40 smooth muscle fibers must depolarize simultaneously before a self-propagating action potential ensues.) Yet, even without an action potential in the multiunit smooth muscle fibers, the local depolarization caused by the nerve transmitter substance itself spreads over the entire fiber and is all that is needed to cause the muscle contraction.

EXCITATION-CONTRACTION COUPLING— ROLE OF CALCIUM IONS

In the previous chapter it was pointed out that the actual contractile process in skeletal muscle is activated by calcium ions. This is also true in smooth muscle. However, the major source of the calcium ions differs in smooth muscle because the sarcoplasmic reticulum of smooth muscle is poorly developed.

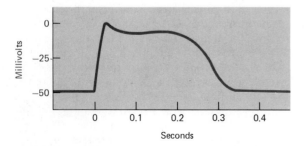

Figure 7–5. Monophasic action potential from a smooth muscle fiber of the rat uterus.

In some types of smooth muscle, almost all the calcium ions that cause contraction enter the muscle cell from the extracellular fluid at the time of the action potential. There is a reasonably high concentration of calcium ions in the extracellular fluid, greater than 10^{-3} molar in comparison with less than 10^{-7} molar in the resting cell, and as was pointed out in the previous section, the smooth muscle action potential is caused to a great extent by influx of calcium ions into the muscle fiber. Because the smooth muscle fibers are extremely small (in contrast to the sizes of the skeletal muscle fibers), these calcium ions can diffuse to all parts of the smooth muscle and elicit the contractile process. The time required for this diffusion to occur is usually 200 to 300 milliseconds and is called the *latent period* before the contraction begins; this latent period is some 50 times as great as that for skeletal muscle contraction.

Yet, in some smooth muscle there is a moderately developed sarcoplasmic reticulum. However, there are no T tubules. Instead, the cisternae of the reticulum abut the cell membrane. Therefore, it is believed that the membrane action potentials in these smooth muscle fibers cause release of calcium ions from these cisternae, thereby providing a greater degree of contraction than would occur on the basis of calcium ions entering through the cell membrane alone.

The Calcium Pump. To cause relaxation of the smooth muscle contractile elements, it is necessary to remove the calcium ions. This removal is achieved by a calcium pump that pumps the calcium ions out of the smooth muscle fiber and back into the extracellular fluid, or pumps the calcium ions into the sarcoplasmic reticulum. However, this pump is very slow-acting in comparison with the fast-acting sarcoplasmic reticulum pump in skeletal muscle. Therefore, the duration of smooth muscle contraction is often in the order of seconds rather than in tens of milliseconds, as occurs for skeletal muscle.

Mechanism by Which Calcium Ions Excite Contraction in Smooth Muscle. The mechanism by which calcium ions excite contraction in smooth muscle fibers is quite different from that in skeletal muscle. In fact, smooth muscle probably does not have an effective troponin complex, the factor that is activated by calcium ions in skeletal muscles to initiate contraction. Instead, the calcium ions excite contraction in smooth muscle fibers by activating the ATPase activity of the myosin heads. When calcium is not present, this ATPase activity in smooth muscle is extremely slight so that ATP cannot be cleaved and the contractile process cannot take place. Calcium ions activate this ATPase activity in the following way:

The first event is the increase in calcium ion concentration as a result of the action potential. Second, the calcium ions bind with a protein, *calmodulin,* that is very similar to the troponin C in skeletal muscle fibers. Third, the bound product of calmodulin and calcium ions in turn binds with or activates one of the light chain polypeptides of the myosin head; this in turn activates the ATPase activity of the myosin head. Fourth, the newly excited ATPase activity of the head then causes cleavage of ATP and the usual conformational changes in the head, leading to the same "walk-along" contractile process in smooth muscle fibers as occurs in skeletal muscle.

NEUROMUSCULAR JUNCTIONS OF SMOOTH MUSCLE

Physiologic Anatomy of Smooth Muscle Neuromuscular Junctions, and Secretion of Acetylcholine or Norepinephrine. Neuromuscular junctions of the type found on skeletal muscle fibers do not occur in smooth muscle. Instead, the nerve fibers generally branch diffusely on top of the muscle fibers, as illustrated in Figure 7–6. In most instances these fibers do not make direct contact with the smooth muscle fibers at all but instead form so-called *diffuse junctions* that secrete their transmitter substance into the interstitial fluid from a few nanometers to a few microns away from the muscle cells; the transmitter substance then diffuses to the cells. Furthermore, where there are many layers of muscle cells, the nerve fibers often innervate only the outer layer, and the muscle excitation then travels from this outer layer to the inner layers by direct action potential conduction or by subsequent diffusion of the transmitter substance.

The axons innervating smooth muscle fibers also do not have typical branching end-feet, as observed in the end-plate on skeletal muscle fibers. Instead, most of the fine terminal axons have multiple varicosities spread along their axes. At these points the Schwann cells are interrupted so that transmitter substance can be secreted through the walls of the varicosities. In the varicosities are vesicles similar to those present in the skeletal muscle end-plate containing transmitter substance. However, in contrast to the vesicles of skeletal muscle junctions that contain only acetylcholine, the vesicles of the autonomic nerve fiber varicosities contain *acetylcholine* in some fibers and *norepinephrine* in others.

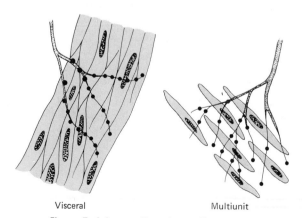

Visceral   Multiunit

Figure 7–6. Innervation of smooth muscle.

Excitation of Some Smooth Muscles, Inhibition of Others. Acetylcholine is an excitatory transmitter substance for smooth muscle fibers in some organs but an inhibitory substance for smooth muscle in other organs. And when acetylcholine excites a muscle fiber, norepinephrine ordinarily inhibits it. Or when acetylcholine inhibits a fiber, norepinephrine usually excites it.

But why these different responses? The answer is that both acetylcholine and norepinephrine excite or inhibit smooth muscle by first binding with a *receptor protein* on the surface of the muscle cell membrane. This receptor in turn controls the opening or closing of ion channels or controls some other means for activating or inhibiting the smooth muscle fiber. Furthermore, some of the receptor proteins are *excitatory receptors* whereas others are *inhibitory receptors*. Thus, it is the type of receptor that determines whether the smooth muscle will be inhibited or excited and also determines which of the two transmitters, acetylcholine or norepinephrine, will be effective in causing the excitation or inhibition.

SMOOTH MUSCLE CONTRACTION WITHOUT ACTION POTENTIALS—EFFECT OF LOCAL TISSUE FACTORS AND HORMONES

Though we have thus far discussed smooth muscle contraction elicited only by nervous signals, probably half or more of all smooth muscle contraction is initiated not by action potentials but by stimulatory factors acting directly on the smooth muscle contractile machinery. The two types of non-nervous and nonaction potential stimulating factors most often involved are (1) local tissue factors, and (2) various hormones.

Smooth Muscle Contraction in Response to Local Tissue Factors. In Chapter 13 we shall discuss the control of contraction of the arterioles, meta-arterioles, and precapillary sphincters. The smaller of these vessels have little or no nervous supply. Yet, the smooth muscle is highly contractile, responding rapidly to changes in local conditions in the surrounding interstitial fluid. In this way a powerful local feedback control system controls the blood flow to the local tissue area. Some of the specific control factors are:

(1) Lack of oxygen in the local tissues causes smooth muscle relaxation and therefore vasodilatation.

(2) Excess carbon dioxide causes vasodilatation.

(3) Increased hydrogen ion concentration also causes increased vasodilatation.

And such factors as lactic acid, increased potassium ions, diminished calcium ion concentration, and decreased body temperature will also cause local vasodilatation.

Effects of Hormones on Smooth Muscle Contraction. Most of the circulating hormones in the body affect smooth muscle contraction at least to some degree, and some have very profound effects. Some of the more important blood-borne hormones are norepinephrine, epinephrine, acetylcholine, angiotensin, vasopressin, oxytocin, serotonin, and histamine.

A hormone will cause contraction of smooth muscle when the smooth muscle cells contain an *excitatory receptor* for the respective hormone. However, the hormone will cause inhibition instead of contraction if the cells contain an *inhibitory receptor* rather than an excitatory receptor. Thus, most of the hormones will cause excitation of some smooth muscle but inhibition of other muscle.

Mechanism of Smooth Muscle Excitation by Local Tissue Factors and Hormones. Hormones or local tissue factors often cause smooth muscle contraction by binding with a specific receptor protein in the membrane, which initiates the contraction, usually by opening calcium ion channels. The flow of calcium ions to the interior of the cell then causes contraction.

In some instances, however, smooth muscle contraction or inhibition is initiated without a change in the membrane potential at all. In these instances it is believed that the exciting hormone binds with a receptor protein that activates a nonvoltage-related mechanism that leads to contraction or inhibition. One such mechanism is activation of the enzyme *adenylcyclase* in the cell membrane; a portion of this enzyme that protrudes into the interior of the cell then causes the formation of *cyclic AMP*, which is a so-called *second messenger*. The cyclic AMP has intracellular effects that inhibit muscle contraction.

MECHANICAL CHARACTERISTICS OF SMOOTH MUSCLE CONTRACTION

From the foregoing discussion of the many different types of smooth muscle and the different ways in which contraction can be elicited, one can readily understand why smooth muscle in different parts of the body has many different characteristics of contraction. For instance, the multiunit smooth muscle of the large blood vessels contracts mainly in response to nerve impulses, whereas in many types of visceral smooth muscle—the smaller blood vessels, the ureter, the bile ducts, and other glandular ducts—a self-excitatory process controlled mainly by local factors and by hormones causes continuous or rhythmic contraction.

Tone of Smooth Muscle. Smooth muscle can maintain a state of long-term, steady contraction that has been called either *tonus* contraction of smooth muscle or simply *smooth muscle tone*. This is an important feature of smooth muscle contraction because it allows prolonged or even indefinite continuance of the smooth muscle function. For instance, the arterioles are maintained in a state of tonic contraction almost throughout the entire life of the person. Likewise, tonic contraction in the gut wall maintains steady pressure on the contents of the gut, and tonic contraction of the urinary bladder wall maintains a moderate amount of pressure on the urine in the bladder.

Tonic contractions of smooth muscle can be caused in either of two ways:

(1) They are sometimes caused by *summation of individual contractile pulses;* each contractile pulse is initiated by a separate action potential in the same way that tetanic contractions are produced in skeletal muscle.

(2) However, most smooth muscle tonic contractions probably result from *prolonged direct smooth muscle excitation* without action potentials, usually caused by local tissue factors or circulating hormones. For instance, prolonged tonic contractions of the blood vessels without the mediation of action potentials are regularly caused by angiotensin, vasopressin, or norepinephrine, and these play an important role in the long-term regulation of arterial pressure, as will be discussed in Chapters 14 and 15.

QUESTIONS

1. Describe the anatomy of a neuromuscular junction.
2. Explain how acetylcholine is secreted by the axon terminals, how it is destroyed by acetylcholine, and how it excites the muscle fiber.
3. What are the characteristics of acetylcholine-gated channels?
4. Approximately what is the voltage of the end-plate potential, and how does it excite the muscle membrane? Describe the disease *myasthenia gravis,* its cause, and its treatment.
5. What are the differences between *multiunit smooth muscle* and *visceral smooth* muscle?
6. How does smooth muscle contraction differ chemically from that of skeletal muscle? How does smooth muscle contraction differ physically from that of skeletal muscle contraction?
7. What are the interrelationships of actin and myosin fibrils during smooth muscle contraction? How do the action potentials of smooth muscle differ from those of skeletal muscle?
8. What is the role of calcium ions in the generation of the smooth muscle action potential?
9. Explain how slow waves cause rhythmical contraction in some smooth muscle masses.
10. What is the difference between the manner in which calcium ions cause contraction of smooth muscle and the manner in which they cause contraction of skeletal muscle?
11. Explain the differences between neuromuscular junctions of smooth muscle and those of skeletal muscle.
12. Why does nervous stimulation of some smooth muscle cause excitation while it causes inhibition of other smooth muscle?
13. Explain how local tissue factors and hormones can cause smooth muscle contraction or inhibition without eliciting action potentials.
14. What causes tone in smooth muscle, and what is the importance of tone in the function of different organs?

References

Bennett, M. R.: Development of neuromuscular synapses. Physiol Rev 63:915, 1983.

Bohr, D. F., and Webb, R. C.: Vascular smooth muscle function and its changes in hypertension. Am J Med 77:3, 1984.

Ceccarelli, B., and Hurlbut, W. P.: Vesicle hypothesis of the release of quanta of acetylcholine. Physiol Rev 60:396, 1980.

Dowben, R. M., ed.: Cell and Muscle Motility. New York, Plenum Publishing Corp., 1983.

Eisenberg, E., and Greene, L. E.: The relation of muscle biochemistry to muscle physiology. Annu Rev Physiol 42:293, 1980.

Furchgott, R. F.: The role of endothelium in the responses of vascular smooth muscle to drugs. Annu Rev Pharmacol Toxicol 24:175, 1984.

Guyton, A. C., and MacDonald, M. A.: Physiology of botulinus toxin. Arch Neurol Psychiat 57:578, 1947.

Hess, G. P., et al.: Acetylcholine receptor-controlled ion translocation: Chemical kinetic investigations of the mechanism. Annu Rev Biophys Bioeng 12:443, 1983.

Johansson, B.: Vascular smooth muscle reactivity. Annu Rev Physiol 43:359, 1981.

Johansson, B., and Somlyo, A. P.: Electrophysiology and excitation-contraction coupling. In Bohr, D. F., et al., eds.: Handbook of Physiology. Sec. 2, Vol. 2. Baltimore, Williams & Wilkins, 1980, p. 301.

Lambert, J. J., et al.: Drug-induced modification of ionic conductance at the neuromuscular junction. Annu Rev Pharmacol Toxicol 23:505, 1983.

Loewenstein, W. R.: Junctional intercellular communication: The cell-to-cell membrane channel. Physiol Rev 61:829, 1981.

McKinney, M., and Richelson, E.: The coupling of neuronal muscarinic receptor to responses. Annu Rev Pharmacol Toxicol 24:121, 1984.

Peper, K., et al.: The acetylcholine receptor at the neuromuscular junction. Physiol Rev 62:1271, 1982.

Popot, J.-L., and Changeux, J.-P.: Nicotinic receptor of acetylcholine: Structure of an oligomeric integral membrane protein. Physiol Rev 64:1162, 1984.

Pumplin, D. W., and Fambrough, D. M.: Turnover of acetylcholine receptors in skeletal muscle. Annu Rev Physiol 44:319, 1982.

Purves, D., and Lichtman, J. W.: Specific connections between nerve cells. Annu Rev Physiol 45:553, 1983.

Somlyo, A. P.: Ultrastructure of vascular smooth muscle. In Bohr, D. F., et al., eds.: Handbook of Physiology. Sec. 2, Vol. 2. Baltimore, Williams & Wilkins, 1980, p. 33.

Vanhoutte, P. M.: Calcium-entry blockers, vascular smooth muscle and systemic hypertension. Am J Cardiol 55:17B, 1985.

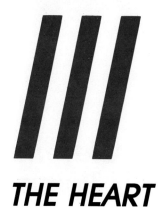

THE HEART

8 ■ Heart Muscle; the Heart As a Pump

9 ■ Rhythmic Excitation of the Heart

10 ■ The Electrocardiogram

8

Heart Muscle; the Heart As a Pump

PHYSIOLOGY OF CARDIAC MUSCLE
    PHYSIOLOGIC ANATOMY OF
        CARDIAC MUSCLE
    ACTION POTENTIALS IN CARDIAC
        MUSCLE
    EXCITATION-CONTRACTION
        COUPLING—FUNCTION OF
        CALCIUM IONS AND THE TUBULES
THE CARDIAC CYCLE
    SYSTOLE AND DIASTOLE
    RELATIONSHIP OF THE
        ELECTROCARDIOGRAM TO THE
        CARDIAC CYCLE
    FUNCTION OF THE ATRIA AS PUMPS
    FUNCTION OF THE VENTRICLES AS
        PUMPS
    FUNCTION OF THE VALVES
    THE AORTIC PRESSURE CURVE
    RELATIONSHIP OF THE HEART
        SOUNDS TO HEART PUMPING

ENERGY FOR CARDIAC
    CONTRACTION
REGULATION OF CARDIAC FUNCTION
    INTRINSIC REGULATION OF
        CARDIAC PUMPING—THE FRANK-
        STARLING LAW OF THE HEART
    CONTROL OF THE HEART RATE AND
        HEART STRENGTH BY
        PARASYMPATHETIC AND
        SYMPATHETIC NERVES
    EFFECT OF HEART DEBILITY ON
        CARDIAC FUNCTION—THE
        HYPOEFFECTIVE HEART
    EFFECT OF EXERCISE ON THE
        HEART—THE HYPEREFFECTIVE
        HEART
    EFFECT OF VARIOUS IONS ON HEART
        FUNCTION
    EFFECT OF TEMPERATURE ON THE
        HEART

In this chapter we explain how the heart operates as a pump—that is, the function of the heart muscle, of the valves, of the various chambers of the heart, and, especially important, how the pumping activity of the heart is regulated.

PHYSIOLOGY OF CARDIAC MUSCLE

PHYSIOLOGIC ANATOMY OF CARDIAC MUSCLE

Figure 8–1 illustrates a typical histologic picture of cardiac muscle, showing the cardiac muscle fibers arranged in a latticework, the fibers dividing, then recombining, and then spreading again. One notes immediately from this figure that cardiac muscle is *striated* in the same manner as typical skeletal muscle. Furthermore, cardiac muscle has typical myofibrils that contain *actin* and *myosin filaments* almost identical to those found in skeletal muscle, and these filaments interdigitate and slide along each other

during the process of contraction in the same manner as occurs in skeletal muscle. (See Chapter 6.)

Cardiac Muscle as a Syncytium. The angulated dark areas crossing the cardiac muscle fibers in Figure 8–1 are called *intercalated discs;* however, they are actually cell membranes that separate individual cardiac muscle cells from each other. That is, cardiac muscle fibers are made up of many cardiac muscle cells connected in series with each other. Yet electrical resistance through the intercalated disc is only one four-hundredth the resistance through the outside membrane of the cardiac muscle fiber, because the cell membranes fuse with each other and form very permeable junctions that allow almost completely free diffusion of ions. Therefore, from a functional point of view, cardiac muscle is a *syncytium*, in which the cardiac muscle cells are so tightly bound that when one of these cells becomes excited, the action potential spreads to all of them, spreading from cell to cell and spreading throughout the latticework interconnections.

The heart is composed of two separate syncytiums,

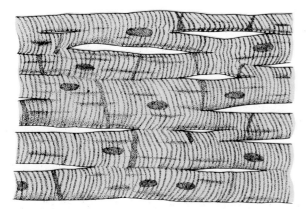

Figure 8-1. The "syncytial," interconnecting nature of cardiac muscle.

the *atrial syncytium* that constitutes the walls of the two atria and the *ventricular syncytium* that constitutes the walls of the two ventricles. These are separated from each other by fibrous tissue that surrounds the valvular openings between the atria and ventricles, but action potentials can be conducted from the atrial syncytium into the ventricular syncytium by way of a specialized conductive system, the *A-V bundle,* which will be discussed in detail in the following chapter. This division of the muscle mass of the heart into two separate functional syncytiums allows the atria to contract a short time ahead of ventricular contraction, which is important for the effectiveness of heart pumping.

ACTION POTENTIALS IN CARDIAC MUSCLE

The *resting membrane potential* of normal cardiac muscle is approximately −85 to −95 millivolt (mv) and approximately −90 to −100 mv in the specialized conductive fibers, the Purkinje fibers, which are discussed in the following chapter.

The *action potential* recorded in ventricular muscle, shown by the bottom record of Figure 8-2, is 105 mv,

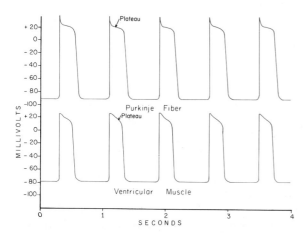

Figure 8-2. Rhythmic action potentials from a Purkinje fiber and from a ventricular muscle fiber, recorded by means of microelectrodes.

which means that the membrane potential rises from its normally very negative value to a slightly positive value of about +20 mv. Because of this change of potential from negative to positive, the positive portion is called the *overshoot potential.* Then, after the initial *spike,* the membrane remains depolarized for about 0.2 second in atrial muscle and about 0.3 second in ventricular muscle, exhibiting a *plateau* as illustrated in Figure 8-2, followed at the end of the plateau by abrupt repolarization. The presence of this plateau in the action potential causes muscle contraction to last 20 to 50 times as long in cardiac muscle as in skeletal muscle.

At this point we must ask the question: Why is the action potential of cardiac muscle so long and why does it have a plateau whereas that of skeletal muscle does not? The principal reason for this difference, as was explained in Chapter 5, is that the membranes of cardiac muscle contain a large population of so-called *slow calcium-sodium channels.* These channels remain open during the action potential for several tenths of a second. During this time large amounts of both calcium and sodium ions continue to flow through the channels to the interior of the cardiac muscle fiber, and this maintains a prolonged period of depolarization. It is this that causes the plateau in the action potential.

Velocity of Conduction in Cardiac Muscle. The velocity of conduction of the action potential in both atrial and ventricular muscle fibers is about 0.3 to 0.5 meter per second, or about one tenth the velocity in skeletal muscle fibers. The velocity of conduction in the specialized conductive system varies from 0.02 to 4 meters per second in different parts of the system, as is explained in the following chapter.

Refractory Period of Cardiac Muscle. Cardiac muscle, like all excitable tissue, is refractory to restimulation during the action potential. The normal refractory period of the ventricle is 0.25 to 0.3 second, which is approximately the duration of the action potential. There is an additional *relative refractory period* of about 0.05 second during which the muscle is more difficult than normal to excite but nevertheless can be excited.

The refractory period of atrial muscle is much shorter than that for the ventricles (about 0.15 second), and the relative refractory period is another 0.03 second. Therefore, the rhythmical rate of contraction of the atria can be much faster than that of the ventricles.

EXCITATION-CONTRACTION COUPLING— FUNCTION OF CALCIUM IONS AND THE T TUBULES

The term *excitation-contraction coupling* refers to the mechanism by which the action potential causes the myofibrils of muscle to contract. This was discussed for skeletal muscle in Chapter 6. However, once again there are differences in this process in cardiac muscle that have important effects on the characteristics of cardiac muscle contraction.

As is true for skeletal muscle, when an action potential passes over the cardiac muscle membrane, the action potential also spreads to the interior of the cardiac muscle fiber along the membranes of the T tubules. The action potentials in turn cause instantaneous release of calcium ions into the muscle sarcoplasm from the cisternae of the sarcoplasmic reticulum. Then the calcium ions diffuse in another few thousandths of a second into the myofibrils where they catalyze the chemical and physical reactions that promote sliding of the actin and myosin filaments along each other; this in turn produces the muscle contraction.

Thus far, this mechanism of excitation-contraction coupling is the same as that for skeletal muscle, but at this point a major difference begins to appear. In addition to the calcium ions that are released into the sarcoplasm from the cisternae of the sarcoplasmic reticulum, large quantities of calcium ions also diffuse into the sarcoplasm from the T tubules at the time of the action potential. The T tubules of cardiac muscle have a diameter five times as great as that of the skeletal muscle tubules and a volume 25 times as great; also, inside the T tubules is a large quantity of mucopolysaccharides that are electronegatively charged and bind an abundant store of calcium ions, keeping this always available for diffusion to the interior of the cardiac muscle fiber when the T tubule action potential occurs.

The strength of contraction of cardiac muscle depends to a great extent on the concentration of calcium ions in the extracellular fluids. The reason for this is that the ends of the T tubules open directly to the outside of the cardiac muscle fibers, allowing the same extracellular fluid that is in the cardiac muscle interstitium to percolate through the T tubules as well. Consequently, the quantity of calcium ions in the T tubule system, as well as the availability of calcium ions to cause cardiac muscle contraction, depends directly on the extracellular fluid calcium ion concentration.

At the end of the plateau of the action potential the influx of calcium ions to the interior of the muscle fiber is suddenly cut off, and the calcium ions in the sarcoplasm are rapidly pumped back into both the sarcoplasmic reticulum and the T tubules. As a result, the contraction ceases until a new action potential occurs.

Duration of Contraction. Cardiac muscle begins to contract after the action potential begins and continues to contract for a few milliseconds after the action potential ends. Therefore, the duration of contraction of cardiac muscle is mainly a function of the duration of the action potential—about 0.2 second in atrial muscle and 0.3 second in ventricular muscle.

THE CARDIAC CYCLE

Figure 8–3 illustrates the physical structure of the heart and also the course of blood flow through the

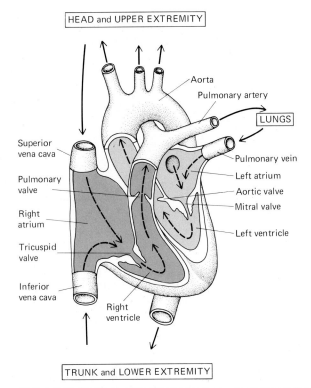

Figure 8–3. Structure of the heart, and course of blood flow through the heart chambers.

heart. It is also clear that the heart is in reality four separate pumps: two *primer pumps*, the *atria*, and two *power pumps*, the *ventricles*.

The period from the end of one heart contraction to the end of the next is called the *cardiac cycle*. Each cycle is initiated by spontaneous generation of an action potential in the S-A node. This node consists of a collection of especially rhythmical muscle located in the anterior wall of the right atrium near the opening of the superior vena cava, and the action potential travels rapidly from here through both atria and then through the A-V bundle into the ventricles. However, because of a special arrangement of the conducting system from the atria into the ventricles, there is a delay of more than 1/10 second between passage of the cardiac impulse from the atria into the ventricles. This allows the atria to contract ahead of the ventricles, thereby pumping blood into the ventricles prior to the very strong ventricular contraction. Thus, the atria act as primer pumps for the ventricles, and the ventricles then provide the major source of power for moving blood through the vascular system.

SYSTOLE AND DIASTOLE

The cardiac cycle consists of a period of relaxation called *diastole* followed by a period of contraction called *systole*.

Figure 8–4 illustrates the different events during the cardiac cycle. The top three curves show the pressure changes in the aorta, the left ventricle, and

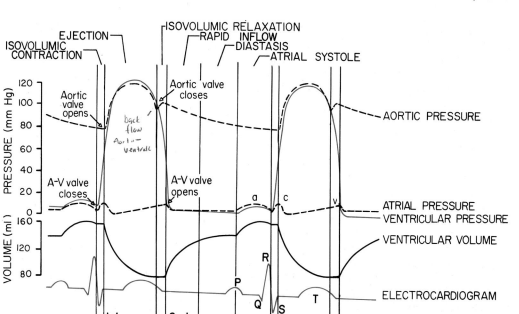

Figure 8-4. The events of the cardiac cycle, showing changes in left atrial pressure, left ventricular pressure, aortic pressure, ventricular volume, the electrocardiogram, and the phonocardiogram.

the left atrium, respectively. The fourth curve depicts the changes in ventricular volume, the fifth the electrocardiogram, and the sixth a phonocardiogram, which is a recording of the sounds produced by the heart as it pumps. It is especially important that the student study in detail the diagram in this figure and understand the causes of all the events illustrated. These are explained as follows:

RELATIONSHIP OF THE ELECTROCARDIOGRAM TO THE CARDIAC CYCLE

The electrocardiogram in Figure 8-4 shows the *P, Q, R, S,* and *T waves,* which will be discussed in Chapter 10. These are electrical voltages generated by the heart and recorded by the electrocardiograph from the surface of the body. The *P wave* is caused by the *spread of depolarization* through the atria, and this is followed by atrial contraction, which causes a slight rise in the atrial pressure curve immediately after the P wave. Approximately 0.16 second after the onset of the P wave, the *QRS waves* appear, resulting from depolarization of the ventricles, which initiates contraction of the ventricles and causes the ventricular pressure to begin rising, as is also illustrated in the figure. Therefore, the QRS complex begins slightly before the onset of ventricular systole.

Finally, one observes the *ventricular T wave* in the electrocardiogram. This represents the stage of repolarization of the ventricles at the time that ventricular muscle fibers begin to relax. Therefore, the T wave occurs slightly prior to the end of ventricular contraction.

FUNCTION OF THE ATRIA AS PUMPS

Blood normally flows continually from the great veins into the atria; approximately 70 per cent of this flows directly through the atria into the ventricles even before the atria contract. Then, atrial contraction causes an additional 20 to 30 per cent filling of the ventricles. Therefore, the atria simply function as primer pumps that increase the ventricular pumping effectiveness by about 30 per cent. Yet, the heart can continue to operate quite satisfactorily under normal resting conditions even without this extra 30 per cent effectiveness because it normally has the capability of pumping 300 to 400 per cent more blood than is required by the body. Therefore, the difference is unlikely to be noticed unless a person exercises; then acute signs of heart failure occasionally develop, especially shortness of breath.

FUNCTION OF THE VENTRICLES AS PUMPS

Filling of the Ventricles. During ventricular systole large amounts of blood accumulate in the atria because of the closed A-V valves. Therefore, just as soon as systole is over and the ventricular pressures fall again to their low diastolic values, the high pressures in the atria immediately push the A-V valves open and cause blood to flow rapidly into the ventricles, as shown by the rise of the *ventricular volume curve* in Figure 8-4. This is called the *period of rapid filling of the ventricles.*

The period of rapid filling lasts approximately the first third of diastole. During the middle third of diastole only a small amount of blood normally flows into the ventricles; this is blood that continues to empty into the atria from the veins and passes on through the atria directly into the ventricles.

During the latter third of diastole, the atria contract and give an additional thrust to the inflow of blood into the ventricles; this accounts for approximately 20 to 30 per cent of the filling of the ventricles during each heart cycle.

Emptying of the Ventricles During Systole

Period of Isovolumic (Isometric) Contraction. Immediately after ventricular contraction begins, the ventricular pressure abruptly rises, as shown in Figure 8–4, causing the A-V valves to close. Then an additional 0.02 to 0.03 second is required for the ventricle to build up sufficient pressure to push the aortic and pulmonary valves open against the pressures in the aorta and pulmonary artery. Therefore, during this period of time, contraction is occurring in the ventricles, but there is no emptying. This period is called the period of *isovolumic* or *isometric contraction,* meaning by these terms that tension is increasing in the muscle but no (or little) shortening of the muscle fibers is occurring.

Period of Ejection. When the left ventricular pressure rises slightly above 80 mm Hg (and the right ventricular pressure slightly above 8 mm Hg), the ventricular pressures push the aortic and pulmonary valves open. Immediately, blood begins to pour out of the ventricles, with about 70 per cent of the emptying occurring during the first third of the period of ejection and the remaining 30 per cent during the next two thirds. Therefore, the first third is called the *period of rapid ejection* and the last two thirds the *period of slow ejection.*

Period of Isovolumic (Isometric) Relaxation.

At the end of systole, ventricular relaxation begins suddenly, allowing the intraventricular pressures to fall rapidly. The elevated pressures in the distended large arteries immediately push blood back toward the ventricles, which snaps the aortic and pulmonary valves closed. For another 0.03 to 0.06 second, the ventricular muscle continues to relax, even though the ventricular volume does not change, giving rise to the period of *isovolumic* (or *isometric*) *relaxation.* During this period the intraventricular pressures fall rapidly back to their very low diastolic levels. Then the A-V valves open to begin a new cycle of ventricular filling.

End-Diastolic Volume, End-Systolic Volume, and Stroke Volume Output.

During diastole, filling of the ventricles normally increases the volume of each ventricle immediately before ventricular contraction begins to about 120 to 130 ml. This volume is known as the *end-diastolic volume.* Then, as the ventricles empty during systole, the volume decreases by about 70 ml, which is called the *stroke volume output.* The remaining volume in each ventricle at the end of systole, about 50 to 60 ml, is called the *end-systolic volume.* The fraction of the end-diastolic volume that

is ejected is called the *ejection fraction*—usually equal to about 60 per cent.

When the heart contracts strongly, the end-systolic volume can fall to as little as 10 to 30 ml. On the other hand, when large amounts of blood flow into the ventricles during diastole, their end-diastolic volumes can become as great as 150 to 180 ml in the normal heart. By both increasing the end-diastolic volume and decreasing the end-systolic volume, the stroke volume output can at times be increased to more than double normal.

FUNCTION OF THE VALVES

The *A-V valves* (the *tricuspid* and the *mitral* valves) prevent backflow of blood from the ventricles to the atria during systole, and the *semilunar valves* (the *aortic* and *pulmonary* valves) prevent backflow from the aorta and pulmonary arteries into the ventricles during diastole. All these valves, which are illustrated in Figure 8–5, close and open *passively.* That is, they close when a backward pressure gradient pushes blood backward, and they open when a forward pressure gradient forces blood in the forward direction. For obvious anatomical reasons, the thin, filmy A-V valves require almost no backflow to cause closure while the much heavier semilunar valves require rather strong backflow for a few milliseconds.

Figure 8–5 also illustrates the *papillary muscles* that attach to the vanes of the A-V valves by the *chordae tendineae.* The papillary muscles contract when the ventricular walls contract, but, contrary to what might be expected, they *do not* help the valves to close. Instead, they pull the vanes of the valves inward toward the ventricles to prevent their bulging too far backward toward the atria during ventricular contraction.

There are differences between the operation of the aortic and pulmonary valves and that of the A-V

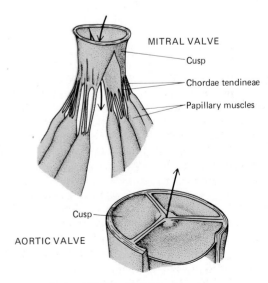

Figure 8–5. Mitral and aortic valves.

valves. First, the high pressures in the arteries at the end of systole cause the semilunar valves to snap to the closed position in comparison with a much softer closure of the A-V valves. Second, the velocity of blood ejection through the aortic and pulmonary valves is far greater than that through the much larger A-V valves. Because of the rapid closure and rapid ejection, the edges of the semilunar valves are subjected to much greater mechanical abrasion than are the A-V valves. It is obvious from the anatomy of the aortic and pulmonary valves, as illustrated in Figure 8–5, that they are well adapted to withstand this extra physical trauma.

THE AORTIC PRESSURE CURVE

During ventricular systole, the entry of blood into the aorta causes the wall of the aorta to stretch and the pressure to rise, as illustrated by the aortic pressure curve in Figure 8–4. Then, at the end of systole, after the left ventricle stops ejecting blood and the aortic valve closes, the elastic stretch of the aorta maintains a high pressure in the aorta even during diastole.

A so-called *incisura* occurs in the aortic pressure curve when the aortic valve closes. This is caused by a short period of backward flow of blood immediately prior to closure of the valve, followed then by sudden cessation of the backflow.

After the aortic valve has closed, pressure in the aorta falls slowly throughout diastole because blood stored in the distended elastic arteries flows continually through the peripheral vessels back to the veins. Before the ventricle contracts again, the aortic pressure usually falls to approximately 80 mm Hg (diastolic pressure), which is two thirds the maximal pressure of 120 mm Hg (systolic pressure) occurring in the aorta during ventricular contraction.

The pressure curve in the pulmonary artery is similar to that in the aorta, except that the pressures are only about one sixth as great.

RELATIONSHIP OF THE HEART SOUNDS TO HEART PUMPING

When listening to the heart with a stethoscope, one does not hear the opening of the valves, for this is a relatively slowly developing process that makes no noise. However, when the valves close, the vanes of the valves and the surrounding fluids vibrate under the influence of the sudden pressure differentials that develop, giving off sound that travels in all directions through the chest.

When the ventricles first contract, one hears a sound that is caused by closure of the A-V valves. The vibration is low in pitch and of relatively long duration and is known as the *first heart sound*. When the aortic and pulmonary valves close, one hears a relatively rapid snap, for these valves close extremely rapidly, and the surroundings vibrate for only a short period of time. This sound is known as the *second*

heart sound. The precise causes of these sounds will be discussed in Chapter 17 in relation to auscultation.

ENERGY FOR CARDIAC CONTRACTION

Heart muscle, like skeletal muscle, utilizes chemical energy to provide the work of contraction. This energy is derived mainly from metabolism of fatty acids and to a lesser extent from metabolism of other nutrients, especially lactate ions and glucose. The different metabolic reactions that liberate this energy will be discussed in Chapters 45 and 46.

Efficiency of Cardiac Contraction. During muscular contraction most of the chemical energy is converted into heat and a small portion into work output. The ratio of work output to chemical energy expenditure is called the efficiency of cardiac contraction, or simply *efficiency of the heart*. The maximum efficiency of the normal heart is between 20 and 25 per cent.

REGULATION OF CARDIAC FUNCTION

When a person is at rest, the heart pumps only 4 to 6 liters of blood each minute. However, during heavy exercise it may be required to pump as much as four to seven times this amount. The present section discusses the means by which the heart can adapt to such extreme increases in cardiac output.

The two basic means by which the volume pumped by the heart is regulated are (1) intrinsic regulation of pumping in response to changes in volume of blood flowing into the heart, and (2) reflex control of the heart rate and heart strength by the autonomic nervous system.

INTRINSIC REGULATION OF CARDIAC PUMPING—THE FRANK-STARLING LAW OF THE HEART

In Chapter 16 we shall see that the major factor determining the amount of blood pumped by the heart each minute is the rate of blood flow into the heart from the veins, which is called *venous return*. That is, each peripheral tissue of the body controls its own blood flow, and whatever amount of blood flows through all the peripheral tissues returns by way of the veins to the right atrium. The heart in turn automatically pumps this incoming blood into the systemic arteries so that it can flow around the circuit again. Thus, the heart must adapt from moment to moment or even second to second to widely varying inputs of blood, sometimes falling as low as 2 to 3 liters per minute and at other times rising to as high as 25 or more liters per minute.

This intrinsic ability of the heart to adapt to changing loads of inflowing blood is called the *Frank-Starling law of the heart*, in honor of Frank and Starling, two great physiologists of nearly a century ago. Basically, the Frank-Starling law states that the more the heart is filled during diastole, the greater will be the quantity of blood pumped into the aorta. Or another way to express this law is: *Within physiological limits, the heart pumps out all the blood that comes to it without allowing excessive damming of blood in the veins.*

Mechanism of the Frank-Starling Law. The principal mechanism by which the heart adapts to changing inflow of blood is the following: When the cardiac muscle becomes stretched an extra amount, as it does when extra amounts of blood enter the heart chambers, the stretched muscle contracts with a greatly increased force, thereby automatically pumping the extra blood into the arteries. This ability of stretched muscle to contract with increased force is characteristic of all striated muscle, not simply of cardiac muscle. Referring back to Chapter 6, one will see that stretching a skeletal muscle, within its physiological limit, also increases its force of contraction. This increased force of contraction is caused by the fact that the actin and myosin filaments are brought to a more nearly optimal degree of interdigitation for achieving contraction.

Constancy of the Cardiac Output Despite Changes in Arterial Pressure Load. One of the most important consequences of the Frank-Starling law of the heart is that, within reasonable limits, changes in arterial pressure load against which the heart pumps have almost no effect on the rate at which blood is pumped by the heart each minute (the cardiac output). This effect is illustrated in Figure 8–6, which shows that up to a pressure of about 170 mm Hg—far above the normal daily pressure range—the cardiac output remains constant whatever the pressure load against which the heart must pump. The significance of this effect is the following: Regardless of the arterial pressure, the most important factor determining the amount of blood pumped by the heart is still the rate of entry of blood into the heart.

Ventricular Function Curves

One of the best ways to express the functional ability of the ventricles to pump blood is by ventricular function curves, as shown in Figures 8–7. This

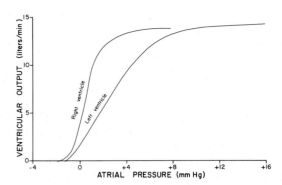

Figure 8–7. Approximate normal right and left ventricular output curves for the human heart as extrapolated from data obtained in dogs.

figure illustrates a type of ventricular function curve called the *ventricular output curve.* The two curves in this figure represent function of the two ventricles of the human heart based on data extrapolated from lower animals. As each atrial pressure rises, the respective ventricular volume output per minute also increases.

Thus, ventricular function curves are another way of expressing the Frank-Starling law of the heart. That is, as the ventricles fill to higher atrial pressures, the strength of cardiac contraction increases, causing the heart to pump increased quantities of blood into the arteries.

CONTROL OF THE HEART RATE AND HEART STRENGTH BY PARASYMPATHETIC AND SYMPATHETIC NERVES

The heart is well supplied with both sympathetic and parasympathetic (vagal) nerves, as illustrated in Figure 8–8. These nerves affect cardiac pumping in two ways: (1) by changing the heart rate, and (2) by changing the strength of contraction of the heart. The effect of nerve stimulation on heart rate and rhythm

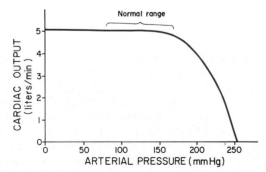

Figure 8–6. Constancy of cardiac output even in the face of wide changes in arterial pressure. Only when the arterial pressure rises above the normal operating pressure range does the pressure load cause the heart to begin to fail.

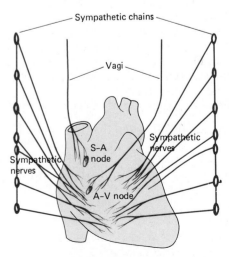

Figure 8–8. The cardiac nerves.

will be discussed more fully in the following chapter. For the present, suffice it to say that parasympathetic stimulation decreases heart rate and sympathetic stimulation increases heart rate. The range of control is from as little as 20 to 30 heart beats per minute with maximum vagal stimulation to as high as 250 beats per minute with maximum sympathetic stimulation.

Effect of Heart Rate on Function of the Heart as a Pump. In general, the more times the heart beats per minute, the more blood it can pump. For instance, when the heart rate is increased by sympathetic stimulation, it reaches its peak ability to pump blood at a rate between 170 and 250 beats per minute.

Nervous Regulation of Contractile Strength of the Heart. In general, sympathetic stimulation increases the strength of heart muscle contraction, whereas parasympathetic stimulation decreases the strength of contraction.

Under normal conditions the sympathetic nerve fibers to the heart continually discharge at a slow rate that maintains a strength of ventricular contraction about 20 per cent above its strength with no sympathetic stimulation at all. Therefore, one method by which the nervous system can decrease the strength of ventricular contraction is simply to slow or stop the transmission of sympathetic impulses to the heart. On the other hand, maximal sympathetic stimulation can increase the strength of ventricular contraction to approximately 100 per cent greater than normal.

Maximal parasympathetic (vagal) stimulation of the heart decreases ventricular contractile strength about 30 per cent. Thus, the parasympathetic effect is, by contrast with the sympathetic effect, relatively small.

EFFECT OF HEART DEBILITY ON CARDIAC FUNCTION—THE HYPOEFFECTIVE HEART

Any factor that damages or depresses the heart, whether it be damage to the myocardium, to the valves, to the conducting system or vagal stimulation of the heart, is likely to make the heart a poorer pump, and the heart under these conditions is called a *hypoeffective heart.* Figure 8–9 illustrates by the very dark curve the normal cardiac function curve and by the three curves below this the effect of different degrees of hypoeffectiveness on cardiac function. Obviously, the more serious the damage or depression, the less will be the cardiac output at any given right atrial pressure.

Different factors that can cause a hypoeffective heart include:

    Myocardial infarction
    Valvular heart disease
    Vagal stimulation of the heart
    Inhibition of the sympathetics to the heart
    Congenital heart disease
    Myocarditis
    Cardiac anoxia
    Diphtheritic or other types of
       myocardial damage

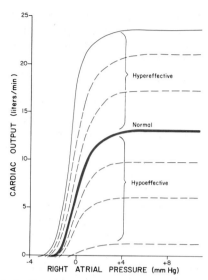

Figure 8–9. Cardiac output curves for various degrees of hypo- and hypereffective hearts. (From Guyton, Jones, and Coleman: Circulatory Physiology: Cardiac Output and Its Regulation. Philadelphia, W. B. Saunders Company, 1973.)

EFFECT OF EXERCISE ON THE HEART— THE HYPEREFFECTIVE HEART

Chronic increase in the work load of the heart, caused by heavy exercise or by some abnormality of the circulation such as high blood pressure, leads to hypertrophy of the cardiac muscle and also to enlargement of the ventricular chambers, which is called *cardiac hypertrophy.* As a result, the overall effectiveness of the heart as a pump increases. The upper three function curves of Figure 8–9 illustrate the effects of different degrees of cardiac hypereffectiveness on the cardiac function curve; maximal degrees of hypereffectiveness can increase pumping by the heart more than 100 per cent.

Other factors besides hypertrophy that can cause a hypereffective heart are

    Sympathetic stimulation (50 to 100 per cent increase)
    Inhibition of parasympathetic stimulation (10 to 20 per cent increase)

EFFECT OF VARIOUS IONS ON HEART FUNCTION

In the discussion of membrane potentials in Chapter 5, it was pointed out that several of the ions have marked effects on membrane potentials and action potentials, and in Chapter 6 it was noted that calcium ions play an especially important role in initiating the muscle contractile process. Therefore, it is to be expected that changes in the concentrations of these certain ions in the extracellular fluids will also have important effects on cardiac function. The most striking effects are caused by changes in the concentrations of potassium and calcium ions.

Effect of Potassium Ions. Excess potassium in the extracellular fluids causes the heart to become extremely dilated and flaccid and slows the heart rate. Very large quantities can also block conduction of the cardiac impulse from the atria to the ventricles through the A-V bundle. Elevation of potassium concentration to only 8 to 12 mEq/liter—two to three times the normal value—can cause such weakness of the heart and abnormal rhythm that this can cause death.

All these effects are caused by the fact that a high extracellular potassium concentration causes a decreased resting membrane potential in the cardiac muscle fibers, as explained in Chapter 5. As the membrane potential decreases, the intensity of the action potential also decreases, which makes the contraction of the heart progressively weaker, because the strength of the action potential determines to a great extent the strength of contraction.

Effect of Calcium Ions. An excess of calcium ions causes effects almost exactly opposite to those of potassium ions, causing the heart to go into spastic contraction. This is caused by the direct effect of calcium ions in exciting the cardiac contractile process, as explained earlier in the chapter. Conversely, a deficiency of calcium ions causes cardiac flaccidity, similar to the effect of excess potassium.

EFFECT OF TEMPERATURE ON THE HEART

Increased temperature causes greatly increased heart rate, and decreased temperature causes greatly decreased rate. For instance, a body temperature of 106° F can sometimes double the heart rate. And a decrease of body temperature to 70° F, caused by immersion in ice water, can decrease the heart rate to as little as one beat every 5 to 15 seconds. These effects presumably result from the heat causing increased permeability of the muscle membrane to the ions, resulting in acceleration of the self-excitation process.

Contractile strength of the heart is often enhanced temporarily by a moderate increase in temperature, but prolonged elevation of the temperature exhausts the metabolic systems of the heart and causes weakness.

QUESTIONS

1. Describe the differences between cardiac muscle and skeletal muscle.
2. What is meant by the *atrial cardiac muscle syncytium* and the *ventricular cardiac muscle syncytium*?
3. How do action potentials of cardiac muscle differ from those in skeletal muscle?
4. How does excitation-contraction coupling in cardiac muscle differ from that in skeletal muscle? Explain especially the importance of calcium ions in the T tubules.
5. Explain what is meant by *systole* and *diastole*.
6. Give the relationships of the waves in the electrocardiogram to the periods of systole and diastole.
7. Explain the role of the atria as "primer" pumps.
8. Describe the different stages of filling of the ventricles during diastole.
9. Describe the stages of ventricular emptying during the pumping cycle.
10. What are meant by *end-diastolic volume, end-systolic volume,* and *stroke volume output*?
11. Explain the function of the valves, pointing out especially the differences in anatomy and function of the A-V valves versus the semilunar valves (aortic and pulmonary valves).
12. Describe the successive stages of the aortic pressure curve and explain the causes of its features.
13. Give the relationship of the heart sounds to the systolic and diastolic periods of the cardiac cycle.
14. Explain the mechanism and importance of the Frank-Starling law of the heart.
15. What is the effect on cardiac output of changing the arterial pressure load?
16. Describe the ventricular function curves for the right and left heart.
17. What is the approximate range of control of heart rate by the parasympathetic and sympathetic nerves?
18. How much can parasympathetic and sympathetic nerve stimulation of the heart change the contractile strength of the heart?
19. Describe the effects of cardiac debility and cardiac hypertrophy on overall heart function as represented by cardiac output curves.
20. What are the respective effects of excess potassium ions and excess calcium ions on heart function?
21. Explain the effect of changes in body temperature on heart rate and heart contraction.

References

Baan, J. et al., eds.: Cardiac Dynamics, Boston, M. Nijhoff, 1979.
Brady, A. J.: Mechanical properties of cardiac fibers. In Berne, R. M. et al., eds.: Handbook of Physiology. Sec. 2, Vol. 1. Baltimore, Williams & Wilkins, 1979, p. 533.
Braunwald, E., and Ross, J., Jr.: Control of cardiac performance. In Berne, R. M. et al., eds.: Handbook of Physiology. Sec. 2, Vol. 1. Baltimore, Williams & Wilkins, 1979, p. 533.

Ellis, D.: Na-Ca exchange in cardiac tissue. Adv Myocardiol 5:295, 1985.
Gadsby, D. C.: The Na/K pump of cardiac cells. Annu Rev Biophys Bioeng 13:373, 1984.
Gilmour, R. F., Jr., and Zipes, D. P.: Slow inward current and cardiac arrhythmias. Am J Cardiol 55:89B, 1985.
Guyton, A. C.: Determination of cardiac output by equating venous return curves with cardiac response curves. Physiol Rev 35:123, 1955.

Guyton, A. C., et al.: Circulatory Physiology: Cardiac Output and Its Regulation, 2nd Ed. Philadelphia, W. B. Saunders Co., 1973.

Langer, G. A., et al.: The myocardium. Int Rev Physiol 9:191, 1976.

Page, E., and Shibata, Y.: Permeable junctions between cardiac cells. Annu Rev Physiol 43:431, 1981.

Sarnoff, S. J.: Myocardial contractility as described by ventricular function curves. Physiol Rev 35:107, 1955.

Starling, E. H.: The Linacre Lecture on the Law of the Heart. London, Longmans Green & Co., 1918.

Sugimoto, T., et al.: Effect of maximal work load on cardiac function. Jpn Heart J 14:146, 1973.

Weisfeldt, M. L., ed.: The Heart in Old Age: Its Function and Response to Stress. New York, Raven Press, 1980.

Winegrad, S.: Calcium release from cardiac sarcoplasmic reticulum. Annu Rev Physiol 44:451, 1982.

Winegard, S.: Regulation of cardiac contractile proteins. Correlations between physiology and biochemistry. Circ Res 55:565, 1984.

9
Rhythmic Excitation of the Heart

**THE SPECIAL EXCITATORY AND
  CONDUCTIVE SYSTEM OF THE HEART**
  THE SINOATRIAL NODE
  *INTERNODAL PATHWAYS AND
    TRANSMISSION OF THE CARDIAC
    IMPULSE THROUGH THE ATRIA*
  *THE ATRIOVENTRICULAR (A-V) NODE
    AND THE PURKINJE SYSTEM*
  *TRANSMISSION THROUGH THE A-V
    BUNDLE AND THE VENTRICLES—
    THE PURKINJE FIBERS*
  *SUMMARY OF THE SPREAD OF THE
    CARDIAC IMPULSE THROUGH THE
    HEART*

**CONTROL OF EXCITATION AND
  CONDUCTION IN THE HEART**
  *THE S-A NODE AS THE PACEMAKER
    OF THE HEART*
  *CONTROL OF HEART RHYTHMICITY
    AND CONDUCTION BY THE
    AUTONOMIC NERVES*
ABNORMAL RHYTHMS OF THE HEART
  *PREMATURE CONTRACTIONS—
    ECTOPIC FOCI*
  HEART BLOCK
  *FLUTTER AND FIBRILLATION—
    RE-ENTRANT PATHWAYS, CIRCUS
    MOVEMENTS*
  CARDIAC ARREST

The heart is endowed with a special system for generating rhythmical impulses to cause rhythmical contraction of the heart muscle, and also for conducting these impulses rapidly throughout the heart. When this system functions normally, the atria contract about one sixth of a second ahead of ventricular contraction, which allows extra filling of the ventricles before they pump the blood through the lungs and peripheral circulation.

Unfortunately, though, this rhythmical and conduction system of the heart is very susceptible to damage by heart disease, especially by ischemia of the heart tissues resulting from poor coronary blood flow. The consequence is often a very bizarre heart rhythm even to the extent of causing death.

THE SPECIAL EXCITATORY AND CONDUCTIVE SYSTEM OF THE HEART

The adult human heart normally contracts at a rhythmic rate of about 72 beats per minute. Figure 9–1 illustrates the special excitatory and conductive system of the heart that controls these cardiac contractions. The figure shows (A) the *S-A node* in which

the normal rhythmic self-excitatory impulse is generated, (B) the *internodal pathways* that conduct the impulse from the S-A node to the A-V node, (C) the *A-V node* in which the impulse from the atria is

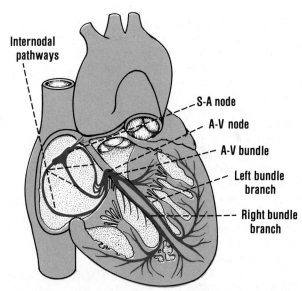

Figure 9–1. The S-A node and the Purkinje system of the heart, showing also the A-V node, the atrial internodal pathways, and the ventricular bundle branches.

delayed before passing into the ventricles, (D) the *A-V bundle,* which conducts the impulse from the atria into the ventricles, and (E) the *left* and *right bundle branches of Purkinje fibers,* which conduct the cardiac impulse to all parts of the ventricles.

THE SINOATRIAL NODE

The sinoatrial (S-A) node is a small, flattened, ellipsoid strip of specialized muscle approximately 3 mm wide, 15 mm long, and 1 mm thick; it is located in the anterosuperior wall of the right atrium immediately anterior and lateral to the opening of the superior vena cava. The fibers of this node are each 3 to 5 microns in diameter, in contrast to a diameter of 15 to 20 microns for the surrounding atrial muscle fibers. However, the S-A fibers are continuous with the atrial fibers so that any action potential that begins in the S-A node spreads immediately into the atria.

Automatic Rhythmicity of the Sinoatrial Fibers

Most cardiac fibers have the capability of *self-excitation,* a process that can cause automatic rhythmical contraction. This is especially true of the S-A node. For this reason, the sinoatrial node ordinarily controls the rate of beat of the entire heart.

Mechanism of S-A Nodal Rhythmicity. The basic biophysics of self-excitatory rhythmicity of excitable tissues was presented in Chapter 5. However, let us review these principles as they apply to the S-A node.

Figure 9–2 illustrates action potentials recorded from an S-A nodal fiber for three heartbeats and, by comparison, a single ventricular muscle fiber action potential, shown to the right. Note that the "resting" potential of the S-A nodal fiber has a maximum negativity of only − 55 to − 60 millivolts in comparison with − 85 to − 90 millivolts for the ventricular fiber.

There is a special feature of the S-A nodal fibers that is essential for their rhythmical self-excitation. This is the fact that they are quite leaky to sodium ions. It is this leakiness that makes the "resting" potential of the S-A nodal fibers less negative than the resting potential of the ventricular muscle fibers, because entry of the positive sodium ions to the interior of the fiber neutralizes much of the fiber negativity. This leakiness to sodium ions also causes the "resting" potential gradually to rise between each two heart beats, as illustrated in Figure 9–2, until it finally reaches the *threshold voltage* of about − 40 millivolts. At this point, this rising voltage suddenly opens the calcium-sodium channels, thus leading to the action potential. Therefore, basically, the inherent leakiness of the S-A nodal fibers to sodium ions causes their self-excitation.

Next, we must answer why this leakiness to sodium ions does not cause the S-A nodal fiber to remain depolarized all the time. The answer to this is that at the termination of the action potential, greatly in-

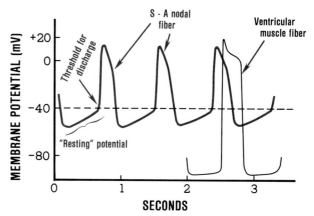

Figure 9–2. Rhythmic discharge of an S-A nodal fiber, and comparison of the S-A nodal action potential with that of a ventricular muscle fiber.

creased numbers of potassium channels have become opened, and these allow far greater quantities of potassium to diffuse out of the fiber than normally. This carries a great excess of positive charges to the exterior and temporarily causes excess negativity inside the fiber, which is called a state of *hyperpolarization.* This hyperpolarization initially carries the "resting" membrane potential down to about − 55 to − 60 millivolts at the termination of the action potential. However, this does not last because the excess potassium channels gradually close. Then the entire process begins again: self-excitation, recovery from the action potential, hyperpolarization after the action potential is over, upward drift of the "resting" potential, then re-excitation again to elicit still another cycle; this process continues indefinitely throughout the life of the person.

INTERNODAL PATHWAYS AND TRANSMISSION OF THE CARDIAC IMPULSE THROUGH THE ATRIA

The ends of the S-A nodal fibers fuse with the surrounding atrial muscle fibers, and action potentials originating in the S-A node travel outward into these fibers. In this way, the action potential spreads through the entire atrial muscle mass and eventually also to the A-V node. However, conduction is somewhat more rapid in several small bundles of atrial muscle fibers called the *internodal pathways,* illustrated in Figure 9–1. These pathways conduct the cardiac impulse directly to the A-V node. The cause of the more rapid velocity of conduction in these bundles is the presence of a number of specialized conduction fibers mixed with the atrial muscle.

THE ATRIOVENTRICULAR (A-V) NODE AND THE PURKINJE SYSTEM

Delay in Transmission at the A-V Node. Fortunately, the conductive system is organized so that the cardiac impulse will not travel from the atria into the ventricles too rapidly; this allows time for the atria

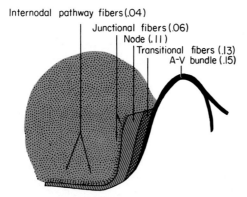

Internodal pathway fibers (.04)
Junctional fibers (.06)
Node (.11)
Transitional fibers (.13)
A-V bundle (.15)

Figure 9-3. Organization of the A-V node. The numbers represent the interval of time from the origin of the impulse in the S-A node. The values have been extrapolated to the human being. (This figure is based on studies in lower animals discussed and illustrated in Hoffman and Cranefield: Electrophysiology of the Heart. Copyright © 1960 by McGraw-Hill, Inc. Used by permission of McGraw-Hill Book Company.)

to empty their contents into the ventricles before ventricular contraction begins. It is primarily the A-V node and its associated conductive fibers that delay this transmission of the cardiac impulse from the atria into the ventricles.

The A-V node is located in the septal wall of the right atrium immediately posterior to the tricuspid valve, as illustrated in Figure 9-1. Figure 9-3 shows diagrammatically the different parts of this node and its connections with the atrial internodal pathway fibers and the A-V bundle. The figure also shows the approximate intervals of time in fractions of a second between the genesis of the cardiac impulse in the S-A node and its appearance at different points in the A-V nodal system. Note that the impulse, after traveling through the internodal pathway, reaches the A-V node approximately 0.04 second after its origin in the S-A node. However, between this time and the time that the impulse emerges in the A-V bundle, another 0.11 second elapses. About one half of this time lapse occurs in the *junctional fibers,* which are *very small fibers* that connect the normal atrial fibers with the fibers of the node itself. The velocity of conduction in these fibers is as little as 0.02 meter per second (about one twentieth that in normal cardiac muscle), which greatly delays entrance of the impulse into the A-V node.

TRANSMISSION THROUGH THE A-V BUNDLE AND THE VENTRICLES— THE PURKINJE FIBERS

The *Purkinje fibers* that lead from the A-V node through the A-V bundle and into the ventricles have functional characteristics quite the opposite of those of the A-V nodal fibers; they are very large fibers, even larger than the normal ventricular muscle fibers, and they transmit impulses at a velocity of 1.5 to 4.0 meters per second, a velocity about 6 times that in the usual cardiac muscle and 150 times that in the

junctional fibers. This allows almost immediate transmission of the cardiac impulse throughout the entire ventricular system. And this transmission in turn causes all parts of the ventricular muscle mass to contract simultaneously, which is necessary for effective pumping.

The very rapid transmission of action potentials by Purkinje fibers is probably caused by increased numbers of ion channels between the successive cardiac cells that make up the Purkinje fibers. At these channels, ions are transmitted easily from one cell to the next, thus enhancing the velocity of transmission.

Distribution of the Purkinje Fibers in the Ventricles. The Purkinje fibers, after originating in the A-V node, form the *A-V bundle,* which then threads through the fibrous tissue between the valves of the heart and thence into the ventricular septum, as shown in Figure 9-1. The A-V bundle divides almost immediately into the *left* and *right bundle branches* that lie beneath the endocardium of the respective sides of the septum. Each of these branches spreads downward toward the apex of the respective ventricle, but also divides into small branches which spread around each ventricular chamber and finally back toward the base of the heart. The terminal Purkinje fibers penetrate about one third of the way into the muscle mass to terminate on the muscle fibers.

From the time that the cardiac impulse first enters the A-V bundle until it reaches the terminations of the Purkinje fibers, the total time that elapses is only about 0.03 second; therefore, once a cardiac impulse enters the Purkinje system, it spreads almost immediately to the entire endocardial surface of the ventricular muscle.

SUMMARY OF THE SPREAD OF THE CARDIAC IMPULSE THROUGH THE HEART

Figure 9-4 illustrates in summary form the transmission of the cardiac impulse through the human heart. The numbers on the figure represent the intervals of time in fractions of a second that lapse between the origin of the cardiac impulse in the S-A node and its appearance at each respective point in the heart.

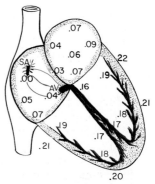

Figure 9-4. Transmission of the cardiac impulse through the heart, showing the time of appearance (in fractions of a second) of the impulse in different parts of the heart.

Note that the impulse spreads at moderate velocity through the atria but is delayed more than 0.1 second in the A-V nodal region before appearing in the A-V bundle. Once it has entered the bundle, it spreads rapidly through the Purkinje fibers to the entire endocardial surfaces of the ventricles. Then the impulse spreads slowly through the ventricular muscle to the epicardial surfaces.

It is extremely important that the student learn in detail the course of the cardiac impulse through the heart *and the times of its appearance* in each separate part of the heart, for a quantitative knowledge of this process is essential to the understanding of electrocardiography, which is discussed in the following chapter.

CONTROL OF EXCITATION AND CONDUCTION IN THE HEART

THE S-A NODE AS THE PACEMAKER OF THE HEART

In the above discussion of the genesis and transmission of the cardiac impulse through the heart, it was stated that the impulse normally arises in the S-A node. However, this need not be the case under abnormal conditions, for other parts of the heart can exhibit rhythmic contraction in the same way that the fibers of the S-A node can; this is particularly true of the A-V nodal and Purkinje fibers.

The A-V nodal fibers, when not stimulated from some outside source, discharge at an intrinsic rhythmic rate of 40 to 60 times per minute, and the Purkinje fibers discharge at a rate of somewhere between 15 and 40 times per minute. These rates are in contrast to the normal rate of the S-A node of 60 to 80 times per minute.

Therefore, the question that we must ask is: Why does the S-A node control the heart's rhythmicity rather than the A-V node or the Purkinje fibers? The answer to this is simply that the discharge rate of the S-A node is considerably faster than that of either the A-V node or the Purkinje fibers. Each time the S-A node discharges, its impulse is conducted into both the A-V node and the Purkinje fibers, discharging their excitable membranes. Then these tissues, as well as the S-A node, begin to recover. But the S-A node recovers much more rapidly than does either of the other two and emits a new impulse before either one of them can reach its own threshold for self-excitation. The new impulse again discharges both the A-V node and Purkinje fibers. This process continues on and on, the S-A node always exciting these other potentially self-excitatory tissues before self-excitation can actually occur.

Thus, the S-A node controls the beat of the heart, because its rate of rhythmic discharge is greater than that of any other part of the heart. Therefore, the S-A node is the normal *pacemaker* of the heart.

Abnormal Pacemakers—The Ectopic Pacemaker.

Occasionally some other part of the heart develops a rhythmic discharge rate that is more rapid than that of the S-A node. For instance, this often occurs as a result of pathology in the A-V node or in the Purkinje fibers. In either of these cases, the pacemaker of the heart shifts from the S-A node to the A-V node or to the excitable Purkinje fibers. Under rare conditions a point in the atrial or ventricular muscle develops excessive excitability and becomes the pacemaker.

A pacemaker located elsewhere than the S-A node is called an *ectopic pacemaker*. Obviously, an ectopic pacemaker causes an abnormal sequence of contraction of the different parts of the heart.

CONTROL OF HEART RHYTHMICITY AND CONDUCTION BY THE AUTONOMIC NERVES

The heart is supplied with both sympathetic and parasympathetic nerves, as discussed in the previous chapter. The parasympathetic nerves are distributed mainly to the S-A and A-V nodes, to a lesser extent to the muscle of the two atria, and even less to the ventricular muscle. The sympathetic nerves, on the other hand, are distributed to all parts of the heart, with a strong representation in the ventricular muscle as well as in all the other areas.

Effect of Parasympathetic (Vagal) Stimulation on Cardiac Rhythm and Conduction—Ventricular Escape. Stimulation of the parasympathetic nerves to the heart (the vagi) causes the hormone *acetylcholine* to be released at the vagal endings. This hormone increases the permeability of cardiac muscle fibers to potassium ions, which has two major effects on the heart. First, it decreases the rate of rhythm of the S-A node, and, second, it decreases the excitability of the A-V junctional fibers between the atrial musculature and the A-V node, thereby slowing transmission of the cardiac impulse into the ventricles.

Very strong stimulation of the vagi can completely stop the rhythmic contraction of the S-A node or completely block transmission of the cardiac impulse through the A-V junction. In either case, rhythmic impulses are no longer transmitted into the ventricles. The ventricles stop beating for 4 to 10 seconds, but then some point in the Purkinje fibers, usually in the A-V bundle, develops a rhythm of its own and causes ventricular contraction at a rate of 15 to 40 beats per minute. This phenomenon is called *ventricular escape*.

Effect of Sympathetic Stimulation on Cardiac Rhythm and Conduction. Sympathetic stimulation causes essentially the opposite effects on the heart to those caused by vagal stimulation, as follows: First, it increases the rate of S-A nodal discharge. Second, it increases the rate of conduction and the excitability in all portions of the heart. Third, it increases greatly the force of contraction of all the cardiac musculature, both atrial and ventricular, as discussed in the previous chapter. All of these results are believed to be caused by the effect of *norepinephrine*, the hormone released at the sympathetic nerve endings to increase the permeability of the muscle fiber membranes to sodium and calcium. This increased permeability has the general effect of increasing the excitability of the fibers.

In short, sympathetic stimulation increases the overall activity of the heart. Maximal stimulation can almost triple the rate of heartbeat and can increase the strength of heart contraction as much as two-fold.

ABNORMAL RHYTHMS OF THE HEART

PREMATURE CONTRACTIONS—ECTOPIC FOCI

Often, a small area of the heart becomes much more excitable than normal and causes abnormal impulses to be generated in between the normal impulses. A depolarization wave spreads outward from the irritable area and initiates *premature contraction* of the heart. The focus at which the abnormal impulse is generated is called an *ectopic focus*.

The usual cause of an ectopic focus is an irritable area of cardiac muscle resulting from a local area of ischemia (too little coronary blood flow to the muscle), overuse of stimulants such as caffeine or nicotine, lack of sleep, anxiety, or some other debilitating state.

HEART BLOCK

Occasionally, transmission of the impulse through the heart is blocked at a critical point in the conductive system. One of the most common of these points is located between the atria and the ventricles; this condition is called *atrioventricular block*. It can result from localized damage or depression of the *A-V junctional* fibers or of the *A-V bundle*. The causes include different types of infectious processes, excessive stimulation by the vagus nerves (which depresses conductivity in the junctional fibers), localized destruction of the A-V bundle as a result of a coronary infarct, pressure on the A-V bundle by arteriosclerotic plaques, or depression caused by various drugs.

When the block occurs in the A-V bundle and the ventricles can no longer receive signals from the atria, a rhythmical signal normally begins in the bundle immediately beyond the block. This then causes the ventricles to beat at a slow rate of 15 to 40 beats per minute. However, the ventricles are no longer coordinated with the atria, so that the heart pumping capability decreases by 20 to 30 per cent.

FLUTTER AND FIBRILLATION—RE-ENTRANT PATHWAYS, CIRCUS MOVEMENTS

Frequently, either the atria or the ventricles begin to contract extremely rapidly and often incoordinately. The low frequency, more coordinate contractions (up to 200 to 300 beats per minute) are generally called *flutter*, and the very high frequency, incoordinate contractions, *fibrillation*. Both of these are usu-

ally caused by a phenomenon called *re-entry* that leads to *a circus movement*.

The Circus Movement. A circus movement occurs when an impulse begins in one part of the heart muscle, spreads in a circuitous pathway through the heart, and then returns to the originally excited muscle and "re-enters" this muscle to stimulate it once more. Thus the excitatory signal continues again and again around the circle, never stopping. This effect is illustrated in Figure 9–5, which depicts several small cardiac muscle strips cut in the form of circles. If such a strip is stimulated at the 12 o'clock position *so that the impulse travels in only one direction,* the impulse spreads progressively around the circle until it returns to the 12 o'clock position. If the originally stimulated muscle fibers are still in a refractory state, the impulse then dies out, for refractory muscle cannot transmit a second impulse. However, three different conditions can cause this impulse to continue to travel around the circle.

First, if the *length of the pathway around the circle is long,* by the time the impulse returns to the 12 o'clock position the originally stimulated muscle will no longer be refractory, and the impulse will continue around the circle again and again.

Second, if the length of the pathway remains constant but the *velocity of conduction becomes decreased* enough, an increased interval of time will elapse before the impulse returns to the 12 o'clock position. By this time the originally stimulated muscle might be out of the refractory state, and the impulse can continue around the circle again and again.

Third, the *refractory period of the muscle might become greatly shortened*. In this case also, the impulse can continue around and around the circle.

All three of these conditions occur in different pathological states of the human heart as follows: (1) A long pathway frequently occurs in dilated hearts. (2) Decreased rate of conduction frequently results from blockage of the Purkinje system, ischemia of the muscle, heart muscle disease, and many other factors. (3) A shortened refractory period frequently

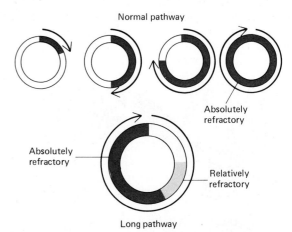

Figure 9–5. The circus movement, showing annihilation of the impulse in the short pathway and continued propagation of the impulse in the long pathway.

occurs in response to various drugs, such as epinephrine, or following repetitive stimulation. Thus, in many different cardiac disturbances circus movements can cause abnormal cardiac rhythmicity that completely ignores the pacesetting effects of the S-A node.

Atrial Flutter and Fibrillation

Atrial Flutter Resulting from a Circus Pathway. The left-hand panel of Figure 9–6 illustrates a circus pathway around and around the atria from top to bottom, the pathway lying to the left of the superior and inferior venae cavae. Such circus pathways often develop in the human heart when the atria become greatly dilated as a result of valvular heart disease. The rate of flutter is usually 200 to 300 times per minute.

Atrial Fibrillation. Atrial fibrillation is completely different from atrial flutter because the circus movement does not travel in a regular pathway. Instead, many simultaneous circus movements occur in multiple areas, causing separate excitation waves that can be seen to travel over the surface of the atria at the same time. Atrial fibrillation occurs frequently when the atria become greatly overdilated—in fact, it occurs many times as frequently as flutter. When flutter does occur, it usually becomes fibrillation after a few days or weeks. To the right in Figure 9–6 are illustrated the pathways of fibrillatory impulses traveling through the atria.

Atrial fibrillation results in complete incoordination of atrial contraction so that atrial pumping ceases entirely. However, the effectiveness of the heart as a pump is reduced only 25 to 30 per cent because blood can flow through the atria into the ventricles without the aid of the "primer" function of atrial pumping, though with less efficiency. For this reason, atrial fibrillation often can continue for many years without serious cardiac debility.

Ventricular Fibrillation. Ventricular fibrillation, like atrial fibrillation, is a state of incoordinate contraction of the ventricular muscle caused by multiple circus movements, as illustrated to the right in Figure 9–7. And as also occurs in atrial fibrillation, ventricular fibrillation provides no effective pumping of

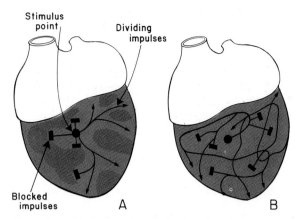

Figure 9–7. *A,* Initiation of fibrillation in a heart when patches of refractory musculature are present. *B,* Continued propagation of *fibrillatory impulses* in the fibrillating ventricle.

blood. Therefore, *ventricular fibrillation invariably causes death within a minute or so* unless some heroic measure is applied to revert the heart back to normal rhythm.

At least one fourth of all persons who die, die in ventricular fibrillation. For instance, the hearts of most patients with coronary infarcts fibrillate shortly before death. In only a few instances on record have fibrillating human ventricles been known to return of their own accord to a rhythmic beat.

The likelihood of circus movements in the ventricles, and consequently of ventricular fibrillation, is greatly increased when the ventricles are dilated or when the rapidly conducting Purkinje system is blocked so that impulses cannot be transmitted rapidly. Also, electric shock, particularly with 60-cycle electric current (as will be discussed later), or the emission of rapid impulses from an ectopic foci are common initiating causes of ventricular fibrillation.

Because ventricular fibrillation is such a dramatic and instantaneous cause of death in so many persons, its basic mechanisms deserve special discussion, as follows:

The "Chain Reaction" Mechanism of Fibrillation. Fibrillation, whether it occurs in the atria or in the ventricles, is a very different condition from flutter. One can see many separate contractile waves spreading in different directions over the cardiac muscle at the same time in either atrial or ventricular fibrillation. One of the best ways to explain the mechanism of fibrillation is to describe the initiation of fibrillation by stimulation with 60-cycle alternating electrical current.

Fibrillation Caused by 60-Cycle Alternating Current. At a central point in the ventricles of heart *A* in Figure 9–7, a 60-cycle electrical stimulus is applied through a stimulating electrode. The first cycle of the electrical stimulus causes a depolarization wave to spread in all directions, leaving all the muscle beneath the electrode in a refractory state. After about 0.25 second, this muscle begins to come out of the refractory state, some portions of the muscle coming out of refractoriness prior to other portions. This state is

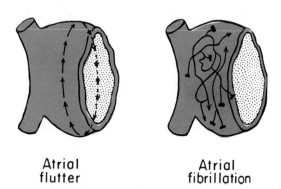

Atrial flutter   **Atrial fibrillation**

Figure 9–6. Pathways of impulses in atrial flutter and atrial fibrillation.

depicted in heart *A*, showing many light patches, which represent excitable cardiac muscle and dark patches, which represent still refractory muscle. The continuing 60-cycle stimulus from the electrode can now cause impulses to travel in certain directions through the heart but not in all directions. Furthermore, when a depolarization wave reaches a refractory area in the heart, it travels to both sides around the area. Thus, a single impulse becomes two impulses. Then when each of these reaches another refractory area it, too, divides to form still two more impulses. In this way many different impulses are continually being formed in the heart by a progressive *chain reaction* until, finally, there are many small depolarization waves traveling in many different directions at the same time. Obviously, this irregular pattern of impulses travels a *circuitous route, which greatly lengthens the conductive pathway, which leads to fibrillation.* One can readily see that a vicious circle has been initiated: More and more impulses are formed, causing more and more patches of refractory muscle, and the refractory patches cause more and more division of the impulses. Thus, heart *B* in Figure 9-7 illustrates the final state that develops in fibrillation.

Electrical Defibrillation of the Ventricles. Though a weak alternating current almost invariably throws the ventricles into fibrillation, a very strong electrical current passed through the ventricles for a short interval of time can actually stop fibrillation. It does this by throwing all the ventricular muscle into refractoriness simultaneously. This is accomplished by passing intense current through electrodes placed on the heart or on the chest wall over the heart as illustrated in Figure 9-8. The current penetrates most of the fibers of the ventricles, thus stimulating essentially all parts of the ventricles simultaneously and causing them to become refractory. As a result, all impulses stop, and the heart then remains quiescent for three to five seconds, after which it begins to beat again, with the S-A node or some other part of the heart becoming the pacemaker. Occasionally, however, the same irritable focus that originally threw the ventricles into fibrillation is still present, and fibrillation begins again immediately.

Unless defibrillated within one minute after fibrillation begins, the heart is usually too weak to be revived. However, it is still possible to revive the heart by preliminarily pumping it by hand and then defibrillating it later. In this way small quantities of

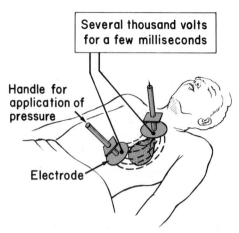

Figure 9-8. Application of electrical current to the chest to stop ventricular fibrillation.

blood are delivered into the aorta, and a renewed coronary blood supply develops. After a few minutes, electrical defibrillation often becomes possible. Indeed, fibrillating hearts have been pumped by hand as long as 90 minutes before defibrillation.

In recent years, a technique of pumping the heart without opening the chest has been developed; this technique consists of intermittent, very powerful thrusts of pressure on the chest wall.

Lack of blood flow to the brain for more than five to ten minutes usually results in permanent mental impairment or even total destruction of the brain. Even though the heart may be revived, the person might die from the effects of brain damage or live with permanent mental impairment.

CARDIAC ARREST

When cardiac metabolism becomes greatly disturbed as a result of any one of many possible conditions, the rhythmic contractions of the heart occasionally stop. One of the most common causes of cardiac arrest is hypoxia of the heart, for severe hypoxia prevents the muscle fibers from maintaining normal ionic differentials across their membranes.

Occasionally, patients with severe myocardial disease develop cardiac arrest, which obviously can lead to death. In many cases, however, rhythmic electrical impulses from an implanted electronic cardiac "pacemaker" have been used successfully to keep patients alive for many years.

QUESTIONS

1. Describe the special excitatory and conductive system of the heart.
2. What is the mechanism of S-A nodal rhymicity?
3. What causes the delay in transmission at the A-V node? And, what is the importance of this delay for cardiac function?
4. Describe the Purkinje system for rapid conduction of the cardiac impulse to all parts of the ventricles.
5. Why is it important that all parts of the ventricles receive the cardiac impulse simultaneously?
6. Why does the S-A node normally function as the pacemaker of the heart?

7. Under what conditions can other areas of the heart besides the S-A node become the pacemaker of the heart?

8. What are the effects of parasympathetic (vagal) stimulation on cardiac rhythmicity and conduction of the cardiac impulse through the conductive system of the heart?

9. What are the effects of sympathetic stimulation on cardiac rhythm, cardiac conduction, and cardiac contractile strength?

10. What types of conditions can cause premature contractions?

11. What happens to cardiac function when conduction of the cardiac impulse through the atrioventricular bundle is blocked?

12. Explain the mechanism of the circus movement.

13. What are the characteristics of *atrial flutter* and *atrial fibrillation*?

14. What happens to the heart in ventricular fibrillation?

15. Explain the "chain reaction" mechanism of fibrillation as well as the means by which 60-cycle alternating current elicits ventricular fibrillation.

16. Why is very strong electric shock to the heart capable of causing defibrillation, whereas weak electric shock is a very common cause of fibrillation?

17. What conditions can cause cardiac arrest?

References

Akera, T., and Brody, T. M.: Myocardial membranes: Regulation and function of the sodium pump. Annu Rev Physiol 44:375, 1982.

Brown, H. F.: Electrophysiology of the sinoatrial node. Physiol Rev 62:505, 1982.

DiFrancesco, D., and Noble, D.: A model of cardiac electrical activity incorporating ionic pumps and concentration changes. Phil Trans R Soc Lond (Biol) 307:353, 1985

Ellis, D.: Na-Ca exchange in cardiac tissues. Adv Myocardiol 5:295, 1985.

Geddes, L. A.: Cardiovascular Medical Devices. New York, John Wiley & Sons, 1984.

Gilmour, R. F., Jr., and Zipes, D. P.: Slow inward current and cardiac arrhythmias. Am J Cardiol 55:89B, 1985

Glitsch, H. G.: Electrogenic Na pumping in the heart. Annu Rev Physiol 44:389, 1982.

Guyton, A. C., and Satterfield, J.: Factors concerned in electrical defibrillation of the heart, particularly through the unopened chest. Am J Physiol 167:81, 1951.

Jacobson, L.: Cardiac Pacing. Principles and Case Studies. New Hyde Park, New York, Medical Examination Publishing Co., 1981.

Josephson, M. E., and Singh, B. N.: Use of calcium antagonists in ventricular dysfunction. Am J Cardiol 55:81B, 1985.

Levy, M. N., et al.: Neural regulation of the heart beat. Annu Rev Physiol 43:443, 1981.

Loewenstein, W. R.: Junctional intercellular communication: The cell-to-cell membrane channel. Physiol Rev 61:829, 1981.

McDonald, T. F.: The slow inward calcium current in the heart. Annu Rev Physiol 44:425, 1982.

Meijler, F. L.: Atrioventricular conduction versus heart size from mouse to whale. J Am Coll Cardiol 5:363, 1985.

Reuter, H.: Ion channels in cardiac cell membranes. Annu Rev Physiol 44:473, 1984.

Sperelakis, N.: Propagation mechanisms in heart. Annu Rev Physiol 41:441, 1979.

Vasselle, M.: Electrogenesis of the plateau and pacemaker potential. Annu Rev Physiol 41:425, 1979.

Verrier, R. L., and Lown, B.: Behavioral stress and cardiac arrhythmias. Annu Rev Physiol 46:155, 1984.

10

The Electrocardiogram

CHARACTERISTICS OF THE NORMAL
  ELECTROCARDIOGRAM
  *DEPOLARIZATION WAVES VERSUS
    REPOLARIZATION WAVES*
  *VOLTAGE AND TIME CALIBRATION
    OF THE ELECTROCARDIOGRAM*
  *RECORDING ELECTROCARDIO-
    GRAMS—THE PEN RECORDER*
  *FLOW OF CURRENT AROUND THE
    HEART DURING THE CARDIAC
    CYCLE*
ELECTROCARDIOGRAPHIC LEADS
  THE THREE STANDARD LIMB LEADS
  CHEST LEADS (PRECORDIAL LEADS)

ELECTROCARDIOGRAPHIC
  INTERPRETATION OF CARDIAC
  ARRHYTHMIAS
  ATRIOVENTRICULAR BLOCK
  PREMATURE CONTRACTIONS
  PAROXYSMAL TACHYCARDIA
  *ABNORMAL RHYTHMS RESULTING
    FROM CIRCUS MOVEMENTS*
ELECTROCARDIOGRAPHIC INTERPRE-
  TATION IN NON-ARRHYTHMIC
  CARDIAC ABNORMALITIES
  *THE MEAN ELECTRICAL AXIS OF THE
    VENTRICLES*
  HYPERTROPHY OF ONE VENTRICLE
  BUNDLE BRANCH BLOCK
  CURRENT OF INJURY

Transmission of the impulse through the heart has been discusssed in detail in Chapter 9. As the impulse passes through the heart, electrical currents spread into the tissues surrounding the heart, and a small proportion of them spreads all the way to the surface of the body. If electrodes are placed on the body surface on opposite sides of the heart, the electrical potentials generated by the heart can be recorded; the recording is the *electrocardiogram*. A normal electrocardiogram for two beats of the heart is illustrated in Figure 10–1.

CHARACTERISTICS OF THE NORMAL ELECTROCARDIOGRAM

The normal electrocardiogram is composed of a P wave, a "QRS complex," and a T wave. The QRS complex is actually three separate waves, the Q wave, the R wave, and the S wave, all of which are caused by passage of the cardiac impulse through the ventricles. In the normal electrocardiogram, the Q and S waves are often much less prominent than the R wave and sometimes are actually absent, but even so, the

wave is still known as the QRS complex, or simply the QRS wave.

The P wave is caused by electrical currents generated as the atria depolarize prior to atrial contraction, and the QRS complex is caused by currents generated when the ventricles depolarize prior to their contraction. Therefore, both the P wave and the QRS complex are *depolarization waves*. The T wave is caused by currents generated as the ventricles recover from the state of depolarization, that is, as they

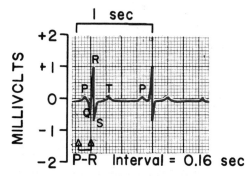

Figure 10–1. The normal electrocardiogram.

repolarize. This process occurs in ventricular muscle about 0.25 second after depolarization, and this wave is known as a *repolarization wave*. Thus, the electrocardiogram is composed of both depolarization and repolarization waves. The principles of depolarization and repolarization were discussed in Chapter 5. However, the distinction between depolarization waves and repolarization waves is so important in electrocardiography that further clarification is needed as follows:

DEPOLARIZATION WAVES VERSUS REPOLARIZATION WAVES

Figure 10–2 illustrates a muscle fiber in four different stages of depolarization and repolarization. During the process of depolarization the normal negative potential inside the fiber is lost and the membrane potential actually reverses; that is, it becomes slightly positive inside and negative outside.

In Figure 10–2A the process of depolarization, illustrated by the positivity inside and negativity outside, is traveling from left to right, and the first half of the fiber is already depolarized while the remaining half is still polarized. This causes the meter to record positively. To the right of the muscle fiber is illustrated a record of the potential between the electrodes as recorded by a high-speed recording meter at this particular stage of depolarization.

In Figure 10–2B depolarization has extended over the entire muscle fiber, and the recording to the right has now returned to the zero base line because both electrodes are in areas of equal negativity. The completed wave is a *depolarization wave* because it has resulted from spread of depolarization along the extent of the muscle fiber.

Figure 10–2C illustrates the repolarization process, during which the recording, as illustrated to the right, is negative.

Finally, in Figure 10–2D the muscle fiber has completely repolarized, and the recording returns once more to the zero level. This completed negative wave is a *repolarization wave* because it has resulted from spread of the repolarization process over the muscle fiber.

Relationship of the Monophasic Action Potential of Cardiac Muscle to the QRS and T Waves. The monophasic action potential of ventricular muscle, which was discussed in the preceding chapter, normally lasts between 0.25 and 0.30 second. The top part of Figure 10–3 illustrates a monophasic action potential recorded from a microelectrode inserted into the inside of a single ventricular muscle fiber. The upsweep of this action potential is caused by *depolarization,* and the return of the potential to the base line is caused by *repolarization.* Note below the simultaneous recording of the electrocardiogram from this same ventricle, which shows the QRS wave appearing at the beginning of the monophasic action potential and the T wave at the end. Note especially that *no potential at all is recorded in the electrocardiogram when the ventricular muscle is either completely polarized or completely depolarized.*

The Electrocardiogram During Ventricular Repolarization—The T Wave. Because the septum and the endocardium depolarize first, it seems logical that they should also repolarize first at the end of ventricular contraction, but this is not the normal case because the septum and endocardium have longer periods of depolarization than other areas of the ventricles. On the other hand, the outer portions of the ventricles have short periods of depolarization. Therefore, *the portion of ventricular muscle to repolarize first is that located exteriorly near the apex of the heart,* and the endocardial surfaces normally re-

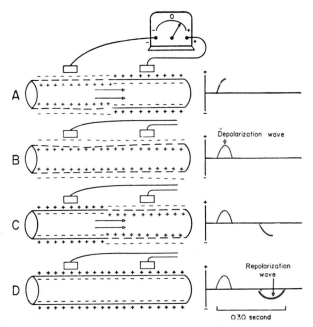

Figure 10–2. Recording the *depolarization wave* and the *repolarization wave* from a cardiac muscle fiber.

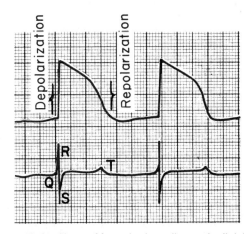

Figure 10–3. *Above:* Monophasic action potential from a ventricular muscle fiber during normal cardiac function, showing rapid depolarization and then repolarization occurring slowly during the plateau stage but very rapidly toward the end. *Below:* Electrocardiogram recorded simultaneously.

polarize last. The reason for this abnormal sequence of repolarization is reputed to be that high pressure in the ventricles during contraction compresses the endocardial blood vessels and greatly reduces coronary blood flow to the endocardium, thereby slowing the repolarization process on the endocardial surfaces. But whatever the cause, *the predominant direction of the potential recorded from the heart during repolarization of the ventricles is from base to apex, which is the same predominant direction of the potential recorded during depolarization. As a result, the T wave in the normal electrocardiogram is positive, which is also the polarity of most of the normal QRS complex.*

VOLTAGE AND TIME CALIBRATION OF THE ELECTROCARDIOGRAM

All recordings of electrocardiograms are made with appropriate calibration in lines on the recording paper.

As illustrated in Figure 10–1, the horizontal lines are spaced so that ten small divisions (1 cm) in the vertical direction in the standard electrocardiogram represent one millivolt.

The vertical lines on the electrocardiogram are time calibration lines. Each inch (2.5 cm) of the standard electrocardiogram is one second. Each inch in turn is usually broken into five segments by dark vertical lines, the distance between which represents 0.20 second. The intervals between the dark vertical lines are broken into five smaller intervals by thin lines, and the distance between each two of the smaller lines represents 0.04 second.

The P-Q Interval. The duration of time between the beginning of the P wave and the beginning of the QRS wave is the interval between the beginning of contraction of the atria and the beginning of contraction of the ventricles. This period of time is called the P-Q interval. The normal P-Q interval is approximately 0.16 second. This interval is sometimes also called the P-R interval, because the Q wave frequently is absent.

The Q-T Interval. Contraction of the ventricle lasts essentially between the Q wave and the end of the T wave. This interval of time is called the Q-T interval and ordinarily is approximately 0.30 second.

RECORDING ELECTROCARDIOGRAMS— THE PEN RECORDER

The electrical currents generated by the cardiac muscle during each beat of the heart regularly change potentials and polarity in less than 0.03 second. Therefore, it is essential that any apparatus for recording electrocardiograms be capable of responding rapidly to these changes in electrical potentials. The most usual type of recorder now used is the pen recorder. This instrument writes the electrocardiogram with a pen directly on a moving sheet of paper. The pen is often a thin tube connected at one end to an inkwell, with its recording end connected to a powerful electromagnet system that is capable of moving the pen back and forth at high speed. As the paper moves forward, the pen records the electrocardiogram. The movement of the pen in turn is controlled by appropriate amplifiers connected to electrocardiographic electrodes on the subject.

FLOW OF CURRENT AROUND THE HEART DURING THE CARDIAC CYCLE

Figure 10–4 illustrates the ventricular muscle mass lying within the chest. Even the lungs, though filled with air, conduct electricity to a surprising extent, and fluids of the other tissues surrounding the heart conduct electricity even more easily. Therefore, the heart is actually suspended in a conductive medium. When one portion of the ventricles becomes electronegative—that is, depolarized—with respect to the remainder, electrical current flows from the depolarized area to the polarized area in large circuitous routes, as noted in the figure.

It will be recalled from the discussion of the Purkinje system in Chapter 9 that the cardiac impulse first arrives in the ventricles in the walls of the septum and almost immediately thereafter along the endocardial surfaces of the remainder of the ventricles, as shown by the shaded areas and the negative signs in Figure 10–4. This provides electronegativity on the insides of the ventricles and electropositivity on the outer walls of the ventricles. If one algebraically averages all the lines of current flow (the elliptical lines in Figure 10–4), he finds that the average current flow is from the base of the heart toward the apex. During most of the cycle of depolarization, the current continues to flow in this direction as the impulse spreads from the endocardial surface outward through the ventricular muscle. However, immediately before the depolarization wave has completed its course

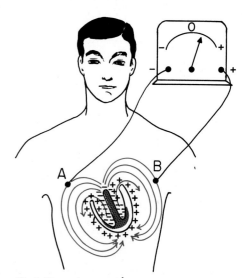

Figure 10–4. Flow of current in the chest around a partially depolarized heart.

through the ventricles, the direction of current flow reverses for about 0.01 second, flowing then from the apex toward the base because the very last part of the heart to become depolarized is the outer walls of the ventricles near their base.

If a meter is connected to the surface of the body as shown in Figure 10–4, the electrode nearer the base will be negative with respect to the electrode nearer the apex, so that the meter shows a potential between the two electrodes. In making electrocardiographic recordings, various standard positions for placement of electrodes are used, and whether the polarity of the recording during each cardiac cycle is positive or negative is determined by the orientation of the electrodes with respect to the current flow in the heart. Some of the conventional electrode systems, commonly called *electrocardiographic leads*, are discussed below.

ELECTROCARDIOGRAPHIC LEADS

THE THREE STANDARD LIMB LEADS

Figure 10–5 illustrates electrical connections between the limbs and the electrocardiograph for recording electrocardiograms from the so-called "standard" limb leads. The electrocardiograph in each instance is illustrated by a mechanical meter in the diagram, though the actual electrocardiograph is a high-speed recording meter.

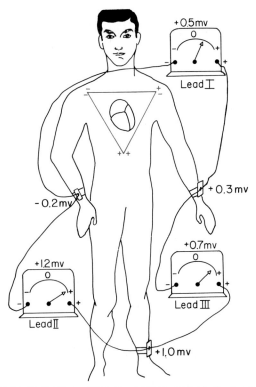

Figure 10–5. Conventional arrangement of electrodes for recording the standard electrocardiographic leads. Einthoven's triangle is superimposed on the chest.

Lead I. In recording limb lead I, the negative terminal of the electrocardiograph is connected to the right arm, and the positive terminal to the left arm. Therefore, when the point on the chest where the right arm connects to the chest is electronegative with respect to the point where the left arm connects, the electrocardiograph records positively—that is, above the zero voltage line in the electrocardiogram. When the opposite is true, the electrocardiograph records below the line.

Lead II. In recording limb lead II, the negative terminal of the electrocardiograph is connected to the right arm and the positive terminal to the left leg. Thus, when the right arm is negative with respect to the left leg, the electrocardiograph records positively.

Lead III. In recording limb lead III, the negative terminal of the electrocardiograph is connected to the left arm and the positive terminal to the left leg. This means that the electrocardiograph records positively when the left arm is negative with respect to the left leg.

Normal Electrocardiograms Recorded by the Three Standard Leads. Figure 10–6 illustrates simultaneous recordings of the normal electrocardiogram in leads I, II, and III. It is obvious from this figure that the electrocardiograms in these three standard leads are very similar to each other, for they all record positive P waves and positive T waves, and the major portion of the QRS complex is also positive in each electrocardiogram.

Because all normal electrocardiograms are very similar to each other, it does not matter greatly which electrocardiographic lead is recorded when one wishes to diagnose the different cardiac arrhythmias, for diagnosis of arrhythmias depends mainly on the time relationships between the different waves of the cardiac cycle. On the other hand, when one wishes

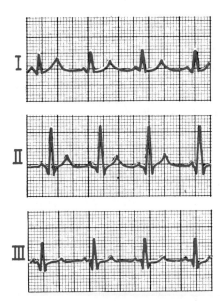

Figure 10–6. Normal electrocardiograms recorded from the three standard electrocardiographic leads.

to determine the extent and type of damage in the ventricles or in the atria, it does matter greatly which leads are recorded, for abnormalities of the cardiac muscle change the patterns of the electrocardiograms markedly in some leads and yet may not affect other leads.

Electrocardiographic interpretation of these two types of conditions—cardiac arrhythmias and cardiac muscle abnormalities—are discussed separately in later sections of this chapter.

CHEST LEADS (PRECORDIAL LEADS)

Often electrocardiograms are recorded with one electrode placed on the anterior chest over the heart, as illustrated by the six separate points in Figure 10–7. The electrode is connected to the positive terminal of the electrocardiograph, and the negative electrode, called the *indifferent electrode,* is normally connected simultaneously through electrical resistances to the right arm, left arm, and left leg, as also shown in the figure. Usually six different standard chest leads are recorded from the anterior chest wall, the chest electrode being placed respectively at each of the six points illustrated in the diagram. The different leads recorded by the method illustrated in Figure 10–7 are known as leads V_1, V_2, V_3, V_4, V_5, and V_6.

Figure 10–8 illustrates the electrocardiograms of the normal heart as recorded in the six standard chest leads. Because the heart surfaces are close to the chest wall, each chest lead records mainly the electrical potential of the cardiac musculature immediately beneath the electrode. Therefore, relatively minute abnormalities in the ventricles, particularly in the anterior ventricular wall, frequently cause marked changes in the electrocardiograms recorded from chest leads.

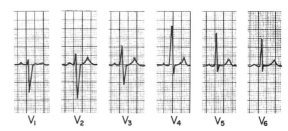

Figure 10–8. Normal electrocardiograms recorded from the six standard chest leads.

ELECTROCARDIOGRAPHIC INTERPRETATION OF CARDIAC ARRHYTHMIAS

The rhythmicity of the heart and some abnormalities of rhythmicity were discussed in Chapter 9. The major purpose of the present section is to describe the electrocardiograms recorded in a few conditions known clinically as "cardiac arrhythmias."

ATRIOVENTRICULAR BLOCK

The only means by which impulses can ordinarily pass from the atria into the ventricles is through the *A-V bundle,* which is also known as the *bundle of His.* Different conditions that can either decrease the rate of conduction of the impulse through this bundle or totally block the impulse are

1. *Ischemia of the A-V junctional fibers.*

2. *Compression of the A-V bundle* by scar tissue or by calcified portions of the heart.

3. *Inflammation of the A-V bundle or fibers of the A-V junction.*

4. *Extreme stimulation of the heart by the vagi.*

Incomplete Heart Block. When conduction through the A-V junction is prolonged from a normal value of 0.16 second to as great as 0.25 to 0.50 second, the action potentials traveling through the A-V junctional fibers are sometimes strong enough to pass on into the A-V node and at other times are not strong enough. Often the impulse passes into the ventricles on one heartbeat and fails to pass on the next one or two beats, thus alternating between conduction and nonconduction. In this instance, the atria beat many times without a corresponding beat of the ventricles, and it is said that there are "dropped beats" of the ventricles. This condition is called *incomplete heart block.*

Figure 10–9 illustrates P-R intervals as long as 0.30 second, and it also illustrates one dropped beat as a result of failure of conduction from the atria to the ventricles.

At times every other beat of the ventricles is dropped, so that a 2:1 rhythm develops in the heart,

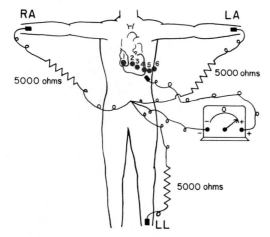

Figure 10–7. Connections of the body with the electrocardiograph for recording chest leads.

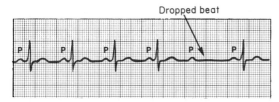

Figure 10–9. Partial atrioventricular block (lead V₃).

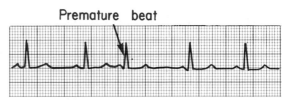

Figure 10–11. Atrial premature contraction (lead I).

with the atria beating twice for every single beat of the ventricles. Sometimes other rhythms, such as 3:2 or 3:1, also develop.

Complete Atrioventricular Block. When the condition causing poor conduction in the A-V bundle becomes extremely severe, complete block of the impulse from the atria into the ventricles occurs. In this instance the P waves become completely dissociated from the QRS-T complexes, as illustrated in Figure 10–10. Note that the rate of rhythm of the atria in this electrocardiogram is approximately 100 beats per minute, while the rate of ventricular beat is less than 40 per minute. Furthermore, there is no relationship whatsoever between the rhythm of the atria and that of the ventricles, for the ventricles have "escaped" from control by the atria, and they are beating at their own natural rate.

Stokes-Adams Syndrome—Ventricular Escape. In some patients with atrioventricular block, total block comes and goes—that is, all impulses are conducted from the atria into the ventricles for a period of time, and then suddenly no impulses at all are transmitted. Particularly does this condition occur in hearts with borderline coronary ischemia.

Immediately after A-V conduction is first blocked, the ventricles stop contracting entirely for about 5 to 10 seconds. Then some part of the Purkinje system beyond the block, usually in the A-V bundle itself, begins discharging rhythmically at a rate of 15 to 40 times per minute and acting as the pacemaker of the ventricles. This is called *ventricular escape*. Because the brain cannot remain active for more than 3 to 5 seconds without blood supply, patients usually faint between block of conduction and "escape" of the ventricles. These periodic fainting spells are known as the Stokes-Adams syndrome.

PREMATURE CONTRACTIONS

A premature contraction is a contraction of the heart prior to the time when normal contraction would have been expected. This condition is also frequently called *premature beat* or *extrasystole*.

Most premature contractions result from *ectopic foci* in the heart, which emit abnormal impulses at odd times during the cardiac rhythm. The possible causes of ectopic foci are (1) local areas of ischemia, (2) small calcified plaques at different points in the heart, which press against the adjacent cardiac muscle so that some of the fibers are irritated, and (3) toxic irritation of the A-V node, Purkinje system, or myocardium caused by drugs, nicotine, caffeine, and so forth.

Atrial Premature Contraction. Figure 10–11 illustrates an electrocardiogram showing a single atrial premature contraction (premature beat). The P wave of this beat is relatively normal and the QRS complex is also normal, but the interval between the preceding beat and the premature beat is shortened. Also, the interval between the premature beat and the next succeeding beat is slightly prolonged. The reason is that the premature beat originated in the atrium at some distance from the S-A node, and the impulse of the premature beat had to travel through a short distance of atrial muscle before it discharged the S-A node. Consequently, the S-A node discharged late in the cycle and made the succeeding heartbeat also late in appearing.

Premature Ventricular Contractions. The electrocardiogram of Figure 10–12 illustrates a series of premature ventricular contractions (called PVCs) alternating with normal beats. Premature ventricular contractions cause several special effects in the electrocardiogram, as follows: First, the QRS complex is usually considerably prolonged. The reason is that the impulse is conducted mainly through the muscle of the ventricles rather than through the Purkinje system.

Second, the QRS complex has a very high voltage, for the following reason: When the normal impulse passes through the heart, it passes through both

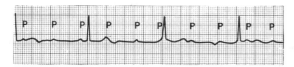

Figure 10–10. Complete atrioventricular block (lead II).

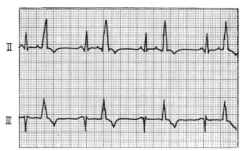

Figure 10–12. Premature ventricular contractions (PVCs) illustrated by the large abnormal QRS-T complexes (leads II and III).

ventricles approximately simultaneously; consequently, the depolarization waves of the two sides of the heart partially neutralize each other. However, when a premature ventricular contraction occurs, the impulse travels in only one direction so that there is no such neutralization effect.

Third, following almost all premature ventricular contractions, the T wave has a potential opposite to that of the QRS complex because the *slow conduction of the impulse* through the cardiac muscle causes the area first depolarized to repolarize first as well. As a result, the direction of the potential in the heart during repolarization is opposite to that during depolarization. This is not true of the normal T wave, as was explained earlier in the chapter.

Some premature ventricular contractions result from simple factors such as cigarettes, coffee, lack of sleep, various mild toxic states, and even emotional irritability. On the other hand, a large share of ventricular premature beats result from some actual pathologic condition of the heart. For instance, many ventricular premature beats occur following coronary thrombosis because of stray impulses originating around the borders of the infarcted area of the heart.

PAROXYSMAL TACHYCARDIA

The term *tachycardia* means rapid rate of heartbeat. Abnormalities in any portion of the heart, including the atria, the Purkinje system, and the ventricles, can sometimes cause rapid rhythmic discharge of impulses which then spread through the heart, thus "pacing" the heart at a rapid rate of contraction.

Atrial Paroxysmal Tachycardia. Figure 10-13 illustrates a sudden increase in rate of heartbeat from approximately 95 beats per minute to approximately 150 beats per minute. Close analysis of the electrocardiogram shows that an inverted P wave occurs before each of the QRS-T complexes during the paroxysm of rapid heartbeat, though this P wave is partially superimposed on the normal T wave of the preceding beat. This indicates that the origin of this particular paroxysmal tachycardia is in the atrium, but because the P wave is abnormal, the origin is not near the S-A node.

Ventricular Paroxysmal Tachycardia. Figure 10-14 illustrates a typical short paroxysm of ventricular tachycardia. The electrocardiogram of ventricular paroxysmal tachycardia has the appearance of a series of ventricular premature beats occurring one after another without any normal beats interspersed.

Ventricular paroxysmal tachycardia is usually a

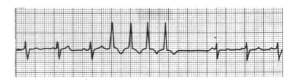

Figure 10-14. Ventricular paroxysmal tachycardia (lead III).

serious condition for two reasons. First, this type of tachycardia usually does not occur unless considerable damage is present in the ventricles. Second, ventricular tachycardia predisposes to ventricular fibrillation, which is almost invariably fatal.

ABNORMAL RHYTHMS RESULTING FROM CIRCUS MOVEMENTS

The circus movement phenomenon was discussed in detail in Chapter 9, and it was pointed out that these movements can cause atrial flutter, atrial fibrillation, and ventricular fibrillation.

Atrial Flutter. Figure 10-15 illustrates the electrocardiogram of atrial flutter. The rate of atrial contraction (P waves) is approximately 300 times per minute, while the rate of ventricular contraction (QRS-T waves) is only 125 times per minute. From the record it will be seen that sometimes a 2:1 rhythm occurs and sometimes a 3:1 rhythm. In other words, the atria beat two or three times for every one impulse that is conducted through the A-V bundle into the ventricles.

Atrial Fibrillation. Figure 10-16 illustrates the electrocardiogram during atrial fibrillation. As was discussed in Chapter 9, numerous impulses spread in all directions through the atria during atrial fibrillation. The intervals between impulses arriving at the A-V node are extremely variable. Therefore, an impulse may arrive at the A-V node immediately after the node itself is out of its refractory period from its previous discharge, or it may not arrive there for several tenths of a second. Consequently, the rhythm of the ventricles is very irregular, many of the ventricular beats falling quite close together and many far apart, the overall ventricular rate being 125 to 150 beats per minute in most instances. On the other hand, the QRS-T complexes are entirely normal unless there is some simultaneous pathological condition of the ventricles.

The pumping effectiveness of the heart in atrial fibrillation is considerably depressed because the ventricles often do not have sufficient time to become filled between beats.

Ventricular Fibrillation. In ventricular fibrillation

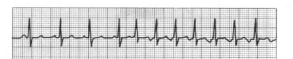

Figure 10-13. Atrial paroxysmal tachycardia—onset in middle of record (lead I).

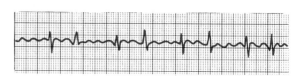

Figure 10-15. Atrial flutter—2:1 and 3:1 rhythm (lead II).

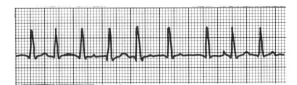

Figure 10-16. Atrial fibrillation (lead I).

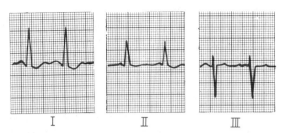

I   II   III

Figure 10-18. Left axis deviation in hypertensive heart disease. Note the slightly prolonged QRS complex.

the electrocardiogram is extremely bizarre, as shown in Figure 10–17, and ordinarily shows no tendency toward a rhythm of any type. The irregularity of this electrocardiogram is what would be expected from multiple impulses traveling in all directions through the heart, as explained in the previous chapter. *Obviously, this condition is immediately lethal.*

ELECTROCARDIOGRAPHIC INTERPRETATION IN NON-ARRHYTHMIC CARDIAC ABNORMALITIES

From the discussion in Chapter 9 of impulse transmission through the heart, it is obvious that any change in the pattern of this transmission can cause abnormal electrical currents around the heart and, consequently, can alter the shapes of the waves in the electrocardiogram. For this reason, almost all serious abnormalities of the heart can be detected by analyzing the contours of the different waves in the different electrocardiographic leads. The purpose of the present section is to present several representative electrocardiograms when the muscle of the heart, especially of the ventricles, contracts abnormally.

THE MEAN ELECTRICAL AXIS OF THE VENTRICLES

It was shown in Figure 10–4 that during most of the cycle of ventricular depolarization, the polarity of the electrical potential is from the base of the ventricle toward the apex—that is, the base of the ventricle is negative, and the apex is positive. This preponderant direction of potential during depolarization is called the *mean electrical axis of the ventricles*. The mean electrical axis of the normal ventricles is 59 degrees (zero degrees is toward the left side of the heart, and the axis is measured clockwise from this direction). However, in certain pathological conditions of the heart, the direction of the potential is changed markedly—sometimes even to opposite poles of the heart.

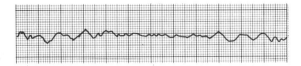

Figure 10-17. Ventricular fibrillation (lead II).

HYPERTROPHY OF ONE VENTRICLE

When one ventricle becomes greatly hypertrophied, the principal direction of the electrical potential in the heart during depolarization—that is, the axis of the heart—shifts toward the hypertrophied ventricle for two reasons. First, far greater quantity of muscle exists on the hypertrophied side of the heart than on the other side, and this allows excess generation of electrical current on that side. Second, more time is required for the depolarization wave to travel through the hypertrophied ventricle than through the normal ventricle. Consequently, the normal ventricle becomes depolarized (negative) considerably in advance of the hypertrophied ventricle, and this causes a strong potential from the normal side of the heart toward the hypertrophied side. Thus the axis deviates toward the hypertrophied ventricle.

Left Axis Deviation Resulting From Hypertrophy of the Left Ventricle. Figure 10–18 illustrates the three standard leads of an electrocardiogram in which the potential is strongly positive in lead I and strongly negative in lead III. This means that the major axis of the potential in the heart is mainly in the direction of lead I, which is from right arm toward left arm; and the potential is opposite to the direction of lead III, which is from left arm toward left leg. That is, the axis of the heart points upward toward the left shoulder. This is called *left axis deviation* because it is to the left of the normal axis of the heart which points downward and only slightly to the left in the chest.

The electrocardiogram of Figure 10–18 is typical of that resulting from increased muscular mass of the left ventricle. In this instance the axis deviation was caused by *high blood pressure*, which caused the left ventricle to hypertrophy in order to pump blood against the elevated systemic arterial pressure. However, a similar picture of left axis deviation occurs when the left ventricle hypertrophies as a result of aortic valvular stenosis, aortic valvular regurgitation, or any of a number of congenital heart conditions in which the left ventricle enlarges while the right side of the heart remains relatively normal in size.

Right axis deviation occurs when the right ventricle enlarges. That is, the potential in lead I then becomes negative while that in lead III becomes strongly positive.

BUNDLE BRANCH BLOCK

Ordinarily, the two lateral walls of the ventricles depolarize at almost the same time, because both the left and right bundle branches transmit the cardiac impulse to the endocardial surfaces of the two ventricular walls at almost the same instant. As a result, the potentials from the walls of the two ventricles almost exactly neutralize each other. However, if one of the major bundle branches is blocked, depolarization of the two ventricles does not occur even nearly simultaneously, and the depolarization potentials do not neutralize each other. As a result, axis deviation occurs, as follows:

Right or Left Bundle Branch Block. When the right bundle branch is blocked, the left ventricle depolarizes far more rapidly than the right ventricle (because the normal left bundle still conducts a rapid signal to the left ventricle), so that the left becomes electronegative while the right remains electropositive. Therefore, a very strong potential develops with its negative end toward the left ventricle and its positive end toward the right ventricle. In other words, intense right axis deviation occurs because the positive end of the axis is to the right of the normal downward direction.

Right axis deviation (denoted especially by the very negative QRS in lead I) caused by right bundle branch block is illustrated in Figure 10–19, which also shows a prolonged QRS complex due to blocked conduction.

Left bundle branch block causes the opposite effect, namely, left axis deviation but also prolonged QRS complex.

CURRENT OF INJURY

Many different cardiac abnormalities, especially those that damage the heart muscle itself, cause part of the heart to remain *depolarized all the time.* When this occurs, current flows between the pathologically depolarized and the normally polarized areas. This is called a *current of injury.* The most common cause

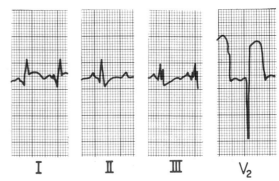

Figure 10–20. Current of injury in acute anterior wall infarction. Note the intense current of injury in lead V_2.

of a current of injury is *ischemia of the muscle caused by coronary occlusion.*

Effect of Current Injury on the QRS Complex—The S-T Segment Shift. It will be recalled that in the normal heart no electrical current flows from the heart when the heart is totally polarized during the T-P interval or when the heart is totally depolarized during the S-T interval. Therefore, in the normal electrocardiogram, both the T-P and the S-T intervals record on the same level. However, when there is a current of injury, the heart cannot completely repolarize during the T-P interval. For this reason, the potential level of the T-P interval is different from that of the S-T interval. This effect is called the *S-T segment shift,* which unfortunately is a misnomer because the abnormality is actually a T-P segment shift.

Acute Anterior Wall Infarction. Figure 10–20 illustrates the electrocardiogram in the three standard leads and in one chest lead recorded from a patient with acute anterior wall cardiac infarction caused by coronary thrombosis. (*Infarction* means loss of coronary blood flow.) The most important diagnostic feature of this electrocardiogram is the current of injury *in the chest lead* (V_2 lead) as denoted by the S-T segment shift (the broad wave at the top of the record following the QRS complex).

Posterior Wall Infarction. Figure 10–21 illustrates the three standard leads and one chest lead from a patient with posterior wall infarction. The major diagnostic feature of this electrocardiogram is the S-T segment shift in the chest lead (V_2 lead) and in leads II and III.

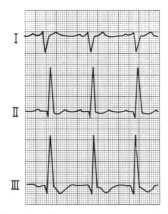

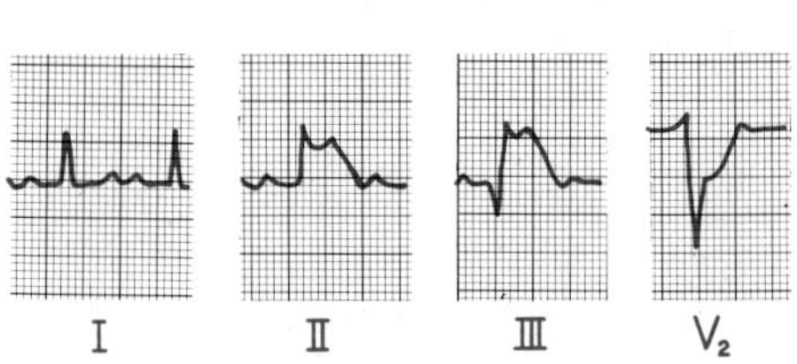

Figure 10–19. Right axis deviation due to right bundle branch block. Note the greatly prolonged QRS complex.

Figure 10–21. Current of injury in acute posterior wall, apical infarction.

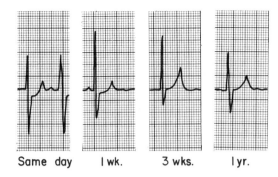

Same day   I wk.   3 wks.   I yr.

Figure 10–22. Recovery of the myocardium following moderate posterior wall infarction, illustrating disappearance of the current of injury (lead V₃).

Recovery from Coronary Thrombosis. Figure 10–22 illustrates the chest lead from a patient with posterior wall infarction, showing the change in this chest lead from the day of the attack to one week later, then three weeks later, and finally one year later. From this electrocardiogram it can be seen that a slight current of injury (S-T segment shift) is present immediately after the acute attack, but after approximately one week the current of injury has diminished considerably and after three weeks it is completely gone. After that, the electrocardiogram changes slightly during the following year because of progressive repair of the damaged muscle.

QUESTIONS

1. Explain what is meant by a *depolarization wave* and by a *repolarization wave* in the electrocardiogram. Which of the normal electrocardiographic waves are depolarization and which are repolarization waves?
2. At what point in the monophasic action potential of ventricular cardiac muscle does the QRS wave occur? At what point does the T wave occur?
3. Explain the voltage and time calibration marks on the electrocardiogram.
4. What is the significance of the *P-Q interval*?
5. Draw a diagram of the heart showing the flow of current around the ventricles when they are approximately half depolarized.
6. Explain the connections of the electrodes to the body for recording the three standard limb leads.
7. Explain how the electrocardiographic chest leads are recorded.
8. What are the characteristics of the electrocardiogram in *incomplete heart block* and *complete heart block*?
9. Describe the characteristics of the electrocardiogram when either *atrial* or *ventricular premature contractions* occur. Explain the differences between the electrocardiographic patterns.
10. Describe the electrocardiogram in *atrial paroxysmal tachycardia*.
11. Describe the electrocardiographic pattern in *atrial fibrillation* and in *ventricular fibrillation*. Explain the irregular timing of the heart beat in atrial fibrillation.
12. What is meant by the mean electrical axis of the ventricles?
13. Explain why the electrical axis deviates to the left in both *hypertrophy* of the left ventricle and *left bundle branch block*.
14. What is the cause of *current of injury* in the electrocardiogram? How can it be used to determine the locus of a myocardial infarct in the heart?

References

Brown, H. F.: Electrophysiology of the sinoatrial node. Physiol Rev 62:505, 1982.

Burch, G. E., and Winsor, T.: A Primer of Electrocardiography, 6th ed. Philadelphia, Lea & Febiger, 1972.

Chou, T.: Electrocardiography in Clinical Practice. New York, Grune & Stratton, 1979.

Chung, E. K.: Electrocardiography: Practical Applications With Vectorial Principles, 2nd ed. Hagerstown, Md., Harper & Row, 1980.

Gilmour, R. F., Jr., and Zipes, D. P.: Slow inward current and cardiac arrhythmias. Am J Cardiol 55:89B, 1985.

Goldman, M. J.: Principles of Clinical Electrocardiography. Los Altos, Calif., Lange Medical Publications, 1982.

Guyton, A. C., and Crowell, J. W.: A stereovectorcardiograph. J Lab Clin Med 40:726, 1952.

Lipman, B.: Clinical Electrocardiography. Chicago, Year Book Medical Publishers, 1984.

Morganroth, J.: Ambulatory Holter electrocardiography: choice of technologies and clinical uses. Ann Intern Med 102:73, 1985.

Narula, O. S., ed.: Cardiac Arrhythmias: Electrophysiology, Diagnosis, and Management. Baltimore, Williams & Wilkins, 1979.

Pick, A., and Langendorf, R.: Interpretation of Complex Arrhythmias. Philadelphia, Lea & Febiger, 1980.

Summerall, C. P.: Monitoring Heart Rhythm. New York, John Wiley & Sons, 1982.

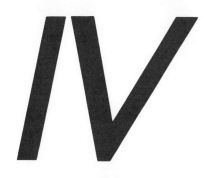

IV

THE CIRCULATION

11 ■ Physics of Blood, Blood Flow, and Pressure: Hemodynamics

12 ■ The Systemic and Pulmonary Circulations

13 ■ Local Control of Blood Flow by the Tissues; Nervous and Humoral Regulation

14 ■ Nervous Reflex and Hormonal Mechanisms for Short-Term Arterial Pressure Control

15 ■ Long-Term Regulation of Mean Arterial Pressure; Hypertension

16 ■ Cardiac Output and Circulatory Shock

17 ■ Coronary Blood Flow: Cardiac Failure; Heart Sounds; Valvular and Congenital Heart Defects

18 ■ Muscle Blood Flow During Exercise; Cerebral, Splanchnic, and Skin Blood Flows

11

Physics of Blood, Blood Flow, and Pressure: Hemodynamics

THE PHYSICAL CHARACTERISTICS OF
  BLOOD
  THE HEMATOCRIT
  PLASMA
INTERRELATIONSHIPS AMONG
  PRESSURE, FLOW, AND RESISTANCE
  BLOOD FLOW
  BLOOD PRESSURE
  RESISTANCE TO BLOOD FLOW

VASCULAR DISTENSIBILITY
  *VASCULAR COMPLIANCE (OR
    CAPACITANCE)*
  *VOLUME-PRESSURE CURVES OF THE
    ARTERIAL AND VENOUS
    CIRCULATIONS*
  *THE MEAN CIRCULATORY FILLING
    PRESSURE*
DELAYED COMPLIANCE (STRESS-
  RELAXATION) OF VESSELS

Figure 11–1 illustrates the general plan of the circulation, showing its two major subdivisions, the *systemic circulation* and the *pulmonary circulation*. In the figure the arteries of each subdivision are represented by a distensible chamber and all the veins by another even larger distensible chamber, and the arterioles and capillaries are shown as very small connections between the arteries and veins. There is almost no resistance to blood flow in all the large vessels of the circulation, but this is not the case in arterioles and capillaries. To cause blood to flow through these small "resistance" vessels, the heart pumps the blood into the arteries under high pressure—normally at a systolic pressure of about 120 mm Hg in the systemic system and 22 mm Hg in the pulmonary system.

As a first step toward explaining the overall function of the circulation, this chapter will discuss the physical characteristics of blood itself and then the physical principles of blood flow through the vessels, especially the interrelationships among pressure, flow, and resistance. The study of these interrelationships and other basic physical principles of blood circulation is called *hemodynamics*.

THE PHYSICAL CHARACTERISTICS OF BLOOD

Blood is a viscous fluid composed of *cells* and *plasma*. More than 99 per cent of the cells are red blood cells; this means that for practical purposes the white blood cells play almost no role in determining the physical characteristics of the blood.

THE HEMATOCRIT

The per cent of the blood that is cells is called the hematocrit. Thus, if a person has a hematocrit of 40, 40 per cent of the blood volume is cells and the remainder is plasma. The hematocrit of the normal man averages about 42, while that of the normal woman averages about 38. These values vary tremendously, depending upon whether or not the person has anemia, the degree of bodily activity, and the altitude at which the person resides.

Effect of Hematocrit on Blood Viscosity. Blood is several times as viscous as water, and this viscosity increases the difficulty with which the blood flows through the small vessels. The greater the percentage

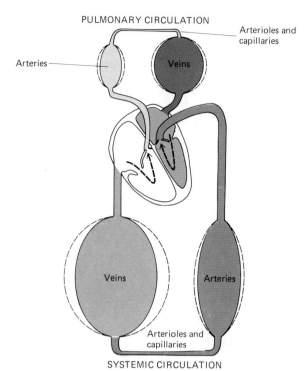

PULMONARY CIRCULATION

SYSTEMIC CIRCULATION

Figure 11–1. Representation of the circulation, showing both the distensible and the resistive portions of the systemic and pulmonary circulations.

of cells in the blood—that is, the greater the hematocrit—the more friction there is between successive layers of blood, and this friction determines viscosity. Therefore, the viscosity of blood increases drastically as the hematocrit increases, as illustrated in Figure 11–2. If we consider the viscosity of water to be 1, then the viscosity of whole blood at normal hematocrit is about 3; this means that three times as much pressure is required to force whole blood in contrast to water through the same tube. Note that when the hematocrit rises to 60 or 70, which it often does in polycythemia as discussed in Chapter 19, the blood viscosity can become as great as ten times that of water, and its flow through blood vessels is greatly retarded.

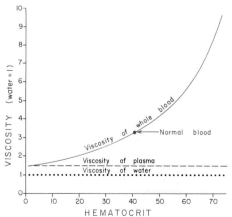

Figure 11–2. Effect of hematocrit on viscosity.

Another factor that affects blood viscosity is the concentration and types of proteins in the plasma, but these effects are so much less important than the effect of hematocrit that they are not significant considerations in most hemodynamic studies. The viscosity of blood plasma is about 1.5 times that of water.

PLASMA

Plasma is part of the extracellular fluid of the body. It is almost identical to the interstitial fluid found between the tissue cells except for one major difference: plasma contains about 7 per cent protein, while interstitial fluid contains an average of only 2 to 3 per cent protein. The reason for this difference is that plasma protein leaks only slightly through the capillary pores into the interstitial spaces. As a result, most of the plasma protein is held in the circulatory system, and that which does leak is soon returned to the circulation by the lymph vessels.

The Types of Protein in Plasma. The plasma protein is divided into three major types, as follows:

	Grams per Deciliter
Albumin	4.5
Globulins	2.5
Fibrinogen	0.3

The primary function of the *albumin* (and of the other types of protein to a lesser extent) is to cause osmotic pressure at the capillary membrane. This pressure, called *colloid osmotic pressure*, prevents the fluid of the plasma from leaking out of the capillaries into the interstitial spaces. This function is so important that it is discussed in detail in Chapter 22.

The globulins are divided into three major types: alpha, beta, and gamma globulins. The *alpha* and *beta globulins* perform diverse functions in the circulation, such as transporting various substances by combining reversibly with them or acting as substrate for formation of other substances. The *gamma globulins,* and to a lesser extent the *beta globulins,* play a special role in protecting the body against infection, for it is these globulins that are mainly the *antibodies* that resist infection and toxicity, thus providing the body with what we call *immunity*. The function of immunity is discussed in detail in Chapter 20.

The *fibrinogen* of plasma is of basic importance in blood clotting and is discussed in Chapter 21.

INTERRELATIONSHIPS AMONG PRESSURE, FLOW, AND RESISTANCE

Flow through a blood vessel is determined entirely by two factors: (1) the *pressure difference* between the two ends of the vessel, which is the net force that pushes the blood through the vessel, and (2) the impediment to blood flow through the vessel, which

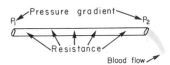

Figure 11–3. Relationships among pressure, resistance, and blood flow.

is called vascular *resistance.* Figure 11–3 illustrates these relationships, showing a blood vessel segment located anywhere in the circulatory system.

P_1 represents the pressure at the origin of the vessel; at the other end the pressure is P_2. The flow through the vessel can be calculated by the following formula, which is called *Ohm's law:*

$$Q = \frac{\Delta P}{R}$$

in which Q is blood flow, ΔP is the pressure difference $(P_1 - P_2)$ between the two ends of the vessel, and R is the resistance. This formula states, in effect, that the blood flow is directly related to the pressure difference but inversely related to the resistance.

It should be noted especially that it is the *difference* in pressure between the two ends of the vessel that determines the rate of flow and not the absolute pressure in the vessel. For instance, if the absolute pressure at both ends of the segment were 100 mm Hg and yet no difference existed between the two ends, there would be no flow despite the presence of 100 mm Hg pressure.

Ohm's law expresses the most important of all the relationships that the student needs to understand to comprehend the hemodynamics of the circulation. Because of the extreme importance of this formula,

the student should also become familiar with its other two algebraic forms:

$$\Delta P = Q \times R$$

$$R = \frac{\Delta P}{Q}$$

BLOOD FLOW

Blood flow means simply the quantity of blood that passes a given point in the circulation in a given period of time. Ordinarily, blood flow is expressed in *milliliters* or *liters per minute,* but it can be expressed in milliliters per second or in any other unit of flow.

The overall blood flow in the circulation of an adult person at rest is about 5000 ml per minute. This is called the *cardiac output* because it is the amount of blood pumped by the heart in a unit period of time.

Methods for Measuring Blood Flow. Many different mechanical or mechanoelectrical devices can be inserted in series with a blood vessel, or in some instances applied to the outside of the vessel, to measure flow. These are called simply *flowmeters.*

The Electromagnetic Flowmeter. One of the most important devices for measuring blood flow is the electromagnetic flowmeter, the principles of which are illustrated in Figure 11–4. Figure 11–4A shows generation of electromotive force in a wire that is moved rapidly through a magnetic field. This is the well-known principle for production of electricity by the electric generator. Figure 11–4B shows that exactly the same principle applies for generation of electrical current in blood when it moves through a magnetic field. In this case, a blood vessel is placed between the poles of a strong magnet, and electrodes

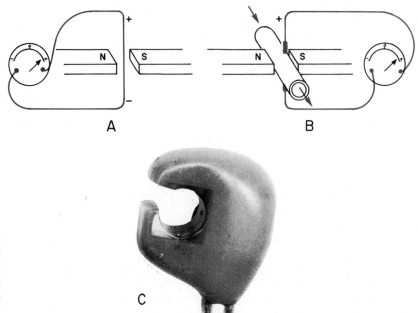

Figure 11–4. A flowmeter of the electromagnetic type, showing *A,* generation of an electromotive force in a wire as it passes through an electromagnetic field; *B,* generation of electromotive force in electrodes on a blood vessel when the vessel is placed in a strong magnetic field and blood flows through the vessel; and *C,* a modern electromagnetic flowmeter "probe" for chronic implantation around blood vessels.

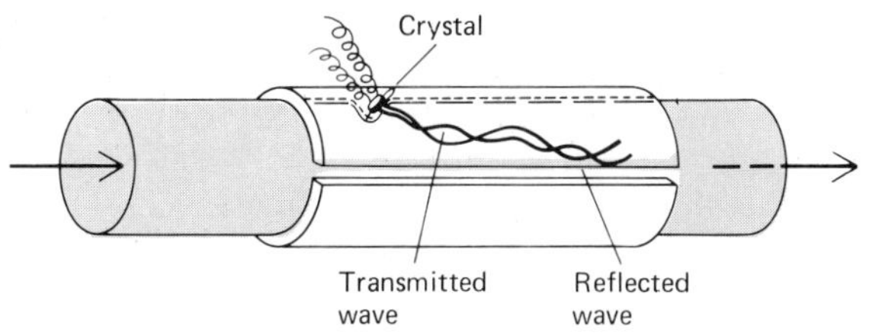

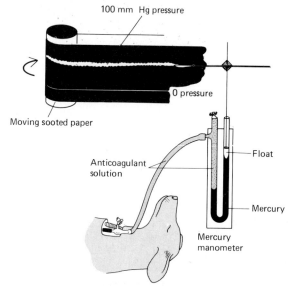

Figure 11–5. An ultrasonic Doppler flowmeter.

are placed on the two sides of the vessel perpendicular to the magnetic lines of force. When blood flows through the vessel, electrical voltage proportional to the rate of flow is generated between the two electrodes, and this is recorded using an appropriate meter or electronic apparatus. Figure 11–4C illustrates an actual "probe" that is placed on a large blood vessel to record its blood flow. This probe contains both the strong magnet and the electrodes.

A special advantage of the electromagnetic flowmeter is that it can record changes in flow that occur in less than 0.01 second, allowing accurate recording of pulsatile changes in flow as well as steady flow.

The Ultrasonic Doppler Flowmeter. Another type of flowmeter that can be applied to the outside of the vessel and that has many of the same advantages as the electromagnetic flowmeter is the ultrasonic Doppler flowmeter illustrated in Figure 11–5. A minute piezoelectric crystal is mounted in the wall of the device. This crystal, when energized with an appropriate electronic apparatus, transmits sound at a frequency of several million cycles per second downstream along the flowing blood. A portion of the sound is reflected by the flowing red blood cells so that reflected sound waves travel backward upstream toward the crystal. However, these reflected waves have a lower frequency than the transmitted wave because the red cells are moving away from the transmitter crystal. This is called the Doppler effect. (It is the same effect that one experiences when a train approaches a listener and passes by while blowing the whistle. Once the whistle has passed by the person, the pitch of the sound from the whistle suddenly becomes much lower than when the train is approaching.) The transmitted wave is intermittently cut off and the reflected wave is received back onto the crystal, then amplified greatly by the electronic apparatus. Another portion of the apparatus determines the frequency difference between the transmitted wave and the reflected wave, thus also determining the velocity of blood flow.

Like the electromagnetic flowmeter, the ultrasonic Doppler flowmeter is capable of recording very rapid, pulsatile changes in flow as well as steady flow.

Laminar Flow of Blood in Vessels. When blood flows at a steady rate through a long, smooth vessel, it flows in *streamlines*, with each layer of blood remaining the same distance from the wall. Also, the central portion of the blood stays in the center of the vessel. This type of flow is called *laminar flow* or *streamline flow,* and it is opposite to *turbulent flow,*

which is blood flowing in all directions in the vessel and continually mixing within the vessel, as will be discussed below.

Turbulent Flow of Blood Under Some Conditions. When the rate of blood flow becomes too great, when it passes an obstruction in a vessel, when it makes a sharp turn, or when it passes over a rough surface, the flow may then become *turbulent* rather than laminar. Turbulent flow means that the blood flows crosswise in the vessel as well as along the vessel, usually forming whorls in the blood called *eddy currents.* These are similar to the whirlpools that one frequently sees in a rapidly flowing river at a point of obstruction.

When eddy currents are present, the resistance to blood flow is much greater than when the flow is streamline because the eddies add tremendously to the overall friction of flow in the vessel.

BLOOD PRESSURE

The Standard Units of Pressure. Blood pressure is almost always measured in *millimeters of mercury (mm Hg)* because the mercury manometer (shown in Figure 11–6) has been used as the standard reference for measuring blood pressure throughout the history of physiology. Actually, blood pressure means the *force exerted by the blood against any unit area of the vessel wall.* When one says that the pressure in a vessel is 50 mm Hg, this means that the force exerted is sufficient to push a column of mercury up to a level 50 mm high. If the pressure is 100 mm Hg, it will push the column of mercury up to 100 mm.

Occasionally, pressure is measured in *centimeters of water.* A pressure of 10 cm of water means a pressure sufficient to raise a column of water to a height of 10 cm. *One millimeter of mercury equals*

Figure 11–6. Recording arterial pressure with a mercury manometer, a method that has been used in the manner shown above for recording pressure throughout the history of physiology.

1.36 cm of water because the specific gravity of mercury is 13.6 times that of water, and 1 cm is 10 times as great as 1 mm.

Measurement of Blood Pressure Using the Mercury Manometer. Figure 11–6 illustrates a standard mercury manometer for measuring blood pressure. A cannula or catheter is inserted into an artery, a vein, or even the heart, and the pressure from the cannula or catheter is transmitted to the left-hand side of the manometer where it pushes the mercury down while raising the right-hand mercury column. The difference between the two levels of mercury is approximately equal to the pressure in the circulation in terms of millimeters of mercury.

High-Fidelity Methods for Measuring Blood Pressure. Unfortunately, the mercury in the mercury manometer has so much *inertia* that it cannot rise and fall rapidly. For this reason the mercury manometer, though excellent for recording steady pressures, cannot respond to pressure changes that occur more rapidly than approximately one cycle every 2 to 3 seconds. Whenever it is desired to record rapidly changing pressures, some other type of pressure recorder is needed. Figure 11–7 demonstrates the basic principles of three electronic pressure *transducers* commonly used for converting pressure into electrical signals and then recording the pressure on a high-speed electrical recorder. Each of these transducers employs a very thin and highly stretched metal membrane which forms one wall of the fluid chamber. The fluid chamber in turn is connected through a needle or catheter with the vessel in which the pres-

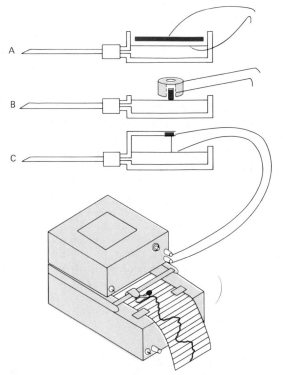

Figure 11–7. Principles of three different types of electronic transducers for recording rapidly changing blood pressures.

sure is to be measured. Pressure variations in the vessel cause changes of pressure in the chamber beneath the membrane. When the pressure is high the membrane bulges outward slightly, and when low it returns toward its resting position.

In Figure 11–7A a simple metal plate is placed a few thousandths of an inch above the membrane. When the membrane bulges outward, the *electrical capacitance* between the plate and membrane increases, and this change in capacitance can be recorded by an appropriate electronic system.

In Figure 11–7B a small iron slug rests on the membrane, and this can be displaced upward into a coil. Movement of the iron changes the *inductance* of the coil, and this, too, can be recorded electronically.

Finally, in Figure 11–7C a very thin, stretched resistance wire is connected to the membrane. When this wire is stretched still more its resistance increases, and when less stretched the resistance decreases. These changes also can be recorded by means of an electronic system.

With some of these high-fidelity types of recording systems, pressure cycles up to 500 cycles per second have been recorded accurately, and in common use are recorders capable of registering pressure changes occurring as rapidly as 20 to 100 cycles per second.

RESISTANCE TO BLOOD FLOW

Units of Resistance. Resistance is the impediment to blood flow in a vessel, but it cannot be measured by any direct means. Instead, resistance must be calculated using Ohm's law, that is, *by dividing the pressure difference by the flow.* If the pressure difference between two points in a vessel is 1 mm Hg and the flow is 1 ml/sec, then the resistance is said to be 1 *peripheral resistance unit,* usually abbreviated *PRU.*

Total Peripheral Resistance and Total Pulmonary Resistance. The rate of blood flow through the circulatory system when a person is at rest is close to 100 ml/sec, and the pressure difference from the systemic arteries to the systemic veins is about 100 mm Hg. Therefore, in round figures the resistance of the entire systemic circulation, called the *total peripheral resistance,* is approximately 100/100 or 1 PRU. In some conditions in which all the blood vessels throughout the body become strongly constricted, the total peripheral resistance rises to as high as 4 PRU, and when the vessels become greatly dilated it can fall to as little as 0.2 PRU.

In the pulmonary system the mean arterial pressure averages 16 mm Hg and the mean left atrial pressure averages 2 mm Hg, giving a net pressure difference of 14 mm. Therefore, in round figures the *total pulmonary resistance* at rest calculates to be about 0.14 PRU. This can increase in disease conditions to as high as 1 PRU and can fall in certain physiological states, such as exercise, to as low as 0.04 PRU.

Conductance of Blood in a Vessel and Its Relationship to Resistance. *Conductance* is a measure of the blood flow through a vessel for a given pressure difference. This is generally expressed in terms of ml/sec/mm Hg pressure, but it can also be expressed in terms of liters/sec/mm Hg or in any other units of blood flow and pressure.

It is immediately evident that conductance is the reciprocal of resistance in accord with the following equation:

$$\text{Conductance} = \frac{1}{\text{Resistance}}$$

Effect of Vascular Diameter on Conductance. Slight changes in the diameter of a vessel cause tremendous changes in its ability to conduct blood when the blood flow is laminar. This is illustrated forcefully by the experiment in Figure 11–8A, which shows three separate vessels with relative diameters of 1, 2, and 4 but with the same pressure difference of 100 mm Hg between the two ends of the vessels. Though the diameters of these vessels increase only fourfold, the respective flows are 1, 16, and 256 ml/mm, which is a 256-fold increase in flow. Thus, the conductance of the vessel increases in proportion to the *fourth power of the diameter,* in accord with the following formula:

$$\text{Conductance} \propto \text{Diameter}^4$$

The cause of this great increase in conductance with an increase in diameter is the following: the blood near the wall of the vessel flows extremely slowly because of the friction of the blood with the vessel wall, whereas blood in the middle of the vessel flows extremely rapidly. In the small vessel essentially all the blood is very near the wall so that the extremely rapidly flowing central stream of blood simply does not exist.

Poiseuille's Law. The quantity of blood that will flow through a vessel in a given period of time is given by the following equation, which is known as *Poiseuille's law:*

$$Q = \frac{\pi \Delta P r^4}{8 \eta l}$$

Note particularly in this equation that the rate of blood flow is directly proportional to the *fourth power of the radius* (r) of the vessel, which illustrates once again that the diameter of a blood vessel plays by far the greatest role of all factors in determining the rate of blood flow through the vessel. Also, the flow is

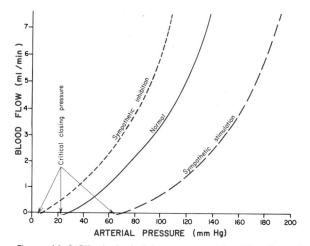

Figure 11–9. Effect of arterial pressure on blood flow through a blood vessel at different degrees of vascular tone caused by increased or decreased sympathetic stimulation of the vessels.

directly proportional to the pressure difference (ΔP) but inversely proportional to the length of the vessel (l) and to the blood viscosity (η).

Effects of Pressure and Sympathetic Nervous Stimulation on Vascular Resistance and Tissue Blood Flow

From the discussions thus far, one would expect that an increase in arterial pressure would cause a direct proportionate increase in blood flow through the various tissues of the body. However, the effect of pressure on blood flow is far greater than one would expect, as illustrated in Figure 11–9. The reason for this is that an increase in arterial pressure not only increases the force that tends to push the blood through the vessels but also distends the vessels at the same time, which increases their conductance, as we shall discuss below. Thus, increased pressure increases the flow in two different ways. Consequently, for most tissues, blood flow at 100 mm Hg arterial pressure is usually about four times as great as the blood flow at 50 mm Hg.

Note also in Figure 11–9 the large changes in blood flow that can be caused by either increased or decreased sympathetic nervous stimulation of the peripheral blood vessels. Thus, inhibition of sympathetic stimulation greatly dilates the vessels and therefore increases the blood flow, sometimes as much as fourfold or more. Conversely, very strong sympathetic stimulation can constrict the vessels so much that blood flow can sometimes be decreased to as low as zero despite high arterial pressure.

VASCULAR DISTENSIBILITY

The diameter of blood vessels, unlike that of metal pipes and glass tubes, increases as the internal pressure increases, because blood vessels are *distensible.* However, the vascular distensibilities differ greatly in

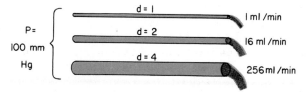

Figure 11–8. Demonstration of the effect of vessel diameter on blood flow.

different segments of the circulation, and, as we shall see in subsequent chapters, this affects significantly the operation of the circulatory system under many changing physiological conditions.

Difference in Distensibility of the Arteries and the Veins. Anatomically, the walls of arteries are far stronger than those of veins. Consequently, the veins, on the average, are about six to ten times as distensible as the arteries. That is, a given rise in pressure will cause about six to ten times as much extra blood to fill a vein as an artery of comparable size.

VASCULAR COMPLIANCE (OR CAPACITANCE)

Usually in hemodynamic studies it is much more important to know the *total quantity of blood* that can be stored in a given portion of the circulation for each mm Hg pressure rise than to know the distensibility of the individual vessels. This value is sometimes called the *total distensibility,* but it is usually expressed still more precisely by either of the terms *compliance* or *capacitance,* which are physical terms meaning the increase in volume that occurs for each given increase in pressure in any vascular area as follows:

$$\text{Vascular compliance} = \frac{\text{Increase in volume}}{\text{Increase in pressure}}$$

Compliance and distensibility are quite different. A highly distensible vessel that has a very slight volume may have far less compliance than a much less distensible vessel that has a very large volume, for *compliance is equal to distensibility × volume.*

The compliance of a vein is about 24 times that of its corresponding artery because it is about 8 times as distensible and it has a volume about 3 times as great ($8 \times 3 = 24$).

VOLUME-PRESSURE CURVES OF THE ARTERIAL AND VENOUS CIRCULATIONS

A convenient method for expressing the relationship of pressure to volume in a vessel or in any specific portion of the circulation is the so-called *volume-pressure curve* (also frequently called the *pressure-volume curve*). The two solid curves of Figure 11–10 represent respectively the volume-pressure curves of the normal arterial and venous systems, showing that when the arterial system, including all the large arteries, the small arteries, and the arterioles, is filled with approximately 750 ml of blood, the mean arterial pressure is 100 mm Hg but when filled with only 500 ml, the pressure falls to zero.

In the entire venous system, on the other hand, the volume of blood normally is about 2500 ml, and tremendous changes in this volume are required to change the venous pressure only a few millimeters of mercury.

Difference in Compliance of the Arterial and Venous Systems. Referring once again to Figure 11–10,

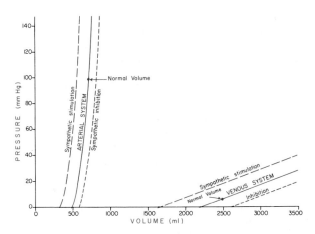

Figure 11–10. Volume-pressure curves of the systemic arterial and venous systems, showing also the effects of sympathetic stimulation to decrease the volume for each pressure level and sympathetic inhibition to increase the volume.

one can see that a change of 1 mm Hg requires a very large change in venous volume but much less change in arterial volume. That is, the *compliance of the venous system is far greater than the compliance of the arterial system—about 24 times as great.*

This difference in compliance is particularly important because it means that tremendous amounts of blood can be stored in the veins with only slight changes in pressure. Therefore, the veins are frequently called *storage areas* of the circulation.

Effect of Sympathetic Stimulation or Sympathetic Inhibition on the Volume-Pressure Relationships of the Arterial and Venous Systems. Also shown in Figure 11–10 are the volume-pressure curves of the arterial and venous systems during moderate sympathetic stimulation and during sympathetic inhibition. It is evident that sympathetic stimulation, with its concomitant increase in smooth muscle tone in the vascular walls, increases the pressure at each volume of the arteries or veins while, on the other hand, sympathetic inhibition decreases the pressure at each respective volume. Obviously, control of the vessels in this manner by the sympathetics is a valuable means for diminishing the dimensions of one segment of the circulation, thus transferring blood to other segments. For instance, an increase in vascular tone throughout the systemic circulation often causes large volumes of blood to shift into the heart, which is a major way in which pumping by the heart is increased.

Sympathetic control of vascular capacity is also especially important during hemorrhage. Enhancement of the sympathetic tone of the vessels, especially of the veins, reduces the dimensions of the circulatory system, and the circulation continues to operate almost normally even when as much as 25 per cent of the total blood volume has been lost.

THE MEAN CIRCULATORY FILLING PRESSURE

The mean circulatory filling pressure (also called the "mean circulatory pressure" or the "static pressure") is a measure of the degree of filling of the entire circulatory system. This is the pressure that one measures everywhere in the circulation if one instantaneously stops all blood flow and brings all the pressures in the circulation immediately to equilibrium. The mean circulatory filling pressure has been estimated reasonably accurately in dogs within 2 to 5 seconds after the heart has been stopped. To do this the heart is thrown into fibrillation by an electrical stimulus, and blood is pumped rapidly from the systemic arteries to the veins to cause pressure equilibration between the two major chambers of the circulation.

The mean circulatory filling pressure measured in the above manner in the normal anesthetized dog is almost exactly 7 mm Hg. It is believed to be about this same value in the human being. However, many different factors can change it, especially change in blood volume and increased or decreased sympathetic stimulation.

The mean circulatory filling pressure is *one of the major factors that determines the rate at which blood flows from the peripheral vascular tree into the right atrium of the heart, which in turn determines the*

cardiac output. This is so important that this relationship will be explained in detail in Chapter 16.

DELAYED COMPLIANCE (STRESS-RELAXATION) OF VESSELS

The term "delayed compliance" means that a vessel exposed to constantly increased pressure will become progressively enlarged because of non-elastic stretch of the vessel wall.

Delayed compliance occurs only slightly in the arteries but to a much greater extent in the veins. As a result, prolonged elevation of venous pressure can often double the blood volume in the venous tree. This is a valuable mechanism by which the circulation can accommodate much extra blood when necessary, such as following too large a transfusion. Also, delayed compliance in the reverse direction is one of the ways in which the circulation automatically adjusts itself over a period of minutes or hours to diminished blood volume after serious hemorrhage.

QUESTIONS

1. What is meant by hematocrit? What is the effect of hematocrit on blood viscosity?
2. Give the characteristics of plasma, especially the types of proteins and their concentrations.
3. State Ohm's law in all of its three different hemodynamic forms.
4. What are the usual units used in expressing blood flow?
5. Explain the function of the electromagnetic flowmeter and of the ultrasonic Doppler flowmeter.
6. Why is laminar flow important in blood vessels?
7. Give the standard units for expressing blood pressure.
8. What are the relative advantages of the mercury monometer versus the high fidelity methods for measuring blood pressure?
9. State the standard units for expressing resistance to blood flow.
10. How does one determine the resistance to blood flow?
11. What is the relationship between resistance to blood flow and conductance of a blood vessel?
12. What is the quantitative relationship between vascular diameter and vascular conductance?
13. How does sympathetic stimulation affect vascular resistance and tissue blood flow?
14. Why is the relationship between pressure and tissue blood flow nonlinear?
15. Explain the difference between vascular distensibility and vascular compliance.
16. How much more compliant is the systemic venous system than the systemic arterial system?
17. Explain what is meant by *mean circulatory filling pressure.*

References

American Physiological Society: Peripheral Circulation and Organ Blood Flow. Washington, D.C., American Physiological Society, 1983.

American Physiological Society: Microcirculation. Washington, D.C., American Physiological Society, 1984.

Chien, S., Usami, S., and Skalak, R.: Blood flow in small tubes. In Renkin, E. M., and Michel, C. C., eds.: Handbook of Physiology. Sec. 2, Vol. 4. Bethesda, American Physiological Society, 1984, p. 217.

Cokelet, G. R.: Rheology and hemodynamics. Annu Rev Physiol 42:311, 1980.

Dobrin, P. B.: Vascular mechanics. In Shepherd, J. T., and Abboud, F. M., eds.: Handbook of Physiology. Sec. 2, Vol. 3. Bethesda, American Physiological Society, 1983, p. 65.

Fukada, E., et al.: Methods to study rheological properties of blood during clotting. Biorheology (Suppl.)1:9, 1984.

Gow, B. S.: Circulation correlates: Vascular impedance, resistance, and capacity. In Bohr, D. F., et al., eds.: Handbook of Physiology. Sec. 2, Vol. 2. Baltimore, Williams & Wilkins, 1980, p. 353.

Guyton, A. C.: Arterial Pressure and Hypertension. Philadelphia, W. B. Saunders Co., 1980.

Guyton, A. C., et al.: Cardiac Output and Its Regulation. Philadelphia, W. B. Saunders Co., 1973.

Kenner, T., ed.: Cardiovascular System Dynamics. Models and Measurements. New York, Plenum Publishing Corp., 1982.

Murphy, R. A.: Mechanics of vascular smooth muscle. In Bohr, D. F., et al., eds.: Handbook of Physiology. Sec. 2, Vol. 2. Baltimore, Williams & Wilkins, 1980, p. 325.

Rodkiewicz, C. M.: Arteries and Arterial Blood Flow. New York, Springer-Verlag, 1983.

Schneck, D. J., and Vawter, D. L., eds.: Biofluid Mechanics. New York, Plenum Press, 1980.

Zweifach, B. W., and Lipowsky, H. H.: Pressure-flow relations in blood and lymph microcirculation. In Renkin, E. M., and Michel, C. C., eds.: Handbook of Physiology. Sec. 2, Vol. 4. Bethesda, American Physiological Society, 1984, p. 251.

12

The Systemic and Pulmonary Circulations

THE SYSTEMIC CIRCULATION
  PRESSURES AND RESISTANCES IN THE
    VARIOUS PORTIONS OF THE
    SYSTEMIC CIRCULATION
  FUNCTION OF THE LARGE ARTERIES
  THE SMALL ARTERIES, ARTERIOLES,
    AND CAPILLARIES
  THE VEINS AND THEIR FUNCTIONS
  PRESSURE PULSES IN THE ARTERIES
THE PULMONARY CIRCULATION
  PHYSIOLOGIC ANATOMY OF THE
    PULMONARY CIRCULATORY
    SYSTEM

PRESSURES IN THE PULMONARY
  SYSTEM
THE BLOOD VOLUME OF THE LUNGS
BLOOD FLOW THROUGH THE LUNGS
  AND ITS DISTRIBUTION
EFFECT OF INCREASED CARDIAC
  OUTPUT ON THE PULMONARY
  CIRCULATION DURING HEAVY
  EXERCISE
SOME PATHOLOGICAL CONDITIONS
  THAT OBSTRUCT BLOOD FLOW
  THROUGH THE LUNGS

The circulation is divided into the *systemic circulation* (also called the peripheral circulation) and the *pulmonary circulation*. Though the vascular system in each separate tissue of the body has its own special characteristics, some general principles of vascular function nevertheless apply in all parts of the system. It is the purpose of the present chapter to discuss these general principles.

The Functional Parts of the Circulation. Before attempting to discuss the details of function in the circulation, it is important to understand the overall role of each of its parts, as follows:

The function of the *arteries* is to transport blood *under high pressure* to the tissues. For this reason the arteries have strong vascular walls, and blood flows rapidly in the arteries.

The *arterioles* are the last small branches of the arterial system, and they act as *control valves* through which blood is released into the capillaries. The arteriole has a strong muscular wall that is capable of closing the arteriole completely or of allowing it to be dilated severalfold, thus having the capability of vastly altering blood flow to the capillaries.

The function of the *capillaries* is to exchange fluid, nutrients, electrolytes, hormones, and other sub-

stances between the blood and the interstitial spaces (or alveoli in the case of the lungs). For this role, the capillary walls are very thin and are permeable to small molecular substances.

The *venules* collect blood from the capillaries; they gradually coalesce into progressively larger veins.

The *veins* function as conduits for transport of blood from the tissues back to the heart. Since the pressure in the venous system is very low, the venous walls are thin. Even so, they are muscular, and this allows them to contract or expand and thereby act as a reservoir for extra blood, either a small or large amount depending upon the needs of the body.

Quantities of Blood in the Different Parts of the Circulation. By far the greater amount of the blood in the circulation is contained in the systemic veins. Figure 12–1 shows this, illustrating that approximately 84 per cent of the entire blood volume of the body is in the systemic circulation, with 64 per cent in the veins, 15 per cent in the arteries, and 5 per cent in the capillaries. The heart contains 7 per cent of the blood, and the pulmonary vessels, 9 per cent. Most surprising is the very low blood volume in the capillaries of the systemic circulation, only about 5 per cent of the total. Yet, it is here that the most

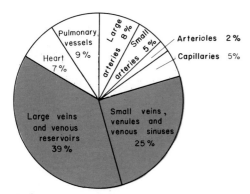

Figure 12–1. Percentage of the total blood volume in each portion of the circulatory system.

important function of the systemic circulation occurs, diffusion of substances back and forth between the blood and the tissues.

THE SYSTEMIC CIRCULATION

PRESSURES AND RESISTANCES IN THE VARIOUS PORTIONS OF THE SYSTEMIC CIRCULATION

Because the heart pumps blood continually into the aorta, the pressure in the aorta is obviously high, averaging almost 100 mm Hg. Also, because the pumping by the heart is pulsatile, the arterial pressure fluctuates between a *systolic level* of 120 mm Hg and a *diastolic level* of 80 mm Hg, as illustrated in Figure 12–2. As the blood flows through the systemic circulation, its pressure falls progressively to approximately 0 mm Hg by the time it reaches the right atrium.

The decrease in arterial pressure in each segment of the systemic circulation is directly proportional to the vascular resistance in the segment. Thus, in the aorta the resistance is almost zero; therefore, the mean arterial pressure at the end of the aorta is still almost 100 mm Hg. Likewise, the resistance in the

large arteries is very slight so that the mean arterial pressure in arteries as small as 3 mm in diameter is still 95 to 97 mm Hg. Then the resistance begins to increase rapidly in the very small arteries, causing the pressure to drop to approximately 85 mm Hg at the beginning of the arterioles.

The resistance of the *arterioles* is greatest of any part of the systemic circulation, accounting for about half the resistance in the entire systemic circulation. Thus, the pressure decreases about 55 mm Hg in the arterioles; therefore, the pressure of the blood as it leaves the arterioles to enter the capillaries is only about 30 mm Hg. Arteriolar resistance is very important in the regulation of blood flow to different tissues of the body and will be discussed in detail later in the chapter and also in the following few chapters.

The pressure at the arterial ends of the *capillaries* is normally about 30 mm Hg and at the venous ends about 10 mm Hg. Therefore, the pressure decrease in the capillaries is only 20 mm Hg, which illustrates that the capillary resistance is only about two fifths that of the arterioles.

The pressure at the beginning of the venous system, that is, at the *venules,* is about 10 mm Hg, and this decreases to almost exactly 0 mm Hg at the right atrium. This considerable decrease in pressure in the veins indicates that the veins have far more resistance than one would expect for vessels of their large sizes. Much of this resistance is caused by compression of the veins from the outside, which keeps many of them, especially the venae cavae, partially collapsed a large share of the time.

FUNCTION OF THE LARGE ARTERIES

The large arteries provide two major functions. The first and most obvious of these is to act as conduits to conduct blood to all the peripheral tissues.

The second important function of the arteries is to serve as a high pressure reservoir to receive the pulsatile output of blood from the heart and to store some of this blood for a few seconds until the next

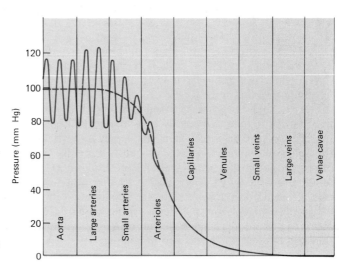

Figure 12–2. Blood pressures in the different portions of the systemic circulatory system.

heartbeat. To serve this function, the large arteries are elastic, which means that they stretch as the pulse of blood from the heart enters the arterial tree. Then they recoil to a smaller size as the blood flows out of the arteries between heartbeats. This elastic nature of the arteries is important for two principal reasons: (1) It prevents the pressure from rising extremely high when the blood is pumped into the arterial tree by ventricular contraction. (2) The elasticity maintains a high arterial pressure between heartbeats so that blood can continue to flow through the tissues without interruption. Therefore, the normal aortic pressure rises only to 120 mm Hg with each heartbeat and falls only to 80 mm Hg between beats.

THE SMALL ARTERIES, ARTERIOLES, AND CAPILLARIES

Upon leaving the small arteries, blood courses through the arterioles, which are only a few millimeters in length and have diameters of from 8 to 50 microns. Each arteriole branches many times to supply 10 to 100 capillaries.

An important characteristic of the small arteries and arterioles is their strong muscular walls. These vessels, as well as the small arteries themselves, are intensely innervated by the sympathetic nervous system and, when stimulated, constrict powerfully. Furthermore, many local factors in the tissues—such as the concentrations of oxygen, carbon dioxide, hydrogen ions, and other factors—can directly affect the degree of constriction of the vessels, especially of the arterioles. Therefore, it is mainly the small arteries and arterioles that control the blood flow to the respective tissues, and this flow is normally controlled almost exactly in proportion to the specific needs of each tissue as will be discussed fully in the following chapter.

There are approximately 10 billion capillaries in the peripheral tissues, and these together have more than 500 square meters of surface area. The thickness of the capillary wall is usually less than 1 micron, and there are small pores in the wall (as will be explained in Chapter 30) through which substances can diffuse.

THE VEINS AND THEIR FUNCTIONS

For years the veins have been considered to be nothing more than passageways for flow of blood into the heart, but it is rapidly becoming apparent that they perform many functions that are necessary to the operation of the circulation. Especially important, they are capable (a) of constricting and enlarging, (b) of storing large quantities of blood and making this blood available when it is required by the remainder of the circulation, (c) of actually propelling blood forward by means of a so-called "venous pump," and even (d) of helping regulate cardiac output, a function that will be described in detail in Chapter 16.

Venous Pressures—Right Atrial Pressure (Central Venous Pressure)

To understand the various functions of the veins, it is first necessary to know something about the pressures in the veins and how they are regulated. Blood from all the systemic veins flows into the right atrium; therefore, the pressure in the right atrium is frequently called the *central venous pressure*. The pressures in the peripheral veins to a great extent depend on the level of this pressure; that is, anything that affects right atrial pressure usually affects venous pressure everywhere in the body.

Right atrial pressure is regulated by a balance between, first, *the ability of the heart to pump blood out of the right atrium* and, second, *the tendency for blood to flow from the peripheral vessels back into the right atrium, which is called venous return.*

If the heart is pumping strongly, the right atrial pressure tends to decrease. On the other hand, weakness of the heart tends to elevate the right atrial pressure. Likewise, any effect that causes rapid inflow of blood into the right atrium from the veins tends to elevate the right atrial pressure. Some of the factors that increase this tendency for venous return (and also to increase the right atrial pressure) are (1) increased blood volume, (2) increased large vessel tone throughout the body with resultant increased peripheral venous pressures, and (3) dilatation of the arterioles, which allows rapid flow of blood from the arteries to the veins.

The *normal right atrial pressure* is approximately 0 mm Hg, which is about equal to the atmospheric pressure around the body. However, it can rise to as high as 20 to 30 mm Hg under very abnormal conditions, such as (a) serious heart failure or (b) following massive transfusion of blood, which will cause excessive quantities of blood to attempt to flow into the heart from the peripheral vessels.

The lower limit to the right atrial pressure is usually about −3 to −5 mm Hg, which is the pressure in the chest cavity surrounding the heart. The right atrial pressure approaches these very low values when the heart pumps with exceptional vigor or when the flow of blood into the heart from the peripheral vessels is greatly depressed, such as following severe hemorrhage.

Effect of Hydrostatic Pressure on Venous Pressure

In any body of water, the pressure at the surface of the water is equal to atmospheric pressure, but the pressure rises 1 mm Hg for each 13.6 mm distance below the surface. This pressure results from the weight of the water and therefore is called *hydrostatic pressure*.

Hydrostatic pressure also occurs in the vascular system of the human being because of the weight of the blood in the vessels, as is illustrated in Figure 12–3. When a person is standing, the pressure in the right

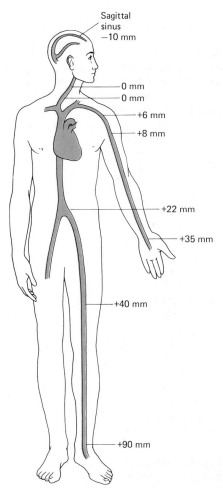

Figure 12-3. Effect of hydrostatic pressure on the venous pressures throughout the body.

atrium remains approximately 0 mm Hg because the heart pumps into the arteries any excess blood that attempts to accumulate at this point. However, in an adult *who is standing absolutely still* the pressure in the veins of the feet is approximately +90 mm Hg simply because of the weight of the blood in the veins between the heart and the feet. The venous pressures at other levels of the body lie proportionately between 0 and 90 mm Hg.

The neck veins collapse almost completely all the way to the skull owing to atmospheric pressure on the outside of the neck. This collapse causes the pressure in these veins to remain zero along their entire extent. The reason for this is that any tendency for the pressure to rise above this level opens the veins and allows the pressure to fall back to zero, and any tendency for the pressure to fall below this level collapses the veins still more, which increases their resistance and again returns the pressure back to zero.

The veins inside the skull, however, are in a noncollapsible chamber, and they will not collapse. Consequently, *negative pressure can exist in the dural sinuses of the head;* in the standing position the venous pressure in the sagittal sinus is approximately −10

mm Hg because of the hydrostatic "suction" between the top of the skull and the base of the skull. Therefore, if the sagittal sinus is opened during surgery, air can be sucked immediately into this vein; the air may even pass downward to cause air embolism in the heart so that the heart valves will not function satisfactorily, and death often ensues.

Effect of the Hydrostatic Factor on Arterial and Other Pressures. The hydrostatic factor also affects the peripheral pressures in the arteries and capillaries as well as in the veins. For instance, a standing person who has an arterial pressure of 100 mm Hg at the level of the heart has an arterial pressure in the feet of about 190 mm Hg. Therefore, any time one states that the arterial pressure is 100 mm Hg, it only means that this is the pressure at the hydrostatic level of the heart.

Venous Valves, the Venous Pump, and Venous Pressure

Because of hydrostatic pressure, the venous pressure in the feet would always be about +90 mm Hg in a standing adult were it not for the valves in the veins. However, every time one moves the legs one tightens the muscles and compresses the veins either in the muscles or adjacent to them, and this squeezes the blood out of the veins. Yet, the valves in the veins, as illustrated in Figure 12-4, are arranged so that the direction of blood flow can be only toward the heart. Consequently, every time a person moves the legs or even tenses the muscles, a certain amount of blood is propelled toward the heart, and the pressure in the veins of the body is lowered. This pumping system is known as the "venous pump" or "muscle pump," and it is efficient enough that under

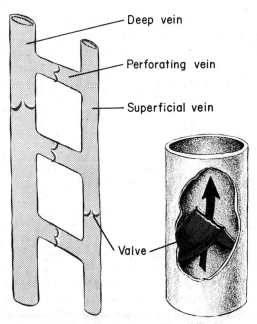

Figure 12-4. The venous valves of the leg.

ordinary circumstances the venous pressure in the feet of a walking adult remains less than 25 mm Hg.

If the human being stands perfectly still, the venous pump does not work, and the venous pressures in the lower part of the leg can then rise to the full hydrostatic value of 90 mm Hg in about 30 seconds. Under such circumstances the pressures within the capillaries also increase greatly, and fluid leaks from the circulatory system into the tissue spaces. As a result, the legs swell, and the blood volume diminishes. Indeed, as much as 15 to 20 per cent of the blood volume is frequently lost from the circulatory system within the first 15 minutes of standing absolutely still, as often occurs when a soldier is made to stand at absolute attention.

Venous Valve Incompetence and Varicose Veins. The valves of the venous system frequently become "incompetent" or sometimes are even destroyed. This is especially true when the veins have been overstretched by an excess of venous pressure for a prolonged period of time, as occurs in pregnancy or when one stands most of the time. Stretching the veins obviously increases their cross-sectional areas, but the valves do not increase in size. Therefore, the valves of the veins will no longer close completely and block reverse blood flow in the enlarged veins. When this develops, the pressure in the veins of the legs increases still more owing to failure of the venous pump; this further increases the size of the veins and finally destroys the function of the valves entirely. Thus, the person develops "varicose veins," which are characterized by large, bulbous protrusions of the veins beneath the skin of the entire leg and particularly of the lower leg.

Blood Reservoir Function of the Veins

It was pointed out earlier in this chapter that over 60 per cent of all the blood in the circulatory system is in the systemic veins. For this reason it is frequently said that the systemic veins act as a *blood reservoir* for the circulation. Also, relatively large quantities of blood are present in the veins of the lungs so that these, too, are considered to be a blood reservoir.

When blood is lost from the body and the arterial pressure begins to fall, pressure reflexes are elicited from the carotid sinuses and other pressure-sensitive areas of the circulation, as will be discussed in Chapter 14; these in turn send sympathetic nerve signals to the veins, causing them to constrict, and this takes up much of the slack in the circulatory system caused by the lost blood. Indeed, even after as much as 20 per cent of the total blood volume has been lost, the circulatory system often functions almost normally because of this variable reservoir system of the veins.

PRESSURE PULSES IN THE ARTERIES

Since the heart is a pulsatile pump, blood enters the arteries intermittently with each heartbeat, caus-

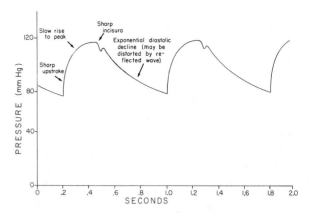

Figure 12–5. A normal pressure pulse contour recorded from the ascending aorta. (From Opdyke: Federation Proceedings, 11:734, 1952.)

ing *pressure pulses* in the arterial system as illustrated in Figure 12–5. In the normal young adult the pressure at the height of a pulse, the *systolic pressure*, is about 120 mm Hg and at its lowest point, the *diastolic pressure*, is about 80 mm Hg. The difference between these two pressures, about 40 mm Hg, is called the *pulse pressure*.

Two major factors affect the pulse pressure: (1) the *stroke volume output* of the heart and (2) the *compliance (total distensibility)* of the arterial tree. A third, less important factor is the character of ejection from the heart during systole.

In general, the greater the stroke volume output, the greater is the amount of blood that must be accommodated in the arterial tree with each heartbeat and, therefore, the greater is the pressure rise and fall during systole and diastole, thus causing a greater pulse pressure.

On the other hand, the less the compliance of the arterial system, the greater will be the rise in pressure for a given stroke volume of blood pumped into the arteries. For instance, the pulse pressure sometimes rises to as much as two times normal in old age because the arteries become hardened with arteriosclerosis and therefore noncompliant.

In effect, then, the pulse pressure is determined approximately by the *ratio of stroke volume output to compliance of the arterial tree*. Therefore, any condition of the circulation that affects either of these two factors will also affect the pulse pressure.

Abnormal Pressure Pulse Contours

Some conditions of the circulation also cause abnormal contours to the pressure pulse wave in addition to altering the pulse pressure, as illustrated in Figure 12–6. Especially distinctive among these are patent ductus arteriosus and aortic regurgitation.

Patent Ductus Arteriosus. The ductus arteriosus is a special artery that carries blood from the pulmonary artery to the aorta during fetal life so that the blood flow can bypass the inactive lungs. Normally, it closes within hours after birth, but in a few persons it

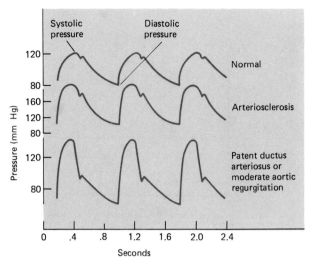

Figure 12–6. Pressure pulse contours in arteriosclerosis, patent ductus arteriosus, and moderate aortic regurgitation.

remains patent (open) indefinitely. Therefore, after birth the blood flows backward from the aorta through the open ductus into the pulmonary artery, allowing very rapid runoff of blood from the arterial tree after each heartbeat and a greatly decreased diastolic pressure. However, this is compensated for by a greater than normal stroke volume output because the blood flowing through the ductus passes rapidly through the lungs a second time and re-enters the left heart as extra inflowing blood. Therefore, the left heart beats with extra force, and the systolic pressure rises much higher than normal. These effects give the pressure pulse contour shown by the lowest curve in Figure 12–6. Here one finds an elevated systolic pressure, a greatly depressed diastolic pressure, and a greatly increased pulse pressure.

Aortic Regurgitation. Aortic regurgitation means backward flow of blood through the aortic valve because of failure of the valve to close. This usually results from heart diseases that destroy the valve, especially rheumatic fever. In aortic regurgitation much of the blood that is pumped into the aorta during systole flows back into the left ventricle during diastole, thus giving a low diastolic pressure. However, this backflow overfills the ventricle before its next beat; therefore, the ventricle pumps a much greater than normal stroke volume output during systole, which causes a high systolic pressure. Thus, the pressure pulse contour is very similar to that of patent ductus arteriosus, as illustrated by the lower curve of Figure 12–6, but is not identical, for in aortic regurgitation the valve sometimes fails to close even partially. When this is true the incisura (the "notch" in the curve that occurs when the valve closes) is entirely absent.

The Radial Pulse

Clinically, it has been the habit for many years for a physician to feel the radial pulse of each patient. This is done to determine the rate of the heartbeat or, frequently, because of the psychic contact that it gives the doctor with the patient. Under certain circumstances, however, the character of the pulse can also be of value in the diagnosis of circulatory diseases.

Weak Pulse. A weak pulse at the radial artery usually indicates either (1) greatly decreased central pulse pressure, such as occurs when the stroke volume output is low, or (2) increased "damping" of the pulse wave caused by vascular spasm; the latter occurs when the sympathetic nervous system becomes overly active following blood loss or when a person is having a chill.

Pulsus Paradoxus. Occasionally the strength of the pulse becomes strong, then weak, then strong, occurring in synchrony with the phases of respiration. This is caused by alternate increase and decrease in cardiac output with each respiration. During inspiration, all the blood vessels of the lungs increase in size because of increased negative pressure in the thorax. Therefore, blood collects in the lungs, and the stroke volume output and pulse strength decrease. During expiration, opposite effects occur. This is a normal phenomenon in all persons, but it becomes extremely distinct in some conditions, such as in very deep breathing or in cardiac tamponade (compression of the heart from the outside by fluid in the pericardial sac or by a constricted pericardium).

Pulse Deficit. The rhythm of the heart is very irregular in atrial fibrillation or in the case of ectopic beats. In these arrhythmias, which were discussed in Chapter 10, two beats of the heart often come so close together that the second beat pumps no blood or very little blood because the left ventricle has too little time to fill between the beats. In this circumstance, one can hear the second beat of the heart with a stethoscope applied directly over the heart but cannot feel a pulse in the radial artery, an effect called a *pulse deficit*. The greater the pulse deficit each minute, the more serious, ordinarily, is the arrhythmia.

THE PULMONARY CIRCULATION

The quantity of blood flowing through the lungs is essentially equal to that flowing through the systemic circulation. However, certain problems related to distribution of blood flow and other hemodynamics are special to the pulmonary circulation and are especially important to the gas exchange function of the lungs. Therefore, the present discussion is concerned specifically with the special features of blood flow in the pulmonary circuit and the function of the right side of the heart in maintaining this flow.

PHYSIOLOGIC ANATOMY OF THE PULMONARY CIRCULATORY SYSTEM

The Right Side of the Heart. As illustrated in Figure 12–7, the right ventricle is wrapped halfway around the left ventricle. The cause of this is the difference in pressures developed by the two ventri-

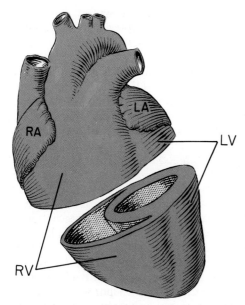

Figure 12–7. The anatomical relationship of the right ventricle to the left ventricle, showing the globular shape of the left ventricle and the half-moon shape of the right ventricle as it drapes around the left ventricle.

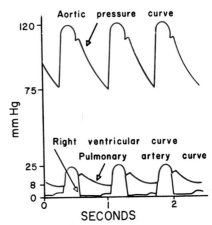

Figure 12–8. Pressure pulse contours in the right ventricle, pulmonary artery, and aorta.

cles during systole. That is, the left ventricle contracts with extreme force in comparison with the right ventricle, which causes the left ventricle to assume a globular shape, and the septum protrudes into the right heart.

The muscle of the right ventricle is slightly more than one third as thick as that of the left ventricle; this also results from the difference in pressures between the two sides of the heart.

The Pulmonary Vessels. The pulmonary artery extends only 5 cm beyond the apex of the right ventricle and then divides into the *right* and *left main branches*, which supply blood to the two respective lungs. The pulmonary artery is also thin, with a wall thickness approximately twice that of the venae cavae and one third that of the aorta. The pulmonary arterial branches are all very short. However, all the pulmonary arteries, even the smaller arteries and arterioles, have much larger diameters than their counterpart systemic arteries. This, combined with the fact that the vessels are very thin and distensible, gives the pulmonary arterial tree a very large compliance, which allows the pulmonary arteries to accommodate most of the stroke volume output of the right ventricle.

PRESSURES IN THE PULMONARY SYSTEM

The Pressure Pulse Curve in the Right Ventricle. The pressure pulse curves of the right ventricle and pulmonary artery are illustrated in the lower portion of Figure 12–8. These are contrasted with the much higher aortic pressure curve shown above. The systolic pressure in the right ventricle of the normal human being averages approximately 25 mm Hg, and the diastolic pressure averages about 0 to 1 mm Hg,

values that are only one fifth those for the left ventricle.

Pressures in the Pulmonary Artery. During systole, the pressure in the pulmonary artery is essentially equal to the pressure in the right ventricle, as also shown in Figure 12–8. However, after the pulmonary valve closes at the end of systole, the ventricular pressure falls precipitously, whereas the pulmonary arterial pressure falls slowly as blood flows through the capillaries of the lungs.

As shown in Figure 12–9, the systolic pulmonary arterial pressure averages approximately 25 mm Hg in the normal human being; the diastolic pulmonary arterial pressure, approximately 8 mm Hg; and the mean pulmonary arterial pressure, 15 mm Hg.

Pulmonary Capillary Pressure. The mean pulmonary capillary pressure, as diagrammed in Figure 12–9, has been estimated by indirect means to be approximately 7 mm Hg. This very low capillary pressure is extremely important in preventing leakage of fluid into the alveoli—that is, in preventing the development of pulmonary edema, as explained in Chapter 23.

Left Atrial and Pulmonary Venous Pressure. The mean pressure in the left atrium and in the major pulmonary veins averages approximately 2 mm Hg in the human being, varying from as low as 1 mm Hg to as high as 5 mm Hg.

It usually is not reasonable to measure the left atrial pressure directly in the normal human being

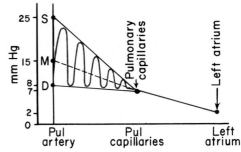

Figure 12–9. Pressures in the different vessels of the lungs.

because it is difficult to pass a catheter through the heart chambers into the left atrium. However, the left atrial pressure often can be estimated closely by measuring the so-called *pulmonary wedge pressure.* This is achieved by inserting a catheter through the right heart and pulmonary artery into one of the small branch pulmonary arteries and then pushing the catheter until it wedges tightly in the artery. The pressure then measured through the catheter, called the "wedge pressure," is about 5 mm Hg. Since all blood flow has been stopped in the small artery and the blood vessels extending from the artery make almost direct connection through the pulmonary capillaries with the blood in the pulmonary veins, this wedge pressure is usually only 1 to 3 mm Hg greater than the left atrial pressure. And when the left atrial pressure rises to high values, so also rises the pulmonary wedge pressure. Wedge pressure measurements are used frequently for studying changes in left atrial pressure in congestive heart failure.

THE BLOOD VOLUME OF THE LUNGS

The blood volume of the lungs is approximately 450 ml, about 9 per cent of the total blood volume of the circulatory system. About 70 ml of this is in the capillaries, and the remainder is divided about equally between the arteries and veins.

The Lungs as a Blood Reservoir. Under different physiological and pathological conditions, the quantity of blood in the lungs can vary from as little as 50 per cent of normal up to as high as 200 per cent of normal. For instance, when a person blows air out so hard that high pressure is built up in the lungs—such as when blowing a trumpet—as much as 250 ml of blood can be expelled from the pulmonary circulatory system into the systemic circulation. Also, loss of blood from the systemic circulation by hemorrhage can be partly compensated for by automatic shift of blood from the lungs into the systemic vessels.

Shift of Blood Between the Pulmonary and Systemic Circulatory Systems as a Result of Cardiac Pathology. Failure of the left side of the heart or increased impediment to blood flow through the mitral valve as a result of mitral stenosis or mitral regurgitation causes blood to dam up in the pulmonary circulation, sometimes increasing the pulmonary blood volume as much as 100 per cent, and also causing corresponding increases in the pulmonary vascular pressures.

On the other hand, exactly the opposite effects take place when the right side of the heart fails.

Because the volume of the systemic circulation is about nine times that of the pulmonary system, a shift of blood from one system to the other affects the pulmonary system greatly but has only mild systemic effects.

BLOOD FLOW THROUGH THE LUNGS AND ITS DISTRIBUTION

The blood flow through the lungs is essentially equal to the cardiac output. Therefore, the factors that control cardiac output—mainly peripheral factors, as discussed in Chapter 16—also control pulmonary blood flow. Under most conditions, the pulmonary vessels act as passive, distensible tubes that enlarge with increasing pressure and narrow with decreasing pressure. But, for adequate aeration of the blood it is important for the blood to be distributed to those segments of the lungs where the alveoli are best oxygenated. This is achieved by the following mechanism:

Effect of Diminished Alveolar Oxygen on Local Alveolar Blood Flow—Automatic Control of Pulmonary Blood Flow Distribution. When the concentration of oxygen in some alveoli becomes very low, the adjacent blood vessels slowly constrict during the ensuing three to ten minutes, the vascular resistance increasing to as much as triple normal. It should be noted specifically that this is *opposite to the effect* normally observed in systemic vessels, which dilate rather than constrict in response to low oxygen. However, it is believed that the low oxygen concentration causes a vasoconstrictor substance to be released from the lung tissue, this substance in turn promoting small arterial and arteriolar constriction. Unfortunately, research workers have not yet been able to isolate the vasoconstrictor substance.

This effect of low oxygen on pulmonary vascular resistance has an important function to distribute blood flow where it is most effective. That is, when some of the alveoli are poorly ventilated so that the oxygen concentration in them becomes low, the local vessels constrict. This in turn causes most of the blood to flow through the other areas of the lungs that are better aerated, thus providing an automatic control system for distributing blood flow through different pulmonary areas in proportion to their degrees of ventilation.

Effect of Hydrostatic Pressure Gradients in the Lungs on Regional Pulmonary Blood Flow

Earlier in this chapter it was pointed out that the pressure in the foot of a standing person can be as much as 90 mm Hg greater than the pressure at the level of the heart. This is caused by *hydrostatic pressure*—that is, by the weight of the blood itself. The same effect, but to a lesser degree, occurs in the lungs. In the normal, upright adult person, the lowest point in the lungs is about 30 cm below the highest point. This represents a 23 mm Hg pressure difference, about 15 mm Hg of which are above the heart and 8 mm Hg below. That is, the pulmonary arterial pressure in the uppermost portion of the lung of a standing person is about 15 mm Hg less than the mean pulmonary arterial pressure, and the pressure in the lowest portion of the lungs is about 8 mm Hg greater. Such pressure differences have profound effects on blood flow through the different areas of the lungs because of the very low pressures in the pulmonary vessels. To help explain this circumstance, the lung is often divided into three different zones,

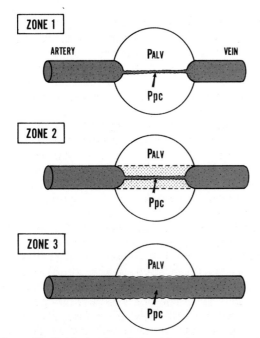

Figure 12–10. Mechanics of blood flow in the three different blood flow zones of the lung: *zone 1*, no flow, because alveolar pressure is greater than arterial pressure; *zone 2*, intermittent flow, because systolic arterial pressure rises higher than alveolar pressure but diastolic pressure falls below alveolar pressure; *zone 3*, continuous flow, because arterial pressure remains greater than alveolar pressure at all times.

as illustrated in Figure 12–10, in which the patterns of blood flow are quite different. Let us explain these differences.

Zone 1 (Area of Zero Flow). When the pulmonary arterial pressure is very low and the person is in a standing position, the pressure in the capillaries at the apices of the lungs may be, because of the hydrostatic pressure effect, 0 mm Hg. In such a condition, the capillaries remain collapsed all the time, as illustrated in the top panel of Figure 12–10 because the pulmonary capillary pressure is not great enough to oppose the tendency of the alveolar air pressure, which normally averages 0 mm Hg, to collapse the capillaries. Therefore, there will be zero blood flow. Thus, *zone 1* is an area of no flow.

Note, however, that a zone 1 area *does not occur in the normal lung* but instead occurs only in abnormal conditions.

Zone 2 (Area of Zero Flow During Part of the Heart Cycle). Recall that the normal pulmonary arterial pressure ranges between 8 mm Hg during diastole and 25 mm Hg during systole. Since the level of the heart is at a hydrostatic pressure level as much as 15 mm Hg below some portions of the normal upright lung, during diastole the pulmonary arterial pressure cannot force blood into the upper portions of the normal lung. Yet, during systole blood does flow. Therefore, as illustrated in the middle panel of Figure 12–10, the alveolar capillaries collapse during the diastolic portion of the heart cycle but open during systole. Thus, in *zone 2*, blood flows intermittently, that is, with zero flow during part of the heart cycle.

In the normal lung under normal standing conditions, the lower part of zone 2 begins 7 to 10 cm above the level of the heart and extends from there all the way to the top of the lungs.

Zone 3 (Area of Continuous Flow). In the lower part of the lung, the pulmonary vascular pressures are always higher than the alveolar pressure, even during diastole. Therefore, as illustrated in the lower part of Figure 12–10, the alveolar capillaries remain distended all the time, and blood flows continuously from the arteries to the veins.

The zone 3 portion of the lung, the portion in which the pulmonary capillaries remain open all the time, normally begins 7 to 10 cm above the level of the heart and extends all the way to the lowermost portions of the lung.

Factors That Can Change the Locations of Zones 1, 2, and 3 in the Lungs. Though normally there is no zone 1 blood flow in the lungs, this very often does occur when the pulmonary arterial pressure falls. This is very common following hemorrhage. However, the most common cause of a zone 1 area in the lungs is breathing against a high air pressure, as occurs when a person is blowing on a musical instrument. Under these conditions, the alveolar pressure rises very high, so high that the pulmonary arterial systolic pressure in the upper part of the lung cannot overcome the compressive effect on the capillaries caused by the high alveolar pressure. Consequently, no blood then flows through this portion of the lungs.

Another factor that affects the zones is position of the body. In the lying position, all portions of the lung become zone 3, and blood flow in the different parts of the lung then becomes rather evenly distributed. In the upside-down position, blood flow to the apices can actually be greater than blood flow to the base of the lung.

EFFECT OF INCREASED CARDIAC OUTPUT ON THE PULMONARY CIRCULATION DURING HEAVY EXERCISE

During heavy exercise the lungs are frequently called upon to absorb up to 20 times as much oxygen into the blood as normally. This absorption is achieved in two ways: (1) by increasing the number of open capillaries so that oxygen can diffuse more readily between the alveolar gas and the blood, and (2) by increasing cardiac output, with its concomitant increase in blood flow through the lungs—the blood thus picking up greater quantities of oxygen.

Fortunately, the cardiac output can increase to four to six times normal before pulmonary arterial pressure becomes excessively elevated because more and more capillaries open up and also because the pulmonary arterioles and capillaries expand. Indeed, the pressure rarely rises more than twofold despite as much as a five- to sixfold increase in flow.

This ability of the lungs to accommodate greatly increased blood flow during exercise with relatively little increase in pulmonary vascular pressure is important for at least two reasons: (1) it obviously conserves the energy of the right heart, and (2) it prevents a significant rise in pulmonary capillary pressure and therefore also prevents development of pulmonary edema during the increased cardiac output.

SOME PATHOLOGICAL CONDITIONS THAT OBSTRUCT BLOOD FLOW THROUGH THE LUNGS

Massive Pulmonary Embolism. One of the most severe postoperative calamities in surgical practice is massive pulmonary embolism. Patients lying immobile in bed tend to develop extensive clots in the veins of the legs because of sluggish blood flow. Also, women frequently develop massive clots in the hypogastric veins after delivery of their babies. Such clots often break away from the initial sites of formation, particularly when the patient first walks after a long period of immobilization. The clots then flow to the right side of the heart and into the pulmonary artery. Such a free-moving clot is called an *embolus.*

Total blockage of only one of the major branches of the pulmonary artery usually is not immediately fatal because the opposite lung can accommodate all the blood flow. However, blood clots have a tendency to grow. Consequently, the embolus becomes larger and larger, and as it extends into the other major branch of the pulmonary artery, the few remaining vessels that do not become plugged are taxed beyond their limit, and death ensues because of an inordinate rise in pulmonary arterial pressure and right-sided heart failure.

Emphysema. Pulmonary emphysema means, literally, too much air in the lungs, and it is usually characterized by destruction of many of the alveolar walls. This causes the adjacent alveoli to become confluent, thereby forming large *emphysematous cavities* rather than the usual small alveoli. Obviously, loss of the alveolar septa greatly decreases the total alveolar surface area of the lungs and hinders gas exchange between the alveoli and the blood.

Emphysema also has an important effect on the pulmonary vasculature, for each time an alveolar wall is destroyed, some of the small blood vessels of the pulmonary system are also destroyed, thus progressively increasing the pulmonary resistance and elevating the pulmonary arterial pressure.

Unfortunately, the prevalence of emphysema is increasing rapidly because of cigarette smoking, which is by far the most common cause of this disease that affects over one tenth of all smokers.

Diffuse Sclerosis of the Lungs. A number of pathological conditions cause excessive fibrosis in the supportive tissues in the lungs, and the fibrous tissue in turn contracts around the vessels. Some of these conditions are *silicosis, tuberculosis, syphilis,* and, to a lesser extent, *anthracosis* (caused by breathing coal dust).

In early stages of diffuse sclerosis, the pulmonary arterial pressure often is normal as long as the person is not exercising, but just as soon as even mild exercise is performed, the pulmonary arterial pressure rises inordinately because the vessels do not have the ability to expand as much as normal pulmonary vessels do. In late stages of diffuse sclerosis the pulmonary arterial pressure remains elevated constantly; as a result, the right ventricle hypertrophies, and it may fail. Diffusion of gases through the alveolar membranes in most instances is impaired either because of decreased surface area or because of diminished blood flow to some alveoli.

Atelectasis. Atelectasis is the clinical term for collapse of a lung or part of a lung. This occurs often when the bronchi become plugged, because the pulmonary blood rapidly absorbs the air in the entrapped alveoli, which causes the alveoli to collapse.

Atelectasis also occurs when the chest cavity is opened to atmospheric pressure, for when air is allowed to enter the pleural space, the elastic nature of the lungs causes them to collapse immediately.

When the elastic tissues of the lungs contract during atelectasis, they constrict not only the alveoli but also the blood vessels. This constriction, in addition to the vasoconstriction caused by oxygen deficiency as discussed earlier in the chapter, automatically decreases blood flow in the atelectatic portions of the lungs to as little as one-fourth normal, shifting the remaining three fourths to the aerated portions. This safety mechanism is important, for it prevents flow of major quantities of blood through collapsed, nonaerated pulmonary areas.

QUESTIONS

1. State approximately the quantities of blood in the different parts of the circulation.
2. Trace the change in the pressure as the blood flows from the arteries to the arterioles, the capillaries, the venules, and the veins in the systemic circulation.
3. What is the importance of the elasticity of the large arteries?
4. What are the specific characteristics of the arterioles and small arteries that make these the main controllers of blood flow through local tissue areas?
5. Explain the factors that control the central venous pressure. How does central venous pressure affect the pressures elsewhere in the veins?
6. What are the effects of hydrostatic pressures on venous and arterial pressures everywhere in the body?
7. What is the function of the venous valves, and how important is this function?
8. How do the veins function as a blood reservoir?
9. What are the principal factors that determine the pulse pressure in the arterial tree?

10. Explain some of the conditions that can give abnormal pressure pulse contours and abnormal radial pulses.
11. Explain the important anatomical differences between the pulmonary circulation and the systemic circulation.
12. What are the quantitative differences between the pulmonary vascular pressures and the systemic pressures?
13. What is the importance of the very low pulmonary capillary pressure?
14. Explain the function of the lungs as a blood reservoir.
15. Describe the mechanism by which low oxygen concentration in the alveoli controls blood flow through the local pulmonary vessels and explain why this is important to function of the lungs.
16. Explain the important effects of hydrostatic pressure gradients on pulmonary vascular function in both normal and abnormal conditions.
17. Why does the pulmonary arterial pressure not rise markedly in the normal person during heavy exercise?
18. How do the following conditions affect blood flow through the lungs: massive pulmonary embolism, emphysema, and atelectasis?

References

Systemic Circulation

American Physiological Society: Peripheral Circulation and Organ Blood Flow. Washington, D.C., American Physiological Society, 1983.

Donald, D. E.: Splanchnic circulation. In Shepherd, J. T., and Abboud, F. M., eds.: Handbook of Physiology. Sec. 2, Vol. 3. Bethesda, American Physiological Society, 1983, p. 219.

Guyton, A. C.: Peripheral circulation. Annu Rev Physiol 21:239, 1959.

Guyton, A. C.: Arterial Pressure and Hypertension. Philadelphia, W. B. Saunders Co., 1980.

Guyton, A. C., et al.: Evidence for tissue oxygen demand as the major factor causing autoregulation. Circ Res 14:60, 1964.

Guyton, A. C., et al.: Cardiac Output and Its Regulation. Philadelphia, W. B. Saunders Co., 1973.

O'Rourke, M. F.: Vascular impedance in studies of arterial and cardiac function. Physiol Rev 62:570, 1982.

Randall, W. C., ed: Nervous Control of Cardiovascular Function. New York, Oxford University Press, 1984.

Rodkiewicz, C. M.: Arteries and Arterial Blood Flow. New York, Springer-Verlag, 1983.

Rothe, C. F.: Reflex control of veins and vascular capacitance. Physiol Rev 63:1281, 1983.

Rothe, C. F.: Venous system: Physiology of the capacitance vessels. In Shepherd, J. T., and Abboud, F. M., eds.: Handbook of Physiology. Sec. 2, Vol. 3. Bethesda, American Physiological Society, 1983, p. 397.

Pulmonary Circulation

Bergofsky, E. H.: Humoral control of the pulmonary circulation. Annu Rev Physiol 42:221, 1980.

Culver, B. H., and Butler, J.: Mechanical influences on the pulmonary microcirculation. Annu Rev Physiol 42:187, 1980.

Dawson, C. A.: Role of pulmonary vasomotion in physiology of the lung. Physiol Rev 64:544, 1984.

Effros, R. M.: Pulmonary microcirculation and exchange. In Renkin, E. M., and Michel, C. C., eds.: Handbook of Physiology. Sec. 2, Vol. 4. Bethesda, American Physiological Society, 1984, p. 865.

Gil, J.: Organization of microcirculation in the lung. Annu Rev Physiol 42:177, 1980.

Grover, R. F., et al.: Pulmonary Circulation. In Shepherd, J. T., and Abboud, F. M., eds.: Handbook of Physiology. Sec. 2, Vol. 3. Bethesda, American Physiological Society, 1983, p. 103.

Guyton, A. C., et al.: Dynamics of subatmospheric pressure in the pulmonary interstitial fluid. In Lung Liquids. Ciba Symposium. New York, Elsevier/North-Holland, 1976, p. 77.

Guyton, A. C., et al.: Forces governing water movement in the lung. In Pulmonary Edema. Washington, D.C., American Physiological Society, 1979, p. 65.

Malik, A. B.: Pulmonary microembolism. Physiol Rev 63:1114, 1983.

Parker, J. C., et al.: Pulmonary transcapillary exchange and pulmonary edema. In Guyton, A. C., and Young, D. B., eds.: International Review of Physiology: Cardiovascular Physiology III, Vol. 18. Baltimore, University Park Press, 1979, p. 261.

Staub, N. C.: Pulmonary edema. Physiol Rev 54:678, 1974.

13

Local Control of Blood Flow by the Tissues; Nervous and Humoral Regulation

---

LOCAL CONTROL OF BLOOD FLOW IN
RESPONSE TO TISSUE NEED
*MECHANISMS OF BLOOD FLOW
CONTROL*
*ACUTE CONTROL OF LOCAL BLOOD
FLOW*
*LONG-TERM BLOOD FLOW
REGULATION*

NERVOUS REGULATION OF THE
CIRCULATION
THE AUTONOMIC NERVOUS SYSTEM
HUMORAL REGULATION OF THE
CIRCULATION

The circulatory system is provided with a complex system for control of blood flow to the different parts of the body. In general, the controls are of three major types:

1. Local control of blood flow in each individual tissue, the flow being controlled mainly in proportion to that tissue's need for blood perfusion.

2. Nervous control of blood flow, which often affects blood flow in large segments of the systemic circulation, such as shifting blood flow from the nonmuscular vascular beds to the muscles during exercise or changing the blood flow in the skin to control body temperature.

3. Humoral control, in which various substances dissolved in the blood such as hormones, ions, or other chemicals can cause either local increase or decrease in tissue flow or widespread generalized changes in flow.

LOCAL CONTROL OF BLOOD FLOW IN RESPONSE TO TISSUE NEED

One of the most fundamental and important characteristics of the circulation is the ability of each tissue to control its own local blood flow in proportion to its need. Furthermore, as the need changes, the flow follows the change.

However, what are some of the specific needs of the tissues for blood flow? The answer to this is manyfold, including especially the following:

(1) Delivery of oxygen to the tissues.

(2) Delivery of other nutrients like glucose, amino acids, fatty acids, and so forth.

(3) Removal of carbon dioxide from the tissues.

(4) Removal of hydrogen ions from the tissues.

Variations in Blood Flow in Different Tissues and Organs. In general, the greater the degree of metabolism in an organ, the greater its blood flow. Note, for instance, in Table 13–1 the very large blood flows in the various glandular organs—for example, several hundred ml/min per 100 grams of thyroid or adrenal gland tissue and a blood flow of 95 ml/min per 100 grams of liver.

Also note the extremely large blood flow through the kidneys, 360 ml/min per 100 grams. This extreme amount of flow is required for the kidneys to perform their function of cleansing the blood of waste products.

On the other hand, most surprising is the low blood flow to the resting muscles of the body, even though they constitute between 30 and 40 per cent of the total body mass. However, in the resting state the metabolic activity of the muscles is very low, and so also is the blood flow, only 4 ml/min per 100 grams. Yet, during very heavy exercise, the metabolic activ-

Table 13–1. BLOOD FLOW TO DIFFERENT ORGANS AND TISSUES UNDER BASAL CONDITIONS

	Per Cent	Ml/min	Ml/min/ 100 gm
Brain	14	700	50
Heart	4	200	70
Bronchial	2	100	25
Kidneys	22	1100	360
Liver	27	1350	95
Portal	(21)	(1050)	
Arterial	(6)	(300)	
Muscle (inactive state)	15	750	4
Bone	5	250	3
Skin (cool weather)	6	300	3
Thyroid gland	1	50	160
Adrenal glands	0.5	25	300
Other tissues	3.5	175	1.3
Total	100.0	5000	—

Based mainly on data compiled by Dr. L. A. Sapirstein.

ity can increase as much as 50-fold and the blood flow as much as 20-fold, rising to as high as 80 ml/min per 100 grams.

MECHANISMS OF BLOOD FLOW CONTROL

Local blood flow control can be divided into two different phases: (1) acute control, and (2) long-term control. Acute control means rapid changes in local blood flow control, occurring within seconds to minutes, to provide a rapid means for maintaining appropriate local tissue conditions. Long-term control, on the other hand, means slow changes in flow over a period of days, weeks, or even months. In general, the long-term changes come about as a result of an increase or decrease in the sizes and numbers of actual blood vessels supplying the tissues.

Functional Anatomy of the Systemic Microcirculation. Though the student will recall that each tissue has its own characteristic vascular system, Figure 13–1 presents a representative local vascular bed. This figure shows that blood enters a capillary bed through a small *arteriole* and leaves by way of a small *venule*. From the arteriole the blood usually divides and flows through several *metarterioles* before entering the *capillaries*. Some of the capillaries are very large, and they course almost directly to the venule. These are called *preferential channels*. However, most of the capillaries, called the *true capillaries*, branch mainly from the metarterioles and then finally terminate in a venule.

The arterioles have a strong muscular coat, and the metarterioles are surrounded by sparse but highly active smooth muscle fibers. In addition, in many tissues, at each point at which a capillary leaves a metarteriole, a small muscular *precapillary sphincter*, consisting of a single spiraling smooth muscle fiber, surrounds the origin of the capillary.

As will be discussed in more detail later in the chapter, the small arteries and arterioles are supplied by extensive innervation from the sympathetic nervous system, and the degree of contraction of these structures is strongly influenced by the intensity of sympathetic signals transmitted from the central nervous system to the blood vessels.

On the other hand, innervation of the metarterioles and the precapillary sphincters is usually very sparse, or even absent in most instances. Instead, the muscle fibers of these two structures are controlled almost entirely by the local factors in the tissues, that is, by the concentrations of oxygen, carbon dioxide, hydrogen ions, electrolytes, and other substances in each individual tissue area. These local factors, therefore, are major controllers of blood flow in the local tissue areas.

ACUTE CONTROL OF LOCAL BLOOD FLOW

Local Blood Flow Regulation When Oxygen Availability Changes. One of the most necessary of the nutrients is oxygen. Whenever the availability of oxygen to the tissues decreases, such as at high altitude, in pneumonia, in carbon monoxide poisoning (which poisons the ability of hemoglobin to transport oxygen), or in cyanide poisoning (which poisons the ability of the tissues to utilize oxygen), the blood flow through the tissues increases markedly. Figure 13–2 shows that as the arterial oxygen saturation falls to about 25 per cent of normal, the blood flow through an isolated leg increases about threefold; that is, the blood flow increases almost enough, but not quite, to

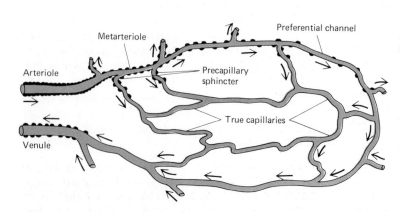

Figure 13–1. Overall structure of a local vascular bed. (From Zweifach: Factors Regulating Blood Pressure. New York, Josiah Macy, Jr., Foundation, 1950.)

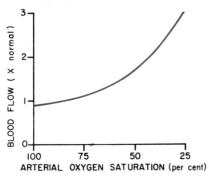

Figure 13-2. Effect of arterial oxygen saturation on blood flow through an isolated dog leg.

make up for the decreased amount of oxygen in the blood, thus automatically maintaining an almost constant supply of oxygen to the tissues. Cyanide poisoning of local tissue areas can cause a local blood flow increase as much as sevenfold, thus illustrating the extreme effect of oxygen deficiency in increasing blood flow.

There are two basic theories for the regulation of local blood flow when either the rate of tissue metabolism changes or the availability of oxygen changes. These are (1) the *vasodilator theory* and (2) the *oxygen demand theory*.

The Vasodilator Theory for Local Blood Flow Regulation. According to this theory, the greater the rate of metabolism, the less the blood flow, or the less the availability of oxygen and other nutrients to a tissue, the greater becomes the rate of formation of a *vasodilator substance*. The vasodilator substance then is believed to diffuse back to the precapillary sphincters, metarterioles, and arterioles to cause dilatation. Some of the different vasodilator substances that have been suggested are *carbon dioxide, lactic acid, adenosine, adenosine phosphate compounds, histamine, potassium ions*, and *hydrogen ions*.

Many physiologists have suggested that the substance *adenosine* is perhaps the most important of the local vasodilators for controlling local blood flow. For instance, vasodilator quantities of adenosine are released from heart muscle cells whenever coronary blood flow becomes too little, and it is believed that this causes local vasodilatation in the heart and thereby returns the blood flow back toward normal. Also, whenever the heart becomes overly active and the heart's metabolism increases, this too causes excessive utilization of oxygen, followed by decreased oxygen concentration in the local tissues, increased degradation of adenosine triphosphate, and, therefore, increased formation of adenosine in the active cells.

The Oxygen Demand Theory for Local Blood Flow Control. Though the vasodilator theory is accepted by most physiologists, several critical facts have made a few physiologists favor still another theory, which can be called either the oxygen demand theory or, more accurately, the *nutrient demand theory* (because probably other nutrients besides oxygen are involved). Oxygen (and other nutrients as well) is required to maintain vascular muscle contraction.

Therefore, in the absence of an adequate supply of oxygen and other nutrients, it is reasonable to believe that the blood vessels would naturally dilate. Also, increased utilization of oxygen in the tissues as a result of increased metabolism would theoretically decrease the local tissue oxygen availability, and this too would cause local vasodilatation.

A mechanism by which the oxygen demand theory could operate is the following: When one observes under a microscope a thin tissue such as a bat's wing, one sees that the precapillary sphincters are normally either completely open or completely closed. The number of precapillary sphincters that are open at any given time is approximately proportional to the requirements of the tissue for nutrition. In addition, the precapillary sphincters often open and close cyclically several times per minute, with the duration of the open phases approximately proportional to the metabolic needs of the tissues. Thus when the oxygen concentration in the tissue rises above a certain level, the precapillary sphincter presumably closes and remains closed until the tissue cells consume the excess oxygen. When the oxygen concentration falls low enough, the sphincter opens once more to begin the cycle again.

However, in most thick tissues, the precapillary sphincters do not open and close rhythmically; instead, a certain proportion of them remain open while the others remain closed. This is the effect that one would expect when several capillaries are supplying the same tissue area, because interference between the capillaries would cause just exactly the right number of capillary sphincters to open to supply the required oxygen, and only occasionally would one of the sphincters close or open.

The evidence against the oxygen demand theory is that many types of smooth muscle can remain contracted for long periods of time in the presence of extremely minute concentrations of oxygen—concentrations even below those normally found in the tissues. A possible answer to this is that the smooth muscle in the microvessels might be genetically more sensitive to oxygen lack than are the types of smooth muscle that have thus far been studied. Indeed, in very small, isolated, perfused arteries (with internal diameters of approximately 0.5 mm), marked vasodilation does occur at oxygen concentrations found even normally in the tissues.

Thus, on the basis of presently available data, either a vasodilator theory or an oxygen demand theory could explain local blood flow regulation in response to the metabolic needs of the tissues. Perhaps the truth lies in a combination of the two mechanisms.

Special Examples of Metabolic Control of Local Blood Flow

The mechanisms that we have described thus far for local blood flow control are frequently called metabolic mechanisms because they function in response to the metabolic needs of the tissues. Two additional special instances of metabolic control of local blood flow are *reactive hyperemia* and *active hyperemia*.

Reactive Hyperemia. When the blood supply to a tissue is blocked for a few seconds to several hours and then is unblocked, the flow through the tissue usually increases to five to eight times normal; the increased flow will continue for a few seconds if the block has lasted a few seconds but sometimes for as long as many hours if the blood flow has been stopped for an hour or more. This phenomenon is called *reactive hyperemia*.

Reactive hyperemia is almost certainly another manifestation of the local "metabolic" blood flow regulation mechanism; that is, lack of flow sets into motion all of those factors that cause vasodilatation. Following short periods of vascular occlusion, the extra blood flow during the reactive hyperemia phase lasts long enough to repay almost exactly the tissue oxygen deficit that has accrued during the period of occlusion. This mechanism emphasizes the close connection between local blood flow regulation and delivery of nutrients to the tissues.

Active Hyperemia. When any tissue becomes highly active, such as a muscle during exercise, a gastrointestinal gland during a hypersecretory period, or even the brain during rapid mental activity, the rate of blood flow through the tissue increases. Here again, by simply applying the basic principles of local blood flow control, one can easily understand this so-called *active hyperemia*. The increase in local metabolism because of the excess activity causes the cells to devour the tissue fluid nutrients extremely rapidly and also to release large quantities of vasodilator substances. The result obviously would be to dilate the local blood vessels, and therefore, to increase local blood flow. In this way, the active tissue will receive the additional nutrients required to sustain its new level of function.

As pointed out earlier, active hyperemia in skeletal muscle can increase the local blood flow as much as 20-fold during intense exercise.

Autoregulation of Blood Flow When the Arterial Pressure Changes from Normal— Metabolic Versus Myogenic Mechanisms

In most tissues of the body, an acute increase or a decrease in arterial pressure will cause an immediate increase or decrease in blood flow. However, within less than a minute, the blood flow usually returns most of the way back toward the normal level. Therefore, if a few minutes are allowed for the local blood flow control mechanisms to function properly, the blood flow will be related to arterial pressure approximately in accord with the *solid curve* labeled *acute* in Figure 13–3. Note that between an arterial pressure of approximately 70 mm Hg and 175 mm Hg the blood flow remains within ± 10 to 25 per cent of the normal value. This maintenance of the flow at nearly normal levels despite marked changes

in arterial pressure is called *autoregulation of blood flow*. For almost a century, two different mechanisms have been proposed to explain the acute autoregulation phenomenon. These have been called (1) the metabolic theory, and (2) the myogenic theory.

The *metabolic theory* can be understood very easily by simply applying the basic principles of local blood flow regulation already discussed in earlier sections. Thus, when the arterial pressure becomes too great, the excess flow provides too many nutrients to the tissues and also flushes vasodilator substances out of the tissues; both these effects will then cause the blood vessels to constrict. Therefore, the increased pressure will not increase flow greatly because the compensatory constriction will mainly nullify the effect of the pressure.

The *myogenic theory*, on the other hand, suggests that still another mechanism besides those related to tissue metabolism at least partially explains the phenomenon of autoregulation. This theory is based on the observation that a sudden stretch of small blood vessels will cause the smooth muscle of the vessel wall to contract. Therefore, it has been suggested that when high arterial pressure stretches the vessel, this in turn causes vascular constriction and reduces the blood flow back near normal. Conversely, at low pressures, the degree of stretch of the vessel is less, so that the smooth muscle relaxes and allows increased flow.

It has been suggested especially that the myogenic mechanism protects the capillaries from excessively high blood pressures. That is, if the pressure in the small arteries and arterioles rises too high, these vessels simply constrict and prevent this high pressure from being transmitted into the capillaries.

LONG-TERM BLOOD FLOW REGULATION

Thus far, all the mechanisms for local blood flow regulation that we have discussed act within a few minutes after the local tissue conditions have changed. Unfortunately, though, even after full function of these acute mechanisms the blood flow usually is adjusted no more than three quarters of the way to the exact requirement of the tissues. However, over a period of hours, days, and weeks a long-term type of local blood flow regulation develops in addition to the acute regulation. This long-term regulation gives far more complete regulation than does the acute mechanism. Figure 13–3 illustrates by the dashed curve the extreme effectiveness of this long-term local blood flow regulation. Note that once the long-term regulation has had time to occur, changes in arterial pressure between 50 and 250 mm Hg have very little effect on the rate of local blood flow.

Long-term regulation also occurs when the metabolic demands of a tissue change. Thus, if a tissue becomes chronically overactive and therefore requires chronically increased quantities of nutrients, the blood supply gradually increases to match the needs of the tissue.

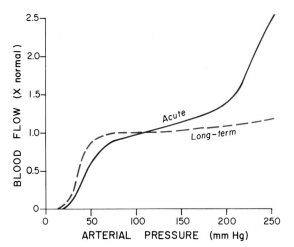

Figure 13–3. Effect of increasing arterial pressure on blood flow through a muscle. The solid curve shows the effect if the arterial pressure is raised over a period of a few minutes. The dashed curve shows the effect if the arterial pressure is raised extremely slowly over a period of many weeks.

Mechanism of Long-Term Regulation—Change in Tissue Vascularity. The mechanism of long-term local blood flow regulation is almost certainly a change in the degree of vascularity of the tissues. That is, if the arterial pressure falls to 60 mm Hg and remains at this level for many weeks, the number and sizes of vessels in the tissue increase; if the pressure then rises to a very high level, the number and sizes of vessels decrease. Likewise, if the metabolism in a given tissue becomes elevated for a prolonged period of time, vascularity increases; or if the metabolism is decreased, vascularity decreases. Thus, there is continual reconstruction of the tissue vasculature to meet the needs of the tissues.

Angiogenesis Factor and Growth of New Vessels. In the past few years, a substance called *angiogenesis factor* has been isolated from several tissues that have excessive metabolic needs, including cancers and the retina of the eye. This factor causes growth of new blood vessels. Furthermore, relative lack of oxygen in relation to the level of metabolism of the tissues is one of the conditions, if not the major condition, that causes angiogenesis factor to be formed in a tissue. Therefore, much belief is developing that this angiogenesis factor is responsible for development of new blood vessels in rapidly growing, highly metabolic, or ischemic tissues.

When angiogenesis factor appears in a tissue, small buds of cells break away from the walls of the venules and small veins, and these cellular masses migrate toward the angiogenesis factor. Then they multiply and form tubular loops that eventually connect with the vascular tree. Thus, new vessels are formed.

If ever enough angiogenesis factor can be isolated or synthesized, it might become an important therapeutic tool for treating ischemic tissues, such as ischemic areas in the heart after a heart attack.

NERVOUS REGULATION OF THE CIRCULATION

Superimposed onto the intrinsic local tissue regulation of blood flow are two additional types of regulation: (1) *nervous* and (2) *humoral*. These regulations are not necessary for most normal functions of the circulation, but they do provide greatly increased effectiveness of control under special conditions such as during exercise or following hemorrhage.

THE AUTONOMIC NERVOUS SYSTEM

The autonomic nervous system is a portion of the nervous system that operates at a subconscious level to control the internal functions of the body. By far the most important part of the autonomic nervous system for regulation of the circulation is the *sympathetic nervous system*. However, the *parasympathetic nervous system* is also important for its regulation of heart function, as we shall see later in the chapter.

The Sympathetic Nervous System. Figure 13–4 illustrates the anatomy of sympathetic nervous control of the circulation. Sympathetic vasomotor nerve fibers leave the spinal cord through all the thoracic and the first one to two lumbar spinal nerves. These pass into the sympathetic chain and thence by two routes to the blood vessels throughout the body: (1) through specific *sympathetic nerves* that innervate mainly the internal viscera, and (2) through the *spinal nerves* that innervate mainly the peripheral areas. The precise pathways of these fibers in the spinal cord and in the sympathetic chains will be discussed in Chapter 38.

The innervation of the small arteries and arterioles allows sympathetic stimulation to increase the *resistance* and thereby to change the rate of blood flow through the tissues. The innervation of large vessels, particularly of the veins, makes it possible for sympathetic stimulation to change the volume of these vessels and thereby to alter the volume of the peripheral circulatory system, which can translocate blood into the heart and thereby play a major role in the regulation of heart pumping.

In addition, sympathetic fibers also go to the heart as was discussed in Chapter 8. It will be recalled that sympathetic stimulation markedly increases the activity of the heart, speeding the heart rate and enhancing its strength of pumping.

Parasympathetic Control of Heart Function, Especially Heart Rate. Though the parasympathetic nervous system is exceedingly important for many other autonomic functions of the body, it plays only a minor role in regulation of the circulation. Its only really important circulatory effect is its control of heart rate by way of parasympathetic fibers carried to the heart in the vagus nerves, shown in Figure 13–4 by the dashed nerve from the medulla directly to the heart.

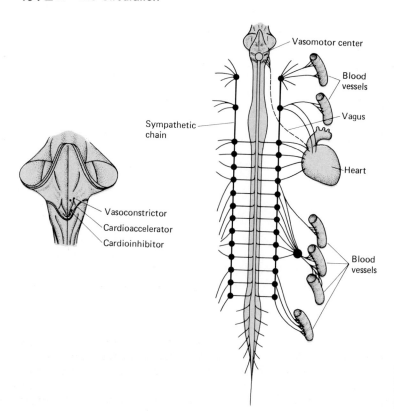

Figure 13-4. The vasomotor center and its control of the circulatory system through the sympathetic nerves and through the vagus nerves to the heart, which are part of the parasympathetic nervous system.

The effects of parasympathetic stimulation on heart function were discussed in detail in Chapter 8. Principally, parasympathetic stimulation causes a marked *decrease* in heart rate and a slight decrease in contractility, an effect that is normally unimportant.

The Sympathetic Vasoconstrictor System and Its Control by the Central Nervous System

The sympathetic nerves carry both vasoconstrictor and vasodilator fibers, but by far the most important of these are the *sympathetic vasoconstrictor* fibers. Sympathetic vasoconstrictor fibers are distributed to essentially all segments of the circulation.

The Vasomotor Center and Its Control of the Vasoconstrictor System—Vasomotor Tone. Located bilaterally in the reticular substance of the medulla and the lower third of the pons, as illustrated in Figure 13–5, is an area called the *vasomotor center*. This center transmits impulses downward through the cord and thence through the sympathetic vasoconstrictor fibers to all or almost all the blood vessels of the body.

Under normal conditions, the vasomotor center transmits signals continuously to the sympathetic vasoconstrictor nerve fibers, causing continuous slow firing of these fibers at a rate of about one half to two impulses per second. This continual firing is called *sympathetic vasoconstrictor tone*. These impulses maintain a partial state of contraction in the blood vessels, a state called *vasomotor tone*.

Figure 13–6 demonstrates the significance of vasoconstrictor tone. In the experiment of this figure, total spinal anesthesia was administered to an animal, which completely blocked all transmission of nerve impulses from the central nervous system to the

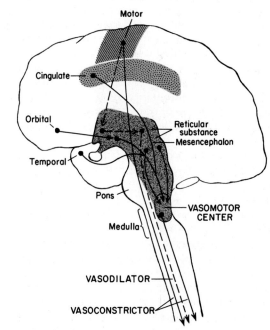

Figure 13–5. Areas of the brain that play important roles in the nervous regulation of the circulation. The dashed lines represent inhibitory pathways.

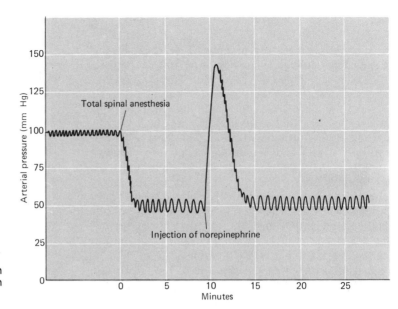

Figure 13-6. Effect of total spinal anesthesia on the arterial pressure, showing a marked fall in pressure resulting from loss of vasomotor tone.

periphery. As a result, the arterial pressure fell from 100 to 50 mm Hg, illustrating the effect of loss of vasoconstrictor tone throughout the body. A few minutes later a small amount of the hormone norepinephrine was injected intravenously—norepinephrine is the substance secreted at the endings of sympathetic nerve fibers throughout the body. As this hormone was transported in the blood to all the blood vessels, the vessels once again became constricted, and the arterial pressure rose to a level even greater than normal for a minute or two until the norepinephrine was destroyed.

Control of Heart Activity by the Vasomotor Center. At the same time that the vasomotor center is controlling the degree of vascular constriction, it also controls heart activity. It sends excitatory impulses through the sympathetic nervous system to the heart to increase heart rate and contractility, or it transmits impulses through the vagus nerve to the heart to decrease heart rate. Therefore, the vasomotor center can either increase or decrease heart activity, this ordinarily increasing at the same time that vasoconstriction occurs throughout the body and ordinarily decreasing at the same time that vasoconstriction is inhibited.

Control of the Vasomotor Center by Higher Nervous Centers. Large numbers of areas throughout the *reticular substance* of the *pons, mesencephalon*, and *diencephalon* can either excite or inhibit the vasomotor center. This reticular substance is illustrated in Figure 13-5 by the diffuse shaded area.

The *hypothalamus* plays a special role in the control of the vasoconstrictor system, for it can exert powerful excitatory or inhibitory effects on the vasomotor center. The *posterolateral portions* of the hypothalamus mainly cause excitation (that is, peripheral vasoconstriction and increased heart pumping), whereas the *anterior part* can cause mild excitation or inhibition, depending on the precise part of the anterior hypothalamus stimulated.

Many different parts of the *cerebral cortex* can also excite or inhibit the vasomotor center. Stimulation of the *motor cortex*, for instance, excites the vasomotor center because of impulses transmitted downward into the hypothalamus and thence to the vasomotor center. Also, stimulation of the *anterior temporal lobe*, the *orbital areas of the frontal cortex*, the *anterior part of the cingulate gyrus*, the *amygdala*, the *septum*, and the *hippocampus* can all either excite or inhibit the vasomotor center, depending on the precise portion of these areas that is stimulated and upon the intensity of the stimulus.

Thus, widespread areas of the brain can have profound effects on the vasomotor center and in turn on the sympathetic vasoconstrictor system of the body, either further enhancing the degree of vasoconstriction or causing vasodilatation by inhibiting the vasoconstrictor tone.

Norepinephrine—The Sympathetic Vasoconstrictor Transmitter Substance. The substance secreted at the endings of the vasoconstrictor nerves is norepinephrine. Norepinephrine acts directly on the so-called "alpha" receptors of the vascular smooth muscle to cause vasoconstriction, as will be discussed in Chapter 38.

HUMORAL REGULATION OF THE CIRCULATION

Humoral regulation of the circulation means regulation by substances in the body fluids, such as by hormones, ions, or so forth. Some of these substances are formed by special glands and then transported in the blood throughout the entire body. Others are formed in local tissue areas and cause only local circulatory effects. Among the most important of the humoral factors that affect circulatory function are the following:

Vasoconstrictor Agents

Epinephrine and Norepinephrine Secreted by the Adrenal Medullae. When the sympathetic nervous system is stimulated to cause direct effects on the blood vessels throughout the body, it also causes the adrenal medullae to secrete large quantities of both *norepinephrine* and *epinephrine* directly into the blood. These hormones then circulate everywhere in the body fluids and act on all vasculature. Norepinephrine has vasoconstrictor effects in almost all vascular beds of the body, and epinephrine has similar effects in most, but not all, beds. For instance, epinephrine often causes mild vasodilatation in both skeletal and cardiac muscle. These two hormones will be discussed in more detail in Chapter 38 in the discussion of the autonomic nervous system.

Angiotensin. Angiotensin is one of the most powerful vasoconstrictor substances known. As little as *one ten millionth* of a gram can increase the arterial pressure of a human being as much as 10 to 20 mm Hg under some conditions. Since this substance is very important in relation to arterial pressure regulation, it will be discussed in detail in the following two chapters.

Briefly, a decrease in arterial pressure will cause the kidneys to secrete the substance *renin*. The renin in turn acts on one of the plasma proteins, *renin substrate*, to split away the vasoactive peptide *angiotensin*. The angiotensin in turn has a number of important effects on the circulation related to arterial pressure control, but most importantly to constrict the blood vessels everywhere in the body, as we shall discuss in the following chapters.

Vasopressin. Vasopressin is formed in the hypothalamus (see Chapter 49) but is transported down the center of nerve axons to the posterior pituitary gland, where it is eventually secreted into the blood. It is even more powerful than angiotensin as a vasoconstrictor, thus making it perhaps the body's most potent constrictor substance. Yet, normally, only very minute amounts of vasopressin are secreted, so that most physiologists have thought that vasopressin plays little role in vascular control. On the other hand, recent experiments have shown that the concentration of circulating vasopressin during severe hemorrhage can rise enough to increase the arterial pressure as much as 60 mm Hg, and in many instances this can by itself bring the arterial pressure almost back up to normal.

Also, vasopressin has an *all-important* function in controlling water reabsorption in the renal tubules, which will be discussed in Chapter 25, and therefore to help control body fluid volume. For this reason, this hormone is also called *antidiuretic* hormone.

Vasodilator Agents

Bradykinin. Several substances called *kinins* that can cause vasodilatation have been isolated from blood and tissue fluids. One of these substances is *bradykinin*.

The kinins are small polypeptides that are split away from alpha$_2$-globulins in the plasma or tissue fluids. Different types of proteolytic enzymes can split the kinins from the globulin. An enzyme of particular importance is *kallikrein*, which is present in the blood and tissue fluids in an inactive form. Kallikrein can be activated in several different ways, such as by maceration of the blood, dilution of the blood, contact of the blood with glass, and other similar chemical and physical effects on the blood. As kallikrein becomes activated, it acts immediately on the alpha$_2$-globulin to release a kinin called *kallidin* that is then converted by tissue enzymes into *bradykinin*. Once formed, the bradykinin persists for only a few minutes, because it is digested by other enzymes.

Bradykinin causes very powerful *arteriolar dilatation* and also *increased capillary permeability*. There is reason to believe that bradykinin and other kinins play special roles in regulating blood flow and capillary leakage of fluids in inflamed tissues. It is also believed that bradykinin plays a role in regulating skin blood flow and also blood flow in the salivary and other gastrointestinal glands.

Serotonin. Serotonin (5-hydroxytryptamine) is present in large concentrations in the chromaffin tissue of the intestine and other abdominal structures. Also, it is present in high concentration in the platelets. Serotonin can have either a vasodilator or vasoconstrictor effect, depending on the condition or the area of the circulation. And, even though these effects can sometimes be powerful, the functions of serotonin in regulation of the circulation are almost entirely unknown. Occasionally, tumors composed of chromaffin tissue develop, called *carcinoid tumors*. These secrete tremendous quantities of serotonin and cause mottled areas of vasodilatation in the skin; but the very fact that these tremendous quantities of serotonin do not drastically disturb the circulation makes it doubtful that serotonin plays a widespread general role in regulation of circulatory function.

Histamine. Histamine is released in essentially every tissue of the body whenever it becomes damaged. Most of the histamine is probably derived from mast cells in the damaged tissues and from basophils in the blood.

Histamine has a powerful vasodilator effect on the arterioles, and like bradykinin, also has the ability to greatly increase capillary porosity, allowing leakage of both fluid and plasma protein into the tissues. Though the role of histamine in normal regulation of the circulation is unknown, in inflamed tissues the intense arteriolar dilatation and increased capillary porosity caused by histamine cause tremendous quantities of fluid to leak out of the circulation into the tissues, inducing edema.

Prostaglandins. Almost every tissue of the body contains small to moderate amounts of several chemically related substances called *prostaglandins*. These substances are released into the local tissue fluids and into the circulating blood under both physiological and pathological conditions. Though some of the prostaglandins cause vasoconstriction, most of the more important ones seem to be mainly vasodilator agents. Thus far, no specific pattern of function of the prostaglandins in circulatory control has been found. However, their widespread prevalence in the tissues and their myriad effects on the circulation make them ideal candidates for special roles in local circulatory control. For this reason, these substances are presently under intensive research investigation, though unequivocal conclusions about their roles in circulatory regulation are still evasive.

Effects of Different Ions and Other Chemical Factors on Vascular Control

Many different ions and other chemical factors can either dilate or constrict local blood vessels. Though the roles of these substances in the overall *regulation* of the circulation generally are not known, their specific effects can be listed as follows:

An increase in *calcium ion* concentration causes vasoconstriction. This results from the general effect of calcium to stimulate smooth muscle contraction, as discussed in Chapter 7.

An increase in *potassium ion* concentration causes vasodilatation. This results from the ability of potassium ions to inhibit smooth muscle contraction.

An increase in *magnesium ion* concentration causes powerful vasodilatation, for magnesium ions inhibit smooth muscle generally.

Increased *sodium ion* concentration causes arteriolar dilatation. This results mainly from an increase in osmolality of the fluids rather than from a specific effect of sodium ion itself. *Increased osmolality* of the blood caused by increased quantities of *glucose* or other nonvasoactive substances also causes arteriolar dilatation. Decreased osmolality causes arteriolar constriction.

An *increase in hydrogen ion* concentration (decrease in pH) causes dilatation of the arterioles. A slight *decrease in hydrogen ion* concentration causes arteriolar constriction, but an intense decrease causes dilatation, the same effect as that which occurs with increased hydrogen ion concentration.

An increase in carbon dioxide concentration causes moderate vasodilatation in most tissues and marked vasodilatation in the brain. However, carbon dioxide, acting on the vasomotor center, has an extremely powerful indirect vasoconstrictor effect that is transmitted through the sympathetic vasoconstrictor system.

QUESTIONS

1. What are some of the special "needs" of the tissues that play a significant role in controlling local tissue blood flow?
2. Describe the typical structure of a microcirculatory bed.
3. What is the specific anatomy of the small arteries and arterioles, and what are their nervous connections that allow these to be especially important in controlling blood flow?
4. What are the specific characteristics of the *metarterioles* and *precapillary sphincters* that allow them to control local blood flow in response to local humoral factors?
5. What is the special importance of oxygen in the control of local blood flow? Explain both the *vasodilator theory* and the *oxygen demand theory* for control of local blood flow.
6. Explain the mechanisms of *reactive hyperemia* and *active hyperemia*.
7. Explain what is meant by *autoregulation*.
8. Explain the difference between long-term blood flow regulation and short-term regulation. What is the function of angiogenesis factor in long-term blood flow regulation?
9. Describe the organization of the autonomic nervous system, especially the sympathetic portion, for circulatory control.
10. What is meant by *vasomotor tone,* and why is this important?
11. What is the role of the higher nervous centers in the control of the circulation?
12. What are the roles of *epinephrine, norepinephrine, angiotensin, vasopressin, bradykinin, serotonin, histamine,* and the *prostaglandins* in the control of blood flow?
13. How do each of the following ions and other chemical factors affect vascular control: *calcium ion, potassium ion, magnesium ion, sodium ion, osmolality of the blood, hydrogen ion, carbon dioxide concentration*?

References

Abboud, F. M., ed.: Disturbances in Neurogenic Control of the Circulation. Baltimore, The Williams & Wilkins Co., 1981.

American Physiological Society: Peripheral Circulation and Organ Blood Flow. Washington, D.C., American Physiological Society, 1983.

Bevan, J. A., et al., eds.: Vascular Neuroeffector Mechanisms. New York, Raven Press, 1980.

Borgstrom, P., et al.: An evaluation of the metabolic interaction with myogenic vascular reactivity during blood flow autoregulation. Acta Physiol Scand 122:275, 1984.

Cowley, A. W., Jr., and Guyton, A. C.: Quantification of intermediate steps in the renin-angiotensin-vasoconstrictor feedback loop in the dog. Circ Res 30:557, 1972.

Duling, B. R., and Klitzman, B.: Local control of microvascular function: role in tissue oxygen supply. Annu Rev Physiol 42:373, 1980.

Guyton, A. C.: Arterial Pressure and Hypertension. Philadelphia, W. B. Saunders Co., 1980.

Guyton, A. C., et al.: Cardiac Output and Its Regulation. Philadelphia, W. B. Saunders Co., 1973.

Hudlicka, O.: Development of microcirculation: capillary growth and adaptation. In Renkin, E. M., and Michel, C. C., eds.: Handbook of Physiology. Sec. 2, Vol. 4. Bethesda, American Physiological Society, 1984, p. 165.

Johansson, B.: Vascular smooth muscle reactivity. Annu Rev Physiol 43:359, 1981.

Olsson, R. A.: Local factors regulating cardiac and skeletal muscle blood flow. Annu Rev Physiol 43:385, 1981.

Randall, W. C., ed.: Nervous Control of Cardiovascular Function. New York, Oxford University Press, 1984.

Renkin, E. M.: Control of microcirculation and blood-tissue exchange. In Renkin, E. M., and Michel, C. C., eds.: Handbook of Physiology. Sec. 2, Vol. 4. Bethesda, American Physiological Society, 1984, p. 627.

Rodkiewicz, C. M.: Arteries and Arterial Blood Flow. New York, Springer-Verlag, 1983.

Rosell, S.: Neuronal control of microvessels. Annu Rev Physiol 42:359, 1980.

Rowell, L. B.: Reflex control of regional circulation in humans. J Autonom Nerv Syst 11:101, 1984.

Vallee, B. L., et al.: Tumor-derived angiogenesis factors from rat Walker 256 carcinoma: an experimental investigation and review. Experientia, 41:1, 1985.

14

Nervous Reflex and Hormonal Mechanisms for Short-Term Arterial Pressure Control

NORMAL ARTERIAL PRESSURES
  THE MEAN ARTERIAL PRESSURE
  CLINICAL METHODS FOR
    MEASURING SYSTOLIC AND
    DIASTOLIC PRESSURES
RELATIONSHIP OF ARTERIAL PRESSURE
  TO CARDIAC OUTPUT AND TOTAL
  PERIPHERAL RESISTANCE
THE OVERALL SYSTEM FOR ARTERIAL
  PRESSURE REGULATION
THE RAPIDLY ACTING NERVOUS
  MECHANISMS FOR ARTERIAL
  PRESSURE CONTROL
  THE ARTERIAL BARORECEPTOR
    CONTROL SYSTEM—
    BARORECEPTOR REFLEXES
  THE CNS ISCHEMIC RESPONSE—
    CONTROL OF ARTERIAL PRESSURE

  BY THE VASOMOTOR CENTER IN
  RESPONSE TO DIMINISHED BRAIN
  BLOOD FLOW
  ATRIAL REFLEX CONTROL OF HEART
  RATE (THE BAINBRIDGE REFLEX)
HORMONAL MECHANISMS FOR RAPID
  CONTROL OF ARTERIAL PRESSURE
  THE NOREPINEPHRINE-EPINEPHRINE
    VASOCONSTRICTOR MECHANISM
  ROLE OF VASOPRESSIN IN RAPID
    CONTROL OF ARTERIAL PRESSURE
  THE RENIN-ANGIOTENSIN
    VASOCONSTRICTOR MECHANISM
    FOR CONTROL OF ARTERIAL
    PRESSURE
THE CAPILLARY FLUID SHIFT
  MECHANISM FOR ARTERIAL
  PRESSURE REGULATION

In the previous chapter we pointed out that each tissue can control its own blood flow by simply dilating or constricting its local arterioles. For this mechanism to work, it is necessary that the arterial pressure remain constant or nearly constant because with a variable arterial pressure one would never know whether dilating the blood vessels would necessarily increase the local blood flow. Fortunately, the circulation has an intricate system for regulation of the arterial pressure. It maintains the normal mean arterial pressure in the young adult within rather narrow limits between 95 mm Hg and 100 mm Hg. Some of the pressure regulatory mechanisms (mainly nervous and hormonal mechanisms) act very rapidly, and some (mainly mechanisms related to kidney function and blood volume regulation) act very slowly. In the present chapter we will discuss the rapid nervous and

hormonal pressure control mechanisms. In the following chapter we will discuss both the long-term regulation of arterial pressure, based primarily on renal and body fluid mechanisms, and the clinical problem of hypertension or "high blood pressure," which is caused by abnormalities of the long-term pressure regulatory mechanisms.

NORMAL ARTERIAL PRESSURES

Arterial Pressures at Different Ages. Figure 14-1 illustrates the typical diastolic, systolic, and mean arterial pressures from birth to 80 years of age. From this figure it can be seen that the systolic pressure of a normal young adult averages about 120 mm Hg and the diastolic pressure about 80 mm Hg—that is,

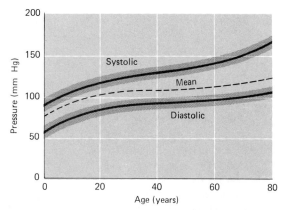

Figure 14–1. Changes in systolic, diastolic, and mean arterial pressures with age. The shaded areas show the normal range.

arterial pressure is said to be 120/80. The shaded areas on either side of the curves depict the normal ranges of systolic and diastolic pressures, showing considerable variation from person to person.

The increase in arterial pressure at older ages is usually associated with developing arteriosclerosis. In this disease the systolic pressure especially increases; in approximately one-tenth of all old people it eventually rises above 200 mm Hg.

THE MEAN ARTERIAL PRESSURE

The mean arterial pressure is the average pressure throughout each cycle of the heartbeat. Offhand one might expect that it would be equal to the average of systolic and diastolic pressures but this is not true because the arterial pressure remains nearer to diastolic level than to systolic level during a greater portion of the pulse cycle, which can be seen in all the pictures of pressure pulses shown in Chapter 12. Therefore, the mean arterial pressure is usually slightly less than the average of systolic and diastolic pressures, as is evident in Figure 14–1.

The mean arterial pressure of the normal young adult averages about 96 mm Hg, which is slightly less than the average of the systolic and diastolic pressures, 120 and 80 mm Hg, respectively. However, for purposes of discussion, the mean arterial pressure is usually considered to be 100 mm Hg because this value is easy to remember. Mean arterial pressure is the average pressure tending to push blood through the systemic circulatory system. Therefore, *from the point of view of tissue blood flow, it is generally the mean arterial pressure that is important.*

CLINICAL METHODS FOR MEASURING SYSTOLIC AND DIASTOLIC PRESSURES

Obviously, it would be impossible to use the various pressure recorders that require needle insertion into an artery, as described in Chapter 12, for making routine pressure measurements in human patients. Instead, the clinician determines systolic and diastolic pressures by indirect means, most usually by the auscultatory method.

The Auscultatory Method. Figure 14–2 illustrates the auscultatory method for determining systolic and diastolic arterial pressures. A stethoscope is placed over the antecubital artery while a blood pressure cuff is inflated around the upper arm. As long as the cuff presses against the arm with so little pressure that the artery remains distended with blood, no sounds whatsoever are heard by the stethoscope despite the fact that the blood within the artery is pulsating. But when the cuff pressure is great enough to close the artery during part of the arterial pressure cycle, a sound is heard in the stethoscope with each pulsation. These sounds are called *Korotkoff's sounds.*

The Korotkoff's sounds are believed to be caused by blood jetting through the partly occluded vessel. The jet causes turbulence in the open vessel beyond the cuff, and this sets up the vibrations heard through the stethoscope.

In determining blood pressure by the auscultatory method, the pressure in the cuff is first elevated well above arterial systolic pressure. As long as this pressure is higher than systolic pressure, the brachial artery remains collapsed and no blood flows into the lower artery during any part of the pressure cycle. Therefore, no Korotkoff's sounds are heard in the lower artery. But then the cuff pressure is gradually reduced. Just as soon as the pressure in the cuff falls below systolic pressure, a small amount of blood slips through the artery beneath the cuff during the peak of systolic pressure, and one begins to hear *tapping* sounds in the antecubital artery in synchrony with the heart beat. As soon as these sounds are heard, the pressure level indicated by the manometer connected to the cuff is approximately equal to the systolic pressure.

As the pressure in the cuff is lowered still more, the Korotkoff's sounds change in quality, having less of the tapping quality but more of a rhythmic, harsher quality. Then, finally, when the pressure in the cuff falls to equal diastolic pressure, the artery no longer

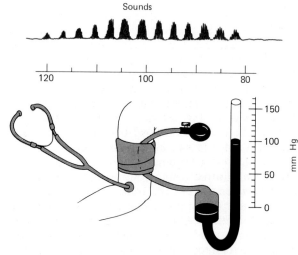

Figure 14–2. The auscultatory method of measuring systolic and diastolic pressures.

closes during diastole, which means that the basic factor causing the sounds (the jetting of blood through a squeezed artery) is no longer present. Therefore, the sounds suddenly change to a muffled quality, and they usually disappear entirely after another 5 to 10 mm drop in cuff pressure. One notes the manometer pressure when the Korotkoff's sounds change to the muffled quality, and this pressure is approximately equal to the diastolic pressure.

The auscultatory method for determining systolic and diastolic pressures is not entirely accurate, but it usually gives values within 10 per cent of those determined by direct measurement from the arteries.

RELATIONSHIP OF ARTERIAL PRESSURE TO CARDIAC OUTPUT AND TOTAL PERIPHERAL RESISTANCE

Before discussing the overall regulation of arterial pressure, it is good to remember the basic relationship between arterial pressure, cardiac output, and total peripheral resistance, as described by Ohm's law which was discussed in detail in Chapter 12, as follows:

Arterial pressure = Cardiac output
$$\times \text{ total peripheral resistance}$$

It is obvious from this formula that any condition that increases either the cardiac output or total peripheral resistance (if the other factor does not change) will cause an increase in mean arterial pressure. Both these factors are often manipulated in the control of arterial pressure, as we shall see in the remainder of this chapter and in the following chapter.

THE OVERALL SYSTEM FOR ARTERIAL PRESSURE REGULATION

Arterial pressure is not regulated by a single pressure controlling system but instead by several interrelated systems that perform specific functions. When a person bleeds severely so that the pressure falls suddenly, two problems immediately confront the pressure control system. The first is to return the arterial pressure immediately to a high enough level that the person can survive through the acute hemorrhagic episode. The second is to return the blood volume eventually to its normal level so that the circulatory system can re-establish full normality, including return of the arterial pressure *all the way back to its normal value*, not merely back to a pressure level required for survival. These two problems characterize two major types of arterial pressure control systems in the body: (1) a system of rapidly acting pressure control mechanisms that are concerned with immediate survival, and (2) a system for long-term control of the basic arterial pressure level.

Rapidly Acting Pressure Control Mechanisms. Several different pressure control mechanisms, all of which are nervous feedback mechanisms, begin to react within seconds. These include the *baroreceptor feedback mechanism* and the *central nervous system ischemic mechanism*. Thus, the first line of defense against abnormal pressures is subserved by the nervous mechanisms for control of arterial pressure.

Within minutes several other pressure control mechanisms also come into play. Three of these are the *renin-angiotensin-vasoconstrictor mechanism, the vasopressin-vasoconstrictor mechanism,* and the *shift of fluid through the capillaries* from the tissues into or out of the circulation to readjust the blood volume as needed. These mechanisms become fully active within 20 minutes to several hours, in contrast to the nervous mechanisms that usually become fully active within a minute or so.

Long-Term Mechanisms for Arterial Pressure Regulation. The nervous regulators of arterial pressure, though acting very rapidly and powerfully to correct acute abnormalities of arterial pressure, generally lose their power to control arterial pressure after a few hours to a few days because most of the nervous pressure receptors "adapt"; that is, they lose their responsiveness. Therefore, except under unusual circumstances, the nervous mechanisms for arterial pressure control do not play a major role in long-term regulation of arterial pressure. Long-term regulation, instead, is vested mainly in a *renal-body fluid-pressure control mechanism*. As we shall discuss in the following chapter, this mechanism involves control of blood volume with its consequent effects on arterial pressure. Part of this mechanism involves control of kidney function by several different hormonal systems, including especially the *renin-angiotensin system* and the hormone *aldosterone* secreted by the adrenal cortex.

THE RAPIDLY ACTING NERVOUS MECHANISMS FOR ARTERIAL PRESSURE CONTROL

THE ARTERIAL BARORECEPTOR CONTROL SYSTEM—BARORECEPTOR REFLEXES

By far the best known of the mechanisms for arterial pressure control is the *baroreceptor reflex*. Basically, this reflex is initiated by stretch receptors, called either *baroreceptors* or *pressoreceptors*, located in the walls of the large systemic arteries. A rise in pressure stretches the baroreceptors and causes them to transmit signals into the central nervous system, and feedback signals are then sent back through the autonomic nervous system to the circulation to reduce arterial pressure downward toward the normal level.

Physiologic Anatomy of the Baroreceptors and Their Innervation. Baroreceptors are spray-type nerve endings lying in the walls of the arteries; they are stimulated when stretched. A few baroreceptors are located in the wall of almost every large artery of the thoracic and neck regions; but, as illustrated in Figure 14–3, baroreceptors are extremely abundant, in (1) the wall of each internal carotid artery slightly above the carotid bifurcation, an area known as the *carotid sinus*, and (2) the wall of the aortic arch.

Figure 14–3 also shows that signals are transmitted from each carotid sinus through the very small *Hering's nerve* to the glossopharyngeal nerve and thence to the *tractus solitarius* in the medullary area of the brain stem. Signals from the arch of the aorta are transmitted through the vagus nerves also into this area of the medulla. Hering's nerve is especially important in physiologic experiments because baroreceptor impulses can be recorded from it with ease.

Response of the Baroreceptors to Pressure. The baroreceptors are not stimulated at all by pressures between 0 and 60 mm Hg, but above 60 mm Hg they respond progressively more and more rapidly and reach a maximum at about 200 mm Hg. However, the increase in number of impulses for each unit change in arterial pressure is greatest at a pressure level near the normal mean arterial pressure. That is, in the normal operating range of arterial pressure, even a slight change in pressure causes strong autonomic reflexes to readjust the arterial pressure back toward normal. Thus, the baroreceptor feedback mechanism functions most effectively in the very pressure range where it is most needed.

The Reflex Initiated by the Baroreceptors. The baroreceptor signals entering the brain stem *inhibit the vasoconstrictor center* of the medulla and *excite the vagal center*. The net effects are (1) *vasodilatation* of the arterioles, (2) *decreased heart rate* and *strength of heart contraction*, (3) *dilatation of the venous system*, which decreases the return of blood to the heart from the veins. Therefore, excitation of the barore-

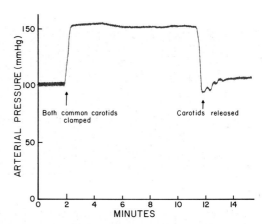

Figure 14–4. Typical carotid sinus reflex effect on arterial pressure caused by clamping both common carotids (after the two vagus nerves have been cut).

ceptors by pressure in the arteries reflexly *causes the arterial pressure to decrease* because of both a decrease in peripheral resistance and a decrease in cardiac output. Conversely, low pressure has opposite effects, reflexly causing the pressure to rise back toward normal.

Figure 14–4 illustrates a typical reflex change in arterial pressure caused by occluding the common carotid arteries. This reduces the carotid sinus pressure; as a result, the baroreceptors become inactive and lose their inhibitory effect on the vasomotor center. The vasomotor center then becomes much more active than usual, causing the arterial pressure to rise and to remain elevated during the ten minutes that the carotids are occluded. Removal of the occlusion allows the pressure to fall immediately to slightly below normal as a momentary overcompensation and then to return to normal in another minute or so.

Function of the Baroreceptors During Changes in Body Posture. The ability of the baroreceptors to maintain relatively constant arterial pressure is extremely important when a person sits or stands after having been lying down. Immediately upon standing, the arterial pressure in the head and upper part of the body obviously tends to fall, and marked reduction of this pressure can cause loss of consciousness. Fortunately, however, the falling pressure at the level of the baroreceptors elicits an immediate reflex, resulting in strong sympathetic discharge throughout the body, and this minimizes the decrease in pressure in the head and upper body.

The Buffer Function of the Baroreceptor Control System. Because the baroreceptor system opposes increases and decreases in arterial pressure, it is often called a *pressure buffer system*, and the nerves from the baroreceptors are called *buffer nerves*.

Figure 14–5 illustrates the importance of this buffer function of the baroreceptors. The upper record in this figure shows an arterial pressure recording for two hours from a normal dog and the lower record from a dog whose baroreceptor nerves from both the carotid sinuses and the aorta had previously been removed. Note the extreme variability of pressure in

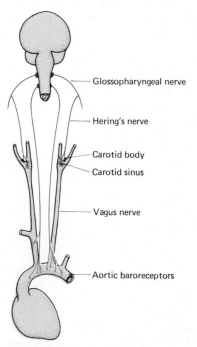

Figure 14–3. The baroreceptor system.

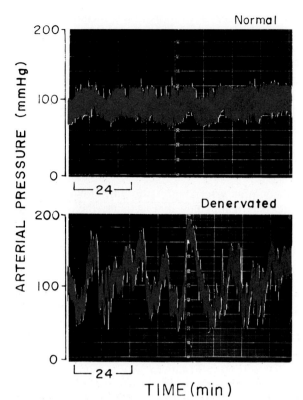

Figure 14–5. Two-hour records of arterial pressure in a normal dog (above) and in the same dog (below) several weeks after the baroreceptors had been denervated. (From Cowley, Liard, and Guyton: *Circ. Res., 32* :564, 1973. By permission of the American Heart Association, Inc.)

the denervated dog caused by simple events of the day such as lying down, standing, excitement, eating, defecating, noises, and so forth. Thus, without the baroreceptor system, the arterial pressure often fell to as low as 50 mm Hg or rose to over 160 mm Hg.

Unimportance of the Baroreceptor System for Long-Term Regulation of Arterial Pressure—"Resetting" of the Baroreceptors

The baroreceptor control system is probably of little or no importance in long-term regulation of arterial pressure for a very simple reason: The baroreceptors themselves "reset" in one to two days to whatever pressure level they are exposed to. That is, if the pressure rises from the normal value of 100 mm Hg to 200 mm Hg, extreme numbers of baroreceptor impulses are at first transmitted. During the next few seconds, the rate of firing diminishes considerably; then it diminishes very slowly during the next one to two days, at the end of which time the rate will have returned essentially to the normal level despite the fact that the arterial pressure remains 200 mm Hg. Conversely, when the arterial pressure falls to a very low value, the baroreceptors at first transmit no impulses at all, but gradually over a day or days the rate of baroreceptor firing returns again to the original control level.

This resetting of the baroreceptors obviously prevents the baroreceptor reflex from functioning as a control system to buffer arterial pressure changes that last longer than a few days at a time. In fact, referring again to Figure 14–5, one can see that the *average* arterial pressure several weeks after removal of the baroreceptor system (lower panel) was almost exactly the same as before removal (upper panel). This illustrates the *unimportance of the baroreceptor system for long-term regulation of the arterial pressure* even though it is a potent mechanism for preventing the rapid changes of arterial pressure that occur moment by moment or hour by hour. Instead, prolonged regulation of arterial pressure requires other control systems, principally the renal-body fluid-pressure control system (along with its associated hormonal mechanisms), to be discussed in the following chapter.

THE CNS ISCHEMIC RESPONSE—CONTROL OF ARTERIAL PRESSURE BY THE VASOMOTOR CENTER IN RESPONSE TO DIMINISHED BRAIN BLOOD FLOW

Normally, most nervous control of blood pressure is achieved by reflexes originating in the baroreceptors or other closely allied receptors, such as *receptors in the atrial walls* and *pulmonary arteries* or *chemoreceptors* in the *aortic* and *carotid bodies*, all of which act in parallel with the baroreceptors. However, when blood flow to the vasomotor center in the lower brain stem becomes decreased enough to cause nutritional deficiency, a condition called *ischemia,* the neurons in the vasomotor center itself respond directly to the ischemia and become strongly excited. When this occurs, the systemic arterial pressure often rises to a level as high as the heart can possibly pump. This effect is believed to be caused by failure of the slowly flowing blood to carry carbon dioxide away from the vasomotor center; the local concentration of the carbon dioxide then increases greatly and has an extremely potent effect in stimulating the sympathetic nervous system. The very great increase in arterial pressure in response to cerebral ischemia is known as the *central nervous system ischemic response* or simply *CNS ischemic response.*

Importance of the CNS Ischemic Response as a Regulator of Arterial Pressure. Despite the extremely powerful nature of the CNS ischemic response, it does not become very active until the arterial pressure falls far below normal, down to 60 mm Hg and below, reaching its greatest degree of stimulation at a pressure of 15 to 20 mm Hg. Therefore, it is not one of the mechanisms for regulating normal arterial pressure. Instead, it operates principally as an *emergency arterial pressure control system that acts rapidly and extremely powerfully to prevent further decrease in arterial pressure whenever blood flow to the brain decreases dangerously close to the lethal level.* It is sometimes called the "last ditch stand" pressure control mechanism.

ATRIAL REFLEX CONTROL OF HEART RATE (THE BAINBRIDGE REFLEX)

An increase in atrial pressure causes an increase in heart rate, sometimes increasing the heart rate as much as 75 per cent. Part of this increase in heart rate is caused by the direct effect of the increased atrial volume to stretch the S-A node, which can increase the heart rate as much as 15 per cent. An additional 40 to 60 per cent increase in rate is caused by a reflex called the *Bainbridge reflex*. The stretch receptors of the atria that elicit the Bainbridge reflex transmit their afferent signals through the vagus nerves to the medulla of the brain. Then, efferent signals are transmitted back through both the vagal and sympathetic nerves to increase the heart's rate and presumably also strength of contraction. Thus, this reflex helps prevent damming of blood in the veins, the atria, and the pulmonary circulation. It obviously has a different purpose from that of controlling arterial pressure and is actually detrimental to pressure control for short periods of time.

HORMONAL MECHANISMS FOR RAPID CONTROL OF ARTERIAL PRESSURE

In addition to the rapidly acting nervous mechanisms for control of arterial pressure, there are at least three hormonal mechanisms that also provide either rapid or moderately rapid control of arterial pressure. These mechanisms are

(1) the norepinephrine-epinephrine vasoconstrictor mechanism;

(2) and vasopressin-vasoconstrictor mechanism;

(3) the the renin-angiotensin vasoconstrictor mechanism.

THE NOREPINEPHRINE-EPINEPHRINE VASOCONSTRICTOR MECHANISM

In the previous chapter it was pointed out that stimulation of the sympathetic nervous system not only causes direct nervous excitation of the blood vessels and heart but also causes release by the adrenal medullae of epinephrine and norepinephrine into the circulating blood. These two hormones circulate to all parts of the body and cause essentially the same effects in controlling arterial pressure as direct sympathetic stimulation. That is, they excite the heart, they constrict most of the blood vessels, and they constrict the veins.

Therefore, the different reflexes that regulate arterial pressure by exciting the sympathetic nervous system cause the pressure to rise in two ways: by direct circulatory stimulation and by indirect stimulation through the release of epinephrine and norepinephrine into the blood.

Epinephrine and norepinephrine circulate in the blood for one to three minutes before being destroyed, thus maintaining a slightly prolonged excitation of the circulation. Also, these hormones can reach some parts of the circulation that have no sympathetic nervous supply at all, including the very minute vessels such as the metarterioles. And these hormones have especially potent actions on some vascular beds, particularly the skin vasculature.

In general, therefore, the epinephrine and norepinephrine system can be considered to be a part of the total sympathetic mechanism for arterial pressure control.

ROLE OF VASOPRESSIN IN RAPID CONTROL OF ARTERIAL PRESSURE

When the arterial pressure falls low, either the same nervous signals that activate the sympathetic nervous system or closely related signals cause the posterior pituitary gland to secrete large quantities of *vasopressin*, as was explained in the previous chapter. The vasopressin in turn has a direct vasoconstrictor effect on the blood vessels, thereby increasing both the total peripheral resistance and the mean circulatory filling pressure, thus raising the arterial pressure back toward normal.

Until recently, most physiologists believed that the amount of vasopressin secreted in low blood pressure states was not sufficient to play a significant role in compensating for the low pressure. However, recent experiments in animals in which the baroreceptor pressure-controlling mechanism has been removed have shown that the circulating amounts of vasopressin found in the blood following hemorrhage can then increase the arterial pressure as much as 35 to 50 mm Hg. In a recent study by Cowley, the vasopressin system was shown to return the blood pressure about 75 per cent of the way toward normal within a few minutes after acute hemorrhage had decreased the arterial pressure to as low as 50 mm Hg.

Therefore, it is almost certain that vasopressin plays a very important role in re-establishing normal arterial pressure when the pressure falls acutely to dangerously low levels.

Vasopressin also plays an indirect role in the long-term control of arterial pressure through its effects on the kidneys in causing decreased excretion of water. Because of this effect, vasopressin is also called *antidiuretic hormone*. When only minute amounts of vasopressin are secreted—in the order of nanograms—the kidney excretion of water decreases to a minimal amount, an effect that helps increase the blood volume any time the arterial pressure remains low for any period of time. The increased blood volume then helps bring the pressure back to normal. Thus, vasopressin not only plays an important role in acute regulation of arterial pressure but also in long-term regulation, which will be discussed in the following chapter.

THE RENIN-ANGIOTENSIN VASOCONSTRICTOR MECHANISM FOR CONTROL OF ARTERIAL PRESSURE

The hormone *angiotensin II* is one of the most potent vasoconstrictors known. It and vasopressin vie

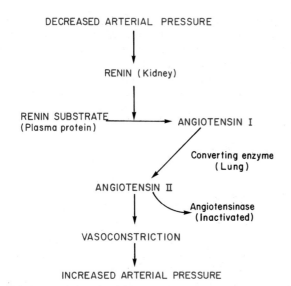

Figure 14–6. The renin-angiotensin-vasoconstrictor mechanism for arterial pressure control.

with each other for this distinction. Whenever the arterial pressure falls very low, large quantities of angiotensin II appear in the circulation. This results from a special mechanism involving the kidneys and the release of the enzyme *renin* from the kidneys when the arterial pressure falls too low.

The overall schema for formation of angiotensin and the effect of angiotensin II to increase arterial pressure are illustrated in Figure 14–6. When blood flow through the kidneys is decreased because of low arterial pressure, the *juxtaglomerular cells* (cells located in the walls of the afferent arterioles immediately proximal to the glomeruli) secrete renin into the blood. In addition, sympathetic nerve signals directly to the juxtaglomerular cells can also cause these cells to release renin whenever the sympathetic nervous system becomes activated. Renin itself is an enzyme that splits the end off one of the plasma proteins, called *renin substrate* (or *angiotensinogen*), to release a decapeptide, *angiotensin I*. The renin persists in the blood for 30 minutes to an hour and continues to cause formation of angiotensin I during this entire time. Within a few seconds after the angiotensin I is formed, two additional amino acids are split from it to form the octapeptide *angiotensin II*. This conversion occurs almost entirely in the small vessels of the lungs, catalyzed by an enzyme called *converting enzyme* that is present in the walls of these vessels. Angiotensin II persists in the blood for a minute or so but is rapidly inactivated by a number of different blood and tissue enzymes collectively called *angiotensinase*.

During its persistence in the blood, angiotensin II has several effects that can elevate arterial pressure. One of these effects occurs very rapidly: vasoconstriction, especially of the arterioles and to a lesser extent of the veins. Constriction of the arterioles increases the peripheral resistance and thereby raises the arterial pressure back toward normal, as illustrated at the

bottom of the schema in Figure 14–6. Also, mild constriction of the veins increases the mean circulatory filling pressure, sometimes as much as 20 per cent, and this promotes increased tendency for venous return of blood to the heart, thereby helping the heart pump against the extra pressure load.

The other effects of angiotensin are mainly related to the body fluid volumes: (1) angiotensin has a direct effect on the kidneys to cause decreased excretion of both salt and water; and (2) angiotensin stimulates the secretion of aldosterone by the adrenal cortex, and this hormone in turn also acts on the kidneys to cause decreased excretion of both salt and water. Both these effects tend to elevate the blood volume— an important factor in long-term regulation of arterial pressure, as will be discussed in the following chapter.

Rapidity of Action and Pressure Controlling Power of the Renin-Angiotensin Vasoconstrictor System. Figure 14–7 illustrates a typical experiment showing the effect of hemorrhage on the arterial pressure under two separate conditions: (1) with the renin-angiotensin system functioning, and (2) without the system functioning (the system was interrupted by a renin-blocking antibody). Note that following hemorrhage, which caused an acute fall of the arterial pressure to 50 mm Hg, the arterial pressure rose back to 83 mm Hg when the renin-angiotensin system was functional. On the other hand, it rose to only 60 mm Hg when the renin-angiotensin system was blocked. This illustrates that the renin-angiotensin system is powerful enough to return the arterial pressure at least halfway back to normal following severe hemorrhage. Therefore, it can sometimes be of lifesaving service to the body, especially in circulatory shock.

Note that the renin-angiotensin vasoconstrictor system requires approximately 20 minutes to become fully active. Therefore, it is far slower to act than are the nervous reflexes and the norepinephrine-epinephrine system; and it also acts only about one half as rapidly as the vasopressin system. However, it also has a correspondingly longer duration of action.

There is reason to believe that the renin-angiotensin vasoconstrictor system is much more powerful

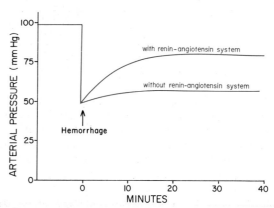

Figure 14–7. Pressure-compensating effect of the renin-angiotensin-vasoconstrictor system following severe hemorrhage. (Drawn from experiments by Dr. Royce Brough.)

under some conditions than others. For instance, some patients with diseased kidneys secrete tremendous quantities of renin, and the pressure control action of the system is then likely to be very powerful.

THE CAPILLARY FLUID SHIFT MECHANISM FOR ARTERIAL PRESSURE REGULATION

In addition to the nervous and hormonal mechanisms for rapid control of arterial pressure, an intrinsic physical mechanism of the circulation also helps to control (or "buffer") arterial pressure, usually beginning to act within a few minutes and reaching full function within a few hours. It is the capillary fluid shift mechanism, which is the following: When the arterial pressure changes, this change is usually accompanied by a similar change in capillary pressure. This causes fluid to begin moving across the capillary membrane between the blood and the interstitial fluid compartment. Within a few minutes to an hour a new state of equilibrium usually will be achieved, but in the meantime this shift of fluid will have played a very beneficial role in the control of arterial pressure. For instance, if the arterial pressure rises too high, loss of fluid through the capillaries into the interstitial spaces causes the blood volume to fall and thereby causes return of arterial pressure back toward normal. This system can return the arterial pressure about three fourths of the way back toward its normal mean value, but it takes effect much more slowly than do the nervous reflex mechanisms.

QUESTIONS

1. What are the approximate values for systolic arterial pressure, diastolic arterial pressure, and mean arterial pressure?
2. Describe the auscultatory method for estimating systolic and diastolic pressures.
3. What are the interrelationships between rapidly acting and long-term mechanisms for control of arterial pressure?
4. Describe the anatomy of the baroreceptor reflex mechanism for controlling arterial pressure.
5. When the arterial pressure rises too high, what are the reflex effects on the circulatory system caused by excitation of the baroreceptors?
6. Explain the role of the baroreceptor pressure control system in relation to body posture, and also explain the buffer function of the baroreceptor system.
7. Why is the baroreceptor system not of importance for long-term regulation of arterial pressure?
8. Explain the CNS ischemic response, and tell why it is frequently called the "last ditch stand" pressure control mechanism.
9. What is the Bainbridge reflex, and why is it sometimes detrimental to pressure control?
10. What is the role of the epinephrine and norepinephrine hormonal system in the reflex control of arterial pressure?
11. How does the vasopressin-vasoconstrictor mechanism contribute to arterial pressure regulation?
12. Describe the sequential events that lead to the formation of angiotensin II when the arterial pressure falls too low?
13. Explain the quantitative value and the timing of the effect of the renin-angiotensin-vasoconstriction system in returning the arterial pressure toward normal following hemorrhage.
14. Explain how a shift of fluid through the capillary membranes helps to buffer arterial pressure changes.

References

Antonaccio, M. J., ed.: Cardiovascular Pharmacology. New York, Raven Press, 1984.

Burattini, R., and Borgdorff, P.: Closed-loop baroreflex control of total peripheral resistance in the cat: identification of gains by aid of a model. Cardiovasc Res 18:715, 1984.

Coleridge, H. M., and Coleridge, J. C. G.: Cardiovascular afferents involved in regulation of peripheral vessels. Annu Rev Physiol 42:413, 1980.

Conway, J.: Hemodynamic aspects of essential hypertension in humans. Physiol Rev 64:617, 1984.

Cushing, H.: Concerning a definite regulatory mechanism of the vasomotor center which controls blood pressure during cerebral compression. Bull Johns Hopkins Hosp 12:290, 1901.

Dampney, R. A., et al.: Identification of cardiovascular cell groups in the brain stem. Clin Exp Hypertens 6:205, 1984.

Edwards, C. R., and Padfield, P. L.: Angiotensin-converting enzyme inhibitors: past, present, and bright future. Lancet, 1:30, 1985.

Guyton, A. C.: Arterial Pressure and Hypertension. Philadelphia, W. B. Saunders Co., 1980.

Guyton, A. C., et al.: Method for studying competence of the body's blood pressure regulatory mechanisms and effect of pressoreceptor denervation. Am J Physiol 164:360, 1951.

Herd, J. A.: Cardiovascular response to stress in man. Annu Rev Physiol 46:177, 1984.

Ludbrook, J.: Reflex control of blood pressure during exercise. Annu Rev Physiol 45:155, 1983.

Mancia, G., and Mark, A. L.: Arterial baroreflexes in humans. In Shepherd, J. T., and Abboud, F. M., eds.: Handbook of Physiology Sec. 2, Vol. 3. Bethesda, American Physiological Society, 1983, p. 755.

Randall, W. C., ed.: Nervous Control of Cardiovascular Function. New York, Oxford University Press, 1984.

Rowell, L. B.: Reflex control of regional circulations in humans. J Autonom Nerv Syst 11:101, 1984.

Sagawa, K.: Baroreflex control of systemic arterial pressure and vascular bed. In Shepherd, J. T., and Abboud, F. M., eds.: Handbook of Physiology. Sec. 2, Vol. 3. Bethesda, American Physiological Society, 1983, p. 453.

15

Long-Term Regulation of Mean Arterial Pressure; Hypertension

THE RENAL–BODY FLUID SYSTEM FOR
   ARTERIAL PRESSURE CONTROL
ROLE OF THE RENIN-ANGIOTENSIN
   SYSTEM AND OF ALDOSTERONE IN
   LONG-TERM ARTERIAL PRESSURE
   REGULATION
HYPERTENSION (HIGH BLOOD
   PRESSURE)
      VOLUME-LOADING HYPERTENSION

VASOCONSTRICTOR HYPERTENSION
TYPES OF HYPERTENSION WITH BOTH
   VOLUME-LOADING AND
   VASOCONSTRICTOR
   COMPONENTS
ESSENTIAL HYPERTENSION
EFFECTS OF HYPERTENSION ON THE
   BODY

The mechanisms for long-term arterial pressure control are considerably different from the short-term mechanisms of control discussed in the previous chapter. The effectiveness of most short-term pressure control mechanisms—the baroreceptor mechanism, for instance—diminishes drastically as time proceeds. On the other hand, the effectiveness of at least one of the long-term pressure control systems is almost zero for the first few hours but then becomes extreme over a period of days and weeks. This is the renal–body fluid pressure control system. Because of this extreme long-term potency, this system plays a central role in long-term pressure control. However, it is aided in this role by a large number of accessory mechanisms, including special effects of the renin-angiotensin system and of the aldosterone system.

THE RENAL–BODY FLUID SYSTEM FOR ARTERIAL PRESSURE CONTROL

By far the most important mechanism for long-term control of arterial pressure is the *renal–body fluid system*. Simply expressed, this system works in the following way: When the arterial pressure rises, the rise in pressure directly causes kidney output of water and salt to increase markedly, which is called *pressure diuresis* and *pressure natriuresis*. This in turn causes decreased extracellular fluid volume and decreased blood volume. The decrease in blood volume decreases the pumping by the heart, which returns the arterial pressure back to normal. Conversely, when the pressure falls too low, the output of water and salt by the kidneys decreases far below normal, so that fluid begins to accumulate in the body, the body fluid volumes increase, the cardiac output increases, and the arterial pressure rises.

An Experiment Demonstrating the Renal–Body Fluid System for Arterial Pressure Control. Figure 15–1 illustrates an experiment in dogs in which all the nervous reflex mechanisms for blood pressure control were blocked and the arterial pressure was then suddenly elevated by infusing about 300 ml of blood. Note the instantaneous increase in cardiac output to approximately double its normal level and the increase in arterial pressure to 115 mm Hg above its resting level. Also shown, by the middle curve, is the effect of this increased arterial pressure on urinary output. The output increased twelvefold, and both the cardiac output and the arterial pressure returned to normal during the subsequent hour. Thus, one sees the extreme capability of the kidneys to readjust the blood volume and in so doing to return the arterial pressure back to normal.

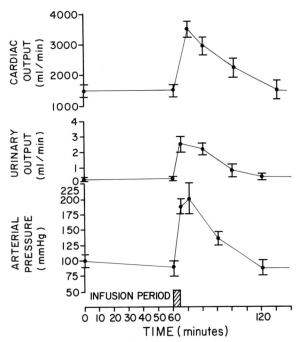

Figure 15–1. Increase in cardiac output, arterial pressure, and urinary output caused by increased blood volume in animals whose nervous pressure control mechanisms had been blocked. This figure shows the return of arterial pressure to normal after about an hour of fluid loss into the urine. (Courtesy of Dr. William Dobbs.)

Quantitation of Pressure Diuresis and Pressure Natriuresis As a Basis for Arterial Pressure Control

Figure 15–2 illustrates the average quantitative effects of pressure diuresis and pressure natriuresis as measured in experimentally perfused isolated kidneys. The curve recorded in this figure is called either a *renal output curve* or a *renal function curve*. Note that at an arterial pressure of 50 mm Hg the urinary output of water and salt is essentially zero. At 100

mm Hg it is normal, and at 200 mm Hg about six to eight times normal. Thus, the effect of arterial pressure on urinary output is a very strong one.

Graphical Analysis of Pressure Control by the Renal–Body Fluid Mechanism, Demonstrating Its "Infinite Gain" Feature. Figure 15–3 illustrates a graphical method that can be used for analyzing arterial pressure control by the renal–body fluid system. This analysis is based on two separate curves that intersect each other: (1) the renal output curve for water and salt, which is the same renal output curve as that illustrated in Figure 15–2, and (2) the curve (or line) that represents the level of water and salt intake.

Obviously, over a long period of time the water and salt must equal the intake. Furthermore, the only place on the graph in Figure 15–3 at which the output equals the intake is where the two curves intersect, which is called the *equilibrium point*. Now, let us see what will happen if the arterial pressure becomes some value that is different from that at the equilibrium point:

First, assume that the arterial pressure rises to 150 mm Hg. At this level, the graph shows that renal output of water and salt is about three times as great as the intake. Therefore, the body loses fluid, the blood volume decreases, and the arterial pressure will decrease. Furthermore, this "negative balance" of fluid will not cease until the pressure falls *all the way* back exactly to the equilibrium point. Indeed, even when the arterial pressure is only 1 mm Hg greater than the equilibrium point, there will still be more loss of water and salt than intake, so that the pressure will still continue to fall that last 1 mm Hg *until it returns exactly to the equilibrium point.*

Now, let us see what will happen if the arterial pressure falls below the equilibrium point. This time, the intake of water and salt is greater than the output. Therefore, the body fluid volume increases, the blood volume increases, and the arterial pressure rises until once again it returns *exactly* to the equilibrium point.

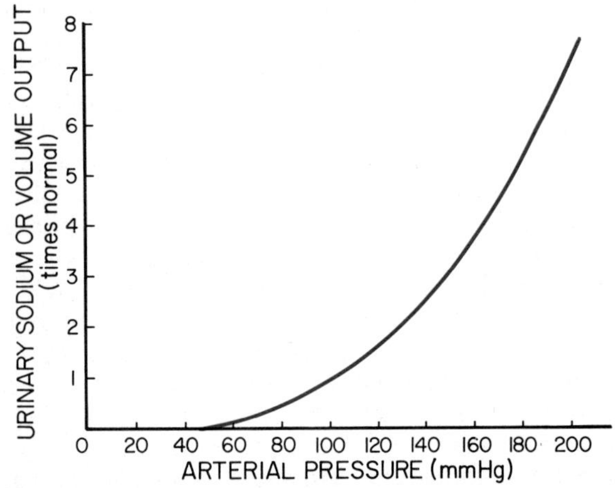

Figure 15–2. A typical renal output curve measured in a perfused isolated kidney, showing both pressure diuresis (excess output of water) and pressure natriuresis (excess output of sodium) when the arterial pressure rises above normal.

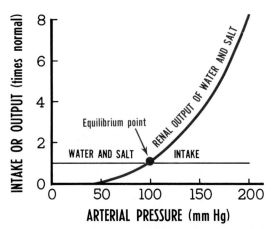

Figure 15–3. Analysis of arterial pressure regulation by equating the renal output curve with the salt and water intake curve. The "equilibrium point" describes the level to which the arterial pressure will be regulated.

This return of the arterial pressure always *all the way* back to the equilibrium point is called the *infinite gain principle* for control of arterial pressure by the renal–body fluid mechanism.

The Two Determinants of the Long-Term Arterial Pressure Level. In Figure 15–3 one can also see that two basic long-term factors determine the long-term arterial pressure level. This can be explained as follows:

As long as the two curves representing (a) renal output of salt and water and (b) salt and water intake remain exactly as they are illustrated in Figure 15–3, the long-term mean arterial pressure level will always readjust exactly to 100 mm Hg, which is the pressure level depicted by the equilibrium point of this figure. Furthermore, there are only two ways in which the pressure of this equilibrium point can be changed from the 100 mm Hg level. One of these is by shifting the renal output curve for salt and water, and the other is by changing the level of the water and salt intake curve. Therefore, expressed very simply, the two primary determinants of the long-term arterial pressure level are

(1) The *degree of shift of the renal output curve* for water and salt along the arterial pressure axis, and

(2) The *level of the water and salt intake curve.*

The operation of these two determinants in the control of arterial pressure is illustrated in Figure 15–4. In Section A of this figure, some abnormality of the kidney has caused the renal output curve to shift 50 mm Hg in the high pressure direction. Note that the equilibrium point has also shifted to 50 mm Hg higher than normal. Therefore, one can state that if the intake of salt and water remains constant but the renal output curve shifts to a new pressure level, so also will the arterial pressure follow to this new pressure level within a few days' time.

Section B of Figure 15–4 illustrates how a change in the level of salt and water intake can change the arterial pressure when the renal output curve remains undisturbed. In this case, the intake has increased four-fold, and the equilibrium point has shifted to a pressure level of 160 mm Hg, 60 mm Hg above the normal level. Conversely, a decrease in the intake level would reduce the arterial pressure.

Therefore, it is *impossible* to change the long-term mean arterial pressure level to a new value without changing one or both of the two basic determinants of the long-term arterial pressure level, either the level of salt and water intake or the degree of shift of the renal function curve along the pressure axis. However, if either of these is changed, one would expect the arterial pressure thereafter to be regulated at a new pressure level.

How Does Increased Fluid Volume Increase the Arterial Pressure? The Role of Autoregulation

The overall mechanism by which increased extracellular volume increases arterial pressure is given in

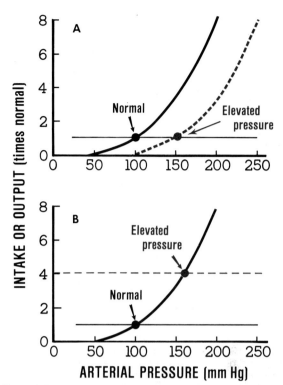

Figure 15–4. Demonstration of the two ways in which the arterial pressure can be increased: *A,* by shifting the renal output curve in the right-hand direction toward a higher pressure level, and *B,* by increasing the intake level of salt and water.

the schema of Figure 15–5. The sequential events are (1) increased extracellular fluid volume, which (2) increases the blood volume, which (3) increases the mean circulatory filling pressure, which (4) increases the venous return of blood to the heart, which (5) increases the cardiac output, which (6) increases the arterial pressure.

Note especially in this schema the two different ways in which an increase in cardiac output can increase the arterial pressure. One of these is (a) the direct effect of increased cardiac output in increasing the pressure, and the other is (b) an indirect effect resulting from local tissue autoregulation of blood flow. This second effect can be explained as follows:

Referring back to Chapter 13, let us recall that whenever an excess amount of blood flows through a tissue, the local vasculature constricts and decreases the blood flow back toward normal. This phenomenon is called "autoregulation," which means simply regulation of blood flow by the tissue itself. When increased blood volume increases the cardiac output, the blood flow increases in all the tissues of the body, so that this autoregulation mechanism will constrict the blood vessels all over the body. This, in turn, will also increase the total peripheral resistance.

Finally, since arterial pressure is equal to cardiac output times total peripheral resistance, the secondary increase in total peripheral resistance that results from the autoregulation mechanism greatly increases

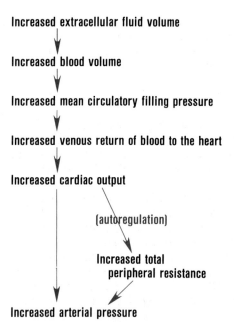

Increased extracellular fluid volume

↓

Increased blood volume

↓

Increased mean circulatory filling pressure

↓

Increased venous return of blood to the heart

↓

Increased cardiac output

(autoregulation)

Increased total
peripheral resistance

Increased arterial pressure

Figure 15–5. The sequential steps by which increased extracellular fluid volume increases the arterial pressure. Note especially that increased cardiac output has both a direct effect of increasing arterial pressure and an indirect effect of increasing the total peripheral resistance.

the rise in arterial pressure that occurs *when only small amounts of excess fluid volume accumulate in the extracellular fluid.*

ROLE OF THE RENIN-ANGIOTENSIN SYSTEM AND OF ALDOSTERONE IN LONG-TERM ARTERIAL PRESSURE REGULATION

The Short-Term and the Long-Term Effects of the Renin-Angiotensin System in Pressure Control. In the last chapter the renin-angiotensin system was discussed as one of the important short-term mechanisms for arterial pressure control. Basically, when the arterial pressure falls too low, the kidneys secrete renin; the renin then causes the formation of angiotensin in the blood; the angiotensin increases the total peripheral resistance; and the increase in total peripheral resistance increases the arterial pressure back most of the way to normal within about 20 minutes.

In addition, angiotensin also has two long-term effects that are potently concerned with long-term arterial pressure regulation. These are as follows:

(1) Angiotensin *directly affects the kidneys to cause salt and water retention* in the body;

(2) Angiotensin *causes the adrenal glands to secrete aldosterone,* and aldosterone in turn also directly affects the kidneys to cause salt and water retention.

Both of these effects shift the renal function curve toward the high-pressure level as illustrated in Figure 15–6.

Therefore, angiotensin can influence the renal–body fluid mechanism for arterial pressure control

and therefore elevate the arterial pressure by two separate mechanisms.

Role of the Renin-Angiotensin System in Maintaining a Normal Arterial Pressure Despite Wide Variations in Salt Intake

Probably the most important function of the renin-angiotensin system is to allow a person to eat either a very small or a very large amount of salt without causing great changes in either extracellular fluid volume or arterial pressure. This function is explained by the schema in Figure 15–7 which shows that the direct effect of increased salt intake is to increase the extracellular fluid volume and this, in turn, to increase the arterial pressure. Then, the increased arterial pressure causes increased blood flow through the kidneys and thereby reduces the rate of secretion of renin to a much lower level; this leads sequentially to decreased renal retention of salt and water, return of the extracellular fluid volume to normal, and finally return of the arterial pressure also to normal. Thus, the renin-angiotensin system is an automatic feedback mechanism that helps maintain the arterial pressure at or near the normal level even when the salt intake is increased. When the salt intake is decreased far below normal, exactly the opposite effects take place.

To emphasize the importance of this effect of the renin-angiotensin system, the arterial pressure rises no more than a few millimeters of Hg in response to greatly increased salt intake when the system functions normally, but, when it fails to function, the pressure rise is about ten times as great, sometimes rising 50 to 60 mm Hg in response to excess salt in the diet.

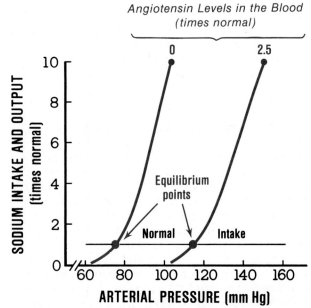

Figure 15–6. Effect of two different angiotensin levels on the renal output curve, showing regulation of the arterial pressure at an "equilibrium point" of 75 mm Hg when the angiotensin level is low and at 115 mm Hg when the angiotensin level is high.

Increased salt intake

↓

Increased extracellular volume

↓

Increased arterial pressure

↓

Decreased renin and angiotensin

↓

Decreased renal retention of salt and water

↓

Return of extracellular volume to normal

↓

Return of arterial pressure to normal

Figure 15–7. The sequential events by which increased salt intake tends to increase the arterial pressure. However, the schema also shows a feedback decrease in activity of the renin-angiotensin system that tends to return the arterial pressure back to the normal level.

HYPERTENSION (HIGH BLOOD PRESSURE)

When a person is said to have hypertension (or "high blood pressure"), it is generally meant that his or her mean arterial pressure is greater than the upper range of accepted normality. Usually, a mean arterial pressure of greater than 110 mm Hg under resting conditions is considered to be hypertensive; this level normally occurs when the diastolic blood pressure is greater than 90 mm Hg and the systolic pressure greater than about 135 to 140 mm Hg. In severe hypertension, the mean arterial pressure often rises to as high as 150 to 170 mm Hg, with diastolic pressures as high as 130 to 150 mm Hg and systolic arterial pressures sometimes as great as 250 mm Hg.

The Basic Causes of Hypertension

Now that we have discussed the principles of long-term arterial pressure regulation, we can call on these principles to discuss the mechanisms by which a person can develop hypertension. Experiments in both animals and human beings have demonstrated that hypertension rarely if ever occurs except when the renal function curve becomes abnormal and is shifted to higher pressure levels. That is, if a greater than normal pressure is required to cause the kidneys to excrete salt and water, then the long-term mechanisms for raising the pressure will become progressively more active until the pressure rises to the high level that is required to make the kidneys excrete normally. This can come about either as a result of salt and water retention, or activation of vascular constrictor mechanisms, or both of these. Therefore, for purposes of discussion, hypertension can be clas-

sified into two very different types (but with many gradations between the two):

(1) *Volume-loading hypertension,* and
(2) *Vasoconstrictor hypertension.*

VOLUME-LOADING HYPERTENSION

Volume-loading hypertension occurs when excess extracellular fluid volume accumulates in the body if all other functions of the circulation are normal.

Let us discuss a typical volume-loading type of hypertension.

The Sequential Effects in the Development of Volume-Loading Hypertension. It is especially instructive to study the sequential changes in circulatory function during the progressive development of volume-loading hypertension. Figure 15–8 illustrates these sequential changes. A week or so prior to the point labeled 0 days, the kidney mass had already been decreased to only 30 per cent of normal. Then at this point, the intake of salt and water was increased to about six times normal. The acute effect was to increase the extracellular fluid volume, the blood volume, and the cardiac output to 20 to 40 per cent above normal. Simultaneously, the arterial pressure began to rise as well, but not nearly so much at first as did the fluid volumes and cardiac output.

After these early acute changes in the circulatory variables had occurred, more prolonged secondary

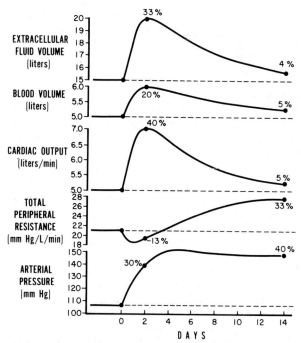

Figure 15–8. Progressive changes in important circulatory system variables during the first few weeks of *volume-loading hypertension.* Note especially the initial rise in cardiac output as the basic cause of the hypertension. Subsequently, the autoregulation mechanism returns the cardiac output almost to normal while at the same time causing a *secondary increase in total peripheral resistance.* (Modified from Guyton: Arterial Pressure and Hypertension. Philadelphia, W. B. Saunders Company, 1980.)

changes occurred during the next few days and weeks. Especially important was the *progressive increase in total peripheral resistance,* while at the same time *the cardiac output decreased almost all the way back to normal.* Multiple experiments have now shown that these changes were almost certainly caused mainly by *the long-term autoregulation* mechanism that was discussed in Chapter 13 and also earlier in this chapter in relation to long-term arterial pressure regulation. That is, after the cardiac output had risen to a high level and had caused hypertension to develop, the excess blood flow through the tissues then caused progressive constriction of the local arterioles, thus returning the cardiac output almost all the way back to normal but simultaneously causing a *secondary increase in total peripheral resistance.*

Note also that the extracellular fluid volume and blood volume returned almost all the way back to normal along with the decrease in cardiac output. This resulted from two factors: First, the increase in arteriolar resistance decreased the capillary pressure, which allowed the fluid in the tissue spaces to be absorbed back into the blood. Second, the elevated arterial pressure caused the kidneys to excrete the excess volume of fluid that accumulated in the blood.

Now, let us take stock of the final state of the circulation several weeks after the initial onset of volume loading. We find the following effects:

(1) *Hypertension,*

(2) *Marked increase in total peripheral resistance,* and

(3) *Almost complete return of the extracellular fluid volume, blood volume, and cardiac output back to normal.*

Therefore, we can divide volume-loading hypertension into two separate sequential stages:

The first stage in volume-loading hypertension results from increased fluid volumes and increased cardiac output. It is this increase in cardiac output that causes the hypertension.

The second stage in volume-loading hypertension is characterized by high blood pressure and high total peripheral resistance but return of the cardiac output so near to normal that the usual measuring techniques most frequently cannot detect an abnormally elevated output.

It should be especially noted that *the increased total peripheral resistance in volume-loading hypertension occurs **after** the hypertension has developed and therefore is **secondary** to the hypertension rather than being the cause of the hypertension.*

Volume-Loading Hypertension Caused by Primary Aldosteronism

Another type of volume-loading hypertension is caused by excess aldosterone in the body or occasionally by excesses of other steroids. A small tumor in one of the adrenal glands occasionally secretes very large quantities of aldosterone, which is the condition called primary aldosteronism. As will be discussed in Chapter 25, the aldosterone increases the rate of reabsorption of salt and water by the tubules of the kidneys, thereby reducing the loss of these in the urine but causing an increase in the extracellular fluid volume. Consequently, mild to moderate hypertension occurs, and when salt intake is increased at the same time, the hypertension becomes greater. Furthermore, if the condition persists for months or years, the excess aldosterone seems to cause pathological changes in the kidneys that make the kidneys then retain still more salt and water in addition to that caused by the aldosterone. Therefore, the hypertension can finally become very severe.

Here again, in the early stages of this type of hypertension, the cardiac output is increased, but in the later stages the cardiac output generally returns almost entirely to normal whereas the total peripheral resistance becomes secondarily elevated.

VASOCONSTRICTOR HYPERTENSION

A second type of hypertension that shows sharp contrasts to the volume-loading type is that caused by continuous infusion of a vasoconstrictor agent into the circulation or by excessive secretion of a vasoconstrictor by one of the endocrine glands. The vasoconstrictors that are especially prone to cause hypertension are (1) angiotensin II, (2) norepinephrine, and (3) epinephrine.

Hypertension Caused by Continuous Infusion of Angiotensin II or Secretion by a Renin-Secreting Tumor

Figure 15–9 illustrates typical development of vasoconstrictor hypertension caused by infusing angiotensin II at a rate approximately six times the rate of normal angiotensin formation in the body. Note especially the marked increases in both total peripheral resistance and arterial pressure but, conversely, a considerable decrease in cardiac output. All these effects can be explained by the basic principles of blood pressure regulation that were presented earlier in the chapter:

The increase in total peripheral resistance obviously results from the very potent effect of angiotensin II in constricting the arterioles. It has usually been stated that it is this increase in total peripheral resistance that causes the hypertension. However, we shall see in the discussion below that it is the effect of the angiotensin II on kidney excretion of salt and water that is critical in the maintenance of the long-term hypertension.

The *decrease in cardiac output* results almost entirely from the intense arteriolar constriction. In the following chapter we shall discuss the regulation of cardiac output, and we will see that an increase in the resistance to peripheral blood flow has a potent effect on decreasing venous return to the heart, which, in turn, causes the decreased cardiac output because the heart automatically adjusts the cardiac output to equal the venous return.

Thus, it is clear from Figure 15–9 that the hyper-

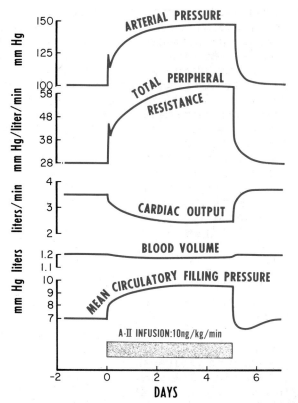

Figure 15–9. Effect of angiotensin infusion at a rate of 10 ng/kg/minute (approximately six times the normal rate of angiotensin formation in the body), illustrating marked increases in total peripheral resistance and arterial pressure, marked decrease in cardiac output, and a slight decrease in blood volume. (Drawn from data obtained in experiments in dogs by D. Young and A. Cowley.)

tension caused by angiotensin-induced vasoconstriction is, like volume-loading hypertension, a high resistance type of hypertension. However, there are subtle differences. In volume-loading hypertension, the total peripheral resistance is not increased quite as much as the increase in pressure, and the cardiac output is slightly above normal. On the other hand, in vasoconstrictor hypertension, the total peripheral resistance is increased somewhat in excess of the increase in arterial pressure, while the cardiac output is decreased to below normal.

Role of the Renal–Body Fluid Pressure Control Mechanism in Determining the Long-Term Arterial Pressure Level in Vasoconstrictor Hypertension. Let us for a moment suppose that angiotensin were infused into a person at a rate high enough to cause a very large increase in total peripheral resistance and therefore also cause an acute rise in arterial pressure. Let us further suppose that the angiotensin had no effect at all on the renal function curve—that is, the angiotensin did not in any way affect the normal capability of the kidneys to excrete salt and water. In such a theoretical instance as this, the initial marked rise in arterial pressure would cause very intense pressure diuresis and pressure natriuresis. Consequently, the blood volume would decrease rapidly and the arterial pressure eventually return to normal,

because it is only at a normal arterial pressure that urinary output would come into balance with the salt and water intake. Therefore, the increase in total peripheral resistance could not sustain a long-term increase in arterial pressure. Instead, to sustain the increased pressure, it is essential that the kidney output curve be shifted to a high pressure level. Thus, strange as it may seem, even in the vasoconstrictor type of hypertension it is the effect of the vasoconstrictor on kidney output of salt and water that determines the arterial pressure level at which the hypertension stabilizes. If the student understands this concept, it will help tremendously in understanding both blood pressure regulation and the different clinical hypertensive conditions.

TYPES OF HYPERTENSION WITH BOTH VOLUME-LOADING AND VASOCONSTRICTOR COMPONENTS

We shall see in subsequent discussions in this chapter that most clinical types of hypertension are rarely of the pure volume-loading type or the pure vasoconstrictor type but instead exhibit various combinations of both of these. Some of these are the following:

Goldblatt Hypertension

When one kidney is removed and a constrictor is placed on the renal artery of the remaining kidney, as illustrated in Figure 15–10, the initial effect is greatly reduced renal arterial pressure, shown by the dashed curve in the lower portion of the figure. However, within a few minutes the systemic arterial pressure begins to rise and continues to rise for several days. The pressure usually rises rapidly for the first hour or so and this is then followed by a slower rise over a period of several days to a much higher pressure level. When the systemic arterial pressure reaches its new stable pressure level, the renal arterial pressure will have returned almost all the way back to normal. The hypertension produced in this way is called *"one-kidney" Goldblatt hypertension* in honor of Dr. Harry Goldblatt, who first studied the important quantitative features of hypertension caused by renal artery constriction.

The early rise in arterial pressure in Goldblatt hypertension is caused by the renin-angiotensin mechanism. Because of the poor blood flow through the kidney after acute application of the constrictor, large quantities of renin are secreted by the kidneys, as illustrated by the lowermost curve in Figure 15–10, and this causes angiotensin to be formed in the blood, as described in the previous chapter; the angiotensin in turn raises the arterial pressure acutely. However, the secretion of renin rises to a peak in a few hours but returns all the way back to normal within five to seven days because the renal arterial pressure by that time has also risen back to normal so that the kidney is no longer ischemic.

The second rise in arterial pressure is caused by

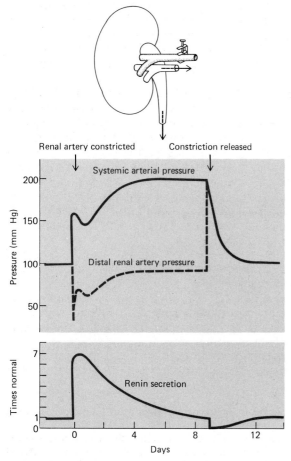

Renal artery constricted   Constriction released

Figure 15–10. Effect of placing a constricting clamp on the renal artery of one kidney after the other kidney has been removed. Note the changes in systemic arterial pressure, renal artery pressure distal to the clamp, and rate of renin secretion. The resulting hypertension is called "one-kidney Goldblatt hypertension."

fluid retention; within five to seven days the fluid volume has increased enough to raise the arterial pressure to its new sustained level. The quantitative value of this sustained pressure level is determined by the degree of constriction of the renal artery. That is, the aortic pressure must now rise to a much higher than normal level in order to make the renal arterial pressure distal to the constrictor rise high enough to cause normal urinary output.

Note especially that one-kidney Goldblatt hypertension has two phases. The first phase is a *vasoconstrictor type of hypertension* caused by angiotensin, but this is only transient. The second stage is a *volume-loading type of hypertension.*

Hypertension in Toxemia of Pregnancy

During pregnancy many patients develop hypertension, which is one of the manifestations of the syndrome called *toxemia of pregnancy.* The pathological abnormality that causes this hypertension is believed to be thickening of the glomerular membranes, which reduces the rate of fluid filtration from the glomeruli into the renal tubules. For obvious reasons, the pressure level of the renal output curve is elevated, and the long-term level of arterial pressure becomes correspondingly elevated. These patients are especially prone to hypertension when they eat large quantities of salt.

Spontaneous Hypertension in Lower Animals

Spontaneous, hereditary hypertension has been observed in a number of different strains of lower animals, including four different strains of rats, at least one strain of rabbits, and at least one strain of dogs. In the strain of rats that has been studied to the greatest extent, the Okamoto strain, there is evidence that in the early development of hypertension the sympathetic nervous system is considerably more active than in normal rats. However, in the late stages of this type of hypertension, structural changes have been observed in the nephrons of the kidneys. Therefore, these structural changes could easily be the basis for the long-term continuance of the hypertension. In two other strains of hypertensive rats, changes in renal function also have been observed.

ESSENTIAL HYPERTENSION

Approximately 90 per cent of all persons who have hypertension are said to have essential hypertension. This term means simply that *the hypertension is of unknown origin.* However, in most patients with essential hypertension, there is a very strong hereditary tendency, the same as occurs in strains of hypertensive lower animals.

Some of the characteristics of severe essential hypertension are the following:

(1) The mean arterial pressure is increased about 40 to 50 per cent.

(2) The renal blood flow in the later stages is decreased to about one half the normal flow.

(3) The resistance to blood flow through the kidneys is increased three- to fourfold.

(4) Despite the great decrease in renal blood flow, the glomerular filtration rate is often very near normal. The reason for this is that the high arterial pressure still causes adequate filtration of fluid through the glomeruli into the renal tubules.

(5) The cardiac output is approximately normal.

(6) The total peripheral resistance is increased about 40 to 50 per cent, about the same amount that the arterial pressure is increased.

And, finally, the most important finding of all in persons with essential hypertension is the following:

(7) *The kidneys will not excrete adequate amounts of salt and water unless the arterial pressure is high.* In other words, if the mean arterial pressure in the essential hypertensive person is 150 mm Hg, reduction of the arterial pressure artificially to the normal value of 100 mm Hg (but without otherwise altering renal function except for the decreased pressure) will cause almost total anuria, and the person will retain salt and water until the pressure rises back to the elevated value of 150 mm Hg.

The exact reason for this failure of the kidneys of essential hypertensive persons to excrete salt and water at normal pressure levels is unknown. However, because of very significant vascular changes in the kidneys, one can surmise that it is the decreased renal blood flow in essential hypertension that is the cause of this failure.

EFFECTS OF HYPERTENSION ON THE BODY

Hypertension can be very damaging because of two primary effects: (1) increased work load on the heart and (2) damage to the arteries themselves by the excessive pressure.

Effects of Increased Work Load on the Heart. Cardiac muscle, like skeletal muscle, hypertrophies when its work load increases. In hypertension, the very high pressure against which the left ventricle must beat causes it to increase in weight as much as two- to threefold. This increase is not accompanied by quite as much increase in coronary blood supply as there is increase in muscle tissue itself. Therefore, *relative ischemia* of the left ventricle develops as the hypertension becomes more and more severe. In the late stages of hypertension, this can become serious enough that the person develops angina pectoris. Also, the very high pressure in the coronary arteries causes rapid development of coronary arteriosclerosis so that hypertensive patients tend to die of coronary occlusion at much earlier ages than do normal persons.

Effects of the High Pressure in the Arteries. High pressure in the arteries not only causes coronary sclerosis but also sclerosis of blood vessels throughout all the remainder of the body. The arteriosclerosis process causes blood clots to develop in the vessels and also causes the blood vessels to become weakened. Therefore, these vessels frequently thrombose, or they rupture and bleed severely. In either case, marked damage can occur in organs throughout the body. Two especially important types of damage that occur in hypertension are

(1) *Cerebral hemorrhage*, which means bleeding of a cerebral vessel with resultant destruction of local areas of brain tissue, and

(2) *Hemorrhage of renal vessels* inside the kidneys, which destroys large areas of the kidneys and therefore causes progressive deterioration of the kidneys and further exacerbation of the hypertension.

QUESTIONS

1. Describe the overall renal–body fluid system for arterial pressure control.
2. Describe the renal function curve.
3. Describe graphical analysis of arterial pressure control by the renal–body fluid mechanism, using the renal function curve and the curve (or line) that represents the level of water and salt intake.
4. What is meant by the *infinite gain principle* for control of arterial pressure by the renal–body fluid mechanism?
5. What are the two determinants of the long-term arterial pressure level?
6. Explain the role of autoregulation in increasing the total peripheral resistance in volume-loading hypertension.
7. Why does the autoregulation mechanism reduce to a very small amount the volume accumulation that is required to cause hypertension?
8. Explain how angiotensin alters the renal function curve and why this causes a long-term increase in arterial pressure.
9. Explain how aldosterone alters the renal function curve and why this causes a long-term increase in arterial pressure.
10. What are the basic differences between volume-loading hypertension and vasoconstrictor hypertension?
11. Explain why the renal–body fluid pressure control mechanism plays an essential role in determining the long-term arterial pressure level even in the vasoconstrictor types of hypertension.
12. Describe Goldblatt hypertension.
13. What are the characteristics of essential hypertension?
14. How is renal function altered in essential hypertension?
15. What are the pathological effects of hypertension on the circulatory system, especially in the brain and in the kidneys?

References

Anderson, D. E.: Interactions of stress, salt, and blood pressure. Annu Rev Physiol 46:143, 1984.

Bianchi, G., et al.: Sodium balance and peripheral resistance in arterial hypertension. J Cardiovasc Pharmacol 6(Suppl. 2):S457, 1984.

Coleman, T. G., and Guyton, A. C.: Hypertension caused by salt loading in the dog. III. Onset transients of cardiac output and other circulatory variables. Circ Res 25:153, 1969.

Coleman, T. G., and Guyton, A. C.: The pressor role of angiotensin in salt deprivation and renal hypertension. Clin Sci 48:458–488, 1975.

Conway, J.: Hemodynamic aspects of essential hypertension in humans. Physiol Rev 64:617, 1984.

Folkow, B.: Physiological aspects of primary hypertension. Physiol Rev 62:347, 1982.

Gibbons, G. H., et al.: Interaction of signals influencing renin release. Annu Rev Physiol 46:291, 1984.

Guyton, A. C.: Arterial Pressure and Hypertension. Philadelphia, W. B. Saunders Co., 1980.

Guyton, A. C., and Coleman, T. G.: Quantitative analysis of the pathophysiology of hypertension. Circ Res 24:1, 1969.

Guyton, A. C., et al.: Arterial pressure regulation: Overriding dominance of the kidneys in long-term regulation and in hypertension. Am J Med 52:584, 1972.

Guyton, A. C., et al.: Salt balance and long-term blood pressure control. Annu Rev Med 31:15–27, 1980.

Haddy, F. J.: The role of a humoral Na^+, K^+–ATPase inhibitor in regulating precapillary vessel tone. J Cardiovasc Pharmacol 6(Suppl. 2):S439, 1984.

Lohmeier, T. E., et al.: Failure of chronic aldosterone infusion to increase arterial pressure in dogs with angiotensin-induced hypertension. Circ Res 43(3):381, 1978.

Manning, R. D., Jr., et al.: Essential role of mean circulatory filling pressure in salt-induced hypertension. Am J Physiol 236:R40, 1979.

Reed, G., and Devous, M.: Cerebral blood flow autoregulation and hypertension. Am J Med Sci 289:37, 1985.

Robinson, B. F.: Calcium-entry blocking agents in the treatment of systemic hypertension. Am J Cardiol 55:102B, 1985.

Vanhoutte, P. M.: Calcium-entry blockers, vascular smooth muscle and systemic hypertension. Am J Cardiol 55:17B, 1985.

16

Cardiac Output and Circulatory Shock

NORMAL VALUES FOR CARDIAC
   OUTPUT
REGULATION OF CARDIAC OUTPUT
   ROLE OF THE HEART IN CARDIAC
      OUTPUT REGULATION—ITS
      "PERMISSIVE" ROLE
   ROLE OF THE PERIPHERAL TISSUES IN
      DETERMINING NORMAL VENOUS
      RETURN AND CARDIAC OUTPUT
**SPECIAL PROBLEMS IN CARDIAC
   OUTPUT REGULATION**
   ROLE OF BLOOD VOLUME AND THE
      MEAN SYSTEMIC FILLING PRESSURE
      IN CARDIAC OUTPUT REGULATION
   REGULATION OF CARDIAC OUTPUT
      IN HEAVY EXERCISE, WHICH
      REQUIRES SIMULTANEOUS
      PERIPHERAL AND CARDIAC
      ADJUSTMENTS

ABNORMALLY LOW AND
   ABNORMALLY HIGH CARDIAC
   OUTPUTS
**METHODS FOR MEASURING CARDIAC
   OUTPUT**
   THE INDICATOR DILUTION METHOD
CIRCULATORY SHOCK
   THE PHYSIOLOGICAL CAUSES OF
      SHOCK
   SHOCK CAUSED BY HYPOVOLEMIA—
      HEMORRHAGIC SHOCK
   HYPOVOLEMIC SHOCK CAUSED BY
      PLASMA LOSS
   HYPOVOLEMIC SHOCK CAUSED BY
      TRAUMA
   ANAPHYLACTIC SHOCK
   SEPTIC SHOCK
   EFFECTS OF SHOCK ON THE BODY

Cardiac output is the quantity of blood pumped by the left ventricle into the aorta each minute. It is perhaps the single most important factor that we have to consider in relation to the circulation, for it is cardiac output that is responsible for transport of substances to and from the tissues.

NORMAL VALUES FOR CARDIAC OUTPUT

The normal cardiac output for the young healthy male adult averages approximately 5.6 liters per minute. However, if we consider all adults, including older people and females, the average cardiac output is very close to 5 liters per minute. In general, the cardiac output of females is about 10 per cent less than that of males of the same body size.

The cardiac output increases approximately in proportion to the surface area of the body. Therefore, the cardiac output is frequently stated in terms of the *cardiac index*, which is the *cardiac output per square meter of body surface area*. The normal human being weighing 70 kg. has a body surface area of approximately 1.7 square meters, which means that the normal average cardiac index for adults of all ages is approximately 3.0 liters per minute per square meter.

Effect of Metabolism and Exercise. The cardiac output usually remains almost proportional to the overall metabolism of the body. That is, the greater the degree of activity of the muscles and other organs, the greater also will be the cardiac output. This relationship is illustrated in Figure 16–1, which shows that as the work output during exercise increases, the cardiac output also increases in almost linear proportion. Note that in very intense exercise the cardiac output can rise to as high as 30 to 35 liters per minute in the young, well-trained athlete, which is about five to seven times the normal control value.

Figure 16–1 also demonstrates that oxygen consumption increases in almost direct proportion to work output during exercise. We shall see later in the chapter that the increase in cardiac output probably results mainly from increased oxygen consumption.

Effect of Age. Figure 16–2 illustrates the change in cardiac index with age. Rising rapidly to a level greater than 4 liters per minute per square meter at

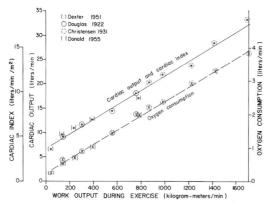

Figure 16–1. Relationships between cardiac output and work output (solid curve) and between oxygen consumption and work output (dashed curve) during different levels of exercise. (From Guyton, Jones, and Coleman: Circulatory Physiology: Cardiac Output and Its Regulation. Philadelphia, W. B. Saunders Company, 1973.)

10 years of age, the cardiac index declines to about 2.4 liters per minute at the age of 80 years. These changes are indicative of the declining bodily activity with age.

REGULATION OF CARDIAC OUTPUT

ROLE OF THE HEART IN CARDIAC OUTPUT REGULATION—ITS "PERMISSIVE" ROLE

It is very tempting to believe that the heart itself controls the cardiac output. However, many experiments have shown that increasing the pumping capability of the heart to greater than normal has very little effect on cardiac output. Also, even a weakened heart will still pump a normal cardiac output if it has not been weakened beyond a lower limit. Therefore, the heart normally plays little role in controlling the

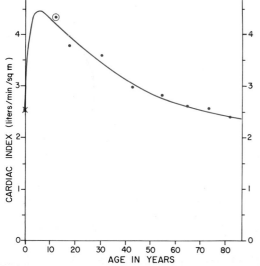

Figure 16–2. Cardiac index at different ages. (From Guyton, Jones, and Coleman: Circulatory Physiology: Cardiac Output and Its Regulation. Philadelphia, W. B. Saunders Company, 1973.)

actual level of cardiac output. Instead, the heart plays a *permissive role* in cardiac output regulation, permitting the output to be regulated at any level up to the limit of its pumping capability. Let us explain this permissive role more fully as follows:

Control of Cardiac Output by Venous Return— The Frank-Starling Law of the Heart. It is worthwhile at this point to recall the Frank-Starling law of the heart, which was discussed in Chapter 8. This law states that, within the physiological limit of the heart, the heart will pump whatever amount of blood enters the right atrium and will do so without significant buildup of back pressure in the right atrium. In other words, the heart is an automatic pump that is capable of pumping far more than the 5 liters per minute that normally returns to it from the peripheral circulation. Consequently, the factor that normally determines how much blood will be pumped by the heart is the amount of blood that flows into the heart from the systemic circulation—which is called the *venous return*—not the pumping capacity of the heart.

Thus, the heart normally will *permit* the cardiac output to be regulated at any value below about 10 to 13 liters per minute, but the actual cardiac output under resting conditions is only approximately 5 liters per minute because this is the normal level of venous return. Therefore, it is the peripheral circulatory system, not the heart, that sets this level of 5 liters per minute.

Increase in Permissive Level of Heart Pumping by Sympathetic Stimulation of the Heart. At times the cardiac output must rise temporarily to levels greater than the normal permissive level of the heart. For instance, in heavy exercise by well-trained athletes, cardiac outputs as high as 35 liters per minute have been measured. Obviously, the resting heart would not be able to pump this amount of blood. On the other hand, *stimulation of the heart by the sympathetic nervous system* (and simultaneous decrease in parasympathetic stimulation) *increases the permissive level of heart pumping to approximately double normal.* This effect comes about by autonomic enhancement of both heart rate and strength of heart contraction. Furthermore, the increase in permissive level of heart pumping occurs within a few seconds after exercise begins, even before most of the increase in venous return occurs.

ROLE OF THE PERIPHERAL TISSUES IN DETERMINING NORMAL VENOUS RETURN AND CARDIAC OUTPUT

Cardiac Output Regulation as the Sum of the Local Blood Flow Regulations Throughout the Body. As long as the arterial pressure remains normal, each local tissue in the body can control its own blood flow by simply dilating or constricting its local blood vessels. This mechanism, which was discussed in detail in Chapter 13, is the means by which each tissue protects its own nutrient supply, controlling the blood flow in response to its own needs.

Therefore, since the venous return to the heart is the sum of all the local blood flows through all the individual tissues of the body, the local blood flow regulatory mechanisms in the peripheral circulation are the true controller of cardiac output under normal conditions. This is an automatic mechanism that allows the heart to respond instantaneously to the needs of each individual tissue. If some tissue needs extra blood flow, its local blood vessels dilate, the venous return increases automatically, and the cardiac output increases by an equivalent amount. If all the tissues throughout the body require increased blood flow at the same time, the venous return becomes very great, and the cardiac output increases accordingly.

Thus, the concept of normal cardiac output regulation is that *the tissues control the output* in accordance with their needs. Again, it must be stated that it is not the heart that controls the cardiac output under normal conditions; instead, the heart plays a permissive role that allows the tissues to do the controlling. The heart does this by maintaining a permissive pumping capacity that is somewhat above the actual venous return—except when the heart fails.

Effect of Local Tissue Metabolism on Cardiac Output Regulation, and Importance of Simultaneous Arterial Pressure Regulation. The most important factor that controls the local blood flows in the individual tissues is the metabolic rates of the respective tissues. Therefore, venous return and cardiac output are normally controlled in relation to the level of metabolism of the body. This effect was illustrated in Figure 16–1, which showed that the cardiac output increases directly in relation to work output during exercise and that the output also increases parallel to the increase in oxygen consumption, which is a measure of the rate of metabolism.

SPECIAL PROBLEMS IN CARDIAC OUTPUT REGULATION

Thus far we have discussed cardiac output regulation when all aspects of circulatory function are normal and when the circulatory system is not stressed beyond moderate limits. Also, we have assumed that the arterial pressure-regulating mechanisms continue to maintain the arterial pressure at a normal level, that the blood volume is normal, and that the heart is normal.

On the other hand, when the cardiac output approaches the limit that the heart can pump, as occurs in very strenuous exercise, or when blood volume or other circulatory factors become abnormal, then it becomes necessary to consider other important effects in cardiac output regulation, as follows:

ROLE OF BLOOD VOLUME AND THE MEAN SYSTEMIC FILLING PRESSURE IN CARDIAC OUTPUT REGULATION

If the quantity of blood in the circulatory system is too little to fill the system adequately, blood will flow very poorly from the peripheral vessels into the heart.

Therefore, the degree of filling of the circulation then becomes a critical factor in determining the venous return to the heart and also in determining the cardiac output.

The student may recall from Chapter 11 that the degree of filling of the circulatory system with blood can be expressed in terms of the *mean circulatory filling pressure;* also, the degree of filling of the systemic portion of the circulation can be expressed in terms of the *mean systemic filling pressure.* The mean systemic filling pressure is the pressure measured in the systemic circulation when blood flow in the circulatory system is suddenly stopped and the blood in the systemic vessels is redistributed so that the pressure in all the vessels is equal. Normally, the mean systemic filling pressure is 7 mm Hg, but an increase in blood volume of 15 to 30 per cent doubles the mean systemic filling pressure, whereas a decrease in blood volume of this same amount reduces the mean systemic filling pressure to zero.

The mean systemic filling pressure is the *average* effective pressure of the blood in the peripheral circulation that tends to push the blood toward the heart. Experiments have demonstrated that, *when the peripheral resistance remains constant,* the rate of *venous return* from the systemic vessels through the veins to the heart is directly proportional to the *mean systemic filling pressure* minus *the right atrial pressure.* Therefore, whenever the mean systemic filling pressure falls to zero, the flow of blood returning to the heart likewise approaches zero.

Consequently, it is very important that the blood volume and its effect on the mean systemic filling pressure remain high enough at all times to supply the peripheral pressure needed to push blood from the peripheral vessels back to the heart.

REGULATION OF CARDIAC OUTPUT IN HEAVY EXERCISE, WHICH REQUIRES SIMULTANEOUS PERIPHERAL AND CARDIAC ADJUSTMENTS

Heavy exercise is one of the most stressful conditions to which the body is ever subjected. The tissues can require as much as 20 times normal amounts of oxygen and other nutrients, so that simply to transport enough oxygen from the lungs to the tissues sometimes demands a minimum cardiac output increase of five- to sixfold. This is greater than the amount of cardiac output the normal, unstimulated heart can pump. Therefore, to insure the massive increase in cardiac output that is required during heavy exercise, almost all factors that are known to increase cardiac output must be called into play as follows:

Muscle Vasodilatation Resulting from Increased Metabolism. By far the most important factor that increases the cardiac output during exercise is the vasodilatation that occurs in the exercising muscles. The cause of the vasodilatation is the large increase in muscle metabolism during exercise. This leads to tremendously increased use of oxygen and other nutrients by the muscles, as well as formation of vasodilator substances, all of which act together to cause marked local vascular dilatation and greatly increased local blood flow. This local vasodilatation requires 5 to 15 seconds to reach full development after a person begins to exercise strongly; but once it does reach full development, the very great decrease in vascular resistance allows extreme quantities of blood to flow into the veins and thence to the heart, thereby markedly increasing venous return and cardiac output.

Role of the Heart in Strenuous Exercise. When large numbers of muscles are exercising simultaneously, the peripheral vasodilatation may be so great and the venous return to the heart so voluminous that the "resting" heart simply cannot pump this extra amount of blood. Therefore, it is essential that the *permissive level of pumping* by the heart be greatly increased from its normal level of 10 to 13 liters per minute. This is achieved mainly by sympathetic stimulation of the heart (but also partly by a *decrease* in parasympathetic stimulation), which increases the permissive level to as high as 20 to 25 liters per minute in a normal person or as high as 35 liters in the trained athlete.

Therefore, in exercise, the cardiac output can increase two- to threefold without stimulation of the heart. But to go above this amount it is absolutely essential that the heart be nervously excited to increase the permissive level of heart pumping.

Increase in Mean Systemic Filling Pressure. Sympathetic stimulation constricts almost all the blood vessels throughout the body besides those in the exercising muscles. The veins, especially, are constricted, which increases the mean systemic filling pressure to as much as 2.5 times normal. This increase in mean systemic filling pressure provides an extra push on the blood in the peripheral vessels to return this blood to the heart. This is absolutely essential to achieve enough venous return, and therefore to achieve enough cardiac output, in heavy exercise.

Summary. It is clear that a complex set of controls comes into play during exercise to allow the heart and the circulation to increase the cardiac output to the tremendous levels required for nutrient supply to the muscles. The increase in cardiac output occurs first when the person begins to anticipate exercise, which stimulates the sympathetic nervous system. Then, tensing of the abdominal muscles gives an additional surge of venous return that also increases the cardiac output. Finally, within seconds after the exercise actually begins, intense local metabolic vasodilatation occurs in the muscles themselves. Combined with the hyperdynamic state of the heart and the increased mean systemic filling pressure, this causes the further surge in the cardiac output up to levels between 20 and 35 liters per minute.

ABNORMALLY LOW AND ABNORMALLY HIGH CARDIAC OUTPUTS

Low Output

Figure 16–3 illustrates the cardiac outputs in different pathological conditions, showing at the far right

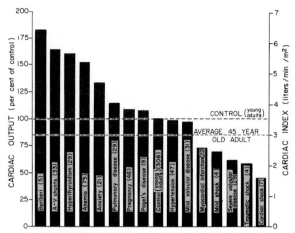

Figure 16–3. Cardiac output in different pathological conditions. The numbers in parentheses indicate number of patients studied in each condition. (From Guyton, Jones, and Coleman: Circulatory Physiology: Cardiac Output and Its Regulation. Philadelphia, W. B. Saunders Company, 1973.)

the conditions that cause abnormally low outputs and at the left the conditions that cause abnormally high outputs.

It is easy to understand those abnormalities of the circulation that cause low cardiac output. These fall into two different categories: (1) those abnormalities that cause the pumping effectiveness of the heart to fall too low, and (2) those that cause venous return to fall too low.

Decreased Cardiac Output Caused by Cardiac Factors. Whenever the heart becomes severely damaged, from whatever cause, its permissive level of pumping may fall below that needed for adequate blood flow to the tissues. Some examples of this include *severe myocardial infarction, severe valvular heart disease, myocarditis, cardiac tamponade,* and certain *cardiac metabolic derangements.* The effect of several of these is illustrated on the right in Figure 16–3, showing the low cardiac outputs that result.

When the cardiac output falls so low that the tissues throughout the body begin to suffer nutritional deficiency, the condition is called *cardiac shock.* This will be discussed in Chapter 17 in relation to cardiac failure.

Decrease in Cardiac Output Caused by Peripheral Factors—Decreased Venous Return. Any factor that interferes with venous return also can lead to decreased cardiac output. Some of these are:

1. *Decreased blood volume.* By far the most common peripheral factor that leads to decreased cardiac output is decreased blood volume, resulting most often from hemorrhage. It is very clear why this decreases the cardiac output: loss of blood decreases the mean systemic filling pressure to such a low level that there simply is not enough blood in the peripheral vessels to create the pressure required to push blood back to the heart. In other words, the mean systemic filling pressure falls to or near to zero, so that venous return also approaches zero.

2. *Acute venous dilatation.* On some occasions the peripheral veins become acutely vasodilated. This

results most often when the sympathetic nervous system suddenly becomes inactive. For instance, fainting often results from sudden loss of sympathetic nervous system activity, which causes the peripheral capacitative vessels, especially the veins, to dilate markedly. This decreases the mean systemic filling pressure because the blood volume can no longer create adequate pressure in the now flaccid peripheral blood vessels. As a result the blood "pools" in the vessels and will not return to the heart.

3. *Obstruction of the veins.* On rare occasions, the large veins leading into the heart become obstructed, in which case the blood in the peripheral vessels cannot flow back into the heart. Consequently the cardiac output falls markedly.

Regardless of the cause of low cardiac output, whether it be a peripheral factor or a cardiac factor, if ever the cardiac output falls below that level required for adequate nutrition of the tissues, the person is said to suffer *circulatory shock*. This can be lethal within a few minutes to a few hours. Circulatory shock will be discussed in detail later in this chapter.

High Cardiac Output—Role of Reduced Total Peripheral Resistance

The left side of Figure 16–3 identifies conditions that commonly cause cardiac outputs higher than normal. One of the distinguishing features of these conditions is that *they all result from chronically reduced total peripheral resistance.* And none of them result from excessive excitation of the heart itself, which we will explain below. For the present, let us look at some of the peripheral factors that can increase the cardiac output to above normal:

(1) *Beriberi.* This is a disease caused by insufficient quantity of the vitamin *thiamine* in the diet. Lack of this vitamin causes diminished ability of the tissues to utilize cellular nutrients, which in turn causes marked peripheral vasodilatation. The total peripheral resistance decreases sometimes to as little as one-half normal. Consequently, the long-term level of cardiac output also often increases to as much as two times normal.

(2) *Arteriovenous fistula (shunt).* Whenever a fistula (also called a shunt) occurs between a major artery and a major vein, tremendous amounts of blood will flow directly from the artery into the vein. This, too, greatly decreases the total peripheral resistance, and likewise increases the venous return and cardiac output.

(3) *Hyperthyroidism.* In hyperthyroidism, the metabolism of all the tissues of the body becomes greatly increased. Oxygen usage increases, and vasodilator products are released from the tissues. Therefore, the total peripheral resistance decreases markedly, and the cardiac output often increases to as much as 40 to 80 per cent above normal.

(4) *Anemia.* In anemia, two peripheral effects greatly decrease the total peripheral resistance. One of these is reduced viscosity of the blood, resulting from the decreased concentration of red blood cells.

The other is diminished delivery of oxygen to the tissues because of the decreased hemoglobin, which causes local vasodilatation. As a consequence, the total peripheral resistance decreases greatly, and the cardiac output increases.

And, any other factor that decreases the total peripheral resistance chronically will also increase the cardiac output.

Failure of Increased Cardiac Pumping to Cause Prolonged Increase of the Cardiac Output. If the heart is suddenly stimulated excessively, the cardiac output often increases as much as 20 to 30 per cent. However, even this small increase is maintained no longer than a few minutes even though the heart continues to be strongly stimulated. There are two reasons for this: (1) Excess blood flow through the tissues causes automatic vasoconstriction of the blood vessels because of the autoregulation mechanism discussed in previous chapters, and this reduces the venous return and cardiac output back toward normal. (2) The slightly increased arterial pressure that results following acute cardiac stimulation raises the capillary pressure, and fluid filters out of the capillaries into the tissues thereby decreasing the blood volume and also decreasing the venous return back toward normal. Also, the increased pressure causes the kidneys to lose fluid volume as well until the arterial pressure and cardiac output return to normal.

Thus, all the known conditions that cause *chronic* elevation of the cardiac output result from decreased total peripheral resistance and not increased cardiac activity.

METHODS FOR MEASURING CARDIAC OUTPUT

In animal experiments, one can cannulate the aorta, the pulmonary artery, or the great veins entering the heart and measure the cardiac output using any type of flowmeter. Also, an electromagnetic or ultrasonic flowmeter can be placed on the aorta or pulmonary artery to measure cardiac output. However, except in rare instances, in the human being cardiac output is measured by indirect methods that do not require surgery. Two of the methods commonly used are the *oxygen Fick method* and the *indicator dilution method.*

Measurement of Cardiac Output by the Oxygen Fick Method

The Fick procedure is best explained by Figure 16–4. This figure shows that 200 ml of oxygen are being absorbed from the lungs into the pulmonary blood each minute. It also illustrates that the blood entering the right side of the heart has an oxygen concentration of 160 ml per liter of blood, whereas that leaving the left side has an oxygen concentration of 200 ml per liter of blood. From these data one can calculate that each liter of blood passing through the lungs picks up 40 ml of oxygen. And, since the total quantity of

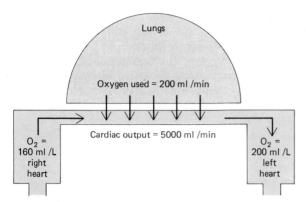

Figure 16–4. The Fick principle for determining cardiac output.

oxygen absorbed into the blood from the lungs each minute is 200 ml, a total of 5 1-liter portions of blood must pass through the pulmonary circulation each minute to absorb this amount of oxygen. Therefore, the quantity of blood flowing through the lungs each minute is 5 liters, which is also a measure of the cardiac output. Thus, the cardiac output can be calculated by the following formula:

Cardiac output (liters/min) =

$$\frac{O_2 \text{ absorbed per minute by the lungs (ml/min)}}{\text{Arteriovenous } O_2 \text{ difference (ml/liter of blood)}}$$

In applying the Fick procedure, accurate determination of venous oxygen concentration can be achieved only by sampling blood directly from the right ventricle or preferably even the pulmonary artery, for blood in any one vein usually has a concentration of oxygen different from that in other veins. To obtain such a sample of mixed venous blood a catheter is usually inserted up the brachial vein of the forearm, through the subclavian vein, down to the right atrium, and finally into the right ventricle or pulmonary artery.

Blood used for determining the oxygen saturation in the arterial blood can be obtained from any artery in the body, because all arterial blood is thoroughly mixed before it leaves the heart and therefore has the same oxygen concentration.

The rate of oxygen absorption by the lungs is usually measured by a "respirometer," which will be described in Chapter 27. In essence, this device is a floating chamber containing oxygen that sinks in the water as oxygen is removed from it, thus measuring the rate of oxygen usage by the rate at which it falls.

THE INDICATOR DILUTION METHOD

In measuring the cardiac output by the indicator dilution method, a small amount of *indicator,* such as a dye, is injected into a large vein or preferably into the right side of the heart itself. This passes rapidly through the right heart, the lungs, the left heart, and finally into the arterial system. Then one records the

concentration of the dye as it passes through one of the peripheral arteries, giving a curve such as one of the two colored curves illustrated in Figure 16–5. In each of these instances, 5 mg of Cardio-Green dye was injected at zero time. In the top recording none of the dye passed into the arterial tree until approximately three seconds after the injection, but then the arterial concentration of the dye rose rapidly to a maximum in approximately six to seven seconds. After that, the concentration fell rapidly. However, before the concentration reached the zero point, some of the dye had already circulated all the way through some of the peripheral vessels and returned through the heart for a second time. Consequently, the dye concentration in the artery began to rise again. For the purpose of calculation, however, it is necessary to extrapolate the early downslope of the curve to the zero point, as shown by the dashed portion of the curve. In this way, the *time-concentration* curve of the dye in an artery can be measured in its first portion and estimated reasonably accurately in its latter portion.

Once the time-concentration curve has been determined, one can then calculate the mean concentration of dye in the arterial blood for the duration of the curve. In Figure 16–5, this was done by measuring the area under the entire curve, and then averaging the concentration of dye for the duration of the curve; one can see from the shaded rectangle straddling the upper curve of the figure that the average concentration of dye was approximately 0.25 mg/deciliter of blood and that the duration of this average value was 12 seconds. A total of 5 mg of dye was injected at the beginning of the experiment. In order for blood carrying only 0.25 mg of dye in each deciliter to carry the entire 5 mg of dye through the heart and lungs in 12 seconds, it would be necessary for a total of 20 1-deciliter portions of blood to pass through the heart during this time, which would be the same as a cardiac output of 2 liters per 12 seconds, or 10 liters per minute.

In the bottom curve of Figure 16–5, the blood flow

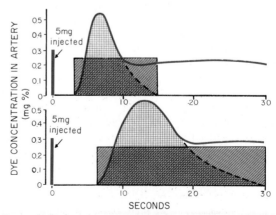

Figure 16–5. Dye concentration curves used to calculate the cardiac output by the dilution method. (The rectangular areas are the calculated average concentrations of dye in the arterial blood for the durations of the respective curves.)

through the heart was considerably slower, and the cardiac output calculated to be 5 liters per minute.

To summarize, the cardiac output can be determined from the following formula.

$$\text{Cardiac output (ml/min)} = \frac{\text{Milligrams of dye injected} \times 60}{\left(\begin{array}{l}\text{Average concentration of dye}\\\text{in each milliliter of blood}\\\text{for the duration of the curve}\end{array}\right) \times \left(\begin{array}{l}\text{Duration of}\\\text{the curve}\\\text{in seconds}\end{array}\right)}$$

CIRCULATORY SHOCK

Circulatory shock means generalized inadequate blood flow throughout the body, to the extent that the tissues are damaged because of too little flow, especially too little delivery of oxygen and other nutrients to the tissue cells. Even the cardiovascular system itself—the heart musculature, the walls of the blood vessels, the vasomotor system, and other circulatory parts—begins to deteriorate so that the shock becomes progressively worse.

THE PHYSIOLOGICAL CAUSES OF SHOCK

Circulatory Shock Caused by Decreased Cardiac Output

Shock usually results from inadequate cardiac output. Therefore, any factor that reduces the cardiac output will likely lead to circulatory shock. Basically, two types of factors can severely reduce the cardiac output; these are

(1) *Cardiac abnormalities that decrease the ability of the heart to pump blood.* These include especially *myocardial infarction* but also *toxic states of the heart, severe heart valve dysfunction,* heart *arrhythmias,* and other conditions. The circulatory shock that results from diminished cardiac pumping ability is called *cardiogenic shock.* This is discussed in the following chapter, where it is pointed out that about 85 per cent of persons who develop cardiogenic shock do not survive.

(2) *Factors that decrease the venous return.* The most common cause of this is *diminished blood volume,* but venous return also can be reduced as a result of decreased *vasomotor tone* or *obstruction to blood flow* at some point in the circulation, especially in the venous return pathway to the heart.

What Happens to Arterial Pressure in Circulatory Shock?

In the minds of many physicians, the arterial pressure is the principal measure of the adequacy of circulatory function. However, the arterial pressure often can be seriously misleading, because many times a person may be in severe shock and still have a normal pressure because powerful nervous reflexes often keep the pressure from falling. Yet at other times the arterial pressure can fall to as low as one-half normal, but the person still has normal tissue perfusion and is not in shock.

Nevertheless, it is true that in most types of shock, especially that caused by severe blood loss, the arterial blood pressure usually does decrease at the same time that the cardiac output decreases, though usually not as much as the decrease in output.

The End-Stages of Circulatory Shock, Whatever the Cause

Once circulatory shock reaches a critical state of severity, regardless of its initiating cause, *the shock itself breeds more shock.* That is, the inadequate blood flow causes the circulatory system itself to begin to deteriorate. This in turn causes even more decrease in cardiac output, and a vicious circle ensues, with progressively increasing circulatory shock, still less adequate tissue perfusion, still more shock, and so forth until death. It is with this late stage of circulatory shock that we are especially concerned, because appropriate physiologic treatment can often reverse the rapid slide to oblivion.

The Stages of Shock. Because the characteristics of circulatory shock change at different degrees of severity, shock is generally divided into three major stages:

(1) A *nonprogressive stage* (sometimes called the *compensated stage*) from which the normal circulatory compensatory mechanisms will eventually cause full recovery if the initiating cause does not become any worse.

(2) A *progressive stage,* in which the shock becomes steadily worse until death.

And (3) an *irreversible stage,* in which the shock has progressed to such an extent that all forms of known therapy will be inadequate to save the life of the person even though for the moment the person is still alive.

Now, let us discuss the different stages of circulatory shock caused by decreased blood volume, which will illustrate the basic principles. Then we can consider the special characteristics of other initiating causes of shock.

SHOCK CAUSED BY HYPOVOLEMIA— HEMORRHAGIC SHOCK

Hypovolemia means diminished blood volume, and hemorrhage is perhaps the most common cause of hypovolemic shock.

Hemorrhage *decreases the mean systemic filling pressure* and as a consequence decreases venous return. As a result, the cardiac output falls below normal, and shock ensues. Obviously, all degrees of shock can result from hemorrhage, from the mildest diminishment of cardiac output to almost complete cessation of output.

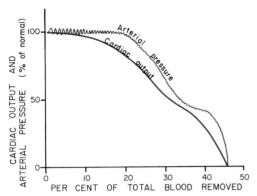

Figure 16–6. Effect of hemorrhage on cardiac output and arterial pressure.

Relationship of Bleeding Volume to Cardiac Output and Arterial Pressure

Figure 16–6 illustrates the effect on both cardiac output and arterial pressure of removing blood from the circulatory system over a period of about half an hour. Approximately 10 per cent of the total blood volume can be removed with no significant effect on arterial pressure or cardiac output, but greater blood loss usually diminishes the cardiac output first and later the pressure, both of these falling to zero when about 35 to 45 per cent of the total blood volume has been removed.

Sympathetic Reflex Compensation in Shock. Fortunately, the decrease in arterial pressure caused by blood loss initiates powerful sympathetic reflexes (initiated mainly by the baroreceptors) that stimulate the sympathetic vasoconstrictor system throughout the body, resulting in three important effects: (1) The arterioles constrict in most parts of the body, thereby greatly increasing the total peripheral resistance. (2) The veins and venous reservoirs constrict, thereby helping to maintain adequate venous return despite diminished blood volume. And (3) heart activity increases markedly, sometimes increasing the heart rate from the normal value of 72 beats per minute to as high as 200 beats per minute.

Value of the Reflexes. In the absence of the sympathetic reflexes, only 15 to 20 per cent of the blood volume can be removed over a period of half an hour before a person will die; this is in contrast to a 30 to 40 per cent loss of blood volume that a person can sustain when the reflexes are intact. Therefore, the reflexes extend the amount of blood loss that can occur without causing death to about two times that which is possible in their absence.

Protection of Coronary and Cerebral Blood Flow by the Reflexes. A special value of the maintenance of normal arterial pressure even in the face of decreasing cardiac output is protection of blood flow through the coronary and cerebral circulatory systems. Fortunately, sympathetic stimulation does not cause significant constriction of either the cerebral or cardiac vessels. In addition, in both these vascular beds local autoregulation is excellent, which prevents

moderate decreases in arterial pressure from significantly affecting their blood flows. Therefore, blood flow through the heart and brain, both of which are essential for continued life, is maintained almost at normal levels as long as the arterial pressure does not fall below about 70 mm Hg, despite the fact that blood flow in many other areas of the body might be decreased almost to zero by this time because of vasospasm.

Nonprogressive and Progressive Hemorrhagic Shock

Figure 16–7 illustrates an experiment that we performed in dogs to demonstrate the effects of different degrees of hemorrhage on the subsequent course of arterial pressure. The dogs were bled rapidly until their arterial pressures fell to different levels. Those dogs whose pressures fell immediately to no lower than 45 mm Hg (Groups I, II, and III) all eventually recovered; the recovery occurred rapidly if the pressure fell only slightly (Group I) but occurred slowly if it fell almost to the 45 mm Hg level (Group III). On the other hand, when the arterial pressure fell below 45 mm Hg (Groups IV, V, and VI), all the dogs died, though many of them hovered between life and death for many hours before the circulatory system began to deteriorate.

This experiment demonstrates that the circulatory system can recover as long as the degree of hemorrhage is no greater than a certain critical amount. However, crossing this critical amount by even a few milliliters of blood loss makes the eventual difference between life and death. Thus, hemorrhage beyond a certain critical level causes shock to become *progressive.* That is, *the shock itself causes still more shock,* the condition becoming a vicious circle that leads eventually to complete deterioration of the circulation and to death.

Nonprogressive Shock—Compensated Shock. If shock is not severe enough to cause its own progression, the person eventually recovers. Therefore, shock of this lesser degree can be called *nonprogressive shock.* It is also frequently called *compensated shock,* meaning that the sympathetic reflexes and other factors have compensated enough to prevent deterioration of the circulation.

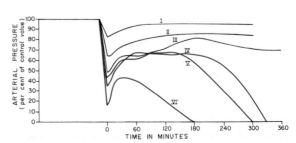

Figure 16–7. Course of arterial pressure in dogs after different degrees of acute hemorrhage. Each curve represents the average results from six dogs.

The factors that cause a person to recover from moderate degrees of shock are the negative feedback control mechanisms of the circulation that attempt to return cardiac output and arterial pressure to normal levels. These include:

1. The *baroreceptor reflexes,* which elicit powerful sympathetic stimulation of the circulation;

2. The *central nervous system ischemic response,* which elicits even more powerful sympathetic stimulation throughout the body but is not activated until the arterial pressure falls below 60 mm Hg;

3. *Reverse stress-relaxation of the circulatory system,* which causes the blood vessels to contract down around the diminished blood volume so that the blood volume that is available will more adequately fill the circulation;

4. *Formation of angiotensin,* which constricts the peripheral arteries and causes increased conservation of water and salt by the kidneys, both of which help prevent progression of the shock;

5. *Formation of vasopressin (antidiuretic hormone),* which constricts the peripheral arteries and veins and also causes greatly increased water retention by the kidneys;

6. *Compensation mechanisms that return the blood volume back toward normal,* including absorption of large quantities of fluid from the intestinal tract, absorption of fluid from the interstitial spaces of the body, conservation of water and salt by the kidneys, and increased thirst and increased appetite for salt which make the person drink water and eat salty foods if able.

The sympathetic reflexes provide immediate help toward bringing about recovery, for they become maximally activated within 30 seconds after hemorrhage. The angiotensin and vasopressin mechanisms, as well as the reverse stress-relaxation that causes contraction of the blood vessels and venous reservoirs around the blood, all require 10 minutes to an hour to occur completely, but, nevertheless, these aid greatly in increasing the arterial pressure or increasing the mean systemic filling pressure and thereby increasing the return of blood to the heart.

Progressive Shock—The Vicious Circle of Cardiovascular Deterioration. Once shock has become severe enough, the structures of the circulatory system themselves begin to deteriorate, and various types of positive feedback develop that can cause a vicious circle of progressively decreasing cardiac output. Figure 16–8 illustrates different types of positive feedback that further depress the cardiac output in shock. Some of the more important of these are the following:

Cardiac Depression. When the arterial pressure falls low enough, *coronary blood flow decreases below that required for adequate nutrition of the myocardium* itself. This obviously weakens the heart and thereby decreases the cardiac output still more. As a consequence, the arterial pressure falls still further, and the coronary blood flow decreases more, making the heart still weaker. Thus, a positive feedback cycle has developed whereby the shock becomes more and more severe.

Figure 16–9 illustrates cardiac output curves from experiments in dogs, showing progressive deterioration of the heart at different times following the onset of shock. A dog was bled until the arterial pressure fell to 30 mm Hg, and the pressure was held at this level by further bleeding or retransfusion of blood as required. Note that there was little deterioration of

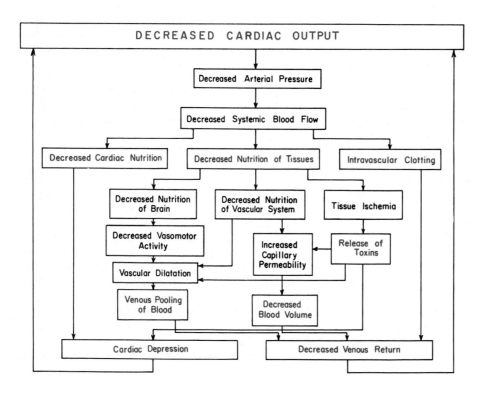

Figure 16–8. Different types of feedback that can lead to progression of shock.

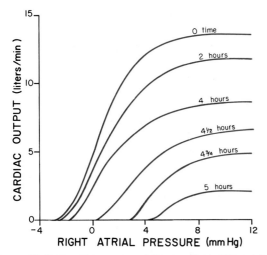

Figure 16–9. Function curves of the heart at different times after hemorrhagic shock begins. (These curves are extrapolated to the human heart from data obtained in dog experiments by Dr. J. W. Crowell.)

the heart during the first two hours, but by four hours the heart had deteriorated about 40 per cent; then, rapidly, during the last hour of the experiment the heart deteriorated almost completely.

Vasomotor Failure. In the early stages of shock various circulatory reflexes cause intense activation of the sympathetic nervous system. This, as discussed previously, helps delay depression of the cardiac output and especially helps prevent decreased arterial pressure. However, there comes a point at which diminished blood flow to the vasomotor center itself so depresses the center that it becomes progressively less active and finally totally inactive.

Increased Capillary Permeability. After many hours of capillary hypoxia the permeability of the capillaries gradually increases and large quantities of fluid begin to transude into the tissues. This further decreases the blood volume, with resultant further decrease in cardiac output, thus making the shock still more severe.

Release of Toxins by Ischemic Tissues. Throughout the history of research in the field of shock, it has been suggested time and again that shock causes tissues to release toxic substances like histamine, serotonin, tissue enzymes, and so forth that then cause further deterioration of the circulatory system. Quantitative studies have especially proved the significance of at least one toxin, *endotoxin*, in some types of shock.

Endotoxin. Endotoxin is a toxin released from the bodies of dead gram-negative bacteria in the intestines. Diminished blood flow to the intestines causes enhanced absorption of this toxic substance from the intestines, and it then causes extensive vascular dilatation, greatly increased cellular metabolism despite the inadequate nutrition of the cells, and cardiac depression. This toxin can play a major role in some types of shock, especially septic shock discussed later in the chapter.

Generalized Cellular Deterioration. As shock becomes very severe, many signs of generalized cellular deterioration occur throughout the body. One organ especially affected is the *liver*, primarily because of the lack of enough nutrients to support the normally high rate of metabolism in liver cells, but also partly because of the extreme vascular exposure of the liver cells to any toxic or other abnormal metabolic factors in shock. Among the different effects that are known to occur are:

1. Active transport of sodium and potassium through the cell membrane is greatly diminished. As a result, sodium and chloride accumulate in the cells and potassium is lost from the cells. In addition the cells begin to swell.

2. Mitochondrial activity in the liver cells, as well as in many other tissues of the body, becomes severely depressed.

3. Lysosomes begin to split in widespread tissue areas, with intracellular release of hydrolases that cause further intracellular deterioration.

4. Cellular metabolism of nutrients such as glucose eventually becomes greatly depressed in the last stages of shock. The activities of some hormones are depressed as well, including as much as 200-fold depression in the action of insulin.

Obviously, all these effects contribute to further deterioration of many different organs of the body, including especially (1) the *liver*, with depression of its many metabolic and detoxification functions; (2) the lungs, with eventual development of pulmonary edema and poor ability to oxygenate the blood; and (3) the heart, thereby further depressing the contractility of the heart.

Irreversible Shock

After shock has progressed to a certain stage, transfusion or any other type of therapy becomes incapable of saving the life of the person. Therefore, the person is then said to be in the *irreversible stage of shock.* Ironically, even in this irreversible stage, therapy can on occasion still return the arterial pressure and even the cardiac output to normal for short periods of time, but the circulatory system nevertheless continues to deteriorate and death ensues in another few minutes to few hours.

Figure 16–10 illustrates this effect, showing that transfusion during the irreversible stage can sometimes cause the cardiac output (as well as the arterial pressure) to return to normal. However, the cardiac output soon begins to fall again, and subsequent transfusions have less and less effect. Thus, something has changed in the overall function of the circulatory system that may not necessarily affect the *immediate* ability of the heart to pump blood but over a long period of time does depress this ability and results in death. Now the question remains: What factor or factors lead to the eventual total deterioration of circulatory function?

The answer to this question seems to be, simply,

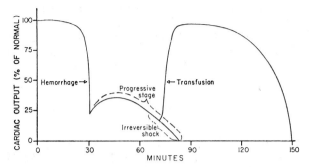

Figure 16–10. Failure of transfusion to prevent death in irreversible shock.

that beyond a certain point so much cellular damage has occurred, so many destructive enzymes have been released into the body fluids, so much acidosis has developed, and so many other destructive factors are now in progress that even a normal cardiac output cannot reverse the continuing deterioration. Therefore, in severe shock a stage is eventually reached beyond which the person is destined to die even though vigorous therapy can still return the cardiac output to normal for short periods of time.

HYPOVOLEMIC SHOCK CAUSED BY PLASMA LOSS

Loss of plasma from the circulatory system, even without the loss of whole blood, can sometimes be severe enough to reduce the total blood volume markedly, in this way causing typical hypovolemic shock similar in almost all details to that caused by hemorrhage. Severe plasma loss commonly occurs in the following conditions:

1. *Intestinal obstruction* is often a cause of reduced plasma volume. The resulting distention of the intestine causes fluid to leak from the intestinal capillaries into the intestinal walls and intestinal lumen. This loss of fluid might result from elevated capillary pressure caused by increased resistance in the stretched veins over the surface of the intestine, or it might be caused by direct damage to the capillaries themselves. Nevertheless, the lost fluid has a very high content of protein, thereby reducing the total plasma protein as well as the plasma volume.

2. Often, in patients who have *severe burns* or other denuding conditions of the skin, so much plasma is lost through the exposed areas that the plasma volume becomes markedly reduced.

The hypovolemic shock that results from plasma loss has almost the same characteristics as the shock caused by hemorrhage, except for one additional complicating factor—the blood viscosity increases greatly as a result of plasma loss, and this further exacerbates the sluggishness of blood flow.

Loss of fluid from all fluid compartments of the body is called *dehydration;* this, too, can reduce the blood volume and cause hypovolemic shock very similar to that resulting from hemorrhage. Some of the causes of this type of shock are: (a) excessive

sweating; (b) fluid loss in severe diarrhea or vomiting; (c) excess loss of fluid by nephrotic kidneys; (d) inadequate intake of fluid and electrolytes; and (e) destruction of the adrenal cortices, with consequent failure of the kidneys to reabsorb sodium, chloride, and water because of the absence of the hormone aldosterone.

HYPOVOLEMIC SHOCK CAUSED BY TRAUMA

One of the most common causes of circulatory shock is trauma to the body. Often the shock results simply from hemorrhage caused by the trauma, but it can also occur even without hemorrhage, for contusion of the body can often damage the capillaries sufficiently to allow excessive loss of plasma into the tissues. This results in greatly reduced plasma volume with resultant hypovolemic shock. Thus, whether or not hemorrhage occurs when a person is severely traumatized, the blood volume can still be markedly reduced.

The *pain* associated with serious trauma can be an additional aggravating factor in traumatic shock, for pain sometimes strongly inhibits the vasomotor center, thereby increasing the vascular capacitance and reducing the venous return.

ANAPHYLACTIC SHOCK

Anaphylaxis is an allergic condition in which the cardiac output and arterial pressure often fall drastically. This is discussed in Chapter 20. It results primarily from an antigen-antibody reaction that takes place all through the body immediately after an antigen to which the person is sensitive has entered the circulatory system. Such a reaction is detrimental to the circulatory system in several important ways. First, if the antigen-antibody reaction takes place in direct contact with the vascular walls or cardiac musculature, damage to these tissues presumably can result directly. Second, cells damaged anywhere in the body by the antigen-antibody reaction release several highly toxic substances into the blood. Among these is *histamine* or *histamine-like substance,* released mainly from the circulating basophils and the mast cells outside the capillaries. The histamine in turn causes (1) an increase in vascular capacity because of venous dilatation, (2) dilatation of the arterioles with resultant greatly reduced arterial pressure, and (3) greatly increased capillary permeability with rapid loss of fluid into the tissue spaces. Unfortunately, all the precise relationships of the above factors in anaphylaxis have not been determined, but the sum total is a great reduction in venous return and often such serious shock that the person dies within minutes.

SEPTIC SHOCK

The condition that was formerly known by the popular name *blood poisoning* is now called *septic shock* by most clinicians. This simply means widely disseminated infection in many areas of the body, with the infection being borne through the blood from one tissue to another and causing extensive damage. Actually, there are many different varieties of septic shock because of the many different types of bacterial infection that can cause it and also because infection in one part of the body will produce different effects from those caused by infection elsewhere in the body.

Septic shock is extremely important to the clinician because it is this type of shock that, more frequently than any other kind of shock besides cardiogenic shock, causes patient death in the modern hospital. Some of the typical causes of septic shock include:

1. Peritonitis caused by spread of infection from the uterus and fallopian tubes, frequently resulting from instrumental abortion.

2. Peritonitis resulting from rupture of the gut, sometimes caused by intestinal disease and sometimes by wounds.

3. Generalized infection resulting from spread of a simple skin infection such as streptococcal or staphylococcal infection.

4. Generalized gangrenous infection resulting specifically from gas gangrene bacilli, spreading first through the tissues themselves and finally by way of the blood to the internal organs, especially to the liver.

5. Infection spreading into the blood from the kidney or urinary tract, often caused by colon bacilli.

Special Features of Septic Shock. Some features often seen in septic shock are the following:

1. High fever.

2. Marked vasodilatation throughout the body, especially in the infected tissues.

3. High cardiac output in perhaps half of the patients, caused by vasodilatation in the infected tissues and also by high metabolic rate and vasodilatation elsewhere in the body resulting from bacterial toxin stimulation of cellular metabolism and from the high body temperature.

4. Sludging of the blood, presumably caused by red cell agglutination in response to degenerating tissues.

5. Development of microclots in widespread areas of the body, a condition called *disseminated intravascular coagulation.* Also this causes the blood clotting factors to be used up so that hemorrhages occur into many tissues, especially into the gut wall and into the intestinal tract.

In the early stages of septic shock the patient usually does not have signs of circulatory collapse but, instead, only signs of the bacterial infection itself. However, as the infection becomes more severe, the circulatory system usually becomes involved either directly or as a secondary result of toxins from the bacteria, and *there finally comes a point at which deterioration of the circulation becomes progressive in the same way that progression occurs in all other types of shock. Therefore, the end stages of septic shock are not greatly different from the end stages of hemorrhagic shock,* even though the initiating factors are markedly different in the two conditions.

EFFECTS OF SHOCK ON THE BODY

Decreased Metabolism in Hypovolemic Shock. The decreased cardiac output in hypovolemic shock reduces the amount of oxygen and other nutrients available to the different tissues, and this in turn reduces the level of metabolism that can be maintained by the different cells of the body. Usually a person can continue to live for only a few hours if the cardiac output falls to as low as 40 per cent of normal.

Muscular Weakness. One of the earliest symptoms of shock is severe muscular weakness which is also associated with profound and rapid fatigue whenever patients attempt to use their muscles. This obviously results from the diminished supply of nutrients—especially oxygen—to the muscles.

Body Temperature. Because of the depressed metabolism in shock, the amount of heat liberated in the body is reduced (except in septic shock in which the infection may cause an opposite effect). As a result, the body temperature tends to decrease if the body is exposed to even the slightest cold.

Mental Function. In the early stages of shock the person is usually conscious, though signs of mental haziness may be noted. As the shock progresses, the person falls into a state of stupor, and in the last stages of shock even the subconscious mental functions, including vasomotor control and respiration, fail.

A person who recovers from shock usually exhibits no permanent impairment of mental functions. However, *following complete circulatory arrest, in which the blood flow is completely cut off from the brain for more than five minutes,* the brain does often suffer severe permanent impairment.

Reduced Renal Function. The very low blood flow during shock greatly diminishes urine output or even causes cessation of output, because glomerular pressure falls below the critical value required for filtration of fluid into Bowman's capsule, as explained in Chapter 24. Also, the kidney has such a high rate of metabolism and requires such large amounts of nutrients that the reduced blood flow often causes *tubular necrosis,* which means death of the tubular epithelial cells, with subsequent sloughing and blockage of the tubules, causing total loss of function of the respective nephrons. This is often a serious aftereffect of shock that occurs during a major surgical operation; the patient sometimes survives the shock associated with the surgical procedure and then dies a week or so later of uremia.

QUESTIONS

1. What are the approximate normal values for cardiac output both at rest and during very heavy exercise?
2. What is meant by the "permissive" role of the heart in the regulation of cardiac output?
3. Explain why increased metabolism in any given tissue of the body increases both the local blood flow and the cardiac output by approximately the same amount?
4. What happens to the cardiac output when the mean systemic filling pressure falls to zero? What conditions can cause the mean systemic filling pressure to fall below normal?
5. List and explain the different factors that cause the extreme increases in cardiac output during strenuous exercise.
6. Discuss the different conditions that can cause greatly decreased cardiac output.
7. Discuss the different conditions that can cause high cardiac outputs.
8. Why does increased pumping activity by the heart fail to cause a prolonged increase in cardiac output?
9. If the amount of oxygen absorbed by the lungs per minute is 150 ml and the arteriovenous oxygen difference (arterial oxygen minus venous oxygen) is 60 ml per liter of blood, what is the cardiac output?
10. Explain the indicator dilution method for measuring cardiac output.
11. Give a definition of "circulatory shock."
12. What are the relationships of arterial pressure and cardiac output to circulatory shock?
13. List and explain the different *negative* feedback mechanisms that help to compensate for circulatory shock.
14. List and explain the important *positive* feedback mechanisms that occur in circulatory shock and can lead to progressive shock.
15. What are some of the cellular effects in circulatory shock that lead to generalized cellular deterioration?
16. What causes shock in its extremely severe stages to become irreversible?
17. What causes the development of *anaphylactic shock?*
18. Explain the causes and special features of *septic shock.*
19. What are the important effects of circulatory shock on bodily function?

References

Cardiac Output

Dodge, H. T., and Kennedy, J. W.: Cardiac output, cardiac performance, hypertrophy, dilatation, valvular disease, ischemic heart disease, and pericardial disease. In Sodeman, W. A., Jr., and Sodeman, T. M., eds.: Pathologic Physiology: Mechanisms of Disease, 6th ed. Philadelphia, W. B. Saunders Co., 1979, p. 271.

Green, J. F.: Determinants of systemic blood flow. In Guyton, A. C., and Young, D. B., eds.: International Review of Physiology: Cardiovascular Physiology, III. Vol. 18. Baltimore, University Park Press, 1979, p. 33.

Guyton, A. C.: Determination of cardiac output by equating venous return curves with cardiac response curves. Physiol Rev 35:123, 1955.

Guyton, A. C.: Essential cardiovascular regulation—the control linkages between bodily needs and circulatory function. In Dickinson, C. J., and Marks, J., eds.: Developments in Cardiovascular Medicine. Lancaster, England, MTP Press, 1978, p. 265.

Guyton, A. C., et al.: Autoregulation of the total systemic circulation and its relation to control of cardiac output and arterial pressure. Circ Res 28 (Suppl. 1):93, 1971.

Guyton, A. C., et al.: Systems analysis of arterial pressure regulation and hypertension. Ann Biomed Eng 1:254, 1972.

Guyton, A. C., et al.: Cardiac Output and Its Regulation. Philadelphia, W. B. Saunders Co., 1973.

Jones, C. E., et al.: Cardiac output and physiological mechanisms in circulatory shock. In MTP International Review of Science: Physiology. Vol. 1. Baltimore, University Park Press, 1974, p. 233.

Rothe, C. F.: Reflex control of veins and vascular capacitance. Physiol Rev 63:1281, 1983.

Rothe, C. F.: Venous system: Physiology of the capacitance vessels. In Shepherd, J. T., and Abboud, F. M., eds.: Handbook of Physiology. Sec. 2, Vol. III. Bethesda, American Physiological Society, 1983, p. 397.

Sarnoff, S., and Mitchell, J. H.: The regulation of the performance of the heart. Am J Med 30:747, 1961.

Circulatory Shock

Bernton, E. W., et al.: Opioids and neuropeptides: Mechanisms in circulatory shock. Fed Proc 44:290, 1985.

Bond, R. F., and Johnson, G., III: Vascular adrenergic interactions during hemorrhagic shock. Fed Proc 44:281, 1985.

Crowell, J. M., and Guyton, A. C.: Evidence favoring a cardiac mechanism in irreversible hemorrhagic shock. Am J Physiol 201:893, 1961.

Crowell, J. W., and Smith, E. E.: Oxygen deficit and irreversible hemorrhagic shock. Am J Physiol 206:313, 1964.

Filkins, J. P.: Monokines and the metabolic pathophysiology of septic shock. Fed Proc 44:300, 1985.

Guyton, A. C., et al.: Cardiac Output and Its Regulation. Philadelphia, W. B. Saunders Co., 1973.

Intensive Care of the Surgical Cardiopulmonary Patient, 2nd ed. Chicago, Year Book Medical Publishers, 1983.

Jones, C. E., et al.: Cardiac output and physiological mechanisms in circulatory shock. In MTP International Review of Science: Physiology. Vol. 1. Baltimore. University Park Press, 1974, p. 233.

Lefer, A. M.: Eicosanoids as mediators of ischemia and shock. Fed Proc 44:275, 1985.

Movat, H. Z.: Microcirculation in disseminated intravascular coagulation induced by endotoxins. In Renkin, E. M., and Michel, C. C., eds.: Handbook of Physiology. Sec. 2, Vol. 4. Bethesda, American Physiological Society, 1984, p. 1047.

17

Coronary Blood Flow; Cardiac Failure; Heart Sounds; Valvular and Congenital Heart Defects

CORONARY BLOOD FLOW
    NORMAL CORONARY BLOOD FLOW
    CONTROL OF CORONARY BLOOD
      FLOW
    NERVOUS CONTROL OF CORONARY
      BLOOD FLOW
    ISCHEMIC HEART DISEASE
    CAUSES OF DEATH FOLLOWING
      ACUTE CORONARY OCCLUSION
    PAIN IN CORONARY DISEASE
CARDIAC FAILURE
    ACUTE EFFECTS OF MODERATE
      GENERALIZED CARDIAC FAILURE
    SUMMARY OF THE CHANGES THAT
      OCCUR FOLLOWING ACUTE
      CARDIAC FAILURE—
      COMPENSATED HEART FAILURE
    DYNAMICS OF SEVERE CARDIAC
      FAILURE—DECOMPENSATED
      HEART FAILURE
    UNILATERAL LEFT HEART FAILURE
    CARDIOGENIC SHOCK
    PHYSIOLOGICAL CLASSIFICATION OF
      CARDIAC FAILURE
    CARDIAC RESERVE

THE HEART SOUNDS AND VALVULAR
  DYSFUNCTION
    NORMAL HEART SOUNDS
    AREAS FOR AUSCULTATION OF
      NORMAL HEART SOUNDS
    THE PHONOCARDIOGRAM
    RHEUMATIC VALVULAR LESIONS
    DYNAMICS OF THE CIRCULATION IN
      AORTIC STENOSIS AND AORTIC
      REGURGITATION
    CIRCULATORY DYNAMICS IN MITRAL
      STENOSIS AND MITRAL
      REGURGITATION
    CIRCULATORY DYNAMICS DURING
      EXERCISE IN PATIENTS WITH
      VALVULAR LESIONS
ABNORMAL CIRCULATORY DYNAMICS
  IN CONGENITAL HEART DEFECTS
    PATENT DUCTUS ARTERIOSUS—A
      LEFT-TO-RIGHT SHUNT
    TETRALOGY OF FALLOT—A RIGHT-
      TO-LEFT SHUNT

CORONARY BLOOD FLOW

Approximately one third of all deaths result from coronary artery disease, and almost all elderly persons have at least some impairment of the coronary artery circulation. The purpose of this chapter is to present this subject, emphasizing also the physiology of coronary occlusion and myocardial infarction.

Figure 17–1 illustrates the heart with its coronary blood supply. Note that the main coronary arteries lie on the surface of the heart, and small arteries penetrate into the cardiac muscle mass. The *left coronary artery* supplies mainly the anterior part of the left ventricle, while the *right coronary artery* supplies most of the right ventricle as well as the posterior part of the left ventricle in most persons.

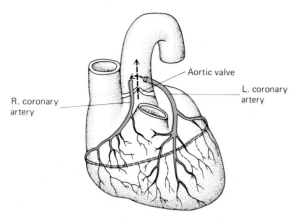

Figure 17–1. The coronary vessels.

NORMAL CORONARY BLOOD FLOW

The resting coronary blood flow in the human being averages approximately 225 ml per minute, which is about 4 to 5 per cent of the total cardiac output.

In strenuous exercise the heart increases its cardiac output as much as four- to sixfold, and it pumps this blood against a higher than normal arterial pressure. Consequently, the work output of the heart under severe conditions may increase as much as six- to eightfold. The coronary blood flow increases three- to fourfold to supply the extra nutrients needed by the heart. Obviously, this increase is not as much as the increase in work load, which means that the ratio of coronary blood flow to energy expenditure by the heart decreases. However, the "efficiency" of cardiac utilization of energy increases to make up for this relative deficiency of blood supply.

Phasic Changes in Coronary Blood Flow—Effect of Cardiac Muscle Compression. Figure 17–2 illustrates the average blood flow *through the small nutrient vessels* of the left ventricular coronary system in milliliters per minute in the human heart during systole and diastole as *calculated* from experiments in lower animals. Note from this diagram that the blood flow in the left ventricle falls to a low value during

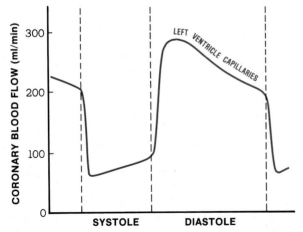

Figure 17–2. Phasic flow of blood through the coronary capillaries of human left ventricle (as extrapolated from studies in dogs).

systole, which is opposite to the flow in all other vascular beds of the body. The reason is the strong compression of the left ventricular muscle around the intramuscular vessels during systole.

During *diastole*, the cardiac muscle relaxes completely and no longer obstructs the blood flow through the left ventricular capillaries, so that blood now flows rapidly during all diastole.

Blood flow through the coronary capillaries of the right ventricle undergoes phasic changes similar to those in the coronary capillaries of the left ventricle during the cardiac cycle, but because the force of contraction of the right ventricle is far less than that of the left ventricle, the inverse phasic changes are only partial in contrast with those in the left ventricle.

CONTROL OF CORONARY BLOOD FLOW

Oxygen Demand as a Major Factor in Local Blood Flow Regulation. Blood flow in the coronaries is regulated almost exactly in proportion to the need of the cardiac musculature for oxygen. Even in the normal resting state, 65 to 70 per cent of the oxygen in the arterial blood is removed as the blood passes through the heart; and because not much oxygen is left, little additional oxygen can be removed from the blood unless the blood flow increases. Fortunately, the blood flow does increase, almost in proportion to the metabolic consumption of oxygen by the heart.

Yet, the exact means by which increased oxygen consumption causes coronary dilatation has not been determined. However, in the presence of very low concentrations of oxygen in the muscle cells, a small proportion of the cell's adenosine triphosphate degrades to *adenosine*, which is a powerful vasodilator and perhaps is the major cause of the vasodilatation. Another possible cause of the dilatation may be that the oxygen deficiency itself could easily cause local vasodilatation because of lack of the required energy (derived from the oxygen) to keep the coronary vessels contracted against the high arterial pressure.

NERVOUS CONTROL OF CORONARY BLOOD FLOW

Stimulation of the autonomic nerves to the heart can affect coronary blood flow in two ways—directly and indirectly. The direct effects result from direct action of the nervous transmitter substances, acetylcholine and norepinephrine, on the coronary vessels themselves. Usually, acetylcholine causes mild dilatation, and norepinephrine mild constriction.

However, the indirect effects play by far the more important role in normal control of coronary blood flow. *Sympathetic stimulation* increases both heart rate and heart contractility as well as its rate of metabolism. In turn, the increased activity of the heart sets off local blood flow regulatory mechanisms for dilating the coronary vessels, the blood flow increasing approximately in proportion to the need of the heart muscle for oxygen. In contrast, *parasym-*

pathetic stimulation slows the heart and also has a slight depressive effect on cardiac contractility, which decreases cardiac oxygen consumption and therefore indirectly constricts the coronaries.

ISCHEMIC HEART DISEASE

The single most common cause of death is ischemic heart disease, which results from insufficient coronary blood flow. Approximately 35 per cent of all human beings in the United States die of this cause. Some deaths occur suddenly as a result of an acute coronary occlusion or of fibrillation of the heart, while others occur slowly over a period of weeks to years as a result of progressive slow occlusion of the coronary vessels.

Atherosclerosis as the Cause of Ischemic Heart Disease. The most frequent cause of diminished coronary blood flow is atherosclerosis; this process is the following: In certain persons who have a genetic predisposition to atherosclerosis or in persons who eat excessive quantities of cholesterol and fats, large quantities of cholesterol gradually become deposited beneath the intima at many points in the arteries. Later, these areas of deposit become invaded by fibrous tissue, and they also frequently become calcified. The net result is the development of atherosclerotic plaques that protrude into the vessels and either block or partially block blood flow.

Acute Coronary Occlusion. Acute occlusion of the coronary artery frequently occurs in a person who already has serious underlying atherosclerotic coronary heart disease. Usually, an atherosclerotic plaque protrudes into the flowing blood and causes a local blood clot called a *thrombus*, which in turn occludes the artery. The thrombus usually begins where the plaque has grown so much that it has broken through the intima, thus coming in contact with the flowing blood. Because the plaque presents an unsmooth surface to the blood, platelets begin to adhere to it, fibrin begins to be deposited, and blood cells become entrapped and form a clot that grows until it occludes the vessel. Or occasionally the clot breaks away from its attachment on the atherosclerotic plaque and flows to a more peripheral branch of the coronary arterial tree, where it blocks the artery at that point.

Collateral Circulation in the Heart. The degree of damage to the heart caused either by slowly developing atherosclerotic constriction of the coronary arteries or by sudden occlusion is determined to a great extent by the degree of collateral circulation that is already developed or that can develop within a short period of time after the occlusion.

Unfortunately, in the normal heart, relatively few communications exist among the larger coronary arteries. But many anastomoses do exist among the smaller arteries of 20 to 250 microns in diameter, as shown in Figure 17–3.

When a sudden occlusion occurs in one of the larger coronary arteries, the sizes of the minute anastomoses increase to their maximum physical di-

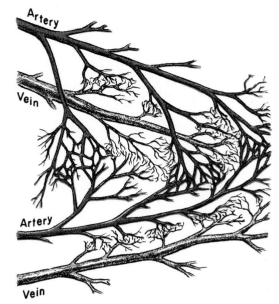

Figure 17–3. Minute anastomoses of the coronary arterial system.

ameters within a few seconds. The blood flow through these minute "collaterals" is usually less than that needed to keep alive the cardiac muscle that they supply, but the collaterals double in size by the second or third day and often provide normal or almost normal coronary supply within about one month. It is because of these developing collateral channels that a patient recovers from the various types of coronary occlusion.

When atherosclerosis constricts the coronary arteries slowly over a period of many years rather than suddenly, collateral vessels can develop at the same time that the atherosclerosis does. Therefore, the person may never experience an acute episode of cardiac dysfunction. Eventually, however, the sclerotic process develops beyond the limits of even the collateral blood supply to provide the needed blood flow, and even the collaterals develop atherosclerosis. When this occurs, the heart muscle becomes severely limited in its work output, sometimes so much that the heart cannot pump even the normally required amounts of blood flow. This is the most common cause of heart failure.

Myocardial Infarction. Immediately after an acute coronary occlusion, blood flow ceases in the coronary vessels beyond the occlusion except for small amounts of collateral flow from surrounding vessels. The area of muscle that has either zero flow or so little flow that it cannot sustain cardiac muscle function is said to be *infarcted*. The overall process is called a *myocardial infarction*.

Soon after the onset of the infarction small amounts of collateral blood seep into the infarcted area, and this, combined with progressive dilatation of the local blood vessels, causes the area to become overfilled with stagnant blood. Simultaneously, the muscle fibers utilize the last vestiges of the oxygen in the blood, causing the hemoglobin to become very dark blue in color. Therefore, the infarcted area takes on a dark bluish hue, and the blood vessels of the area appear to be engorged despite the lack of blood flow. Also, the cardiac muscle cells begin to swell because of diminished cellular metabolism. Finally, after a few hours, much of the muscle dies if enough collateral vessels do not open.

CAUSES OF DEATH FOLLOWING ACUTE CORONARY OCCLUSION

The four major causes of death following acute myocardial infarction are (1) decreased cardiac output; (2) damming of blood in the pulmonary or systemic veins with death resulting from edema, especially pulmonary edema; (3) fibrillation of the heart; and (4) occasionally rupture of the heart.

Decreased Cardiac Output—Cardiogenic Shock. When some of the cardiac muscle mass is not functioning at all and other portions are too weak to contract with great force, the overall pumping ability of the affected ventricle is proportionately depressed. When the pumping is depressed enough, the heart fails acutely and the peripheral tissues become severely damaged as a result of too little blood flow. This condition is called *cardiogenic* or *cardiac shock*. It will be discussed later in the chapter.

Damming of Blood in the Venous System. When the heart is not pumping blood forward, it must be damming blood in the venous system of the lungs or of the systemic circulation. These effects often cause very little difficulty during the first few hours after the myocardial infarction. Instead, the symptoms develop a few days later for the following reason: The diminished cardiac output leads to diminished blood flow to the kidneys, and for reasons that will be discussed in Chapter 25, the kidneys retain large quantities of fluid. This adds progressively to the venous congestive symptoms. Therefore, many patients who seemingly are getting along well will suddenly develop acute pulmonary edema several days after onset of a myocardial infarction and often will die within a few hours after appearance of the initial edema symptoms.

Rupture of the Infarcted Area. During the first day of an acute infarct there is little danger of rupture of the ischemic portion of the heart, but a few days after a large infarct occurs, the dead muscle fibers begin to degenerate, and the dead heart musculature is likely to become very thin and then to rupture.

When a ventricle does rupture, the loss of blood into the pericardial space causes rapid development of *cardiac tamponade*—that is, compression of the heart from the outside by blood collecting in the pericardial cavity. Because the heart is compressed, blood cannot flow into the right atrium with ease, and the patient dies of suddenly decreased cardiac output.

Fibrillation of the Ventricles Following Myocardial Infarction. Many persons who die of coronary occlusion die because of ventricular fibrillation. At least four different factors enter into the tendency for the heart to fibrillate:

First, acute loss of blood supply to the cardiac muscle causes rapid depletion of potassium from the ischemic musculature. This increases the irritability of the cardiac musculature.

Second, ischemia of the muscle causes an "injury current," which can elicit abnormal impulses that cause fibrillation.

Third, powerful sympathetic reflexes develop following massive infarction, principally because the heart does not pump an adequate volume of blood into the arterial tree; therefore the arterial pressure falls, which causes the baroreceptors to excite the sympathetics. The sympathetic stimulation also increases irritability of the cardiac muscle and thereby predisposes to fibrillation.

Fourth, the myocardial infarction itself often causes the ventricle to dilate excessively. This increases the pathway length for impulse conduction in the heart and also frequently causes abnormal conduction pathways around the infarcted area of the cardiac muscle. Both of these effects predispose to development of circus movements. As was discussed in Chapter 9, this is the basic cause of fibrillation.

PAIN IN CORONARY DISEASE

Normally, a person cannot "feel" his or her heart, but the ischemic heart does exhibit pain sensation. Exactly what causes this pain is not known, but it is believed that ischemia causes the muscle to release acidic substances such as lactic acid or other pain-promoting products such as histamine or kinins that are not removed rapidly enough by the slowly moving blood.

The pain impulses are conducted mainly through the sympathetic afferent nerve fibers into the central nervous system.

Angina Pectoris. In most persons who develop progressive constriction of their coronary arteries, cardiac pain, called *angina pectoris*, begins to appear whenever the load on the heart becomes too great in relation to the coronary blood flow. This pain is usually felt beneath the upper sternum and is often also referred to surface areas of the body, most often down the left arm and to the left shoulder but also frequently to the neck and even to the side of the face or to the opposite arm and shoulder. The reason for this distribution of pain is that the heart originates during embryonic life in the neck, as do the arms. Therefore, both of these structures receive pain nerve fibers from the same spinal cord segments.

In general, most persons who have chronic angina pectoris feel the pain when they exercise and also when they experience emotions that increase metabolism of the heart or temporarily constrict the coronary vessels because of sympathetic vasoconstrictor nerve signals. Usually the pain lasts only a few minutes.

Treatment with Vasodilator Drugs. Several vasodilator drugs, when administered during an acute anginal attack, will often give immediate relief from the pain. Two commonly used drugs are nitroglycerin and amyl nitrite.

Surgical Treatment—Aortic-Coronary Bypass. In many patients with coronary ischemia, the constricted areas of the coronary vessels are located at only a few discrete points, and the coronary vessels beyond these points are of normal or almost normal size. A surgical procedure has been developed in the past few years, called *aortic-coronary bypass*, for anastomosing small vein grafts to the aorta and to the sides of the more peripheral coronary vessels. Usually, two to six such grafts are performed during the operation, each of which supplies a peripheral coronary artery beyond a block.

The results from this type of surgery have been good in over half of the patients, causing this to be the most common cardiac operation performed. Anginal pain is relieved in most patients. Also, in patients whose hearts have not become too severely damaged prior to the operation, the coronary bypass procedure often can provide the patient with normal survival expectation. On the other hand, if the heart has already been severely damaged, the bypass procedure is likely to be of little value.

Coronary Angioplasty. During the past ten years, a procedure has been employed to open partially blocked coronary vessels before they become totally occluded. This procedure, called *coronary artery angioplasty*, is the following: A very small catheter, about 1 millimeter in diameter, has a balloon surrounding it, beginning a few millimeters from its tip and extending backward along its shaft for 2 to 3 centimeters. The tip of this catheter is passed under x-ray guidance into the coronary system and pushed through the almost occluded artery until the balloon portion of the catheter straddles the partially occluded point. Then the balloon is inflated with several atmospheres of pressure, which stretches the diseased artery almost to the point of bursting. After this procedure is performed, the blood flow through the vessel usually increases as much as three- to fourfold, and more than three quarters of the patients who undergo the procedure are relieved of the coronary ischemic symptoms for at least several years, though many of the patients still will require coronary bypass surgery eventually.

CARDIAC FAILURE

Perhaps the most important ailment that must be treated by the physician is cardiac failure, which can result from any heart condition that reduces the ability of the heart to pump blood. Usually the cause is decreased contractility of the myocardium caused by diminished coronary blood flow, but failure to pump adequate quantities of blood can also be caused by damage to the heart valves, external pressure around the heart, vitamin deficiency, primary cardiac

muscle disease, or any other abnormality that makes the heart a hypoeffective pump.

ACUTE EFFECTS OF MODERATE GENERALIZED CARDIAC FAILURE

If a heart suddenly becomes severely damaged in any way, such as by myocardial infarction, the pumping ability of the heart is immediately depressed. As a result, two essential effects occur: (a) reduced cardiac output and (b) damming of blood in the veins resulting in increased systemic venous pressure.

Figure 17–4 illustrates the sequential changes in heart function immediately following an acute myocardial infarction, showing, first, a normal cardiac output curve, depicting the state of the circulation prior to the infarction. Point A represents the normal state of the circulation, showing that the normal cardiac output under resting conditions is 5 liters per minute and the right atrial pressure 0 mm Hg.

Immediately after the heart becomes damaged, the cardiac output curve becomes greatly reduced, falling to the lower, long-dashed curve. Within a few seconds after the acute heart attack, a new circulatory state is established at point B rather than point A, showing that the cardiac output has fallen to 2 liters per minute, about two fifths normal, while the right atrial pressure has risen to 4 mm Hg because blood returning to the heart is dammed up in the right atrium. This low cardiac output is still sufficient to sustain life, but it is likely to be associated with fainting. Fortunately, this acute stage lasts for only a few seconds because sympathetic reflexes occur immediately that can compensate to a great extent for the damaged heart, as follows:

Compensation for Acute Cardiac Failure by Sympathetic Reflexes. When the cardiac output falls precariously low, many of the different circulatory reflexes discussed in Chapter 14 are immediately achieved. The best known of these is the baroreceptor reflex, which is activated by diminished arterial pres-

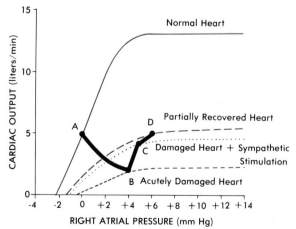

Figure 17–4. Progressive changes in the cardiac output curve following acute myocardial infarction. The cardiac output and right atrial pressure change progressively from point A to point D, as explained in the text.

sure. It is probable that the chemoreceptor reflex, the central nervous system ischemic response, and possibly even reflexes originating in the damaged heart itself also contribute to a lesser extent to the nervous response. But whatever all the reflexes might be, the sympathetics become strongly stimulated within a few seconds.

Strong sympathetic stimulation has two major effects on the circulation: First, even the damaged heart responds to the sympathetic stimulation with increased force of contraction. Thus, *the heart becomes a stronger pump, often as much as 100 per cent stronger, under the influence of the sympathetic impulses.* This effect is also illustrated in Figure 17–4, which shows elevation of the cardiac output curve after sympathetic compensation (the dotted curve). Second, sympathetic stimulation increases the tendency for venous return, for it increases the tone of most of the blood vessels of the circulation, especially of the veins, *raising the mean systemic filling pressure* to 12 to 14 mm Hg, almost 100 per cent above normal. As will be recalled from the discussion in Chapter 16, this greatly increases the tendency of blood to flow back to the heart. Therefore, the damaged heart becomes primed with more inflowing blood than usual, and the right atrial pressure rises still further, which helps the heart to pump larger quantities of blood. Thus, in Figure 17–4 the new circulatory state is depicted by Point C, showing a cardiac output of 4.2 liters per minute and a right atrial pressure of 5 mm Hg.

The sympathetic reflexes become maximally developed in about 30 seconds. Therefore, a person who has a sudden moderate heart attack may experience nothing more than cardiac pain and a few seconds of fainting. Shortly thereafter, with the aid of the sympathetic reflex compensations described above, the cardiac output may return to a level entirely adequate to sustain the person who remains quiet, though the pain may persist.

The Chronic Stage of Failure. After the first few minutes of an acute heart attack, a prolonged secondary state begins. This is characterized mainly by two events: (1) retention of fluid by the kidneys and (2) progressive recovery of the heart itself over a period of several weeks to months.

Compensation by Renal Retention of Fluid. A low cardiac output has a profound depressant effect on renal function. In general, the urinary output does not return to normal after an acute heart attack until the cardiac output rises either all the way back to normal or almost to normal. This relationship of renal function to cardiac output is one of the most important of all the factors affecting the dynamics of the circulation in chronic cardiac failure.

There are several known causes of the reduced renal output during cardiac failure, all of which are perhaps equally important but in different ways.

1. A decrease in cardiac output has a tendency to *reduce glomerular filtration* by the kidneys because of (a) *reduced arterial pressure* and (b) *intense sympathetic constriction of the arterioles of the kidney.*

2. The reduced blood flow to the kidneys causes *marked increase in renin output*, and this in turn causes the formation of angiotensin by the mechanism described in Chapter 14. The angiotensin has a direct effect on the arterioles of the kidneys to decrease further the blood flow through the kidneys. Therefore, the net loss of water and salt into the urine is greatly decreased, and the quantities of salt and water in the body fluids increase.

3. In the chronic stage of heart failure, *large quantities of aldosterone are secreted* by the adrenal cortex. This further increases the reabsorption of sodium from the renal tubules and in turn leads to a secondary increase in water reabsorption as well.

The Beneficial Effects of Moderate Fluid Retention in Cardiac Failure. A moderate amount of fluid retention with consequent increase in blood volume is a very important factor helping to compensate for the diminished pumping ability of the heart. The venous return increases mainly because the increased blood volume increases the mean systemic filling pressure, which *increases the pressure gradient for flow of blood toward the heart.*

Detrimental Effects of Excess Fluid Retention in the Severe Stages of Cardiac Failure. In contrast with the beneficial effects of moderate fluid retention in cardiac failure, in severe failure with extreme excess of fluid retention the fluid then begins to have very serious detrimental consequences. They include overstretching of the heart, thus weakening the heart still more; filtration of fluid into the lungs, causing pulmonary edema and consequent deoxygenation of the blood; and, often, development of extensive edema in all of the peripheral tissues of the body as well.

Recovery of the Myocardium Following Myocardial Infarction. After a heart becomes suddenly damaged as a result of myocardial infarction, the natural reparative processes of the body begin immediately to help restore normal cardiac function. A new collateral blood supply begins to penetrate the peripheral portions of the infarcted area, often completely restoring the muscle function. Also, the undamaged musculature hypertrophies, in this way offsetting much of the cardiac damage.

Obviously, the degree of recovery depends on the degree and type of cardiac damage, and it varies from no recovery at all to almost complete recovery. Ordinarily, after myocardial infarction the heart recovers rapidly during the first few days and weeks and will have achieved most of its final state of recovery within four to six months.

The second curve of Figure 17–4 illustrates function of the partially recovered heart a week or so after the acute myocardial infarction. By this time, considerable fluid has been retained in the body, and the tendency toward venous return has increased markedly; therefore, the right atrial pressure has also risen. As a result, the state of the circulation is now changed from Point C to Point D, which represents a *normal* cardiac output of 5 liters per minute but with the right atrial pressure elevated to 6 mm Hg.

Since the cardiac output has returned to normal,

renal output also has returned to normal and no further fluid retention will occur. Therefore, except for the high right atrial pressure represented by Point D in this figure, the person now has essentially normal cardiovascular dynamics *as long as he remains at rest.*

SUMMARY OF THE CHANGES THAT OCCUR FOLLOWING ACUTE CARDIAC FAILURE—COMPENSATED HEART FAILURE

To summarize the events discussed in the past few sections describing the moderate heart attack, we may divide the stages into (1) the instantaneous effect of the cardiac damage to depress cardiac function, (2) compensation by the sympathetic nervous system, and (3) chronic compensations resulting from partial heart recovery and renal retention of fluid. All these changes are shown graphically by the very heavy line in Figure 17–4. The progression of this line shows the normal state of the circulation (point A), the state a few seconds after the heart attack but before sympathetic reflexes have occurred (point B), the rise in cardiac output toward normal caused by sympathetic stimulation (point C), and final return of the cardiac output to normal following several days to several weeks of cardiac recovery and fluid retention (point D). This final state is called compensated heart failure.

Compensated Heart Failure. Note especially in Figure 17–4 that the pumping ability of the heart, as depicted by the cardiac function curve, is still depressed to less than one-half normal. This illustrates that factors that increase the right atrial pressure (principally retention of fluid) can maintain the cardiac output at a normal level despite continued weakness of the heart itself. However, one of the results of chronic cardiac weakness is this chronic increase in right atrial pressure itself; in Figure 17–4 it is shown to be 6 mm Hg. There are many persons, especially in old age, who have completely normal resting cardiac outputs but mildly to moderately elevated right atrial pressures because of compensated heart failure. These persons may not know that they have cardiac damage because the damage more often than not has occurred a little at a time, and the compensation has occurred concurrently with the progressive stages of damage.

DYNAMICS OF SEVERE CARDIAC FAILURE—DECOMPENSATED HEART FAILURE

If the heart becomes severely damaged, then no amount of compensation, either by sympathetic nervous reflexes or by fluid retention, can cause this weakened heart to pump a normal cardiac output. As a consequence, the cardiac output cannot rise to a high enough value to bring about return of normal renal function. Therefore *fluid continues to be retained indefinitely and the person develops progressively more and more edema;* this state of events eventually leads to death. This is called *decompensated heart failure.*

The main basis of decompensated heart failure is *failure of the heart to pump sufficient blood to make the kidneys function adequately.*

Treatment of Decompensation. The two ways in which the decompensation process can often be stopped are (1) strengthening the heart in any one of several ways, especially by administration of a cardiotonic drug, such as digitalis, so that it can pump adequate quantities of blood to make the kidneys function normally again, or (2) administering diuretics and reducing water and salt intake, which brings about a balance between fluid intake and output despite the low cardiac output.

Both methods stop the decompensation process by re-establishing normal fluid balance so that the progressive edema is blocked.

UNILATERAL LEFT HEART FAILURE

In the discussions thus far, we have considered failure of the heart as a whole. Yet in a large number of patients, left-sided failure predominates over right-sided failure, though in rare instances, especially in congenital heart disease, the right side may fail without significant failure of the left side. The effects of right heart failure are much the same as those of failure of the whole heart, but the effects of unilateral left heart failure are different, as follows:

When the left side of the heart fails without concomitant failure of the right side, blood continues to be pumped into the lungs with usual right heart vigor while it is not pumped adequately out of the lungs into the systemic circulation. As a result, large volumes of blood shift from the systemic circulation into the pulmonary circulation.

As the volume of blood in the lungs increases, the pulmonary vessels enlarge, and if the pulmonary capillary pressure rises above about 28 mm Hg, that is, above the colloid osmotic pressure of the plasma, fluid begins to filter out of the capillaries into the interstitial spaces and alveoli, resulting in *pulmonary edema.*

Thus, among the most important problems of left heart failure are *pulmonary vascular congestion* and *pulmonary edema.* Pulmonary edema sometimes can occur so rapidly that it causes death by suffocation after only 20 to 30 minutes of severe acute left heart failure.

Course of Events for Several Days After Acute Left Heart Failure. During the several days after the onset of left heart failure, one additional feature must be added to the acute picture. This is progressive increase in the volume of extracellular fluid. This increase is caused by the effect of the heart failure to decrease kidney excretion of salt and water. In moderate acute left heart failure the pulmonary capillary pressure does not rise high enough to cause pulmonary edema. Yet, following renal retention of fluid for the next few days, the blood volume increases and more blood is pumped into the lungs by the right ventricle. Then, the pulmonary capillary pressure rises still more, often rising above the plasma colloid osmotic pressure level (about 28 mm Hg), resulting in severe pulmonary edema. Indeed, this is a common occurrence: The patient suddenly develops severe pulmonary edema a few days after the acute attack and dies a respiratory death, not a death resulting from diminished cardiac output.

CARDIOGENIC SHOCK

In very severe heart failure, the cardiac output often falls too low to supply the body with adequate blood flow. As a result, the tissues deteriorate rapidly and death ensues. Sometimes death comes in less than an hour; at other times, it comes over a period of several days. The circulatory shock that is caused by inadequate cardiac pumping is called *cardiogenic shock* or *cardiac shock*; it is sometimes also called the *power failure syndrome*.

Cardiogenic shock is extremely important to the clinician because approximately one-tenth of all patients who have acute myocardial infarction will have enough power failure to die of circulatory shock before the physiologic compensatory measures can come into play to save life. Once cardiac shock has become well established after myocardial infarction, all the typical progressive events occur that also occur in the late stages of other types of circulatory shock, as described in the previous chapter, especially rapid, progressive deterioration of almost all bodily functions.

Vicious Circle of Cardiac Deterioration in Cardiogenic Shock. The discussion of circulatory shock in Chapter 16 emphasized the tendency of the heart itself to become progressively damaged during the course of shock. That is, the low arterial pressure that occurs during shock reduces the coronary supply, which makes the heart still weaker, which makes the shock still worse, the process eventually becoming a vicious circle of cardiac deterioration. In cardiogenic shock caused by myocardial infarction, this problem is greatly compounded by the already existing coronary thrombosis. For instance, in a normal heart, the arterial pressure usually must be reduced below about 45 mm Hg before cardiac deterioration sets in. However, in a heart that already has a major coronary vessel blocked, deterioration will set in when the arterial pressure falls as low as 80 to 90 mm Hg.

Unfortunately, even with the best therapy, once the shock syndrome has begun, with the arterial pressure remaining as much as 20 mm Hg below normal for as long as an hour, 85 per cent of the patients die.

PHYSIOLOGICAL CLASSIFICATION OF CARDIAC FAILURE

From the above discussions, it is apparent that the symptoms of cardiac failure fall into the following three physiological classifications: (1) low cardiac output, (2) pulmonary congestion, and (3) systemic congestion.

Low cardiac output usually occurs immediately after a heart attack. If the attack is mainly right sided, this may be the only symptom. If the acute heart attack is mainly left-sided, concurrent pulmonary congestion almost always occurs along with the low cardiac output, but the pulmonary congestion may be mild (without pulmonary edema) until after considerable fluid has been retained by the kidneys. If the cardiac output is low enough, cardiac shock ensues, with death being likely.

Pulmonary congestion may be the only effect in patients with pure left-sided *chronic* heart failure, because in the chronic stage enough fluid will have been retained to return the cardiac output to normal despite the weak left ventricle—but this occurs at the expense of greatly elevated pulmonary vascular pressures. And since the right heart is not failing, pulmonary congestive symptoms alone can occur with essentially no systemic congestion and no low cardiac output.

Systemic congestion alone can occur in pure right-sided *chronic* heart failure. In this condition there is no pulmonary congestion, and if sufficient fluids have been retained in the blood to prime the heart sufficiently, the heart may pump a normal cardiac output.

Obviously, all the above classes of heart failure can occur together or in any combination.

CARDIAC RESERVE

Fortunately, the normal heart can increase its output to four to five times normal under conditions of stress in most younger persons and to six to seven times normal in endurance athletes. The maximum percentage that the cardiac output can increase above normal is called the *cardiac reserve*. Thus, in the normal young adult the cardiac reserve is 300 to 400 per cent. In the athletically trained person, it is occasionally as high as 500 to 600 per cent, while in the asthenic person it may be as low as 200 per cent. As an example, during severe exercise the cardiac output of the normal healthy young adult can rise to about five times normal; this is an increase above normal of 400 per cent—that is, a cardiac reserve of 400 per cent.

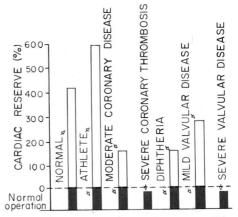

Figure 17–5. Cardiac reserve in different conditions.

Any factor that prevents the heart from satisfactorily pumping blood decreases the cardiac reserve. This can result from ischemic heart disease, primary myocardial disease, vitamin deficiency, damage to the myocardium, valvular heart disease, and many other factors, some of which are illustrated in Figure 17–5.

THE HEART SOUNDS AND VALVULAR DYSFUNCTION

The function of the heart valves was discussed in Chapter 8, and it was pointed out that closure of the valves is associated with audible sounds, though no sounds usually occur when the valves open. The purpose of the present section is to discuss the factors that cause the sounds in the heart, under both normal and abnormal conditions.

NORMAL HEART SOUNDS

Listening with a stethoscope to a normal heart, one hears a sound usually described as "lub, dub, lub, dub. . . ." The "lub" is associated with closure of the A-V valves at the beginning of systole and the "dub," with closure of the semilunar valves (the aortic and pulmonary valves) at the end of systole. The "lub" sound is called the *first heart sound* and the "dub" the *second heart sound*, because the normal cycle of the heart is considered to start with the beginning of systole.

Causes of the First and Second Heart Sounds. Closure of the valves in any pump system usually causes a certain amount of noise, because the valves close solidly and suddenly over some opening, setting up vibrations in the fluid or walls of the pump. In the heart, the cause of the first heart sound is *vibration of the taut A-V valves immediately after closure*, as well as *vibration of the adjacent blood, the walls of the heart, and the major vessels around the heart.* That is, contraction of the ventricle causes sudden backflow of blood against the A-V valves, causing them to bulge toward the atria until the chordae tendineae abruptly stop the backbulging. The elastic tautness of the valves then causes the backsurging blood to bounce forward again into the ventricles. This sets the blood, the ventricles, and the valves all into vibration. The vibrations then travel to the chest wall, where they can be heard as sound by the stethoscope.

The second heart sound results from vibration of the semilunar valves, the blood, and the walls of the pulmonary artery, aorta, and, to a much lesser extent, ventricles. When the semilunar valves close, they bulge backward toward the ventricles, and their elastic stretch recoils the blood back into the arteries, which causes a short period of reverberation of blood back and forth between the walls of the arteries and the valves. The vibrations set up in the arterial walls are then transmitted along the arteries to the chest wall, where they create sound that can be heard.

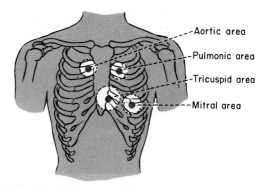

Figure 17–6. Chest areas from which each valve sound is best heard.

AREAS FOR AUSCULTATION OF NORMAL HEART SOUNDS

Listening to the sounds of the body, usually with the aid of a stethoscope, is called *auscultation.* Figure 17–6 illustrates the areas of the chest wall from which the sounds from the respective valves can best be distinguished. With the stethoscope placed in any one of the special valvular areas, not only the sound from the particular valve being studied, but the sounds from all the other valves can also be heard. However, the sound from the special valve is as loud *relative to the other sounds* as it ever will be. The cardiologist distinguishes the sounds from the different valves by a process of elimination; he moves the stethoscope from one area to another, noting the loudness of the sounds in different areas and gradually picking out the sound components from each valve.

The areas for listening to the different heart sounds are not directly over the valves themselves. The aortic area is upward along the aorta, the pulmonic area is upward along the pulmonary artery, the tricuspid area is over the right ventricle, and the mitral area is over the apex of the heart.

THE PHONOCARDIOGRAM

If a microphone specially designed to detect low-frequency sound waves is placed on the chest, the heart sounds can be amplified. Recording is possible by a high-speed recording apparatus, such as an oscilloscope or a high-speed pen recorder; these devices, described in Chapters 5 and 10, record nerve potentials and electrocardiograms. The recording is called a *phonocardiogram*, and the heart sounds appear as waves, as illustrated schematically in Figure 17–7. Record A is a recording of normal heart sounds, showing especially the vibrations of the first and second heart sounds.

RHEUMATIC VALVULAR LESIONS

By far the greatest number of valvular lesions results from rheumatic fever. Rheumatic fever is an autoimmune or allergic disease in which the heart valves are likely to be damaged or destroyed. It is

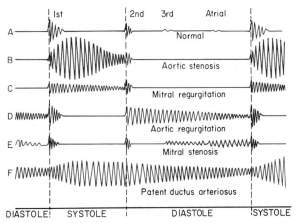

Figure 17-7. Phonocardiograms from normal and abnormal hearts.

initiated by streptococcal toxin in the following manner:

The entire sequence of events almost always begins with a preliminary streptococcal infection (caused by Group A hemolytic streptococci), such as a sore throat, scarlet fever, or middle ear infection. The streptococci release several different proteins against which antibodies are formed, the most important of which seems to be a protein called the "M" antigen. The antibodies then react with many different tissues of the body, causing either immunological or allergic damage. These reactions continue to take place as long as the antibodies persist in the blood—six months or more. As a result, rheumatic fever causes damage in many parts of the body but especially in certain very susceptible areas such as the heart valves.

In rheumatic fever, large hemorrhagic, fibrinous, bulbous lesions grow along the inflamed edges of the heart valves. Because the mitral valve receives more trauma during valvular action than any of the other valves, this valve is the one most often seriously damaged, and the aortic valve is the second most frequently damaged. The tricuspid and pulmonary valves are much less severely involved, probably because the stresses acting on these valves are slight compared with those in the left ventricle.

Scarring of the Valves. The lesions of acute rheumatic fever frequently occur on adjacent valve leaflets simultaneously so that the edges of the leaflets become stuck together. Then weeks, months, or years later, the lesions become scar tissue, permanently fusing portions of the leaflets. Also, the free edges of the leaflets, which are normally filmy and free-flapping, become solid, scarred masses.

A valve in which the leaflets adhere to each other so extensively that blood cannot flow through satisfactorily is said to be *stenosed*. On the other hand, when the valve edges are so destroyed by scar tissue that they cannot close when the ventricles contract, *regurgitation*, or backflow, of blood occurs when the valve should be closed.

Abnormal Heart Sounds Caused by Valvular Lesions

As illustrated by the phonocardiograms of Figure 17-7, many abnormal heart sounds, known as murmurs, occur when there are abnormalities of the valves, as follows:

The Murmur of Aortic Stenosis. In aortic stenosis, blood is ejected from the left ventricle through only a small opening of the aortic valve. Because of the resistance to ejection, the pressure in the left ventricle rises sometimes to as high as 300 mm Hg while the pressure in the aorta is still normal. Thus, a nozzle effect is created *during systole*, with blood jetting at tremendous velocity through the small opening of the valve. This causes *severe turbulence* of the blood in the root of the aorta. The turbulent blood impinging against the aortic walls causes intense vibration, and a loud murmur is transmitted throughout the upper aorta and even into the larger arteries of the neck. This sound is harsh and occasionally so loud that it can be heard several feet away from the patient.

The Murmur of Aortic Regurgitation. In aortic regurgitation, no sound is heard during systole, but *during diastole* blood flows backward from the aorta into the left ventricle, causing a "blowing" murmur of relatively high pitch and with a swishing quality heard maximally over the left ventricle. This murmur results from *turbulence* of blood jetting backward into the blood already in the left ventricle.

The Murmur of Mitral Stenosis. In mitral stenosis, blood passes with difficulty from the left atrium into the left ventricle, and because the pressure in the left atrium rarely rises above 35 mm Hg except for short periods of time, no great pressure differential ever develops to force blood from the left atrium into the left ventricle. Consequently, the abnormal sounds in mitral stenosis are usually weak, rumbling sounds heard during diastole over the left ventricle. Despite the weakness of these sounds, mitral stenosis can be severely debilitating.

Phonocardiograms of Valvular Murmurs. Phonocardiograms B, C, D, and E of Figure 17-7 illustrate, respectively, idealized records obtained from patients with aortic stenosis, mitral regurgitation, aortic regurgitation, and mitral stenosis. It is obvious from these phonocardiograms that the aortic stenotic lesion causes the loudest of all these murmurs, and the mitral stenotic lesion causes the weakest, a murmur of very low frequency and rumbling quality. The phonocardiograms show how the intensity of the murmurs varies during different portions of systole and diastole, and the relative timing of each murmur is also evident. Note especially that the murmurs of aortic stenosis and mitral regurgitation occur only during systole, while the murmurs of aortic regurgitation and mitral stenosis occur only during diastole—if a student does not understand this timing, a moment's pause should be taken until it is understood.

DYNAMICS OF THE CIRCULATION IN AORTIC STENOSIS AND AORTIC REGURGITATION

In aortic stenosis the left ventricle fails to empty adequately, whereas in aortic regurgitation blood returns to the ventricle after the ventricle has been emptied. Therefore, in either case, the *net* stroke volume output of the heart is reduced.

Eventual Failure of the Left Ventricle, and Development of Pulmonary Edema. In the early stages of aortic stenosis or aortic regurgitation, the intrinsic ability of the left ventricle to adapt to increasing loads prevents significant abnormalities in circulatory function other than increased work output required of the left ventricle. Therefore, marked degrees of aortic stenosis or aortic regurgitation often occur before the person knows that he has serious heart disease.

However, beyond critical stages of development of these two aortic lesions, the left ventricle finally cannot keep up with the work demand, and as a consequence the left ventricle dilates and cardiac output begins to fall while blood simultaneously dams up in the left atrium and lungs behind the failing left ventricle. The left atrial pressure rises progressively, and at pressures above 30 to 40 mm. Hg, edema appears in the lungs, often leading to death.

CIRCULATORY DYNAMICS IN MITRAL STENOSIS AND MITRAL REGURGITATION

In mitral stenosis blood flow from the left atrium into the left ventricle is impeded, and in mitral regurgitation much of the blood that has flowed into the left ventricle leaks back into the left atrium during systole rather than being pumped into the aorta. Therefore, the effect is a great increase in the blood in the left atrium as well as reduced net movement of blood from the left atrium into the left ventricle.

Pulmonary Edema in Mitral Valvular Disease. Obviously, the buildup of blood in the left atrium causes progressive increase in left atrial pressure, which can result eventually in the development of serious pulmonary edema. Ordinarily, lethal edema will not occur until the mean left atrial pressure rises at least above 30 mm Hg; more often it must rise to as high as 40 mm Hg, because the lung lymphatic vasculature enlarges manyfold and can carry fluid away from the lung tissues extremely rapidly.

Enlarged Left Atrium and Atrial Fibrillation. The high left atrial pressure also causes progressive enlargement of the left atrium, which increases the distance that the cardiac impulse must travel in the atrial wall. Eventually, this pathway becomes so long that it predisposes the atria to the development of circus movements. Therefore, in late stages of mitral valvular disease, especially stenosis, atrial fibrillation almost always occurs. This state further reduces the pumping effectiveness of the heart and therefore causes still further cardiac debility.

CIRCULATORY DYNAMICS DURING EXERCISE IN PATIENTS WITH VALVULAR LESIONS

During exercise very large quantities of venous blood are returned to the heart from the peripheral circulation. Therefore, all of the dynamic abnormalities that occur in the different types of valvular heart disease become tremendously exacerbated. Even in mild valvular heart disease in which the symptoms may be completely unrecognizable at rest, severe symptoms often develop during heavy exercise. For instance, in patients with aortic valvular lesions, exercise can cause acute left ventricular failure followed by acute pulmonary edema. Also, in patients with severe mitral disease, exercise can cause so much damming of blood in the lungs that serious pulmonary edema ensues within minutes.

Even in less severe cases of valvular disease, the patient finds that his cardiac reserve is diminished in proportion to the severity of the valvular dysfunction. That is, the cardiac output does not increase as it should during exercise. Therefore, the muscles of the body fatigue rapidly.

ABNORMAL CIRCULATORY DYNAMICS IN CONGENITAL HEART DEFECTS

Occasionally, the heart or its associated blood vessels are malformed during fetal life; the defect is called a *congenital anomaly*. One of the common causes of congenital heart defects is a virus infection in the mother during the first trimester of pregnancy when the fetal heart is being formed. Defects are particularly prone to develop when the mother contracts German measles at this time—so often indeed that obstetricians advise termination of pregnancy if German measles does occur in the first trimester. However, some congenital defects of the heart are hereditary; the same defect has been known to occur in identical twins and also in succeeding generations. Children of patients surgically treated for congenital heart disease have ten times as much chance of having congenital heart disease as do other children. Congenital defects of the heart are also frequently associated with other congenital defects of the body.

Though there are many different types of congenital heart defects, two that illustrate important effects on cardiac function are *patent ductus arteriosus* and *tetralogy of Fallot*.

PATENT DUCTUS ARTERIOSUS—A LEFT-TO-RIGHT SHUNT

During fetal life a large blood vessel called the *ductus arteriosus* connects directly between the aorta

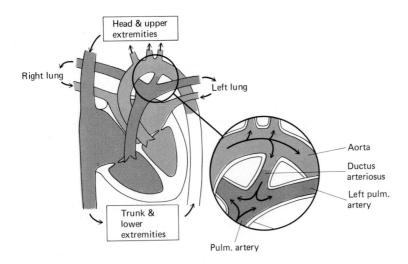

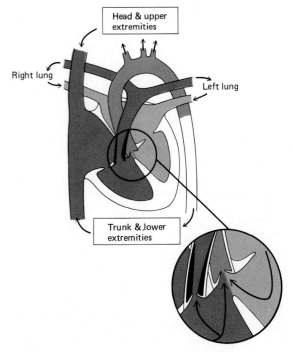

Figure 17–8. Patent ductus arteriosus, illustrating the degree of blood oxygenation in the different parts of the circulation.

and the pulmonary artery. And because the pulmonary arterial pressure in the fetus is higher than the aortic pressure, almost all the pulmonary arterial blood flows directly into the aorta rather than through the lungs. This allows immediate recirculation of the blood through the systemic arteries of the fetus. Obviously, this lack of blood flow through the lungs is of no detriment to the fetus, because the blood is oxygenated by the placenta of the mother.

Closure of the Ductus. As soon as the baby is born its lungs inflate; and not only do the alveoli fill, but also the resistance to blood flow through the pulmonary vascular tree decreases tremendously, allowing pulmonary arterial pressure to fall. Simultaneously, the aortic pressure rises because of sudden cessation of blood flow through the placenta. Thus, the pressure in the pulmonary artery falls, while that in the aorta rises. As a result, blood flow through the ductus reverses at birth, now flowing backward from the aorta to the pulmonary artery. This new state of blood flow causes the ductus arteriosus to become occluded within a few hours to a few days in most babies, so that blood flow through the ductus does not persist. The ductus closes because the aortic blood now flowing through the ductus has about two times as high an oxygen concentration as the pulmonary blood and the oxygen constricts the ductus muscle. In a few instances it takes several months for the ductus to close completely, and in about 1 of every 5500 babies the ductus never closes, causing the condition known as *patent ductus arteriosus*, which is illustrated in Figure 17–8.

Dynamics of Persistent Patent Ductus. During the early months of an infant's life a patent ductus usually does not cause severely abnormal dynamics because the blood pressure of the aorta then is not much higher than the pressure in the pulmonary artery, and only a small amount of blood flows backward into the pulmonary system. However, in most instances, as the child grows older the differential between the pressure in the aorta and that in the pulmonary artery progressively increases, with corresponding increase

in the backward flow of blood from the aorta to the pulmonary artery. Also, the diameter of the partially closed ductus often increases with time, making the condition worse.

Recirculation Through the Lungs. In the older child with a patent ductus, as much as half to two thirds of the aortic blood flows through the ductus into the pulmonary artery, then through the lungs, into the left atrium, and finally back into the left ventricle, passing through this lung circuit two or more times for every one time that it passes through the systemic circulation.

Diminished Cardiac and Respiratory Reserve. The major effects of patent ductus arteriosus on the patient are low cardiac and respiratory reserve. The left

Figure 17–9. Tetralogy of Fallot, illustrating the degree of blood oxygenation in the different parts of the circulation.

ventricle is already pumping approximately two or more times the normal cardiac output, and the maximum that it can possibly pump is about four to six times normal. Therefore, during exercise the cardiac output can be increased much less than usual. With even moderately strenuous exercise, therefore, the patient is likely to become weak and occasionally even faint from momentary heart failure. Also, the high pressures in the pulmonary vessels often lead to *pulmonary congestion.*

As a result of the increased load on the heart and especially because pulmonary congestion and pulmonary vascular sclerosis effects become progressively more severe with age, most patients with uncorrected patent ductus die between the ages of 20 and 40.

The Machinery Murmur. In the infant with patent ductus arteriosus, occasionally no abnormal heart sounds are heard because the quantity of reversed blood flow may be insufficient. As the baby grows older, at the age of one to three years, a harsh, blowing murmur begins to be heard in the pulmonic area of the chest. This sound is continuous during the entire heart cycle, but it is much more intense during systole, when the aortic pressure is high, and much less intense during diastole, when the aortic pressure falls very low, so that the murmur waxes and wanes with each beat of the heart, creating the so-called machinery murmur. The idealized phonocardiogram of this murmur is shown in Figure 17–7F.

Surgical Treatment. Surgical treatment of patent ductus arteriosus is extremely simple, for all one needs to do is to ligate the patent ductus or to divide it and sew the two ends closed.

TETRALOGY OF FALLOT—A RIGHT-TO-LEFT SHUNT

Tetralogy of Fallot is illustrated in Figure 17–9, from which it will be noted that four different abnormalities of the heart occur simultaneously.

First, the *aorta originates from the right ventricle* rather than the left, or it overrides the septum as shown in the figure.

Second, the *pulmonary artery is stenosed*, so that much less than normal amounts of blood pass from the right ventricle into the lungs; instead, the blood passes into the aorta.

Third, *blood from the left ventricle flows through a ventricular septal defect* into the right ventricle and then into the aorta or directly into the overriding aorta.

Fourth, because the right side of the heart must pump large quantities of blood against the high pressure in the aorta, its musculature is highly developed, causing an *enlarged right ventricle.*

Abnormal Dynamics. It is readily apparent that the major physiological difficulty caused by tetralogy of Fallot is the shunting of blood past the lungs without its becoming oxygenated. As much as 75 per cent of the venous blood returning to the heart may pass directly from the right ventricle into the aorta without becoming oxygenated. Tetralogy of Fallot is the major cause of cyanosis in babies ("blue babies").

Surgical Treatment. In recent years tetralogy of Fallot has been treated successfully by surgery. The operation is to open the pulmonary stenosis, to close the septal defect, and to reconstruct the flow pathway into the aorta. This surgery increases the average life expectancy from 5 or 6 years up to 60 or more years.

QUESTIONS

1. What is the normal blood flow through the coronary system, and how much can this increase during exercise?
2. Why is blood flow through the left ventricular coronary vessels greater during diastole than during systole?
3. What factors control the coronary blood flow?
4. What causes *atherosclerosis?*
5. Describe what happens when an *acute coronary occlusion* occurs? Describe recovery from this occlusion by the development of collateral vessels.
6. What are the various effects of coronary occlusion that frequently lead to death?
7. What are the causes of *angina pectoris?*
8. Describe the surgical treatment for coronary disease using the *aortic-coronary bypass* operation or *coronary angioplasty.*
9. Describe the sequential changes that occur in circulation function after an *acute myocardial infarction* and the development of acute cardiac failure and subsequent recovery of circulatory function.
10. Explain why moderate fluid retention can be of value in helping the circulatory system to compensate for moderate degrees of heart failure, whereas extreme

retention of fluid in severe degrees of heart failure can be lethal.
11. What are the specific characteristics of *unilateral left heart failure?* Explain why pulmonary edema is usually worse in unilateral left heart failure than in generalized heart failure?
12. What is meant by *cardiogenic shock?* Why does this condition frequently lead to a vicious circle of cardiac deterioration?
13. Name the three different types of cardiac failure in the physiological classification of failure, and state the cause of each of these types.
14. What is meant by *cardiac reserve?* What are some of the causes of very low cardiac reserve?
15. What causes the normal first and second heart sounds?
16. What is the cause of rheumatic valvular heart disease? What is the difference between a *stenosed valve* and a *regurgitating valve?*
17. Describe the *heart murmurs* caused by different valvular lesions.
18. Describe the dynamics of the circulation in *aortic stenosis, aortic regurgitation, mitral stenosis,* and *mitral regurgitation.*

19. Why do fatigue and pulmonary edema frequently occur in valvular heart disease patients during exercise?
20. Describe the cause and circulatory effects of *patent ductus arteriosus.*

21. Describe the congenital abnormality of the heart called *tetrology of Fallot.* Explain why this is called a *right-to-left shunt* and why it is so detrimental to the circulatory system.

References

Coronary Blood Flow

Conti, C. R.: Large vessel coronary vasospasm: Diagnosis, natural history and treatment. Am J Cardiol 55:41B, 1985.

Feigl, E. O.: Coronary physiology. Physiol Rev 63:1, 1983.

Gensini, G. G., ed.: Coronary Arteriography. Mt. Kisco, N. Y., Futura Publishing Co., 1985.

Gregg, D. E.: Coronary Circulation in Health and Disease. Philadelphia, Lea & Febiger, 1950.

Guyton, R. A., and Daggett, W. M.: The evolution of myocardial infarction: Physiological basis for clinical intervention. Int Rev Physiol 9:305, 1976.

Hutchinson: Prevention of Coronary Heart Disease. Chicago, Year Book Medical Publishers, 1985.

Kalsner, S., ed.: The Coronary Artery. New York, Oxford University Press, 1982.

Reimer, K. A., and Jennings, R. B.: Effects of calcium-channel blockers on myocardial preservation during experimental acute myocardial infarction. Am J Cardiol 55:107B, 1985.

Rigotti, N. A., et al.: Exercise and coronary heart disease. Annu Rev Med 34:391, 1983.

Stone, H. L.: Control of the coronary circulation during exercise. Annu Rev Physiol 45:213, 1983.

Cardiac Failure

Francis, G. S.: Neurohumoral mechanisms involved in congestive heart failure. Am J Cardiol 55:15A, 1985.

Guyton, A. C.: The systemic venous system in cardiac failure. J Chronic Dis 9:465, 1959.

Guyton, A. C., et al.: Cardiac Output and Its Regulation. Philadelphia, W. B. Saunders Co., 1973.

Kones, R. J.: Cardiogenic Shock: Mechanisms and Management. New York, Futura Publishing Co., 1975.

Lange, L. G., and Sobel, B. E.: Pharmacological salvage of myocardium. Annu Rev Pharmacol Toxicol 22:115, 1982.

Norris, R. M.: Myocardial Infarction. Its Presentation, Pathogenesis and Treatment. New York, Churchill Livingstone, Inc., 1982.

Orrego, F.: Calcium and the mechanism of action of digitalis. Gen Pharmacol 15:273, 1984.

Silver, M. D.: Cardiovascular Pathology. New York, Churchill Livingstone, Inc., 1983.

Swan, H. J. C., and Parmley, W. W.: Congestive heart failure. In Sodeman, W. A., Jr., and Sodeman, T. M., eds.: Pathologic Physiology: Mechanisms of Disease, 6th Ed. Philadelphia, W. B. Saunders Co., 1979, p. 313.

Zelis, R., et al.: Cardiocirculatory dynamics in the normal and failing heart. Annu Rev Physiol 43:455, 1981.

Heart Sounds, Valvular and Congenital Heart Defects

Barry, A.: Aortic and Tricuspid Valvular Disease. New York, Appleton-Century-Crofts, 1980.

Cooley, D. A., and Hallman, G. L.: Surgical Treatment of Congenital Heart Disease. Philadelphia, Lea & Febiger, 1966.

DePace, N. L., et al.: Acute severe mitral regurgitation. Pathophysiology, clinical recognition, and management. Am J Med 78:293, 1985.

Grossman, W., ed.: Cardiac Catheterization and Angiography, 2nd ed. Philadelphia, Lea & Febiger, 1980.

Kremkau, F. W.: Diagnostic Ultrasound; Physical Principles and Exercises. New York, Grune & Stratton, 1980.

Lear, M. W.: Heartsounds. New York, Simon & Schuster, 1979.

Mair, D. D., and Ritter, D. G.: The physiology of cyanotic congenital heart disease. Int Rev Physiol 9:275, 1976.

Perloff, J. K.: The Clinical Recognition of Congenital Heart Disease. Philadelphia, W. B. Saunders Co., 1978.

Rapaport, E., ed.: Current Controversies in Cardiovascular Disease. Philadelphia, W. B. Saunders Co., 1980.

Shah, P. M., and Roberts, D. L.: Diagnosis and Treatment of Aortic Valve Stenosis. Chicago, Year Book Medical Publishers, 1977.

Stapleton, J. F., and Harvey, W. P.: Heart sounds, murmurs, and precordial movements. In Sodeman, W. A., Jr., and Sodeman, T. M., eds.: Pathologic Physiology: Mechanisms of Disease, 6th Ed. Philadelphia, W. B. Saunders Co., 1979, p. 335.

Taussig, H.: Congenital Malformations of the Heart. Vol. 1: General Considerations, 2nd ed. Vol. 2: Specific Malformations, 2nd ed. Cambridge, Mass., Harvard University Press, 1960.

Weisfeldt, L., and Chandra, N.: Physiology of cardiopulmonary resuscitation. Annu Rev Med 32:435, 1981.

18

Muscle Blood Flow During Exercise; Cerebral, Splanchnic, and Skin Blood Flows

BLOOD FLOW THROUGH SKELETAL
MUSCLES AND ITS REGULATION IN
EXERCISE
RATE OF BLOOD FLOW THROUGH
THE MUSCLES
CONTROL OF BLOOD FLOW
THROUGH THE SKELETAL MUSCLES
CIRCULATORY ADJUSTMENTS
DURING EXERCISE
THE CEREBRAL CIRCULATION
NORMAL RATE OF CEREBRAL BLOOD
FLOW
REGULATION OF CEREBRAL BLOOD
FLOW

THE SPLANCHNIC CIRCULATION
BLOOD FLOW THROUGH THE LIVER
BLOOD FLOW THROUGH THE
INTESTINAL VESSELS
PORTAL VENOUS PRESSURE
THE SPLENIC CIRCULATION
CIRCULATION IN THE SKIN
PHYSIOLOGIC ANATOMY OF THE
CUTANEOUS CIRCULATION
REGULATION OF BLOOD FLOW IN
THE SKIN

The blood flow in many special areas of the body, such as the lungs and the heart, has already been discussed in previous chapters. In the present chapter the characteristics of blood flow in some of the other important vascular areas, such as the muscles, the brain, the splanchnic system, and the skin, are presented.

BLOOD FLOW THROUGH SKELETAL MUSCLES AND ITS REGULATION IN EXERCISE

Very strenuous exercise is the most stressful condition that the normal circulatory system faces. This is true because the blood flow in muscles can increase more than 20-fold (a greater increase than in any other tissue of the body) and also because there is such a very large mass of skeletal muscle in the body. The product of these two factors is so great that the total muscle blood flow in the normal young adult can increase during heavy exercise from the normal level of less than 1 liter per minute to as great as 20 liters per minute, high enough to increase the cardiac output to as much as five times normal and in the well-trained athlete to as much as six to seven times normal.

RATE OF BLOOD FLOW THROUGH THE MUSCLES

During rest, blood flow through skeletal muscle averages 3 to 4 ml per minute per 100 grams of muscle. However, during extreme exercise this rate can increase as much as 15- to 25-fold, rising to 50 to 80 ml per 100 grams of muscle.

Intermittent Flow During Muscle Contraction. Figure 18–1 illustrates a study of blood flow changes in the calf muscles of the human leg during strong rhythmic muscular exercise. Note that the flow increases and decreases with each muscle contraction, decreasing during the contraction phase and increasing between contractions. At the end of the rhythmic contractions, the blood flow remains very high for a few seconds longer but then gradually fades toward normal during the next few minutes.

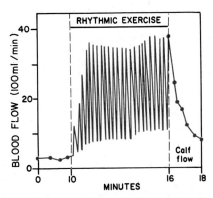

Figure 18–1. Effects of muscle exercise on blood flow in the calf of a leg during strong rhythmic contraction. The blood flow was much less during contraction than between contractions. (From Barcroft and Dornhorst: *J. Physiol., 109*:402, 1949.)

The cause of the decreased flow during muscle contraction is compression of the blood vessels by the contracted muscle. During strong *tetanic* contraction, which causes sustained compression of the blood vessels, the blood flow can be almost totally stopped.

Opening of Muscle Capillaries During Exercise. During rest, only 20 to 25 per cent of the muscle capillaries are open. But during strenuous exercise all the capillaries open up. This opening of dormant capillaries also diminishes the distance that oxygen and other nutrients must diffuse from the capillaries to the muscle fibers and contributes a much increased surface area through which nutrients can diffuse from the blood.

CONTROL OF BLOOD FLOW THROUGH THE SKELETAL MUSCLES

Local Regulation. The tremendous increase in muscle blood flow that occurs during skeletal muscle activity is caused primarily by local factors in the muscles acting directly on the arterioles to cause vasodilatation.

This local increase in flow during muscle contraction is probably caused by several different factors all operating at the same time. One of the most important of these is reduction of oxygen in the muscle tissues. That is, during muscle activity the muscle utilizes oxygen very rapidly, thereby decreasing the oxygen concentration in the tissue fluids. This in turn causes vasodilatation either because the vessel walls cannot maintain contraction in the absence of oxygen or because oxygen deficiency causes release of vasodilator substances. The vasodilator substance that has been suggested most widely in recent years has been *adenosine,* but recent experiments have shown that adenosine probably cannot cause long-sustained vasodilation in skeletal muscle.

Other vasodilator substances released during muscle contraction include potassium ions, acetylcholine, adenosine triphosphate, lactic acid, and carbon dioxide.

Nervous Control of Muscle Blood Flow. In addition to the local tissue regulatory mechanism, the skeletal muscles are also provided with sympathetic vasoconstrictor nerves and, in some species of animals, possibly some sympathetic vasodilator nerves as well, though these are probably of little importance.

Sympathetic Vasoconstrictor Nerves. The sympathetic vasoconstrictor nerve fibers secrete norepinephrine and when maximally stimulated can decrease blood flow through the muscles to perhaps one-half to one-fourth normal. This vasoconstriction is of physiological importance in circulatory shock and during other periods of stress when it is desirable to reduce blood flow through the many muscles of the body.

In addition to the norepinephrine secreted at the sympathetic vasoconstrictor nerve endings, the adrenal medullae secrete large amounts of additional norepinephrine and epinephrine into the circulating blood during strenuous exercise. The circulating norepinephrine acts on the muscle vessels to cause a vasoconstrictor effect similar to that caused by direct sympathetic nerve stimulation. The epinephrine, on the other hand, has a vasodilator effect because epinephrine excites the *beta* receptors of the vessels, which are vasodilator receptors, in contrast to the *alpha* vasoconstrictor receptors excited by the norepinephrine.

CIRCULATORY ADJUSTMENTS DURING EXERCISE

In addition to the increased blood flow through the exercising muscles, three other major effects occur during exercise that are essential for the circulatory system to supply the tremendous flow required by the muscles. These effects are (1) mass discharge of the sympathetic nervous system throughout the body with consequent stimulatory effects on the circulation, (2) increase in cardiac output, and (3) increase in arterial pressure.

Mass Sympathetic Discharge. At the onset of exercise, signals are transmitted not only from the brain to the muscle to cause muscle contraction but also from the higher levels of the brain into the vasomotor center to initiate mass sympathetic discharge. Simultaneously, the parasympathetic signals to the heart are greatly attenuated. Therefore, two major circulatory effects result. First, the heart is stimulated to greatly increased heart rate and pumping strength as a result of the sympathetic drive to the heart, as well as release of the heart from the normal parasympathetic inhibition. Second, all the blood vessels of the peripheral circulation are strongly contracted except the vessels in the active muscles, which are strongly vasodilated by the local vasodilator effects in the muscles themselves. Thus, the heart is stimulated to supply the increased blood flow required by the muscles, and blood flow through most nonmuscular areas of the body is temporarily reduced, thereby temporarily "lending" their blood supply to the muscles. However, two of the organ circulatory systems, the *coronary* and *cerebral systems, are spared this vasoconstrictor effect* because both these circulatory areas have very poor vasoconstrictor innervation—fortunately so because both the heart and the brain are as essential to exercise as are the skeletal muscles themselves.

Increase in Cardiac Output. The increase in cardiac output during exercise results mainly from the intense, locally induced vasodilatation in active muscles. As was explained in Chapter 16 in relation to the basic theory of cardiac output regulation, local vasodilatation increases the venous return of blood back to the heart. The heart in turn pumps this extra returning blood and sends it immediately back to the muscles through the arteries. Thus, it is mainly the muscles themselves that determine the amount of increase in cardiac output—up to the limit of the heart's ability to respond.

However, another factor that increases the venous return is the *strong sympathetic stimulation of the veins.* This stimulation greatly increases the mean systemic filling pressure, sometimes to as high as 30 mm Hg (four times normal), and is therefore important in increasing venous return.

Mechanisms by Which the Heart Increases Its Output. One of the mechanisms by which the heart increases its output during exercise is the Frank-Starling mechanism, which was discussed in Chapter 8. Via this mechanism, when increased quantities of blood flow from the veins into the heart and dilate its chambers, the heart muscle contracts with increased force, thus pumping an increased volume of blood with each heart beat. However, in addition to this basic intrinsic cardiac mechanism, the heart is also strongly stimulated by the sympathetic nervous system, and the normal parasympathetic inhibition is reduced or eliminated. The net effects are greatly increased heart rate (occasionally to as high as 200 beats per minute) and almost doubling of the cardiac muscle strength of contraction. These two effects combine to make the heart capable of pumping at least 100 per cent more blood than would be true based on the Frank-Starling mechanism alone.

Increase in Arterial Pressure—Importance of Increased Sympathetic Activity. The mass sympathetic discharge during exercise and the resultant vasoconstriction of most of the blood vessels besides those in the active muscles almost always increase the arterial pressure during exercise. This increase can be as little as 20 or as great as 80 mm Hg, depending on the conditions under which the exercise is performed. When a person performs exercise under very tense conditions but uses only a few muscles, the sympathetic response occurs everywhere in the body but vasodilatation occurs in only a few muscles. Therefore, the net effect is mainly one of vasoconstriction, often increasing the mean arterial pressure to as high as 180 mm Hg. Such a condition occurs in a person standing on a ladder and nailing with a hammer on the ceiling above.

On the other hand, when a person performs whole-body exercise, such as running or swimming, the increase in arterial pressure is often only 20 to 40 mm Hg. The lack of a tremendous rise in pressure results from the extreme vasodilatation occurring in large masses of muscle.

Importance of the Arterial Pressure Rise During Exercise. In the well-trained athlete the muscle blood flow can increase at least 20-fold. Though almost half of this increase results from vasodilatation in the active muscles, the increase in arterial pressure also plays an important role. The reason is that an increase in pressure stretches the arteries, thus doubling the flow increase.

THE CEREBRAL CIRCULATION

NORMAL RATE OF CEREBRAL BLOOD FLOW

The normal blood flow through the brain tissue of the adult averages 50 to 55 ml per 100 grams of brain per minute. For the entire brain of the average adult, this is approximately 750 ml per minute, or 15 per cent of the total resting cardiac output.

REGULATION OF CEREBRAL BLOOD FLOW

As in most other vascular areas of the body, cerebral blood flow is highly related to the metabolism of the cerebral tissue. At least three different metabolic factors have been shown to have potent effects on cerebral blood flow. These are carbon dioxide concentration, hydrogen ion concentration, and oxygen concentration. An *increase* in either the carbon dioxide or the hydrogen ion concentration increases cerebral blood flow, whereas a *decrease* in oxygen concentration increases the flow.

Regulation of Cerebral Blood Flow in Response to Excess Carbon Dioxide or Hydrogen Ion Concentration. An increase in carbon dioxide concentration in the arterial blood perfusing the brain greatly increases cerebral blood flow. This is illustrated in Figure 18–2, which shows that doubling the arterial P_{CO_2} by breathing carbon dioxide also approximately doubles the flow.

Carbon dioxide increases cerebral blood flow by combining with water in the body fluids to form

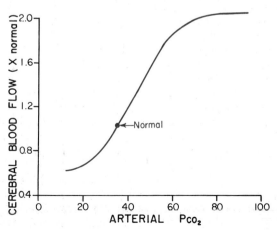

Figure 18–2. Relationship between arterial P_{CO_2} and cerebral blood flow.

carbonic acid, with subsequent dissociation to form hydrogen ions. The hydrogen ions then, are the basic cause of the vasodilatation of the cerebral vessels—the dilatation being almost directly proportional to the increase in hydrogen ion concentration.

Any other substance that increases the acidity of the brain tissue, and therefore also increases the hydrogen ion concentration, increases blood flow as well. Such substances include lactic acid, pyruvic acid, or any other acidic material formed during the course of metabolism.

Importance of the Carbon Dioxide and Hydrogen Control of Cerebral Blood Flow. Increased hydrogen ion concentration greatly depresses neuronal activity. Therefore, it is fortunate that an increase in hydrogen ion concentration causes an increase in the blood flow, which in turn carries both carbon dioxide and other acidic substances away from the brain tissues. Thus, this mechanism helps maintain a constant hydrogen ion concentration in the cerebral fluids and therefore also maintains a normal level of neuronal activity.

Oxygen Deficiency as a Regulator of Cerebral Blood Flow. Except during periods of intense brain activity, the utilization of oxygen by the brain tissue remains within very narrow limits—within a few per cent of 3.5 ml of oxygen per 100 grams of brain tissue per minute. If the blood flow to the brain ever becomes insufficient to supply this needed amount of oxygen, the oxygen deficiency mechanism for vasodilatation, which was discussed in Chapter 13 and which functions in essentially all tissues of the body, immediately causes vasodilatation, returning the blood flow and transport of oxygen to the cerebral tissues to near normal. Thus, this local blood flow regulatory mechanism is much the same as that existing in the coronary and skeletal muscle circulations and in many other circulatory areas of the body.

Experiments have shown that a decrease in cerebral *tissue* P_{O_2} below approximately 30 mm Hg (normal value is 35 to 40 mm Hg) will begin to increase cerebral blood flow. This is very fortuitous because brain function becomes deranged at not much lower values of P_{O_2}, especially so at P_{O_2} levels below 20 mm Hg. Even coma can result at these low levels. Thus, the oxygen mechanism for local regulation of cerebral blood flow is a very important protective response against diminished cerebral neuronal activity and, therefore, against derangement of mental capability.

Measurement of Cerebral Blood Flow and Effect of Cerebral Activity on the Flow. A method has recently been developed to record blood flow in as many as 256 isolated segments of the human cerebral cortex simultaneously. A radioactive substance, usually radioactive xenon, is injected into the carotid artery; then the radioactivity of the cortex is recorded as the radioactive substance passes through the brain tissue. Two hundred and fifty-six small radioactive scintillation detectors are focused on the same number of separate parts of the cortex; the rate of decay of the radioactivity after it once appears in each tissue segment is a direct measure of the rate of blood flow through the segment.

Using this technique, it has become clear that the blood flow in each individual segment of the brain changes within seconds in response to changes in local neuronal activity. For instance, simply clasping the hand causes an immediate increase in blood flow in the motor cortex of the opposite side of the brain. Reading a book increases the blood flow in multiple areas of the brain, especially in the occipital cortex and in the language areas of the temporal cortex. This measuring procedure can also be used to localize the origin of epileptic attacks, for the blood flow increases acutely and markedly (as much as sevenfold!) in the focal point of the attack at its very onset.

Role of the Sympathetic Nervous System in Regulating Cerebral Blood Flow. The cerebral circulatory system has a strong sympathetic innervation that passes upward from the superior cervical sympathetic ganglia along with the cerebral arteries. This innervation supplies both the large superficial arteries and the small arteries that penetrate into the substance of the brain. However, neither transection of these sympathetic nerves nor stimulation of them normally causes significant change in the cerebral blood flow. Therefore, it was long stated that the sympathetic nerves play essentially no role in regulating cerebral blood flow.

However, recent experiments have shown that sympathetic stimulation can, under some conditions, constrict the cerebral arteries markedly. The reason that this usually does not occur is that the local blood flow regulatory mechanisms are so powerful that they normally compensate almost entirely for the effects of the sympathetic stimulation. Yet, in those conditions in which these mechanisms fail to compensate enough, then sympathetic control of cerebral blood flow becomes quite important. For instance, when the arterial pressure rises to a very high level during strenuous exercise and during other states of excessive circulatory activity, the sympathetic nervous system constricts the large and intermediate-sized arteries and prevents the very high pressure from ever reaching the smaller blood vessels. Experiments have shown that this is important in preventing the occurrence of a vascular hemorrhage into the brain—that is, for preventing the occurrence of cerebral stroke.

Brain Edema

One of the most serious complications of abnormal cerebral hemodynamics is the development of brain edema. Because the brain is encased in a solid vault, the accumulation of edema fluid compresses the blood vessels, with eventual depression of blood flow and destruction of brain tissue.

The usual cause of brain edema is either greatly increased capillary pressure or damage to the capillary endothelium. The most common cause is brain concussion, in which the brain tissues and capillaries are traumatized and capillary fluid leaks into the traumatized tissues. Once brain edema begins, it often initiates a vicious cycle because of the following positive feedback: The edema compresses the vasculature. This in turn decreases the blood flow and causes brain ischemia. The ischemia causes arteriolar dilatation with increased capillary pressure. The increased capillary pressure then causes more edema fluid, so that the edema becomes progressively worse. Once this vicious cycle has begun, heroic measures must be used to prevent total destruction of the brain.

THE SPLANCHNIC CIRCULATION

A large share of the cardiac output flows through the vessels of the intestines and through the spleen, finally coursing into the portal venous system and then through the liver, as illustrated in Figure 18–3. This is called the *portal circulatory system,* and it, plus the arterial blood flow into the liver, is called the *splanchnic circulation.*

BLOOD FLOW THROUGH THE LIVER

About 1100 ml of portal blood enter the liver each minute. This flows through the *hepatic sinuses* in close contact with the cords of liver parenchymal cells. Then it enters the *central venules* of the liver lobules and from there flows into the vena cava.

In addition to the portal blood flow, approximately 350 ml of blood flows into the liver each minute through the hepatic artery, making a total hepatic flow of about 1450 ml per minute, or an average of 29 per cent of the total cardiac output.

Control of Liver Blood Flow. Because three quarters of the blood flow through the liver is derived from the portal blood flow into the liver, it is the

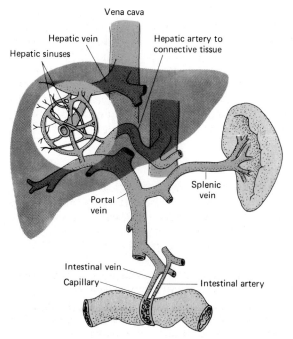

Figure 18–3. The portal and hepatic circulations.

various factors that determine flow through the gastrointestinal tract and spleen that mainly control liver blood flow, as will be discussed in subsequent sections of this chapter.

Reservoir Function of the Liver. Because the liver is an expandable and compressible organ, large quantities of blood can be stored in its blood vessels. Its normal blood volume, including both that in the hepatic veins and hepatic sinuses, is 450 ml, or almost 10 per cent of the total blood volume. However, when high pressure in the right atrium causes back pressure in the liver, the liver expands, and as much as 1 liter of extra blood occasionally is thereby stored in the hepatic veins and sinuses. Thus, in effect, the liver is a large, expandable, venous organ capable of acting as a valuable blood reservoir in times of excess blood volume and capable of supplying extra blood in times of diminished blood volume.

Permeability of the Hepatic Sinuses. The hepatic sinuses are lined with an endothelium similar to that of the capillaries, but its permeability is extreme in comparison with that of usual capillaries—so much so that even the proteins of the blood diffuse into the extravascular spaces of the liver almost as easily as fluids. Fortunately, the pressure in the sinuses is only 6 to 8 mm Hg so that most of the proteins that diffuse out of the sinuses also diffuse back in. Yet, the remainder passes into the liver lymphatics, so that liver lymph normally contains almost as great a protein concentration as that of the plasma itself.

This extreme permeability of the liver sinuses brings the fluids of the hepatic blood into extremely close contact with the liver parenchymal cells, thus facilitating rapid exchange of nutrient materials between the blood and the liver cells.

The Blood-Cleansing Function of the Liver. Blood flowing through the intestinal capillaries picks up many bacteria from the intestines. Indeed, a sample of blood from the portal system almost always grows colon bacilli when cultured, whereas growth of colon bacilli from blood in the systemic circulation is extremely rare. Special high-speed motion pictures of the action of Kupffer cells, which are large phagocytic reticuloendothelial cells that line the hepatic sinuses, have demonstrated that these cells can cleanse blood extremely efficiently as it passes through the sinuses; when a bacterium comes into momentary contact with a Kupffer cell, in less than 0.01 second the bacterium passes inward through the wall of the Kupffer cell to become permanently lodged therein until it is digested. Probably not over 1 per cent of the bacteria entering the portal blood from the intestines succeeds in passing through the liver into the systemic circulation.

BLOOD FLOW THROUGH THE INTESTINAL VESSELS

About four fifths of the portal blood flow originates in the intestines and stomach (about 850 ml per minute), and the remaining one fifth originates in the spleen and pancreas. Over two thirds of the intestinal flow is to the mucosa to supply the energy needed for forming the intestinal secretions and for absorbing the digested food.

Control of Gastrointestinal Blood Flow. Blood flow in the gastrointestinal tract is controlled in almost exactly the same way as in most other areas of the body: mainly by local regulatory mechanisms. Furthermore, blood flow to the mucosa and submucosa, where the glands are located and where absorption occurs, is controlled separately from blood flow to the musculature. When glandular secretion increases, so does mucosal and submucosal blood flow—sometimes as much as eightfold! Likewise, when motor activity of the gut increases, blood flow in the muscle layers increases.

However, the precise mechanisms by which alterations in gastrointestinal activity alter the blood flow are not completely understood. It is known that decreased availability of oxygen to the gut increases local blood flow in the same way that this occurs elsewhere in the body; therefore local regulation of blood flow in the gut might occur almost entirely secondarily to changes in metabolic rate. On the other hand, it is also known that various peptide hormones are released from the mucosa of the intestinal tract during the digestive process and that some of these also cause mucosal vasodilatation. The best known of these hormones are *vasoactive intestinal peptide, gastrin, secretin,* and *cholecystokinin.* Also, it has been claimed that some or all of the gastrointestinal glands form two *kinins,* the substances *kallidin* and *bradykinin,* at the same time that they release their secretions. These kinins are powerful vasodilators and have been postulated to cause much of the mucosal vasodilatation.

Sympathetic Nervous Control of Gastrointestinal Blood Flow. Sympathetic stimulation has a direct effect on essentially all the gastrointestinal blood vessels to cause intense vasoconstriction of the arterioles with greatly decreased blood flow. However, after a few minutes of this vasoconstriction, the flow returns almost to normal via a mechanism called autoregulatory escape. That is, the local metabolic vasodilator mechanisms that are elicited by ischemia become prepotent over the sympathetic vasoconstriction and, therefore, redilate the arterioles, thus causing return of the necessary nutrient blood flow to the gastrointestinal glands and muscle.

A major value of sympathetic vasoconstriction in the gut is that it allows the shutting off of splanchnic blood flow for short periods of time during heavy exercise when increased flow is needed by the skeletal muscle and heart.

Sympathetic stimulation causes especially strong vasoconstriction of the intestinal and mesenteric *veins.* Furthermore, this vasoconstriction does not "escape." Instead, it decreases the volume of these veins and thereby displaces large amounts of blood into other parts of the circulation. In hemorrhagic shock or other states of low blood volume, this mechanism can provide probably 200 to 300 milliliters of extra blood to sustain the general circulation.

PORTAL VENOUS PRESSURE

The liver offers a moderate amount of resistance to blood flow from the portal system to the vena cava. As a result, the pressure in the portal vein averages 8 to 10 mm Hg, which is considerably higher than the almost zero pressure in the vena cava. Because of this high portal venous pressure, the pressures in the intestinal venules and capillaries have a much greater tendency to become abnormally high than is true elsewhere in the body.

Blockage of the Portal System—Cirrhosis of the Liver. Frequently, extreme amounts of fibrous tissue develop within the liver structure, destroying many of the parenchymal cells and eventually contracting around the blood vessels, thereby greatly impeding the flow of portal blood through the liver. This disease process is known as *cirrhosis of the liver.* It results most frequently from alcoholism, but it can also follow ingestion of poisons such as carbon tetrachloride, virus diseases such as infectious hepatitis, or infectious processes in the bile ducts.

The portal system is also occasionally blocked by a large clot developing in the portal vein or in its major branches.

When the portal system is suddenly blocked, the return of blood from the intestines and spleen to the systemic circulation is tremendously impeded, the capillary pressure rising as much as 15 to 20 mm Hg, and the patient often dies within a few hours because of excessive loss of fluid from the capillaries into the lumina and walls of the intestines.

Ascites as a Result of Portal Obstruction. Ascites is free fluid in the peritoneal cavity, sometimes in quantities of many liters. It results from exudation of fluid either from the surface of the liver or from the surfaces of the gut and its mesentery. Ascites usually will develop only in case outflow of blood from the liver into the inferior vena cava is blocked. This causes extremely high pressure in the liver sinusoids, which in turn causes fluid to weep from the surfaces of the liver. The weeping fluid is almost pure plasma, containing tremendous quantities of protein. The protein, because it causes a high colloid osmotic pressure in the abdominal fluid, then pulls by osmosis additional fluid from the surfaces of the gut and mesentery.

THE SPLENIC CIRCULATION

The Spleen as a Blood Reservoir. The spleen is a globular-shaped organ located behind the stomach. It is highly vascular, containing about 100 to 150 ml of blood.

Figure 18–4 illustrates a small section of the spleen showing that it has two areas for the storage of blood: the *venous sinuses* and the *pulp.* Many small vessels flow directly into the venous sinuses. In the splenic pulp, the capillaries are very permeable, so much so that much of the blood leaks out of these capillaries into the pulp and oozes through the pulp before entering the venous sinuses. Many of the red blood

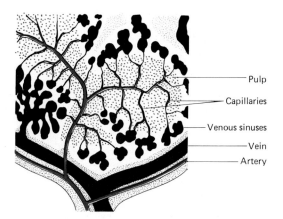

Figure 18–4. The functional structures of the spleen. (Modified from Bloom and Fawcett: A Textbook of Histology. 10th ed. Philadelphia, W. B. Saunders Company, 1975.)

- Pulp
- Capillaries
- Venous sinuses
- Vein
- Artery

cells become entrapped within the pulp and thus are stored in a concentrated form. When the sympathetic nervous system constricts the blood vessels throughout the body, the vessels of the spleen also constrict. As a result, the spleen releases much of its stored blood, including the stored red blood cells of the pulp; this release sometimes increases the hematocrit as much as 1 to 2 per cent in lower aminals, though the effect in the human being is questionable.

The Blood-Cleansing Function of the Spleen— Removal of Old Cells. Blood passing through the splenic pulp before it enters the sinuses undergoes thorough squeezing. Therefore, fragile red blood cells do not withstand the trauma. For this reason, many of the red blood cells destroyed in the body have their final demise in the spleen. After the cells rupture, the released hemoglobin and the cell stroma are ingested by the reticuloendothelial cells of the spleen.

Reticuloendothelial Cells of the Spleen. The pulp of the spleen contains many large phagocytic reticuloendothelial cells, and the venous sinuses are lined with similar cells. These cells are large macrophages that act as a cleansing system for the blood, similar to that in the venous sinuses of the liver. When the blood is invaded by infectious agents, the reticuloen-

dothelial cells of the spleen rapidly remove debris, bacteria, parasites, etc.

CIRCULATION IN THE SKIN

PHYSIOLOGIC ANATOMY OF THE CUTANEOUS CIRCULATION

Circulation through the skin subserves two major functions: first, *nutrition of the skin tissues* and, second, *conduction of heat* from the internal structures of the body to the skin so that the heat can be removed from the body. To perform these two functions the circulatory apparatus of the skin is characterized by two major types of vessels, diagrammed in Figure 18–5: (1) the usual nutritive arteries, capillaries, and veins and (2) vascular structures concerned with heating the skin, consisting principally of (a) an extensive *subcutaneous venous plexus,* which holds large quantities of blood that can heat the surface of the skin, and (b) in some skin areas, *arteriovenous anastomoses,* which are large vascular communications directly between the arteries and the venous plexuses. The walls of these anastomoses have strong muscular coats innervated by sympathetic vasoconstrictor nerve fibers that secrete norepinephrine. When constricted, they reduce the flow of blood into the venous plexuses to almost nothing; or when maximally dilated, they allow extremely rapid flow of warm blood into the plexuses. The arteriovenous anastomoses are found principally in the volar surfaces of the hands and feet, the lips, the nose, and the ears, which are areas of the body most often exposed to maximal cooling. In the other areas of the skin where arteriovenous anastomoses do not occur, large arterioles and capillaries serve a similar role in providing blood flow, though not as much, into the venous plexus.

Rate of Blood Flow Through the Skin. The rate of blood flow through the skin is among the most variable of any part of the body, because the flow required to regulate body temperature changes markedly in response to, first, the rate of metabolic activity

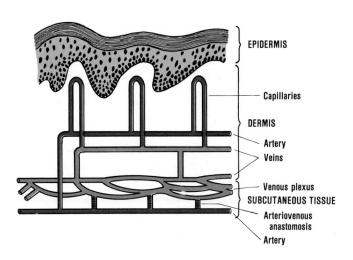

Figure 18–5. The skin circulation.

- EPIDERMIS
- Capillaries
- DERMIS
- Artery
- Veins
- Venous plexus
- SUBCUTANEOUS TISSUE
- Arteriovenous anastomosis
- Artery

of the body, and, second, the temperature of the surroundings. This will be discussed in detail in Chapter 47. The blood flow required for nutrition is slight, so that this plays almost no role in controlling normal skin blood flow. At ordinary skin temperatures, the amount of blood flowing through the skin vessels to provide heat regulation is about ten times as much as that needed to supply the nutritive needs of the tissues.

Under ordinary cool conditions the blood flow to the skin is about 0.25 liter/sq meter of body surface area, or a total of about 400 ml per minute in the average adult. This can decrease to as little as 50 ml per minute in severe cold, and, when the skin is heated until maximal vasodilatation has resulted, the blood flow can be as much as 2 to 3 liters per minute, thus illustrating both the extreme variability of skin blood flow and the great drain on cardiac output that can occur under hot conditions.

REGULATION OF BLOOD FLOW IN THE SKIN

Nervous Control of Cutaneous Blood Flow. Since most of the blood flow through the skin is to control body temperature, and since this function in turn is regulated by the nervous system, the blood flow through the skin is principally regulated by nervous mechanisms rather than by local regulation, which is opposite to the regulation in most parts of the body.

Temperature Control Center of the Hypothalamus. Located in the preoptic region of the anterior hypothalamus is a small center that is capable of controlling body temperature. Heating this area causes vasodilation of essentially all the skin vessels of the body and also causes sweating. Cooling of the center causes vasoconstriction and cessation of sweating. The detailed function of this control system will be discussed in Chapter 47 in relation to body temperature. The important point in the present discussion is that the hypothalamus controls blood flow in the skin in response to changes in body temperature by two mechanisms: (1) a vasoconstrictor mechanism and (2) a vasodilator mechanism.

The Vasoconstrictor Mechanism. The skin throughout the body is supplied with sympathetic vasoconstrictor fibers that secrete norepinephrine at their endings. This constrictor system is extremely powerful in the feet, hands, lips, nose, and ears, which are the areas most frequently exposed to severe cold and which are also the areas where large numbers of arteriovenous anastomoses are found. At normal body temperature the sympathetic vasoconstrictor nerves keep these anastomoses almost totally closed, but when the body becomes overly heated the number of sympathetic impulses is greatly reduced so that the anastomoses dilate and allow large quantities of warm blood to flow into the venous plexuses, thereby promoting loss of heat from the body.

In the remainder of the body—that is, over the surfaces of the arms, legs, and body trunk—almost no arteriovenous anastomoses are present, but nevertheless vasoconstrictor control of the nutritive vessels can still effect major decreases in blood flow by constricting the local arterioles. On the other hand, when the body becomes overheated, the sympathetic vasoconstrictor impulses cease, and the blood flow to the skin increases about twofold.

The Vasodilator Mechanism. When the body temperature becomes excessive and sweating begins to occur, the blood flow through the skin of the forearms and trunk increases an additional severalfold, which occurs as a result of so-called active vasodilatation of the vessels. However, the basic mechanism by which this active dilation occurs is not completely known. This additional increase in blood flow does not occur except in the presence of sweating, and it does not occur in lower animals that do not have sweat glands. Therefore, it has been postulated that the sympathetic fibers that secrete acetylcholine to activate the sweat glands cause a secondary vasodilatation as follows: The increased activity of the sweat glands is postulated to cause these glands to release an enzyme called *kallikrein,* which in turn splits the polypeptide *bradykinin* from globulin in the interstitial fluids. Bradykinin in turn is a powerful vasodilator substance that could account for the greatly increased blood flow when sweating begins to occur. In opposition to this theory, however, is the fact that inhibition of the bradykinin mechanism does not completely block the increased blood flow associated with sweating. Therefore, other vasodilator peptides have also been suggested as the cause of the vasodilation.

Shift of Blood from the Skin to the Remainder of the Circulation in Times of Circulatory Stress. The skin venous plexuses of the entire body, including those of the hands, feet, arms, legs, and trunk, are all strongly supplied with sympathetic vasoconstrictor innervation. In times of circulatory stress, such as during exercise, following severe hemorrhage, or even in states of anxiety, sympathetic stimulation of these venous plexuses can force large quantities of blood, estimated to be as much as 5 to 10 per cent of the total blood volume, into the internal vessels. Thus, the subcutaneous veins of the skin act as an important blood reservoir, often providing blood to serve other circulatory functions when needed.

QUESTIONS

1. Approximately how much can the blood flow through an exercising muscle increase above the normal resting level?
2. What proportion of the muscle capillaries are open during rest? What happens to the capillary blood flow during exercise?
3. What causes the blood vessels of the muscles to dilate during exercise?

4. What other circulatory adjustments besides the local vasodilation of the muscles must occur if the circulatory system is to be able to cope with the increased flow required by the muscles?
5. Discuss the role of the sympathetic nervous system during exercise.
6. Explain the relative roles of tissue carbon dioxide, tissue hydrogen ion concentration, and tissue oxygen concentration in the control of cerebral blood flow.
7. Explain how brain edema can occur and why it is frequently very destructive to the brain.
8. What proportion of the total cardiac output at rest passes through the liver?
9. Explain the *blood reservoir function* of the liver.
10. What is the permeability of hepatic sinuses relative to other vascular beds of the body? How does this affect the function of the liver?
11. Explain the blood-cleansing functions of the liver and the spleen.
12. How do local factors in the gastrointestinal tract control local blood flow?
13. What is the role of resistance to blood flow through the liver in determining portal venous pressure?
14. What is cirrhosis of the liver, and how does it affect portal venous pressure?
15. What is *ascites,* and under what conditions does it develop?
16. Why is blood flow through the skin so variable?
17. Why is blood flow through the skin controlled almost entirely by the nervous system in contrast with most other tissues, in which blood flow is controlled mainly by local regulatory factors?
18. Explain the control of skin temperature by the temperature control center of the hypothalamus.
19. Describe the vasoconstrictor and the vasodilator mechanisms for skin blood flow control.

References

American Physiological Society: Peripheral Circulation and Organ Blood Flow. Washington, D.C., American Physiological Society, 1983.

Anderson, P. O.: Vascular control in the colon and rectum. Scand J Gastroenterol 93:65, 1984.

Bissonnette, J. M., et al.: Regulation of cerebral blood flow in the fetus. J Dev Physiol 6:275, 1984.

Fox, E. L.: Sports Physiology. Philadelphia, W. B. Saunders Co., 1979.

Gisvold, S. E., and Steen, P. A.: Drug therapy in brain ischaemia. Br J Anaesthesiol 57:96, 1985.

Guth, P. H.: Stomach blood flow and acid secretion. Annu Rev Physiol 44:3, 1982.

Harrison, M. H.: Effects of thermal stress and exercise on blood volume in humans. Physiol Rev 65:149, 1985.

Heistad, D. D., and Kontos, H. A.: Cerebral circulation. In Shepherd, J. T., and Abboud, F. M., eds.: Handbook of Physiology. Sec. 2, Vol. 3. Bethesda, American Physiological Society, 1983, p. 137.

Jarrett, A.: Physiology and Pathophysiology of the Skin. New York, Academic Press, 1984.

Kontos, H. A.: Regulation of the cerebral circulation. Annu Rev Physiol 43:397, 1981.

Lassen, N. A.: Study of local cerebral blood flow. In Dickinson, C. J., and Marks, J., eds.: Developments in Cardiovascular Medicine. Lancaster, England, MTP Press, 1978, p. 9.

McDowall, D. G.: Induced hypotension and brain ischaemia. Br J Anaesthesiol 57:110, 1985.

Najarian, J. S.: Advances in Vascular Surgery. Chicago, Year Book Medical Publishers, 1983.

Rappaport, A. M.: Hepatic blood flow: Morphologic aspects and physiologic regulation. In Javitt, N. B., ed.: International Review of Physiology: Liver and Biliary Tract Physiology I. Vol. 21. Baltimore, University Park Press, 1980, p. 1.

Reed, G., and Devous, M.: Cerebral blood flow autoregulation and hypertension. Am J Med Sci 289:37, 1985.

Roddie, I. C.: Circulation to skin and adipose tissue. In Shepherd, J. T., and Abboud, F. M., eds.: Handbook of Physiology. Sec. 2, Vol. 3. Bethesda, American Physiological Society, 1983, p. 285.

Shepherd, A. P.: Local control of intestinal oxygenation and blood flow. Annu Rev Physiol 44:13, 1982.

Shepherd, J. T.: Circulation to skeletal muscle. In Shepherd, J. T., and Abboud, F. M., eds.: Handbook of Physiology. Sec. 2, Vol. 3. Bethesda, American Physiological Society, 1983, p. 319.

Strauss, R. H., ed.: Sports Medicine and Physiology. Philadelphia, W. B. Saunders Co., 1979.

Tepperman, B. L., and Jacobson, E. D.: Measurement of gastrointestinal blood flow. Annu Rev Physiol 44:71, 1982.

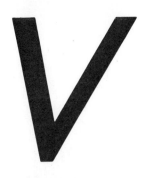

BLOOD CELLS, IMMUNITY, AND BLOOD CLOTTING

19 ■ Red Blood Cells, White Blood Cells, and Resistance of the Body to Infection

20 ■ Immunity, Allergy, Blood Groups, Transfusion, and Transplantation

21 ■ Hemostasis and Blood Coagulation

19

Red Blood Cells, White Blood Cells, and Resistance of the Body to Infection

THE RED BLOOD CELLS
GENESIS OF THE RED BLOOD CELL
FORMATION OF HEMOGLOBIN
IRON METABOLISM
DESTRUCTION OF RED BLOOD CELLS
THE ANEMIAS
*EFFECTS OF ANEMIA ON THE
CIRCULATORY SYSTEM*
**WHITE BLOOD CELLS AND RESISTANCE
OF THE BODY TO INFECTION**
*THE LEUKOCYTES (WHITE BLOOD
CELLS)*

*PROPERTIES OF NEUTROPHILS,
MONOCYTES, AND
MACROPHAGES*
*THE TISSUE MACROPHAGE SYSTEM
(THE RETICULOENDOTHELIAL
SYSTEM)*
*INFLAMMATION AND FUNCTION OF
NEUTROPHILS AND
MACROPHAGES*
THE EOSINOPHILS
THE BASOPHILS
THE LEUKEMIAS
AGRANULOCYTOSIS

With this chapter we begin a discussion of the blood cells and of other cells closely related to those of the blood: the cells of the reticuloendothelial system and of the lymphatic system.

THE RED BLOOD CELLS

The major function of red blood cells is to transport hemoglobin, which in turn carries oxygen from the lungs to the tissues. Normal red blood cells are biconcave disks having a mean diameter of approximately 8 microns and a thickness at the thickest point of 2 microns and in the center of 1 micron or less. The shapes of red blood cells can change remarkably as the cells pass through capillaries. Actually, the red blood cell is a "bag" that can be deformed into almost any shape. Furthermore, because the normal cell has a great excess of cell membrane for the quantity of material inside, deformation does not stretch the membrane and consequently does not rupture the cell as would be the case with many other cells.

In normal men the average number of red blood cells per cubic millimeter is 5,200,000 and in normal women 4,700,000. Also, the altitude at which the person lives affects the number of red blood cells; this is discussed later.

Quantity of Hemoglobin in the Cells and Transport of Oxygen. When the hematocrit (defined as the percentage of the blood that is red cells—normally 40 to 45 per cent) and the quantity of hemoglobin in each respective cell are normal, the blood contains an average of 15 grams of hemoglobin in every 100 ml. As will be discussed in connection with the transport of oxygen in Chapter 28, each gram of pure hemoglobin is capable of combining with approximately 1.39 ml of oxygen. Therefore, in a normal person, over 20 ml of oxygen can be carried in combination with hemoglobin in each 100 ml of blood.

GENESIS OF THE RED BLOOD CELL

The red blood cells are produced in the bone marrow from a cell known as the *proerythroblast*, illustrated in Figure 19–1. New proerythroblasts are continually being formed from primordial stem cells located throughout the bone marrow.

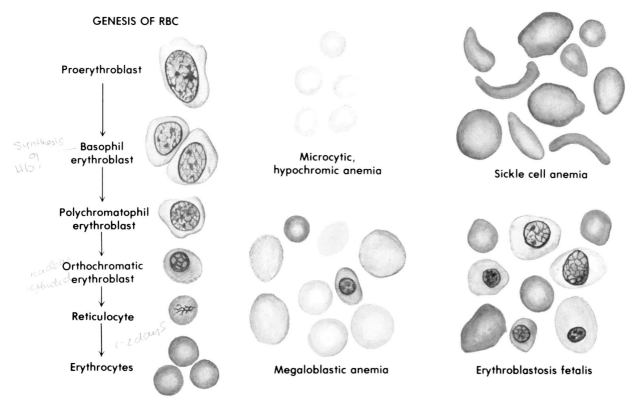

GENESIS OF RBC

Proerythroblast

Basophil erythroblast

Polychromatophil erythroblast

Orthochromatic erythroblast

Reticulocyte

Erythrocytes

Microcytic, hypochromic anemia

Sickle cell anemia

Megaloblastic anemia

Erythroblastosis fetalis

Figure 19–1. Genesis of red blood cells, and red blood cells in different types of anemias.

As illustrated in Figure 19–1, the proerythroblast first forms the *basophil erythroblast,* which begins the synthesis of hemoglobin. This cell gives rise to the *polychromatophil erythroblast,* so called because of a mixture of basophilic material and the red hemoglobin. Following this, the nucleus of the cell shrinks while still greater quantities of hemoglobin are formed, and the cell becomes an *orthochromatic erythroblast.* Finally, after the cytoplasm of this cell has become filled with hemoglobin the nucleus becomes extremely small and is extruded. At the same time, the endoplasmic reticulum is being reabsorbed. The cell at this stage of development is called a *reticulocyte* because it still contains a small amount of basophilic Golgi apparatus and mitochondria interspersed among the hemoglobin in the cytoplasm. While the cells are in this reticulocyte stage, they pass into the blood capillaries by *diapedesis* (squeezing through the pores of the endothelium).

The remaining basophilic material disappears in another one to two days, and the cell is then the mature erythrocyte. In normal blood, the total proportion of reticulocytes among all the cells is slightly less than 1 per cent.

Tissue Oxygenation as the Basic Regulator of Red Blood Cell Production

Any condition that decreases the quantity of oxygen transported to the tissue ordinarily increases the rate of red blood cell production. Thus, when a person becomes extremely *anemic* as a result of

hemorrhage or any other condition, the bone marrow immediately begins to produce large quantities of red blood cells. Also, destruction of major portions of the bone marrow by any means, especially x-ray therapy, causes hyperplasia of the remaining bone marrow in an attempt to supply the demand for red blood cells in the body.

At very *high altitudes,* where the quantity of oxygen in the air is greatly decreased, insufficient oxygen is transported to the tissues, and red cells are produced so rapidly that their number in the blood is considerably increased.

Erythropoietin, Its Formation in Response to Hypoxia, and Its Function in Regulating Red Blood Cell Production. The principal factor that stimulates red blood cell production is a circulating hormone called *erythropoietin,* a glycoprotein with a molecular weight of about 40,000. In the absence of erythropoietin, hypoxia has either no effect or very little effect in stimulating red blood cell production. On the other hand, when the erythropoietin system is functional, hypoxia causes marked increase in erythropoietin production, and the erythropoietin in turn enhances red blood cell production until the hypoxia is relieved. This mechanism is illustrated by the system diagram in Figure 19–2.

Role of the Kidneys in the Formation of Erythropoietin. In the normal person, 90 to 95 per cent of all erythropoietin is formed in the kidneys. Though, it is not known exactly where in the kidney it is formed, some research has suggested that erythropoietin might be formed by the *juxtaglomerular cells,*

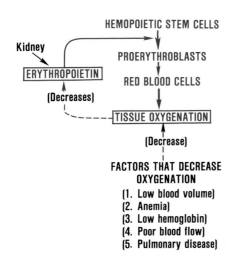

Figure 19–2. Function of the erythropoietin mechanism to increase the production of red blood cells when extraneous factors decrease tissue oxygenation.

cells in the walls of the afferent arterioles adjacent to the glomeruli. Regardless of where erythropoietin is formed in the kidney, when both kidneys are removed from a person or when the kidneys are destroyed by renal disease, the person invariably becomes very anemic because the 5 to 10 per cent of erythropoietin formed in other tissues (mainly in the liver but perhaps also in macrophages) is sufficient to cause only one third to one half as much red blood cell formation as needed by the body.

Effect of Erythropoietin on Erythrogenesis. Upon placing an animal or person in an atmosphere of low oxygen, erythropoietin begins to be formed within minutes or hours, and it reaches maximum production within 24 hours. Yet, almost no new red blood cells appear in the circulating blood until about five days later. From this fact, it has been determined that the important effect of erythropoietin is to stimulate the production of proerythroblasts from hemopoietic stem cells in the bone marrow. In addition, once the proerythroblasts are formed, the erythropoietin causes these cells also to pass more rapidly through the different erythroblastic stages than normally, thus speeding up the production of new cells. The rapid production of cells continues as long as the person remains in the low oxygen state or until enough red blood cells are produced to carry adequate amounts of oxygen to the tissues despite the low oxygen; at this time the rate of erythropoietin production decreases to a level that will maintain the required number of red cells.

Upon removal of a person from a state of low oxygen, the rate of oxygen transport to the tissues rises above normal, which causes his rate of erythropoietin formation to decrease to zero almost instantaneously and his rate of red blood cell production to fall essentially to zero within several days. Red cell production remains at this extremely low level until enough cells have lived out their life spans and degenerated, so that the tissues again receive only their normal complement of oxygen.

In the complete absence of erythropoietin, few red blood cells are formed by the bone marrow. At the other extreme, when extreme quantities of erythropoietin are formed, the rate of red blood cell production can rise to as high as ten or more times normal. Therefore, the erythropoietin control mechanism for red blood cell production is an extremely powerful one.

Vitamins Needed for Formation of Red Blood Cells

The Maturation Factor—Vitamin B$_{12}$ (Cyanocobalamin). Vitamin B$_{12}$ is an essential nutrient for all cells of the body, and growth of tissues in general is greatly depressed when this vitamin is lacking. This results from the fact that vitamin B$_{12}$ is required for synthesis of DNA. Therefore, lack of this vitamin causes failure of nuclear maturation and division. Since tissues that produce red blood cells are among the most rapidly growing and proliferating of all the body's tissues, lack of vitamin B$_{12}$ especially inhibits the rate of red blood cell production. Furthermore, the erythroblastic cells of the bone marrow, in addition to failing to proliferate rapidly, become larger than normal, developing into so-called *megaloblasts,* and the adult erythrocyte, called a *macrocyte,* has a flimsy membrane and is often irregular, large, and oval instead of the usual biconcave disc. These poorly formed macrocytes, after entering the circulating blood, are capable of carrying oxygen normally but their fragility causes them to have a short life, one half to one third of normal. Therefore, it is said that vitamin B$_{12}$ deficiency causes *maturation failure* in the process of erythropoiesis.

Maturation Failure Caused by Poor Absorption of Vitamin B$_{12}$—Pernicious Anemia. The most common cause of maturation failure is not lack of vitamin B$_{12}$ in the diet but instead failure to absorb vitamin B$_{12}$ from the gastrointestinal tract. This often occurs in the disease called *pernicious anemia,* in which the basic abnormality is an *atropic gastric mucosa* that fails to secrete normal gastric secretions. The parietal cells of the gastric glands secrete a glycoprotein called *intrinsic factor,* which combines with vitamin B$_{12}$ of the food and makes the B$_{12}$ available for absorption by the gut. It does this in the following way: First, the intrinsic factor binds tightly with the vitamin B$_{12}$. In this bound state the B$_{12}$ *is protected from digestion by the gastrointestinal enzymes.* Second, still in the bound state, the intrinsic factor binds to specific receptor sites on the brush border membranes of the mucosal cells in the ileum. Third, vitamin B$_{12}$ is transported into the blood during the next few hours, probably by the process of pinocytosis carrying the intrinsic factor and the vitamin together through the membrane.

Lack of intrinsic factor, therefore, causes loss of much of the vitamin because of both enzyme action in the gut and failure of its absorption.

Effect of Folic Acid (Pteroylglutamic Acid) on Red Cell Maturation. Occasionally a patient with maturation failure anemia responds to folic acid therapy instead of to vitamin B_{12}, so it is apparent that this vitamin is also concerned with the maturation of red blood cells. Folic acid, like B_{12}, is required for formation of DNA but in a different way. It promotes the methylation of deoxyuridylate to form deoxythymidylate, one of the nucleotides required for DNA synthesis.

FORMATION OF HEMOGLOBIN

Synthesis of hemoglobin begins in the erythroblasts and continues slightly even into the reticulocyte stage. Figure 19–3 shows the basic chemical steps in the formation of hemoglobin. The heme portion of hemoglobin is synthesized mainly from acetic acid and glycine; most of this synthesis occurs in the mitochondria. The acetic acid is changed in the Krebs cycle, which will be explained in Chapter 45, into succinyl-CoA, and then two molecules of this combine with two molecules of glycine to form a pyrrole compound. In turn, four pyrrole compounds combine to form a protoporphyrin compound. One of the protoporphyrins, known as protoporphyrin IX, then combines with iron to form the heme molecule. Finally, the heme molecule combines with a very long polypeptide chain synthesized by the ribosomes, forming a subunit of hemoglobin called a *hemoglobin chain*. Each of these chains has a molecular weight of about 16,000, and four of them in turn bind together loosely to form the whole hemoglobin molecule (Fig. 19–4).

There are slight variations in the subunit hemoglobin chains, depending on the amino acid composition of its polypeptide portion. The different types of chains are designated *alpha chains, beta chains, gamma chains*, and so forth. The most common form of hemoglobin in the adult human being, *hemoglobin A*, is a combination of *two alpha chains* and *two beta chains*.

Since each chain has a heme prosthetic group, there are four separate iron atoms in each hemoglobin molecule; each of these can bind with 1 molecule of oxygen, making a total of 4 molecules of oxygen (or 8 atoms) that can be transported by each hemoglobin molecule. Hemoglobin has a molecular weight of 64,458.

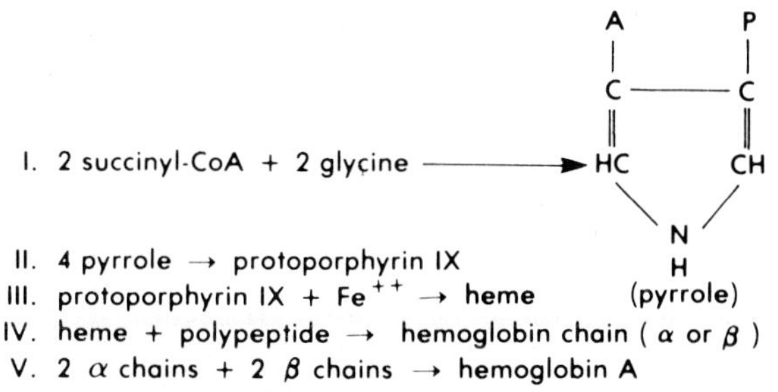

I. 2 succinyl-CoA + 2 glycine ⟶

II. 4 pyrrole ⟶ protoporphyrin IX

III. protoporphyrin IX + Fe^{++} ⟶ heme   (pyrrole)

IV. heme + polypeptide ⟶ hemoglobin chain (α or β)

V. 2 α chains + 2 β chains ⟶ hemoglobin A

Figure 19–3. Formation of hemoglobin.

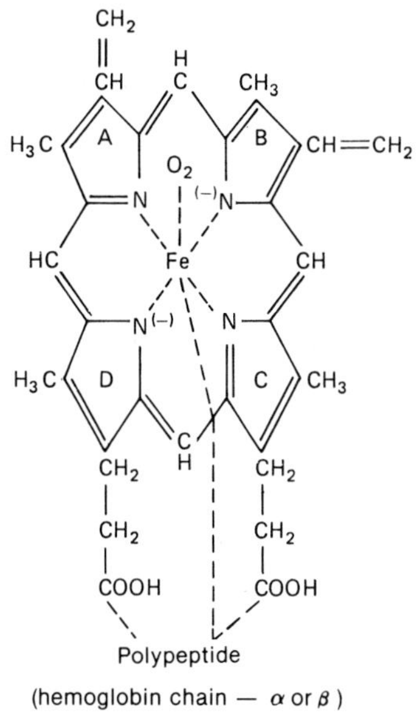

Figure 19–4. Basic structure of the hemoglobin molecule, showing one of the four heme complexes bound with the central globin core of the hemoglobin molecule.

Combination of Hemoglobin with Oxygen. The most important feature of the hemoglobin molecule is its ability to combine loosely and reversibly with oxygen. This ability will be discussed in detail in Chapter 28 in relation to respiration, for the primary function of hemoglobin in the body is to combine with oxygen in the lungs and then to release this oxygen in the tissue capillaries where the gaseous tension of oxygen is much lower than in the lungs.

Oxygen *does not* combine with the two positive valences of the ferrous iron in the hemoglobin molecule. Instead, it binds loosely with one of the six "coordination" valences of the iron atom. This is an extremely loose bond so that the combination is easily reversible.

IRON METABOLISM

Because iron is important for formation of hemoglobin, myoglobin, and other substances such as the cytochromes, cytochrome oxidase, peroxidase, and catalase, it is essential to understand the means by which iron is utilized in the body.

The total quantity of iron in the body averages about 4 grams, approximately 65 per cent of which is present in the form of hemoglobin. About 4 per cent is present in the form of myoglobin, 1 per cent in the form of the various heme compounds that promote intracellular oxidation, 0.1 per cent combined with the protein transferrin in the blood plasma, and 15 to 30 per cent stored mainly in the liver in the forms of ferritin and hemosiderin.

Transport and Storage of Iron. Transport, storage, and metabolism of iron in the body are illustrated in Figure 19–5, which may be explained as follows: When iron is absorbed from the small intestine, it immediately combines with a beta globulin, *apotrans-*

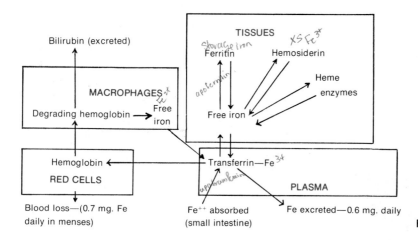

Figure 19–5. Iron transport and metabolism.

ferrin, to form *transferrin*, which is then transported in the blood plasma. The iron is loosely combined and, consequently, can be released to any of the tissue cells at any point in the body. Excess iron in the blood is deposited in all cells of the body *but especially in the liver cells*, where about 60 per cent of the excess is stored. There it combines mainly with another protein, *apoferritin*, to form *ferritin*. Apoferritin has a molecular weight of approximately 460,000, and varying quantities of iron can combine in clusters of iron radicals with this large molecule. This iron stored in ferritin is called *storage iron*.

When the quantity of iron in the plasma falls very low, iron is removed from ferritin quite easily. The iron is then transported again by the transferrin in the plasma to the portions of the body where it is needed.

A unique characteristic of the transferrin molecule is that it binds with receptors in the cell membranes of erythroblasts in the bone marrow. Then it, along with its bound iron, is ingested into the erythroblasts by endocytosis. Finally, the transferrin delivers the iron directly to the mitochondria where heme is synthesized. In persons who do not have adequate quantities of transferrin in their blood, failure to transport iron to the erythroblasts in this manner causes severe hypochromic anemia—that is, decreased numbers of red cells and even those cells containing very little hemoglobin.

When red blood cells have lived their life span and are destroyed, the hemoglobin released from the cells is ingested by the cells of the macrophage-monocyte system. There free iron is liberated, and it can then either be stored in the ferritin pool or be reused for formation of hemoglobin.

Daily Loss of Iron. About 1 milligram of iron is excreted each day by men, mainly into the feces. Additional quantities of iron are lost whenever bleeding occurs. Thus, in women, the menstrual loss of blood brings the average iron loss to a value of approximately 2 milligrams per day.

Absorption of Iron from the Gastrointestinal Tract. Iron is absorbed in all parts of the small intestine by an active absorptive process, though the precise mechanism of this active absorption is unknown. The rate of iron absorption is extremely slow, with a maximum rate of only a few milligrams per day. This means that when tremendous quantities of iron are present in the food, only small proportions of this will be absorbed. On the other hand, if only minute quantities are present, far greater proportions will be absorbed.

Regulation of Total Body Iron by Alteration of Rate of Absorption. When the body has become saturated with iron so that essentially all of the apoferritin in the iron storage areas is already combined with iron, the rate of absorption of iron from the intestinal tract becomes greatly decreased. This probably results mainly from the fact that once all the apoferritin in the body has become saturated with iron, it becomes difficult for transferrin to release iron to the tissues. As a consequence, the transferrin, which is normally only one third saturated with iron, now becomes almost fully bound with iron so that the transferrin accepts almost no new iron from the mucosal cells.

DESTRUCTION OF RED BLOOD CELLS

When red blood cells are delivered from the bone marrow into the circulatory system they normally circulate an average of 120 days before being destroyed. Even though mature red cells do not have a nucleus and also have neither mitochondria nor endoplasmic reticulum, nevertheless they do still have cytoplasmic enzymes that are capable of metabolizing glucose and forming small amounts of ATP. The ATP in turn serves the red cell in several important ways such as (1) to maintain pliability of the cell membrane, and (2) to maintain membrane transport of ions. However, these metabolic systems of the red cell become progressively less active with time. As the cells become older they become progressively more fragile, presumably because their life processes simply wear out.

Once the red cell membrane becomes very fragile, the cell may rupture during passage through some tight spot of the circulation. Many of the red cells fragment in the spleen where the cells squeeze through the red pulp of the spleen. Here the spaces between the structural trabeculae of the pulp are only 3 microns wide, in comparison with the 8 micron diameter of the red cell. When the spleen is removed, the number of abnormal cells and old cells circulating in the blood increases considerably.

Destruction of Hemoglobin. The hemoglobin released from the cells when they burst is phagocytized almost immediately by macrophages in many parts of the body, but especially in the liver (the Kupffer cells), spleen, and bone marrow. During the next few hours to days, the macrophages release the iron from the hemoglobin back into the blood to be carried by transferrin either to the bone marrow for production of new red blood cells or to the liver and other tissues for storage in the form of ferritin. The porphyrin portion of the hemoglobin molecule is converted by the macrophages, through a series of stages, into the bile pigment *bilirubin*, which is released into the blood and later secreted by the liver into the bile; this will be discussed in relation to liver function in Chapter 43.

THE ANEMIAS

Anemia means a deficiency of red blood cells, which can be caused either by too rapid loss or too slow production of red blood cells. Some types of anemia and their physiological causes are the following:

Blood Loss Anemia. After rapid hemorrhage the body replaces the plasma within one to three days, but this leaves a low concentration of red blood cells. If a second hemorrhage does not occur, the red blood cell concentration returns to normal within three to four weeks.

Aplastic Anemia. *Bone marrow aplasia* means lack of a functioning bone marrow. For instance, the person exposed to gamma ray radiation from a nuclear bomb blast is likely to sustain complete destruction of the bone marrow, followed in a few weeks by lethal anemia. Likewise, excessive x-ray treatment, certain industrial chemicals, and even drugs to which the person might be sensitive can cause the same effect.

Megaloblastic Anemia. From the earlier discussion in this chapter of vitamin B_{12}, folic acid, and intrinsic factor from the stomach mucosa, one can readily understand that loss of any one of these factors can lead to very slow reproduction of the erythroblasts in the bone marrow; as a result, these grow too large, with odd shapes, and are called *megaloblasts*. Thus, atrophy of the stomach mucosa, as occurs in *pernicious anemia*, or loss of the entire stomach as the result of total gastrectomy can lead to megaloblastic anemia.

Hemolytic Anemia. Many different abnormalities of the red blood cells, many of which are hereditarily acquired, make the cells very fragile, so that they rupture easily as they go through the capillaries, especially through the spleen. Therefore, even though the number of red blood cells formed is completely normal, or even vastly excessive in some hemolytic

diseases, the red cell life span is so short that serious anemia results. One of these types of anemia that is highly prevalent is *sickle cell anemia.*

In sickle cell anemia, which is present in 0.3 to 1.0 per cent of West African and American blacks, the cells contain an abnormal type of hemoglobin called *hemoglobin S*, caused by abnormal composition of amino acids in the beta chains of the hemoglobin. When this hemoglobin is exposed to low concentrations of oxygen, it precipitates into long crystals inside the red blood cell. These crystals elongate the cell and give it the appearance of being a sickle rather than a biconcave disc. The precipitated, sharp-pointed hemoglobin crystals also damage the cell membrane so that the cells become highly fragile, leading to serious anemia. Such patients frequently go into a vicious cycle called a sickle cell disease "crisis" in which low oxygen tension in the tissues causes sickling, which causes impediment of blood flow through the tissues, causing still further decrease in oxygen tension. Thus, once the process starts, it progresses rapidly, leading to a serious decrease in red blood cell mass within a few hours and, often, to death.

EFFECTS OF ANEMIA ON THE CIRCULATORY SYSTEM

The viscosity of the blood, which was discussed in detail in Chapter 11, depends almost entirely on the concentration of red blood cells. In severe anemia the blood viscosity may fall to as low as 1.5 times that of water rather than the normal value of approximately 3 times the viscosity of water. The greatly decreased viscosity decreases the resistance to blood flow in the peripheral vessels so that far greater than normal quantities of blood return to the heart. Moreover, hypoxia due to diminished transport of oxygen by the blood causes the tissue vessels to dilate, allowing further increase in the return of blood to the heart, increasing the cardiac output to a still higher level. Thus, one of the major effects of anemia is greatly *increased work load on the heart*. This can be especially serious when the person begins to exercise, for the heart is not capable of pumping much greater quantities of blood than it is already pumping. Consequently, during exercise, which greatly increases the tissue demand for oxygen, extreme tissue hypoxia results, and acute cardiac failure often ensues.

WHITE BLOOD CELLS AND RESISTANCE OF THE BODY TO INFECTION

Our bodies normally are exposed to bacteria, viruses, fungi, and parasites, which occur especially in the skin, the mouth, the respiratory passageways, the intestinal tract, the lining membranes of the eyes, and even the urinary tract. Many of these agents are capable of causing serious disease if they invade the deeper tissues. In addition, we are exposed intermittently to other highly infectious bacteria and viruses besides those that are normally present in our bodies, and these cause lethal diseases such as pneumonia, streptococcal infection, and typhoid fever.

Fortunately, our bodies have a special system for combatting the different infectious and toxic agents. This is composed of the *leukocytes* (also called white blood cells), the *macrophage system* (frequently but incorrectly called the reticuloendothelial system), and the *lymphoid tissue*. These tissues function in two different ways to prevent disease: (1) by actually destroying invading agents by the process of phagocytosis and (2) by forming antibodies and sensitized lymphocytes, one or both of which may destroy the invader. The present discussion is concerned with the first of these methods, whereas the following chapter is concerned with the second.

THE LEUKOCYTES (WHITE BLOOD CELLS)

The leukocytes are the *mobile units* of the body's protective system. They are formed partially in the bone marrow (the *granulocytes* and *monocytes*, and a few *lymphocytes*) and partially in the lymph tissue (*lymphocytes* and *plasma cells*). The real value of the white blood cells is that most of them are specifically transported to areas of serious inflammation, thereby providing a rapid and potent defense against any infectious agent that might be present.

General Characteristics of Leukocytes

The Types of White Blood Cells. Six different types of white blood cells are normally found in the blood. These are *polymorphonuclear neutrophils, polymorphonuclear eosinophils, polymorphonuclear basophils, monocytes, lymphocytes,* and *plasma cells*. In addition, there are large numbers of *platelets*, which are important in blood coagulation and are fragments of a seventh type of white cell found in the bone marrow, the *megakaryocyte*. The three types of polymorphonuclear cells have granular appearance, as illustrated in Figure 19–6, for which reason they are called *granulocytes,* or in clinical terminology they are often called simply "polys."

The granulocytes and the monocytes protect the body against invading organisms by ingesting them—that is, by the process of *phagocytosis*. The lymphocytes function mainly in connection with the immune system; this will be discussed in the following chapter.

Concentrations of the Different White Blood Cells in the Blood. The adult human being has approximately 7000 white blood cells per cubic millimeter of blood. The normal percentages of the different types of white blood cells are approximately the following:

Polymorphonuclear neutrophils	62.0%
Polymorphonuclear eosinophils	2.3%
Polymorphonuclear basophils	0.4%
Monocytes	5.3%
Lymphocytes	30.0%

Genesis of the Leukocytes

Figure 19–6 illustrates the stages in the development of white blood cells. The polymorphonuclear cells and monocytes are normally formed only in the bone marrow. On the other hand, lymphocytes and plasma cells are produced in the various lymphogenous organs, as we shall discuss in the following chapter.

The white blood cells formed in the bone marrow are stored until they are needed in the circulatory system. Then when the need arises, various factors

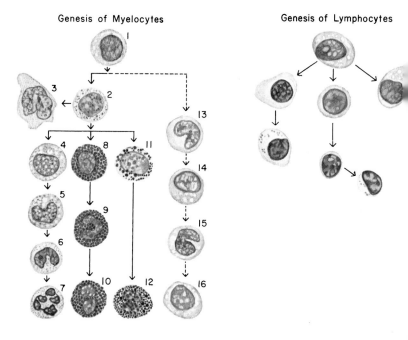

Genesis of Myelocytes   Genesis of Lymphocytes

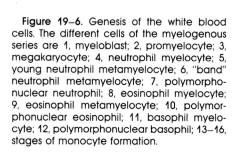

Figure 19–6. Genesis of the white blood cells. The different cells of the myelogenous series are 1, myeloblast; 2, promyelocyte; 3, megakaryocyte; 4, neutrophil myelocyte; 5, young neutrophil metamyelocyte; 6, "band" neutrophil metamyelocyte; 7, polymorphonuclear neutrophil; 8, eosinophil myelocyte; 9, eosinophil metamyelocyte; 10, polymorphonuclear eosinophil; 11, basophil myelocyte; 12, polymorphonuclear basophil; 13–16, stages of monocyte formation.

that are discussed later cause them to be released. Normally, about three times as many granulocytes are stored in the marrow as circulate in the entire blood. This represents about a six-day supply of granulocytes.

Materials Needed for Formation of White Blood Cells. In general, the white blood cells need essentially the same vitamins and amino acids as most of the other cells of the body for their formation. Especially does lack of folic acid, a compound of the vitamin B complex, block the formation of white blood cells as well as prevent maturation of red blood cells, which was pointed out earlier.

Life Span of the White Blood Cells

The life of the granulocytes in the blood, once released from the bone marrow, is normally four to eight hours and another four to five days in the tissues. In times of serious tissue infection, this total life span is often shortened to only a few hours because the graunulocytes then proceed rapidly to the infected area, ingest the invading organisms, and in the process are themselves destroyed.

The monocytes also have a short transit time in the blood before wandering through the capillary membranes into the tissues. However, once in the tissues they swell to much larger sizes to become *tissue macrophages* and in this form can live for months or even years unless destroyed by performing phagocytic function. These tissue macrophages form the basis of the tissue macrophage system that provides a first line of defense in the tissues against infection, as we shall discuss later in the chapter.

PROPERTIES OF NEUTROPHILS, MONOCYTES, AND MACROPHAGES

It is mainly the neutrophils and the monocytes that attack and destroy invading bacteria, viruses, and other injurious agents. The neutrophils are mature cells that can attack and destroy bacteria and viruses even in the circulating blood. On the other hand, the blood monocytes are immature cells that have very little ability to fight infectious agents. However, once they enter the tissues they begin to swell, often increasing their diameters as much as fivefold, to as great as 80 microns, a size that can be seen with the naked eye. Also, extremely large numbers of lysosomes and mitochondria develop in the cytoplasm, giving the cytoplasm the appearance of a bag filled with granules. These cells are now called *macrophages*, and they are extremely capable of combating disease agents.

Diapedesis. Neutrophils and monocytes can squeeze through the pores of the blood vessels by the process of diapedesis. That is, even though a pore is much smaller than the size of the cell, a small portion of the cell slides through the pore at a time, the portion sliding through being momentarily constricted to the size of the pore.

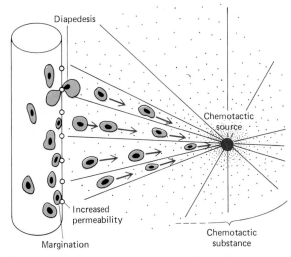

Figure 19–7. Movement of neutrophils by the process of *chemotaxis* toward an area of tissue damage.

Ameboid Motion. Both neutrophils and macrophages move through the tissues by ameboid motion, which was described in Chapter 2. Some of the cells can move through the tissues at rates as great as 40 microns per minute—that is, they can move several times their own length each minute.

Chemotaxis. A number of different chemical substances in the tissues cause both neutrophils and macrophages to move toward the source of the chemical. This phenomenon is known as *chemotaxis* (Fig. 19–7). When a tissue becomes inflamed, a number of different products of the inflammation can cause chemotaxis of both neutrophils and macrophages. These include (a) some of the bacterial toxins, (b) degenerative products of the inflamed tissues themselves, (c) several reaction products of the "complement complex" (discussed in the following chapter), and (d) several reaction products caused by plasma clotting in the inflamed area.

Phagocytosis. The most important function of the neutrophils and macrophages is phagocytosis.

Obviously, the phagocytes must be selective of the material that is phagocytized, or otherwise some of the normal cells and other structures of the body would be ingested. Whether or not phagocytosis will occur depends especially upon three selective procedures. First, if the surface of a particle is rough, the likelihood of phagocytosis is increased. Second, most natural substances of the body have protective coats that repel the phagocytes. On the other hand, dead tissues and foreign particles frequently have no protective coats, and many are also strongly electrically charged, which also makes them subject to phagocytosis. Third, the body has a specific means for recognizing certain foreign materials. This is the function of the immune system that will be described in the following chapter. That is, the immune system develops antibodies against infectious agents like bacteria. These antibodies then adhere to the bacterial membranes and thereby make the bacteria especially susceptible to phagocytosis.

Phagocytosis by Neutrophils. The neutrophils entering the tissues are already mature cells that can immediately begin phagocytosis. On approaching a particle to be phagocytized, the neutrophil first attaches to receptors on the particle, then projects pseudopodia in all directions around the particle, and the pseudopodia meet each other on the opposite side and fuse. This creates an enclosed chamber containing the phagocytized particle. Then the chamber invaginates to the inside of the cytoplasmic cavity and breaks away from the outer cell membrane to form a free-floating *phagocytic vesicle* (also called a *phagosome*) inside the cytoplasm.

A neutrophil can usually phagocytize 5 to 20 bacteria before the neutrophil itself becomes inactivated and dies.

Phagocytosis by Macrophages. Macrophages, when activated by the immune system as described in the following chapter, are much more powerful phagocytes than the neutrophils, often capable of phagocytizing as many as 100 bacteria. They have the ability to engulf much larger particles and often five or more times as many particles as the neutrophils. And they can even phagocytize whole red blood cells or malarial parasites, whereas neutrophils are not capable of phagocytizing particles much larger than bacteria. Also, macrophages have the ability to phagocytize necrotic tissue and even dead neutrophils, which is a very important function performed by these cells in chronic infection.

Enzymatic Digestion of the Phagocytized Particles. Once a foreign particle has been phagocytized, lysosomes immediately come in contact with the phagocytic vesicle, and their membranes fuse with those of the vesicle, thereby dumping many digestive enzymes of the lysosomes into the vesicle. Thus, the phagocytic vesicle now becomes a *digestive vesicle,* and digestion of the phagocytized particle begins immediately. Both neutrophils and macrophages have an abundance of lysosomes filled with *proteolytic enzymes* especially geared for digesting bacteria and other foreign protein matter.

THE TISSUE MACROPHAGE SYSTEM (THE RETICULOENDOTHELIAL SYSTEM)

In the preceding paragraphs we have described the macrophages mainly as mobile cells that are capable of wandering through the tissues. However, a large portion of the monocytes, on entering the tissues and after becoming macrophages, become attached to the tissues and remain attached for months or perhaps even years unless they are called upon to perform specific protective functions. They have the same capabilities as the mobile macrophages to phagocytize large quantities of bacteria, viruses, necrotic tissue, or other foreign particles in the tissue. And, when appropriately stimulated, they can break away from their attachments and become mobile macrophages that respond to chemotaxis and all the other stimuli related to the inflammatory process.

The combination of mobile macrophages and fixed tissue macrophages is collectively called the *reticu-*

loendothelial system. The reason for this name is that it was formerly believed that a major share of the blood vessel endothelial cells could perform phagocytic functions similar to those performed by the macrophage system. However, recent studies have disproved this. Therefore, the reticuloendothelial system is actually a misnomer. Yet, because the term is so widely used, it should be remembered to be almost synonymous with the tissue macrophage system.

The tissue macrophages in various tissues differ in appearances because of environmental differences, and they are known by different names: *Kupffer's cells* in the liver; *tissue macrophages* in the lymph nodes, spleen, and bone marrow; *alveolar macrophages* in the alveoli of the lungs; *tissue histiocytes, clasmatocytes,* or *fixed macrophages* in the subcutaneous tissues; and *microglia* in the brain.

Macrophages of the Lymph Nodes. Essentially no particulate matter that enters the tissues can be absorbed directly through the capillary membranes into the blood. Instead, if the particles are not destroyed locally in the tissues, they enter the lymph and flow through the lymphatic vessels to the lymph nodes located intermittently along the course of the lymphatic. The foreign particles are trapped there in a meshwork of sinuses lined by *tissue macrophages.*

Figure 19–8 illustrates the general organization of the lymph node, showing lymph entering by way of the *afferent lymphatics,* flowing through the *medullary sinuses,* and finally passing out of the *hilus* into the *efferent lymphatics.* Large numbers of macrophages line the sinuses, and if any particles enter the sinuses the macrophages phagocytize them and prevent general dissemination throughout the body.

INFLAMMATION AND FUNCTION OF NEUTROPHILS AND MACROPHAGES

When tissue injury occurs, whether it be caused by bacteria, trauma, chemicals, heat, or any other phenomenon, multiple substances that cause dramatic secondary changes in the tissues are released by the injured tissues. These secondary changes are called *inflammation.* Inflammation is characterized by (1) vasodilatation of the local blood vessels with conse-

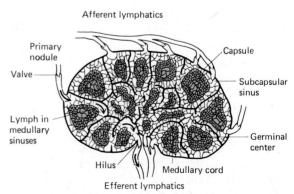

Figure 19–8. Functional diagram of a lymph node. (Redrawn from Ham: Histology. Philadelphia, J. B. Lippincott Company, 1971.)

quent excess local blood flow, (2) increased permeability of the capillaries with leakage of large quantities of fluid into the interstitial spaces, (3) often clotting of the fluid in these spaces because of excessive amounts of fibrinogen and other proteins leaking from the capillaries, and (4) swelling of the cells. Some of the many tissue products that cause these reactions include *histamine, bradykinin, serotonin, prostaglandins,* several different *reaction products of the immune system* (that are described in the following chapter), and *reaction products of the blood-clotting system.* Several of these substances strongly activate the machrophage system, and within a few hours the macrophages begin to devour the destroyed tissues—but at times the macrophages also further injure the still-living tissue cells.

The "Walling Off" Effect of Inflammation. One of the first results of inflammation is to "wall off" the area of injury from the remaining tissues. That is, the tissue spaces and the lymphatics in the inflamed area are blocked by fibrinogen clots so that fluid barely flows through the spaces. Therefore, this walling-off process delays the spread of bacteria or toxic products.

The Macrophage and Neutrophil Response to Inflammation

The Tissue Macrophages as the First Line of Defense. The macrophages that are already present in the tissues, whether they be the histiocytes in the subcutaneous tissues, the alveolar macrophages in the lungs, the microglia in the brain, or so forth, immediately begin their phagocytic actions. Therefore, they are the first line of defense against infection during the first hour or so.

Neutrophilia and Neutrophil Invasion of the Inflamed Area—The Second Line of Defense. The term *neutrophilia* means an increase in the number of neutrophils in the blood. The term *leukocytosis* is also often used to mean the same as neutrophilia, though this term actually means excess number of all white cells, whatever their types.

Within a few hours after the onset of acute inflammation, the number of neutrophils in the blood sometimes increases as much as four- to fivefold—to as high as 15,000 to 25,000 per cubic millimeter. This results from a combination of chemical substances that are released from the inflamed tissues, collectively called *leukocytosis-inducing factor* or *granulocyte-releasing factor.* This factor diffuses from the inflamed tissue into the blood and is carried to the bone marrow. There it mobilizes large numbers of leukocytes, mainly neutrophils, that are already preformed and stored in the marrow tissue. In this way large numbers of neutrophils are almost immediately transferred from the bone marrow storage pool into the circulating blood and then are attracted by chemotaxis into the inflamed tissue.

Thus, within several hours after tissue damage begins, the area becomes well supplied with neutrophils. Since neutrophils are already mature cells, they are ready to begin immediately their scavenger functions for removal of foreign matter from the inflamed tissues.

Increased Production of Neutrophils by the Bone Marrow—Colony-Stimulating Factor. Inflammation not only causes release of leukocytes from the bone marrow's storage pool but causes an increased rate of production of leukocytes as well. A number of different factors seem to cause this; several of these have been isolated and characterized and collectively are called *colony-stimulating factor* because they all cause colonies of leukocytes to proliferate in tissue culture as well as causing increased leukocyte production in the bone marrow.

Macrophage Proliferation and the Monocyte Response—The Third Line of Defense. Though the first and second lines of defense in tissue infection are the already present tissue macrophages and the rapid production and movement of neutrophils into the inflamed area, still a third line of defense is a slow but long-continuing increase in the number of macrophages as well. This results partly from reproduction of the already present tissue macrophages but also from migration of large numbers of monocytes into the inflamed area. Though the monocytes are still immature cells and do not have the capability of phagocytosis when they first enter the tissues, over a period of 8 to 12 hours they swell markedly, form greatly increased quantities of cytoplasmic lysosomes, exhibit increased ameboid motion, and move chemotactically toward the damaged tissues.

Next, the rate of production of monocytes by the bone marrow also increases. This possibly results partly from stimulation by colony-stimulating factor, but there seem to be other, yet undefined stimulating factors as well, because in long-term chronic infection there is progressively increasing production of monocytes, thereby increasing the ratio of macrophages to neutrophils in the tissues. Therefore, the long-term chronic defense against infection is often mainly a macrophage response rather than a neutrophil response.

As has already been pointed out, the macrophages can phagocytize far more bacteria and far larger particles, including even neutrophils and large quantities of necrotic tissue. Also, the macrophages play an important role in initiating the development of antibodies, as we shall discuss in the following chapter.

Formation of Pus

When the neutrophils and macrophages engulf large numbers of bacteria and necrotic tissue, essentially all the neutrophils and many if not most of the macrophages themselves eventually die. After several days, a cavity is often excavated in the inflamed tissues containing varying portions of necrotic tissue, dead neutrophils, and dead macrophages. Such a mixture is commonly known as *pus.*

THE EOSINOPHILS

The eosinophils normally comprise 2 to 3 per cent of all the blood leukocytes. Eosinophils are weak phagocytes, and they exhibit chemotaxis, but in comparison with the neutrophils it is doubtful that the eosinophils are of significant importance in protection against usual types of infection.

On the other hand, eosinophils are often produced in very large numbers in persons with parasitic infections, and they migrate into tissues diseased by parasites. Though most of the parasites are too large to be phagocytized by the eosinophils or by any other phagocytic cells, nevertheless the eosinophils attach to the parasites and release substances that kill many of them. For instance, one of the most widespread infections of the world is *schistosomiasis,* a parasitic infection found in as many as one third of the population of some tropical countries; the parasite invades literally any part of the body. Eosinophils can attach to the juvenile forms of the parasite and can kill many of them.

Eosinophils also have a special propensity to collect in tissues in which allergic reactions have occurred, such as in the peribronchial tissues of the lungs in asthmatic persons. The eosinophils are believed to detoxify some of the inflammation-inducing substances released during allergic reactions.

THE BASOPHILS

The basophils in the circulating blood are very similar to though not identical with the large *mast* cells located immediately outside many of the capillaries in the body. Both these cells liberate *heparin* into the blood, a substance that can prevent blood coagulation and that can also speed the removal of fat particles from the blood after a fatty meal.

The mast cells and basophils play an exceedingly important role in some types of allergic reactions because the type of antibody that causes allergic reactions, the IgE type (see Chapter 20), has a special propensity to become attached to mast cells and basophils. Then, when the specific antigen subsequently reacts with the antibody, this causes the mast cell or basophil to rupture and release exceedingly large quantities of *histamine, bradykinin, serotonin, heparin,* and a number of *lysosomal enzymes.* These in turn cause local vascular and tissue reactions that cause the allergic manifestations.

THE LEUKEMIAS

Uncontrolled production of white blood cells is caused by cancerous mutation of a myelogenous or a lymphogenous cell. This causes *leukemia,* which is usually characterized by greatly increased numbers of abnormal white blood cells in the circulating blood. These can be either *myelogenous cells* produced in the bone marrow, *lymphogenous cells* produced in the lymphoid tissue, or bizarre and undifferentiated cells not identical with any of the normal white blood cells. Usually the more undifferentiated the cells the more *acute* is the leukemia, often leading to death within a few months. But with some of the more differentiated cells, the process can be quite *chronic,* sometimes developing slowly over a period of 10 to 20 years.

Perhaps the most important effect of leukemia on the body is the excessive use of metabolic substrates by the growing cancerous cells. The leukemic tissues reproduce new cells so rapidly that tremendous demands are made on the body fluids for foodstuffs, especially the amino acids and vitamins. Consequently, the energy of the patient is greatly depleted, and the excessive utilization of amino acids causes rapid deterioration of the normal protein tissues of the body. Thus, while the leukemic tissues grow, the other tissues are debilitated. Obviously, after metabolic starvation has continued long enough, this alone is sufficient to cause death.

AGRANULOCYTOSIS

A clinical condition known as "agranulocytosis" occasionally occurs, in which the bone marrow stops producing white blood cells, leaving the body unprotected against bacteria and other agents that might invade the tissues. The cause may be x-ray or nuclear irradiation or reaction to a drug.

Normally, the human body lives in symbiosis with many bacteria, for all the mucous membranes of the body are constantly exposed to large numbers of bacteria. The mouth almost always contains various spirochetal, pneumococcal, and streptococcal bacteria, and these same bacteria are present to a lesser extent in the entire respiratory tract. The gastrointestinal tract is especially loaded with colon bacilli. Furthermore, one can almost always find bacteria in the eyes, the urethra, and the vagina. Therefore, any decrease in the number of neutrophils immediately allows invasion of the tissues by the bacteria that are already present in the body. Within two days after the bone marrow stops producing white blood cells, ulcers may appear in the mouth and colon, or the person develops some form of severe respiratory infection. Bacteria from the ulcers then rapidly invade the surrounding tissues and the blood. Without treatment, death often ensues three to six days after acute agranulocytosis begins.

QUESTIONS

1. Describe the functions of the red blood cells.
2. Where are the red blood cells formed, and what are the stages of their formation?
3. Explain the role of tissue oxygenation and *erythropoietin* in the regulation of red blood cell production.
4. What important vitamins are required for proper formation of red blood cells and why?
5. List the important features of the hemoglobin molecule, and describe its chemical method for transporting oxygen to the tissues.
6. Describe the mechanisms of absorption of iron from the gut, its transport in the blood, and its storage in the liver.
7. How is the total body iron controlled?
8. What is the average life of the red blood cell, and how are the old cells destroyed? What happens to the hemoglobin and the iron of the destroyed cells?
9. Describe the characteristics of several types of anemia.
10. Describe the different types of white blood cells, and state their relative percentages in the blood.
11. Describe the formation and life span of the different white blood cells.
12. List the specific properties of *neutrophils* and *macrophages* for the *phagocytosis* of bacteria and tissue debris.
13. Describe the anatomy and the function of the *macrophage system* of the body.
14. Discuss the roles of the neutrophils and macrophages in *inflammation*.
15. What controls the numbers of neutrophils and macrophages?
16. Discuss the role of the *eosinophils* for protection against parasites and the role of these white blood cells in allergy.
17. Discuss the roles of the *basophils* in blood coagulation and in allergy.
18. What types of *leukemic cells* are frequently formed, and what are the effects of leukemia on the body?
19. What is *agranulocytosis,* and what does this do to the body?

References

Red Blood Cells

Benz, E. H., Jr., and Forget, B. G.: The thalassemia syndromes: models for the molecular analysis of human disease. Annu Rev Med 33:363, 1982.

Charlton, R. W., and Bothwell, T. H.: Iron absorption. Annu Rev Med 34:55, 1983.

Eaves, A. C., and Eaves, C. J.: Erythropoiesis in culture. Clin Haematol 13:371, 1984.

Eaves, C. J., and Eaves, A. C.: Factors and hemopoiesis: Pandora's box revisited. Prog Clin Biol Res 148:83, 1984.

Harrison, P. R.: Molecular analysis of erythropoiesis. A current appraisal. Exp Cell Res 155:321, 1984.

Johnson, G. R.: Haemopoietic multipotential stem cells in culture. Clin Haematol 13:309, 1984.

Mackinney, A. A., Jr.: The Pathophysiology of Blood. New York, John Wiley & Sons, 1984.

Metcalf, D., and Nicola, N. A.: The regulatory factors controlling murine erythropoiesis in vitro. Prog Clin Biol Res 148:93, 1984.

Ogawa, M., et al.: Differentiation and proliferative kinetics of hemopoietic stem cells in culture. Prog Clin Biol Res 148:35, 1984.

Schmid-Schonbein, H., et al.: Biology of red cells: Non-nucleated erythrocytes as fluid drop-like cell fragments. Int J Microcirc Clin Exp 3:161, 1984.

Stanley, E. R., and Jubinsky, P. T.: Factors affecting the growth and differentiation of haemopoietic cells in culture. Clin Haematol 13:329, 1984.

Thompson, R. B.: A Short Textbook of Haematology. Baltimore, Urban & Schwarzenberg, 1984.

White Blood Cells and Resistance to Infection

Barrett, K. E., and Metcalfe, D. D.: Mast cell heterogeneity: evidence and implications. J Clin Immunol 4:253, 1984.

Ford-Hutchinson, A. W.: Leukotrienes: their formation and role as inflammatory mediators. Fed Proc 44:25, 1985.

Freedman, M. H.: Congenital failure of hematopoiesis in the newborn infant. Clin Perinatol 11:417, 1984.

Galli, S. J., et al.: Basophils and mast cells: morphologic insights into their biology, secretory patterns, and function. Prog Allergy 34:1, 1984.

Johnson, G. R.: Haemopoietic multipotential stem cells in culture. Clin Haematol 13:309, 1984.

Mackinney, A. A., Jr.: The Pathophysiology of Blood. New York, John Wiley & Sons, 1984.

May, M. E., and Waddell, C. C.: Basophils in peripheral blood and bone marrow. A retrospective review. Am J Med 76:509, 1984.

Ogawa, M., et al.: Differentiation and proliferative kinetics of hemopoietic stem cells in culture. Prog Clin Biol Res 148:35, 1984.

Rebuck, J. W., et al., eds.: The Reticuloendothelial System. Huntington, N.Y., R. E. Krieger Publishing Co., 1980.

Shiffmann, E.: Leukocyte chemotaxis. Annu Rev Physiol 44:553, 1982.

Stanley, E. R., and Jubinsky, P. T.: Factors affecting the growth and differentiation of haemopoietic cells in culture. Clin Haematol 13:329, 1984.

Thompson, R. B.: A Short Textbook of Haematology. Baltimore, Urban & Schwarzenberg, 1984.

20

Immunity, Allergy, Blood Groups, Transfusion, and Transplantation

INNATE IMMUNITY
ACQUIRED IMMUNITY
    TWO BASIC TYPES OF ACQUIRED
       IMMUNITY
    ANTIGENS
    ROLE OF LYMPHOID TISSUE IN
       ACQUIRED IMMUNITY
    SPECIFICITY OF ANTIBODIES AND T
       LYMPHOCYTES—ROLE OF
       LYMPHOCYTE CLONES
    SPECIFIC ATTRIBUTES OF THE B
       LYMPHOCYTE SYSTEM—THE
       ANTIBODIES AND HUMORAL
       IMMUNITY
    SPECIAL ATTRIBUTES OF THE T
       LYMPHOCYTE SYSTEM—ACTIVATED
       CELLS AND CELL-MEDIATED
       IMMUNITY

TOLERANCE OF THE ACQUIRED
    IMMUNITY SYSTEM TO ONE'S OWN
    TISSUES—ROLE OF THE THYMUS
    AND THE BURSA
    VACCINATION
ALLERGY
BLOOD GROUPS AND BLOOD
   TRANSFUSION
    ANTIGENICITY AND IMMUNE
       REACTIONS OF BLOOD
    O-A-B BLOOD GROUPS
    THE Rh BLOOD TYPES
    ACUTE KIDNEY SHUTDOWN
       FOLLOWING TRANSFUSION
       REACTIONS
TRANSPLANTATION OF TISSUES AND
   ORGANS

INNATE IMMUNITY

The human body has the ability to resist almost all types of organisms or toxins that tend to damage the tissues and organs. This capacity is called *immunity*. Much of the immunity is caused by a special immune system that forms *antibodies* and *activated lymphocytes* that attack and destroy the specific organisms or toxins. This type of immunity is *acquired immunity*. However, an additional portion of the immunity results from general processes rather than from processes directed at specific disease organisms. This is called *innate immunity*. It includes the following:

1. Phagocytosis of bacteria and other invaders by white blood cells and cells of the tissue macrophage system, as described in the previous chapter.

2. Destruction by the acid secretions of the stomach and by the digestive enzymes of organisms swallowed into the stomach.

3. Resistance of the skin to invasion by organisms.

4. Presence in the blood of certain chemical compounds that attach to foreign organisms or toxins and destroy them.

This innate immunity makes the human body resistant to such diseases as some paralytic virus infections of animals, hog cholera, cattle plague, and distemper—a viral disease that kills a large percentage of dogs that become afflicted with it. On the other hand, lower animals are resistant or even completely immune to many human diseases, such as poliomyelitis, mumps, human cholera, measles, and syphilis, which are very destructive or even lethal to the human being.

ACQUIRED IMMUNITY

In addition to its innate immunity, the human body also has the ability to develop extremely powerful specific immunity against individual invading agents such as lethal bacteria, viruses, toxins, and even foreign tissues from other animals. This is called *acquired immunity*.

Acquired immunity can often bestow extreme protection. For instance, certain toxins such as the paralytic toxin of botulinum or the tetanizing toxin of tetanus, can be protected against in doses as high as 100,000 times the amount that would be lethal without immunity. For this reason, the process known as "vaccination" is extremely important in protecting human beings against diseases and against toxins, as will be explained in the course of this chapter.

TWO BASIC TYPES OF ACQUIRED IMMUNITY

Two basic, but closely allied, types of acquired immunity occur in the body. In one of these the body develops circulating *antibodies*, which are globulin molecules that are capable of attacking the invading agent. This type of immunity is called *humoral immunity*. The second type of acquired immunity is achieved through the formation of large numbers of *activated lymphocytes* that are specifically designed to destroy the foreign agent. This type of immunity is called *cell-mediated immunity*.

We shall see shortly that both the antibodies and the activated lymphocytes are formed in the lymphoid tissue of the body. First, let us discuss the initiation of the immune process by *antigens*.

ANTIGENS

Since acquired immunity does not occur until after first invasion by a foreign organism or toxin, it is clear that the body must have some mechanism for recognizing the initial invasion. Each toxin or each type of organism almost always contains one or more specific chemical compounds in its makeup that are different from all other compounds. In general, these are proteins or large polysaccharides, and it is they that cause the acquired immunity. These substances are called *antigens*.

For a substance to be antigenic it usually must have a high molecular weight, 8000 or greater. Furthermore, the process of antigenicity usually depends upon regularly recurring prosthetic radicals on the surface of the large molecule, which perhaps explains why proteins and polysaccharides are almost always antigenic, for they both have this type of stereochemical characteristic.

ROLE OF LYMPHOID TISSUE IN ACQUIRED IMMUNITY

Acquired immunity is the product of the body's lymphoid tissue. In persons who have a genetic lack of lymphoid tissue or whose lymphoid tissue has been destroyed by radiation or by chemicals, no acquired immunity whatsoever can develop. And almost immediately after birth such a person dies of fulminating infection unless treated by heroic measures. There-

fore, it is clear that the lymphoid tissue is essential to survival of the human being.

The lymphoid tissue is located most extensively in the *lymph nodes*, but it is also found in special lymphoid tissues such as that of the *spleen, submucosal areas of the gastrointestinal tract*, and the *bone marrow*. The lymphoid tissue is distributed very advantageously in the body to intercept the invading organisms or toxins before they can spread too widely. For instance, the lymphoid tissue of the gastrointestinal tract is exposed immediately to antigens invading through the gut. The lymphoid tissue of the throat and pharynx (the tonsils and adenoids) is extremely well located to intercept antigens that enter by way of the upper respiratory tract. The lymphoid tissue in the lymph nodes is exposed to antigens that invade the peripheral tissues of the body. And, finally, the lymphoid tissue of the spleen and bone marrow plays the specific role of intercepting antigenic agents that have succeeded in reaching the circulating blood.

Two Types of Lymphocytes That Promote, Respectively, Cell-Mediated Immunity and Humoral Immunity—the T and the B Lymphocytes. Though most of the lymphocytes in normal lymphoid tissue look alike when studied under the microscope, these cells are distinctly divided into two major populations. One of the populations is responsible for forming the activated lymphocytes that provide cell-mediated immunity and the other for forming the antibodies that provide humoral immunity.

Both of these types of lymphocytes are derived originally in the embryo from *pluripotent hemopoietic stem cells* that differentiate and become committed to form lymphocytes. The lymphocytes that are formed eventually end up in the lymphoid tissue, but before doing so they are further differentiated or "preprocessed" in the following ways:

Those lymphocytes that are eventually destined to form activated lymphocytes first migrate to and are preprocessed in the *thymus* gland, for which reason they are called T lymphocytes. These are responsible for cell-mediated immunity.

The other population of lymphocytes—those that are destined to form antibodies—are preprocessed in some unknown area of the body, probably in the liver during midfetal life and in the bone marrow in late fetal life and after birth. However, this population of cells was first discovered in birds, in which the preprocessing occurs in the *bursa of Fabricius*, a structure not found in mammals. For this reason these lymphocytes are called B lymphocytes, and they are responsible for humoral immunity.

Figure 20–1 illustrates the two separate lymphocyte systems for the formation, respectively, of the activated T lymphocytes and the antibodies.

Role of the Thymus Gland for Preprocessing the T Lymphocytes. Most of the preprocessing of the T lymphocytes of the thymus gland occurs shortly before the birth of the baby and for a few months after birth. Therefore, beyond this period of time, removal of the thymus gland usually will not seriously impair

CELL – MEDIATED IMMUNITY

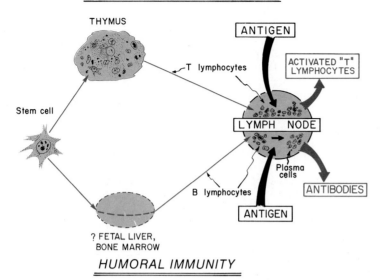

Figure 20–1. Formation of antibodies and sensitized lymphocytes by a lymph node in response to antigens. This figure also shows the origin of *thymic* ("T") and *bursal* ("B") lymphocytes that are responsible for the cell-mediated and humoral immune processes of the lymph nodes.

the T lymphocytic immune system, the system necessary for cell-mediated immunity. However, removal of the thymus several months before birth can completely prevent development of all cell-mediated immunity. Since it is this cellular type of immunity that is mainly responsible for rejection of transplanted organs such as hearts and kidneys, one can transplant organs with little likelihood of rejection if the thymus is removed from an animal a reasonable period of time before birth.

Role of the Bursa of Fabricius for Preprocessing B Lymphocytes in Birds. During the latter part of fetal life the bursa of Fabricius preprocesses the B lymphocytes and prepares them to manufacture antibodies. Here again, this preprocessing continues for a while after birth. In mammals, it is believed that the B cells are preprocessed during midfetal life in the liver but thereafter in the bone marrow.

Spread of Processed Lymphocytes to the Lymphoid Tissue. After formation of processed lymphocytes in both the thymus and the bursa, these first circulate freely in the blood for a few hours but then become entrapped in the lymphoid tissue. Thus, the lymphocytes do not originate primordially in the lymphoid tissue but, instead, are transported to this tissue by way of the preprocessing areas of the thymus and probably fetal liver and bone marrow.

SPECIFICITY OF ANTIBODIES AND T LYMPHOCYTES—ROLE OF LYMPHOCYTE CLONES

When either antibodies or activated T lymphocytes, called T cells, are formed in the lymphoid tissue, these then can react highly specifically against the particular type of antigen that initiated their development. The mechanism for this is almost certainly the following:

Millions of Preformed Specific Lymphocytes in the Lymphoid Tissue. We now know that there are at least a million different types of preformed B lymphocytes and equally as many preformed T lymphocytes that are capable of forming the highly specific antibodies, or T cells, when activated by the appropriate antigens. Each one of these preformed lymphocytes is capable of forming only one type of antibody or one type of T cell with a single type of specificity. And only the specific type of antigen with which it can react can activate it. However, once the specific lymphocyte is activated by its antigen, it reproduces wildly, forming tremendous numbers of duplicate lymphocytes. If it is a B lymphocyte, its progeny will eventually secrete antibodies that then circulate throughout the body. If it is a T lymphocyte, its progeny are activated T cells that are released into the lymph and carried to the blood and tissues.

All the different lymphocytes that are capable of forming one specific antibody or T cell are called a *clone of lymphocytes.* That is, the lymphocytes in each clone are alike and are derived originally from one or a few early lymphocytes of its specific type.

Mechanism for Activating a Clone of Lymphocytes

Each clone of lymphocytes is responsive to only a single type of antigen (or to similar antigens that have almost exactly the same stereochemical characteristics). The reason for this is the following: In the case of the B lymphocytes, each one of them has in its cell membrane about 100,000 antibody molecules that will react highly specifically with only the one specific type of antigen. Therefore, when the appropriate antigen comes along, it immediately attaches to the cell membrane; this leads to the activation process, which we will describe in more detail subsequently. In the case of the T lymphocytes, molecules very similar to antibodies, called *surface receptor proteins* (or T cell markers), are in the cell membrane, and these too are highly specific for the one specified activating antigen.

Role of Macrophages in the Activation Process. Aside from the lymphocytes in lymphoid tissue, literally millions of macrophages are also present in the same lymphoid tissue. These line the sinusoids of the lymph nodes, spleen, and other lymphoid tissue, and they lie in apposition to many of the lymph node lymphocytes. Most invading organisms are first phagocytized and partially digested by the macrophages, and the antigenic products are liberated into the macrophage cytosol. It is believed that the macrophages then pass these antigens directly to the lymphocytes, thus leading to activation of the specified clones. The macrophages also secrete an activating substance that promotes the growth and reproduction of the specific lymphocytes. This substance is called *interleukin 1.*

Role of the T cells in the Activation of the B Lymphocytes. Most antigens activate both T lymphocytes and B lymphocytes at the same time. Some of the T cells that are formed, called *helper cells,* in turn secrete specific substances (collectively called *lymphokines*) that further activate the B lymphocytes. Indeed, without the help of these T cells, the quantity of antibodies formed by the B lymphocytes is usually very slight.

SPECIFIC ATTRIBUTES OF THE B LYMPHOCYTE SYSTEM—THE ANTIBODIES AND HUMORAL IMMUNITY

Formation of Antibodies by the Plasma Cells. Prior to exposure to a specific antigen, the clones of B lymphocytes remain dormant in the lymphoid tissue. However, upon entry of a foreign antigen, those B lymphocytes specific for the antigen immediately enlarge and take on the appearance of *lymphoblasts.* Some of these then further differentiate to form *plasmablasts,* which divide rapidly and form about 500 mature *plasma cells* in about four days. The mature plasma cell then produces gamma globulin antibodies at an extremely rapid rate—about 2000 molecules per second for each plasma cell. The antibodies are secreted into the lymph and are carried to the circulating blood. This process continues for several days or weeks until death of the plasma cells.

The Nature of the Antibodies

The antibodies are gamma globulins called *immunoglobulins,* and they have molecular weights between approximately 150,000 and 900,000. Usually they constitute about 20 per cent of all the plasma proteins.

All the immunoglobulins are composed of combinations of *light* and *heavy polypeptide chains.* Most have two light and two heavy chains, as illustrated in Figure 20–2. Each heavy chain is paralleled by a light chain at one of its ends, thus forming a heavy-light

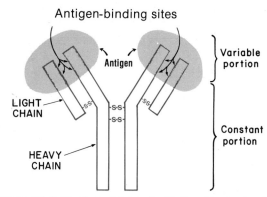

Figure 20–2. Structure of the typical IgG antibody, showing it to be composed of two heavy polypeptide chains and two light polypeptide chains. The antigen binds at two different sites on the variable portions of the chains.

pair, and there are always at least two such pairs in each immunoglobulin molecule.

Figure 20–2 shows a designated end of each of the light and each of the heavy chains, called the "variable portion," and the remainder of each chain is called the "constant portion." The variable portion is different for each specificity of antibody, it is this portion that attaches specifically to a particular type of antigen. The constant portion of the antibody determines much of the gross physical and chemical properties of the antibody, establishing such factors as diffusivity of the antibody in the tissues, adherence of the antibody to specific structures within the tissues, attachment to the *complement complex,* and other biological properties of the antibody.

Specificity of Antibodies. Each antibody that is specific for a particular antigen has a different organization of amino acid residues *in the variable portions* of both the light and heavy chains. These have a different steric shape for each antigen specificity, so that when an antigen comes in contact with it the prosthetic radicals of the antigen fit as a mirror image with those of the antibody, thus allowing a rapid bonding between the antibody and the antigen.

Mechanisms of Action of Antibodies

Antibodies act mainly in two different ways to protect the body against invading agents: (1) by direct attack on the invader, or (2) by activation of the *complement system* that then destroys the invader.

Direct Action of Antibodies on Invading Agents. Because of the bivalent nature of the antibodies and the multiple antigen sites on most invading agents, the antibodies can inactivate the invading agent in one of several ways, as follows:

1. *Agglutination,* in which multiple large structures with antigens on their surfaces, such as bacteria or red cells, are bound together into a clump.

2. *Precipitation,* in which the molecular complex of soluble antigen (such as tetanus toxin) and antibody becomes so large that it is rendered insoluble and precipitates.

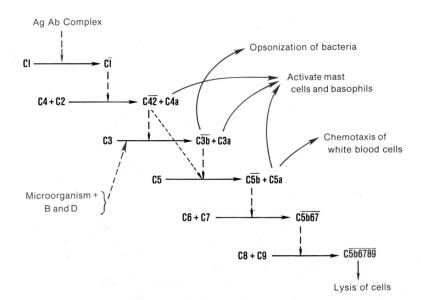

Figure 20–3. Cascade of reactions during activation of the classical pathway of complement. (Modified from Alexander and Good: Fundamentals of Clinical Immunology. Philadelphia, W. B. Saunders Company, 1977, by permission.)

3. *Neutralization,* in which the antibodies cover the toxic sites of the antigenic agent.

4. *Lysis,* in which some very potent antibodies are occasionally capable of directly attacking membranes of cellular agents and thereby causing rupture of the cell.

However, the direct actions of antibodies attacking the antigenic invaders probably, under normal conditions, are not strong enough to play a major role in protecting the body against the invader. Most of the protection comes through the *amplifying* effects of the complement system described below.

The Complement System for Antibody Action. "Complement" is a collective term to describe a system of about 20 different proteins, in the blood and tissue fluids, many of which are enzyme precursors. The principal actors in this system are 11 proteins, designated C1 through C9, B, and D, illustrated in Figure 20–3. The enzyme precursors are normally inactive, but they can be activated by an antigen-antibody reaction. That is, when an antibody binds with an antigen, a specific reactive site on the "constant" portion of the antibody becomes uncovered, or activated, and this in turn binds directly with the C1 molecule of the complement system, setting into motion a "cascade" of sequential reactions, illustrated in Figure 20–3, beginning with activation of the proenzyme C1 itself. Only a few antigen-antibody combinations are required to activate many molecules in this first stage of the complement system. The C1 enzymes thus formed then activate successively increasing quantities of enzymes in the later stages of the system, so that from a very small beginning a very large reaction occurs. Multiple end-products are formed as illustrated in the figure, and several of these cause important effects that help to prevent damage by the invading organism or toxin. Among the more important effects are the following:

(1) *Opsonization* and *phagocytosis.* One of the products of the complement cascade, C3b, strongly activates phagocytosis by both neutrophils and mac-

rophages, causing them to engulf the bacteria to which the antigen-antibody complexes are attached. This process is called *opsonization*. It often enhances the number of bacteria that can be destroyed by many hundredfold.

(2) *Lysis.* One of the most important of all the products of the complement cascade is called the *lytic complex,* which is a combination of multiple complement factors and is designated C5b6789. This has a direct effect of rupturing the cell membranes of bacteria or other invading organisms.

(3) *Agglutination.* The complement products also change the surfaces of the invading organisms, causing them to adhere to each other, thus promoting agglutination.

(4) *Neutralization of viruses.* The complement enzymes and other complement products can attack the structures of some viruses and thereby render them nonvirulent.

(5) *Chemotaxis.* Fragment C5a causes chemotaxis of neutrophils and macrophages, thus causing large numbers of these phagocytes to migrate into the local region of the antigenic agent.

SPECIAL ATTRIBUTES OF THE T LYMPHOCYTE SYSTEM—ACTIVATED CELLS AND CELL-MEDIATED IMMUNITY

Release of Activated T Cells from Lymphoid Tissue. Upon exposure to the proper antigens, the T lymphocytes of the lymphoid tissue proliferate and release large numbers of activated T cells in ways that parallel antibody release by the B lymphocytes. The only real difference is that instead of releasing antibodies, whole activated T cells are formed and released into the lymph. These then pass into the circulation and are distributed throughout the body fluids, sometimes lasting for months or even years.

Antigen Receptors on the T Lymphocytes. Antigens bind with *receptor molecules* on the surfaces of T cells in the same way that they bind with antibodies.

These receptor molecules are composed of a variable unit similar to the variable portion of the humoral antibody, but its stem section is firmly bound to the cell membrane. Therefore, it is never secreted from the cell into the body fluids. There are as many as 100,000 receptor sites on a single T cell.

Multiple Types of T Cells and Their Functions

In the last few years it has become clear that there are several different types of T cells. These are classified into three major groups: (1) *cytotoxic T cells,* (2) *helper T cells,* and (3) *suppressor T cells.* The functions of each of these are quite distinct.

Cytotoxic T Cells. The cytotoxic T cell is a direct attack cell, capable of killing microorganisms and at times even some of the body's own cells. For this reason, these cells are frequently called *killer cells.* The receptor proteins on the surfaces of the cytotoxic cells cause them to bind tightly to those organisms or cells that contain their binding-specific antigen. Then, they kill the attacked cell in the manner illustrated in Figure 20–4. The immediate effect of the binding is swelling of the T cell and release of cytotoxic substances directly into the attacked cell. The cytotoxic substances are probably mainly lysosomal enzymes manufactured in the T cell.

The "killer" cells can attack many different microorganisms one after another, killing many separate organisms instead of merely one, often without the killer cells themselves being harmed.

These cells are especially lethal to tissue cells that have been invaded by viruses because many virus particles become entrapped in the membranes of these cells and attract the T cells because of the viral antigenicity. The cytotoxic cells also play an important role in destroying cancer cells, heart transplant cells, or other types of cells that are "foreign" to the person's own body.

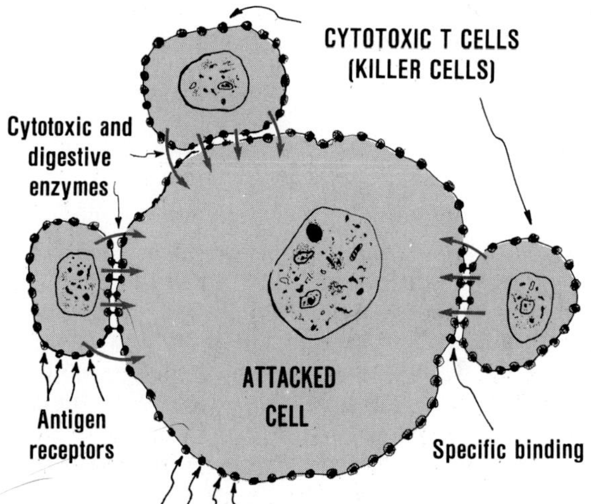

The Helper T Cells. The helper T cells are by far the most numerous of the T cells. As their name implies they "help" in the functions of the immune system in multiple ways. Some of their important functions are as follows:

(1) *Increasing the activation of B cells, cytotoxic T cells, and suppressor T cells by antigens.* The B lymphocyte clones in the lymphoid tissue, as well as the cytotoxic T cells and suppressor T cell clones, are usually activated poorly by most antigens in the absence of helper T cells. In contrast, the helper T cell clones can be activated by very small quantities of antigens. Once the helper T cells have been activated, they in turn secrete "lymphokines" that enhance the response of the other types of lymphoid cells to the antigen as well.

(2) *Stimulation of the activity of other T cells.* The helper T cells secrete a substance called *interleukin 2,* one of the lymphokines, that increases the activity of other T cells, including cytotoxic T cells, some suppressor T cells, and probably even some of the other helper T cells.

(3) *Activation of the macrophage system.* The helper T cells secrete another lymphokine, called *macrophage migration inhibition factor,* that plays two important roles in the macrophage response to invading organisms. First, it slows or stops the migration of macrophages that have been chemotactically attracted into the infected tissue area, thus causing a great accumulation of macrophages. Second, it activates the macrophages to cause far more efficient phagocytosis, allowing them to attack and destroy greatly increased numbers of invading organisms.

Suppressor T Cells. Much less is known about the suppressor T cells than about the others, but they are capable of suppressing the functions of both cytotoxic and helper T cells. It is believed that these suppressor functions serve the purpose of regulating the activities of the other cells, keeping them from causing excessive immune reactions that might be severely damaging to the body. For this reason, the suppressor cells are frequently also called *regulatory T cells.* The suppressor T cells probably play an important role in limiting the ability of the immune system to attack a person's own body tissues, called *immune tolerance,* as we shall discuss in the following section.

TOLERANCE OF THE ACQUIRED IMMUNITY SYSTEM TO ONE'S OWN TISSUES—ROLE OF THE THYMUS AND THE BURSA

Obviously, if a person should become immune to his or her own tissues, the process of acquired immunity would destroy the individual's own body. Fortunately, the immune mechanism normally "recognizes" a person's own tissues as being completely distinctive from those of invaders, and his immunity system forms very few antibodies or activated T cells against his own antigens. This phenomenon is known as *tolerance* to the body's own tissues.

CYTOTOXIC T CELLS (KILLER CELLS)

Cytotoxic and digestive enzymes

Antigen receptors

ATTACKED CELL

Specific binding

Antigens

Figure 20–4. Direct destruction of an invading cell by sensitized lymphocytes.

Mechanism of Tolerance. It is believed that most of the phenomenon of tolerance develops during the processing of the T lymphocytes in the thymus and the B lymphocytes in the B lymphocyte processing area. The reason for this belief is that injecting a strong antigen into a fetus at the time that the lymphocytes are being processed in these two areas will prevent the development of clones of lymphocytes in the lymphoid tissue that are specific for the injected antigen.

Therefore, it is believed that during the processing of lymphocytes in the thymus and in the B lymphocyte processing area, all those clones of lymphocytes that are specific for the body's own tissues are self-destroyed because of their continual exposure to the body's antigens.

However, still another method by which tolerance might occur has recently been suggested, based on the suppressor function of the suppressor T cells. In a few instances it has been noted that increase in the number of suppressor cells is associated with reduced immunity against some antigens. Therefore, it is theoretically possible that immunity against the body's own antigens might be suppressed by strong development of specific suppressor T cells; as yet, this is not entirely clear.

Failure of the Tolerance Mechanism—Autoimmune Diseases. Unfortunately, people frequently lose some of their immune tolerance to their own tissues—that is, they do form immunity against certain of their own tissues. This is called *autoimmunity*. This occurs to a greater extent the older a person becomes. It usually occurs after destruction of some of the body's tissues, which releases considerable quantities of antigens that circulate in the body and presumably cause acquired immunity in the form of either activated T cells or antibodies.

Diseases that result from autoimmunity include *rheumatic fever*, in which the body becomes immunized against tissues in the joints and heart, especially the heart valves, following exposure to a specific type of streptococcal toxin; one type of *glomerulonephritis*, in which the person becomes immunized against the basement membranes of the glomeruli; *myasthenia gravis*, in which immunity develops against the acetylcholine receptor proteins of the neuromuscular junction, causing paralysis; and *lupus erythematosus*, in which the person becomes immunized against many different body tissues at the same time, a disease that causes extensive damage and often rapid death.

VACCINATION

The process of vaccination has been used for many years to cause acquired immunity against specific diseases. A person can be vaccinated by injecting dead organisms that are no longer capable of causing disease but which still have their chemical antigens. This type of vaccination is used to protect against typhoid fever, whooping cough, diphtheria, and many other types of bacterial diseases. Also, immunity can be achieved against toxins that have been treated with chemicals so that their toxic nature has been destroyed even though their antigens for causing immunity are still intact. This procedure is used in vaccinating against tetanus, botulism, and other similar toxic diseases. And, finally, a person can be vaccinated by infecting him with live organisms that have been "attenuated." That is, these organisms either have been grown in special culture mediums or have been passed through a series of animals until they have mutated enough that they will not cause disease but do still carry the specific antigens. This procedure is used to protect against poliomyelitis, yellow fever, measles, smallpox, and many other viral diseases.

ALLERGY

One of the important side effects of immunity is the development, under some conditions, of allergy. There are several different types of allergy, some of which can occur in any person. However, most allergies occur only in persons who have a specific allergic tendency.

The "allergic tendency" is genetically passed on from parent to child, and it is characterized by the presence of large quantities of the type of antibodies called IgE *antibodies*. These antibodies are called *reagins* or *sensitizing antibodies* to distinguish them from the more common IgG antibodies. When an *allergen* (defined as an antigen that reacts specifically with a specific type of IgE reagin antibody) enters the body, an allergen-reagin reaction takes place, and a subsequent allergic reaction takes place.

A special characteristic of the IgE antibodies (the reagins) is a strong propensity to attach to mast cells and basophils. Indeed, these cells can bind as many as half a million molecules of IgE antibodies. Then, when an antigen (an allergen) binds with the IgE antibodies attached to the mast cells or basophils, this causes an immediate change in the membrane of the cells, causing many of the mast cells and basophils to rupture; others release their granules without rupturing and also secrete additional substances not already preformed in the granules. Some of the many different substances that are either released immediately or secreted shortly thereafter include *histamine, slow-reacting substance of anaphylaxis, eosinophil chemotactic substance,* a *protease,* a *neutrophil chemotactic substance, heparin,* and *platelet activating factors.* These substances cause such phenomena as dilatation of the local blood vessels, attraction of eosinophils and neutrophils to the reactive site, damage to the local tissues by the protease, increased permeability of the capillaries with loss of fluid into the tissues, and contraction of local smooth muscle cells. Therefore, any number of different types of abnormal tissue responses can occur, depending upon the type of tissue in which the allergen-reagin reaction occurs. Among the different types of allergic reactions caused in this manner are:

Anaphylaxis. When a specific allergen is injected

directly into the circulation it can react in widespread areas of the body with the basophils of the blood and the mast cells located immediately outside the small blood vessels. Therefore, a widespread allergic reaction occurs throughout the vascular system and in closely associated tissues. This is called *anaphylaxis.* The *histamine* released into the circulation causes widespread peripheral vasodilatation as well as increased permeability of the capillaries and marked loss of plasma from the circulation. Often, persons experiencing this reaction die of circulatory shock within a few minutes unless treated with norepinephrine to oppose the effects of the histamine. But also released from the cells is the substance called *slow-reacting substance of anaphylaxis,* which sometimes causes spasm of the smooth muscle of the bronchioles, eliciting an asthma-like attack and sometimes causing death by suffocation.

Urticaria. Urticaria results from antigen entering specific skin areas and causing localized anaphylactoid reactions. *Histamine* released locally causes (a) vasodilatation that induces an immediate *red flare* and (b) increased permeability of the capillaries that leads to swelling of the skin in another few minutes. The swellings are commonly called "hives."

Hay Fever. In hay fever, the allergen-reagin reaction occurs in the nose. *Histamine* released in response to this causes rapid fluid leakage into the tissues of the nose, and the nasal linings become swollen and secretory.

Asthma. In asthma, the allergen-reagin reaction occurs in the bronchioles of the lungs. Here, the most important product released from the mast cells seems to be the *slow-reacting substance of anaphylaxis,* which causes spasm of the bronchiolar smooth muscle. Consequently, the person has difficulty breathing until the reactive products of the allergic reaction have been removed.

BLOOD GROUPS AND BLOOD TRANSFUSION

ANTIGENICITY AND IMMUNE REACTIONS OF BLOOD

When blood transfusions from one person to another were first attempted the transfusions were successful in some instances, but in many more immediate or delayed agglutination and hemolysis of the red blood cells occurred. Soon it was discovered that the bloods of different persons usually have different antigenic and immune properties, so that antibodies in the plasma of one blood react with antigens on the surfaces of the red cells of another. Furthermore, the antigens and the antibodies are almost never precisely the same in one person as in another. For this reason, it is easy for blood from a donor to be mismatched with that of a recipient. Fortunately, if proper precautions are taken, one can determine ahead of time whether or not appropriate antibodies and antigens are present in the donor and recipient bloods to cause

a reaction, but, on the other hand, lack of proper precautions often results in varying degrees of red cell agglutination and hemolysis, resulting in a typical *transfusion reaction* that can lead to death.

Multiplicity of Antigens in the Blood Cells. At least 30 commonly occurring antigens, each of which can at times cause antigen-antibody reactions, have been found in human blood cells, especially on the surfaces of the cell membranes.

Two particular groups of antigens are more likely than the others to cause blood transfusion reactions. These are the so-called *O-A-B* system of antigens and the *Rh* system. Bloods are divided into different *groups* and *types* in accordance with the types of antigens present in the cells.

O-A-B BLOOD GROUPS

The A and B Antigens, Called Agglutinogens

Two related antigens—type A and type B—occur on the surfaces of the red blood cells in a large proportion of the population. Because of the way these antigens are inherited, people may have neither of them on their cells, they may have one, or they may have both simultaneously.

Strong antibodies that react specifically with either the type A or type B antigen almost always occur in the plasmas of persons who do not have the antigens on their red cells. These antibodies bind with the red cell antigens to cause agglutination of the red cells. Therefore, the type A and type B antigens are called *agglutinogens,* and the plasma antibodies that cause the agglutination are called *agglutinins.* It is on the basis of the presence or absence of the agglutinogens in the red blood cells that blood is grouped for the purpose of transfusion.

The Four Major O-A-B Blood Groups. In transfusing blood from one person to another, the bloods of donors and recipients are normally classified into four major O-A-B groups, as illustrated in Table 20–1, depending on the presence or absence of the two agglutinogens. When neither A nor B agglutinogen is present, the blood group is *group O.* When only type A agglutinogen is present, the blood is *group A.* When only type B agglutinogen is present, the blood is *group B.* And when both A and B agglutinogens are present, the blood is *group AB.*

Table 20–1. THE BLOOD GROUPS WITH THEIR GENOTYPES AND THEIR CONSTITUENT AGGLUTINOGENS AND AGGLUTININS

Genotypes	Blood Groups	Agglutinogens	Agglutinins
O O	O	—	Anti-A and Anti-B
OA or AA	A	A	Anti-B
OB or BB	B	B	Anti-A
AB	AB	A and B	—

The Agglutinins

When type A agglutinogen *is not present* in a person's red blood cells, antibodies known as *anti-A agglutinins* develop in his plasma. Also, when type B agglutinogen *is not present* in the red blood cells, antibodies known as *anti-B agglutinins* develop in the plasma.

Thus referring once again to Table 20–1, it will be observed that group O blood, though containing no agglutinogens, does contain both *anti-A* and *anti-B agglutinins,* while group A blood contains type A agglutinogens and *anti-B agglutinins,* and group B blood contains type B agglutinogens and *anti-A agglutinins.* Finally, group AB blood contains both A and B agglutinogens but no agglutinins at all.

Origin of Agglutinins in the Plasma. The agglutinins are gamma globulins, as are other antibodies, and are produced by the same cells that produce antibodies to any other antigens.

But why are these agglutinins produced in individuals who do not have the antigenic substances in their red blood cells? The answer to this seems to be that small amounts of group A and B antigens enter the body in the food, in bacteria, and in other ways, and these substances initiate the development of the anti-A or anti-B agglutinins. The newborn baby has few if any agglutinins, showing that agglutinin formation occurs almost entirely after birth.

The Agglutination Process in Transfusion Reactions

When bloods are mismatched so that anti-A or anti-B agglutinins are mixed with red blood cells containing A or B agglutinogens respectively, the red cells agglutinate by the following process: The agglutinins attach themselves to the red blood cells. Because the agglutinins have at least two binding sites, a single agglutinin can attach to two or more different red blood cells at the same time, thereby causing the cells to adhere to each other. This causes the cells to clump. Then these clumps plug small blood vessels throughout the circulatory system. During the ensuing few hours to few days, the phagocytic white blood cells destroy the agglutinated cells, releasing hemoglobin into the plasma.

Hemolysis in Transfusion Reactions. Sometimes, when recipient and donor bloods are mismatched, immediate hemolysis of red cells occurs in the circulating blood. In this case the antibodies cause lysis of the red blood cells by activating the complement system. This in turn releases proteolytic enzymes (the *lytic complex*) that rupture the cell membranes, as was described earlier in the chapter.

However, immediate intravascular hemolysis is far less common than agglutination, because not only does there have to be a very high titer of antibodies for this to occur but also a different type of antibody seems to be required, mainly the IgM antibodies; these antibodies are called *hemolysins.* However, even agglutination eventually leads to hemolysis of

Table 20–2. BLOOD TYPING—SHOWING AGGLUTINATION OF CELLS OF THE DIFFERENT BLOOD GROUPS WITH ANTI-A AND ANTI-B AGGLUTININS

Red Blood Cells	Sera	
	Anti-A	Anti-B
O	–	–
A	+	–
B	–	+
AB	+	+

the agglutinated red cells because the phagocytic white blood cells rupture the agglutinated cells within a few hours after agglutination has taken place.

Blood Typing

Prior to giving a transfusion, it is necessary to determine the blood group of the recipient and the group of the donor blood so that the bloods will be appropriately matched. This is called *blood typing,* and it is performed in the following way: The red blood cells are first diluted with saline. One portion is then mixed with anti-A agglutinin while another portion is mixed with anti-B agglutinin. After several minutes, each mixture is observed under a microscope. If the red blood cells have become clumped—that is, "agglutinated"—one knows that an antibody-antigen reaction has resulted.

Table 20–2 illustrates the reactions that occur with each of the four different types of blood. Group O red blood cells have no agglutinogens and, therefore, do not react with either the anti-A or the anti-B serum. Group A blood has A agglutinogens and therefore agglutinates with anti-A agglutinins. Group B blood has B agglutinogens and agglutinates with anti-B serum. Group AB blood has both A and B agglutinogens and agglutinates with both types of serum.

THE Rh BLOOD TYPES

In addition to the O-A-B blood group system, several other systems are sometimes important in the transfusion of blood. The most important of these is the Rh system. The one major difference between the O-A-B system and the Rh system is the following: In the O-A-B system, the agglutinins responsible for causing transfusion reactions develop spontaneously, whereas in the Rh system spontaneous agglutinins almost never occur. Instead, the person must first be massively exposed to an Rh antigen, usually by transfusion of blood, before enough agglutinins to cause a significant transfusion reaction will develop.

The Rh Antigens—"Rh Positive" and "Rh Negative" Persons. There are six common types of Rh antigens, each of which is called an Rh factor. However, one of these, called the *type D antigen,* is widely prevalent in the population and is also considerably more antigenic than the other Rh antigens. Therefore, anyone who has this type of Rh antigen is said to be *Rh positive,* whereas those persons who do not have type D antigen are said to be *Rh negative*. However, it must be noted that even in Rh negative persons some of the other Rh antigens can still cause transfusion reactions.

The Rh Immune Response

Formation of Anti-Rh Agglutinins. When red blood cells containing Rh factor, or even protein breakdown products of such cells, are injected into a person without the factor—that is, into the Rh negative person—anti-Rh agglutinins develop very slowly, the maximum concentration of agglutinins occurring approximately two to four months later. This immune response occurs to a much greater extent in some people than in others. On multiple exposure to the Rh factor, the Rh negative person eventually becomes strongly "sensitized" to the Rh factor—that is, he or she develops a very high titer of anti-Rh agglutinins.

Characteristics of Rh Transfusion Reactions. If an Rh negative person has never before been exposed to Rh positive blood, transfusion of Rh positive blood into him causes no immediate reaction at all. However, in some of these persons anti-Rh antibodies develop in sufficient quantities during the next two to four weeks to cause agglutination of the transfused cells that are still in the blood. These cells are then hemolyzed by the tissue macrophage system. Thus, a delayed transfusion reaction occurs, though it is usually mild. Yet, on subsequent transfusion of Rh positive blood into the same person, who is now immunized against the Rh factor, the transfusion reaction is greatly enhanced and can be as severe as the reactions that occur with types A and B bloods.

Erythroblastosis Fetalis

Erythroblastosis fetalis is a disease of the fetus and newborn infant characterized by progressive agglutination and subsequent phagocytosis of the red blood cells. In most instances of erythroblastosis fetalis the mother is Rh negative, and the father is Rh positive; the baby has inherited the Rh positive characteristic from the father, and the mother has developed anti-Rh agglutinins that have diffused through the placenta into the fetus to cause red blood cell agglutination.

Incidence of the Disease. An Rh negative mother having her first Rh positive child usually does not develop sufficient anti-Rh agglutinins to cause any harm. However, an Rh negative mother having her second Rh positive child often will have become "sensitized" by the first child and therefore will often develop anti-Rh agglutinins rapidly upon becoming pregnant with the second child. Approximately 3 per cent of these second babies exhibit some signs of erythroblastosis fetalis; approximately 10 per cent of the third babies exhibit the disease; and the incidence rises progressively with subsequent pregnancies.

The Rh negative mother develops anti-Rh agglutinins only when the fetus is Rh positive. Therefore,

after an erythroblastotic child has been born, it is not certain that future children will also be erythroblastotic.

Effect of the Mother's Antibodies on the Fetus. After anti-Rh antibodies have formed in the mother, they diffuse very slowly through the placental membrane into the fetus' blood. There they cause slow agglutination of the fetus' blood. The agglutinated red blood cells gradually hemolyze, releasing hemoglobin into the blood. The macrophages then convert the hemoglobin into bilirubin, which causes yellowness (jaundice) of the skin. The antibodies probably also attack and damage many of the other cells of the body.

Clinical Picture of Erythroblastosis. The newborn, jaundiced, erythroblastotic baby is usually anemic at birth, and the anti-Rh agglutinins from the mother usually circulate in the baby's blood for one to two months after birth, destroying more and more red blood cells.

The hemopoietic tissues of the baby attempt to replace the hemolyzing red blood cells. The liver and the spleen become greatly enlarged and produce red blood cells in the same manner that they normally do during the middle of gestation. Because of the very rapid production of cells, many early forms, including many nucleated blastic forms, are emptied into the circulatory system, and it is because of the presence of these in the blood that the disease has been called "erythroblastosis fetalis."

Though the severe anemia of erythroblastosis fetalis is usually the cause of death, many children who barely survive from the anemia exhibit permanent mental impairment or damage to motor areas of the brain because of precipitation of bilirubin in the neuronal cells, causing their destruction, a condition called *kernicterus*.

Treatment of the Erythroblastotic Baby. The usual treatment for erythroblastosis fetalis is to replace the newborn infant's blood with Rh negative blood. Approximately 400 ml of Rh negative blood is infused over a period of 1.5 or more hours while the baby's own Rh positive blood is being removed.

ACUTE KIDNEY SHUTDOWN FOLLOWING TRANSFUSION REACTIONS

One of the most lethal effects of transfusion reactions is acute kidney shutdown, which can begin within a few minutes to a few hours and continue until the person dies of renal failure.

The kidney shutdown seems to result from three different causes: First, the antigen-antibody reaction of the transfusion reaction releases toxic substances from the hemolyzing blood that cause powerful renal vasoconstriction. Second, the loss of circulating red cells along with production of toxic substances from the hemolyzed cells and from the immune reaction often causes circulatory shock; the arterial blood pressure falls very low and the renal blood flow and urinary output decrease. Third, if the total amount of free hemoglobin in the circulating blood rises above a critical level, much of it leaks through the glomerular membranes into the kidney tubules. If this amount is still slight, it can be reabsorbed through the tubular epithelium into the blood and will cause no harm, but, if it is great, then only a small percentage is reabsorbed. Yet water continues to be reabsorbed, causing the tubular hemoglobin concentration to rise so high that it precipitates and blocks many of the tubules. Thus, renal vasoconstriction, circulatory shock, and tubular blockage all add together to cause acute renal shutdown. If the shutdown is complete, the patient can die within a week to 12 days, as explained in Chapter 26, unless treated with the artificial kidney.

TRANSPLANTATION OF TISSUES AND ORGANS

In this modern age of surgery, many attempts are being made to transplant tissues and organs from one person to another, or, occasionally, from lower animals to the human being. Many of the different antigenic proteins of red blood cells that cause transfusion reactions plus still many more are present in the other cells of the body as well. Consequently, any foreign cells transplanted into a recipient can cause immune responses and immune reactions. In other words, most recipients are just as able to resist invasion by foreign cells as to resist invasion by foreign bacteria.

Except for transplantations between identical twins, who have identical antigen types, immune reactions almost always occur, causing death of all the cells in the graft within two to five weeks after transplantation unless some specific therapy is used to prevent the immune reaction. However, when the tissues are properly "typed" and are very similar prior to transplant, completely successful transplantations occasionally result.

Some of the different cellular tissues and organs that have been transplanted either experimentally or for therapeutic benefit from one person to another are skin, kidney, heart, liver, glandular tissue, bone marrow, and lung. Many kidney transplants have been successful for as long as five to ten years and a few liver and heart transplants for one to ten years.

Tissue Typing

In the same way that red blood cells can be typed to prevent reactions between recipient and donor, so also is it possible to "type" tissues to help prevent graft rejection, though thus far this procedure has met with far less success than has been achieved in red blood cell typing.

The most important antigens that cause transplant rejection are a group of antigens called the HLA antigens. This is a group of about 100 different antigens, which occur in the white blood cells as well as in the tissue cells. Therefore, tissues can be typed by typing these antigens in the membranes of lymphocytes that have been separated from the person's blood, using methods similar to those used for blood typing.

Prevention of Graft Rejection by Suppressing the Immune System

Obviously, if the immune system were completely suppressed, graft rejection would not occur. In fact, in an occasional person who has serious depression of the immune system, grafts can be successful without the use of any therapy at all to prevent rejection. However, in the normal person, even with the best possible tissue typing, grafts will rarely resist rejection for more than a few weeks to few months without the employment of some therapeutic procedure to suppress the immune system. Some of the therapeutic agents that have been used for this purpose include the following:

(1) *Glucocorticoid hormones (or drugs with glucocorticoid activity)*, which suppress the growth of all lymphoid tissue.

(2) *Various drugs that have a toxic effect on the lymphoid system* and therefore block the formation of antibodies and T cells, especially the drug azathioprine (Imuran).

(3) *Cyclosporin A*, which has a specific cytotoxic effect on T cells and therefore is especially efficacious in blocking the rejection reaction.

Unfortunately, use of these agents leaves the person unprotected from disease; therefore, bacterial and viral infections sometimes become rampant. In addition, the incidence of cancer is several times greater in an immunosuppressed person, presumably because the immune system is important in destroying many early cancers before they can begin to develop.

QUESTIONS

1. What is the difference between *innate immunity* and *acquired immunity*?
2. Characterize the two different types of acquired immunity.
3. What is an *antigen*, and what are its characteristics?
4. What are the roles of lymphoid tissue in acquired immunity?
5. What are the differences between *T lymphocytes* and *B lymphocytes*?
6. Explain the preprocessing of T lymphocytes in the thymus gland.
7. Explain the preprocessing of B lymphocytes in other tissues of the body, probably the liver.
8. What is meant by a *lymphocyte clone*?

9. Explain how a clone of lymphocytes is activated. What is the role of macrophages in this activation?
10. Describe the antibodies. What are the *light* and *heavy polypeptide chains?* Also, what is meant by the *variable portion* and the *constant portion* of the light and heavy polypeptide chains?
11. What are the different actions of antibodies?
12. How does the complement system enter into antibody actions?
13. What are the three different types of T cells?
14. Explain how *cytotoxic T cells* kill microorganisms.
15. Explain how *helper T cells* help other portions of the immune system to become activated.
16. What are possible regulatory functions of the *suppressor T cells?*
17. What is the mechanism of *tolerance?*
18. Explain how *autoimmune diseases* develop.
19. What type of antibodies frequently causes allergy, and what is the relationship of these antibodies to mast cells and basophils?
20. What are some of the allergic conditions experienced by different persons?
21. Characterize the *O-A-B blood group system.*
22. What are the *agglutinogens* and the *agglutinins?*
23. Explain how transfusion reactions occur.
24. Explain the differences between transfusion reactions caused by the Rh blood types and the O-A-B blood types.
25. Explain the development of *erythroblastosis fetalis.*
26. Why do transfusion reactions occasionally cause acute kidney shutdown?
27. Explain *tissue typing* for the transplantation of tissues and organs.
28. What is the importance of suppressing the immune system in the prevention of transplant rejection?

References

Immunity

Atassi, M. Z.: Antigenic structures of proteins. Eur J Biochem 145:1, 1984.

Beer, D. J., et al.: The influence of histamine on immune and inflammatory responses. Adv Immunol 35:209, 1984.

Bloch, E. F., and Malveaux, F. J.: The significance of immunoglobulin E in resistance to parasitic infections. Ann Allergy 54:83, 1985.

Caterson, B., et al.: Production and characterization of monoclonal antibodies directed against connective tissue proteoglycans. Fed Proc 44:386, 1985.

Cooper, J., et al.: Network regulation among T cells: Qualitative and quantitative studies on suppression in the non-immune state. Immunol Rev 79:63, 1984.

Coutinho, A., et al.: T-cell–dependent B cell activation. Immunol Rev 78:211, 1984.

Ford-Hutchinson, A. W.: Leukotrienes: their formation and role as inflammatory mediators. Fed Proc 44:25, 1985.

Gatenby, P. A., et al.: T cells, T cell subsets and immunoregulation. Aust NZ J Med 14:89, 1984.

Kendall, M. D.: Have we underestimated the importance of the thymus in man? Experientia 40:1181, 1984.

McNamara, M., et al.: T-cell helper circuits. Immunol Rev 79:87, 1984.

Muraguchi, A., et al.: Regulation of human B-cell activation, proliferation, and differentiation by soluble factors. J Clin Immunol 4:337, 1984.

Piper, P. J.: Formation and actions of leukotrienes. Physiol Rev 64:744, 1984.

Takemore, T., and Rajewsky, K.: Mechanism of neonatally induced idiotype suppression and its relevance for the acquisition of self-tolerance. Immunol Rev 79:103, 1984.

Vitetta, E. S., et al.: T-cell–derived lymphokines that induce IgM and IgG secretion in activated murine B cells. Immunol Rev 78:137, 1984.

Blood Groups, Transfusion, and Transplantation

Ascher, N. L., et al.: Cellular basis of allograft rejection. Immunol Rev 77:217, 1984.

Colvin, R. B.: Flow cytometric analysis of T cells: diagnostic applications in transplantation. Ann NY Acad Sci 428:5, 1984.

Demetris, A. J., et al.: Pathology of hepatic transplantation: a review of 62 adult allograft recipients immunosuppressed with a cyclosporin/steroid regimen. Am J Pathol 118:151, 1985.

Hancock, W. W.: Analysis of intragraft effector mechanisms associated with human renal allograft rejection: immunohistological studies with monoclonal antibodies. Immunol Rev 77:61, 1984.

Hobbs, J. R., ed.: Thymic Factor Therapy. New York, Raven Press, 1985.

Hunt, S. A., and Stinson, E. B.: Cardiac transplantation. Annu Rev Med 32:213, 1981.

Kahan, B. D., et al.: Clinical and experimental studies with cyclosporine in renal transplantation. Surgery 97:125, 1985.

Mohn, J. F., et al., eds.: Human Blood Groups. New York, S. Karger, 1977.

Wood, R. F.: Renal Transplantation. A Clinical Handbook. Philadelphia, W. B. Saunders Co., 1984.

21

Hemostasis and Blood Coagulation

EVENTS IN HEMOSTASIS
  VASCULAR SPASM
  FORMATION OF THE PLATELET PLUG
  BLOOD COAGULATION IN THE
    RUPTURED VESSEL
  FIBROUS ORGANIZATION OR
    DISSOLUTION OF THE BLOOD
    CLOT
MECHANISM OF BLOOD
  COAGULATION
  GENERAL MECHANISM
  CONVERSION OF PROTHROMBIN TO
    THROMBIN
  CONVERSION OF FIBRINOGEN TO
    FIBRIN—FORMATION OF THE
    CLOT
  THE VICIOUS CIRCLE OF CLOT
    FORMATION
  INITIATION OF COAGULATION:
    FORMATION OF PROTHROMBIN
    ACTIVATOR

PREVENTION OF BLOOD CLOTTING
  IN THE NORMAL VASCULAR
  SYSTEM—THE INTRAVASCULAR
  ANTICOAGULANTS
LYSIS OF BLOOD CLOTS—PLASMIN
CONDITIONS THAT CAUSE EXCESSIVE
  BLEEDING IN HUMAN BEINGS
  DECREASED PROTHROMBIN, FACTOR
    VII, FACTOR IX, AND FACTOR X
    CAUSED BY VITAMIN K
    DEFICIENCY
  HEMOPHILIA
  THROMBOCYTOPENIA
THROMBOEMBOLIC CONDITIONS IN
  THE HUMAN BEING
  FEMORAL THROMBOSIS AND
    MASSIVE PULMONARY EMBOLISM
  DISSEMINATED INTRAVASCULAR
    CLOTTING

EVENTS IN HEMOSTASIS

The term *hemostasis* means prevention of blood loss. Whenever a vessel is severed or ruptured, hemostasis is achieved by several different mechanisms, including (1) vascular spasm, (2) formation of a platelet plug, (3) blood coagulation, and (4) eventual growth of fibrous tissue into the blood clot to close the hole in the vessel permanently.

VASCULAR SPASM

Immediately after a blood vessel is cut or ruptured, the stimulus of the traumatized vessel causes the wall of the vessel to contract; this instantaneously reduces the flow of blood from the vessel rupture. The contraction results from both nervous reflexes and local myogenic spasm. The nervous reflexes presumably are initiated by pain or other impulses originating from the traumatized vessel or from nearby tissues. However, most of the spasm probably results from local myogenic contraction of the blood vessel initiated by direct damage to the vascular wall, which presumably causes transmission of action potentials along the vessel wall for several centimeters and results in constriction of the vessel. The more of the vessel that is traumatized, the greater the degree of spasm; this means that a sharply cut blood vessel usually bleeds much more than does a vessel ruptured by crushing. This local vascular spasm can last for many minutes or even hours, during which time the ensuing processes of platelet plugging and blood coagulation can take place.

FORMATION OF THE PLATELET PLUG

If the rent in the blood vessel is very small—and many very small vascular holes do develop each day—it is often sealed by a *platelet plug* rather than by a blood clot. To understand this, it is important that we first discuss the nature of platelets themselves.

Physical and Chemical Characteristics of Platelets

Platelets are minute round or oval discs 2 to 4 microns in diameter. They are formed in the bone marrow from *megakaryocytes*, which are extremely large cells of the hemopoietic series in the bone marrow that do not themselves leave the marrow to enter the blood. Instead, platelets form as buds on the surfaces of the megakaryocytes and pinch off to be released into the blood. The normal concentration of platelets in the blood is between 150,000 and 350,000 per cubic millimeter.

In the cytoplasm of platelets are such active factors as (1) *actin* and *myosin molecules*, similar to those found in muscle cells, that can cause the platelets to contract; (2) enzyme systems that are capable of forming *ATP* and *ADP*; (3) enzyme systems that synthesize *prostaglandins*, which are local hormones that cause many different types of vascular and other local tissue reactions; (4) an important protein called *fibrin-stabilizing factor*, which we will discuss later in relation to blood coagulation; and (5) a *growth factor* that can cause vascular endothelial cells, vascular smooth muscle cells, and fibroblasts to multiply and grow, thus causing cellular growth that helps repair damaged vascular walls.

The cell membrane of the platelets is also important. On the surface is a coat of *glycoproteins* that causes the membrane to adhere to injured areas of the vessel wall, especially to injured endothelial cells and even more so to any exposed collagen from deeper in the vessel wall. In addition, the membrane contains large amounts of *phospholipids* that can activate one of the blood-clotting systems, the so-called intrinsic system that we shall discuss later.

Mechanism of the Platelet Plug. Platelet repair of vascular openings is based on several important functions of the platelet itself: When platelets come in contact with a damaged vascular surface, such as the collagen fibers in the vascular wall or even damaged endothelial cells, they immediately change their characteristics drastically. They begin to swell; they assume irregular forms with numerous irradiating processes protruding from their surfaces; they become sticky so that they stick to the collagen fibers; and they secrete large quantities of *ADP*, and their enzymes form *thromboxane A*, a type of prostaglandin, that is also secreted by the platelets into the blood. The ADP and thromboxane A, in turn, act on nearby platelets to activate them as well, and the stickiness of these additional platelets causes them to adhere to the originally activated platelets. Therefore, at the site of any rent in a vessel, the damaged vascular wall or extravascular tissues elicit a vicious cycle of activation of successively increasing numbers of platelets; these accumulate to form a *platelet plug*. This is a fairly loose plug, but it is usually successful in blocking the blood loss if the vascular opening is small. Then, during the subsequent process of blood coagulation, to be described in subsequent paragraphs, *fibrin threads* form that attach to the platelets, thus forming a tight and unyielding plug.

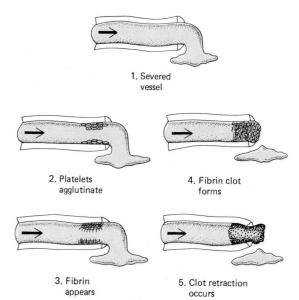

1. Severed vessel

2. Platelets agglutinate

3. Fibrin appears

4. Fibrin clot forms

5. Clot retraction occurs

Figure 21–1. The clotting process in the traumatized blood vessel. (Modified from Seegers: Hemostatic Agents. Courtesy of Charles C Thomas Publisher, Springfield, Illinois.)

BLOOD COAGULATION IN THE RUPTURED VESSEL

The third mechanism for hemostasis is formation of the blood clot. The clot begins to develop in 15 to 20 seconds if the trauma of the vascular wall has been severe and in 1 to 2 minutes if the trauma has been minor. Activator substances from the traumatized vascular wall, from platelets, and blood proteins adhering to the traumatized vascular wall initiate the clotting process. The physical events of this process are illustrated in Figure 21–1, and the chemical events will be discussed in detail later in the chapter.

Within three to six minutes after rupture of a vessel, if the vessel opening is not too large, the entire opening is filled with clot. After 30 minutes to an hour, the clot retracts; this closes the vessel still further. Platelets play an important role in this clot retraction, as will also be discussed later in the chapter.

FIBROUS ORGANIZATION OR DISSOLUTION OF THE BLOOD CLOT

Once a blood clot has formed, it can follow two separate courses: it can become invaded by fibroblasts, which subsequently form connective tissue all through the clot; or it can dissolve. The usual course for a clot that forms in a small hole of a vessel wall is invasion by fibroblasts, beginning within a few hours after the clot is formed (which is promoted at least partially by a *growth factor* secreted by platelets) and continuing to complete organization of the clot into fibrous tissue within approximately seven to ten days. On the other hand, when a large amount of blood coagulates to form one large blood clot, such as blood that has leaked into tissues, special substances within the clot itself become activated, and these then function as enzymes to dissolve the clot itself, as will be discussed later in the chapter.

MECHANISM OF BLOOD COAGULATION

Basic Theory. Over 40 different substances that affect blood coagulation have been found in the blood and tissues, some promoting coagulation, called *procoagulants*, and others inhibiting coagulation, called *anticoagulants*. Whether or not the blood will coagulate depends on the balance between these two groups of substances. Normally the anticoagulants predominate and the blood does not coagulate, but when a vessel is ruptured the activity of the procoagulants in the area of damage becomes much greater than that of the anticoagulants, and then a clot does develop.

GENERAL MECHANISM

All research workers in the field of blood coagulation agree that clotting takes place in three essential steps:

First, a substance or complex of substances called *prothrombin activator* is formed in response to rupture of the vessel or damage to the blood itself.

Second, the prothrombin activator catalyzes the conversion of *prothrombin* into *thrombin*.

Third, the thrombin acts as an enzyme to convert *fibrinogen* into *fibrin threads* that enmesh platelets, blood cells, and plasma to form the clot itself.

Let us first discuss the mechanism by which the blood clot itself is formed, beginning with the second of the above steps, the conversion of prothrombin to thrombin; then we will come back to the first stage in the clotting process in which prothrombin activator is formed.

CONVERSION OF PROTHROMBIN TO THROMBIN

After prothrombin activator has been formed as a result of rupture of the blood vessel or as a result of damage to special activator substances in the blood itself, the prothrombin activator can then cause conversion of prothrombin to thrombin, which in turn causes polymerization of fibrinogen molecules into fibrin threads within another 10 to 15 seconds. Thus the rate-limiting factor in causing blood coagulation is usually the formation of prothrombin activator and not the subsequent reactions beyond that point, for these normally occur very rapidly to form the clot itself.

Prothrombin and Thrombin. Prothrombin is a plasma protein formed by the liver, an alpha$_2$-globulin, having a molecular weight of 68,700. It is present in normal plasma in a concentration of about 15 mg/dl. It is an unstable protein that can easily split into smaller compounds, one of which is *thrombin*, with a molecular weight of 33,700, almost exactly half that of prothrombin.

Effect of Prothrombin Activator on Forming Thrombin from Prothrombin. Figure 21–2 illus-

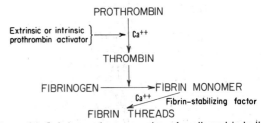

Figure 21–2. Schema for conversion of prothrombin to thrombin, and polymerization of fibrinogen to form fibrin threads.

trates the conversion of prothrombin to thrombin under the influence of prothrombin activator and calcium ions. The rate of formation of thrombin from prothrombin is almost directly proportional to the quantity of prothrombin activator available, which itself is approximately proportional to the degree of trauma to the vessel wall or to the blood.

CONVERSION OF FIBRINOGEN TO FIBRIN—FORMATION OF THE CLOT

Fibrinogen. Fibrinogen is a high molecular weight protein (340,000) also formed in the liver and occurring in the plasma in quantities of 100 to 700 mg/dl.

Action of Thrombin on Fibrinogen to Form Fibrin. Thrombin is a protein *enzyme* with proteolytic capabilities. It acts on fibrinogen to remove four low molecular weight peptides from each molecule of fibrinogen, forming a molecule of *fibrin monomer* that has the automatic capability of polymerizing with other fibrin monomer molecules. Therefore, many fibrin monomer molecules polymerize within seconds into *long fibrin threads* that form the *reticulum* of the clot.

In the early stages of this polymerization, the fibrin monomer molecules are held together by weak noncovalent bonds, and the threads also are not cross-linked with each other; therefore, the resultant clot is weak and can be broken apart with ease. However, still another process occurs during the following few minutes that greatly strengthens the fibrin reticulum. This process involves a substance called *fibrin-stabilizing factor* that is normally present in small amounts in the plasma globulins but that is also released from platelets entrapped in the clot. This substance operates as an enzyme to cause *covalent* bonds between the fibrin monomer molecules as well as multiple cross-linkages between the adjacent fibrin threads, thus adding tremendously to the three-dimensional strength of the fibrin meshwork.

The Blood Clot. The clot is composed of a meshwork of fibrin threads running in all directions and entrapping blood cells, platelets, and plasma. The fibrin threads adhere to damaged surfaces of blood vessels; therefore, the blood clot becomes adherent to any vascular opening and thereby prevents blood loss.

Clot Retraction—Serum. Within a few minutes after a clot is formed, it begins to contract and usually expresses most of the fluid from the clot within 30 to 60 minutes. The fluid expressed is called *serum*, because all its fibrinogen and most of the other clotting factors have been removed; in this way, serum differs from plasma. Serum obviously cannot clot because of lack of these factors.

Platelets are necessary for clot retraction to occur. Therefore, failure of clot retraction is an indication that the number of platelets in the circulating blood is low. Electron micrographs of platelets in blood clots show that they become attached to the fibrin threads in such a way that they actually bond different threads together. Furthermore, platelets entrapped in the clot continue to release procoagulant substances, one of which is fibrin-stabilizing factor that causes more and more cross-linking bonds between the adjacent fibrin threads. In addition, the platelets themselves contribute directly to clot contraction by activating the platelet actin and myosin molecules, which are contractile proteins and cause strong contraction of the platelet spicules attached to the fibrin.

As the clot retracts, the edges of the broken blood vessel are pulled together, thus probably contributing to the ultimate state of hemostasis.

THE VICIOUS CIRCLE OF CLOT FORMATION

Once a blood clot has started to develop, it normally extends within minutes into the surrounding blood. That is, the clot itself initiates a vicious circle to promote more clotting. One of the most important causes of this reaction is the proteolytic action of thrombin which activates many of the other blood-clotting factors in addition to fibrinogen. For instance, thrombin has a direct proteolytic effect on prothrombin itself, tending to split this into still more thrombin, and it also acts on some of the blood-clotting factors responsible for the formation of prothrombin activator.

INITIATION OF COAGULATION: FORMATION OF PROTHROMBIN ACTIVATOR

Now that we have discussed the clotting process initiated by the formation of thrombin from prothrombin, we must turn to the more complex mechanisms that activate the prothrombin. These mechanisms all lead to the formation of *prothrombin activator*, which then causes prothrombin conversion to thrombin.

Prothrombin activator can be formed in two basic ways: (1) by the *extrinsic pathway* that begins with trauma to the vascular wall and surrounding tissues, or (2) by the *intrinsic pathway* that begins with trauma of the blood itself.

In both the extrinsic and intrinsic pathways a series of different plasma proteins, especially beta-globulins, play major roles. These, along with the other factors already discussed that enter into the clotting process, are called *blood-clotting factors* and for the most part they are inactive forms of proteolytic enzymes. When converted to the active forms, their enzymatic actions cause the successive, cascading reactions of the clotting process.

Table 21–1. CLOTTING FACTORS IN THE BLOOD AND THEIR SYNONYMS

Clotting Factor	Synonym
Fibrinogen	Factor I
Prothrombin	Factor II
Tissue thromboplastin	Factor III; tissue factor
Calcium	Factor IV
Factor V	Proaccelerin; labile factor; Ac-globulin; Ac-G
Factor VII	Serum prothrombin conversion accelerator; proconvertin; SPCA; stable factor
Factor VIII	Antihemophilic factor, AHF; antihemophilic globulin, AHG; antihemophilic factor A
Factor IX	Plasma thromboplastin component, PTC; Christmas factor; antihemophilic factor B
Factor X	Stuart factor; Stuart-Prower factor
Factor XI	Plasma thromboplastin antecedent, PTA; antihemophilic factor C
Factor XII	Hageman factor
Factor XIII	Fibrin-stabilizing factor
Platelets	

Most of the clotting factors are designated by Roman numerals, as listed in Table 21–1.

The Extrinsic Mechanism for Initiating Clotting

The extrinsic mechanism for initiating the formation of prothrombin activator begins with blood coming in contact with traumatized vascular wall or extravascular tissues and occurs according to the following three basic steps, as illustrated in Figure 21–3.

(1) *Release of tissue thromboplastin.* Traumatized tissue releases a complex of several factors called *tissue thromboplastin.* This includes especially *phospholipids* from the membranes of the tissues and at least one important *glycoprotein*, which functions as a *proteolytic enzyme.*

(2) *Activation of factor X to form activated factor X—role of factor VII and tissue factor.* The tissue glycoprotein complexes with blood coagulation factor VII, and this complex, in the presence of tissue phospholipids, acts enzymatically on factor X to form *activated factor X.*

(3) *Effect of activated factor X to form prothrombin activator—role of factor V.* The activated factor X complexes immediately with the tissue phospholipids released as part of the tissue thromboplastin and also with factor V to form the complex called *prothrombin activator.* Within a few seconds this splits prothrombin to form thrombin, and the clotting process proceeds as has already been explained.

The Intrinsic Mechanism for Initiating Clotting

The second mechanism for initiating the formation of prothrombin activator, and therefore for initiating clotting, begins with trauma to the blood itself and

EXTRINSIC PATHWAY

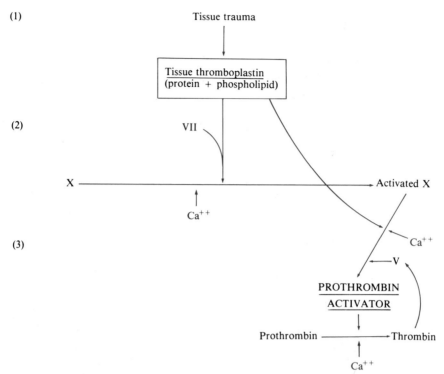

Figure 21–3. The extrinsic pathway for initiating blood clotting.

continues through the following series of cascading reactions, as illustrated in Figure 21–4.

(1) *Activation of factor XII and release of platelet phospholipids by blood trauma.* Trauma to the blood alters two important clotting factors in the blood—factor XII and the platelets. When factor XII is disturbed, for example, by coming into contact with collagen or with a wettable surface such as glass, it takes on a new configuration that converts it into a proteolytic enzyme called activated factor XII.

Simultaneously, the blood trauma also damages the platelets, either because of adherence to collagen or to a wettable surface (or by damage in other ways), and this releases platelet phospholipid which also plays a role in subsequent clotting reactions.

(2) *Activation of factor XI.* The activated factor XII acts enzymatically on factor XI to activate this as well, which is the second step in the intrinsic pathway.

(3) *Activation of factor IX by activated factor XI.* The activated factor XI then acts enzymatically on factor IX to activate this factor, also.

(4) *Activation of factor X—role of factor VIII.* The activated factor IX, acting in concert with factor VIII and with the platelet phospholipids from the traumatized platelets, activates factor X. When either factor VIII or platelets are in short supply, this step is deficient. Factor VIII is the factor that is missing in the person who has classic *hemophilia*, for which reason it is called *antihemophilic factor*. Platelets are the clotting factor that is lacking in the bleeding disease called *thrombocytopenia*.

(5) *Action of activated factor X to form prothrombin activator—role of factor V.* This step in the intrinsic pathway is essentially the same as the last step in the extrinsic pathway. That is, activated factor X combines with factor V and platelet phospholipids to form the complex called *prothrombin activator*. The prothrombin activator in turn initiates within seconds the cleavage of prothrombin to form thrombin, thereby setting into motion the final clotting process, as described earlier.

Role of Calcium Ions in the Intrinsic and Extrinsic Pathways

Except for the first two steps in the intrinsic pathway, calcium ions are required for promotion of all the reactions. Therefore, in the absence of calcium ions, blood clotting will not occur.

When blood is removed from a person, it can be prevented from clotting by reducing the calcium ion concentration below the threshold level for clotting, either by deionizing the calcium by reacting it with substances such as *citrate ion* or by precipitating the calcium with substances such as *oxalate ion*.

Summary of Blood Clotting Initiation

It is clear from the above schemas of the intrinsic and extrinsic systems for initiating blood clotting that clotting is initiated after rupture of blood vessels by both the pathways. The tissue thromboplastin initiates

INTRINSIC PATHWAY

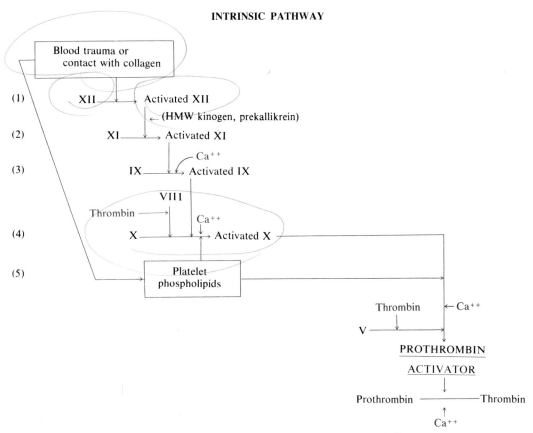

Figure 21-4. The intrinsic pathway for initiating blood clotting.

the extrinsic pathway, whereas contact of factor XII and the platelets with collagen in the vascular wall initiates the intrinsic pathway.

In contrast, when blood is removed from the body and held in a test tube, the intrinsic pathway alone must elicit the clotting. This usually results from contact of factor XII and platelets with the wall of the tube, which activates both of these and initiates the intrinsic mechanism. If the surface of the container is very "nonwettable," such as a siliconized surface, blood clotting can sometimes be prevented for an hour or more.

PREVENTION OF BLOOD CLOTTING IN THE NORMAL VASCULAR SYSTEM—THE INTRAVASCULAR ANTICOAGULANTS

Endothelial Surface Factors. Probably the two most important factors for preventing clotting in the normal vascular system are, first, the smoothness of the endothelium that prevents contact activation of the intrinsic clotting system and, second, a monomolecular layer of protein adsorbed to the inner surface of the endothelium that repels the clotting factors and platelets, thereby preventing activation of clotting. When the endothelial wall is damaged, its smoothness and protein layer are both lost, which activates both factor XII and the platelets, thus setting off the intrinsic pathway of clotting.

Antithrombin III. Among the most important anticoagulants in the blood itself are those that remove

thrombin from the blood. The most powerful of these is an alpha-globulin called *antithrombin III* or also *antithrombin-heparin cofactor*.

The thrombin that is not decomposed in the clotting process itself soon combines with antithrombin III, which blocks the effect of the thrombin on the fibrinogen and then inactivates the bound thrombin during the next 12 to 20 minutes.

Heparin. Heparin is another powerful anticoagulant. Yet, its concentration in the blood is normally very slight, so that only under some physiological conditions does it have significant anticoagulant effects. On the other hand, it is used very widely in medical practice to prevent intravascular clotting.

The heparin molecule is a highly negatively charged conjugated polysaccharide. By itself it has little or no anticoagulant property, but it combines with antithrombin III and increases as much as a thousandfold the effectiveness of antithrombin III to remove thrombin and thus to act as an anticoagulant. Therefore, in the presence of excess heparin the removal of thrombin from the circulating blood is almost instantaneous.

Heparin is produced by many different cells of the human body, though especially large quantities are formed by the basophilic *mast cells* located in the pericapillary connective tissue throughout the body. These cells continually secrete small quantities of heparin, and minute quantities also diffuse into the circulatory system. The *basophil cells* of the blood, which seem to be functionally almost identical with the mast cells, also release small quantities of heparin into the plasma.

Mast cells are extremely abundant in the tissue surrounding the capillaries of the lungs and to a lesser extent the capillaries of the liver. It is easy to understand why large quantities of heparin might be needed in these areas, for the capillaries of the lungs and liver receive many embolic clots formed in the slowly flowing venous blood; sufficient formation of heparin might prevent further growth of the clots.

LYSIS OF BLOOD CLOTS—PLASMIN

The plasma proteins contain a euglobulin called *plasminogen* or *profibrinolysin* which, when activated, becomes a substance called *plasmin* or *fibrinolysin*. Plasmin is a proteolytic enzyme that resembles trypsin, the most important digestive enzyme of pancreatic secretion. It digests the fibrin threads of the blood clot.

Formation of Plasmin and Lysis of Clots. When a clot is formed a large amount of plasminogen is incorporated in the clot along with other plasma proteins. However, this will not become plasmin and will not cause lysis of the clot until it is activated. Fortunately, the tissues and blood contain substances that can activate plasminogen to plasmin, including (1) thrombin, (2) activated factor XII, (3) lysosomal enzymes from damaged tissues, and (4) factors from the vascular endothelium. Within a day or two after blood has leaked into a tissue and clotted, these activators usually cause the formation of enough plasmin that it then begins to dissolve the clot.

Clots that occur inside blood vessels can also be dissolved, though this occurs more readily in the small vessels than in the large ones.

Significance of the Fibrinolysin System. The lysis of blood clots allows slow clearing (over a period of several days) of extraneous blood in the tissues and sometimes allows reopening of clotted vessels. Unfortunately, reopening of large vessels occurs only rarely. But an important function of the fibrinolysin system is to remove very minute clots from the millions of tiny peripheral vessels that eventually would all become occluded were there no way to cleanse them.

CONDITIONS THAT CAUSE EXCESSIVE BLEEDING IN HUMAN BEINGS

Excessive bleeding can result from deficiency of any one of the many different blood clotting factors. Three particular types of bleeding tendencies that have been studied to the greatest extent will be discussed: (1) bleeding caused by vitamin K deficiency, (2) hemophilia, and (3) thrombocytopenia (platelet deficiency).

DECREASED PROTHROMBIN, FACTOR VII, FACTOR IX, AND FACTOR X CAUSED BY VITAMIN K DEFICIENCY

With few exceptions, almost all the blood-clotting factors are formed by the liver. Therefore, diseases of the liver such as *hepatitis, cirrhosis,* and *acute yellow atrophy* all can depress the clotting system so greatly that the patient develops a severe tendency to bleed.

Another cause of depressed formation of clotting factors by the liver is vitamin K deficiency. Vitamin K is necessary to promote the formation of four of the most important clotting factors, *prothrombin, factor VII, factor IX,* and *factor X.* In the absence of vitamin K, insufficiency of these coagulation factors can also lead to a serious bleeding tendency.

Fortunately, vitamin K is continually synthesized in the intestinal tract by bacteria so that vitamin K deficiency rarely if ever occurs simply because of its absence from the diet, except in newborn children before they establish their intestinal bacterial flora. However, vitamin K deficiency does often occur as a result of poor absorption of fats from the gastrointestinal tract, because vitamin K is fat-soluble and ordinarily is absorbed into the blood along with the fats.

HEMOPHILIA

Hemophilia is a bleeding tendency that occurs almost exclusively in men. In 85 per cent of cases it is caused by *deficiency of factor VIII;* this type of hemophilia is called *hemophilia A* or *classic hemophilia.* About one of every 10,000 males in the United States has classic hemophilia. In the other 15 per cent of the patients, the bleeding tendency is caused by deficiency of factor IX. Both these factors are transmitted genetically by way of the female chromosome as a recessive trait. Therefore, almost never will a woman have hemophilia because at least one of her two X chromosomes will have the appropriate genes. However, if one of her X chromosomes is deficient, she will be a *hemophilia carrier,* transmitting the disease to half her male offspring and transmitting the carrier state to half her female offspring.

The bleeding trait in hemophilia can have various degrees of severity, depending upon the severity of the genetic deficiency. Usually, bleeding will not occur except after trauma, but the degree of trauma required to cause severe and prolonged bleeding may be so mild that it is hardly noticeable. For instance, even falling on a knee may cause severe bleeding into the knee joint. Likewise, a mild blow to the head can frequently cause intracranial bleeding, or bleeding can occur in fascial compartments in the arm or leg and compress both nerves and blood vessels to the extent of causing severe atrophy of the limbs. And bleeding can often last for literally weeks after extraction of a tooth.

When a person with classic hemophilia develops severe, prolonged bleeding, almost the only therapy that is truly effective is injection of clotting factor VIII purified at great expense only from human blood.

THROMBOCYTOPENIA

Thrombocytopenia means the presence of a very low quantity of platelets in the circulatory system. Persons with thrombocytopenia have a tendency to bleed as do hemophiliacs, except that the bleeding is usually from many small capillaries rather than from larger vessels, as in hemophilia. As a result, small punctate hemorrhages occur throughout all the body tissues. The skin of such a person displays many small, purplish blotches, giving the disease the name *thrombocytopenic purpura*. It will be remembered that platelets are especially important for repair of minute breaks in capillaries and other small vessels. Indeed, platelets can aggregate to fill such ruptures without actually causing clots.

Ordinarily, bleeding does not occur until the number of platelets in the blood falls below a value of approximately 50,000 per cubic millimeter rather than the normal 150,000 to 350,000. Levels as low as 10,000 per cubic millimeter are frequently lethal.

Most persons with thrombocytopenia have the disease known as *idiopathic thrombocytopenia*, which means simply thrombocytopenia of unknown cause. However, in the past few years it has been discovered that in most of these persons specific antibodies are destroying the platelets. Occasionally these have developed because of transfusions from other persons, but usually they result from development of autoimmunity to the person's own platelets, the cause of which, however, is not known.

THROMBOEMBOLIC CONDITIONS IN THE HUMAN BEING

Thrombi and Emboli. An abnormal clot that develops in a blood vessel is called a *thrombus*. Once a clot has developed, continued flow of blood past the clot is likely to break it away from its attachment, and such freely flowing clots are known as *emboli*. Emboli generally do not stop flowing until they come to a narrow point in the circulatory system. Thus, emboli originating in large arteries or in the left side of the heart eventually plug either smaller systemic arteries or arterioles, maybe in the brain, the kidneys, or elsewhere. On the other hand, emboli originating in the venous system and in the right side of the heart flow into the vessels of the lung to cause pulmonary arterial embolism.

Causes of Thromboembolic Conditions. The causes of thromboembolic conditions in the human being are usually twofold: First, any *roughened endothelial surface of a vessel*—as may be caused by arteriosclerosis—is likely to initiate the clotting process. Second, blood often clots *when it flows very slowly* through blood vessels, for small quantities of thrombin and other procoagulants are always being formed. These are generally removed from the blood by the macrophage system, mainly the Kupffer's cells of the liver. If the blood is flowing too slowly, the concentrations of the procoagulants in local areas often rise high enough to initiate clotting, but when the blood flows rapidly, these are rapidly mixed with large quantities of blood and are removed during passage through the liver.

FEMORAL THROMBOSIS AND MASSIVE PULMONARY EMBOLISM

Because clotting almost always occurs when blood flow is blocked for many hours in any vessel of the body, the immobility of bed patients plus the practice of propping the knees with underlying pillows often causes intravascular clotting because of blood stasis in one or more of the leg veins for hours at a time. Then the clot grows, mainly in the direction of the slowly moving blood, sometimes growing the entire length of the leg veins and occasionally even up into the common iliac vein and inferior vena cava. Then, about one time out of every ten, a large part of the clot disengages from its attachments to the vessel wall and flows freely with the venous blood into the right side of the heart and thence into the pulmonary arteries to cause *massive pulmonary embolism*. If the clot is large enough to occlude both the pulmonary arteries, immediate death ensues. If only one pulmonary artery or a smaller branch is blocked, death may not occur, or the embolism may lead to death a few hours to several days later because of further growth of the clot within the pulmonary vessels.

DISSEMINATED INTRAVASCULAR CLOTTING

Occasionally, the clotting mechanism becomes activated in widespread areas of the circulation, giving rise to the condition called *disseminated intravascular clotting*. This often results from the presence of large amounts of traumatized or dying tissue in the body that releases tissue thromboplastin into the blood. Frequently, the clots are small but numerous, and they plug a large share of the small peripheral blood vessels. This occurs especially in septicemic shock, in which either circulating bacteria or bacterial toxins—especially *endotoxins*—activate the clotting mechanisms. The plugging of the small peripheral vessels greatly diminishes the delivery of oxygen and other nutrients to the tissues—a situation which exacerbates the shock picture. It is partly for this reason that full-blown septicemic shock is lethal in 85 per cent or more of the patients.

A peculiar effect of disseminated intravascular clotting is that the patient frequently begins to bleed. The reason for this is that so many of the clotting factors are removed by the widespread clotting that too few procoagulants remain to allow normal hemostasis of the remaining blood.

QUESTIONS

1. Explain the role of *vascular spasm* in hemostasis.
2. How do *platelet plugs* contribute to hemostasis?
3. Name the three principal stages of the blood coagulation mechanism.
4. What is the source of *prothrombin,* and what causes it to be converted to thrombin?
5. How does thrombin convert *fibrinogen* into fibrin? What is the role of *fibrin-stabilizing factor?*
6. What is the role of *platelets* in clot retraction?
7. Why does clot formation become a vicious circle?
8. What are the principal differences between the *extrinsic* and *intrinsic mechanisms* for the formation of *prothrombin activator?*
9. What are the special roles of *Factor XII* and *platelets* in the intrinsic mechanism for initiating clotting?
10. What is the relationship of *Factor VIII* to *hemophilia?*
11. Explain how tissue trauma leads to clotting.
12. Explain how each of the following factors helps to prevent clotting in the normal vascular system: *epithelial surface factors, antithrombin III,* and *heparin.*
13. What is the role of *plasmin* in the lysis of blood clots?
14. Explain the bleeding in each of the following conditions: vitamin K deficiency, hemophilia, and thrombocytopenia.
15. What are the basic causes of *thromboembolic conditions?*
16. Explain the genesis of *pulmonary embolism* and *disseminated intravascular clotting.*

References

Carpentier, A.: Low molecular weight (LMW) heparin derivatives in experimental extra-corporeal circulation (ECC). Haemostasis 14:325, 1984.

Chavin, S. I.: Factor VIII: Structure and function in blood clotting. Am J Hematol 16:297, 1984.

Frojmovic, M. M., and Milton, J. G.: Human platelet size, shape, and related functions in health and disease. Physiol Rev 62:185, 1982.

Fukada, E., et al.: Methods to study rheological properties of blood during clotting. Biorheology, Suppl. 1:9, 1984.

Kline, D. L., and Reddy, K. N. N., eds.: Fibrinolysis. Boca Raton, Fla., CRC Press, 1980.

Mann, K. G.: The biochemistry of coagulation. Clin Lab Med 4:207, 1984.

Murano, G., and Bick, R. L., eds.: Basic Concepts of Hemostasis and Thrombosis: Clinical Laboratory Evaluation of Thrombohemorrhagic Phenomena. Boca Raton, Fla., CRC Press, 1980.

Nemerson, Y., and Nossel, H. L.: The biology of thrombosis. Annu Rev Med 33:479, 1982.

Olson, R. E.: The function and metabolism of vitamin K. Annu Rev Nutr 4:281, 1984.

Ratnoff, O. D.: Thrombosis and the hypercoagulable state. Circulation 70:III72, 1984.

Wall, R. T., and Harker, L. A.: The endothelium and thrombosis. Annu Rev Med 31:361, 1980.

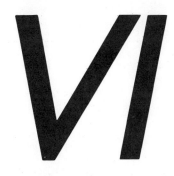

THE BODY FLUIDS AND
THE KIDNEYS

22 ■ Capillary Dynamics; Exchange of Fluid Between the Blood and the Interstitial Fluid

23 ■ The Lymphatic System, Interstitial Fluid Dynamics, Edema, the Pulmonary Fluid, and the Special Fluid Systems

24 ■ Formation of Urine by the Kidneys

25 ■ Regulation of Blood Fluids and Their Constituents by the Kidneys and the Thirst Mechanism

26 ■ Regulation of Acid-Base Balance; Renal Disease; Micturition

22

Capillary Dynamics; Exchange of Fluid Between the Blood and the Interstitial Fluid

STRUCTURE OF THE CAPILLARY
    SYSTEM
FLOW OF BLOOD IN THE
    CAPILLARIES—VASOMOTION
EXCHANGE OF NUTRIENTS AND OTHER
    SUBSTANCES BETWEEN THE BLOOD
    AND THE INTERSTITIAL FLUID
    DIFFUSION THROUGH THE CAPILLARY
        MEMBRANE
THE INTERSTITIUM AND THE
    INTERSTITIAL FLUID
DISTRIBUTION OF FLUID VOLUME
    BETWEEN THE PLASMA AND

INTERSTITIAL FLUID
CAPILLARY PRESSURE
INTERSTITIAL FLUID PRESSURE
PLASMA COLLOID OSMOTIC
    PRESSURE
INTERSTITIAL FLUID COLLOID
    OSMOTIC PRESSURE
EXCHANGE OF FLUID VOLUME
    THROUGH THE CAPILLARY
    MEMBRANE
THE STARLING EQUILIBRIUM FOR
    CAPILLARY EXCHANGE

In the capillaries the most purposeful function of the circulation occurs, namely, interchange of nutrients and cellular excreta between the tissues and the circulating blood. About 10 billion capillaries, which have a total surface area of probably 500 to 700 square meters, provide this function. Indeed, it is rare that any single functional cell of the body is more than 20 to 30 microns away from a capillary.

The purpose of this chapter is to discuss the transfer of substances between the blood and interstitial fluid and especially to discuss the factors that affect the transfer of fluid volume itself between the circulating blood and the interstitial fluids.

STRUCTURE OF THE CAPILLARY SYSTEM

The microcirculation of each organ is specifically organized to serve that organ's own special needs. However, Figure 22–1 illustrates the structure of a representative capillary bed as seen in the mesentery, illustrating that blood enters the capillaries through an *arteriole* and leaves by way of a *venule*. Blood from the arteriole passes into a series of *metarterioles,* which are called by some physiologists *terminal arterioles* and which have a structure midway between that of arterioles and capillaries. After leaving the metarteriole, the blood enters the *capillaries,* some of which are large and are called *preferential channels* and others of which are small and are *true capillaries.* After passing through the capillaries the blood enters the venule and returns to the general circulation.

The arterioles are highly muscular, and their diameters can be manyfold, as discussed in Chapter 12. The metarterioles (the terminal arterioles) do not have a continuous muscular coat, but smooth muscle fibers encircle the vessel at intermediate points, as illustrated in Figure 22–1 by the large black dots to the sides of the metarteriole.

At the point where the true capillaries originate from the metarterioles a smooth muscle fiber usually encircles the capillary. This is called the *precapillary sphincter.* This sphincter can open and close the entrance to the capillary.

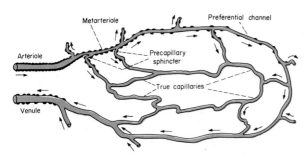

Figure 22–1. Structure of the mesenteric capillary bed. (From Zweifach: Factors Regulating Blood Pressure. New York, Josiah Macy, Jr., Foundation, 1950.)

The venules are considerably larger than the arterioles and have a much weaker muscular coat. Yet, it must be remembered that the pressure in the venules is much less than that in the arterioles so that the venules can still contract considerably.

Structure of the Capillary Wall. Figure 22–2 illustrates the ultramicroscopic structure of a typical capillary wall as found in most organs of the body, especially in the muscles and connective tissue. Note that the wall is composed of a unicellular layer of endothelial cells and is surrounded by a basement membrane on the outside. The total thickness of the wall is about 0.5 micron.

The diameter of the capillary is 4 to 9 microns, barely large enough for red blood cells and other blood cells to squeeze through.

"Pores" in the Capillary Membrane. Studying Figure 22–2, one sees two minute passageways connecting the interior of the capillary with the exterior. One of these is the *intercellular cleft*, which is a thin slit that lies between adjacent endothelial cells. The cells are held apart approximately 6 to 7 nanometers (60 to 70 Angstroms) by loose reticular fibrillae composed of proteoglycans, mainly hyaluronic acid. These intercellular clefts represent no more than one thousandth of the total surface area of the capillary. Nevertheless, it is believed that most water-soluble ions and molecules pass between the interior and exterior of the capillary through these *slit-pores*.

Also present in the endothelial cells are many *pinocytic vesicles*. These form at one surface of the

cell and move to the opposite surface where they discharge their contents, often carrying large molecules and even solid particles through the capillary membrane. Note also in Figure 22–2 that some of these pinocytic vesicles occasionally coalesce with each other and form a continuous channel through the endothelial membrane as illustrated by the so-called *pinocytic channel* shown to the right in the figure. However, it is still doubted whether large amounts of substances pass through the capillary membrane via such channels.

FLOW OF BLOOD IN THE CAPILLARIES—VASOMOTION

Blood usually does not flow continuously through the capillaries. Instead, it flows intermittently, turning on and off every few seconds or minutes. The cause of this intermittency is the phenomenon called *vasomotion*, which means intermittent contraction of the metarterioles and precapillary sphincters.

Regulation of Vasomotion. The most important factor found thus far to affect the degree of opening and closing of the metarterioles and precapillary sphincters is the concentration of *oxygen* in the tissues. When the oxygen concentration is very low, the intermittent periods of blood flow occur more often, and the duration of each period of flow lasts for a longer time, thereby allowing the blood to carry increased quantities of oxygen (as well as other nutrients) to the tissues. It follows also that the greater the use of oxygen by the tissue, the greater will be the amount of blood that flows. Thus, by this intermittent opening and closing of the precapillary sphincters and metarterioles, the blood flow to the tissue is *autoregulated*. This was discussed in Chapter 13.

EXCHANGE OF NUTRIENTS AND OTHER SUBSTANCES BETWEEN THE BLOOD AND THE INTERSTITIAL FLUID

DIFFUSION THROUGH THE CAPILLARY MEMBRANE

By far the most important means by which substances are transferred between the plasma and interstitial fluids is by *diffusion*. Figure 22–3 illustrates this process, showing that as the blood traverses the capillary, tremendous numbers of water molecules and dissolved particles diffuse back and forth through the capillary wall, providing continual mixing between the interstitial fluids and the plasma, as was explained in Chapter 4. Diffusion results from thermal motion of the water molecules and the dissolved substances in the fluid, the different particles moving first in one direction, then another, moving randomly in every direction.

Diffusion of Lipid-Soluble Substances Through the Capillary Membrane. If a substance is lipid-soluble,

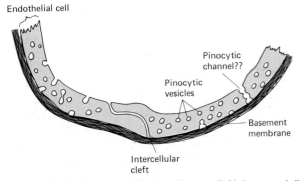

Figure 22–2. Structure of the capillary wall. Note especially the *intercellular cleft* at the junction between adjacent endothelial cells; it is believed that most water-soluble substances diffuse through the capillary membrane along this cleft.

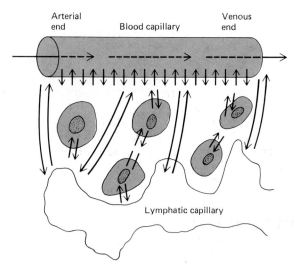

Figure 22–3. Diffusion of fluid and dissolved substances between the capillary and interstitial fluid spaces.

it can diffuse directly through the cell membranes of the capillary without having to go through the pores. Such substances include especially oxygen and carbon dioxide. Since these can permeate all areas of the capillary membrane, their rates of transport through the capillary membrane are many times the rates for most lipid-insoluble substances such as sodium ions, glucose, and so forth.

Diffusion of Water Molecules Through the Capillary Membrane. After the lipid-soluble molecules, water molecules are the next most rapid to diffuse through the capillary membrane. A small amount of water diffusion occurs directly through the endothelial cell wall, first into the intracellular fluid of the endothelial cell and then out the membrane on the other side of the cell. However, far more water diffuses through the "pores" in the capillary membrane, especially through the intercellular clefts.

Diffusion of Water-Soluble, Lipid-Insoluble Substances Through the Capillary Membrane. Many substances needed by the tissues are soluble in water but cannot pass through the lipid membranes of the endothelial cells; such substances include sodium ions, chloride ions, glucose, and so forth. These substances diffuse between the plasma and interstitial fluids only through the capillary pores.

Despite the fact that not over 1/1000 of the surface area of the capillaries is represented by the intercellular junctions, the velocity of thermal motion is so great that even this small area is sufficient to allow tremendous diffusion of water and water-soluble substances through these pores. To give one an idea of the extreme rapidity with which substances diffuse, *the rate at which water molecules diffuse through the capillary membrane is approximately 80 times as great as the rate at which plasma itself flows linearly along the capillary.* That is, the water of the plasma is exchanged with the water of the interstitial fluids 80 times before the plasma can go the entire distance through the capillary.

Effect of Molecular Size on Passage Through the Pores. The width of the capillary intercellular slit-pores, 6 to 7 nanometers, is about 20 times the diameter of the water molecule. On the other hand, the diameters of plasma protein molecules are slightly greater than the width of the pores. Other substances, such as sodium ions, chloride ions, glucose, and urea, have intermediate diameters. Therefore, it is obvious that the permeability of the capillary pores for different substances will vary according to their molecular diameters.

Table 22–1 gives the relative permeabilities of the capillary pores in muscle for substances commonly encountered by the capillary membrane, illustrating, for instance, that the permeability for glucose molecules is 0.6 times as great as that for water molecules, while the permeability for albumin molecules is less than 1/10,000 that for water molecules. Thus, the membrane is almost impermeable to albumin, which causes a significant concentration difference to develop between the albumin of the plasma and that of the interstitial fluid, as will become evident later in the chapter.

Fortunately, the rates of diffusion through the capillary membranes of most *nutritionally* important substances are so great that only slight concentration differences suffice to cause more than adequate transport between the plasma and interstitial fluid. For instance, the concentration of oxygen in the interstitial fluid immediately outside the capillary is probably no more than 1 per cent less than the concentration in the blood, and yet this 1 per cent difference causes enough oxygen to move from the blood into the interstitial spaces to provide all the oxygen required for tissue metabolism.

THE INTERSTITIUM AND THE INTERSTITIAL FLUID

Approximately one sixth of the body consists of spaces between cells, which collectively are called the *interstitium.* The fluid in these spaces is the *interstitial fluid.*

The structure of the interstitium is illustrated in Figure 22–4. It has two major types of solid structures:

Table 22–1. RELATIVE PERMEABILITY OF MUSCLE CAPILLARY PORES TO DIFFERENT-SIZED MOLECULES

Substance	Molecular Weight	Permeability
Water	18	1.00
NaCl	58.5	0.96
Urea	60	0.8
Glucose	180	0.6
Sucrose	342	0.4
Inulin	5,000	0.2
Myoglobin	17,600	0.03
Hemoglobin	68,000	0.01
Albumin	69,000	<0.0001

Modified from Pappenheimer.

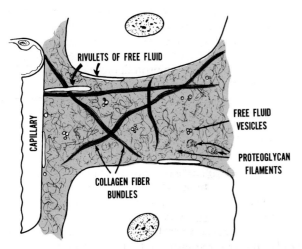

Figure 22–4. Structure of the interstitium. Proteoglycan filaments fill the spaces between the collagen fiber bundles. Free fluid vesicles are seen and small amounts of free fluid in the form of rivulets.

(1) collagen fiber bundles and (2) proteoglycan filaments. Figure 22–4 illustrates that the collagen fiber bundles extend long distances in the interstitium. They are extremely strong and therefore provide most of the tensional strength of the tissues. The proteoglycan filaments, on the other hand, are extremely thin, coiled molecules composed of about 98 per cent hyaluronic acid and 2 per cent protein. These molecules are so thin that they can never be seen with a light microscope and are very difficult to demonstrate even with the electron microscope. Nevertheless, they form a mat of very fine reticular filaments aptly described as a "brush pile." This brush pile of proteoglycan filaments is everywhere in the interstitium. It fills all the spaces between the collagen fibers, the crannies between the cells, and almost all the other minute spaces of the tissues.

"Tissue Gel" in the Interstitium. The fluid in the interstitium is an ultrafiltrate of plasma derived from the capillaries. In the interstitium this fluid is mainly entrapped in the minute spaces among the proteoglycan filaments. This combination of the proteoglycan filaments and the fluid entrapped within them has the characteristics of a *gel*, and therefore is often called the *tissue gel*.

Because of the large number of proteoglycan filaments, fluid *flows* through the tissue gel only very poorly. Instead, it mainly *diffuses* through the gel; that is, it moves molecule by molecule from one place to another by the process of kinetic motion rather than by large numbers of molecules moving together.

In contrast to the severe impediment of flow through the gel, diffusion through the gel occurs about 95 to 99 per cent as rapidly as it does through free fluid. This diffusion allows rapid transport through the interstitium not only of the water molecules, but also electrolytes, nutrients, cellular excreta, oxygen, carbon dioxide, and so forth.

"Free" Fluid in the Interstitium. Though almost all the fluid in the interstitium is normally entrapped within the tissue gel, occasionally small *rivulets of "free" fluid* and also small *free fluid vesicles* are also present, which means fluid that is free of the proteoglycan molecules and therefore can flow freely. When a dye is injected into the circulating blood, it can often be seen to flow through the interstitium in small rivulets, usually coursing along the surfaces of collagen fibers or surfaces of cells. However, the amount of free fluid present in *normal* tissues is very slight. On the other hand, when the tissues develop *edema, it is the small pockets and rivulets of free fluid that expand tremendously*.

DISTRIBUTION OF FLUID VOLUME BETWEEN THE PLASMA AND INTERSTITIAL FLUID

The pressure in the capillaries continuously tends to force fluid and its dissolved substances through the capillary pores into the interstitial spaces. But, in contrast, osmotic pressure caused by the plasma proteins (called *colloid* osmotic pressure) tends to cause fluid movement by osmosis from the interstitial spaces into the blood; it is mainly this osmotic pressure that prevents continual loss of fluid volume from the blood into the interstitial spaces. Yet, the process is much more complicated than this and includes the role of the lymphatic system to return back to the circulation the small amounts of protein and fluid that do leak continuously into the interstitial spaces. In the following few paragraphs we will discuss all of the factors that play a significant role in the movement of fluid volume through the capillary membrane, and in the following chapter we will discuss the role of the lymphatic system in this overall mechanism.

The Four Primary Forces That Determine Fluid Movement Through the Capillary Membrane. Figure 22–5 illustrates the four primary forces that determine whether fluid will move out of the blood into the interstitial fluid or in the opposite direction; these are as follows:

1. The *capillary pressure* (Pc), which tends to move fluid outward through the capillary membrane.

2. The *interstitial fluid pressure* (Pif), which tends to move fluid inward through the capillary membrane when Pif is positive but outward when Pif is negative.

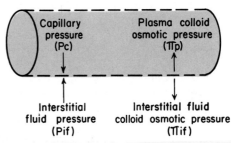

Figure 22–5. Forces operative at the capillary membrane tending to move fluid either outward or inward through the membrane.

3. The *plasma colloid osmotic pressure* (IIp), which tends to cause osmosis of fluid inward through the membrane.

4. The *interstitial fluid colloid osmotic pressure* (IIif), which tends to cause osmosis of fluid outward through the membrane.

The regulation of fluid volumes in the blood and interstitial fluid is so important that each of these factors is discussed in turn in the following sections.

CAPILLARY PRESSURE

Two different methods have been used to estimate the capillary pressure: (1) *direct cannulation of the capillaries,* which has given an average mean capillary pressure of about 25 mm Hg, and (2) *indirect functional measurement of the capillary pressure,* which has given a capillary pressure averaging about 17 mm Hg. These methods are the following:

Cannulation Method for Measuring Capillary Pressure. To measure pressure in a capillary by cannulation, a microscopic glass pipet is thrust directly into the capillary, and the pressure is measured by an appropriate micromanometer system. Using this method, capillary pressures have been measured in capillaries of exposed tissues of lower animals and in large capillary loops of the eponychium at the base of the fingernail in human beings. These measurements have given pressures of 30 to 40 mm Hg in the arterial ends of the capillaries, 10 to 15 mm Hg in the venous ends, and about 25 mm Hg in the middle.

Isogravimetric and Isovolumetric Methods for Indirectly Measuring Mean Capillary Pressure. Figure 22–6 illustrates an *isogravimetric* method for estimat-

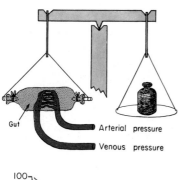

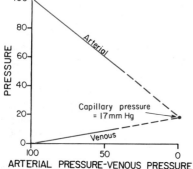

Figure 22–6. Isogravimetric method for measuring capillary pressure (explained in the text).

ing capillary pressure. This figure shows a section of gut held by one arm of a gravimetric balance. Blood is perfused through the gut. When the arterial pressure is decreased, the resulting decrease in capillary pressure allows the osmotic pressure of the plasma proteins to cause absorption of fluid out of the gut wall and makes the weight of the gut decrease. This immediately causes displacement of the balance arm. However, to prevent this weight decrease, the venous pressure is raised an amount sufficient to overcome the effect of decreasing the arterial pressure. In other words, the capillary pressure is kept constant by raising the venous pressure.

In the lower part of the figure, the changes in arterial and venous pressures that exactly nullify all weight changes are illustrated. The arterial and venous lines meet each other at a value of 17 mm Hg. Therefore, the capillary pressure must have remained at this same level of 17 mm Hg throughout these maneuvers, or otherwise filtration or absorption of fluid through the capillary walls would have occurred. Thus, in a roundabout way, the "functional" capillary pressure is measured to be about 17 mm Hg.

The *isovolumetric* method for measuring capillary pressure is essentially the same as the isogravimetric method, except that the *volume* of the tissue is recorded rather than the weight. The arterial and venous pressures are gradually brought toward each other and are continually adjusted so that the tissue neither gains nor loses volume. On extrapolating the arterial and venous pressures, one again finds that the capillary pressure estimated by this means is considerably lower than that measured by direct cannulation, again averaging about 17 mm Hg.

Functional Capillary Pressure. Since the cannulation method does not give the same pressure measurement as the isogravimetric and isovolumetric methods, one must decide which of these measurements is probably the true functional capillary pressure of the tissues. The isovolumetric and isogravimetric measurements are probably much nearer to the normal values for capillary pressure than are the micropipet measurements, for several reasons:

First, the metarterioles and precapillary sphincters of the capillary system are normally more often closed during a greater part of the vasomotion cycle than they are open. When they are closed, the pressure in the entire capillary system beyond the closures should be almost exactly equal to the pressure at the venous ends of the capillaries, about 10 mm Hg. Therefore, if one considers a *weighted* average of the pressures in all capillaries, one would expect the *functional* mean capillary pressure to be much nearer to the pressure in the venous ends of the capillaries than to the pressure in the arterial ends.

Second, the surface area of the venous capillaries is several times as great as the surface area of the arterial capillaries. Therefore, the mean pressure in the venous capillaries, 10 mm Hg, plays a far greater role in determining the *functional* capillary pressure than does the mean arterial capillary pressure, 35 mm Hg.

Third, the venous capillaries are several times as permeable as the arterial capillaries. Therefore, for determining fluid movement through the capillary membrane, the venous capillary pressures are much more important than the arterial capillary pressures.

Thus, there are many reasons for believing *that the normal functional mean capillary pressure is about 17 mm Hg.*

INTERSTITIAL FLUID PRESSURE

The interstitial fluid pressure, like capillary pressure, has been difficult to measure, primarily because the maximum width of the spaces between the reticular fibers that make up the solid structure of the interstitium is only 10 to 40 nanometers, much too small to cannulate for direct measurement of the pressure. Therefore, most frequently, indirect methods have been used for measuring this pressure.

Prior to 1961, it had been believed universally that the interstitial fluid pressure was always slightly greater than atmospheric pressure. However, on the basis of measurements made in our laboratory in 1961, we concluded that the interstitial fluid pressure is probably subatmospheric in most tissues of the body, usually 2 to 7 mm Hg less than the pressure of the surrounding air. Since that time, a continuing controversy has existed concerning whether or not the interstitial fluid pressure is truly less than the atmospheric level.

With this as background, let us now summarize some of the methods that have been used for measuring the interstitial fluid pressure.

Measurement of Interstitial Fluid Pressure in Implanted Perforated Hollow Capsules. Figure 22–7 illustrates an indirect method for measuring interstitial fluid pressure which may be explained as follows: A small hollow plastic capsule perforated by several hundred small holes is implanted in the tissues, and the surgical wound is allowed to heal for approximately one month. At the end of that time, tissue will have grown inward through the holes to line the inner surface of the sphere. Furthermore, the cavity is filled with fluid that flows freely through the per-

forations back and forth between the fluid in the interstitial spaces and the fluid in the cavity. Therefore, the pressure in the cavity should equal the fluid pressure in the interstitial fluid spaces. A needle is inserted through the skin and through one of the perforations to the interior of the cavity, and the pressure is measured by use of an appropriate manometer.

Interstitial fluid pressure measured by this method in normal loose subcutaneous tissue averages −5 to −6 mm Hg. That is, the pressure is *less than atmospheric pressure* or, in other words, is a semivacuum or a suction.

The significance of the negativity of interstitial fluid pressure is that it causes *suction of fluid out of the capillaries,* as we shall see in subsequent sections of this chapter. The mechanism for development of the negative interstitial fluid pressure is discussed in the following chapter in relation to interstitial fluid dynamics.

Measurement of the Interstitial Fluid Pressure Using a Micropipet. Recently, microscopic pipets have been placed into tissue spaces in attempts to measure the interstitial fluid pressure. Earlier measurements in this way suggested slightly positive pressures of +1 to +2 mm Hg in the connective tissue of the bat wing, but negative pressures of −1 to −3 mm Hg have more recently also been made using this same method. Since the pipets are 30 to 50 times as large as the spaces between the reticular fibrillae of the interstitium, one wonders how much the distortion of the tissues that is caused by the method affects the measurement.

Is the True Interstitial Fluid Pressure in Subcutaneous Tissue Subatmospheric?

The concept that the interstitial fluid pressure is subatmospheric in many tissues of the body began with clinical observations that could not be explained by the previously held concept that interstitial fluid pressure was always positive. However, in addition to the clinical observations, many different special experiments in both animals and human beings have supported the concept that the interstitial fluid pressure is usually negative in loose subcutaneous tissue and in most other soft tissues that are not surrounded by high pressure containments. Some of the pertinent observations are the following:

(1) When a skin graft is placed on a concave surface of the body, such as an eye socket after removal of the eye, before the skin becomes attached to the sublying socket, fluid tends to collect underneath the graft. Also, the skin attempts to shorten, and tries to pull away from the concavity. Nevertheless, some negative force underneath the skin causes absorption of the fluid and usually literally pulls the skin back into the concavity.

(2) In most natural cavities of the body where there is free fluid in dynamic equilibrium with the surrounding interstitial fluids, the pressures that have been

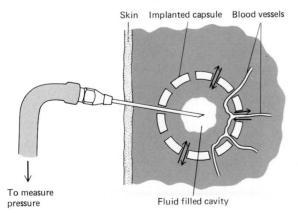

Figure 22–7. The perforated capsule method for measuring interstitial fluid pressure.

measured have been negative. Some of these are the following:

> Intrapleural space: −8 mm Hg;
> Joint synovial spaces: −4 to −8 mm Hg;
> Epidural space: −4 to −7 mm Hg.

(3) The implanted capsule method for measuring the interstitial fluid pressure can be used to record dynamic changes in this pressure. The changes are approximately those that one would calculate to occur when (a) the arterial pressure is increased or decreased, (b) fluid is injected into the surrounding tissue spaces, or (c) a highly concentrated colloid osmotic agent is injected into the blood to absorb fluid from the tissue spaces. None of the other methods for measuring interstitial fluid pressure have shown this dynamic capability. Therefore, we tend to trust the capsule measurements much more than the other measurements of interstitial fluid pressure. The capsule measurements are usually more negative than the measurements made in other ways.

Therefore, in the remainder of this chapter and in the following two chapters, we will frequently speak of the concept of negative interstitial fluid pressures and will consider the pressure in the loose subcutaneous connective tissue to be an average value of −5.3 mm Hg, a value typical for the capsule measurements. Yet, the student should remember that some physiologists still believe that all tissues have strong enough connective tissue fibers to maintain positive compression of the fluids in the interstitial spaces all the time.

PLASMA COLLOID OSMOTIC PRESSURE

Colloid Osmotic Pressure Caused by Plasma Proteins. The proteins are the only dissolved substances of the plasma and interstitial fluid that do not diffuse readily through the capillary membrane. Furthermore, when small quantities of protein do diffuse into the interstitial fluid, these are soon removed from the interstitial spaces by way of the lymph vessels. Therefore, the concentration of protein in the plasma averages about three times as much as that in the interstitial fluid, 7.3 gm/dl in the plasma versus 2 to 3 gm/dl in the interstitial fluid.

In the discussion of osmotic pressure in Chapter 4, it was pointed out that only those substances that fail to pass through the pores of a semipermeable membrane exert osmotic pressure. Since the proteins are the only dissolved constituents that do not readily penetrate the pores of the capillary membrane, it is the dissolved proteins of the plasma and interstitial fluids that are responsible for the osmotic pressure at the capillary membrane. To distinguish this osmotic pressure from that which occurs at the cell membrane, it is called either *colloid osmotic pressure* or *oncotic pressure*. The term *colloid* osmotic pressure is derived from the fact that a protein solution resembles a colloidal solution despite the fact that it is actually a true solution. (The osmotic pressure that results at the cell membrane is often called *total osmotic pressure* to distinguish it from the colloid osmotic pressure because essentially all dissolved substances of the body fluids exert osmotic pressure at the cell membrane.)

Normal Values for Plasma Colloid Osmotic Pressure. The colloid osmotic pressure of normal human plasma averages approximately 28 mm Hg; 19 mm of this is caused by the dissolved protein, and 9 mm by the cations held in the plasma by the negative electrical charges of the proteins.

Note particularly that the 28 mm Hg colloid osmotic pressure that can develop at the capillary membrane is only 1/200 the total osmotic pressure that would develop at a *cell* membrane if normal interstitial fluid were on one side of the cell membrane and pure water on the other side. Thus, the colloid osmotic pressure of the plasma is actually a weak osmotic force; but, even so, it plays an exceedingly important role in the maintenance of normal blood and interstitial fluid volumes.

Effect of the Different Plasma Proteins on Colloid Osmotic Pressure. The plasma proteins are a mixture of proteins that contains albumin, with an average molecular weight of 69,000; globulins, 140,000; and fibrinogen, 400,000. Thus, 1 gram of globulin contains only half as many molecules as 1 gram of albumin, and 1 gram of fibrinogen contains only one sixth as many molecules as 1 gram of albumin. (It will be recalled from the discussion of osmotic pressure in Chapter 4 that the osmotic pressure is determined by the *number of molecules* dissolved in a fluid rather than by the weight of these molecules.) The average relative concentrations of the different types of proteins in the plasma and their respective colloid osmotic pressures are:

	gm/dl	Πp (mm Hg)
Albumin	4.5	21.8
Globulins	2.5	6.0
Fibrinogen	0.3	0.2
TOTAL	7.3	28.0

Thus, about 75 per cent of the total colloid osmotic pressure of the plasma results from the albumin fraction, 25 per cent from the globulins and almost none from the fibrinogen. Therefore, from the point of view of capillary dynamics, it is mainly albumin that is important.

INTERSTITIAL FLUID COLLOID OSMOTIC PRESSURE

Though the size of the usual capillary pore is smaller than the molecular sizes of the plasma proteins, this is not true of all the pores. Therefore, small amounts of plasma proteins do leak through the pores into the interstitial spaces.

The total quantity of protein in the entire 12 liters of interstitial fluid of the body is slightly greater than the total quantity of protein in the plasma itself, but since this volume is four times the volume of plasma the average protein *concentration* of the interstitial fluid is only a little more than one fourth that in plasma, or approximately 2 grams per dl. The average colloid osmotic pressure for this concentration of proteins in the interstitial fluids is approximately 6 mm Hg.

EXCHANGE OF FLUID VOLUME THROUGH THE CAPILLARY MEMBRANE

Now that the different factors affecting capillary membrane dynamics have been discussed, it is possible to put all these together to see how normal capillaries function.

The capillary pressure at the arterial ends of the capillaries is 15 to 25 mm Hg greater than at the venous ends. Because of this difference, fluid "filters" out of the capillaries at their arterial ends and then is reabsorbed into the capillaries at their venous ends. Thus, a small amount of fluid actually "flows" through the tissues from the arterial ends of the capillaries to the venous ends. The dynamics of this flow are the following:

Analysis of the Forces Causing Filtration at the Arterial End of the Capillary. The forces operative at the arterial end of the capillary that cause movement through the capillary membrane are as follows:

	mm Hg
Forces tending to move fluid outward:	
Capillary pressure	30.0
Negative interstitial fluid pressure pulling the fluid	5.3
Interstitial fluid colloid osmotic pressure	6.0
TOTAL OUTWARD FORCE	41.3
Force tending to move fluid inward:	
Plasma colloid osmotic pressure	28.0
TOTAL INWARD FORCE	28.0
Summation of forces:	
Outward	41.3
Inward	28.0
NET OUTWARD FORCE	13.3

Thus, the summation of forces at the arterial end of the capillary shows a net *filtration pressure* of 13.3 mm Hg, tending to move fluid in the outward direction.

This 13.3 mm Hg filtration pressure causes, on the average, about 0.5 per cent of the plasma to filter out of the arterial end of the capillaries into the interstitial spaces.

Analysis of Reabsorption at the Venous End of the Capillary. The low pressure at the venous end of the capillary changes the balance of forces in favor of absorption as follows:

	mm Hg
Force tending to move fluid inward:	
Plasma colloid osmotic pressure	28.0
TOTAL INWARD FORCE	28.0

	mm Hg
Forces tending to move fluid outward:	
Capillary pressure	10.0
Negative interstitial fluid pressure	5.3
Interstitial fluid colloid osmotic pressure	6.0
TOTAL OUTWARD FORCE	21.3
Summation of forces:	
Inward	28.0
Outward	21.3
NET INWARD FORCE	6.7

Thus, the force that causes fluid to move into the capillary, 28 mm Hg, is greater than that opposing reabsorption, 21.3 mm Hg. The difference, 6.7 mm Hg, is the *reabsorption pressure*. This reabsorption pressure is considerably less than the filtration pressure, but remember that the venous capillaries are more numerous and more permeable than the arterial capillaries so that less pressure is required to cause the inward movement of fluid.

The reabsorption pressure causes about nine tenths of the fluid that has filtered out of the arterial ends of the capillaries to be reabsorbed at the venous ends. The other one tenth flows into the lymph vessels, as is discussed in the following chapter.

Flow of Fluid Through the Interstitial Spaces

The 0.3 per cent of the plasma fluid that filters out of the arterial ends of the capillaries *flows* through the tissue spaces to the venous ends of the capillaries where all but about one tenth of it is reabsorbed. (A much higher proportion than this is reabsorbed in the muscles where very little protein leaks through the capillary membranes, and much less is reabsorbed in the liver where tremendous amounts of protein leak.)

THE STARLING EQUILIBRIUM FOR CAPILLARY EXCHANGE

E. H. Starling pointed out almost a century ago that under normal conditions a state of near-equilibrium exists at the capillary membrane whereby the amount of fluid filtering outward through the arterial capillaries equals that quantity of fluid that is returned to the circulation by reabsorption at the venous ends of the capillaries. This near-equilibrium is caused by near-equilibration of the *mean* forces tending to move fluid through the capillary membranes. If we assume that the mean *functional* capillary pressure is 17 mm Hg, the normal mean dynamics of the capillary are the following:

	mm Hg
Mean forces tending to move fluid outward:	
Mean capillary pressure	17.0
Negative interstitial fluid pressure	5.3
Interstitial fluid colloid osmotic pressure	6.0
TOTAL OUTWARD FORCE	28.3

Mean force tending to move fluid inward:

Plasma colloid osmotic pressure	28.0
TOTAL INWARD FORCE	28.0

Summation of mean forces:

Outward	28.3
Inward	28.0
NET OUTWARD FORCE	0.3

Thus, we find a near-equilibrium but nevertheless a slight imbalance of forces, 0.3 mm Hg, that causes slightly more filtration of fluid into the interstitial spaces than reabsorption. This slight excess of filtration is called the *net filtration,* and it is balanced by fluid return to the circulation through the lymphatics. The normal rate of net filtration in the entire body is about 2 ml/min. This figure also represents the average rate of fluid flow into the lymphatics each minute.

The Filtration Coefficient. In the above example an average net imbalance of forces at the capillary membranes of 0.3 mm Hg causes a net rate of fluid filtration in the entire body of 2 ml/min. Expressing this per millimeter of mercury, one finds a net filtration rate of 6.67 ml fluid/min/mm Hg for the entire body. This is called the *filtration coefficient.* It can be used to calculate the total filtration for any degree of imbalance of forces at the capillary membranes. For instance, for an imbalance of 6 mm Hg, the filtration would be 40 ml/min, a twentyfold increase above normal.

QUESTIONS

1. Describe the structure of a representative capillary bed, such as that in the mesentery.
2. Describe the pores in the capillary membrane.
3. Explain how nutrients and other substances pass from the capillaries to the tissues by diffusion.
4. What is the relative permeability of the capillary membrane to plasma proteins in comparison with water and the electrolytes of plasma?
5. Characterize the *interstitium* and the *interstitial fluid.*
6. Name the four *primary forces* that determine fluid movement through the capillary membrane, and explain why each of these causes fluid movement.
7. What is the normal *capillary pressure?* How is it measured?
8. What is the normal *interstitial fluid pressure?* How is it measured?
9. What are some of the reasons for believing that the true interstitial fluid pressure in the soft tissues of the body is subatmospheric?
10. What is the normal plasma colloid osmotic pressure?
11. What is the normal interstitial fluid colloid osmotic pressure.
12. State the quantitative values for the four forces that cause fluid absorption at the arterial ends of the capillaries.
13. State the quantitative values for the four primary forces that cause fluid absorption at the venous ends of the capillaries.
14. State quantitative values for the balance of the mean forces in the entire capillary bed.
15. What is meant by the *filtration coefficient?* How is it calculated?

References

Barry, P. H., and Diamond, J. M.: Effects of unstirred layers on membrane phenomena. Physiol Rev 64:763, 1984.

Bundgaard, M.: Transport pathways in capillaries—in search of pores. Annu Rev Physiol 42:325, 1980.

Crone, C., and Levitt, D. G.: Capillary permeability to small solutes. In Renkin, E. M., and Michel, C. C., eds.: Handbook of Physiology. Sec. 2, Vol. 4. Bethesda, American Physiological Society, 1984, p. 411.

Gore, R. W., and McDonagh, P. E.: Fluid exchange across single capillaries. Annu Rev Physiol 42:337, 1980.

Guyton, A. C.: Concept of negative interstitial pressure based on pressures in implanted perforated capsules. Circ Res 12:399, 1963.

Guyton, A. C., et al.: Interstitial fluid pressure. Physiol Rev 51:527, 1971.

Guyton, A. C., et al.: Circulatory Physiology II. Dynamics and Control of the Body Fluids. Philadelphia, W. B. Saunders Co., 1975.

Landis, E. M.: Capillary pressure and capillary permeability. Physiol Rev 14:404, 1934.

Michel, C. C.: Fluid movements through capillary walls. In Renkin, E. M., and Michel, C. C., eds.: Handbook of Physiology. Sec. 2, Vol. 4. Bethesda, American Physiological Society, 1984, p. 375.

Simionescu, M., and Simionescu, N.: Ultrastructure of the microvascular wall: Functional correlations. In Renkin, E. M., and Michel, C. C., eds.: Handbook of Physiology. Sec. 2, Vol. 4. Bethesda, American Physiological Society, 1984, p. 41.

Simionescu, N.: Cellular aspects of transcapillary exchange. Physiol Rev 63:1536, 1983.

Taylor, A. E., and Granger, D. N.: Exchange of macromolecules across the microcirculation. In Renkin, E. M., and Michel, C. C., eds.: Handbook of Physiology. Sec. 2, Vol. 4. Bethesda, American Physiological Society, 1984, p. 467.

23

The Lymphatic System, Interstitial Fluid Dynamics, Edema, the Pulmonary Fluid, and the Special Fluid Systems

THE LYMPHATIC SYSTEM
  THE LYMPH CHANNELS OF THE BODY
  FORMATION OF LYMPH
  TOTAL RATE OF LYMPH FLOW
  REGULATION OF INTERSTITIAL FLUID
    PROTEIN BY LYMPHATIC PUMPING
  MECHANISM OF NEGATIVE
    (SUBATMOSPHERIC) INTERSTITIAL
    FLUID PRESSURE

EDEMA
  PRESSURE-VOLUME CURVE OF THE
    INTERSTITIAL FLUID SPACES
PULMONARY INTERSTITIAL FLUID
  DYNAMICS
  PULMONARY EDEMA
SPECIAL FLUID SYSTEMS OF THE BODY
  THE CEREBROSPINAL FLUID SYSTEM
  THE INTRAOCULAR FLUID

THE LYMPHATIC SYSTEM

The lymphatic system represents an accessory route by which fluids can flow from the interstitial spaces into the blood. And, most important of all, the lymphatics can carry proteins and large particulate matter away from the tissue spaces, neither of which can be removed by absorption directly into the blood capillary.

THE LYMPH CHANNELS OF THE BODY

All tissues of the body, with the exception of a very few, have lymphatic channels or other channels similar to lymphatics that drain excess fluid directly from the interstitial spaces. Essentially all the lymph from the lower part of the body—even most of that from the legs—flows up the *thoracic duct* and empties into the venous system at the juncture of the *left* internal jugular vein and subclavian vein, as illus- trated in Figure 23–1. However, small amounts of lymph from the lower part of the body can enter the veins in the inguinal region and perhaps also at various points in the abdomen.

Lymph from the left side of the head, the left arm, and the left chest region also enters the thoracic duct before it empties into the veins. Lymph from the right side of the neck and head, from the right arm, and from parts of the right thorax enters the *right lymph duct*, which then empties into the venous system at the juncture of the *right* subclavian vein and internal jugular vein.

The Lymphatic Capillaries and Their Permeability

The minute quantity of fluid that returns to the circulation by way of the lymphatics is extremely important, because substances of high molecular weight such as proteins cannot pass with ease through

237

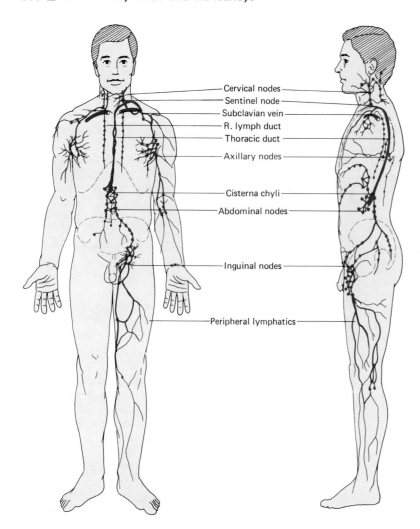

Figure 23-1. The lymphatic system.

Cervical nodes
Sentinel node
Subclavian vein
R. lymph duct
Thoracic duct
Axillary nodes
Cisterna chyli
Abdominal nodes
Inguinal nodes
Peripheral lymphatics

the pores of the venous capillaries, but they can enter the lymphatic capillaries almost completely unimpeded. The reason for this is a special structure of the lymphatic capillaries, illustrated in Figure 23-2. This figure shows the endothelial cells of the capillary attached by *anchoring filaments* to the connective tissue between the surrounding tissue cells. However, at the junctions of adjacent endothelial cells there are usually very loose connections between the cells. Instead, the edge of one endothelial cell usually overlaps the edge of the adjacent one in such a way that the overlapping edge is free to flap inward, thus forming a minute valve that opens to the interior of the capillary. Interstitial fluid, along with its suspended particles, can push the valve open and flow directly into the capillary. But this fluid has difficulty leaving the capillary once it has entered because any backflow will close the flap valve. Thus, the lymphatics have valves at the very tips of the terminal lymphatic capillaries as well as valves along their larger vessels up to the point where they empty into the blood circulation.

FORMATION OF LYMPH

Lymph is interstitial fluid that flows into the lymphatics. Therefore, lymph has almost the same com-

position as the tissue fluid in the part of the body from which the lymph flows.

The protein concentration in the interstitial fluid averages about 2 gm per 100 ml, and the protein concentration of lymph flowing from most of the peripheral tissues is near to this value. On the other hand, lymph formed in the liver has a protein concentration as high as 6 gm per 100 ml, and lymph

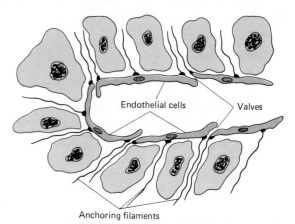

Endothelial cells
Valves
Anchoring filaments

Figure 23-2. Special structure of the lymphatic capillaries that permits passage of substances of high molecular weight back into the circulation.

formed in the intestines has a protein concentration as high as 3 to 5 gm per 100 ml. Since more than half of the lymph is derived from the liver and intestines, the thoracic duct lymph, which is a mixture of lymph from all areas of the body, usually has a protein concentration of 3 to 5 gm per 100 ml.

The lymphatic system is also one of the major routes for absorption of nutrients from the gastrointestinal tract, being responsible principally for the absorption of fats, as will be discussed in Chapter 44.

TOTAL RATE OF LYMPH FLOW

Approximately 100 ml of lymph flows through the thoracic duct of a resting person per hour, and perhaps another 20 ml of lymph flows into the circulation each hour through other channels, making a total estimated lymph flow of about 120 ml per hour, illustrating that the flow of lymph is relatively small in comparison with the total two-way exchange of fluid by diffusion between the plasma and the interstial fluid.

Factors That Determine the Rate of Lymph Flow

Interstitial Fluid Pressure. Elevation of interstitial *free* fluid pressure above its normal level of −5.3 mm Hg increases the flow of interstitial fluid into the lymphatic capillaries and consequently also increases the rate of lymph flow. The increase in flow becomes progressively greater until the interstitial fluid pressure reaches a value slightly greater than zero mm Hg; at that point the flow rate reaches a maximum, but by that time it has risen to 10 to 50 times normal. Therefore, any factor that increases the net filtration out of the capillaries will also increase the rate of lymph flow. Such factors include

Elevated capillary pressure
Decreased plasma colloid osmotic pressure
Increased interstitial fluid protein
Increased permeability of the capillaries

The Lymphatic Pump. Valves exist periodically all along the lymph channels; typical valves are illus-

trated in Figure 23–3 in a *collecting lymphatic* into which the lymphatic capillaries empty. Therefore, every time a lymph vessel or a lymphatic capillary is compressed by pressure from any source, lymph is squeezed forward along the lymphatics. The lymph vessels can be compressed either by contraction of the walls of the lymphatics or by pressure from surrounding structures.

Motion pictures taken of exposed lymph vessels, both in animals and in human beings, have shown that any time a lymph vessel becomes stretched with fluid the smooth muscle in the wall of the vessel automatically contracts. Furthermore, each segment of the lymph vessel between successive valves functions as a separate automatic pump. That is, filling of a segment causes it to contract, and the fluid is then pumped through the next valve into the following lymphatic segment. This fills the subsequent segment so that within a few seconds it too contracts, the process continuing all along the lymphatic until the fluid is finally emptied. In a large lymph vessel this lymphatic pump can generate pressure as high as 25 to 50 mm Hg if the outflow from the vessel becomes blocked.

In addition to the pumping caused by intrinsic contraction of the lymph vessel walls, any external factor that compresses the lymph vessel can also cause pumping. In order of their importance, such factors are

Contraction of muscles
Movements of the parts of the body
Arterial pulsations
Compression of the tissue by objects outside the body

The lymphatic pump becomes very active during exercise, often increasing lymph flow as much as 5- to 15-fold. On the other hand, during periods of rest, lymph flow is very sluggish.

REGULATION OF INTERSTITIAL FLUID PROTEIN BY LYMPHATIC PUMPING

Since protein continually leaks from the capillaries into the interstitial fluid spaces, it must also be

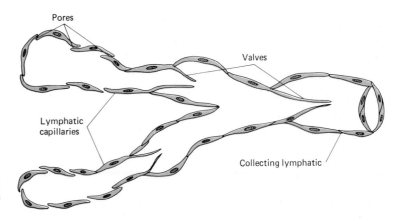

Figure 23–3. Structure of lymphatic capillaries and a collecting lymphatic, showing also the lymphatic valves.

continually removed, or otherwise the tissue colloid osmotic pressure will become so high that normal capillary dynamics can no longer continue. Therefore, by far the most important of all the lymphatic functions is the maintenance of low protein concentration in the interstitial fluid. The mechanism of this maintenance is the following:

As fluid leaks from the arterial ends of the capillaries into the interstitial spaces, only small quantities of protein accompany it, but then, as fluid is reabsorbed at the venous ends of the capillaries, most of the protein is left behind. Therefore, *protein progressively accumulates in the interstitial fluid* and this in turn *increases the tissue colloid osmotic pressure*. This osmotic pressure decreases reabsorption of fluid by the capillaries, thereby *promoting increased tissue fluid volume* and *increased interstitial fluid pressure*. The increased pressure then causes the lymphatic pump to pump the interstitial fluid into the lymphatic capillaries, carrying with it the excess protein that has accumulated. This continued *washout* of the protein keeps its concentration at a low level in the interstitial fluid.

To summarize, an increase in tissue fluid protein increases the rate of lymph flow, and this washes the proteins out of the tissue spaces, automatically decreasing the protein concentration back to its normal low level.

The importance of this function of the lymphatics cannot be stressed too strongly, for *there is no other route besides the lymphatics through which excess proteins can return to the circulatory system*. If it were not for this continual removal of proteins, the dynamics of fluid exchange at the blood capillaries would become so abnormal within about a day that life could no longer continue.

MECHANISM OF NEGATIVE (SUBATMOSPHERIC) INTERSTITIAL FLUID PRESSURE

Until recent measurements of the interstitial fluid pressure demonstrated that it is negative—that is, less than atmospheric pressure—rather than positive, as explained in the preceding chapter, it was taught that the normal interstitial fluid pressure ranges between +1 and +4 mm Hg, and it has still been difficult to understand how negative pressure can develop in the interstitial fluid spaces. However, we can explain this negative interstitial fluid pressure by the following considerations:

First, the lymph fluid can flow into lymphatic vessels from the interstitial spaces even when the interstitial fluid pressure is negative, mainly because the lymphatic pump can create slight degrees of suction. And this lymph flow keeps the protein concentration of the interstitial fluid at a low value, thereby keeping the colloid osmotic pressure also at a low value, usually at about 6 mm Hg in most peripheral tissues such as the muscles.

Second, the negativity of the interstitial fluid pressure can then be explained mainly on the basis of the

balance of forces at the capillary membrane. If we add all the other forces besides the interstitial fluid pressure that cause movement of fluid across the capillary membrane, we find the following:

	mm Hg
Outward force:	
Capillary pressure	17
Interstitial fluid colloid osmotic pressure	6
TOTAL	23
Inward force:	
Colloid osmotic pressure	28
DIFFERENCE (Interstitial fluid pressure)	−5

Thus, we see that the interstitial fluid pressure required to balance the other forces across the capillary membrane is −5 mm Hg. Indirectly, this results from the continual pumping of *protein* into the lymphatic vessels. Another −0.3 mm Hg is caused by the continual pumping of *fluid* into the lymphatic vessels, giving a total calculated negativity of −5.3 mm Hg.

Significance of the Normally "Dry" State of the Interstitial Spaces. The normal tendency of the capillaries to absorb fluid from the interstitial spaces and thereby to create a partial vacuum causes all the minute structures of the interstitial spaces to be *compacted*. This represents a "dry" state; that is, no *excess* fluid is present besides that required simply to fill the crevices between the tissue elements plus that held in the interstices of the tissue gel, as will be discussed later in the chapter.

This compacted state of the tissues is particularly important for optimal nutrition of the tissues, because nutrients pass from the blood to the cells by diffusion, and the rate of diffusion between two points is inversely proportional to the distance between the cells and the capillaries.

EDEMA

Edema means the presence of excess interstitial fluid in the tissues. Obviously, any factor that increases the interstitial fluid pressure high enough can cause excess interstitial fluid volume and thereby cause edema. However, to explain the conditions under which edema develops, we must first characterize the *pressure-volume curve* of the interstitial fluid spaces.

PRESSURE-VOLUME CURVE OF THE INTERSTITIAL FLUID SPACES

Figure 23–4 illustrates the average relationship between pressure and volume in the interstitial fluid spaces in the human body as extrapolated from measurements in the dog.

One of the most significant features of the curve is the flat portion of this curve at the bottom—that is,

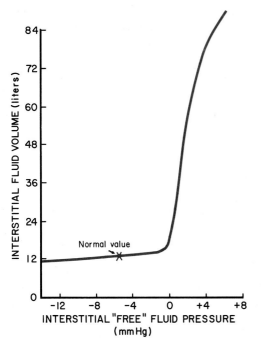

Figure 23–4. Pressure-volume curve of the interstitial spaces. (Extrapolated to the human being from data obtained in dogs.)

so long as the interstitial fluid pressure remains in the negative range, there is little change in interstitial fluid volume despite marked change in pressure. Therefore, edema will not occur so long as the interstitial free fluid pressure remains negative. The reason is that the negative pressure keeps the tissue spaces compacted all the time to almost the smallest volume possible. Indeed, in several hundred measurements of interstitial fluid pressure made in experimental animals, no edema has ever been recorded in the presence of negative interstitial pressure.

Tremendous Increase in Interstitial Fluid Volume When the Interstitial Free Fluid Pressure Becomes Positive. Note in Figure 23–4 that just as soon as the interstitial free fluid pressure rises above atmospheric pressure (above zero pressure), the slope of the pressure-volume curve suddenly changes and the volume increases precipitously. An additional increase in interstitial free fluid pressure of only 1 to 3 mm Hg now causes the interstitial fluid volume to increase several hundred per cent. Finally, at the very top of the figure, the skin begins to be stretched, so that the volume now increases much less rapidly.

Positive Interstitial Fluid Pressure as the Physical Basis for Edema

After studying the pressure-volume curve of Figure 23–4, one can readily see that whenever the interstitial free fluid pressure rises above the surrounding atmospheric pressure, the tissue spaces begin to swell. Therefore, *the physical cause of edema is positive pressure (that is, supra-atmospheric pressure) in the interstitial fluid spaces.*

Edema usually is not detectable in tissues until the interstitial fluid volume has risen to about 30 per cent above normal. But note that the interstitial fluid volume increases to several hundred per cent above normal in seriously edematous tissues.

Edema Resulting From Abnormal Capillary Dynamics

From the discussions of capillary and interstitial fluid dynamics in the preceding and present chapters, it is already evident that several different abnormalities in these dynamics can increase the tissue pressure and in turn cause extracellular fluid edema. The different causes of extracellular fluid edema are

1. *Increased capillary pressure*, which causes excess filtration of fluid through the capillaries.

2. *Decreased plasma protein*, which causes reduced plasma colloid osmotic pressure and therefore failure to retain fluid in the capillaries.

3. *Lymphatic obstruction*, which causes protein to accumulate in the tissue spaces and therefore causes osmosis of fluid out of the capillaries.

4. *Increased capillary permeability*, which allows leakage of excess fluid and protein into the tissue spaces.

Edema Caused by Kidney Retention of Fluid

When the kidney fails to excrete adequate quantities of urine, but the person continues to drink normal amounts of water and ingest normal amounts of electrolytes, the total amount of extracellular fluid in the body increases progressively. This fluid is absorbed from the gut into the blood and elevates the capillary pressure. This is turn causes most of the fluid to pass into the interstitial fluid spaces, elevating the interstitial fluid pressure as well. Therefore, simple retention of fluid by the kidneys can result in extensive edema.

Edema Caused by Heart Failure

Heart failure is one of the most frequent causes of edema, for when the heart no longer pumps blood out of the veins with ease, blood dams up in the venous system. The capillary pressure rises, and serious "cardiac edema" occurs. In addition, the kidneys also function poorly in heart failure, and this leads to even more edema as described above and as discussed in detail in Chapter 17.

PULMONARY INTERSTITIAL FLUID DYNAMICS

The dynamics of the pulmonary interstitial fluid are essentially the same as those of the fluid in the peripheral tissues except for the following important quantitative differences:

1. The pulmonary capillary pressure is very low in comparison with the systemic capillary pressure, approximately 7 mm Hg in comparison with 17 mm Hg.

2. The interstitial fluid pressure in the lung interstitium has been measured to be −8 mm Hg in comparison with −5 mm Hg in subcutaneous tissue.

3. The pulmonary capillaries are relatively leaky to protein molecules, so that the protein concentration of lymph leaving the lungs is relatively high, averaging about 4 gm per 100 ml, instead of 2 gm per 100 ml in the peripheral tissues.

4. The rate of lymph flow from the lungs is also very high, mainly because of the continuous pumping motion of the lungs.

Now let us see how these quantitative differences affect pulmonary fluid dynamics.

Interrelationship Between Interstitial Fluid Pressure and Other Pressures in the Lung. Figure 23–5 illustrates a pulmonary capillary, a pulmonary alveolus, and a lymphatic capillary draining the interstitial space between the capillary and the alveolus. Note that the balance of forces at the capillary membrane is such that the interstitial pressure is normally −8 mm Hg.

The Mechanism for Keeping the Alveoli "Dry." How is it that the fluid normally present in the interstitial spaces is prevented from flooding the alveoli? The answer to this question is the negative fluid pressure of approximately −8 mm Hg in the interstitial spaces between the capillary and the alveolar membrane. This continually tends to pull fluid inward through the alveolar membrane and therefore also prevents fluid loss in the outward direction.

PULMONARY EDEMA

Pulmonary edema occurs in the same way that edema occurs elsewhere in the body. Any factor that

PRESSURES CAUSING FLUID MOVEMENT

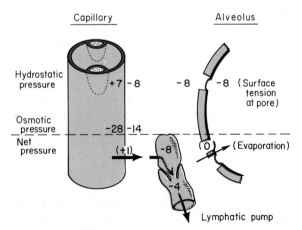

Figure 23–5. Hydrostatic and osmotic forces at the capillary (left) and alveolar membrane (right) of the lungs. Also shown is a lymphatic (center) that pumps fluid from the pulmonary interstitial spaces. (Modified from Guyton, Taylor, and Granger: Dynamics and Control of the Body Fluids. Philadelphia, W. B. Saunders Company, 1975.)

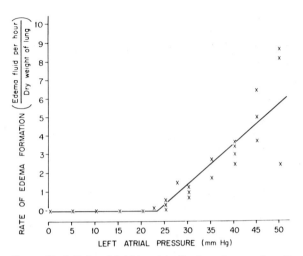

Figure 23–6. Rate of fluid loss into the lung tissues when the left atrial pressure (and also pulmonary capillary pressure) is increased. (From Guyton and Lindsey: Circ Res 7:649, 1959, by permission of the American Heart Association, Inc.)

causes the pulmonary interstitial fluid pressure to rise from the negative range into the positive range will cause sudden filling of the pulmonary interstitial spaces, and in more severe cases even the alveoli, with large amounts of free fluid—occasionally as much as 1 liter of fluid that literally suffocates the person.

Pulmonary "Interstitial Fluid" Edema Versus Pulmonary "Alveolar" Edema. The interstitial fluid volume of the lungs usually cannot increase more than about 50 per cent (representing less than 100 ml of fluid) before the alveolar epithelial membranes rupture and fluid begins to pour from the interstitial spaces into the alveoli. The cause of this occurrence is simply the almost infinitesmal tensional strength of the pulmonary alveolar epithelium; that is, any positive pressure in the interstitial fluid spaces seems to cause immediate rupture of the alveolar epithelium.

Therefore, except in the mildest cases of pulmonary edema, most of the fluid enters the alveoli.

Safety Factor Against Pulmonary Edema. The most common cause of pulmonary edema is greatly elevated pulmonary capillary pressure resulting from *failure of the left heart*, which causes damming of blood in the lungs. However, the pulmonary capillary pressure usually must rise to very high values before serious pulmonary edema develops. This effect is illustrated in Figure 23–6, which shows development of lung edema in dogs subjected to progressively increasing left atrial pressure. In this experiment, no edema fluid developed in the lungs until left atrial pressure rose from the normal level of about 2 mm Hg to above 23 mm Hg, which was approximately 3 mm Hg greater than the colloid osmotic pressure of dog blood, about 20 mm Hg. In the human being, the colloid osmotic pressure is about 28 mm Hg, so that pulmonary edema will rarely develop below 30 mm Hg pulmonary capillary pressure. Thus, if the capillary pressure in the lungs is normally 7 mm Hg and this pressure must usually rise above 30 mm Hg before edema occurs, the lungs have a *safety factor against edema* of approximately 23 mm Hg.

Pulmonary Edema as a Result of Capillary Damage. Pulmonary edema can also result from local capillary damage in the lungs. This effect is often caused by bacterial infection such as occurs in pneumonia, by irritant gases such as chlorine or sulfur dioxide, or by war gases—mustard gas, for instance. All these directly damage the alveolar epithelium and the endothelium of the capillaries, allowing rapid transudation of both fluid and protein into the interstitial spaces and alveoli.

Rapidity of Death in Acute Pulmonary Edema. When the pulmonary capillary pressure does rise above the safety factor level, lethal pulmonary edema can occur within hours if it is only slightly above the safety factor, and within 20 to 30 minutes if it is as much as 25 to 30 mm Hg above the safety factor level. Thus, in acute left heart failure, in which the pulmonary capillary pressure occasionally rises to as high as 50 mm Hg, death from acute pulmonary edema frequently ensues within 30 minutes.

SPECIAL FLUID SYSTEMS OF THE BODY

Several special fluid systems exist in the body, each performing functions peculiar to itself. For instance, the cerebrospinal fluid supports the brain in the cranial vault; the intraocular fluid maintains distension of the eyeballs so that the optical dimensions of the eye remain constant; and the potential spaces, such as the pleural and pericardial spaces, provide lubricated chambers in which the internal organs can move. All these fluid systems have some characteristics that are similar to each other and that are also similar to those of the interstitial fluid system. However, to emphasize their special characteristics, we will discuss the cerebrospinal and ocular fluid systems.

THE CEREBROSPINAL FLUID SYSTEM

The entire cavity enclosing the brain and spinal cord has a volume of approximately 1650 ml, and about 150 ml of this volume is occupied by cerebrospinal fluid. This fluid, as shown in Figure 23–7, is found in the ventricles of the brain, in the cisterns around the brain, and in the subarachnoid space around both the brain and the spinal cord. All these chambers are connected with each other, and the pressure of the fluid is regulated at a constant level.

Cushioning Function of the Cerebrospinal Fluid. A major function of the cerebrospinal fluid is to cushion the brain within its solid vault. Were it not for this fluid, any blow to the head would cause the brain to be shaken around and severely damaged. However, the brain and the cerebrospinal fluid have approximately the same specific gravity, so that the brain simply floats in the fluid. Therefore, blows on the head move the entire skull and brain at once, causing

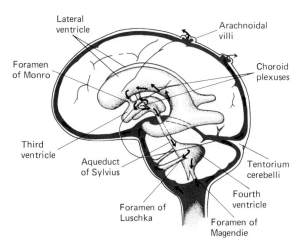

Figure 23–7. Pathway of cerebrospinal fluid flow from the choroid plexuses in the lateral ventricles to the arachnoidal villi protruding into the dural sinuses.

no one portion of the brain to be momentarily contorted by the blow.

Formation, Flow, and Absorption of Cerebrospinal Fluid. Cerebrospinal fluid is formed at a rate of approximately 500 ml each day, which is about three times as much as the total volume of fluid in the entire cerebrospinal fluid cavity. Essentially all of this fluid is formed by the choroid plexus, which is a cauliflower-like growth of blood vessels covered by a thin coat of epithelial cells. This plexus projects into (1) the temporal horns of the lateral ventricles, (2) the posterior portions of the third ventricle, and (3) the roof of the fourth ventricle.

Cerebrospinal fluid is continually secreted by the choroid plexus. This secretion occurs from the epithelial cells by the process of *active secretion*, which was explained in Chapter 4. The fluid then flows out of the fourth ventricle into the subarachnoid space through small openings adjacent to the cerebellum, the *foramina of Luschka* and the *foramen of Magendie*. From here, it flows throughout the entire subarachnoid space but mainly up over the surface of the brain, where it is reabsorbed into the blood through special structures called *arachnoidal villi* or *granulations*. These project from the subarachnoid spaces into the venous sinuses of the brain. The arachnoidal villi are actually arachnoidal trabeculae that have penetrated through the venous walls, resulting in extremely permeable areas that allow relatively free flow of cerebrospinal fluid into the venous blood.

Cerebrospinal Fluid Pressure

The normal pressure in the cerebrospinal fluid system when one is lying in a horizontal position averages 130 mm water (10 mm Hg). The pressure is regulated by the combination of, first, the *rate of fluid formation* and, second, the *resistance to absorption through the arachnoidal villi*. When either of these is increased, the pressure rises; and when either is

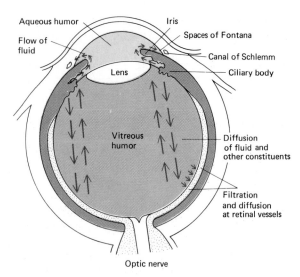

Figure 23–8. Formation and flow of fluid in the eye.

decreased, the pressure falls. A common cause of elevated cerebrospinal fluid is a large *brain tumor* that increases the cerebrospinal fluid pressure by compressing the brain against the subarachnoid spaces and against the veins, thereby decreasing the rate of absorption of fluid.

Hydrocephalus. *Hydrocephalus* means excess water in the cranial vault. This condition is caused by (1) blockage of flow out of one or more of the ventricles, which leads to ventricular swelling or (2) overdevelopment of the choroid plexus in the newborn infant, so that far more fluid is formed than can re-enter the venous system through the arachnoidal villi; fluid therefore collects both inside the ventricles and on the outside of the brain. In the hydrocephalic infant, whose skull remains very pliable until the bones fuse at the age of 3 to 4 years, the head swells tremendously, often damaging the brain severely.

THE INTRAOCULAR FLUID

The eye is filled with intraocular fluid, which maintains sufficient pressure in the eyeball to keep it distended. Figure 23–8 illustrates that this fluid can be divided into two portions, the *aqueous humor*, which lies in front and to the sides of the lens, and the *vitreous humor*, which lies between the lens and the retina. The aqueous humor is a freely flowing clear fluid, while the vitreous humor, sometimes called the *vitreous body*, is a gelatinous mass held together by a fine fibrillar network of proteoglycan molecules. Substances can *diffuse* slowly in the vitreous humor, but there is little *flow* of fluid.

Aqueous humor is continually being formed and reabsorbed. The balance between formation and reabsorption of aqueous humor regulates the total volume and pressure of the intraocular fluid.

Formation and Absorption of Aqueous Humor— The Ciliary Body. Aqueous humor is formed in the human eye *at an average rate of 1 to 2 ml each minute.*

Essentially all of this fluid is *actively* secreted by the *ciliary processes*, which are linear folds projecting from the *ciliary body* into the space behind the iris, as seen in Figure 23–8. Because of their folding architecture, the total surface area of the ciliary processes is approximately 6 sq cm in each eye, a large area, considering the small size of the ciliary body. The surfaces of these processes are covered by epithelial secretory cells, and immediately beneath these is a highly vascular area.

After the aqueous humor is secreted by the ciliary processes, it flows, as shown in Figure 23–8, *between the ligaments of the lens*, then *through the pupil*, and finally *into the anterior chamber of the eye*. Here, the fluid flows into the *angle between the cornea and the iris*, thence through a meshwork of *trabeculae* and finally into the *canal of Schlemm*. Figure 23–9 illustrates the anatomical structures at the iridocorneal angle, showing that the spaces between the trabeculae extend all the way from the anterior chamber to the canal of Schlemm. The canal of Schlemm in turn is a thin-walled vein that extends circumferentially all the way around the eye. Its endothelial membrane is so porous that even large protein molecules, as well as small particulate matter, can pass from the anterior chamber into the canal of Schlemm.

Intraocular Pressure

The average normal intraocular pressure is approximately 16 mm Hg, with a range from 12 to 20 mm Hg.

The intraocular pressure of the normal eye remains almost exactly constant throughout life, illustrating that the pressure-regulating mechanism is very effective. The pressure is regulated mainly by the outflow resistance from the anterior chamber into the canal of Schlemm, presumably in the following way:

The wall of the canal of Schlemm consists of multiple layers, and the intraocular fluid penetrates through the iridocorneal angle to the outer surface of this wall. When the pressure of the intraocular fluid is low, the thickness of the wall is very slight, and the

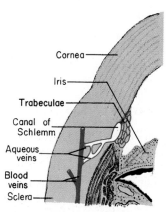

Figure 23–9. Anatomy of the iridocorneal angle, showing the system for outflow of aqueous humor into the conjunctival veins.

multiple layers remain compacted against each other in such a way that the fluid cannot flow readily into the canal of Schlemm. However, when the intraocular pressure rises higher than about 15 mm Hg, much of the intraocular fluid then penetrates into the wall of the canal of Schlemm, pushing the layers of the cells apart and opening large fluid channels about 2 to 3 microns in size. These, in turn, allow large quantities of intraocular fluid then to enter the canal of Schlemm. Thus, this valvelike opening of the spaces through the wall of the canal of Schlemm provides an automatic regulatory system for keeping the intraocular pressure at a nearly constant level day in and day out.

Glaucoma. Glaucoma is a disease of the eye in which the intraocular pressure becomes pathologically high. As the pressure rises, the retinal artery, which enters the eyeball at the optic disc, is compressed, thus reducing the nutrition to the retina. Pressures above as little as 25 to 30 mm Hg, when maintained for long periods of time, often result in permanent atrophy of the retina and optic nerve with consequent blindness.

Glaucoma is one of the most common causes of blindness. Very high pressures lasting only a few days can at times cause total and permanent blindness, but in cases with only mildly elevated pressures, blindness may develop progressively over a period of many years.

In essentially all cases of glaucoma, the abnormally high pressure results from increased resistance to fluid outflow at the iridocorneal junction. In most patients, the cause of this is unknown, but in others it results from infection or trauma to the eye. In these persons large quantities of red blood cells, white blood cells, and tissue debris collect in the aqueous humor and then pass into the trabecular spaces of the iridocorneal angle, where they block the outflow of fluid, thereby greatly increasing the intraocular pressure.

QUESTIONS

1. Describe the anatomy of the lymphatic system. How are the *lymphatic capillaries* different from *blood capillaries*?
2. What is the relationship between *interstitial fluid pressure* and lymph flow?
3. Describe the lymphatic pump. What are the different external effects that can compress the lymph vessels and cause lymphatic pumping?
4. Why is the concentration of proteins higher in the lymph than in the fluid that filters out of the arterial ends of the capillaries?
5. Why does leakage of protein out of the capillaries into the interstitial spaces increase lymph flow?
6. Explain the mechanism and the importance of lymph flow in regulating tissue fluid protein concentration.
7. What causes *negative* interstitial fluid pressure?
8. Why is it important for the interstitial spaces to be normally compacted in a so-called "dry" state?
9. What is the relationship between *positive* tissue pressure and edema?
10. List the types of functional abnormalities of capillary dynamics that can cause edema.
11. Describe the quantitative differences between pulmonary interstitial fluid dynamics and peripheral interstitial fluid dynamics, beginning with the differences between the forces active at the capillary membrane.
12. What is the mechanism for keeping the alveoli normally "dry"?
13. Why does positive pressure in the pulmonary interstitium usually cause fluid to flood the alveoli?
14. Explain the concept of *safety factor against pulmonary edema.*
15. Describe the formation, flow, and absorption of fluid in the cerebrospinal fluid system. What are the factors that control the *cerebrospinal fluid pressure?*
16. What can lead to *hydrocephalus?*
17. Describe the formation, flow, and absorption of fluid in the eyeball.
18. Explain the factors that control the *intraocular pressure.*
19. What is *glaucoma?* Describe its usual cause and its effects on the eye.

References

Lymphatic System, Interstitium, Pulmonary Fluid

Aukland, K., and Nicolaysen, G.: Interstitial fluid volume: Local regulatory mechanisms. Physiol Rev 61:556, 1981.
Bert, J. L., and Pearce, R. H.: The interstitium and microvascular exchange. In Renkin, E. M., and Michel, C. C., eds.: Handbook of Physiology. Sec. 2, Vol. 4. Bethesda, American Physiological Society, 1984, p. 521.
Curry, F.-R. E.: Mechanics and thermodynamics of transcapillary exchange. In Renkin, E. M., and Michel, C. C., eds.: Handbook of Physiology. Sec. 2, Vol. 4. Bethesda, American Physiological Society, 1984, p. 309.
Gross, J. F., and Popel, A., eds.: Mathematics of Microcirculation Phenomena. New York, Raven Press, 1980.

Guyton, A. C.: Interstitial fluid pressure: II. Pressure-volume curves of interstitial space. Circ Res 16:452, 1965.
Guyton, A. C., and Lindsey, A. W.: Effect of elevated left atrial pressure and decreased plasma protein concentration on the development of pulmonary edema. Circ Res 7:649, 1959.
Guyton, A. C., et al.: Interstitial fluid pressure. Physiol Rev 51:527, 1971.
Guyton, A. C., et al.: Dynamics and Control of the Body Fluids. Philadelphia, W. B. Saunders Co., 1975.
Kinmonth, J. G.: The Lymphatics. Surgery, Lymphography and Diseases of the Chyle and Lymph Systems. Baltimore, E. Arnold, 1982.

Notter, R. H., and Finkelstein, J. N.: Pulmonary surfactant: An interdisciplinary approach. J Appl Physiol 57:1613, 1984.

Parker, J. C., et al.: Pulmonary transcapillary exchange and pulmonary edema. In Guyton, A. C., and Young, D. B., eds.: International Review of Physiology: Cardiovascular Physiology III. Vol. 18. Baltimore, University Park Press, 1979, p. 261.

Yoffey, J. M., and Courtice, F. C., eds.: Lymphatics, Lymph and Lymphomyeloid Complex. New York, Academic Press, 1970.

Special Fluid Systems

Agostoni, E.: Mechanics of the pleural space. Physiol Rev 52:57, 1972.

Bill, A.: Blood circulation and fluid dynamics in the eye. Physiol Rev 55:383, 1975.

Bill, A.: Circulation in the eye. In Renkin, E. M., and Michel, C. C., eds.: Handbook of Physiology. Sec. 2, Vol. 4. Bethesda, American Physiological Society, 1984, p. 1001.

Davson, H.: The Physiology of the Cerebrospinal Fluid. Boston, Little, Brown, 1967.

Fenstermacher, J. D., and Rapoport, S. I.: Blood-brain barrier. In Renkin, E. M., and Michel, C. C., eds.: Handbook of Physiology. Sec. 2, Vol. 4. Bethesda, American Physiological Society, 1984, p. 969.

Hills, B. A.: The pleural interface. Thorax 40:1, 1985.

Notter, R. H., and Finkelstein, J. N.: Pulmonary surfactant: An interdisciplinary approach. J Appl Physiol 57:1613, 1984.

Shulman, K., ed.: Intracranial Pressure IV. New York, Springer-Verlag, 1980.

Siesjo, B. K.: Cerebral circulation and metabolism. J Neurosurg 60:883, 1984.

24

Formation of Urine by the Kidneys

Part 1 ■ Glomerular Filtration, Tubular Function, and Plasma Clearance

PHYSIOLOGIC ANATOMY OF THE KIDNEYS

BASIC THEORY OF NEPHRON FUNCTION

RENAL BLOOD FLOW AND PRESSURES

BLOOD FLOW THROUGH THE KIDNEYS

PRESSURES IN THE RENAL CIRCULATION

GLOMERULAR FILTRATION AND THE GLOMERULAR FILTRATE

THE GLOMERULAR FILTRATION RATE

DYNAMICS OF GLOMERULAR FILTRATION

REABSORPTION AND SECRETION IN THE TUBULES

BASIC MECHANISMS OF ABSORPTION AND SECRETION IN THE TUBULES

REABSORPTION AND SECRETION OF DIFFERENT TYPES OF SUBSTANCES IN DIFFERENT SEGMENTS OF THE TUBULES

CONCENTRATIONS OF DIFFERENT SUBSTANCES IN THE URINE

THE CONCEPT OF PLASMA CLEARANCE

INULIN CLEARANCE AS A MEASURE OF GLOMERULAR FILTRATION RATE

PARA-AMINOHIPPURIC ACID (PAH) CLEARANCE AS A MEASURE OF PLASMA FLOW THROUGH THE KIDNEYS

Part 2 ■ Control of Excretion of Water and Individual Solutes by the Kidneys

THE DILUTING MECHANISM OF THE KIDNEYS: THE MECHANISM FOR EXCRETING EXCESS WATER

THE MECHANISM FOR EXCRETING EXCESS SOLUTES: THE COUNTERCURRENT MECHANISM FOR EXCRETING A CONCENTRATED URINE

UREA EXCRETION

SODIUM EXCRETION

POTASSIUM EXCRETION

FLUID VOLUME EXCRETION

AUTOREGULATION OF GLOMERULAR FILTRATION RATE

AUTOREGULATION OF RENAL BLOOD FLOW

ROLES OF THE RENIN-ANGIOTENSIN SYSTEM AND THE EFFERENT VASOCONSTRICTOR MECHANISM IN CONSERVING WATER AND SALT BUT ELIMINATING UREA DURING ARTERIAL HYPOTENSION

Part 1 ■ Glomerular Filtration, Tubular Function, and Plasma Clearance

The kidneys perform two major functions: first, they excrete most of the end-products of bodily metabolism, and second, they control the concentrations of most of the constituents of the body fluids. The purpose of the present chapter is to discuss the principles of urine formation and especially the mechanisms by which the kidneys excrete the end-products of metabolism.

PHYSIOLOGIC ANATOMY OF THE KIDNEY

The two kidneys together contain about 2,400,000 nephrons, and each nephron is capable of forming urine by itself. The nephron is composed basically of (1) a *glomerulus* from which fluid is filtered and (2) a long *tubule* in which the filtered fluid is converted into urine on its way to the *pelvis* of the kidney.

Figure 24–1 shows the general organizational plan of the kidney, illustrating especially the distinction between the *cortex* of the kidney and the *medulla*. And Figure 24–2 illustrates the basic anatomy of the nephron, which may be described as follows: Blood

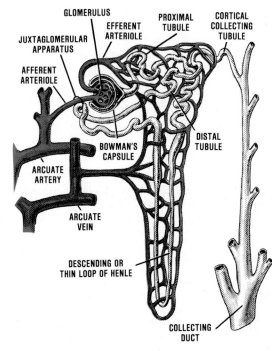

Figure 24–2. The nephron. (From Smith: The Kidney: Structure and Functions in Health and Disease. New York, Oxford University Press, 1951.)

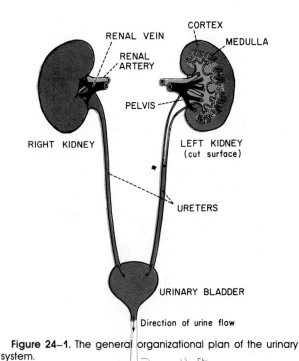

Figure 24–1. The general organizational plan of the urinary system.

enters the glomerulus through the *afferent arteriole* and then leaves through the *efferent arteriole*. The glomerulus is a network of up to 50 branching capillaries covered by epithelial cells. Pressure of the blood in the glomerulus causes fluid to filter through the glomerular capillaries into *Bowman's capsule,* from which it flows first into the *proximal tubule.* From here the fluid passes into the *loop of Henle,* which loops downward toward the renal medulla; about a third to a fifth of the loops penetrate deeply into the medulla. The lower portion of the loop has a very thin wall and therefore is called the *thin segment* of the loop of Henle. From the loop of Henle the fluid flows through the *distal tubule.* Thence, it flows first into the *collecting tubule* and finally, into the *collecting duct,* which collects fluid from many nephrons. The collecting duct passes from the cortex back downward through the medulla, paralleling the loops of Henle. Then it empties into the pelvis of the kidney.

As the glomerular filtrate flows through the tubules, over 99 per cent of its water and varying amounts of its solutes are reabsorbed into the peritubular capillaries, and small amounts of other solutes are secreted into the tubules. The remaining tubular water and solutes become urine.

The Peritubular Capillary Network and the Vasa Recta. Surrounding the entire tubular system of the kidney is an extensive network of capillaries called the *peritubular capillary network*. This network is supplied with blood from the *efferent arterioles,* blood that has already passed through the glomerulus. Most of the peritubular capillary network lies in the renal cortex alongside the proximal tubules, distal tubules, and collecting tubules. However, from the deeper portions of this peritubular network, long and straight capillary loops called *vasa recta* extend downward into the medulla to lie side by side with the lower parts of the thin segments of the loops of Henle all the way to the renal papillae. Then, like the loops of Henle, they also turn back toward the cortex and empty into the cortical veins.

Functional Diagram of the Nephron. Figure 24–3 illustrates a simplified diagram of the "physiologic nephron." This diagram contains most of the nephron's functional structures, and it is used in subsequent discussions to explain many aspects of renal function.

BASIC THEORY OF NEPHRON FUNCTION

The basic function of the nephron is to clean, or "clear," the blood plasma of unwanted substances as it passes through the kidney. The substances that must be cleared include particularly the end-products of metabolism, such as urea, creatinine, uric acid, and urates. In addition, many other substances, such as sodium ions, potassium ions, chloride ions, and hydrogen ions, tend to accumulate in the body in excess quantities; it is the function of the nephron also to clear the plasma of these excesses.

The principal mechanism by which the nephron clears the plasma of unwanted substances is: (1) It filters a large proportion of the plasma, usually about one fifth of it, through the glomerular membrane into the tubules of the nephron. (2) Then, as this filtered fluid flows through the tubules, the *unwanted substances fail to be reabsorbed* while the *wanted substances, especially the water and many of the electrolytes, are reabsorbed* back into the plasma of the peritubular capillaries. In other words, the wanted portions of the tubular fluid are returned to the blood and the unwanted portions pass into the urine.

A second mechanism by which the nephron clears the plasma of other unwanted substances is by *secretion.* That is, substances are secreted from the plasma directly through the epithelial cells lining the tubules into the tubular fluid. Thus, the urine that is eventually formed is composed mainly of *filtered* substances but also of small amounts of *secreted* substances.

RENAL BLOOD FLOW AND PRESSURES

BLOOD FLOW THROUGH THE KIDNEYS

The rate of blood flow through both kidneys of a 70 kg man is about 1200 ml/min.

The portion of the total cardiac output that passes through the kidneys is called the *renal fraction.* Since the normal cardiac output of a 70 kg adult man is about 5600 ml/min and the blood flow through both kidneys is about 1200 ml/min, one can calculate that the normal renal fraction is about 21 per cent. This can vary from as little as 12 per cent to as high as 30 per cent in the normal resting person.

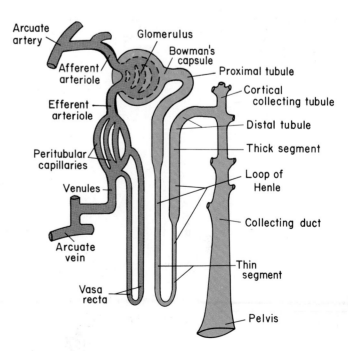

Figure 24–3. The functional nephron.

PRESSURES IN THE RENAL CIRCULATION

Figure 24–4 gives the approximate pressures in the different parts of the renal circulation and tubules, showing an initial pressure of approximately 100 mm Hg in the large arteries and about 8 mm Hg in the veins into which the blood finally drains. The two major areas of resistance to blood flow in the nephron are (1) the *afferent arteriole* and (2) the *efferent arteriole*. In the afferent arteriole the pressure falls from 100 mm Hg at its arterial end to a mean pressure of about 60 mm Hg in the glomerulus. As the blood flows through the efferent arterioles from the glomerulus to the peritubular capillary system, the pressure falls another 47 mm Hg to a mean peritubular capillary pressure of about 13 mm Hg.

Thus, the *high-pressure capillary bed* in the glomerulus operates at a mean pressure of about 60 mm Hg and therefore causes rapid filtration of fluid into Bowman's capsule. By contrast, the *low-pressure capillary bed* in the peritubular capillary system operates at a mean capillary pressure of about 13 mm Hg, which allows rapid absorption of fluid because of the high osmotic pressure of the plasma.

GLOMERULAR FILTRATION AND THE GLOMERULAR FILTRATE

The Glomerular Membrane and Glomerular Filtrate. The fluid that filters through the glomerulus

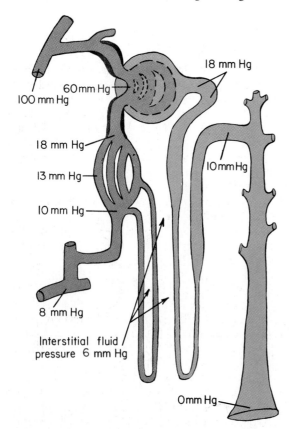

Figure 24–4. Approximate pressures at different points in the vessels and tubules of the functional nephron and in the interstitial fluid.

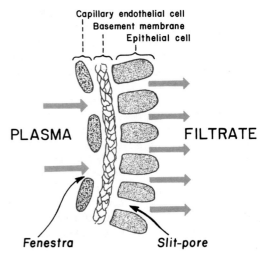

Figure 24–5. Functional structure of the glomerular membrane.

into Bowman's capsule is called *glomerular filtrate,* and the membrane of the glomerular capillaries is called the *glomerular membrane.* Though, in general, this membrane is similar to that of other capillaries throughout the body, it has several differences. Most important, as illustrated in Figure 24–5, it has three major layers: (1) the endothelial layer of the capillary itself, (2) a basement membrane, and (3) a layer of epithelial cells on the outer surfaces of the glomerular capillaries. Yet, despite the number of layers, the permeability of the glomerular membrane is over 100 times greater than that of the usual capillary.

The tremendous permeability of the glomerular membrane is caused by its special structure, which is illustrated in Figure 24–5. The capillary *endothelial cells* lining the glomerulus are perforated by literally thousands of small holes called *fenestrae*. Then, outside the endothelial cells is a basement membrane composed mainly of a meshwork of proteoglycan fibrillae. A final layer of the glomerular membrane is a layer of epithelial cells that line the outside of the glomerulus. However, these cells are not continuous but instead consist mainly of finger-like projections that cover the outer surface of the basement membrane. These fingers form slits called *slit-pores*, through which the glomerular filtrate filters. Thus, the glomerular filtrate must pass through three different layers before entering Bowman's capsule, but each of these layers is several hundred times as permeable as the usual capillary membrane, which accounts for the tremendous volume of glomerular filtrate that can be formed each minute. Yet, despite the tremendous permeability of the glomerular membrane, it has an extremely high degree of selectivity for the sizes of molecules that it allows to pass. In general, all molecules with a molecular weight of less than about 60,000 to 70,000 pass through the membrane with ease, whereas almost all larger molecules are blocked almost completely.

There are two basic reasons for the high degree of molecular selectivity by the glomerular membrane.

First is the sizes of the pores in the membrane itself. That is, the pores of the membrane are large enough to allow molecules with diameters up to about 8 nanometers (80Å) to pass through. Yet the molecular diameter of the plasma protein albumin molecule, with a molecular weight of 69,000, is only about 6 nanometers, which is somewhat smaller than the sizes of these large pores. Therefore, why do the protein molecules not pass through in great quantity? The answer is the second factor that determines the permeability of the membrane: The *glomerular pores are lined with a complex of glycosylated proteins that have very strong negative electrical charges.* The plasma proteins also have strong negative electrical charges. Therefore, electrostatic repulsion of the protein molecules by the pore walls keeps these molecules from passing through.

Composition of the Glomerular Filtrate. The glomerular filtrate has almost exactly the same composition as the fluid that filters from the arterial ends of the capillaries into the interstitial fluids. It contains no red blood cells and about 0.003 per cent protein, or about one two-thousandth of the protein in the plasma. The electrolyte and other solute composition of glomerular filtrate is also similar to that of the interstitial fluid.

To summarize: For all practical purposes, glomerular filtrate is the same as plasma except that it has no significant amount of proteins.

THE GLOMERULAR FILTRATION RATE

The quantity of glomerular filtrate formed each minute in all nephrons of both kidneys is called the *glomerular filtration rate.* In the normal person this averages approximately 125 ml/min; however, in different normal functional states of the kidneys, it can vary from a few to 200 ml/min. To express this differently, the total quantity of glomerular filtrate formed each day averages about 180 liters, or more than two times the total weight of the body. Over 99 per cent of the filtrate is normally reabsorbed in the tubules, the remainder passing into the urine, as explained later in the chapter.

DYNAMICS OF GLOMERULAR FILTRATION

Glomerular filtration occurs in almost exactly the same manner that fluid filters out of any high pressure capillary in the body. This is, *pressure inside the glomerular capillaries* causes fluid to filter through the capillary membrane into Bowman's capsule. On the other hand, *colloid osmotic pressure of the blood and pressure in Bowman's capsule* oppose the filtration.

Glomerular Pressure. As stated earlier, *the glomerular pressure is about 60 mm Hg.*

Pressure in Bowman's Capsule. In lower animals, pressure measurements have been made in Bowman's capsule and at different points along the renal tubules by inserting micropipets into the lumen. On the basis of these studies, *capsular pressure in the human being is estimated to be about 18 mm Hg.*

Colloid Osmotic Pressure in the Glomerular Capillaries. Because approximately one fifth of the plasma in the capillaries filters into the capsule, the protein concentration increases about 20 per cent as the blood passes from the arterial to the venous ends of the glomerular capillaries. If the normal colloid osmotic pressure of blood entering the capillaries is 28 mm Hg, it rises to approximately 36 mm Hg by the time the blood reaches the venous ends of the capillaries, and *the average colloid osmotic pressure is about 32 mm Hg.*

Filtration Pressure, Filtration Coefficient, and Glomerular Filtration Rate. The filtration pressure is the net pressure forcing fluid through the glomerular membrane, and this is *equal to the glomerular pressure minus glomerular colloid osmotic pressure and capsular pressure.* Therefore, the *normal filtration pressure is about 60 − 32 − 18, or 10 mm Hg.*

The filtration coefficient, called K_f, is the glomerular filtration rate for both kidneys per mm Hg of filtration pressure. Therefore, the glomerular filtration rate is equal to the filtration pressure times the filtration coefficient, or

$$GFR = \text{Filtration pressure} \cdot K_f$$

The normal filtration coefficient is 12.5 ml per min per mm Hg of filtration pressure. Thus, at a normal mean filtration pressure of 10 mm Hg, the total filtration rate of both kidneys is 125 ml per min.

Factors That Affect Glomerular Filtration Rate

Arterial Pressure. When the arterial pressure rises, this obviously increases the pressure in the glomerulus as well. Therefore, the glomerular filtration rate increases. The increase in filtration is not as great as would be expected, however, because arterioles are automatically controlled by a mechanism called *autoregulation* (which is discussed later in the chapter) to keep the glomerular pressure from rising as much as it otherwise would.

Effect of Afferent Arteriolar Constriction on Glomerular Filtration Rate. Constricting the afferent arterioles decreases the rate of blood flow into the glomeruli and therefore also decreases glomerular pressure. Consequently, there is a corresponding decrease in glomerular filtration.

Effect of Efferent Arteriolar Constriction. Constriction of the efferent arterioles increases the resistance to outflow of blood from the glomeruli. This obviously increases the glomerular pressure and usually increases the glomerular filtration rate. However, as discussed below, when efferent arteriolar constriction becomes too great and blood flow is greatly impeded, then the glomerular filtration rate decreases.

Effect of Glomerular Blood Flow on Glomerular Filtration Rate. When either the afferent or the efferent arterioles is constricted, the amount of blood flowing into the glomerulus each minute becomes reduced. Then, as fluid is filtered from the glomeruli, the plasma protein concentration and the colloid osmotic pressure of the plasma in the glomeruli rise. These changes, in turn, oppose filtration. Therefore, when the glomerular blood flow falls significantly below normal, the glomerular filtration rate is likely to be seriously depressed despite a high glomerular pressure.

REABSORPTION AND SECRETION IN THE TUBULES

The glomerular filtrate entering the tubules of the nephron flows (1) through the *proximal tubule*, (2) through the *loop of Henle*, (3) through the *distal tubule*, (4) through the *collecting tubule*, and (5) through the *collecting duct* into the pelvis of the kidney. Along this course, substances are selectively reabsorbed or secreted by the tubular epithelium, and the resultant fluid entering the pelvis is *urine*. Reabsorption plays a much greater role than does secretion in this formation of urine, but secretion is especially important in determining the amounts of potassium ions, hydrogen ions, and a few other substances in the urine, as discussed later.

Ordinarily, more than 99 per cent of the water in the glomerular filtrate is reabsorbed as it passes through the tubules. Therefore, if some dissolved constituent of the glomerular filtrate is not reabsorbed at all along the entire course of the tubules, this reabsorption of water obviously concentrates the substance more than 99-fold. On the other hand, some constituents, such as glucose and amino acids, are reabsorbed almost entirely so that their concentrations decrease almost to zero before the fluid becomes urine. In this way the tubules separate substances that are to be conserved in the body from those that are to be eliminated in the urine.

BASIC MECHANISMS OF ABSORPTION AND SECRETION IN THE TUBULES

The basic mechanisms for transport through the tubular membrane are essentially the same as those for transport through other membranes of the body. These can be divided into *active transport* and *passive transport*. The basic essentials of these mechanisms are described here, but for additional details the reader should refer to Chapter 4.

Active Transport Through the Tubular Wall

Figure 24–6 illustrates, by way of example, the mechanism for active transport of sodium from the lumen of the proximal tubule into the peritubular capillary. Note first the character of the epithelial cells that line the tubule. Each cell has a "brush" border on its luminal surface. This brush is composed of literally thousands of very minute microvilli that increase the surface area of luminal exposure of the cell about 20-fold.

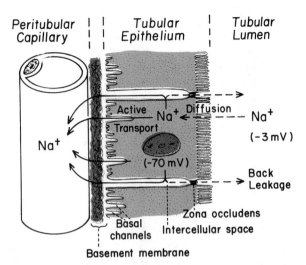

Figure 24–6. Mechanism for active transport of sodium from the tubular lumen into the peritubular capillary, illustrating active transport at the base and sides of the epithelial cell and diffusion through the luminal border of the cell.

Sodium ions are actively transported only through the lateral and basal membranes of the epithelial cell, passing from inside the cell into *basal channels* beneath the cell and into spaces between the cells. This transport outward from the cell diminishes the sodium concentration inside the cell and also decreases the electrical potential inside the cell to a low value of approximately −70 millivolts. The low concentration and the negative potential inside the cell establish a sodium ion concentration gradient and an electrical gradient from the lumen of the tubule to the inside of the cell, and this gradient then causes sodium ions to diffuse from the tubule through the brush border into the cell. Once inside the cell, the sodium is carried by the active transport process the rest of the way into the peritubular fluid.

Other substances besides sodium that are actively absorbed through the tubular epithelial cells include *glucose, amino acids, calcium ions, potassium ions, chloride ions, phosphate ions, urate ions,* and others.

In addition, some substances are actively *secreted* into all or some portions of the tubules; these include especially *hydrogen ions* and *potassium ions*. Active secretion occurs in the same way as active absorption except that the cell membrane transports the secreted substance in the opposite direction.

Passive Absorption of Water: Osmosis of Water Through the Tubular Epithelium

When the different solutes are transported out of the tubule and through the tubular epithelium, their total concentration decreases inside the tubular lumen and increases outside. These changes obviously create a concentration difference that causes osmosis of water in the same direction that the solutes have been transported.

However, some portions of the tubular system are far more permeable to water than are others. In those portions that are highly permeable, such as the proximal tubules, osmosis of water occurs so rapidly that the osmolar concentration of solutes on the peritubular side of the membrane is almost never more than a few milliosmoles greater than on the intratubular side. On the other hand, portions of the ascending limb of the loop of Henle are an example of a tubular area that is almost completely impermeable to water, a fact that plays a very important role in the mechanism for controlling urine concentration (discussed later in this chapter).

Passive Absorption of Urea and Other Nonactively Transported Solutes by the Process of Diffusion

When water is reabsorbed by osmosis, the concentration of urea in the tubular fluid rises, which obviously establishes a concentration difference for urea between the tubular and peritubular fluids. This in turn causes urea also to diffuse from the tubular fluid into the peritubular fluid. This same effect also occurs for other tubular solutes that are not actively reabsorbed but that can diffuse through the tubular membrane.

The rate of resorption of a nonactively reabsorbed solute is determined by (1) the amount of water that is reabsorbed, because this determines the tubular concentration of the solute, and (2) the permeability of the tubular membrane for the solute. The permeability of the membrane for urea in most parts of the tubules is far less than that for water, which means that far less urea is reabsorbed than water. Therefore, a large proportion of the urea remains in the tubules and is lost in the urine—usually about 50 per cent of all that enters the glomerular filtrate. The permeability of the tubular membrane for reabsorption of creatinine, inulin (a large polysaccharide), mannitol (a monosaccharide), and sucrose is zero, which means that once these substances have filtered into the glomerular filtrate, 100 per cent of that which enters the glomerular filtrate passes on into the urine.

REABSORPTION AND SECRETION OF DIFFERENT TYPES OF SUBSTANCES IN DIFFERENT SEGMENTS OF THE TUBULES

Transport of Water and Flow of Tubular Fluid at Different Points in the Tubular System. Water transport occurs entirely by osmotic diffusion. That is, whenever some solute in the glomerular filtrate is absorbed by any means, the resulting decreased concentration of solute in the tubular fluid and increased concentration in the peritubular fluid cause osmosis of water out of the tubules.

However, because the permeabilities of the different tubular segments vary tremendously for water, the amount of the glomerular filtrate water reabsorbed in the different segments also varies tremendously, as follows:

	Per Cent
Proximal tubules	65
Loop of Henle	15
Distal tubules	10
Collecting tubules and ducts	9.3
Passing into the urine	0.7

We shall see later in the chapter that these values vary greatly under different operational conditions of the kidney, particularly when the kidney is forming very dilute or very concentrated urine.

Note especially the very large proportion of the glomerular filtrate that is absorbed in the proximal tubules.

Reabsorption of Substances of Nutritional Value to the Body—Glucose, Proteins, Amino Acids, Acetoacetate Ions, and Vitamins. Five different substances in the glomerular filtrate of particular importance to bodily nutrition are glucose, proteins, amino acids, acetoacetate ions, and the vitamins. Normally all of these are completely or almost completely reabsorbed by active processes in the *proximal tubules* of the kidney. Therefore, almost none of these substances remain in the tubular fluid entering the loop of Henle.

Most of the nutritionally important substances such as glucose and amino acids are absorbed by the mechanism of *sodium-cotransport,* described in Chapter 4. That is, as sodium is absorbed, during one step in the transport process both the sodium ion and the glucose molecule attach to a common "carrier molecule," and the glucose is thus conveyed along with the sodium.

Special Mechanism for Absorption of Protein. As much as 30 grams of protein filters into the glomerular filtrate every day. This would be a great metabolic drain on the body if the protein were not returned to the body fluids. Because the protein molecule is much too large to be transported by the usual transport processes, protein is reabsorbed through the brush border of the proximal tubular epithelium by pinocytosis, which means simply that the protein attaches itself to the membrane and this portion of the membrane then invaginates to the interior of the cell. Once inside the cell, the protein is digested into its constituent amino acids, which are then absorbed through the base and sides of the cell into the peritubular fluids. Details of the pinocytosis mechanism were discussed in Chapter 4.

Poor Reabsorption of the Metabolic End-Products: Urea, Creatinine, and Others. Only moderate quantities of *urea*—about 50 per cent of the total—are reabsorbed during the entire course through the tubular system.

Creatinine is not reabsorbed in the tubules at all; indeed, small quantities of creatinine are actually secreted into the tubules by the proximal tubules, so that the total quantity of creatinine increases about 20 per cent.

The *urate ion* is absorbed much more than urea—about 86 per cent reabsorption. But even so, large quantities of urate remain in the fluid that finally issues into the urine. Several other end-products, such as *sulfates, phosphates,* and *nitrates,* are transported in much the same way as urate ions. All of these are normally reabsorbed to a far less extent than is water, so that their concentrations become greatly increased as they flow along the tubules. Yet, *each is actively absorbed to some extent,* which keeps their concentrations in the extracellular fluid from ever falling too low.

Transport of Different Ions by the Tubular Epithelium—Sodium, Chloride, Bicarbonate, and Potassium. In most segments of the tubules, positive ions are transported through the tubular epithelium by active transport processes, while negative ions are usually transported passively as a result of electrical differences developed across the membrane when the positive ions are transported. For instance, when sodium ions are transported out of the proximal tubular fluid, the resulting electronegativity that develops in the tubular fluid causes chloride ions to follow in the wake of the sodium ions. But, despite this general rule, some physiologists believe that chloride ions are absorbed actively from the ascending limb of the loop of Henle and from a portion of the distal tubule.

Secretion of Potassium and Hydrogen Ions. Potassium ions are actively secreted into the tubular fluid as it passes through the distal tubules and collecting tubules. This will be discussed at greater length in the following chapter in relation to the regulation of potassium concentration in the extracellular fluids.

Hydrogen ions are actively secreted in the proximal tubules, distal tubules, collecting tubules, and collecting ducts. This secretion plays an exceedingly important role in controlling the hydrogen ion concentration of the extracellular fluid, as will be discussed in Chapter 26.

Special Aspects of Bicarbonate Ion Transport. Bicarbonate ion is mainly reabsorbed in the form of carbon dioxide rather than in the form of bicarbonate ion itself. This occurs as follows: The bicarbonate ions in the tubular fluid first combine with hydrogen ions that are secreted into the fluid by the epithelial cells. The chemical reaction that occurs forms carbonic acid, which then dissociates into water and carbon dioxide. The carbon dioxide, being highly lipid-soluble, diffuses rapidly through the tubular membrane into the peritubular capillary blood.

Transport of Other Ions. Though we know much less about the specific means of transport of other ions besides the four discussed above, in general essentially all of them can be reabsorbed either by active transport or as a result of electrical differences across the membrane. Thus, calcium, magnesium, and other positive ions are actively reabsorbed, and many of the negative ions are reabsorbed as a result of electrical differences that develop when the positive ions are reabsorbed. In addition, certain negative ions—urate, phosphates, sulfates, and nitrates—can be reabsorbed by active transport, this occurring to the greatest extent in the proximal tubules.

CONCENTRATIONS OF DIFFERENT SUBSTANCES IN THE URINE

Whether or not a substance becomes concentrated in the tubular fluid as it moves along the tubules is determined by the *relative reabsorption (or secretion) of the substance versus the reabsorption of water.* If a greater percentage of water is reabsorbed, the substance becomes more concentrated. Conversely, if a greater percentage of the substance is reabsorbed, it becomes more diluted. In general, there are three different classes of substances:

First, the nutritionally important substances—glucose, protein, and amino acids—are reabsorbed much more rapidly than water, and their concentrations fall extremely rapidly in the proximal tubules and remain essentially zero throughout the remainder of the tubular system as well as in the urine.

Second, the concentrations of the metabolic end-products become progressively greater throughout the tubular system, because all these substances are reabsorbed to a far less extent than is water.

Third, many of the ions are normally excreted into the urine in concentrations not greatly different from those in the glomerular filtrate and extracellular fluid. For instance, sodium and chloride ions, on the average, are normally reabsorbed from the tubules in proportions not too dissimilar from that of water.

Table 24–1 summarizes the concentrating ability of the tubular system for different substances. It also gives the actual quantities of the different substances normally filtered through the glomeruli into the tubules each minute.

THE CONCEPT OF PLASMA CLEARANCE

The term *plasma clearance* is used to express the ability of the kidneys to clean, or "clear," the plasma of various substances. Thus, if the plasma passing through the kidneys contains 0.1 g of a substance in each 100 ml and 0.1 g of this substance also passes into the urine each minute, then 100 ml of the plasma is cleaned or "cleared" of the substance per minute.

Plasma clearance for any substance can be calculated by the following formula:

Plasma clearance (ml/min) =
$$\frac{\text{Quantity of urine (ml/min)} \times \text{Concentration in urine}}{\text{Concentration in plasma}}$$

The concept of plasma clearance is important because it is an excellent measure of kidney function. The clearance of different substances can be determined by simply analyzing the concentrations of the substances simultaneously in the plasma and in the urine while also measuring the rate of urine formation.

Table 24–1. RELATIVE CONCENTRATIONS OF SUBSTANCES IN THE GLOMERULAR FILTRATE AND IN THE URINE

	Glomerular Filtrate (125 ml/min)		Urine (1 ml/min)		Conc. Urine/ Conc. Plasma (Plasma Clearance per Min)
	Quantity/min	Concentration	Quantity/min	Concentration	
Na$^+$	17.7 mEq	142 mEq/L	0.128 mEq	128 mEq/L	0.9
K$^+$	0.63	5	0.06	60	12
Ca^{++}	0.5	4	0.0048	4.8	1.2
Mg^{++}	0.38	3	0.015	15	5.0
Cl$^-$	12.9	103	0.134	134	1.3
HCO$_3^-$	3.5	28	0.014	14	0.5
H$_2$PO$_4^-$ HPO$_4^{--}$ }	0.25	2	0.05	50	25
SO$_4^{--}$	0.09	0.7	0.033	33	47
Glucose	125 mg	100 mg/100 ml	0 mg	0 mg/100 ml	0.0
Urea	33	26	18.2	1820	70
Uric acid	3.8	3	0.42	42	14
Creatinine	1.4	1.1	1.96	196	140

INULIN CLEARANCE AS A MEASURE OF GLOMERULAR FILTRATION RATE

Inulin is a polysaccharide that has the specific attributes of not being reabsorbed to a significant extent by the tubules of the nephron and yet being of small enough molecular weight (about 5200) that it passes through the glomerular membrane as freely as the water of the plasma. Also, inulin is not actively secreted even in the minutest amount by the tubules. Consequently, glomerular filtrate contains the same concentration of inulin as does plasma, and as the filtrate flows through the tubules all the inulin continues on into the urine. Thus, *all the glomerular filtrate is cleared of inulin* even though almost all of the water of the filtrate is reabsorbed back into the blood. Therefore, *the amount of glomerular filtrate formed is exactly equal to the amount of plasma that is simultaneously cleared.* Therefore, the plasma clearance per minute of inulin is also equal to the glomerular filtration rate.

As an example, let us assume that it is found by chemical analysis that the inulin concentration in the plasma is 0.1 g in each 100 ml, and that 0.125 g of inulin passes into the urine per minute. Therefore, by dividing 0.1 into 0.125, one finds that 1.25 *100-ml portions* of glomerular filtrate must be formed each minute in order to deliver to the urine the analyzed quantity of inulin. In other words, 125 ml of glomerular filtrate is formed per minute, and this is also the plasma clearance of inulin.

PARA-AMINOHIPPURIC ACID (PAH) CLEARANCE AS A MEASURE OF PLASMA FLOW THROUGH THE KIDNEYS

PAH, like inulin, passes through the glomerular membrane with perfect ease along with the remainder of the glomerular filtrate. However, it is different from inulin in that almost all the PAH remaining in the plasma after the glomerular filtrate is formed is secreted into the tubules by the tubular epithelium if the plasma concentration of PAH is very low. Indeed, only about one-tenth of the original PAH remains in the plasma when the blood leaves the kidneys.

Therefore, one can use the clearance of PAH for estimating the *flow of plasma* through the kidneys, because the amount of plasma flow must always be about 10 per cent greater than the PAH clearance. Thus, if the PAH clearance is 600 ml per minute, then one can calculate that the plasma flow is about 660 ml per minute.

QUESTIONS, PART 1

1. Describe the functional anatomy of the kidney, paying special attention to the arrangements of the separate segments of the nephron.
2. What is meant by the *high-pressure capillary system* of the kidney and by the *low-pressure capillary system*?
3. Describe the relationship of the *vasa recta* to the loops of Henle.
4. State approximate values in the human being for *rate of blood flow* through the kidneys, *glomerular filtration rate,* and *rate of urine excretion.*
5. Approximately what proportion of the glomerular filtrate is normally reabsorbed during the formation of urine?
6. Explain the effects on glomerular filtration of afferent arteriolar constriction and of efferent arteriolar constriction.
7. Describe the characteristics of the glomerular membrane and its permeability to various substances.
8. Compare the composition of glomerular filtrate with that of plasma.

9. State approximate values for the forces at the glomerular membrane that determine glomerular filtration.
10. Describe the chemical and physical events causing active transport of sodium ions through the tubular epithelium.
11. Why does absorption of osmotic substances through the tubular epithelium cause osmosis of water through the epithelium as well?
12. Explain why urea and other waste products become concentrated as they pass through the tubular system.
13. What are the specific characteristics of absorption of each of the following substances through the tubular epithelium: glucose; proteins; amino acids; and sodium, chloride, bicarbonate, and potassium ions?
14. What important ions are secreted into the tubular fluid through the tubular epithelium?
15. Explain the concept of *plasma clearance*.
16. If the concentration of inulin in the blood is 0.05 g in each 100 ml of plasma and a total of 0.02 g of inulin passes into the urine per minute, what is the glomerular filtration rate?

Part 2 ■ Control of Excretion of Water and Individual Solutes by the Kidneys

THE DILUTING MECHANISM OF THE KIDNEYS: THE MECHANISM FOR EXCRETING EXCESS WATER

One of the most important functions of the kidney is to control the osmolality of the body fluids. It does so by excreting excessive amounts of water in the urine when the body fluids are too dilute or by excreting excessive amounts of solutes when the body fluids are too concentrated.

Whether the kidneys excrete excess water or excess solutes is controlled by *antidiuretic hormone,* a hormone secreted by the posterior pituitary gland, which will be discussed in more detail in the following chapter. In the absence of antidiuretic hormone the kidneys excrete excessive amounts of water, but when the blood concentration of antidiuretic hormone is high the kidneys excrete excessive amounts of solutes. Let us explain first the mechanism for excreting excess water—that is, the mechanism for excreting a dilute urine.

When the glomerular filtrate is formed in the glomerulus, its osmolality is almost exactly the same as that of the plasma, approximately 300 milliosmoles per liter. To excrete excess water, it is necessary to dilute the filtrate as it passes through the tubules. This is achieved by reabsorbing a lower proportion of water than solutes. Figure 24-7 illustrates this process. The colored arrows in this figure represent rapid reabsorption of tubular solute, and the thickened walls of the more distal tubular segments indicate that these portions are relatively impermeable to water when antidiuretic hormone is *not* present in the circulating body fluids.

In almost all of these tubular areas, beginning in the ascending limb of the loop of Henle and going all the way through the remaining tubular segments, the major driving force is active transport of sodium ions. This then causes electrogenic passive absorption of the anions, mainly chloride ions. However, there is also active reabsorption of other ions as well, as explained earlier in the chapter. Consequently, most of the ionic substances of the tubular fluids are reabsorbed from these late segments of the tubular system before the fluid empties as urine, but large amounts of the water remain and the urine is dilute. Note in Figure 24-7 that, in the ascending limb of the loop of Henle, the osmolality of the fluid falls rapidly to about 100 milliosmoles per liter, and to as

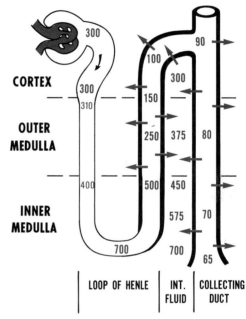

Figure 24-7. The renal mechanism for forming a dilute urine. The darkened walls of the distal portions of the tubular system indicate that these portions of the tubules are relatively impermeable to the reabsorption of water in the absence of antidiuretic hormone. The solid arrows indicate active processes for absorption of most of the solutes besides the urinary waste products. (Numerical values are in milliosmoles per liter.)

low as 65 to 70 milliosmoles (mOsm) per liter in the last portions of the collecting duct and in the urine.

To summarize, the process for excreting a dilute urine is simply one of absorbing solutes from the latter segments of the tubules while water fails to be reabsorbed. However, this failure to reabsorb the water occurs only when antidiuretic hormone is *not* being secreted by the posterior pituitary gland.

THE MECHANISM FOR EXCRETING EXCESS SOLUTES: THE COUNTERCURRENT MECHANISM FOR EXCRETING A CONCENTRATED URINE

The process for concentrating urine is not nearly so simple as for diluting it. Yet, at times it is exceedingly important to concentrate the urine as much as possible so that excess solutes can be eliminated with as little loss of water as possible—for instance, when one is exposed to desert conditions with an inadequate supply of water. Fortunately, the kidneys have developed a special mechanism for concentrating the urine called the *countercurrent mechanism*.

The countercurrent mechanism depends on a peculiar anatomical arrangement of the loops of Henle and the vasa recta. In the human being, the loops of Henle of one third to one fifth of the nephrons dip deep into the medulla and then return to the cortex; some dip all the way to the tips of the papillae that project into the renal pelvis. This group of nephrons with the long loops of Henle is called the *juxtamedullary nephrons*. Paralleling the long loops of Henle are loops of peritubular capillaries called the *vasa recta*; these also loop down into the medulla from the cortex and then back out to the cortex. These arrangements of the different parts of the juxtamedullary nephron and the vasa recta are diagrammed in Figure 24–8.

Hyperosmolality of the Medullary Interstitial Fluid and Mechanisms for Achieving It

The first step in the excretion of excess solutes in the urine—that is, for excretion of a concentrated urine—is to create hyperosmolality of the medullary interstitial fluid, which is necessary for concentrating the urine.

The normal osmolality of the fluids in almost all parts of the body is about 300 mOsm/liter. However, as shown by the numbers in Figure 24–8, the osmolality of the interstitial fluid in the medulla of the kidney is much higher than this, and it becomes progressively greater the deeper one goes into the

medulla, increasing from 300 mOsm/liter in the cortex to 1200 mOsm/liter (occasionally as high as 1400 mOsm/liter) in the pelvic tip of the medulla. Three different solute-concentrating mechanisms are mainly responsible for this hyperosmolality; these are the following:

First, the principal cause of the greatly increased medullary osmolality is active transport of sodium ions (plus cotransport of potassium and chloride ions) out of the thick portion (the upper portion with thick epithelial cells) of the ascending limb of the loop of Henle. The large colored arrows shown in this tubular segment in Figure 24–8 illustrate this transport especially of sodium and chloride ions (as well as potassium, calcium, and magnesium ions to a lesser extent) out of the loop of Henle and into the medullary interstitial fluid. All these solutes become concentrated in this fluid.

Second, ions are also transported into the medullary interstitial fluid from the collecting duct, mainly resulting from active transport of sodium ions and electrogenic passive absorption of chloride ions along with the sodium ions.

And, third, when the concentration of antidiuretic hormone is high in the blood, large amounts of urea are also absorbed into the fluid of the inner medulla from the collecting duct. The reason is: In the presence of antidiuretic hormone, the inner medullary portion of the collecting duct becomes moderately permeable to urea and highly permeable to water. The fact that it becomes highly permeable to water causes rapid reabsorption of water out of the collecting duct, and this greatly increases the concentration of urea in the duct. Now, because of this high urea concentration, the urea too diffuses through the collecting duct wall into the medullary interstitium.

In summary, at least three different factors contrib-

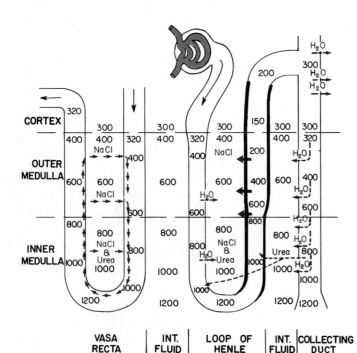

Figure 24–8. The countercurrent mechanism for concentrating the urine. (Numerical values are in milliosmoles per liter.)

ute to the marked increase in osmolality in the medullary interstitial fluid. These are (1) active transport of the ions into the interstitium by the ascending limb of the loop of Henle, (2) active transport of ions from the collecting duct into the interstitium, and (3) passive diffusion of large amounts of urea from the collecting duct into the interstitium. The net result is an increase in the osmolality of the medullary interstitial fluid, when adequate amounts of antidiuretic hormone are present, to as high as 1200 to 1400 mOsm/liter near the tips of the papillae.

Mechanism for Excreting a Concentrated Urine—Role of Antidiuretic Hormone

Now that we have explained how the kidney creates hyperosmolality in the medullary interstitium, it becomes a simple matter to explain the mechanism for excreting a concentrated urine, thus causing loss of excess solutes from the body fluids while at the same time retaining as much water as possible.

When the concentration of *antidiuretic hormone* in the blood is high, the epithelium of the cortical collecting tubule, the collecting duct, and in some species of animals the late distal tubule as well become highly permeable to water. This is illustrated in Figure 24–8 by the thin walls of these segments of the tubular system. Most importantly, as the tubular fluid flows through the collecting duct, water is pulled by osmosis into the highly concentrated fluid of the medullary interstitium. Thus, the collecting duct fluid also becomes highly concentrated, and it issues from the papilla into the pelvis of the kidney at a concentration of about 1200 mOsm/liter, almost exactly equal to the osmolal concentration of the solutes in the medullary interstitium near the papilla.

Mechanism by Which Antidiuretic Hormone Increases Water Reabsorption. The precise mechanism by which antidiuretic hormone increases water reabsorption by the late distal tubules, collecting tubules, and collecting ducts is not known. However, several established facts about the mechanism are the following: Antidiuretic hormone itself acts not on the luminal membrane of the tubular epithelial cells but instead on the basolateral membrane of these cells. It activates the enzyme *adenyl cyclase* in this membrane, which then causes formation of *cyclic adenosine monophosphate* (cyclic AMP) in the cell cytoplasm. The cyclic AMP then diffuses to the luminal membrane of the cells where it greatly increases the permeability to water. The exact way in which this happens is not known, but electron micrographs have shown increased numbers of microtubules in the vicinity of this luminal membrane after antidiuretic hormone stimulation. Regardless of the mechanism, it is the increase in permeability of the luminal membrane that is responsible for the increased water reabsorption by the late distal tubules, collecting tubules, and collecting ducts.

Countercurrent Exchange Mechanism in the Vasa Recta

We have now discussed the mechanisms by which high concentrations of solutes are achieved in the medullary interstitium and in the urine. However, without a special medullary vascular system as well, the flow of blood through the interstitium would rapidly remove the excess solutes and keep the concentration from rising very high. Fortunately, the medullary blood flow has two characteristics, both exceedingly important, for maintaining the high solute concentration in the medullary interstitial fluids. These are:

First, the medullary blood flow is very slow, amounting to only 1 to 2 per cent of the total blood flow of the kidney. Because of this very sluggish blood flow, removal of solutes is minimized.

Second, the vasa recta function as a *countercurrent exchanger* that also minimizes the washout of solutes from the medulla. This can be explained as follows: A countercurrent fluid exchange mechanism is one in which fluid flows through a long U-tube, with the two arms of the U lying in close proximity to each other so that fluid and solutes can exchange readily between the two arms. This obviously also requires that each of the two arms of the U be highly permeable, which is true for the vasa recta. When the fluids and solutes in the two parallel streams of flow can exchange rapidly, tremendous concentrations of solute can be maintained at the tip of the loop with negligible washout of solute.

For instance, in Figure 24–8, as blood flows down the descending limbs of the vasa recta, sodium chloride and urea diffuse into the blood from the interstitial fluid while water diffuses outward into the interstitium; these two effects cause the osmolal concentration in the capillary blood to rise to a maximum concentration of 1200 mOsm/liter at the tips of the vasa recta. Then, as the blood flows back up the ascending limbs, the extreme diffusibility of all molecules through the capillary membrane allows essentially all the extra sodium chloride and urea to diffuse back out of the blood into the interstitial fluid while water diffuses back into the blood. Therefore, by the time the blood finally leaves the medulla, its osmolal concentration has fallen back to be only slightly greater than that of the blood that had initially entered the vasa recta. As a result, blood flowing through the vasa recta carries only a minute amount of the medullary interstitial solutes away from the medulla despite the high medullary concentration of these solutes. This is essential for maintaining the high osmolality in the medulla, which in turn is essential for concentrating the urine.

UREA EXCRETION

The body forms an average of 25 to 30 grams of urea each day—more than this in persons who eat a

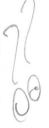

very high protein diet and less in persons who are on a low protein diet. All this urea must be excreted in the urine; otherwise, it will accumulate in the body fluids. Its normal concentration in plasma is approximately 26 mg/dl, but patients with renal insufficiency frequently have levels as high as 200 mg/dl, and it has been recorded as high as 800 mg/dl.

The two major factors that determine the rate of urea excretion are (1) the concentration of urea in the plasma, and (2) the glomerular filtration rate. These factors increase urea excretion mainly because the "load" of urea entering the proximal tubules is equal to the *plasma urea concentration times the glomerular filtration rate*. And, in general, the quantity of urea that passes on through the tubules into the urine averages between 40 and 60 per cent of the urea load that enters the proximal tubules.

SODIUM EXCRETION

The role of the kidney in sodium excretion is quite different from its role in urea excretion. The kidney attempts to eliminate as much urea as possible from the blood. To do this, large amounts of glomerular filtrate must be formed simply to supply the necessary tubular load of urea. By contrast, for sodium excretion the great amount of glomerular filtrate formed each day creates a serious problem. The reason for this is that the glomerular filtrate normally contains about 26,000 mEq of sodium each day, and yet the average intake of sodium per day is only 150 mEq. Therefore, the kidneys can be allowed to excrete only about 150 of the total 26,000 mEq. Consequently, the principal role of the tubular system in sodium excretion is to reabsorb sodium, not to excrete it. Indeed, it must reabsorb about 99.3 per cent of the total sodium load, and also must adjust the final amount of sodium that issues into the urine hour by hour or day by day so that it will balance the daily intake of sodium. Thus, the two jobs that the tubular system must perform for sodium excretion are (1) to reabsorb nearly all of it, and (2) to adjust very carefully the remaining amount that is excreted for maintaining appropriate amounts of sodium in the body fluids.

Reabsorption of Most of the Tubular Sodium in the Proximal Tubules and Loops of Henle. By the time the tubular fluid reaches the distal tubules, all but about 8 per cent of the sodium has already been reabsorbed. About 65 per cent of this is reabsorbed in the proximal tubules because of the active transport of sodium by the proximal tubular epithelial cells. Then, in the ascending limb of the loop of Henle, approximately another 27 per cent of the sodium is reabsorbed, leaving only 8 per cent to enter the distal tubules.

Thus, the proximal tubules and the loops of Henle are responsible for returning most of the sodium in the glomerular filtrate back to the plasma, thereby conserving the sodium for the body.

Variable Reabsorption of Sodium in the Late Distal Tubules and Cortical Collecting Tubules. Sodium reabsorption in the late distal tubules, the cortical collecting tubules, and the collecting ducts is highly variable. Its rate of reabsorption is controlled mainly by the concentration in the blood of *aldosterone*, a hormone secreted by the adrenal cortex. In the presence of large amounts of aldosterone, almost the last vestiges of tubular sodium are reabsorbed from these portions of the tubular system so that essentially none of the sodium enters the urine. On the other hand, in the absence of aldosterone, a large proportion of the sodium that enters the distal tubules is not reabsorbed and does then pass into the urine. Thus, the sodium excretion may be as little as 0.1 gram per day or as great as 30 grams per day, depending on the amount of aldosterone that is secreted.

Mechanism by Which Aldosterone Enhances Sodium Transport. Upon entering a tubular epithelial cell, aldosterone combines with a *receptor protein* in the cell cytoplasm; this combination diffuses within minutes into the nucleus where it activates the DNA molecules to form one or more types of messenger RNA. The RNA is then believed to cause formation of carrier proteins or protein enzymes that are necessary for the sodium transport process. Various theories have suggested (a) that a specific protein increases the permeability of the luminal border of the cell to sodium, (b) that an increased quantity of sodium-potassium-ATPase (which is the sodium pumping protein) develops in the basolateral membrane of the epithelial cell, or (c) that a protein enzyme or enzymes increase the availability of ATP to the sodium-ATPase so that it can function more actively as a sodium pump. Unfortunately, the precise mechanism is yet unknown.

Ordinarily, aldosterone has no effect on sodium transport for the first 45 minutes after it is administered; after this time the specific proteins important for transport begin to appear in the epithelial cells, followed by progressive increase in transport during the ensuing few hours.

POTASSIUM EXCRETION

The amount of potassium entering the glomerular filtrate each day is about 800 mEq, whereas the daily intake of potassium is only about 100 mEq. Therefore, to maintain normal body potassium balance, only one eighth of the total daily tubular load of potassium can be excreted. Furthermore, as is true for sodium excretion, the rate of potassium excretion must be carefully controlled so that it will exactly match the daily potassium intake.

Absorption of Large Amounts of Potassium from the Proximal Tubules and Loops of Henle. Large amounts of potassium are reabsorbed in the same manner that sodium is reabsorbed by the proximal tubules and the loops of Henle. Thus, active transport of potassium by the proximal tubular epithelial cells reabsorbs about 65 per cent of all the filtered potassium. Then, approximately another 27 per cent is reabsorbed by active transport in the ascending limbs of the loops of Henle, leaving about 8 per cent of the original filtered potassium to enter the distal tubules. This represents only about 65 mEq of potassium per day, which is actually less than the average daily intake of potassium for most people.

Active Secretion of Potassium in the Late Distal Tubules and Collecting Tubules and Ducts. Normally, considerable amounts of potassium are *secreted* into the distal tubules, and some also into the collecting tubules and ducts. That is, as sodium is transported through the epithelial cell into the peritubular fluid, potassium is simultaneously transported in the opposite direction into the tubular lumen.

In the absence of tubular secretion of potassium, death will eventually ensue from potassium toxicity. Indeed, cardiac arrhythmias usually appear when the plasma potassium concentration rises from the normal value of 4.5 mEq per liter to a level of 8 mEq per liter. A still higher potassium concentration than this can end in cardiac arrest or fibrillation.

Control of the Rate of Potassium Secretion. The rate of tubular secretion of potassium is controlled in proportion to the need to eliminate potassium from the extracellular fluid. To achieve this, two major factors determine the rate of tubular secretion of potassium:

(1) Control of potassium secretion by aldosterone. Earlier, we noted that aldosterone has a potent effect in controlling sodium transport through the epithelial cells in the terminal portions of the tubular system, beginning in the late distal tubules. And it was also pointed out that as sodium is transported into the interstitium, potassium is transported from the interstitium into the tubule. Therefore, aldosterone controls potassium secretion at the same time that it controls sodium reabsorption. Indeed, aldosterone is actually much more important for controlling extracellular fluid potassium concentration than for controlling sodium concentration, as we discuss in the following chapter.

(2) Effect of plasma potassium concentration on rate of potassium secretion. When the plasma potassium concentration rises too high, the rate of potassium transport into the tubular lumen increases markedly. The probable reason is that the increased potassium concentration gradient from the interstitial fluid to the tubular lumen now allows extra potassium ions to be pumped by the tubular cells. In fact, this increased gradient of potassium has far more effect on potassium excretion than would be expected from the increase in gradient alone, but the reason is unknown.

FLUID VOLUME EXCRETION

Up to this point we have considered the intrarenal mechanisms that determine the *concentrations* of various substances in the urine—water, urea, sodium, and potassium. Now it is important to consider the different factors that determine the rate of fluid *volume* excretion.

Importance of Conserving Body Fluid, and the Concept of Glomerulotubular Balance. The kidney's problem in fluid volume excretion is much the same as for sodium excretion, that is, not to lose too much volume from the body. To achieve this, over 99 per cent of the glomerular filtrate volume must be reabsorbed by the tubules. Also, when the glomerular filtration rate increases, the tubules, especially the proximal tubules, automatically adjust their rates of volume reabsorption almost to keep step with the increased rate of filtration. This phenomenon is called glomerulotubular balance.

The reason that the glomerulotubular balance principle holds true (or at least nearly holds true) is that increased flow of filtrate into the tubular system markedly activates most of the tubular reabsorptive mechanisms so that they almost keep up with the increased volume of fluid to be processed.

Glomerulotubular Imbalance and Its Importance in Fluid Volume Regulation. Though the concept of glomerulotubular balance is important to explain the way in which glomerular filtration rate and rate of tubular reabsorption automatically adjust to one another, precise measurements show that 100 per cent glomerulotubular balance for the entire tubular system almost never occurs. For instance, the following table gives approximate values for glomerular filtration rates, total rates of tubular fluid reabsorption, and rates of urine output for the average human adult, as extrapolated mainly from data for dogs:

Glomerular Filtration Rate	Rate of Tubular Reabsorption	Rate of Urine Output
ml	*ml*	*ml*
50	49.8	0.2
75	74.7	0.3
100	99.5	0.5
125	124.0	1.0
150	145.0	5.0
175	163.0	12.0

If we examine these figures critically, we see that glomerular filtration rate and rate of tubular reabsorption actually do appear to parallel each other very closely. On the other hand, the slight degree of imbalance that does occur causes far greater change, proportionately, in urine output than in either glomerular filtration rate or tubular reabsorption rate. For instance, let us study the increase in glomerular filtration rate from 100 to 150 ml/min. The rate of reabsorption increases from 99.5 to 145 ml/min, representing only slight glomerulotubular imbalance. Nevertheless, this 50 per cent increase in glomerular filtration rate causes a 1000 per cent increase in rate of urine output! Thus, even a very slight degree of glomerulotubular imbalance can lead to a tremendous increase in urine output when the glomerular filtration rate is increased. Also, very slight changes in rate of reabsorption of tubular fluid can cause equally as great alterations in urine output.

Therefore, the various factors that can alter either glomerular filtration rate or rate of tubular reabsorption are also the factors that play significant roles in determining the rate of fluid volume excretion. The four most important of these are

(1) *Rate of Tubular Reabsorption of Osmotic Substances.* The greater the reabsorption of osmotic substances such as glucose, sodium, and so forth, the greater is the osmotic reabsorption of water and, therefore the less urine volume output.

(2) *Degree of Sympathetic Stimulation of the Kidneys.* The greater the degree of sympathetic stimulation, the less the renal blood flow, which decreases glomerular filtration and increases tubular reabsorption, both of which decrease the volume of urine output.

(3) *Effect of Antidiuretic Hormone to Increase Tubular Reabsorption of Water.* As already explained, the greater the amount of antidiuretic hormone, the greater is the rate of tubular reabsorption of water. Therefore the urine volume decreases.

(4) *Effect of Arterial Pressure on Urine Volume Excretion.* The effect of arterial pressure on urine volume excretion is especially important because this effect forms the basis for long-term arterial pressure regulation, which is explained in detail in Chapter 15. In that chapter, it is pointed out that an increase in arterial pressure increases urine output drastically. This effect is illustrated in Figure 24–9, showing that when the pressure rises from 100 mm Hg to 200 mm Hg, the urine output increases approximately 7-fold. Conversely, when the pressure falls from 100 mm Hg to 50 mm Hg, urine output falls to either zero or near zero. There are two principal reasons for this exceedingly strong effect of arterial pressure on urine volume output:

(a) An increase in arterial pressure increases the

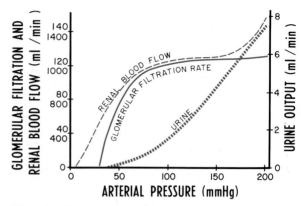

Figure 24–10. Autoregulation of glomerular filtration rate (GFR) and renal blood flow (RBF) when the arterial pressure is increased, but there is lack of autoregulation of urine flow.

glomerular capillary pressure and therefore increases the glomerular filtration rate as well.

(b) An increase in arterial pressure increases the flow of blood through the peritubular capillaries at the same time that it increases glomerular pressure. The increased peritubular flow raises the peritubular capillary pressure, which decreases fluid reabsorption from the renal tubules into the blood. This obviously is another important way that increased arterial pressure increases the volume output from the kidney.

One must remember that this effect of arterial pressure on volume output is one of the most important of all of the circulatory control mechanisms. As explained in Chapter 15, when the arterial pressure rises above normal, the resulting increase in urine volume output continues to deplete the body until the arterial pressure falls back to the normal level. Conversely, when the arterial pressure becomes too low, the kidneys excrete less volume than is ingested each day. Therefore, the body fluid volume increases until the arterial pressure rises once again back to the normal level.

AUTOREGULATION OF GLOMERULAR FILTRATION RATE

Even though a change in arterial pressure causes a marked change in urinary output, this pressure can change from as little as 75 mm. Hg to as high as 160 mm Hg while causing very little change in glomerular filtration rate. This effect is illustrated in Figure 24–10 and is called *autoregulation of glomerular filtration rate.* It is important because the nephron requires an optimal rate of glomerular filtration if it is to perform its function. Even a 5 per cent too great or too little rate of glomerular filtration can have profound effects in causing either excess fluid loss in the urine or too little excretion of the necessary waste products.

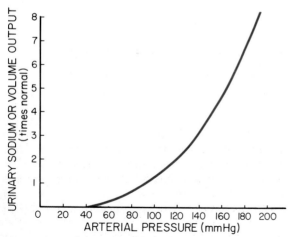

Figure 24–9. Effect of arterial pressure change on urinary output.

Mechanism of Autoregulation of Glomerular Filtration Rate— Tubuloglomerular Feedback

Fortunately, each nephron is provided with not one but *two* special feedback mechanisms that add together to provide the necessary degree of glomerular filtration autoregulation. These two mechanisms are (1) an *afferent arteriolar vasodilator feedback mechanism* and (2) an *efferent arteriolar vasoconstrictor feedback mechanism.* The combination of these two feedback mechanisms is called *tubuloglomerular feedback.* And the feedback process probably occurs either entirely or almost entirely at the *juxtaglomerular complex,* which has the following characteristics:

The Juxtaglomerular Complex. Figure 24–11 illustrates the juxtaglomerular complex, showing that the distal tubule passes in the angle between the afferent and efferent arterioles, actually abutting each of these two arterioles. Furthermore, those epithelial cells of the distal tubule that come in contact with the arterioles are more dense than the other tubular cells and are collectively called the *macula densa.* The point where the macula densa is located is at the beginning of the distal tubule, at the upper end of the ascending limb of the loop of Henle. The smooth muscle cells of the afferent and, to a lesser extent, of the efferent arterioles where they come in contact with the macula densa contain dark granules. These cells are called *juxtaglomerular cells* (JG cells), and the granules are composed mainly of inactive *renin.*

The Afferent Arteriolar Vasodilator Feedback Mechanism. A low rate of glomerular filtration allows over-reabsorption of sodium and chloride ions in the tubules and therefore decreases the concentration of these ions at the macula densa. This decrease in ions in turn initiates a signal from the macula densa to dilate the afferent arterioles. Putting these two facts together, the following is the mechanism by which the afferent arteriolar vasodilator feedback mechanism controls glomerular filtration rate:

(1) Too little flow of glomerular filtrate into the tubules causes decreased sodium and chloride ion concentration at the macula densa.

(2) The decreased ion concentration causes afferent arteriolar dilatation.

(3) This in turn increases the rate of blood flow into the glomerulus and increases the glomerular pressure.

(4) The increased glomerular pressure increases the glomerular filtration rate back toward the required level.

The Efferent Arteriolar Vasoconstrictor Feedback Mechanism. Too low an ion concentration at the macula densa is believed to cause the juxtaglomerular cells to release renin, and this in turn causes formation of angiotensin. The angiotensin then constricts mainly the efferent arteriole because it is more sensitive to angiotensin than is the afferent arteriole.

With these facts in mind, we can now describe the efferent arteriolar vasoconstrictor mechanism that helps to maintain a constant glomerular filtration rate:

(1) A too low glomerular filtration rate causes excess reabsorption of sodium and chloride ions from the filtrate, reducing the concentration of these ions at the macula densa.

(2) The low concentration of ions then causes the JG cells to release renin from their granules.

(3) The renin causes formation of angiotensin II.

(4) The angiotensin II constricts the efferent arterioles, which causes the pressure in the glomerulus to rise.

(5) The increased pressure then causes the glomerular filtration rate to return back toward normal.

Thus, this is still another negative feedback mechanism that helps to maintain a very constant glomerular filtration rate; it does so by constricting the efferent arterioles at the same time that the afferent vasodilator mechanism described above dilates the afferent arterioles. When both of these mechanisms function together, the glomerular filtration rate increases only a few per cent even though the arterial pressure increases between the limits of 75 mm Hg and 160 mm Hg.

AUTOREGULATION OF RENAL BLOOD FLOW

When the arterial pressure is changed for only a few minutes at a time, renal blood flow is autoregulated at the same time that the glomerular filtration rate is autoregulated. This is illustrated in Figure 24–10, which shows a relatively constant renal blood flow between the limits of 70 and 160 mm Hg arterial pressure.

It is mainly the afferent arteriolar vasodilator feedback mechanism described above that causes this renal blood flow autoregulation. This can be explained as follows: When the renal blood flow becomes too little, the glomerular pressure falls and the glomerular filtration rate also becomes too little. As a consequence, the feedback mechanism causes afferent arteriolar dilatation to return the glomerular filtration rate back toward normal. At the same time, the dilatation also increases the blood flow back toward normal despite the low arterial pressure.

ROLES OF THE RENIN-ANGIOTENSIN SYSTEM AND THE EFFERENT VASOCONSTRICTOR MECHANISM IN CONSERVING WATER AND SALT BUT ELIMINATING UREA DURING ARTERIAL HYPOTENSION

The efferent arteriolar vasoconstrictor mechanism not only helps to maintain normal glomerular filtration when the arterial pressure falls too low but also provides a means for controlling urea excretion separately from the excretion of water and salt. In arterial hypotension it is very important to conserve as much water and salt as possible. On the other hand, it is equally important to continue excreting the body's waste products, the most abundant of which is urea. Therefore, let us explain this:

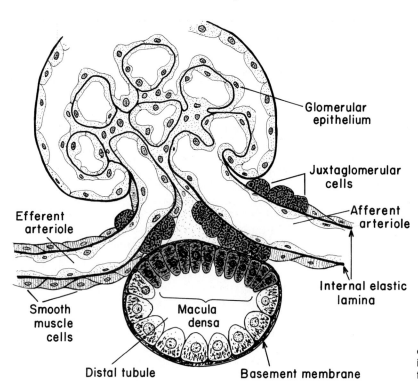

Figure 24–11. Structure of the juxtaglomerular apparatus, illustrating its possible feedback role in the control of nephron function. (Modified from Ham: Histology. J. B. Lippincott Co.)

Earlier in the chapter it was pointed out that the rate of urea excretion is almost directly proportional to the rate of glomerular filtration. In prolonged periods of low arterial pressure (hypotension) the efferent arteriolar vasoconstrictor mechanism can often maintain a high glomerular filtration rate despite the low pressure; as a result, almost normal amounts of urea will be excreted in the urine. Therefore, hypotension down to arterial pressure levels as low as 65 to 75 mm Hg usually does not cause significant retention of urea in the body fluids.

On the other hand, as angiotensin II increases within the kidneys and also in the circulating blood during arterial hypotension, this accumulation causes marked retention by the kidney of water and of the various ions—sodium, chloride, potassium, and others. Thus, this angiotensin mechanism provides a means for conserving water and ions despite the fact that urea continues to be excreted.

The angiotensin probably causes water and ion conservation mainly by the following mechanism: It increases renal arteriolar resistance, which reduces renal blood flow and therefore also reduces peritubular capillary pressure. This in turn increases the rate of reabsorption of water and electrolytes from the tubular system, as explained earlier in this chapter. Angiotensin also stimulates the secretion of aldosterone, which is still another factor in causing reabsorption of sodium and chloride ions from the distal segments of the tubular system.

QUESTIONS, PART 2

1. Explain how the kidney excretes a dilute urine.
2. Explain how the kidney excretes a concentrated urine.
3. Explain the concept of the *countercurrent phenomenon* that occurs in the renal medulla.
4. What is the role of antidiuretic hormone in shifting renal function from excreting a dilute urine to excreting a concentrated urine?
5. Describe the manner in which the kidneys excrete urea.
6. Describe what happens to sodium at each stage of its passage through the tubular system.
7. Describe what happens to potassium at each stage in its passage through the tubular system.
8. What is the effect of aldosterone on potassium secretion?
9. Discuss the concept of glomerulotubular balance and its relationship to control of the volume of fluid excretion by the kidneys.
10. Explain the effect of arterial pressure on the volume of urine excretion. Why is this relationship very important to the overall control of circulatory function?
11. Describe the *juxtaglomerular complex* and its relationship to the autoregulation of glomerular filtration rate.
12. Explain the differences between the afferent and the efferent arteriolar feedback mechanisms for control of glomerular filtration rate.
13. Why is the *renin-angiotensin system* of importance in allowing a person to conserve water and electrolytes in low blood pressure states while at the same time continuing to excrete waste products?

References

Andersson, B.: Regulation of body fluids. Annu Rev Physiol 39:185, 1977.

Beeuwkes, R., III: The vascular organization of the kidney. Annu Rev Physiol 42:531, 1980.

Berry, C. A.: Heterogeneity of tubular transport processes in the nephron. Annu Rev Physiol 44:181, 1982.

Bulger, R. E., and Dobyan, D. C.: Recent advances in renal morphology. Annu Rev Physiol 44:147, 1982.

Burg, M., and Good, D.: Sodium chloride coupled transport in mammalian nephrons. Annu Rev Physiol 45:533, 1983.

Churg, J., ed.: The Kidney. Baltimore, Williams & Wilkins, 1979.

Glynn, I. M., and Karlish, S. J. D.: The sodium pump. Annu Rev Physiol 37:13, 1975.

Katz, A. I., and Lindheimer, M. D.: Actions of hormones on the kidney. Annu Rev Physiol 39:97, 1977.

Knox, F. G., and Spielman, W. S.: Renal circulation. In Shepherd, J. T., and Abboud, F. M., eds.: Handbook of Physiology. Sec. 2, Vol. 3. Bethesda, American Physiological Society, 1983, p. 183.

Koeppen, B. M., et al.: Electrophysiology of mammalian renal tubules: Inferences from intracellular microelectrode studies. Annu Rev Physiol 45:497, 1983.

Lassiter, W. E.: Kidney. Annu Rev Physiol 37:371, 1975.

Maude, D. L.: Mechanism of tubular transport of salt and water. In MTP International Review of Science: Physiology. Vol. 6. Baltimore, University Park Press, 1974, p. 39.

Ross, C. R., and Holohan, P. D.: Transport of organic anions and cations in isolated renal plasma membranes. Annu Rev Pharmacol Toxicol 23:65, 1983.

Smith, H. W.: The Kidney: Structure and Function in Health and Disease. New York, Oxford University Press, 1951.

Vander, A. J.: Renal Physiology. New York, McGraw-Hill, 1980.

Walker, L. A., and Valtin, H.: Biological importance of nephron heterogeneity. Annu Rev Physiol 44:203, 1982.

25

Regulation of the Body Fluids and Their Constituents by the Kidneys and the Thirst Mechanism

TOTAL BODY WATER
BODY FLUID COMPARTMENTS
    BLOOD VOLUME
CONSTITUENTS OF EXTRACELLULAR
    AND INTRACELLULAR FLUIDS
OSMOTIC EQUILIBRIA AND FLUID
    VOLUME SHIFTS BETWEEN THE
    EXTRACELLULAR AND
    INTRACELLULAR FLUIDS
    BASIC PRINCIPLES OF OSMOSIS AND
        OSMOTIC PRESSURE
    OSMOLARITY OF THE BODY FLUIDS
    MAINTENANCE OF OSMOTIC
        EQUILIBRIUM BETWEEN
        EXTRACELLULR AND
        INTRACELLULAR FLUIDS
CONTROL OF BLOOD VOLUME
    BASIC MECHANISM FOR BLOOD
        VOLUME CONTROL
CONTROL OF EXTRACELLULAR FLUID
    VOLUME
CONTROL OF EXTRACELLULAR FLUID

SODIUM CONCENTRATION AND
EXTRACELLULAR FLUID OSMOLARITY
THE OSMOSODIUM RECEPTOR–
    ANTIDIURETIC HORMONE
    FEEDBACK CONTROL SYSTEM
THIRST AND ITS ROLE IN
    CONTROLLING SODIUM
    CONCENTRATION AND
    OSMOLARITY
COMBINED ROLES OF THE
    ANTIDIURETIC AND THIRST
    MECHANISMS FOR CONTROL OF
    EXTRACELLULAR FLUID SODIUM
    CONCENTRATION AND
    OSMOLARITY
CONTROL OF SODIUM INTAKE–
    APPETITE AND CRAVING FOR SALT
CONTROL OF EXTRACELLULAR
POTASSIUM CONCENTRATION
CONTROL OF THE EXTRACELLULAR
CONCENTRATIONS OF OTHER IONS

The principal function of the kidneys is to control almost all the characteristics of the body fluids, especially of the extracellular fluid—such characteristics as volume, composition, and osmolarity. This chapter will discuss these fluids and the role of the kidneys and the thirst mechanism in their control.

TOTAL BODY WATER

The total amount of water in a man of average weight (70 kg total) is approximately 40 liters (see Fig. 25–1), averaging 57 per cent of his total body weight.

Most of our daily intake of water enters by the oral route, but a small amount is also synthesized in the body as the result of oxidation of hydrogen in the food; this quantity ranges between 150 and 250 ml per day, depending on the rate of metabolism. The normal intake of fluid, including that synthesized in the body, averages about 2300/ml per day.

Table 25–1 shows the routes by which water is lost from the body under different conditions. Normally, at an atmospheric temperature of about 68°F approximately 1400 ml of the 2300 ml of water intake is lost in the *urine*, 100 ml is lost in the *sweat*, and 200 ml in the *feces*. The remaining 700 ml is lost by *evaporation from the respiratory tract* and by *diffusion*

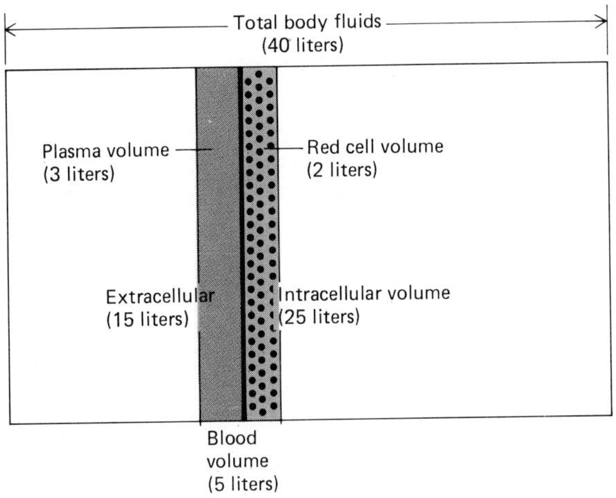

Figure 25–1. The body fluids diagrammed, showing the extra-cellular fluid volume, intracellular fluid volume, blood volume, and total body fluids.

Table 25–1. DAILY LOSS OF WATER (in Milliliters)

	Normal Temperature	Hot Weather	Prolonged Heavy Exercise
Insensible loss:			
Skin	350	350	350
Respiratory tract	350	250	650
Urine	1400	1200	500
Sweat	100	1400	5000
Feces	100	100	100
Total	2300	3300	6600

The extracellular fluid can be divided into *interstitial fluid, plasma, cerebrospinal fluid, intraocular fluid, fluids of the gastrointestinal tract,* and *fluids of the potential spaces.*

BLOOD VOLUME

Blood contains both extracellular fluid (the fluid of the plasma) and intracellular fluid (the fluid in the red blood cells). However, since blood is contained in a closed chamber all its own—the circulatory system—its volume and its special dynamics are exceedingly important.

The average blood volume of a normal adult is almost exactly 5000 ml. Approximately 3000 ml of this is plasma, and the remainder, 2000 ml, is red blood cells. However, these values vary greatly in different individuals, and sex, weight, and many other factors affect the blood volume.

Measurement of Blood Volume—The Dilution Principle. The blood volume can be measured by (1) injecting into the blood a substance that cannot escape from the blood compartment, (2) allowing the substance to disperse evenly throughout the blood, and (3) then measuring the extent to which the substance has become diluted. For instance, radioactive red blood cells can be injected. The greater the blood volume, the less is the concentration of these radioactive cells after complete dispersion of the cells throughout the vascular tree. Thus, the volume can be determined by the formula at the bottom of the page.

Note that all one needs to know is (1) the total quantity of the test substance put into the blood and (2) the concentration in the blood after dispersement.

In a similar way the plasma volume can be measured by injecting a substance that will disperse evenly in the plasma but will neither leave the blood compartment nor enter the red blood cells. The blood is centrifuged and the concentration of the test substance in the plasma is determined. One of the most widely used substances for measuring plasma volume is a dye called T–1824. This dye attaches to the

through the skin, which together are called *insensible water loss* because we do not know that we are actually losing water at the time that it is leaving the body.

In very hot weather, additional water loss in the sweat occasionally rises to as much as 1.5 liters an hour, which obviously can rapidly deplete the body fluids. Sweating will be discussed in Chapter 47.

Exercise increases the loss of water in two ways: First, it increases the rate of respiration, which promotes increased water loss through the respiratory tract in proportion to the increased ventilatory rate. Second, and much more important, exercise increases the body heat and consequently is likely to result in excessive sweating.

BODY FLUID COMPARTMENTS

The Intracellular Compartment. About 25 of the 40 liters of fluid in the body are inside the approximately 75 trillion cells of the body and are collectively called the *intracellular fluid*. The fluid of each cell contains its own individual mixture of different constituents, but the concentrations of these constituents are reasonably similar from one cell to another. For this reason, the intracellular fluid of all the different cells is considered to be one large fluid compartment, though in reality it is an aggregate of trillions of minute compartments.

The Extracellular Fluid Compartment. All the fluids outside the cells are called *extracellular fluid*, and these fluids are constantly mixing, as was explained in Chapter 1. The total amount of fluid in the extracellular compartment averages 15 liters in a 70-kg adult.

$$\text{Volume in milliliters} = \frac{\text{Quantity of test substance injected}}{\text{Concentration per milliliter of blood}}$$

plasma proteins and therefore will not leave the plasma. Also, radioactive albumin is often injected for the same purpose. Once the plasma volume has been determined, the blood volume can be determined by measuring the hematocrit (the ratio of red cells to plasma) and then using this to calculate the blood volume from the plasma volume.

CONSTITUENTS OF EXTRACELLULAR AND INTRACELLULAR FLUIDS

Figure 25–2 illustrates diagrammatically the major constituents of the extracellular and intracellular fluids. The quantities of the different substances are represented in *milliequivalents* or *millimoles per liter*. However, the protein molecules and some of the nonelectrolyte molecules are extremely large compared with the more numerous small ions. Therefore, *in terms of mass,* the proteins and nonelectrolytes actually constitute about 90 per cent of the dissolved constituents in the plasma, about 60 per cent in the interstitial fluid, and about 97 per cent in the intracellular fluid.

Figure 25–3 illustrates the distribution of the nonelectrolytes in the plasma; most of these same substances are also present in almost equal concentrations in the interstitial fluid, except for some of the

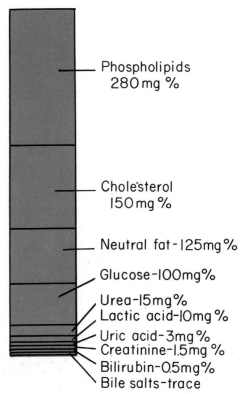

Figure 25–3. The nonelectrolytes of the extracellular fluid.

fatty compounds that are present in the plasma in large suspended particles, the *lipoproteins*.

The Extracellular Fluid. Referring again to Figure 25–2, one sees that extracellular fluid, both that of the blood plasma and that of the interstitial fluid, contains large quantities of *sodium* and *chloride ions*, reasonably large quantities of *bicarbonate ions*, but only small quantities of other ions. However, plasma has about three times the concentration of protein as that in interstitial fluid. (The proteins in these fluids and their significance are discussed in detail in Chapter 22.)

In Chapter 1 it was pointed out that the extracellular fluid is called the *internal environment* of the body and that its constituents are accurately regulated so that the cells remain bathed continuously in a fluid containing the proper electrolytes and nutrients for continued cellular function. The regulation of these constituents will be presented later in this chapter.

The Intracellular Fluid. From Figure 25–2 it is also readily apparent that the intracellular fluid contains only small quantities of sodium and chloride ions and almost no calcium ions; but it does contain large quantities of *potassium* and *phosphate* and moderate quantities of *magnesium* and *sulfate ions,* all of which are present in only small concentrations in the extracellular fluid. In addition, the cells contain especially large amounts of protein, approximately four times as much as the plasma.

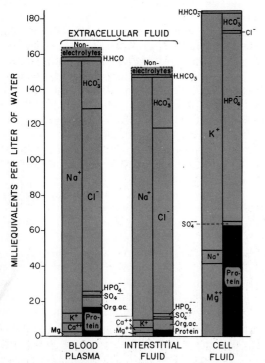

Figure 25–2. The compositions of plasma, interstitial fluid, and intracellular fluid. (Modified and reprinted by permission from Gamble: Chemical Anatomy, Physiology, and Pathology of Extracellular Fluid: A Lecture Syllabus. Harvard University Press, 1954.)

OSMOTIC EQUILIBRIA AND FLUID VOLUME SHIFTS BETWEEN EXTRACELLULAR AND INTRACELLULAR FLUIDS

One of the most troublesome of all problems in clinical medicine is maintenance of adequate body fluids and proper balance between the extracellular and intracellular fluid volumes in seriously ill patients. The purpose of the following discussion, therefore, is to explain the interrelationships between extracellular and intracellular fluid volumes and the osmotic factors that cause shifts of fluid between the extracellular and intracellular compartments.

BASIC PRINCIPLES OF OSMOSIS AND OSMOTIC PRESSURE

The basic principles of osmosis and osmotic pressure were presented in Chapter 4. However, these principles are important enough to the following discussion that they are reviewed here briefly.

Whenever a membrane between two fluid compartments is permeable to water but not to some of the dissolved solutes (this is called a *selectively permeable membrane*) and the concentration of the solutes is greater on one side of the membrane than on the other, water moves by the phenomenon called *osmosis* through the membrane toward the side with the greater concentration of solutes.

Osmosis results from the kinetic motion of the molecules (and ions) in the solutions on the two sides of the membrane and can be explained in the following way: The individual molecules on both sides of the membrane are equally active because the temperature, which is a measure of the kinetic activity of the molecules, is the same on both sides. However, the nondiffusible solute on one side of the membrane displaces some of the water molecules, thereby reducing the concentration of water molecules. As a result, the so-called *chemical potential* (which means the total activity) of water molecules on this side is less than on the other side, so that fewer water molecules strike each pore of the membrane each second on the solute side of the pore than on the pure water side. This causes more diffusion of water molecules from the water side to the solute side than in the other direction, and the difference between the diffusions in the two directions is called *net* diffusion. This net diffusion is osmosis.

Osmosis of water molecules can be opposed by applying a pressure across the membrane in the direction opposite to that of the osmosis. The amount of pressure required to oppose the osmosis exactly is called the *osmotic pressure*.

Relationship of the Molecular Concentration of a Solution to Its Osmotic Pressure. The *molecular concentration* of a solution means the number of molecules, not the weight of the solute, in each volume of solution. Each nondiffusible molecule dissolved in water reduces the chemical potential of the water by exactly the same amount. Consequently, the tendency for the water in the solution to diffuse through a membrane is reduced in direct proportion to the number of nondiffusible molecules. And, as a corollary, the osmotic pressure of the solution is also proportional to the number of nondiffusible molecules in the solution. This relationship holds true for all nondiffusible molecules almost regardless of their molecular weight. For instance, one molecule of albumin with a molecular weight of 70,000 has the same osmotic effect as a molecule of glucose with a molecular weight of 180.

Osmotic Effect of Ions. Nondiffusible ions cause osmosis and osmotic pressure in exactly the same manner as do nondiffusible molecules. Furthermore, when a molecule dissociates into two or more ions, each of the ions then exerts osmotic pressure individually. Therefore, to determine the osmotic effect, all the nondiffusible ions must be added to all the nondiffusible molecules; but note that a bivalent ion, such as calcium, exerts no more osmotic pressure than does a univalent ion, such as sodium.

Osmoles. The ability of solutes to cause osmosis and osmotic pressure is measured in terms of "osmoles"; the osmole is a measure of the total number of particles. *One mole of nondiffusible and nonionizable substance is equal to 1 osmole.* On the other hand, if a substance ionizes into two ions (sodium chloride into sodium and chloride ions, for instance), then 0.5 mole of the substance equals 1 osmole. The obvious reason for using the osmole is that osmotic pressure is determined by the number of particles instead of the mass of the solute.

In general, the osmole is too large a unit for satisfactory use in expressing osmotic activity of solutes in the body. Therefore, the term *milliosmole*, which equals 0.001 osmole, is commonly used.

Osmolarity. The osmolar concentration of a solution is called its *osmolarity*, and it is expressed as osmoles per liter of solution. For instance, the osmolarity of the interstitial fluid is approximately 300 milliosmoles. The osmotic pressure of a solution *at body temperature* can be determined approximately from the following formula:

Osmotic pressure (mm Hg)
$$= 19.3 \times \text{osmolarity (milliosmoles/liter)}$$

Using this formula, one calculates the osmotic pressure of the interstitial fluid to be over 5000 mm Hg.

OSMOLARITY OF THE BODY FLUIDS

Table 25–2 lists the osmotically active substances in plasma, interstitial fluid, and intracellular fluid. The milliosmoles of each of them per liter are given. Note especially that approximately four fifths of the total osmolarity of the interstitial fluid and plasma is caused by sodium and chloride ions, while approxi-

Table 25–2. OSMOLAR SUBSTANCES IN EXTRACELLULAR AND INTRACELLULAR FLUIDS

	Plasma (mOsmole/l of H_2O)	Interstitial (mOsmole/l of H_2O)	Intracellular (mOsmole/l of H_2O)
Na^+	146	142	14
K^+	4.2	4.0	140
Ca^{++}	2.5	2.4	0
Mg^{++}	1.5	1.4	31
Cl^-	105	108	4
HCO_3^-	27	28.3	10
$HPO_4^{--}, H_2PO_4^-$	2	2	11
SO_4	0.5	0.5	1
Phosphocreatine			45
Carnosine			14
Amino acids	2	2	8
Creatine	0.2	0.2	9
Lactate	1.2	1.2	1.5
Adenosine triphosphate			5
Hexose monophosphate			3.7
Glucose	5.6	5.6	
Protein	1.2	0.2	4
Urea	4	4	4
TOTAL mOsmole/l	302.9	301.8	302.2
Corrected for ionic interaction (mOsmole/l)	282.6	281.3	281.3
Total osmotic pressure at 37° C (mm Hg)	5453	5430	5430

mately half of the intracellular osmolarity is caused by potassium ions, the remainder being divided among the many other intracellular substances.

As noted at the bottom of the table, the total osmolarity of each of the three compartments is approximately 300 milliosmoles per liter, with that of the plasma being 1.3 milliosmoles greater than that of the interstitial and intracellular fluids. This slight difference between plasma and interstitial fluid is caused by the osmotic effect of the plasma proteins, which maintains a pressure in the capillaries about 22 mm Hg greater than in the surrounding interstitial fluid spaces, as was explained in Chapter 22.

MAINTENANCE OF OSMOTIC EQUILIBRIUM BETWEEN EXTRACELLULAR AND INTRACELLULAR FLUIDS

The tremendous osmotic pressure that can develop across the cell membrane when one side is exposed to pure water—more than 5400 mm Hg—illustrates how much osmotic force can become available to push water molecules through the membrane when the solutions of the two sides of the membrane are not in osmotic equilibrium. As an example, in Figure 25–4A a cell is placed in a solution that has an osmolarity far less than that of the intracellular fluid. As a result, osmosis of water begins immediately from the extracellular fluid to the intracellular fluid, causing the cell to swell and diluting the intracellular fluid while concentrating the extracellular fluid. When the fluid inside the cell becomes diluted sufficiently to equal the osmolar concentration of the fluid on the outside, further osmosis then ceases. This final condition is shown in Figure 25–4B. In Figure 25–4C, a cell is placed in a solution having a much higher concentration outside the cell than inside. This time,

water passes by osmosis to the exterior, diluting the extracellular fluid and concentrating the intracellular fluid. In this process the cell shrinks until the two osmolar concentrations become equal, as shown in Figure 25–4D.

Rapidity of Attaining Extracellular and Intracellular Osmotic Equilibrium. The transfer of water through the cell membrane by osmosis occurs so rapidly that any lack of osmotic equilibrium between the two fluid compartments in any given tissue is usually corrected within a few seconds to within a minute or so at most. However, this rapid transfer of water through the cell membrane does not mean that

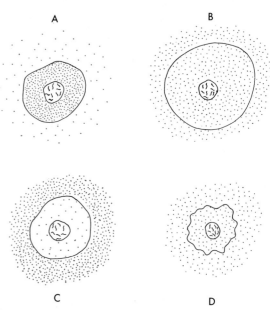

Figure 25–4. Establishment of osmotic equilibrium when cells are placed in a hypo- or hypertonic solution.

complete equilibration occurs between the extracellular and intracellular compartments throughout the whole body within this same short period of time. The reason is that fluid usually enters the body through the gut and must then be transported by the blood to all tissues before complete equilibration can occur. In the normal person it may take as long as 30 minutes for the fluid to be transported everywhere in the body after drinking water.

Isotonicity, Hypotonicity, and Hypertonicity. A fluid into which normal body cells can be placed without causing either swelling or shrinkage of the cells is said to be *isotonic* with the cells. A 0.9 per cent solution of sodium chloride or a 5 per cent glucose solution is approximately isotonic.

A solution that will cause the cells to swell is said to be *hypotonic;* any solution of sodium chloride with less than 0.9 per cent concentration is hypotonic.

A solution that will cause the cells to shrink is said to be *hypertonic;* sodium chloride solutions of greater than 0.9 per cent concentration are all hypertonic.

CONTROL OF BLOOD VOLUME

Constancy of the Blood Volume. The extreme degree of precision with which the blood volume is controlled is illustrated in Figure 25–5, which shows that tremendous changes in fluid intake, from very low values to very high values, cause almost no change in blood volume (except when the intake becomes so low that it is not sufficient to make up for even the slightest fluid losses). To state this another way, even when the intake of water and salt is increased many-fold, the blood volume is hardly altered. Conversely, a decrease in fluid intake to as little as one-third normal also causes very little change.

BASIC MECHANISM FOR BLOOD VOLUME CONTROL

The basic mechanism for blood volume control is essentially the same as the basic mechanism for ar-

terial pressure control that was presented in Chapter 15. It was pointed out in this earlier chapter that extracellular fluid volume, blood volume, cardiac output, arterial pressure, and urine output are all mainly or partially controlled by a single common basic feedback mechanism. Therefore, let us explain again the basic principles of this mechanism:

When the blood volume becomes too great, the cardiac output and arterial pressure increase. This pressure increase, in turn, profoundly increases kidney excretion of fluid from the body. This excretion returns the blood volume back to normal. Conversely, if the blood volume falls below normal, the cardiac output and arterial pressure decrease, the kidneys now retain fluid, and progressive accumulation of the fluid intake eventually builds the blood volume back to normal. (Obviously, parallel processes also occur to reconstitute red cells, plasma proteins, and other blood constituents.)

Role of the Volume Receptors in Blood Volume Control. It was pointed out in Chapter 17 that "volume receptor" reflexes help to control blood volume. The volume receptors are stretch receptors located in the walls of the right and left atria. When the blood volume becomes excessive, a large share of this volume accumulates in the central veins of the thorax and causes increased pressure in the two atria. The resultant stretch of the atrial walls transmits nerve signals into the brain, and these in turn elicit responses that accelerate the return of blood volume to normal. The two most important responses are the following:

1. The sympathetic nervous signals to the kidneys are inhibited, thus slightly to moderately increasing the rate of urinary output.

2. The secretion of antidiuretic hormone by the supraopticohypophyseal system is reduced, allowing increased water excretion by the kidneys.

Possible Role of Atrial Natriuretic Factor in Volume Control. Large numbers of cells in the walls of the two atria, but especially in the right atrium, contain a hormone-like substance called *atrial natriuretic factor*. When this factor is infused into the circulating blood, it causes as much as a three to ten

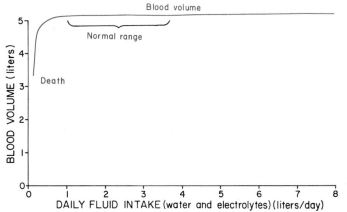

Figure 25–5. Effect on blood volume of marked changes in daily fluid intake. Note the precision of blood volume control in the normal range.

times increase in renal excretion of sodium. And, concomitant with the sodium loss is loss of water as well, and both the extracellular fluid volume and blood volume decrease slightly. Therefore, it has been suggested that atrial natriuretic factor may play a role in the regulation of blood volume. That is, excess blood volume stretches the atrial walls, and this promotes the release of atrial natriuretic factor that in turn causes sodium excretion and reduction of the blood volume. Unfortunately, the quantitative aspects of this mechanism are yet unclear, but it could operate in parallel with the volume receptor mechanism to help regulate blood volume.

In most instances, the volume receptor reflex effects, possibly operating in association with atrial natriuretic factor as well, can cause the blood volume to return almost all the way to normal within an hour or so, but the final determination of the precise level to which the blood volume will be adjusted is still a function of the basic volume control mechanism discussed above. The reason is that over a period of one to three days the volume receptors, and possibly the natriuretic mechanism, adapt so completely that they no longer transmit any corrective signals. Therefore, they appear to be of value only to help readjust the volume during the first few hours or days after an abnormality occurs, but not for long-term monitoring of volume or for precise adjustments of the long-term level of blood volume.

CONTROL OF EXTRACELLULAR FLUID VOLUME

It is already clear from the above discussion of the basic mechanism for blood volume control that extracellular fluid volume is controlled at the same time as the blood volume. That is, when fluid is reabsorbed by the kidney or is ingested by mouth, the fluid first goes into the blood, but it rapidly becomes distributed between the interstitial spaces and the plasma. Though it is the blood volume that raises the arterial pressure and thereby causes increased urinary output and not increased interstitial fluid volume, fluid will not remain in the blood without also appropriately filling the interstitial spaces with fluid at the same time. Yet, the relative distribution of volume between the interstitial spaces and the blood can vary greatly, depending on the physical characteristics of the circulatory system and of the interstitial spaces.

Under normal conditions, the approximate relationship between extracellular fluid volume and blood volume is that illustrated in Figure 25–6. The curve of this figure shows that at the lower extracellular fluid volumes, an increase in extracellular fluid volume is associated with a parallel increase in blood volume. However, when the extracellular fluid volume rises above 20 to 22 liters, very little of the additional fluid will remain in the blood, almost all of it instead going into the interstitial spaces. This is caused by the fact that the interstitial fluid pressure

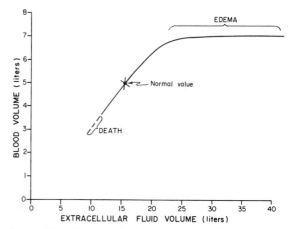

Figure 25–6. Relationship between extracellular fluid volume and blood volume, showing a nearly linear relationship in the normal range but indicating failure of the blood volume to continue rising when the extracellular fluid volume becomes excessive.

rises from its normal negative value (subatmospheric) to a positive value. When this occurs, the compliance of the tissue spaces becomes tremendous, so that they can then hold as much as 20 to 40 liters of fluid with very little additional rise in interstitial pressure. Therefore, the interstitial fluid spaces, under these conditions, literally become an "overflow" reservoir for excess fluid from the blood. This obviously causes edema, but it also acts as an important overflow release valve for the circulatory system, a well-known phenomenon that is utilized daily by the clinician to allow him to administer almost unlimited quantities of intravenous fluid and yet not force the heart into cardiac failure.

CONTROL OF EXTRACELLULAR FLUID SODIUM CONCENTRATION AND EXTRACELLULAR FLUID OSMOLARITY

Relationship of Sodium Concentration to Extracellular Fluid Osmolarity. The osmolarity of the extracellular fluids (and also of the intracellular fluids, since they remain in osmotic equilibrium with the extracellular fluids) is determined almost entirely by the extracellular fluid sodium concentration. The reason is that sodium is by far the most abundant positive ion of the extracellular fluid. Furthermore, the acid-base control mechanisms of the kidneys, which will be discussed in the following chapter, adjust the negative ion concentrations of the body fluids to equal those of the positive ions. Therefore, in effect, the sodium ion concentration of the extracellular fluid determines 90 to 95 per cent of the *effective* osmotic pressure of the extracellular fluid. Consequently, we can generally talk in terms of control of sodium concentration and control of osmolarity at the same time.

Two separate control systems operate in close association to regulate extracellular sodium concentration and osmolarity. These are (1) the osmosodium receptor–antidiuretic hormone system and (2) the thirst mechanism.

THE OSMOSODIUM RECEPTOR–ANTIDIURETIC HORMONE FEEDBACK CONTROL SYSTEM

Figure 25–7 illustrates the osmosodium receptor–antidiuretic hormone system for control of extracellular fluid sodium concentration and osmolarity. It is a typical feedback control system that operates by the following steps:

1. An increase in osmolarity (excess sodium and the negative ions that go with it) excites neuronal cells called *osmoreceptors* located in the *supraoptic nuclei of the hypothalamus.*

2. Excitation of the osmoreceptors causes release of antidiuretic hormone.

3. The antidiuretic hormone *increases the permeability of the late distal tubules, collecting tubules, and collecting ducts,* as explained in the previous chapter, and therefore causes increased conservation of water by the kidneys.

4. The conservation of water but loss of sodium and other osmolar substances in the urine causes dilution of the sodium and other substances in the extracellular fluid, thus correcting the initial excessively concentrated extracellular fluid.

Conversely, when the extracellular fluid becomes too dilute (hypo-osmotic), less antidiuretic hormone is formed, and excess water is lost along with very few extracellular fluid solutes, thus concentrating the body fluids back toward normal.

Mechanism for Exciting the Osmoreceptors (or Osmosodium Receptors). Located in the supraoptic nuclei of the anterior hypothalamus, as shown in Figure 25–8, are the specialized neuronal cells called *osmoreceptors.* These respond to changes in osmolarity of the extracellular fluid. When the extracellular osmolarity becomes low, osmosis of water into the osmoreceptors causes them to swell. This *decreases* their rate of impulse discharge. Conversely, increased osmolarity in the extracellular fluid pulls water out of the osmoreceptors, causing them to shrink and thereby to *increase* their rate of discharge.

The osmoreceptors respond to changes in extracellular fluid sodium concentration but not to changes in potassium concentration and only slightly to changes in urea and glucose concentrations. The reason probably is that these other substances can penetrate the osmoreceptor cell membranes and therefore cause little or no osmotic effect. Therefore, for all practical purposes, the osmoreceptors are actually sodium concentration receptors—hence the name *osmosodium receptors.*

The nerve signals from the osmoreceptors are transmitted from the supraoptic nuclei through the pituitary stalk into the posterior pituitary gland, where they promote the release of antidiuretic hormone (ADH).

Thus, ADH secretion is controlled by the osmolarity (or sodium concentration) of the extracellular fluid—the greater the osmolarity, the greater the rate of ADH secretion.

Water Diuresis. When a person drinks a large amount of water, a phenomenon called *water diuresis* ensues very shortly thereafter, a typical record of which is shown in Figure 25–9. In this example, a man drank 1 liter of water, and approximately 30 minutes later his urine output increased to 8 times normal. It remained at this level for two hours—that is, until the osmolarity of the extracellular fluid had returned essentially to normal. The delay in onset of water diuresis is caused partly by delay in absorption of the water from the gastrointestinal tract and partly by the time required for destruction of the antidiuretic hormone that had already been released by the pituitary gland prior to drinking the water.

Diabetes Insipidus. Destruction of the supraoptic nuclei or high level destruction of the nerve tract from the supraoptic nuclei to the posterior pituitary gland causes antidiuretic hormone secretion to cease or at least to become greatly reduced. When this happens, the person thereafter excretes a dilute urine, and the daily urine volume is increased to 3 to 10 times normal, which is 5 to 15 liters per day. This condition is called *diabetes insipidus.* In diabetes insipidus, the body fluid volumes remain almost normal so long as the thirst mechanism in still functional,

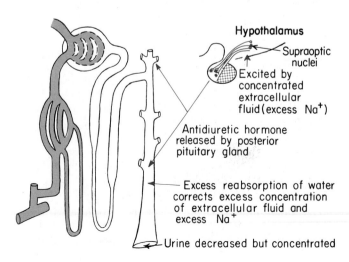

Hypothalamus
Supraoptic nuclei
Excited by concentrated extracellular fluid (excess Na^+)

Antidiuretic hormone released by posterior pituitary gland

Excess reabsorption of water corrects excess concentration of extracellular fluid and excess Na^+

Urine decreased but concentrated

Figure 25–7. Control of extracellular fluid osmolality and sodium ion concentration by the osmosodium receptor-antidiuretic hormone feedback control system.

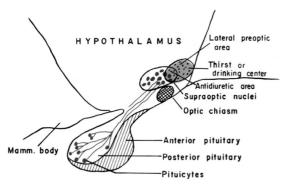

Figure 25–8. The supraopticopituitary antidiuretic system and its relationship to the thirst center in the hypothalamus.

because this ordinarily makes the person drink enough water to make up for the increased loss of water in the urine. On the other hand, any factor that prevents adequate intake of fluid, such as unconsciousness, results rapidly in a state of dehydration, tremendous hyperosmolarity, and excessive concentration of sodium in the extracellular fluid.

Syndrome of Inappropriate ADH Secretion. Certain types of tumors, especially bronchogenic tumors of the lungs or tumors of the basal regions of the brain, often secrete large quantities of antidiuretic or a similar hormone. This condition is called the *syndrome of inappropriate ADH secretion.* This excess ADH causes only a slight increase in extracellular fluid volume; instead, its principal effect is *to decrease greatly the sodium concentration of the extracellular fluid.* The explanation of this effect is the following: The ADH at first causes a decrease in urine output and a simultaneous slight increase in blood volume. This in turn activates the basic mechanism for blood volume control. That is, a slight rise in arterial pressure occurs, and this causes a secondary *increase* in urinary output. Furthermore, the urine that is excreted is tremendously concentrated because of the concentrating action of the ADH as explained in the previous chapter. Consequently, the kidneys excrete extreme amounts of sodium into the urine but retain excessive amounts of water in the extracellular fluid. Therefore, the sodium concentration becomes seriously reduced, sometimes falling from a normal value of 142 mEq/liter down to as low as 110 to 120 mEq/liter. At values this low, patients frequently die sudden deaths because of coma and convulsions.

This disease is especially instructive because it illustrates both the extreme importance of the antidiuretic hormone mechanism for control of sodium concentration and its relatively mild effect on control of body fluid volume.

THIRST AND ITS ROLE IN CONTROLLING SODIUM CONCENTRATION AND OSMOLARITY

The phenomenon of thirst is as important for regulating body water and sodium concentration as is the osmoreceptor-ADH–renal mechanism discussed above, because the amount of water in the body at any one time is determined by the balance between both *intake* and *output* of water. Thirst, the primary regulator of the intake of water, is defined as the *conscious desire for water.*

Neural Integration of Thirst—the Thirst Center. Referring again to Figure 25–8, one sees a small area located slightly anterior to the supraoptic nuclei in the lateral preoptic area of the hypothalamus called the *thirst center.* Electrical stimulation of this center by implanted electrodes causes an animal to begin drinking within seconds and to continue drinking until the electrical stimulus is stopped. Injection of hypertonic salt solutions into the area, which causes osmosis of water out of the neuronal cells and shrinkage of the cells, also causes drinking. Thus, the neuronal cells of the thirst center function in almost the identical way as the osmoreceptors of the supraoptic nuclei.

Temporary Relief of Thirst Caused by the Act of Drinking. A thirsty person receives relief from thirst immediately after drinking water, even before the water has been absorbed from the gastrointestinal tract. In fact, in persons with esophageal fistula (a condition in which the water passes to the exterior from the esophagus and never goes into the gastrointestinal tract), partial relief of thirst still occurs following the act of drinking, but this relief is only temporary, and the thirst returns after 15 minutes or more. If the water does enter the stomach, distention of the stomach and other portions of the upper gastrointestinal tract provides still further temporary relief from thirst. For instance, simple inflation of a balloon in the stomach can relieve thirst for 5 to 30 minutes.

One might wonder what the value of this temporary relief from thirst could be, but there is good reason for it. After a person has drunk water, as long as one-half to one hour may be required for all of the water to be absorbed and distributed throughout the

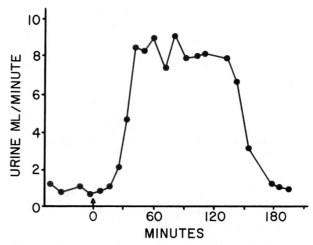

Figure 25–9. Water diuresis in a human being following ingestion of 1000 ml of water. (Redrawn from Smith: The Kidney: Structure and Functions in Health and Disease. Oxford University Press, 1951.)

body. Were the thirst sensation not temporarily relieved after drinking water, the person would continue to drink more and more. When all this water was finally absorbed, the body fluids would be far more diluted than normal, and an abnormal condition opposite to that which the person was attempting to correct would be created. It is well known that a thirsty animal almost never drinks more than the amount of water needed to relieve the state of dehydration. Indeed, it is uncanny that the animal usually drinks almost exactly the right amount.

Role of Thirst in Controlling Osmolarity and Sodium Concentration of the Extracellular Fluid—The Tripping Mechanism. The kidneys are continually excreting fluid, and water is also lost by evaporation from the skin and lungs. Therefore, a person is continually being dehydrated which causes the volume of extracellular fluid to decrease and its concentration of sodium and other osmolar elements to rise. When the sodium concentration rises to approximately 2 mEq/liter above normal (or the osmolarity rises to approximately 4 mOsm/liter above normal) the drinking mechanism becomes "tripped" because the person by then reaches a level of thirst that is strong enough to activate the motor effort necessary to cause drinking. The person ordinarily drinks precisely the required amount of fluid to bring the extracellular fluids back to normal—that is, to a state of *satiety*. Then the process of dehydration and sodium concentration begins again, and the drinking mechanism is tripped again, the process continuing on and on indefinitely.

In this way, both the sodium concentration and osmolarity of the extracellular fluid are very precisely controlled.

COMBINED ROLES OF THE ANTIDIURETIC AND THIRST MECHANISMS FOR CONTROL OF EXTRACELLULAR FLUID SODIUM CONCENTRATION AND OSMOLARITY

When either the antidiuretic hormone mechanism or the thirst mechanism fails, the other ordinarily can still control both sodium concentration and extracellular fluid osmolarity with reasonable effectiveness. On the other hand, if both of them fail simultaneously, neither sodium nor osmolarity is then adequately controlled.

Figure 25–10 dramatically demonstrates the overall capability of the ADH-thirst system to control extracellular fluid sodium concentration. This figure demonstrates the ability of the same animal to control its extracellular fluid sodium concentration in two different conditions: (1) in the normal state and (2) after both the antidiuretic hormone and thirst mechanisms had been blocked. Note that in the normal animal a six-fold increase in sodium intake caused the sodium concentration to change only two-thirds of 1 per cent (from 142 mEq/liter up to 143 mEq/liter)—an excellent degree of sodium concentration control. Now note the dashed curve of the figure, which shows the

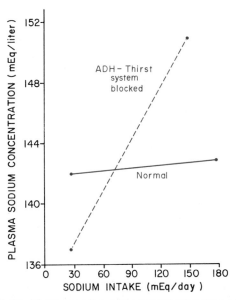

Figure 25–10. Effect on the extracellular fluid sodium concentration in dogs caused by tremendous changes in sodium intake (1) under normal conditions, and (2) after the antidiuretic hormone and thirst feedback systems had been blocked. This figure shows lack of sodium ion control in the absence of these systems. (Courtesy of Dr. David B. Young.)

change in sodium concentration when the ADH-thirst system was blocked. In this case, sodium concentration increased 10 per cent with only a fivefold increase in sodium intake (a change in sodium concentration from 137 mEq/liter up to 151 mEq/liter), which is an extreme change in sodium concentration when one realizes that the normal sodium concentration rarely rises or falls more than 1 per cent from day to day.

Therefore, the major feedback mechanism for control of sodium concentration (and also for extracellular osmolarity) is the ADH-thirst mechanism. In the absence of this mechanism there is no feedback mechanism that will cause the body to increase water ingestion or to conserve water by the kidneys when excess sodium enters the body. Therefore, the sodium concentration simply increases.

CONTROL OF SODIUM INTAKE— APPETITE AND CRAVING FOR SALT

Maintenance of normal extracellular sodium requires not only the control of sodium excretion but also the control of sodium intake. Unfortunately, we know very little about this except that salt-depleted persons (or persons who have lost blood) develop a desire for salt; as an example, this occurs in persons who have *Addison's disease*, a condition in which the adrenal cortices no longer secrete aldosterone, so that the salt stores of the body become depleted. Likewise, it is well known that animals living in areas far removed from the seashore actively search out "salt licks." This craving for salt is analogous to thirst, and it is also analogous to *appetite* for other types of foods, which is still another homeostatic mechanism that will be discussed in Chapter 48.

CONTROL OF EXTRACELLULAR POTASSIUM CONCENTRATION

It is especially important to control the extracellular fluid potassium concentration because very slight changes in concentration often can alter nervous and cardiac functions seriously, as discussed in Chapter 5 for peripheral nerves, in Chapter 31 for the central nervous system, and Chapter 8 for the heart. The normal concentration is about 4.5 mEq/liter, and this rarely rises or falls more than ± 0.3 mEq.

Two major factors play important roles in controlling the potassium ion concentration: (1) a direct effect of increased extracellular fluid potassium concentration in causing increased secretion of potassium into the tubules and (2) an effect of aldosterone in increasing potassium secretion.

The Direct Effect of Extracellular Fluid Potassium Concentration on Potassium Secretion Into the Tubules

Potassium is secreted into the tubular fluid in the late distal tubules and cortical collecting tubules. For reasons that are not clear, the rate of secretion is determined strongly by the concentration of the potassium ions in the interstitial fluid of the kidneys, which is part of the body's extracellular fluid. Consequently, as the extracellular fluid potassium concentration increases, the rate of potassium secretion into the tubules also increases markedly. This increase obviously functions as an automatic means for reducing the extracellular fluid potassium ion concentration back toward normal.

Effect of Aldosterone on Tubular Secretion of Potassium Ions

In the previous chapter, it was pointed out that aldosterone not only causes increased sodium reabsorption by the tubules but also causes greatly *increased tubular secretion of potassium* as well, and therefore increased loss of potassium in the urine. Though the antidiuretic hormone and thirst mechanisms can override aldosterone control of extracellular fluid sodium concentration, this is not true for the control of potassium concentration. Therefore, aldosterone plays an exceedingly important role in the control of extracellular fluid potassium ion concentration. We will explain this control system in the following sections.

Effect of Potassium Ion Concentration on Rate of Aldosterone Secretion. In a properly functioning feedback system, the factor that is controlled almost invariably has a feedback effect to control the controller; this is precisely true for the aldosterone-potassium control system because the rate of aldosterone secretion is controlled very strongly by the extracellular fluid potassium concentration. Figure 25–11 illustrates the tremendous increases in aldosterone secretion rate caused by very minute increases in potassium ion concentration.

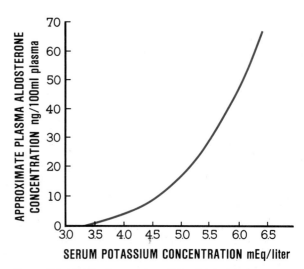

Figure 25–11. Effect on extracellular fluid aldosterone concentration of potassium ion concentration changes. Note the extreme change in aldosterone concentration for very minute changes in potassium concentration.

Basic Mechanism for Aldosterone Control of Potassium Concentration. Putting the effects illustrated in Figure 25–11 together with the fact that aldosterone greatly increases renal excretion of potassium, one can construct a very simple system for negative feedback control of potassium concentration. That is, (1) an increase in potassium concentration causes an increase in aldosterone in the circulating blood. (2) The increase in aldosterone causes a marked increase in potassium excretion by the kidneys. (3) The increased potassium excretion then decreases the extracellular fluid potassium concentration back toward normal.

Importance of the Aldosterone Feedback System for Control of Potassium Concentration. Without a functioning aldosterone feedback system, an animal can easily die from either hypopotassemia (hypokalemia) or hyperpotassemia (hyperkalemia).

Figure 25–12 illustrates the potent effect of the aldosterone feedback system in controlling potassium concentration. In the experiment in this figure, dogs were subjected to an almost sevenfold increase in potassium intake in two different states: (1) the normal state and (2) after the capability of the aldosterone feedback system to respond to changing potassium concentration had been blocked by removing the adrenal glands and the animals had been given a fixed rate of aldosterone infusion.

Note that in the normal animal the sevenfold increase in potassium intake caused an increase in plasma potassium concentration of only 2.4 per cent—from a concentration of 4.2 mEq/liter to 4.3 mEq/liter. Thus, when the aldosterone feedback system was functioning normally, the potassium concentration remained precisely controlled despite the tremendous change in potassium intake.

On the other hand, the dashed curve in the figure shows the effect after the aldosterone system had been blocked. Note that the same increase in potassium intake then caused a 26 per cent increase in

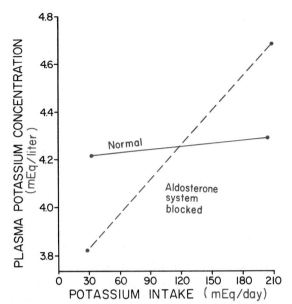

Figure 25–12. Effect on extracellular fluid potassium concentration of tremendous changes in potassium intake (1) under normal conditions, and (2) after the aldosterone feedback system had been blocked. This figure demonstrates that potassium concentration is very poorly controlled after block of the aldosterone system. (Courtesy of Dr. David B. Young.)

potassium concentration. Thus, the control of potassium concentration in the normal animals was many times more effective in the animals without an aldosterone feedback mechanism.

Effect of Primary Aldosteronism and Addison's Disease on Extracellular Fluid Potassium Concentration. Primary aldosteronism is caused by a tumor of the zona glomerulosa of one of the adrenal glands, the tumor secreting tremendous quantities of aldosterone. One of the most important effects of this disease is a severe decrease in extracellular fluid potassium concentration, so much so that many of these patients experience paralysis caused by failure of nerve transmission.

Conversely, in the patient with Addison's disease, whose adrenal glands have been destroyed, the extracellular fluid potassium concentration frequently rises to as high as twice normal, resulting in cardiac debility that leads to cardiac arrest, which is often the cause of death in these patients.

CONTROL OF THE EXTRACELLULAR CONCENTRATIONS OF OTHER IONS

Regulation of Calcium Ion Concentration. The role of calcium in the body and the control of its concentration in the extracellular fluid are discussed in detail in Chapter 53 in relation to the endocrinology of parathyroid hormone, calcitonin, and bone, but are briefly considered here.

The day-by-day calcium ion concentration is controlled principally by the effect of parathyroid hormone on bone reabsorption. When the extracellular fluid concentration of calcium falls too low, the parathyroid glands are directly stimulated to promote increased secretion of parathyroid hormone, and this hormone in turn acts directly on the bones to increase the reabsorption of bone salts, thus releasing large amounts of calcium into the extracellular fluid and elevating the calcium level back to normal.

However, the bones are not an inexhaustible supply and eventually will run out of calcium. Therefore, long-term control of calcium ion concentration results from the action of parathyroid hormone to control the reabsorption of calcium from the kidney tubules and the absorption of calcium from the gut through the gastrointestinal mucosa. Both of these effects are markedly increased by parathyroid hormone until the calcium ion concentration returns to normal. These results will be discussed in more detail in Chapter 53.

Regulation of Phosphate Concentration. Phosphate concentration is regulated primarily by an *overflow* mechanism, which can be explained as follows: The renal tubules have a normal capability to reabsorb a maximum of 0.1 millimole of phosphate per minute. When less than this "load" of phosphate is present in the glomerular filtrate, all of it is reabsorbed. When more is present, the excess is excreted. Therefore, phosphate ion normally spills into the urine when its concentration in the plasma is above the threshold value of approximately 0.8 millimole/liter. Any time the concentration falls below this value, the phosphate is conserved in the plasma, and the daily ingested phosphate accumulates in the extracellular fluid until its concentration rises above the threshold.

Since most people ingest large quantities of phosphate day in and day out, either in milk or in meat, the concentration of phosphate is usually maintained at a level of about 1.0 millimole/liter, a level barely great enough for there to be continual overflow of excess phosphate into the urine.

Regulation of Other Negative Ions. The regulation of chloride and bicarbonate ions are discussed in the following chapter in connection with acid-base balance of the body. But other important negative ions in the body fluid include sulfates, nitrates, urates, lactates, and the amino acids. Essentially all of these, like phosphate, have definite maximum rates of tubular reabsorption. When the concentration of each is below its respective threshold, it is conserved in the extracellular fluid, but above this threshold the excess spills into the urine. Thus, the concentrations of most of these negative ions are regulated by the overflow mechanism in the same way that phosphate ion concentration is regulated.

QUESTIONS

1. State the approximate rates of water loss in the body by way of the urine and other routes.
2. What are the approximate normal values in the adult for blood volume, plasma volume, extracellular fluid volume, and intracellular fluid volume?
3. Explain the dilution principle for measuring blood volume.
4. What are the principal differences between the constituents of the extracellular fluid and those of intracellular fluid?
5. Explain why a difference in osmolar concentration of two solutions will cause osmosis of water through a selectively permeable membrane between the solutions.
6. What is meant by osmotic pressure, and how can it be determined for any given solution?
7. What is meant by osmolarity of fluids?
8. What is the quantitative relationship between the milliosmolar concentration of a solution and its osmotic pressure?
9. Explain the tremendous quantitative difference between the colloid osmotic pressure of plasma and the total osmotic pressure of the extracellular fluid. Why is the first of these important for osmotic effects at the capillary membrane, whereas the second is of importance for osmotic effects at the cell membrane?
10. What is meant by isotonicity, hypotonicity, and hypertonicity?
11. Explain overall control of the blood volume.
12. What is the relationship of the extracellular fluid volume to the blood volume?
13. Explain the antidiuretic hormone and thirst mechanisms for controlling the sodium concentration in the extracellular fluid.
14. Why does the sodium concentration in the extracellular fluid determine most of the osmolar concentration of the body fluids?
15. What is meant by the tripping mechanism of thirst control?
16. Explain the feedback mechanisms by which the body controls the extracellular potassium concentration. Why is aldosterone especially involved with potassium concentration control but not to a great extent with sodium concentration control?
17. Explain the overflow mechanism for control of extracellular fluid phosphate concentration.

References

Altura, B. M., and Altura, B. T.: Magnesium, electrolyte transport and coronary vascular tone. Drugs 28(Suppl.1):120, 1984.

Andersson, B., and Rundgren, M.: Thirst and its disorders. Annu Rev Med 33:231, 1982.

Angus, Z. S., et al.: PTH, calcitonin, cyclic nucleotides, and the kidney. Annu Rev Physiol 43:583, 1981.

Baer, P. G., and McGiff, J. C.: Hormonal systems and renal hemodynamics. Annu Rev Physiol 42:589, 1980.

Brownstein, M. J.: Biosynthesis of vasopressin and oxytocin. Annu Rev Physiol 45:129, 1983.

Buckalew, V. M., Jr., and Gruber, K. A.: Natriuretic hormone. Annu Rev Physiol 46:343, 1984.

Fanestil, D. D., and Park, C. S.: Steroid hormones and the kidney. Annu Rev Physiol 43:637, 1981.

Fregley, M. J., and Rowland, N. E.: Role of renin-angiotensin-aldosterone system in NaCl appetite of rats. Am J Physiol 248:R1, 1985.

Gibbons, G. H., et al.: Interaction of signals influencing renin release. Annu Rev Physiol 46:291, 1984.

Guyton, A. C., et al.: Theory for renal autoregulation by feedback at the juxtaglomerular apparatus. Circ Res 14:187, 1964.

Handler, J. S., and Orloff, J.: Antidiuretic hormone. Annu Rev Physiol 43:611, 1981.

Harrison, M. H.: Effects of thermal stress and exercise on blood volume in humans. Physiol Rev 65:149, 1985.

Menninger, R. P.: Current concepts of volume receptor regulation of vasopressin release. Fed Proc 44:55, 1985.

Miller, M.: Assessment of hormonal disorders of water metabolism. Clin Lab Med 4:729, 1984.

Navar, L. G., et al.: Distal tubular feedback control of renal hemodynamics and autoregulation. Annu Rev Physiol 42:557, 1980.

O'Connor, W. J.: Normal Renal Function. The Excretion of Water and Electrolytes Derived from Food and Drink. New York, Oxford University Press, 1982.

Sklar, A. H., and Schrier, R. W.: Central nervous system mediators of vasopressin release. Physiol Rev 63:1243, 1983.

Sutton, R. A.: Diuretics and calcium metabolism. Am J Kidney Dis 5:4, 1985.

Swanson, L. W., and Sawchenko, P. E.: Hypothalamic integration: Organization of the paraventricular and supraoptic nuclei. Annu Rev Neurosci 6:269, 1983.

Young, D. B., et al.: Effectiveness of the aldosterone-sodium and -potassium feedback control system. Am J Physiol 231:945, 1976.

Young, D. B., et al.: Control of extracellular sodium concentration by antidiuretic hormone-thirst feedback mechanism. Am J Physiol 232:R145, 1977.

Zerbe, R. et al.: Vasopressin function in the syndrome of inappropriate antidiuresis. Annu Rev Med 31:315, 1980.

26

Regulation of
Acid-Base Balance;
Renal Disease;
and Micturition

DEFENSE AGAINST CHANGES IN
    HYDROGEN ION
    CONCENTRATION
FUNCTION OF ACID-BASE BUFFERS
RESPIRATORY REGULATION OF
    ACID-BASE BALANCE
    RENAL REGULATION OF HYDROGEN
        ION CONCENTRATION
    RENAL REGULATION OF PLASMA
        CHLORIDE CONCENTRATION—THE
        CHLORIDE TO BICARBONATE
        RATIO

CLINICAL ABNORMALITIES OF
    ACID-BASE BALANCE
RENAL DISEASE
    RENAL FAILURE
    THE NEPHROTIC SYNDROME—
        INCREASED GLOMERULAR
        PERMEABILITY
MICTURITION
    THE MICTURITION REFLEX

When one speaks of the regulation of acid-base balance, he actually means regulation of hydrogen ion concentration in the body fluids. The hydrogen ion concentration in different solutions can vary from less than 10^{-14} equivalents per liter to higher than 10^0, which means a total variation of more than a quadrillionfold.

Merely slight changes in hydrogen ion concentration from the normal value can cause marked alterations in the rates of chemical reactions in the cells, some being depressed and others accelerated. For this reason, the regulation of hydrogen ion concentration is one of the most important aspects of homeostasis.

Normal Hydrogen Ion Concentration and Normal pH of the Body Fluids—Acidosis and Alkalosis. The hydrogen concentration in the extracellular fluid is normally regulated at a constant value of approximately 4×10^{-8} Eq/liter; this value can vary from as low as 1.0×10^{-8} to as high as 1.0×10^{-7} without causing death.

From these values, it is already apparent that expressing hydrogen ion concentration in terms of actual concentrations is a cumbersome procedure.

Therefore, the symbol *pH* has come into use for expressing the concentration; pH is related to actual hydrogen ion concentration by the following formula (when H^+ concentration is expressed in equivalents per liter):

$$pH = \log \frac{1}{H^+ \text{ conc.}} = -\log H^+ \text{ conc.} \quad (1)$$

Note from this formula that a low pH corresponds to a high hydrogen ion concentration, which is called *acidosis*; and, conversely, a high pH corresponds to a low hydrogen ion concentration, which is called *alkalosis*.

The normal pH of arterial blood is 7.4, and the pH of venous blood and of interstitial fluids is about 7.35 because of extra quantities of carbon dioxide that form carbonic acid in these fluids.

Since the normal pH of the arterial blood is 7.4, a person is considered to have acidosis whenever the pH is below this value and to have alkalosis when it rises above 7.4. The lowest limit at which a person can live more than a few hours is about 7.0, and the highest limit approximately 8.0.

279

DEFENSE AGAINST CHANGES IN HYDROGEN ION CONCENTRATION

To prevent acidosis or alkalosis, three principal control systems are available: (1) All the body fluids are supplied with acid-base *buffer systems* that immediately combine with any acid or alkali to prevent excessive changes in hydrogen ion concentration. (2) If the hydrogen ion concentration does change measurably, the *respiratory center is immediately stimulated* to alter the rate of breathing. This changes the rate of carbon dioxide removal from the body fluids, which, for reasons that will be presented later, causes the hydrogen ion concentration to return toward normal. (3) When the hydrogen concentration changes from normal, *the kidneys excrete either an acid or an alkaline urine,* thereby also helping to readjust the hydrogen ion concentration of the body fluids back toward normal.

The buffer systems can act within a fraction of a second to prevent excessive changes in hydrogen ion concentration. On the other hand, it takes 3 to 12 minutes for the respiratory system to function fully to readjust the hydrogen ion concentration after a sudden change has occurred. Finally, the kidneys, though providing the most powerful of all the acid-base regulatory systems, require several hours to several days to readjust fully the hydrogen ion concentration.

FUNCTION OF ACID-BASE BUFFERS

An acid-base buffer is a solution containing a combination of two or more chemical compounds that prevent marked changes in hydrogen ion concentration when either an acid or a base is added to the solution. An *acid* is defined as a substance that can contribute hydrogen ions to a solution. A *base* is defined as a substance that will combine with hydrogen ions in a solution and will thereby remove them. The alkaline chemicals are types of bases, which gives rise to the term *alkalosis,* a state in which there are too few hydrogen ions in the body fluids.

If only a few drops of concentrated hydrochloric acid are added to a beaker of pure water, the pH of the water might immediately fall to as low as 1.0. However, if a satisfactory buffer system is present, the hydrochloric acid combines instantaneously with the buffer, and the pH falls only slightly. Perhaps the best way to explain the action of an acid-base buffer is to consider an actual simple buffer system, such as the bicarbonate buffer, which is extremely important in regulation of acid-base balance in the body.

The Bicarbonate Buffer System. A typical bicarbonate buffer system consists of a *mixture* of carbonic acid (H_2CO_3) and sodium bicarbonate ($NaHCO_3$) in the same solution. It must first be noted that carbonic acid is a very weak acid.

When a strong acid, such as hydrochloric acid, is added to a bicarbonate buffer, the following reaction takes place:

$$HCl + NaHCO_3 \rightarrow H_2CO_3 + NaCl \qquad (2)$$

From this equation it can be seen that the strong hydrochloric acid is converted into the very weak carbonic acid. Therefore, the HCl lowers the pH of the solution only slightly.

On the other hand, if a strong base, such as sodium hydroxide, is added to the same bicarbonate buffer solution, the following reaction takes place:

$$NaOH + H_2CO_3 \rightarrow NaHCO_3 + H_2O \qquad (3)$$

This equation shows that the hydroxyl ion of the sodium hydroxide combines with a hydrogen ion from the carbonic acid to form water and that the other product formed is sodium bicarbonate. The net result is exchange of the strong base NaOH for the very weak base $NaHCO_3$.

Thus, the mixture of carbonic acid and sodium bicarbonate act as a buffer to prevent either a marked rise or fall in pH. Fortunately, this buffer is present in all the fluids of the body, both extracellular and intracellular, and it plays an important role in maintaining normal acid-base balance.

Relationship of Bicarbonate and Carbon Dioxide Concentrations to pH—the Henderson-Hasselbalch Equation. There is always a definite mathematical relationship between the ratio of the concentrations of the acidic and basic elements of each buffer system on the one hand and the pH of the solution on the other hand. The following equation, called the *Henderson-Hasselbalch equation,* gives this relationship for the bicarbonate buffer system:

$$pH = 6.1 + \log \frac{HCO_3^-}{CO_2} \qquad (4)$$

In this equation, the carbon dioxide concentration represents the acidic element—because carbon dioxide (CO_2) combines with water to form carbonic acid, H_2CO_3—and the bicarbonate ion (HCO_3^-) represents the basic element. Note that the pH changes in direct proportion to the change in the *logarithm of the ratio* between the basic and acid elements of the buffer system. Thus, when the ratio is in favor of the basic element (HCO_3^-), the pH increases, denoting alkalosis. When the ratio is in favor of the acidic element (CO_2), the pH decreases, denoting acidosis.

The Phosphate Buffer System. Another buffer system, the phosphate buffer system, acts in almost the same manner as the bicarbonate buffer system, but it is composed of the following combination: NaH_2PO_4, which is the acidic component because of the two hydrogen atoms, and Na_2HPO_4, which is the basic component because of the two sodium atoms. This system is especially important in the tubular fluids of the kidneys because phosphate usually becomes greatly concentrated in the tubules. The phosphate buffer is also very important in the intracellular fluids because the concentration of phosphate in these fluids is many times that in the extracellular fluids.

The Protein Buffer System. By far the most plentiful buffer in the body is the protein of the cells and plasma consisting of the following combination: H-protein and Na-protein, which are a weak acid and a weak base respectively. There is a slight amount of diffusion of hydrogen ions through the cell membrane; even more important, carbon dioxide can diffuse readily through cell membranes, and bicarbonate ions can diffuse to some extent (they require several hours to come to equilibrium in most cells other than the red blood cells). The diffusion of these causes the pH in the intracellular fluids to change approximately in proportion to the changes in pH in the extracellular fluids. Therefore, all the buffer systems inside the cells help to buffer the extracellular fluids as well. Indeed, experimental studies have shown that about three quarters of all the buffering power of the body fluids is inside the cells and most of this results from the intracellular proteins. However, except for the red blood cells, the slowness of movement of hydrogen and bicarbonate ions through the cell membranes often delays the ability of the intracellular buffers to buffer extracellular acid-base abnormalities for several hours.

RESPIRATORY REGULATION OF ACID-BASE BALANCE

Because carbon dioxide combines with water to form carbonic acid, an *increase in carbon dioxide* concentration in the body fluids *decreases the pH* toward the acidic side, whereas a decrease in carbon dioxide raises the pH toward the alkaline side. It is on the basis of this effect that the respiratory system is capable of altering the pH either up or down.

Balance Between Metabolic Formation of Carbon Dioxide and Pulmonary Expiration of Carbon Dioxide. Carbon dioxide is continually being formed in the body by the different intracellular metabolic processes, the carbon in the foods being oxidized by oxygen to form carbon dioxide. This in turn diffuses into the interstitial fluids and blood and is transported to the lungs, where it diffuses into the alveoli and is transferred to the atmosphere by pulmonary ventilation. However, several minutes are required for this passage of carbon dioxide from the cells to the atmosphere, so that an average of 1.2 millimoles/liter of dissolved carbon dioxide is normally in the extracellular fluids at all times.

If the rate of metabolic formation of carbon dioxide becomes increased, its concentration and also the hydrogen ion concentration in the extracellular fluids is increased. Conversely, decreased metabolism decreases the carbon dioxide and hydrogen ion concentrations.

On the other hand, if the rate of pulmonary ventilation is increased, the rate of expiration of carbon dioxide becomes increased, and this decreases both the amount of accumulated carbon dioxide and the hydrogen ion concentration in the extracellular fluids.

Effect of Hydrogen Ion Concentration to Control Alveolar Ventilation. Not only does the rate of alveolar ventilation affect the hydrogen ion concentration of the body fluids, but, in turn, the hydrogen ion concentration controls the rate of alveolar ventilation. This results from a *direct action of hydrogen ions on the respiratory center in the medulla oblongata,* which controls breathing, discussed in detail in Chapter 29.

Figure 26–1 illustrates the changes in alveolar ventilation caused by changing the pH of arterial blood from 7.0 to 7.6. From this graph it is evident that a decrease in pH from the normal value of 7.4 to the strongly acidic range can increase the rate of alveolar ventilation to as much as four to five times normal, while an increase in pH into the alkaline range can decrease the rate of alveolar ventilation to as little as 50 to 75 per cent of normal.

Feedback Regulation of Hydrogen Ion Concentration by the Respiratory System. Because of the ability of the respiratory center to respond to hydrogen ion

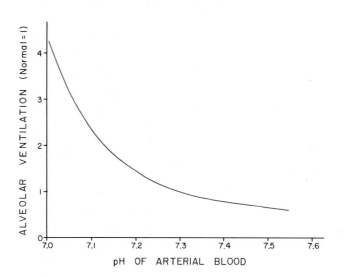

Figure 26–1. Effect of blood pH on the rate of alveolar ventilation. (Constructed from data obtained by Gray: Pulmonary Ventilation and its Regulation. Courtesy of Charles C Thomas, Publisher, Springfield, Illinois.)

concentration, and because changes in alveolar ventilation in turn alter the hydrogen ion concentration in the body fluids, the respiratory system acts as a typical feedback regulatory system for controlling hydrogen ion concentration. That is, when the hydrogen ion concentration becomes high, the respiratory system becomes more active, and alveolar ventilation increases. As a result the carbon dioxide concentration in the extracellular fluids decreases, thus reducing the hydrogen concentration back toward a normal value. Conversely, if the hydrogen ion concentration falls too low, the respiratory center becomes depressed, alveolar ventilation also decreases, and the carbon dioxide and hydrogen ion concentrations rise back toward normal.

Effectiveness of Respiratory Regulation of Hydrogen Ion Concentration. Unfortunately, respiratory control cannot return the hydrogen ion concentration all the way to the normal value of 7.4 when some abnormality outside the respiratory system has altered the pH. The reason is that as the pH returns toward normal the stimulus, the abnormal pH that has been causing either increased or decreased respiration, will itself begin to be lost. Ordinarily the respiratory mechanism for regulation of hydrogen ion concentration has a control effectiveness of between 50 and 75 per cent. That is, if the hydrogen ion concentration should suddenly be decreased from 7.4 to 7.0 by some extraneous factor, the respiratory system, in 3 to 12 minutes, returns the pH to a value of about 7.2 to 7.3.

RENAL REGULATION OF HYDROGEN ION CONCENTRATION

The kidneys regulate hydrogen ion concentration principally by increasing or decreasing the bicarbonate ion concentration in the body fluid. To do this, a complex series of reactions occurs in the renal tubules, as described in the following sections.

Tubular Secretion of Hydrogen Ions. The epithelial cells of the proximal tubules, ascending limbs of the loop of Henle, distal tubules, collecting tubules, and collecting ducts all secrete hydrogen ions into the tubular fluid. The mechanism by which this occurs is illustrated in Figure 26–2. The secretory process *begins with carbon dioxide* in the tubular epithelial cells. The carbon dioxide, under the influence of an enzyme, *carbonic anhydrase*, combines with water inside the cells to form carbonic acid, which then dissociates into *bicarbonate ions*, and *hydrogen ions*. Finally, the hydrogen ions are secreted by the mechanism of Na^+-H^+ *countertransport*. That is, as sodium moves from the lumen of the tubule to the interior of the cell, it combines with a *carrier protein* in the luminal border of the cell membrane, and at the same time a hydrogen ion inside the cell combines with the opposite side of the same carrier protein. Then, because the concentration of sodium is much lower inside the cell than in the tubular lumen, this causes movement of the sodium down the concentration

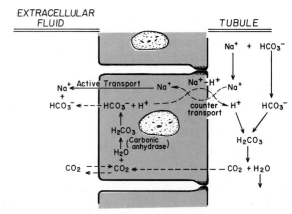

Figure 26–2. Chemical reactions for (1) hydrogen ion secretion, (2) sodium ion absorption in exchange for a hydrogen ion, and (3) combination of hydrogen ions with bicarbonate ions in the tubules.

gradient to the interior, providing at the same time the energy for moving the hydrogen ion in the opposite direction (the counter direction) into the tubular lumen. This process can transport the hydrogen ions against their concentration gradient.

In the collecting ducts hydrogen ion secretion can continue until the concentration of hydrogen ions in the tubules becomes as much as 900 times that in the extracellular fluid or, in other words, until the pH of the tubular fluids falls to about 4.5. This represents a limit to the ability of the tubular epithelium to secrete hydrogen ions.

About 84 per cent of all the hydrogen ions secreted by the tubules are secreted in the proximal tubules, but the maximum concentration gradient that can be achieved here is only about 3- to 4-fold instead of the 900-fold that can be achieved in the collecting ducts.

Regulation of Hydrogen Ion Secretion by the Carbon Dioxide Concentration in the Extracellular Fluid. Since the chemical reactions for secretion of hydrogen ions begin with carbon dioxide, the greater the carbon dioxide concentration in the extracellular fluid, the more rapidly the reactions proceed and the greater becomes the rate of hydrogen ion secretion. Therefore, any factor that increases the carbon dioxide concentration in the extracellular fluids also increases the rate of hydrogen ion secretion.

Interaction of Bicarbonate Ions with Hydrogen Ions in the Tubules—Reabsorption of Bicarbonate Ions. The renal tubules are not very permeable to the bicarbonate ion because it is a large ion and also is electrically charged. However, the bicarbonate ion can, in effect, be reabsorbed by a special process, which is illustrated in Figure 26–2.

The reabsorption of bicarbonate ions is initiated by a reaction in the tubules between the bicarbonate ions and the hydrogen ions secreted by the tubular cells, as illustrated in the figure. This reaction causes the formation of carbonic acid, which then dissociates into carbon dioxide and water. The water becomes part of the tubular fluid, while the carbon dioxide, having the capability to diffuse extremely readily through the cellular membranes, instantaneously diffuses into epithelial cells or even all the way into the blood and is expired in the usual way by the lungs. *If an excess of hydrogen ions is secreted by the tubules, the bicarbonate ions will be almost completely removed from the tubules,* so that for practical purposes *none* will remain to pass into the urine.

If we now note in Figure 26–2 the chemical reactions that are responsible for formation of hydrogen ions in the epithelial cells, we see that each time a hydrogen ion is formed and secreted into the tubule, a bicarbonate ion is formed at the same time by the dissociation of H_2CO_3. The bicarbonate ion then enters the extracellular fluid.

The net effect of all these reactions is a mechanism for reabsorption of bicarbonate ions from the tubules, though the bicarbonate ions that enter the extracellular fluid are not the same bicarbonate ions that are removed from the tubular fluid.

Normal Rates of Bicarbonate Ion Filtration and Hydrogen Ion Secretion into the Tubules—"Titration" of Bicarbonate Ions Against Hydrogen Ions. Under normal conditions, the rate of hydrogen ion secretion is about 3.50 millimoles/minute, and the rate of filtration of bicarbonate ions in the glomerular filtrate is about 3.49 millimoles/minute. Thus, the quantities of the two ions entering the tubules are almost equal, and they combine with each other and actually annihilate each other, the end-products being carbon dioxide and water. Therefore, it is said that the bicarbonate ions and hydrogen ions normally "titrate" each other in the tubules.

However, note also that this titration process is not quite exact, for usually a slight excess of hydrogen ions (the acidic component) remains in the tubules to be excreted in the urine. The reason is that under normal conditions a person's metabolic processes continually form a small amount of excess acid that gives rise to the slight excess of hydrogen ions over bicarbonate ions in the tubules.

On rare occasions the bicarbonate ions are in excess, as we shall see in subsequent discussions. When this circumstance occurs, the titration process again is not quite complete; this time, excess bicarbonate ions (the basic component) are left in the tubules to pass into the urine.

Thus, the basic mechanism by which the kidney corrects either acidosis or alkalosis is incomplete titration of hydrogen ions against bicarbonate ions, leaving one or the other of these to pass into the urine and therefore to be removed from the extracellular fluid.

Renal Correction of Alkalosis—Decrease in Bicarbonate Ions in the Extracellular Fluid

Now that we have described the mechanisms by which the renal tubules secrete hydrogen ions and reabsorb bicarbonate ions, we can explain the manner in which the kidneys readjust the pH of the extracellular fluids when it becomes abnormal.

The initial step in this explanation is to understand what happens to the concentrations of carbon dioxide and bicarbonate ions in the extracellular fluids in alkalosis and acidosis. First, let us consider *alkalosis*. The *ratio* of bicarbonate ions to dissolved carbon dioxide molecules increases when the pH rises into the alkalosis range above 7.4. The effect of this on the titration process in the tubules is also to increase the *ratio* of bicarbonate ions filtered into the tubules to the hydrogen ions secreted. This increase occurs because the high extracellular bicarbonate ion concentration increases its filtration in the glomerular filtrate, and the low carbon dioxide concentration decreases the secretion of hydrogen ions. Therefore, the fine balance that normally exists in the tubules between the hydrogen and bicarbonate ions no longer occurs. Instead, far greater quantities of bicarbonate ions than hydrogen ions now enter the tubules. Since no bicarbonate ions can be reabsorbed without first reacting with hydrogen ions, all the excess bicarbonate ions pass into the urine and carry with them sodium ions or other positive ions. Thus, in effect, sodium bicarbonate is removed from the extracellular fluid.

Loss of sodium bicarbonate from the extracellular fluid decreases the bicarbonate ion portion of the bicarbonate buffer system, and this shifts the pH of the body fluids back in the acid direction. Thus the alkalosis is corrected.

Renal Correction of Acidosis—Increase in Bicarbonate Ions in the Extracellular Fluid

In acidosis the *ratio* of carbon dioxide to bicarbonate ions in the extracellular fluid increases, which is exactly opposite to the effect in alkalosis. Therefore, in acidosis, the *rate of hydrogen ion secretion* rises to a level far greater than the *rate of bicarbonate ion filtration* into the tubules. As a result, a great excess of hydrogen ions is secreted into the tubules, and they have far too few bicarbonate ions to react with. These excess hydrogen ions combine with the buffers in the tubular fluid, as explained in the following paragraphs, and are excreted into the urine.

Hydrogen ions are thus lost from the extracellular fluid. At the same time, an excess of bicarbonate ions enters this fluid and combines with sodium to form the weak base $NaHCO_3$. The net result is correction of the acidosis.

Transport of Excess Tubular Hydrogen Ions into the Urine by the Phosphate Buffer. The phosphate buffer is composed of a mixture of Na_2HPO_4 and NaH_2PO_4. Both become more concentrated in the tubular fluid than in the plasma because of their relatively poor reabsorption and because of removal of water from the tubular fluid. Therefore, even though the phosphate buffer is very weak in the blood, it is a much more powerful buffer in the tubular fluid and is responsible for transporting a major share of excess hydrogen ions into the urine.

Excess hydrogen ions entering the tubules combine with the Na_2HPO_4 to form NaH_2PO_4 plus a sodium ion. The NaH_2PO_4 passes on into the urine, while the sodium ion is absorbed into the extracellular fluid in place of the hydrogen ion, and at the same time a *bicarbonate ion,* formed in the process of secreting the hydrogen ion, is also released into the extracellular fluid. Thus, the net effect of this reaction is to increase the amount of sodium bicarbonate in the extracellular fluids, which is the kidney's way of reducing the degree of acidosis in the body fluids.

Transport of Excess Hydrogen Ions into the Urine by the Tubular Ammonia Buffer System. Another very potent buffer system of the tubular fluid is composed of ammonia (NH_3) and the ammonium ion (NH_4^+). The epithelial cells of all the tubules besides those of the thin segment of the loop of Henle continually synthesize ammonia, which diffuses into the tubules. The ammonia then reacts with hydrogen ions, as illustrated in Figure 26–3, to form ammonium ions. These are then excreted into the urine in combination with chloride ions and other tubular anions. Note in the figure that the net effect of these reactions, again, is *to increase the sodium bicarbonate concentration* in the extracellular fluid.

This ammonium ion mechanism for transport of excess hydrogen ions in the tubules is especially important for two reasons: (1) Each time an ammonia molecule combines with a hydrogen ion to form an ammonium ion, the concentration of ammonia in the tubular fluid decreases, which has an automatic effect on the tubular epithelial cells, causing them to secrete still more ammonia. Thus, the rate of ammonia secretion into the tubular fluid is actually controlled by the amount of excess hydrogen ions to be transported. (2) Most of the negative ions of the tubular fluid are chloride ions. Only a few hydrogen ions can be transported into the urine in direct combination with chloride, because hydrochloric acid is a very strong acid and the tubular pH would otherwise fall rapidly below the critical value of 4.5, so that further hydrogen ion secretion would cease. However, when hydrogen ions combine with ammonia and the resulting ammonium ions then combine with chloride, the pH does not fall significantly because ammonium chloride is only very weakly acidic. Therefore, this ammonia buffer system allows the tubules to secrete many times the hydrogen ions that would otherwise be possible and also enhances manyfold the ability of the kidneys to correct acidosis in the body fluids.

Rapidity of Acid-Base Regulation by the Kidneys

The total amount of buffers in the entire body (within the range of pH 7.0 to 7.8) is approximately 1000 millimoles. If all of them should be suddenly shifted to the alkaline or acidic side by the injection of an alkali or an acid, the kidneys would be able to return the pH of the body fluids back almost to normal in one to three days. Though this mechanism is slow to act, it continues acting until the pH returns almost exactly to normal rather than a certain percentage of the way. Therefore, the real value of the renal mechanism for regulating hydrogen ion concentration is not rapidity of action but instead its ability in the end to neutralize completely any excess acid or alkali that enters the body fluids, unless the excess continues to enter.

Ordinary, the kidneys can remove up to about 500 millimoles of acid or alkali each day. If greater quantities than this enter the body fluids, the kidneys are unable to cope with the extra load, and severe and lethal acidosis or alkalosis ensues.

Range of Urinary pH. In the process of adjusting the hydrogen ion concentration of the extracellular fluid, the kidneys often excrete urine at a pH as low as 4.5 or as high as 8.0. When acid is being excreted the pH falls, and when alkali is being excreted the pH rises. Even when the pH of the arterial blood is at the normal value of 7.4, a fraction of a millimole of acid is still lost each minute. The reason is that about 50 to 80 millimoles more acid than alkali are formed in the body each day, and this acid must be removed continually. Because of the presence of this excess acid in the urine, the normal urine pH is about 6.0 instead of 7.4, the pH of the blood.

RENAL REGULATION OF PLASMA CHLORIDE CONCENTRATION—THE CHLORIDE TO BICARBONATE RATIO

In the above discussions we have emphasized the ability of the kidneys to increase bicarbonate ion in the extracellular fluid whenever a state of acidosis develops, or to remove bicarbonate ions in a state of alkalosis. Thus, the bicarbonate ion is shuttled back and forth between high and low values as one of the principal means of adjusting the acid-base balance of the extracellular buffer systems and therefore also for adjusting the extracellular fluid pH.

However, in the process of juggling the extracellular fluid concentration of bicarbonate ion, it is essential to remove some other anion from the extracellular fluids each time the bicarbonate is increased, or to increase some other anion when the bicarbonate concentration is decreased. In general, the anion that is reciprocally juggled up or down with the bicarbo-

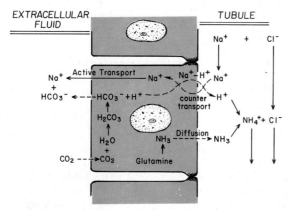

Figure 26–3. Secretion of ammonia by the tubular epithelial cells, and reaction of the ammonia with hydrogen ions in the tubules.

nate ion is the chloride ion because this is the anion in greatest concentration in the extracellular fluid.

Function of the Ammonia Buffer System in Controlling the Bicarbonate Ion to Chloride Ion Ratio. It was pointed out above that the ammonia buffer system plays an extremely important role in removing excess hydrogen ions from the tubules. Now, let us study Figure 26–3 once again. We see that in the process of transporting excess hydrogen ions into the urine in combination with ammonia, for each hydrogen ion transported a chloride ion also passes into the urine as NH_4Cl, and a bicarbonate ion simultaneously enters the extracellular fluid. Consequently, this ammonia system substitutes a bicarbonate ion in the extracellular fluid for a chloride ion that is lost from the extracellular fluids. Conversely, when a person is alkalotic, the ammonia system becomes inoperative; bicarbonate ions instead of chloride ions then pass into the urine, and a concomitant excess of chloride is reabsorbed.

Thus, in the process of controlling the pH of the body fluids, the renal acid-base regulating system also regulates the ratio of chloride ions to bicarbonate ions in the extracelluar fluid.

CLINICAL ABNORMALITIES OF ACID-BASE BALANCE

Respiratory Acidosis and Alkalosis

From the discussions earlier in the chapter it is obvious that any factor that decreases the rate of pulmonary ventilation increases the concentration of dissolved carbon dioxide in the extracellular fluid, which in turn leads to increased carbonic acid and hydrogen ions, thus resulting in acidosis. Because this type of acidosis is caused by an abnormality of respiration, it is called *respiratory acidosis.*

On the other hand, excessive pulmonary ventilation reverses the process and decreases the hydrogen ion concentration, thus resulting in alkalosis; this condition is called *respiratory alkalosis.*

A person can cause respiratory acidosis in himself by simply holding his breath, which he can do until the pH of the body fluids falls to as low as perhaps 7.0. On the other hand, he can voluntarily overbreathe and cause alkalosis to a pH of about 7.9.

Respiratory acidosis frequently results from pathological conditions. For instance, damage to the respiratory center in the medulla oblongata that causes reduced breathing, obstruction of the passageways in the respiratory tract, pneumonia, decreased pulmonary membrane surface area, and any other factor that interferes with the exchange of gases between the blood and alveolar air, results in respiratory acidosis.

On the other hand, only rarely do pathological conditions cause *respiratory alkalosis.* However, occasionally a psychoneurosis causes overbreathing to the extent that a person becomes alkalotic. A physiological type of respiratory alkalosis occurs when a person ascends to a *high altitude.* The low oxygen content of the air stimulates respiration, which causes excess loss of carbon dioxide and development of mild respiratory alkalosis.

Metabolic Acidosis and Alkalosis

The terms *metabolic acidosis* and *metabolic alkalosis* refer to all other abnormalities of acid-base balance besides those caused by excess or insufficient carbon dioxide in the body fluids. Use of the word "metabolic" in this instance is unfortunate, because carbon dioxide is also a metabolic product. Yet, by convention, carbonic acid resulting from dissolved carbon dioxide is called a *respiratory acid,* while any other acid in the body, whether it be formed by metabolism or simply ingested by the person, is called a *metabolic acid,* or a *fixed acid.*

Causes of Metabolic Acidosis

Diarrhea. Severe diarrhea is one of the most frequent causes of metabolic acidosis for the following reasons: The gastrointestinal secretions normally contain large amounts of sodium bicarbonate. Therefore, excessive loss of these secretions during a bout of diarrhea is exactly the same as excretion of large amounts of sodium bicarbonate into the urine. This causes a shift of the bicarbonate buffer system toward the acid side and results in metabolic acidosis. In fact, acidosis resulting from severe diarrhea can be so serious that it is one of the most common causes of death in young children.

Uremia. A second type of acidosis is uremic acidosis, which occurs in severe renal disease. The cause is failure of the kidneys to rid the body of even the normal amounts of acid formed each day by the metabolic processes of the body.

Diabetes Mellitus. A third and extremely important cause of metabolic acidosis is diabetes mellitus. In this condition, lack of insulin secretion by the pancreas prevents normal use of glucose for metabolism. Instead, fat is split into acetoacetic acid, which in turn is metabolized by the tissues for energy in place of glucose. Simultaneously, the concentration of acetoacetic acid in the extracellular fluids often rises very high, causing acidosis, and large quantities of it are excreted in the urine, sometimes as much as 500 to 1000 millimoles per day.

Causes of Metabolic Alkalosis. Metabolic alkalosis does not occur nearly as often as metabolic acidosis. However, there are several common causes of metabolic alkalosis, as follows:

Excessive Ingestion of Alkaline Drugs. One of the most common causes of alkalosis is excessive ingestion of alkaline drugs, such as sodium bicarbonate, for the treatment of gastritis or peptic ulcer.

Alkalosis Caused by Loss of Chloride Ions. Excessive vomiting of gastric contents without vomiting of lower gastrointestinal contents causes excessive loss of hydrochloric acid secreted by the stomach mucosa. This loss leads to reduction of chloride ions and enhancement of bicarbonate ions in the extracellular fluid. The bicarbonate ions are derived from the stomach glandular cells that secrete the hydrogen ions; these form bicarbonate ion in the same way that the tubular cells do when they secrete hydrogen ions. The net result is loss of acid from the extracellular fluids and development of metabolic alkalosis.

Alkalosis Caused by Excess Aldosterone. When excess quantities of aldosterone are secreted by the adrenal glands, the extracellular fluid becomes slightly alkalotic. This is caused in the following way: the aldosterone promotes extensive reabsorption of sodium ions from the distal segments of the tubular system, but coupled with this is increased secretion of hydrogen ions and loss from the extracellular fluids, thus promoting alkalosis.

Effects of Acidosis and Alkalosis on the Body

Acidosis. The major effect of acidosis is depression of the *central nervous system*. When the pH of the blood falls below 7.0, the nervous system becomes so depressed that the person first becomes disoriented and later comatose. Therefore, patients dying of diabetic acidosis, uremic acidosis, and other types of acidosis usually die in a state of coma.

In metabolic acidosis the high hydrogen ion concentration causes increased rate and depth of respiration. Therefore, one of the diagnostic signs of *metabolic* acidosis is increased pulmonary ventilation. On the other hand, *in respiratory acidosis, respiration is usually depressed* because this is the cause of the acidosis, which is opposite to the effect in metabolic acidosis.

Alkalosis. The major effect of alkalosis on the body is *overexcitability of the nervous system*. This occurs both in the central nervous system and in the peripheral nerves, but usually the peripheral nerves are affected before the central nervous system. The nerves often become so excitable that they automatically and repetitively fire even when they are not stimulated by normal stimuli. As a result, the muscles go into a state of *tetany*, which means a state of tonic spasm. This tetany usually appears first in the muscles of the forearm and then spreads rapidly to the muscles of the face and finally all over the body. Extremely alkalotic patients may die from tetany of the respiratory muscles.

Occasionally an alkalotic person develops severe symptoms of central nervous system overexcitability. The symptoms may manifest themselves as extreme nervousness or, in susceptible persons, as convulsions. For instance, in persons who are predisposed to epileptic fits, simply over-breathing often results in an attack. Indeed, this is one of the clinical methods for assessing one's degree of epileptic predisposition.

Physiology of Treatment in Acidosis or Alkalosis

Obviously, the best treatment for acidosis or alkalosis is to remove the condition causing the abnormality, but, if this cannot be effected, different drugs can be used to neutralize the excess acid or alkali.

To neutralize excess acid, large amounts of sodium bicarbonate can be ingested by mouth. It is absorbed into the blood and increases the bicarbonate ion portion of the bicarbonate buffer, thereby shifting the pH to the alkaline side.

For treatment of alkalosis, ammonium chloride is often administered by mouth. When it is absorbed into the blood, the ammonia portion of the ammonium chloride is converted by the liver into urea; this reaction liberates hydrochloric acid, which immediately reacts with the buffers of the body fluids to shift the hydrogen ion concentration in the acid direction.

RENAL DISEASE

It will not be possible to discuss here the great numbers of kidney diseases. However, especially important are (1) renal failure and (2) the nephrotic syndrome.

RENAL FAILURE

Renal Failure Caused by Acute Glomerular Nephritis. Acute glomerular nephritis is a disease that results from an antigen-antibody reaction in which the glomeruli become markedly inflamed. Large numbers of white blood cells collect in the inflamed glomeruli, and the endothelial cells on the vascular side of the glomerular membrane, as well as the epithelial cells on the Bowman's capsule side of the membrane, proliferate, sometimes completely filling the glomeruli and the capsule. These inflammatory reactions can cause total or partial blockage of large numbers of glomeruli, and many of those glomeruli that are not blocked develop greatly increased permeability of the glomerular membrane, allowing large amounts of protein to leak into the glomerular filtrate. Also, rupture of the membrane in severe cases often allows large numbers of red blood cells to pass into the glomerular filtrate. In the severest cases total renal shutdown occurs.

The inflammation of acute glomerular nephritis almost invariably occurs one to three weeks following, elsewhere in the body, an infection caused by certain types of group A beta streptococci, such infections as a streptococcal sore throat, streptococcal tonsillitis, scarlet fever, or even streptococcal infection of the skin. The infection itself does not cause damage to the kidneys, but when antibodies develop against the streptococcal antigen, the antibodies and antigen react with each other to form a precipitate that becomes entrapped in the middle of the glomerular membrane. The reactivity of this precipitated complex leads to inflammation of the glomeruli.

The acute inflammation of the glomeruli most often subsides in ten days to two weeks, and the nephrons may return to normal function. Sometimes, however, the inflammatory reactions are so severe that many of the glomeruli are destroyed permanently.

Chronic Glomerulonephritis. Chronic glomerulonephritis is caused by any one of several different diseases that damage principally the glomeruli. The basic glomerular lesion is usually very similar to that which occurs in acute glomerulonephritis. It normally begins with accumulation of precipitated antigen-antibody complex in the glomerular membrane followed by inflammation of the glomeruli. The glomerular membrane becomes progressively thickened and is eventually invaded by fibrous tissue. In the later stages of the disease, glomerular filtration becomes greatly reduced because of decreased numbers of filtering capillaries in the glomerular tufts and because of thickened glomerular membranes. In the final stages of the disease many of the glomeruli are completely replaced by fibrous tissue, and the function of these nephrons is thereafter lost.

Pyelonephritis. Pyelonephritis is an infectious and inflammatory process that usually begins in the renal pelvis but extends progressively into the renal parenchyma. The infection can result from many different types of bacteria but especially from the colon bacillus that originates from fecal contamination of the urinary tract. Invasion of the kidneys by these bacteria results in progressive destruction of renal tubules, glomeruli, and any other structures in the path of the invading organisms. Consequently, large portions of the functional renal tissue are lost.

A particularly interesting feature of pyelonephritis is that the invading infection usually affects the medulla of the kidney before it affects the cortex. Since one of the primary functions of the medulla is to provide the countercurrent mechanism for concentrating the urine, patients with pyelonephritis frequently have reasonably normal renal function except for inability to concentrate their urine.

Abnormal Excretory Function in Renal Failure

The most important effect of renal failure is the inability of the kidneys to cope with large loads of urea, acids, or other substances that must be excreted. Normally, one half of the nephrons can eliminate essentially all the normal load of waste products from the body without serious accumulation of these in the body fluids. However, further reduction of numbers of nephrons leads to unwarranted urinary retention, and death ensues when the number of nephrons falls below 10 to 20 per cent of normal.

Effects of Renal Failure on the Body Fluids—Uremia

The effect of acute or chronic renal failure on the body fluids depends to a great extent on the water and food intake of the person. Assuming that the person continues to ingest moderate amounts of water and food, the concentration changes of different substances in the extracellular fluid are approximately those that follow acute renal shutdown, shown in

Figure 26–4. The most important effects are (1) *generalized edema* resulting from water and salt retention; (2) *acidosis* resulting from failure of the kidneys to rid the body of normal acidic products; (3) *high concentrations of the nonprotein nitrogens* (NPN), especially *urea*, resulting from failure of the body to excrete the metabolic end-products, and (4) *high concentration of other urinary retention products* including *creatinine, uric acid, phenols, guanidine bases, sulfates, phosphates,* and *potassium.* This condition is called *uremia* because of the high concentrations of normal urinary excretory products that collect in the body fluids.

Acidosis in Renal Failure. Each day the metabolic processes of the body normally produce 50 to 80 millimoles more metabolic acid than metabolic alkali. Therefore, any time the kidneys fail to function, acid begins to accumulate in the body fluids. Normally, the buffers of the fluids can buffer up to a total of 500 to 1000 millimoles of acid without severe depression of the extracellular fluid pH, but gradually this buffering power is used up, so that the pH eventually falls drastically. The patient becomes *comatose* at about this same time, and it is believed that this coma is mainly caused by the acidosis, as is discussed below.

Increase in Urea and Other Nonprotein Nitrogens in Uremia. The nonprotein nitrogens include urea, uric acid, creatinine, and a few less important compounds. These, in general, are the end-products of protein metabolism and must be removed from the body continually to insure continued protein metabolism in the cells. The concentrations of these, particularly of urea, can rise to as high as ten times normal during one to two weeks of renal failure. However, even these high levels do not seem to affect physiological function nearly so much as the high concentrations of hydrogen and potassium ions and some of the other less obvious substances, such as very toxic guanidine bases, ammonium ions, and others. Yet one of the most important means for assessing the degree of renal failure is to measure the concentration of the nonprotein nitrogens.

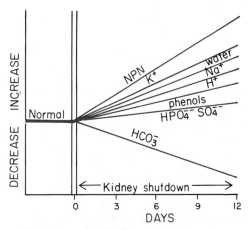

Figure 26–4. Effect of kidney shutdown on extracellular fluid constituents.

Uremic Coma. After a few days of complete renal failure the sensorium of the patient becomes clouded, and he soon progresses into a state of coma. Acidosis is one of the principal factors responsible for the coma; acidosis caused by other conditions, such as severe diabetes mellitus, also causes coma. However, many other abnormalities could also be contributory—the generalized edema, the high potassium concentration, and possibly even the high nonprotein nitrogen concentration.

Because of the effect of a low pH to stimulate the respiratory control center in the brain stem, the respiration usually is deep and rapid in coma, a characteristic that is a respiratory attempt to compensate for the metabolic acidosis. In addition, the arterial pressure falls progressively during the last day or so before death, then rapidly in the last few hours. Death occurs usually when the pH of the blood falls to about 6.9.

Dialysis of Uremic Patients with the Artificial Kidney

Artificial kidneys have now been used for about 35 years to treat patients with severe renal failure. They have been developed to such a point that many thousands of persons with permanent renal failure or even total kidney removal are being maintained in health for years at a time, their lives depending entirely on the artificial kidney.

The basic principle of the artificial kidney is to pass blood through very minute blood channels bounded by thin membranes. On the other sides of the membranes is a *dialyzing fluid* into which unwanted substances in the blood pass by diffusion.

Figure 26–5 illustrates diagrammatically an artificial kidney in which blood flows continually between two thin sheets of cellophane; on the outside of the sheets is the dialyzing fluid. The cellophane is porous enough to allow all constituents of the plasma except the plasma proteins to diffuse freely in both directions—from plasma into the dialyzing fluid and from the dialyzing fluid back into the plasma. If the concentration of a substance is greater in the plasma than in the dialyzing fluid, there is net transfer of the substance from the plasma into the dialyzing fluid. The amount of the substance that is transferred depends on (1) the difference between the concentrations on the two sides of the membrane, (2) molecular size, the smaller molecules diffusing more rapidly than larger ones, and (3) the length of time that the blood and the fluid remain in contact with the membrane.

In normal operation of the artificial kidney, blood continually flows from an artery, through the kidney, and back into a vein. The total amount of blood in the artificial kidney at any one time is usually less than 500 ml, the rate of flow may be several hundred ml per minute, and the total diffusing surface is usually between 10,000 and 20,000 square centimeters. To prevent coagulation of blood, a small amount

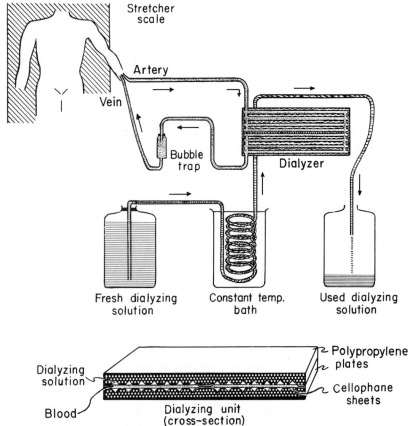

Figure 26–5. Principles of the artificial kidney.

of heparin is infused into the blood as it enters the artificial kidney.

The Dialyzing Fluid. Table 26–1 compares the constituents of a typical dialyzing fluid with those in normal plasma and uremic plasma. Note that sodium, potassium, and chloride concentrations in the dialyzing fluid and in normal plasma are identical, but in uremic plasma the potassium concentration is considerably greater. This ion diffuses through the dialyzing membrane so rapidly that its concentration falls to equal that in the dialyzing fluid within only three to four hours' exposure to the dialyzing fluid.

On the other hand, there is no phosphate, urea, urate, sulfate, or creatinine in the dialyzing fluid. Therefore, when the uremic patient is dialyzed, these substances are lost in large quantities into the dialyzing fluid, thereby removing major proportions of them from the plasma.

Therefore, the constituents of the dialyzing fluid are chosen so that those substances in excess in the extracellular fluid in uremia can be removed at rapid rates, while the normal electrolytes remain essentially normal.

THE NEPHROTIC SYNDROME—INCREASED GLOMERULAR PERMEABILITY

Large numbers of patients with renal disease develop a so-called *nephrotic syndrome*, which is characterized especially by *loss of large quantities of plasma proteins into the urine*. In some instances this loss occurs without evidence of any other abnormality of renal function, but more often it is associated with some degree of renal failure.

The cause of the protein loss in the urine is increased permeability of the glomerular membrane. Therefore, any disease condition that increases the permeability of this membrane can cause the nephrotic syndrome. Such diseases include some types of *chronic glomerulonephritis* (in the previous discus-

sion, it was noted that this disease primarily affects the glomeruli and causes a greatly increased permeability of the glomerular membrane), *amyloidosis*, which results from deposition of an abnormal proteinoid substance in the walls of blood vessels and seriously damages the basement membrane of the glomerulus, and *lipoid nephrosis*, a disease found mainly in young children.

Lipoid Nephrosis. Lipoid nephrosis deserves special comment because it is very common in children, occurring most often before the age of four but occasionally in adults as well. Its basic cause is unknown, but the resulting renal lesion increases the permeability of the glomerular membrane and causes massive loss of proteins into the urine. This lesion develops in the following way: The epithelial cells that line the outer surface of the glomerulus are defective. They are greatly swollen, and they fail to form the usual foot processes that cover the Bowman's capsule surface of the glomerulus. It will be recalled from the discussion of the glomerular membrane in Chapter 24 that the openings between these foot processes are very small, and this smallness contributes to preventing the passage of protein through the glomerular membrane. Therefore, in the absence of the foot processes, tremendous quantities of protein leak into the glomerular filtrate though even larger elements of the blood, such as red cells, are still completely prevented from leaking.

The name *lipoid nephrosis* is derived from the fact that large quantities of lipid droplets are found in the epithelial cells lining the tubules and also from the fact that the concentration of lipid substances in the blood is usually increased. The lipid deposits in the tubules apparently play no role in the loss of proteins.

Administration of glucocorticoids such as prednisone usually causes complete remission of lipoid nephrosis although these hormones will not cause remission of most other types of nephrotic syndrome.

Protein Loss. In the nephrotic syndrome, as much as 30 grams of plasma proteins can be lost into the urine each day. Though the resulting low plasma protein concentration stimulates the liver to produce far more plasma proteins than usual, nevertheless, the liver often cannot keep up with the loss. Therefore, in severe nephrosis the colloid osmotic pressure of the plasma sometimes falls extremely low, often from the normal level of 28 mm Hg to as low as 6 to 8 mm Hg.

Edema. The low plasma colloidal osmotic pressure in turn allows large amounts of fluid to filter into the interstitial spaces and also into the potential spaces of the body, thus causing serious *edema*. The nephrotic person has been known on occasion to develop as much as 40 liters of excess extracellular fluid, and as much as 15 liters of this has been *ascites* in the abdomen. Also, the joints swell, and the pleural cavity and the pericardium become partially filled with fluid.

A nephrotic person can be greatly benefited by intravenous infusion of large quantities of concen-

Table 26–1. COMPARISON OF DIALYZING FLUID WITH NORMAL AND UREMIC PLASMA

Constituent	Normal Plasma	Dialyzing Fluid	Uremic Plasma
Electrolytes (mEq/Liter)			
Na^+	142	142	142
K^+	5	4	7
Ca^{++}	3	3	2
Mg^{++}	1.5	1.5	1.5
Cl^-	107	107	107
HCO_3^-	27	27	14
Lactate$^-$	1.2	1.2	1.2
HPO_4^{--}	3	0	9
Urate$^-$	0.3	0	2
Sulfate^{--}	0.5	0	3
Nonelectrolytes (mg %)			
Glucose	100	125	100
Urea	26	0	200
Creatinine	1	0	6

trated plasma proteins. Yet this is of only temporary benefit because enough protein can be lost into the urine in only a day to return the person to his original predicament.

MICTURITION

Micturition is the process by which the urinary bladder empties when it becomes filled. Basically the bladder (1) progressively fills until the tension in its walls rises above a threshold value, at which time (2) a nervous reflex called the *micturition reflex* occurs that either causes micturition or, if it fails in this, at least causes excess pressure in the bladder and a conscious desire to urinate.

Physiologic Anatomy of the Bladder

The urinary bladder, illustrated in Figure 26–6, is a smooth muscle chamber composed of two principal parts: (1) the *body*, which is the major part of the bladder, in which the urine collects, and (2) the *neck*, which is a funnel-shaped extension of the body.

The smooth muscle of the bladder is known as the *detrusor muscle*. Its muscle fibers extend in all directions and, when contracted, can increase the pressure in the bladder sometimes to as high as 40 to 60 mm Hg. Thus, it is the detrusor muscle that empties the bladder.

On the posterior wall of the bladder, lying immediately above the bladder neck, is a small, smooth triangular area called the *trigone*. The lowermost apex of the trigone lies at the bladder neck, and the two ureters enter the bladder at the uppermost angles of the trigone. Where each ureter enters the bladder, it courses obliquely through the detrusor muscle and then passes still another 1 to 2 centimeters underneath the bladder mucosa before emptying into the bladder. This oblique passage of the ureter acts as a valve to prevent reflux of urine into the ureter when the bladder pressure rises.

The muscle of the bladder neck is frequently called the *internal sphincter*. Its natural tone normally keeps the bladder neck empty of urine, and therefore pre-

vents emptying of the bladder until the pressure in the body of the bladder rises above a critical threshold.

Beyond the bladder neck, the urethra passes through the *urogenital diaphragm*, which contains a layer of muscle called the *external sphincter* of the bladder. This muscle is a voluntary skeletal muscle in contrast to the smooth muscle of the bladder body and bladder neck. This external muscle is under voluntary control of the nervous system and can be used to prevent urination even when the involuntary controls are attempting to empty the bladder.

Innervation of the Bladder. The principal nerve supply to the bladder is by way of the *pelvic nerves*, which connect with the spinal cord through the sacral plexus, mainly connecting with cord segments S-2 and S-3. Coursing through the pelvic nerves are both *sensory nerve fibers* and *motor fibers*. The sensory fibers mainly detect the degree of stretch of the bladder walls. Stretch signals from the bladder neck are especially strong and are mainly responsible for initiating the reflexes that cause bladder emptying.

The motor nerve fibers transmitted in the pelvic nerves are *parasympathetic fibers*. These terminate on ganglion cells located in the wall of the bladder. Short postganglionic nerves then innervate the *detrusor muscle*.

Aside from the pelvic nerves, two other types of innervation are important to bladder function: (1) *pudendal nerve fibers* that innervate the skeletal muscle of the external bladder sphincter and (2) *sympathetic innervation* from the sympathetic chain through the hypogastric nerves.

Transport of Urine Through the Ureters

The ureters are small smooth muscle tubes that originate in the pelves of the two kidneys and pass downward to enter the bladder. Each ureter is innervated by both sympathetic and parasympathetic nerves, and each also has an intramural plexus of neurons and nerve fibers that extends along its entire length.

As urine collects in the kidney pelvis, the pressure in the pelvis increases and initiates a peristaltic contraction that spreads downward along the ureter to force urine toward the bladder. The peristaltic wave can move urine against an obstruction with a pressure as high as 50 to 100 mm Hg. Transmission of the peristaltic wave is probably caused mainly by nerve impulses passing along the intramural plexus in the same manner that the intramural plexus functions in the gut.

Tone of the Bladder Wall and the Cystometrogram During Bladder Filling

The solid curve depicted in Figure 26–7 is called the *cystometrogram* of the bladder. It shows the changes in intravesical pressure as the bladder fills with urine. When no urine at all is in the bladder, the intravesical pressure is approximately zero, but

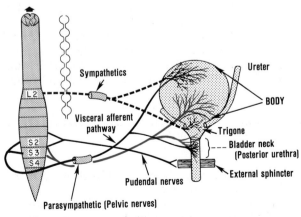

Figure 26–6. The urinary bladder and its innervation.

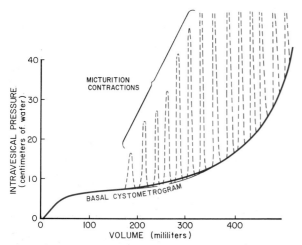

Figure 26–7. A normal cystometrogram showing also acute pressure waves (the dashed curves) caused by micturition reflexes.

by the time 30 to 50 milliliters of urine has collected, the pressure will have risen to 5 to 10 cm water. Additional urine up to 200 to 300 milliliters can collect with only a small amount of additional rise in pressure; this is caused by *intrinsic tone* of the bladder wall itself. Beyond 400 to 500 milliliters, collection of more urine causes the pressure to rise very rapidly.

Superimposed on the tonic pressure changes during filling of the bladder are periodic acute increases in pressure, which last from a few seconds to more than a minute. The pressure can rise only a few centimeters of water or it can rise to over 100 cm water. These are *micturition waves* in the cystometrogram caused by the micturition reflex, which is discussed next.

THE MICTURITION REFLEX

Referring again to Figure 26–7, one sees that as the bladder fills, many superimposed *micturition contractions* begin to appear. These are the result of a stretch reflex initiated by stretch receptors in the bladder wall, especially in the bladder neck. Sensory signals are conducted to the sacral segments of the cord through the pelvic nerves and then back again to the bladder through the parasympathetic fibers in these same nerves.

Once a micturition reflex begins, it is self-regenerative. That is, initial contraction of the bladder further activates the receptors, causing still further increase in afferent impulses from the bladder, which causes further increase in reflex contraction of the bladder, the cycle thus repeating itself again and again until

the bladder has reached a strong degree of contraction. Then, after a few seconds to more than a minute, the reflex begins to fatigue, and the regenerative cycle of the micturition reflex ceases, allowing rapid cessation of the bladder contraction. In other words, the micturition reflex is a single complete cycle of (a) progressive and rapid increase in pressure, (b) a period of sustained pressure, and (c) return of the pressure to the basal tonic pressure of the bladder. Once a micturition reflex has occurred and has not succeeded in emptying the bladder, the nervous elements of this reflex usually remain in an inhibited state for at least a few minutes to sometimes as long as an hour or more before another micturition reflex occurs. However, as the bladder becomes still more filled, micturition reflexes occur more and more often and more and more powerfully.

Once the micturition reflex becomes powerful enough and the fluid pressure in the bladder great enough to force the bladder neck open despite the tonic contraction of the bladder neck muscle, stretch of the neck then strongly exacerbates the micturition reflex and also causes still another reflex. This reflex passes to the sacral portion of the spinal cord and then *back to the external sphincter to inhibit it.* If this inhibition is more potent than the voluntary constrictor signals from the brain, then urination will occur. If not, urination still will not occur until the bladder fills still more and the micturition reflex becomes more powerful.

Control of Micturition by the Brain. The micturition reflex is a completely automatic cord reflex, but it can be inhibited or facilitated by centers in the brain. These include (a) strong *facilitatory and inhibitory centers in the brain stem,* probably located in the pons and (b) several *centers located in the cerebral cortex* that are mainly inhibitory but can at times become excitatory.

The micturition reflex is the basic cause of micturition, but the higher centers normally exert final control of micturition by the following means:

1. The higher centers keep the micturition reflex partially inhibited all the time except when micturition is desired.

2. The higher centers prevent micturition, even if a micturition reflex occurs, by continual tonic contraction of the external urinary sphincter until a convenient time presents itself.

3. When the time to urinate arrives, the cortical centers can (a) facilitate the sacral micturition centers to initiate a micturition reflex and (b) inhibit the external urinary sphincter so that urination can occur.

QUESTIONS

1. What is the relationship between the hydrogen ion concentration and the pH of a fluid?
2. Explain how the bicarbonate buffer system buffers the hydrogen ion concentration.
3. Give the Henderson-Hasselbalch equation for the re-

lationship between pH and the two elements of the bicarbonate buffer system.
4. Explain how the phosphate and protein systems buffer the hydrogen ion concentration.
5. What is the feedback mechanism controlling respiration

that also helps to control the hydrogen ion concentration of the extracellular fluids?

6. Explain the mechanism for hydrogen ion secretion by the renal tubular epithelium.
7. How does the reaction of hydrogen ions with bicarbonate ions in the tubules provide an indirect method for reabsorption of bicarbonate ions?
8. Explain the "titration" of hydrogen ions against bicarbonate ions in the renal tubules as a means for controlling extracellular fluid hydrogen ion concentration.
9. Why is the phosphate buffer system of special importance for transport of hydrogen ions from the tubules into the urine?
10. How does the ammonia buffer system increase the transport of hydrogen ions from the tubules into the urine as much as tenfold?
11. Explain the mechanism by which the ratio of the concentrations of bicarbonate ions and chloride ions is controlled in the extracellular fluid.
12. What is the difference between metabolic acidosis and respiratory acidosis?
13. Explain the various causes of respiratory acidosis and alkalosis and of metabolic acidosis and alkalosis.
14. Why can either acidosis or alkalosis be fatal?
15. Give the sequence of events in the development of acute renal failure caused by acute glomerulonephritis.
16. How does pyelonephritis differ in its effects on renal function from glomerular nephritis?
17. What are the effects on the body of uremia?
18. Explain the manner in which the artificial kidney removes unwanted substances from the body fluids.
19. What is *lipoid nephrosis*, and how does it affect renal function?
20. Explain the mechanism by which the ureters transport urine from the kidneys to the urinary bladder.
21. Describe the anatomy and the function of the *micturition reflex*.
22. How is micturition controlled?

References

Acid-Base Balance

Catto, G. R.: Clinical Aspects of Renal Physiology. Philadelphia, W. B. Saunders Company, 1981.
Goldberger, E.: A Primer of Water, Electrolyte, and Acid-Base Syndromes. Philadelphia, Lea & Febiger, 1980.
Halperin, M. L., et al.: Distal renal tubular acidosis syndromes: a pathophysiological approach. Am J Nephrol 5:1, 1985.
Ives, H. E., and Rector, F. C., Jr.: Proton transport and cell function. J Clin Invest 73:285, 1984.
Jones, N. L.: Blood Gases and Acid-base Physiology. New York, B. C. Decker, 1980.
Kovacevic, A., and McGivan, J. D.: Mitochondrial metabolism of glutamine and glutamate and its physiological significance. Physiol Rev 63:547, 1983.
Rose, B. D.: Clinical Physiology of Acid-Base and Electrolyte Disorders. New York, McGraw-Hill Book Co., 1984.
Tannen, R. L.: Control of acid secretion by the kidney. Annu Rev Med 31:35, 1980.
White, F. N., and Somero, G.: Acid-base regulation and phospholipid adaptations to temperature: time courses and physiological significance of modifying the milieu for protein function. Physiol Rev 62:40, 1982.

Renal Disease; Micturition

Adler, S. G., et al.: Hypersensitivity phenomena and the kidney: role of drugs and environmental agents. Am J Kidney Dis 5:75, 1985.
Bernstein, K. N., and O'Connor, D. T.: Antiadrenergic antihypertensive drugs: their effect on renal function. Annu Rev Pharmacol Toxicol 24:105, 1984.
Bricker, N. S.: The Kidney. Diagnosis and Management. New York, John Wiley & Sons, 1984.
Catto, G. E.: Clinical Aspects of Renal Physiology. Philadelphia, W. B. Saunders Company, 1981.
Charlton, C. A.: The Urological System. New York, Churchill Livingstone, 1983.
Cummings, N. B., ed.: Immune Mechanisms in Renal Disease. New York, Plenum Publishing Corp., 1983.
DeFronzo, R. A., et al.: Clinical disorders of hyperkalemia. Annu Rev Med 33:521, 1982.
Herrin, J. T.: Management of children with progressive renal failure. Annu Rev Med 34:21, 1983.
Kanwar, Y. S.: Biophysiology of glomerular filtration and proteinuria. Lab Invest 51:7, 1984.
Leaf, A., and Cotran, R. S.: Renal Pathophysiology. 2nd ed. New York, Oxford University Press, 1980.
Martinez, M. M.: Handbook of Renal Therapeutics. New York, Plenum Publishing Corp., 1983.
Porter, G., ed.: Nephrotoxic Mechanisms of Drugs and Environmental Toxins. New York, Plenum Publishing Corp., 1982.
Walser, M.: Nutrition in renal failure. Annu Rev Nutr 3:125, 1983.
Williams, R. C., Jr.: Immune complexes in human diseases. Annu Rev Med 32:13, 1981.
Wills, M. R.: Uremic toxins, and their effect on intermediary metabolism. Clin Chem 31:5, 1985.

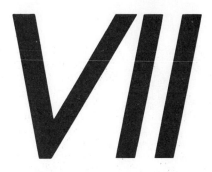

RESPIRATION

27 ■ Pulmonary Ventilation and Physical Principles of Gaseous Exchange

28 ■ Transport of Oxygen and Carbon Dioxide Between the Alveoli and the Tissue Cells

29 ■ Regulation of Respiration and Respiratory Insufficiency

27

Pulmonary Ventilation and Physical Principles of Gaseous Exchange

MECHANICS OF PULMONARY
   VENTILATION
   *BASIC MECHANISMS OF LUNG
      EXPANSION AND CONTRACTION*
   RESPIRATORY PRESSURES
   *EXPANSIBILITY OF THE LUNGS AND
      THORAX: COMPLIANCE*
   THE WORK OF BREATHING
THE PULMONARY VOLUMES AND
   CAPACITIES
   THE PULMONARY VOLUMES
   THE PULMONARY CAPACITIES
THE MINUTE RESPIRATORY
   VOLUME—RESPIRATORY RATE AND
   TIDAL VOLUME

ALVEOLAR VENTILATION
   RATE OF ALVEOLAR VENTILATION
FUNCTIONS OF THE RESPIRATORY
   PASSAGEWAYS
   FUNCTIONS OF THE NOSE
   *THE TRACHEA, BRONCHI, AND
      BRONCHIOLES*
   VOCALIZATION
PHYSICAL PRINCIPLES OF GASEOUS
   EXCHANGE
   THE VAPOR PRESSURE OF WATER
   *DIFFUSION OF GASES THROUGH
      TISSUES*

The process of respiration can be divided into four major mechanistic events: (1) pulmonary ventilation, which means the inflow and outflow of air between the atmosphere and the lung alveoli, (2) diffusion of oxygen and carbon dioxide between the alveoli and the blood, (3) transport of oxygen and carbon dioxide in the blood and body fluids to and from the cells, and (4) regulation of ventilation and other facets of respiration. The present chapter and the two following discuss these four major aspects of respiration. In a fourth chapter the special respiratory problems related to aviation medicine and deep sea diving physiology are discussed to illustrate some of the basic principles of respiratory physiology.

MECHANICS OF PULMONARY VENTILATION

BASIC MECHANISMS OF LUNG EXPANSION AND CONTRACTION

The lungs can be expanded and contracted in two ways, (1) by downward and upward movement of the

diaphragm to lengthen or shorten the chest cavity and (2) by elevation and depression of the ribs to increase and decrease the anteroposterior diameter of the chest cavity. Figure 27–1 illustrates these two methods.

Normal quiet breathing is accomplished almost entirely by inspiratory movement of the *diaphragm*. During inspiration the diaphragm pulls the lower surfaces of the lungs downward. Then, during expiration, the diaphragm simply relaxes and the *elastic recoil* of the lungs, chest wall, and abdominal structures compresses the lungs. During heavy breathing, however, the elastic forces are not powerful enough to cause the necessary rapid expiration, which is achieved by contraction of the abdominal muscles, which squeezes the abdominal contents upward against the bottom of the diaphragm.

The second method of expanding the lungs is to raise the rib cage. This expands the lungs because in the natural resting position, the ribs slant downward, thus allowing the sternum to fall backward toward the spinal column. But when the rib cage is elevated, the ribs project directly foward, so that the sternum

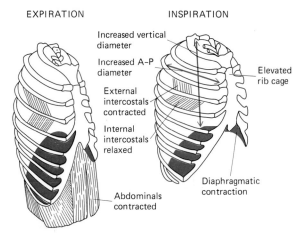

EXPIRATION   INSPIRATION

Increased vertical
diameter

Increased A-P
diameter

External
intercostals
contracted

Internal
intercostals
relaxed

Elevated
rib cage

Diaphragmatic
contraction

Abdominals
contracted

Figure 27–1. Expansion and contraction of the thoracic cage during expiration and inspiration, illustrating especially diaphragmatic contraction, elevation of the rib cage, and function of the intercostals.

now also moves forward away from the spine, making the anteroposterior thickness of the chest about 20 per cent greater during maximum inspiration than during expiration. Therefore, those muscles that elevate the chest cage can be classified as muscles of inspiration. These especially include the *neck muscles* that pull the upper ribs and sternum upward. Those muscles that depress the chest cage are muscles of expiration. These especially include the *abdominal recti* that pull downward on the sternum and lower ribs.

RESPIRATORY PRESSURES

Intra-alveolar Pressure. The respiratory muscles cause pulmonary ventilation by alternately compressing and distending the lungs, which in turn causes the pressure in the alveoli to rise and fall. During inspiration the intra-alveolar pressure becomes slightly negative *with respect to atmospheric pressure,* normally slightly less than −1 mm Hg, and this causes air to flow inward through the respiratory passageways. During normal expiration, on the other hand, the intra-alveolar pressure rises to slightly less than + 1 mm Hg, which causes air to flow outward through the respiratory passageways. Note especially how little pressure is required to move air into and out of the normal lung, though many times as much pressure is required in some types of lung diseases.

During maximum expiratory effort with the glottis closed, the intra-alveolar pressure can be increased to as much as 140 mm Hg in the strong healthy male, and during maximum inspiratory effort it can be reduced to as low as −100 mm Hg.

Recoil Tendency of the Lungs and the Intrapleural Pressure. The lungs have a continual elastic tendency to collapse and therefore to pull away from the chest wall. This is called the recoil tendency of the lungs, and it is caused by two different factors. First, throughout the lungs are many *elastic fibers* that are stretched by lung inflation and therefore attempt to

shorten. Second, and even more important, the *surface tension* of the fluid lining the alveoli also causes a continual elastic tendency for the alveoli to collapse. This effect is caused by intermolecular attraction between the surface molecules of the alveolar fluid; that is, each molecule pulls on the next one so that the whole lining sheet of fluid on the alveolar surfaces acts like many small elastic balloons continually trying to collapse the lung.

Ordinarily, the elastic fibers in the lungs account for about one third of the recoil tendency, and the surface tension phenomenon accounts for about two thirds.

The total recoil tendency of the lungs can be measured by the amount of negative pressure in the pleural space required to prevent collapse of the lungs; this pressure is called the *intrapleural pressure* or, occasionally, the *lung recoil pressure.* It is normally about −4 mm Hg. That is, a *negative* pressure of −4 mm Hg on the outer surfaces of the lungs is required to keep them expanded to normal size. When the lungs are stretched to very large size, such as at the end of deep inspiration, the pleural pressure required then may be as great as −12 to −18 mm Hg.

Surfactant in the Alveoli, and Its Effect on the Collapse Tendency. A lipoprotein mixture called surfactant is secreted by special *surfactant-secreting cells* (the type II granular pneumocytes) that are component parts of the alveolar epithelium. This mixture, containing especially the phospholipid *dipalmitoyl lecithin,* decreases the surface tension of the fluid lining the alveoli. In the absence of surfactant, lung expansion is extremely difficult, often requiring negative pleural pressures as low as −20 to −30 mm Hg to overcome the collapse tendency of the alveoli. This illustrates that surfactant is exceedingly important for minimizing the effect of surface tension in causing collapse of the lungs.

A few newborn babies, especially premature babies, do not secrete adequate quantities of surfactant, which makes lung expansion difficult. Without immediate and very careful treatment, most of these die soon after birth because of inadequate ventilation. This condition is called *hyaline membrane disease* or *respiratory distress syndrome.*

Surfactant acts by decreasing the forces between the surface molecules of the alveolar fluid. In the absence of surfactant, this interface has a surface tension of about 50 dynes/cm. By contrast, with surfactant, the surface tension varies between 5 and 30 dynes/cm, averaging about four times less than in the absence of surfactant.

Surfactant has a special property of decreasing the surface tension more as the alveoli become smaller, which nullifies some of the collapse tendency of the alveoli as they become smaller. Consequently, surfactant is very important in maintaining the equality of size of the alveoli—that is, the large alveoli develop greater surface tension and therefore contract, while the smaller alveoli develop less surface tension and therefore tend to enlarge.

EXPANSIBILITY OF THE LUNGS AND THORAX: COMPLIANCE

Both the lungs and the thorax are viscoelastic structures. The elastic properties of the lungs, as pointed out previously, are caused, first, by the surface tension of the fluids lining the alveoli and, second, by elastic fibers throughout the lung tissue itself. The elastic properties of the thorax are caused by the natural elasticity of the muscles, tendons, and connective tissue of the chest. Therefore, part of the effort expended by the inspiratory muscles during breathing is simply to stretch the elastic structures of the lungs and thorax.

The expansibility of the lungs and thorax is called *compliance*. This is expressed as the *volume increase in the lungs for each unit increase in intra-alveolar pressure*. The compliance of the normal lungs and thorax combined is 0.13 liter per centimeter of water pressure. That is, every time the alveolar pressure is increased by 1 cm water, the lungs expand 130 ml.

Compliance of the Lungs Alone. The lungs alone, when removed from the chest, are almost twice as distensible as the lungs and thorax together, because the thoracic cage itself must also be stretched when the lungs are expanded *in situ*. Thus, the compliance of the normal lungs when removed from the thorax is about 0.22 liter per cm water. This illustrates that the muscles of inspiration must expend energy not only to expand the lungs but also to expand the thoracic cage around the lungs.

Measurement of Lung Compliance. Compliance of the lungs is measured in the following way: The person's glottis must first be completely open and remain so, so that the alveolar pressure will be equal to atmospheric pressure. Then air is inspired in steps of approximately 50 to 100 ml at a time, and pressure measurements are made at the end of each step from an intraesophageal balloon (which measures almost exactly the intrapleural pressure). Then the air is expired, also in steps, until the lung volume returns to the original expiratory resting level. The relationship of lung volume to pressure is then plotted as illustrated in Figure 27–2. This graph shows that the plot during inspiration is a different curve from that during expiration, which is caused by the viscous properties of the lungs. The average compliance is represented by the dashed line in the figure. Thus, in the normal-sized person the lung volume increases about 220 ml for a change in translung pressure (atmospheric pressure in the alveoli of the lung minus intraesophageal pressure) of 1 cm water. Therefore, the compliance in this instance is 0.22 liter per cm water.

Slight modifications of this procedure can be used to measure the compliance of the lungs and thoracic cage together.

Factors That Cause Abnormal Compliance. Any condition that destroys lung tissue, causes it to become fibrotic or edematous, blocks the bronchioles, or in any other way impedes lung expansion and contraction causes decreased lung compliance. When

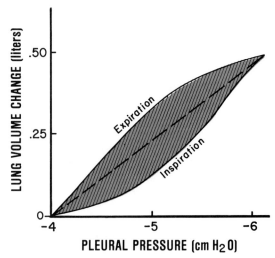

Figure 27–2. Compliance diagram in a normal person. This diagram shows the compliance of the lungs alone.

considering the compliance of both the lung and thorax together, one must also include any abnormality that reduces the expansibility of the thoracic cage. Thus, deformities of the chest cage, such as kyphosis, severe scoliosis, and other restraining conditions such as fibrotic pleurisy or paralyzed and fibrotic muscles can all reduce the expansibility of the chest and thereby reduce the total pulmonary compliance.

THE WORK OF BREATHING

We have already pointed out that during normal quiet respiration, respiratory muscle contraction occurs only during inspiration, while expiration is entirely a passive process caused by elastic recoil of the lung and chest cage structures. Therefore, the respiratory muscles normally perform work only to cause inspiration and not to cause expiration.

The work of inspiration can be divided into three different fractions: (1) that required to expand the lungs against its elastic forces, called *compliance work*, (2) that required to overcome the viscosity of the lung and chest wall structures, called *tissue resistance work*, and (3) that required to overcome airway resistance during the movement of air into the lungs, called *airway resistance work*.

Energy Required for Respiration. During normal quiet respiration, only 2 to 3 per cent of the total energy expended by the body is required to energize the pulmonary ventilatory process. During very heavy exercise, the absolute amount of energy required for pulmonary ventilation can increase as much as 25-fold. However, this still does not represent a significant increase in *percentage* of total energy expenditure, because the total energy release in the body increases at the same time as much as 15- to 20-fold. Thus, even in heavy exercise only 3 to 4 per cent of the total energy expended is used for ventilation.

On the other hand, pulmonary diseases that decrease the pulmonary compliance, that increase air-

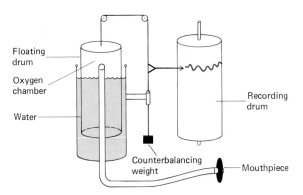

Figure 27–3. A spirometer.

way resistance, or that increase the viscosity of the lung or chest wall can at times increase the work of breathing so much that one-third or more of the total energy expended by the body is for respiration alone. Such respiratory disease can proceed to such a point that this excess work load alone is the cause of death.

THE PULMONARY VOLUMES AND CAPACITIES

Spirometry. A simple method for studying pulmonary ventilation is to record the volume movement of air into and out of the lungs, a process called *spirometry*. A typical spirometer is illustrated in Figure 27–3. This consists of a drum inverted over a chamber of water, with the drum counterbalanced by a weight. In the space above the water in the drum is a breathing mixture of gases, usually air or oxygen; a tube connects the mouth with the gas chamber. When one breathes into and out of the chamber the drum rises and falls, and an appropriate recording is made on a moving sheet of paper.

Figure 27–4 illustrates a spirogram showing changes in lung volume under different conditions of breath-

ing. For ease in describing the events of pulmonary ventilation, the air in the lungs has been subdivided at different points on this diagram into four different *volumes* and four different *capacities*, which are discussed in the following paragraph.

THE PULMONARY VOLUMES

To the left in Figure 27–4 are listed four different pulmonary lung volumes, which when added together equal the maximum volume to which the lungs can be expanded. The significance of each of these volumes is as follows:

1. The *tidal volume* is the volume of air inspired or expired with each normal breath, and it amounts to about 500 ml.

2. The *inspiratory reserve volume* is the extra volume of air that can be inhaled forcefully after the end of a normal tidal inspiration; it is usually equal to approximately 3000 ml.

3. The *expiratory reserve volume* is the amount of air that can still be exhaled forcefully after the end of a normal tidal expiration; it normally amounts to about 1100 ml.

4. The *residual volume* is the volume of air still remaining in the lungs after the most forceful expiration. This volume averages about 1200 ml.

THE PULMONARY CAPACITIES

In describing events in the pulmonary cycle, it is sometimes desirable to consider two or more of the above volumes together. Such combinations are called *pulmonary capacities*. In Figure 27–4 are listed the different pulmonary capacities, which can be described as follows:

1. The *inspiratory capacity* equals the *tidal volume* plus the *inspiratory reserve volume*. This is the amount of air (about 3500 ml) that a person can breathe beginning at the normal expiratory level and then distending his lungs to the maximum amount.

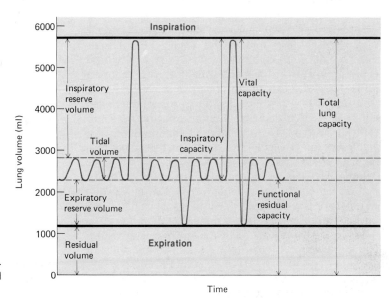

Figure 27–4. Diagram showing respiratory excursions during normal breathing and during maximal inspiration and maximal expiration.

2. The *functional residual capacity* equals the *expiratory reserve volume* plus the *residual volume*. This is the amount of air remaining in the lungs at the end of normal expiration (about 2300 ml).

3. The *vital capacity* equals the *inspiratory reserve volume* plus the *tidal volume* plus the *expiratory reserve volume*. This is the maximum amount of air that a person can expel from the lung after first filling the lungs to their maximum extent and then expiring to the maximum extent (about 4600 ml).

4. The *total lung capacity* is the maximum volume to which the lungs can be expanded with the greatest possible inspiratory effort (about 5800 ml).

All pulmonary volumes and capacities are about 20 to 25 per cent less in the female than in the male, and they obviously are greater in large and athletic persons than in small and asthenic persons.

Resting Expiratory Level. Normal pulmonary ventilation is accomplished almost entirely by the muscles of inspiration. On relaxation of the inspiratory muscles, the elastic properties of the lungs and thorax cause the lungs to contract passively. Therefore, when all inspiratory muscles are completely relaxed the lungs return to a relaxed state, called the *resting expiratory level*. The volume of air in the lungs at this level is equal to the functional residual capacity, or about 2300 ml in the young adult.

Significance of the Residual Volume. The residual volume represents the air that cannot be removed from the lungs even by forceful expiration. This is important because it provides air in the alveoli to aerate the blood even between breaths. Were it not for this residual air, the concentrations of oxygen and carbon dioxide in the blood would rise and fall markedly with each respiration, which would certainly be disadvantageous to the respiratory process.

Significance of the Vital Capacity. Other than the anatomical build of a person, the major factors that affect vital capacity are (1) the position of the person during the vital capacity measurement, (2) the strength of the respiratory muscles, and (3) the distensibility of the lungs and chest cage together, which is called pulmonary compliance.

The average vital capacity in the young adult male is about 4.6 liters, and in the young adult female about 3.1 liters, though these values are much greater in some persons of the same weight than in others.

Paralysis of the respiratory muscles, which occurs often following spinal cord injuries or poliomyelitis, can cause a great decrease in vital capacity, to as low as 500 to 1000 ml—barely enough to maintain life—or even to zero, in which case death ensues. And such conditions as tuberculosis, emphysema, chronic asthma, lung cancer, chronic bronchitis, and fibrotic pleurisy can all reduce the pulmonary compliance and thereby greatly decrease the vital capacity. For this reason vital capacity measurements are among the most important of all clinical respiratory measurements for assessing the progress of different types of diseases.

THE MINUTE RESPIRATORY VOLUME—RESPIRATORY RATE AND TIDAL VOLUME

The *minute respiratory volume* is the total amount of new air breathed each minute; this is equal to the *tidal volume* × the *respiratory rate*. The normal tidal volume is about 500 ml, and the normal respiratory rate is approximately 12 breaths per minute. Therefore, the *minute respiratory volume averages about 6 liters per minute.* A person can live for short periods of time with a minute respiratory volume as low as 1.5 liters per minute and with a respiratory rate as low as two to four breaths per minute.

The respiratory rate occasionally rises to as high as 40 to 50 per minute, and the tidal volume can become as great as the vital capacity, about 4600 ml in the young adult male. However, at rapid breathing rates, a person usually cannot sustain a tidal volume greater than about one half the vital capacity. Combining these factors, a young male adult has a so-called *maximum breathing capacity* of about 100 to 120 liters per minute.

ALVEOLAR VENTILATION

The ultimate importance of the pulmonary ventilatory system is to renew continually the air in the gas exchange areas of the lungs where the air is in close proximity to the pulmonary blood. These areas include the alveoli, the alveolar sacs, the alveolar ducts, and the respiratory bronchioles. The rate at which new air does reach these areas is called *alveolar ventilation*.

The Dead Space, and Its Effect on Alveolar Ventilation. Unfortunately, some of the air that a person breathes never reaches the gas exchange areas but instead only fills the respiratory passages. This air is called *dead space air* because it is not useful for the gas exchange process; the respiratory passages in which no gas exchange takes place are called the *dead space*.

On expiration, the air in the dead space is exhaled first, before any of the air from the alveoli reaches the atmosphere. Therefore, the dead space is equally disadvantageous for removal of the expiratory gases from the lungs.

The normal dead space air in the young adult is about 150 milliliters. This amount increases slightly with age.

Anatomical Versus Physiological Dead Space. All the space of the respiratory system besides the gas exchange areas is called the *anatomic dead space*. On occasion, however, some of the alveoli themselves are not functional or are only partially functional because of absent or poor blood flow through adjacent pulmonary capillaries. Therefore, from a functional point of view, these alveoli must also be considered to be dead space. When the alveolar dead space is included in the total measurement of dead space, it is then called *physiologic dead space*, in contradistinction to the anatomic dead space. In the normal person, the anatomic and the physiologic dead spaces are nearly equal because all alveoli are functional in the normal lung, but in persons with partially functional or nonfunctional alveoli in some parts of the lungs, the physiological dead space is sometimes as much as ten times the anatomical dead space, or as much as 1 to 2 liters. This amount obviously makes it difficult to supply enough alveolar ventilation to aerate the blood.

RATE OF ALVEOLAR VENTILATION

Alveolar ventilation per minute is the total volume of new air entering the alveoli and other gas exchange areas each minute. It is equal to the respiratory rate times the amount of new air that enters the alveoli with each breath

$$\dot{V}_A = Freq \cdot (V_T - V_D)$$

in which $\dot{V}_A$ is the *volume of alveolar ventilation per minute*, Freq is the *frequency of respiration per minute*, V_T is the *tidal volume*, and V_D is the *dead space volume*.

Thus, with a normal tidal volume of 500 milliliters, a normal dead space of 150 milliliters, and a respiratory rate of 12 times per minute, alveolar ventilation equals $12 \times (500 - 150)$, or 4200 milliliters per minute.

Theoretically, when the tidal volume falls to equal the dead space volume, no new air at all should enter the alveoli with each breath, and the alveolar ventilation per minute should become zero however rapidly the person breathes. However, this is not entirely true because the flow patterns in the passageways allow some alveolar air to be expired before all the dead space air is expired. Also, the same is true for inspiration. Therefore, there can be a slight amount of alveolar ventilation even with tidal volumes of as little as 60 to 75 milliliters.

On the other hand, when the tidal volume is several liters, the effect of dead space volume on alveolar ventilation obviously becomes almost insignificant.

Alveolar ventilation is one of the major factors that determines the concentrations of oxygen and carbon dioxide in the alveoli. Therefore, almost all discussions of gaseous exchange in the following chapters emphasize alveolar ventilation. *The respiratory rate, the tidal volume, and the minute respiratory volume are mainly of importance only insofar as they affect alveolar ventilation.*

FUNCTIONS OF THE RESPIRATORY PASSAGEWAYS

FUNCTIONS OF THE NOSE

As air passes through the nose, three distinct functions are performed by the nasal cavities: First, the *air is warmed* by the extensive surfaces of the turbinates and septum, which are illustrated in Figure 27–5. Second, the *air is moistened* to a considerable

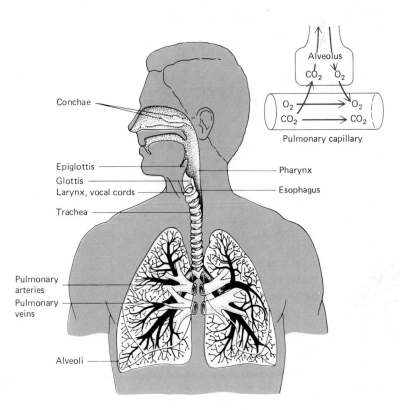

Figure 27–5. The respiratory passages.

extent even before it passes beyond the nose. Third, the *air is filtered* by the hairs and much more so by precipitation of particles on the conchae. All these functions together are called the *air conditioning function* of the upper respiratory passageways. Ordinarily, the air rises to within 2 to 3 per cent of body temperature and to within 2 to 3 per cent of full saturation with water vapor before it reaches the trachea. When a person breathes air through a tube directly into his trachea (as through a tracheostomy), the cooling, and especially the drying, effect in the trachea and the lungs can lead to lung infection.

THE TRACHEA, BRONCHI, AND BRONCHIOLES

After passing through the nose and pharynx, the air is distributed to the lungs by way of the *trachea, bronchi,* and *bronchioles,* as shown in Figure 27–5. To keep the trachea from collapsing during respiration, multiple *cartilage rings* extend above five sixths of the way around the trachea. In the walls of the bronchi are less extensive *cartilage plates* that also maintain a reasonable amount of rigidity yet allow sufficient motion for the lungs to expand and contract. These plates become progressively less extensive in the later generations of bronchi and are completely gone in the bronchioles.

The Muscular Wall of the Bronchiole and Its Control. The walls of the bronchioles are mainly entirely smooth muscle, with the exception of the most terminal bronchiole, called the *respiratory bronchiole,* which has only a few smooth muscle fibers. Many obstructive diseases of the lung cause narrowing of the muscular bronchioles, often because of excessive contraction of the smooth muscle itself.

Under normal respiratory conditions, the bronchioles remain mainly in a relaxed condition, and air flows easily through these so that less than 1 mm Hg air pressure gradient from the alveoli to the trachea is sufficient to cause all the air flow required for quiet breathing. But this is not true during disease. For instance, in asthma the degree of contraction is sometimes so great that 20 times as much pressure may be required to provide adequate air flow; this is especially true during expiration.

Nervous Control of the Bronchioles. The only important nervous control of the bronchioles is by way of parasympathetic nerve fibers carried in the vagus nerves. These nerves secrete acetylcholine and when activated cause mild-to-moderate constriction of the bronchioles. Though it is doubtful that parasympathetic stimulation by itself ever causes serious bronchiolar constriction, nevertheless, when disease processes have already caused some constriction, superimposed nervous stimulation often seems to worsen the condition. In these conditions, administration of drugs that block the effects of acetylcholine, such as the drug *atropine,* often can relax the bronchioles enough to relieve the obstruction.

Humoral Control of the Bronchioles. Several different humoral substances also are quite active in causing bronchiolar constriction. Two of the most important of these are *histamine* and the substance called *slow reactive substance of anaphylaxis.* Both of these are released in the lung tissues by mast cells during allergic reactions, especially allergic reactions to pollen breathed in the air. Therefore, they play key roles in causing the airway obstruction that occurs in allergic asthma. Also, irritants entering the airways—such as smoke, dust, sulfur dioxide, and some of the acidic elements in smog—can all initiate similar local reactions that cause obstructive constriction of the bronchioles.

In contrast with the humoral substances that constrict the bronchioles, two other hormones, epinephrine and norepinephrine, both of which are secreted by the adrenal glands in response to sympathetic stimulation, relax the bronchioles. Therefore, activation of the sympathetic nervous system is often valuable in relaxing the airways and preventing obstruction. For instance, this occurs when the sympathetic nervous system is activated during heavy exercise. In addition, injection of one of these two substances intravenously is often of value in treating severe respiratory obstruction.

The Mucous Coat of the Respiratory Passageways and Action of Cilia to Clear the Passageways

All the respiratory passages, from the nose to the terminal bronchioles, are kept moist by a layer of mucus that coats the entire surface. This mucus is secreted partly by individual goblet cells in the epithelial lining of the passages and partly by small submucous glands. In addition to keeping the surfaces moist, the mucus also traps small particles out of the inspired air and keeps most of these from ever reaching the alveoli. Then, the mucus itself is removed from the passages in the following manner:

The entire surface of the respiratory passages, both in the nose and in the lower passages, is lined with ciliated epithelium, with about 200 cilia on each epithelial cell. These beat continually at a rate of 10 to 20 times per second by the mechanism explained in Chapter 2, and the direction of their "power stroke" is always toward the pharynx. That is, the cilia in the lower respiratory passages beat upward, whereas those in the nose beat downward. This continual beating causes the coat of mucus to flow slowly, at a velocity of about 1 cm per minute, toward the pharynx. Then the mucus and its entrapped particles are either swallowed or coughed to the exterior.

The Cough Reflex

The bronchi and the trachea are so sensitive that any amount of foreign matter or irritation initiates the cough reflex. The *larynx* and *carina* (the point where the trachea divides into the bronchi) are especially sensitive. Afferent impulses pass from the respiratory passages mainly through the vagus nerves to the medulla. There, an automatic sequence of events is triggered by the neuronal circuits of the medulla, causing the following effects:

First, about 2.5 liters of air is inspired. Second, the epiglottis closes, and the vocal cords shut tightly to entrap the air within the lungs. Third, the abdominal muscles contract forcefully, pushing against the diaphragm. Consequently, the pressure in the lungs rises to as high as 100 or more mm Hg. Fourth, the vocal cords and the epiglottis suddenly open widely so that air under pressure in the lungs *explodes* outward. Indeed, the air is sometimes expelled at velocities as high as 75 to 100 miles an hour. Furthermore, and very important, the strong compression of the lungs also collapses the bronchi and trachea by causing the noncartilaginous parts of these to invaginate inward. Therefore, the exploding air actually passes through *bronchial* and *tracheal slits*. The rapidly moving air usually carries with it any foreign matter that is present in the bronchi or trachea.

VOCALIZATION

Speech involves the respiratory system particularly, but it also involves (1) specific speech control systems in the cerebral cortex, which will be discussed in Chapter 36, (2) respiratory control centers of the brain stem, and (3) the articulation and resonance structures of the mouth and nasal cavities. Basically, speech is composed of two separate mechanical functions: (1) *phonation*, which is achieved by the larynx, and (2) *articulation*, which is achieved by the structures of the mouth.

Phonation. The larynx is specially adapted to act as a vibrator. The vibrating element is the *vocal cords*, which are folds along the lateral walls of the larynx that are stretched and positioned by several specific muscles within the confines of the larynx itself.

Figure 27–6A illustrates the basic structure of the larynx, showing that each vocal cord is stretched between the *thyroid cartilage* and an *arytenoid cartilage*. The specific muscles within the larynx that position and control the degree of stretch of the vocal cords are also shown.

Vibration of the Vocal Cords. One might suspect that the vocal cords would vibrate in the direction of the flowing air. However, this is not the case. Instead, they vibrate laterally. The cause of the vibration is the following: When the vocal cords are closed together and air is expired, pressure of the air from below pushes the vocal cords apart, which allows rapid flow of air between their margins. The rapid flow of air then immediately creates a partial vacuum between the vocal cords, which pulls them once again toward each other. This stops the flow of air, pressure builds up behind the cords, and the cords open once more, thus continuing in a vibratory pattern.

The pitch of the sound emitted by the larynx can be changed in two different ways: first, *stretching or relaxing the vocal cords;* second, *changing the shape and mass of the vocal cord edges.* When very high frequency sounds are to be emitted, slips of the muscle in the vocal cords are contracted in such a way that the edges of the cords are sharpened and thinned, whereas when bass frequencies are to be emitted, the muscles are contracted in a different pattern, so that the edges are greatly thickened. Figure 27–6B shows some of the positions and shapes of the vocal cords during different types of phonation.

Articulation and Resonance. The three major organs of articulation are the *lips*, the *tongue*, and the *soft palate*. These need not be discussed in detail because all of us are familiar with their movements during speech and other vocalizations.

The resonators include the *mouth*, the *nose and associated nasal sinuses*, the *pharynx*, and even the *chest cavity* itself. Here again we are all familiar with the resonating qualities of these different structures. For instance, the function of the nasal resonators is illustrated by the change in quality of the voice when a person has a severe cold.

PHYSICAL PRINCIPLES OF GASEOUS EXCHANGE

After the alveoli are ventilated with fresh air, the next step in the respiratory process is *diffusion* of oxygen from the alveoli into the pulmonary blood

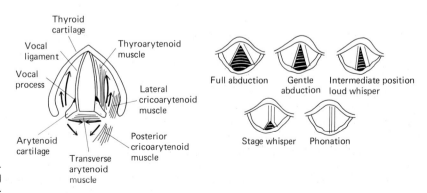

Figure 27–6. Laryngeal function in phonation. (Modified from Greene: The Voice and Its Disorders. 4th ed. Philadelphia, J. B. Lippincott Company, 1980.)

and diffusion of carbon dioxide in the opposite direction—from the pulmonary blood into the alveoli.

All the gases that are of concern in respiratory physiology are simple molecules that are free to move among each other, which is the process called diffusion. This is also true of the gases dissolved in the fluids and tissues of the body.

However, for diffusion to occur, there must be a source of energy. It is provided by the kinetic motion of the molecules themselves. That is, except at absolute zero temperature, all molecules of all matter are continuously undergoing some type of motion. For free molecules that are not physically attached to others, this principle means linear movement of the molecules at high velocity until they strike other molecules. Then they bounce away in new directions and continue moving until they strike still other molecules. In this way, each molecule moves rapidly among the others.

Gas Pressures in a Mixture of Gases— Partial Pressures of Individual Gases

The cause of the pressure that a gas exerts against a surface is constant impaction of the kinetically moving molecules against the surface. Obviously, the greater the concentration of the gas, the greater also is the summated force of impaction of all the molecules striking the surface at any given instant. Therefore, the pressure of a gas is directly proportional to its concentration. It is also directly proportional to the average kinetic energy of the molecules, which in turn is directly proportional to temperature. Therefore, the greater is the temperature, the greater the pressure; however, in the body, the temperature remains relatively constant at 37°C, so this usually is not a factor of major consideration in respiratory problems.

Now, let us consider the pressure exerted by each one of the gases in a mixture of gases. For instance, consider air, which has an approximate composition of 79 per cent nitrogen and 21 per cent oxygen. The total pressure of this mixture at sea level is 760 mm Hg. A portion of this total is caused by nitrogen and another portion by oxygen. It is clear from the above description of the molecular basis of pressure that each gas contributes to the total pressure in direct proportion to its relative concentration. Therefore, 79 per cent of the 760 mm Hg is caused by nitrogen (about 600 mm Hg) and 21 per cent by oxygen (about 160 mm Hg). Thus, the partial pressure of nitrogen in the mixture is 600 mm Hg, and the partial pressure of oxygen is 160 mm Hg, while the total pressure is 760 mm Hg, the sum of the individual partial pressures.

The partial pressures of the individual gases in a mixture are designated by the terms P_{O_2}, P_{CO_2}, P_{N_2}, P_{H_2O}, P_{He}, and so forth.

Partial Pressure of Gases in Water and Tissues

When a gas under pressure is impressed onto a water interface, instead of bouncing back from the interface some of the molecules will move on into the water and become dissolved. However, as more and more molecules become dissolved they also begin to diffuse backward to the interface, and some escape back into the gas phase. Once the concentration of dissolved molecules reaches a certain level, the number of molecules leaving the solution to enter the gas phase becomes exactly equal to the number of molecules moving in the opposite direction from the gas into the solution. Thus, a state of *equilibrium* has occurred. In this equilibrium state the pressure of the dissolved gas is exactly equal to the pressure of the gas in the gas state, each pushing against the other at the interface with equal force. Thus, gases in solution exert pressures in exactly the same way as they do in gas phase mixtures. And the partial pressures of the separate dissolved gases are designated like those of the gases in the gaseous state, i.e., P_{O_2}, P_{CO_2}, P_{N_2}, P_{He}.

Factors That Determine the Concentration of a Gas Dissolved in a Fluid. The concentration of a gas in a solution is determined not only by its pressure but also by the *solubility coefficient* of the gas. That is, some types of molecules, especially carbon dioxide, are physically or chemically attracted to water molecules, which makes them far more soluble than others. Obviously, far more of them can then become dissolved without building up excess pressure within the solution.

These principles can be expressed by the following formula, which is *Henry's law*:

$$\text{Concentration of dissolved gas} = \text{pressure} \times \text{solubility coefficient}$$

When concentration is expressed in volumes of gas dissolved in each volume of water at zero degrees centigrade and pressure is expressed in atmospheres, the solubility coefficients of important respiratory gases at body temperature are the following:

Oxygen	0.024
Carbon dioxide	0.57
Nitrogen	0.012

Note especially how much more carbon dioxide than oxygen—about 20 times as much—dissolves in the fluids of the body for the same amount of pressure.

THE VAPOR PRESSURE OF WATER

All gases in the body are in direct contact with water. Therefore, all gaseous mixtures in the body are saturated with water vapor. This must always be considered when the dynamics of gaseous exchange are discussed.

The vapor pressure of water depends entirely on the temperature. The greater the temperature, the greater is the activity of the water molecules, and the greater is the likelihood these molecules will escape from the surface of the water into the gaseous phase. When dry air is suddenly mixed with water, the water vapor pressure is zero at first, but water molecules immediately begin escaping from the surface of the water into the air. As the air becomes progressively more humidified, an equilibrium pressure is approached at which the rate of condensation of water becomes equal to the rate of water vaporization. This pressure is called the vapor pressure of the water.

The water vapor pressure at room temperature is about 20 mm Hg. However, the most important value to remember is the vapor pressure at body temperature, 47 mm Hg; this value will appear in many of our subsequent discussions.

Diffusion of Gases Through Liquids— The Pressure Gradient for Diffusion

Now, let us return to the problem of diffusion. From the above discussion it is already clear that when the concentration, or pressure, of a gas is greater in one area than in another area, there will be net diffusion from the high-pressure area toward the low-pressure area. For instance, in the chamber shown in Figure 27–7, one can readily see that the molecules in the area of high pressure, because of their greater number, have a greater statistical chance of moving randomly—that is, of *diffusing*—into the area of low pressure than do molecules attempting to go in the other direction. However, a lesser number of molecules diffuse randomly from the area of low pressure toward the area of high pressure. Therefore, the *net diffusion* of gas from the area of high pressure to the area of low pressure is equal to the number of molecules diffusing in this direction *minus* the number diffusing in the opposite direction, and this in turn is proportional to the gas pressure difference between the two areas.

The principle of diffusion from an area of high pressure to an area of low pressure holds true for diffusion of gases in a gaseous mixture, diffusion of dissolved gases in a solution, and even diffusion of gases from the gaseous phase into the dissolved state in liquids. That is, *there is always net diffusion from areas of high pressure to areas of low pressure.*

Quantifying the Net Rate of Diffusion. In addition to the pressure difference, several other factors affect the rate of gas diffusion in a fluid. These are (1) the solubility of the gas in the fluid, (2) the cross-sectional area of the fluid, (3) the distance through which the gas must diffuse, (4) the molecular weight of the gas, and (5) the temperature of the fluid. In the body, the temperature remains reasonably constant and usually need not be considered. All of these factors can be expressed in a single formula, as follows:

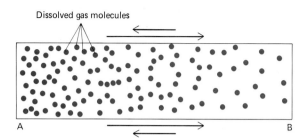

Figure 27–7. Net diffusion of oxygen from one end of a chamber to the other.

$$D \propto \frac{\Delta P \times A \times S}{d \times \sqrt{MW}}$$

in which D is the diffusion rate, ΔP is the pressure difference between the two ends of the chamber, A is the cross-sectional area of the chamber, S is the solubility of the gas, d is the distance of diffusion, and MW is the molecular weight of the gas.

It is obvious from this formula that the characteristics of the gas itself determine two factors of the formula: solubility and molecular weight. Therefore, the *diffusion coefficient*—that is, the rate of diffusion through a given area for a given distance and pressure difference—for any given gas is proportional to $S/\sqrt{MW}$. Considering the diffusion coefficient for oxygen to be 1, the *relative* diffusion coefficients for different gases of respiratory importance in the body fluids are

Oxygen	1.0
Carbon dioxide	20.3
Nitrogen	0.53

DIFFUSION OF GASES THROUGH TISSUES

The gases that are of respiratory importance are highly soluble in lipids and consequently are highly soluble in cell membranes. Because of this, these gases diffuse through the cell membranes with very little impediment. Instead, the major limitation of the movement of gases in tissues is the rate at which the gases can diffuse through the tissue water instead of through the cell membranes. Therefore, diffusion of gases through the tissues, including the respiratory membrane, is almost equal to the diffusion of gases through water, as given in the above list of diffusion rates for the important respiratory gases. Note especially that carbon dioxide diffuses 20 times as rapidly as oxygen.

QUESTIONS

1. Explain the roles of the diaphragm and of the elasticity of the chest cage in expansion and contraction of the lungs.

2. Explain the roles of the neck muscles and the abdominal recti in causing expansion and contraction of the lungs.

3. How much does the intra-alveolar pressure change during normal inspiration and expiration? What are the maximum limits of the intra-alveolar pressure?
4. What are the two factors that cause the lungs to collapse when the thoracic cage is opened?
5. Explain the role of *surfactant* in decreasing the tendency of the lungs to collapse.
6. What is meant by the *compliance* of the lungs? How much greater is the compliance of the lungs alone than the compliance of the lungs and thoracic cage together?
7. Define and give normal values for *tidal volume, inspiratory reserve volume, expiratory reserve volume,* and *residual volume.*
8. Define and give normal quantitative values for *inspiratory capacity, functional residual capacity, vital capacity,* and *total lung capacity.*
9. What is the functional significance of the *residual volume*?
10. Give normal values for the *respiratory rate,* the *minute respiratory volume,* and *alveolar ventilation.*
11. Explain the quantitative difference between *minute respiratory volume* and *alveolar ventilation.*
12. Why is the *physiological dead space* often many times greater than *anatomical dead space*?

13. What are the air conditioning functions of the nose?
14. Explain the different nervous and humoral factors that control the bronchioles.
15. What are the roles of *mucus* and the *cilia* in the respiratory passageways?
16. Explain the mechanism of the cough reflex.
17. How are the vocal cords controlled for the purpose of changing the frequency and quality of the sounds emitted by the larynx?
18. Explain the concept of *partial pressures* of individual gases when they exist in a mixture.
19. Explain why net diffusion of a gas always occurs in the direction of high pressure to low pressure regardless of whether the gas is in the gaseous state, is dissolved in tissues, or is dissolved in the blood.
20. Explain why the *vapor pressure of water* in the alveoli remains very nearly constant under normal conditions at a level of 47 mm Hg.
21. Give the equation for net rate of diffusion of a gas in a fluid or in a tissue, and explain each of the elements of the equation.
22. How much more rapidly does carbon dioxide diffuse through tissues than does oxygen?

References

Pulmonary Ventilation

Bless, D. M., ed.: Vocal Fold Physiology. Contemporary Research and Clinical Issues. San Diego, College-Hill Press, 1983.
Burri, P. H.: Fetal and postnatal development of the lung. Annu Rev Physiol 46:617, 1984.
Culver, B. H., and Butler, J.: Mechanical influences on the pulmonary microcirculation. Annu Rev Physiol 42:187, 1980.
Drazen, J. M., et al.: High-frequency ventilation. Physiol Rev 64:505, 1984.

Physical Principles of Gaseous Exchange

Forster, R. E., and Crandall, E. D.: Pulmonary gas exchange. Annu Rev Physiol 38:69, 1976.

Forster, R. E.: Pulmonary ventilation and blood gas exchange. In Sodeman, W. A., Jr., and Sodeman, W. A., eds.: Pathologic Physiology: Mechanisms of Disease, 5th ed. Philadelphia, W. B. Saunders Company, 1974, p. 371.
Glass, M. L., and Wood, S. C.: Gas exchange and control of breathing in reptiles. Physiol Rev 63:232, 1983.
Jones, N. L.: Blood Gases and Acid-Base Physiology. New York, B. C. Decker, 1980.
Rahn, H., and Farhi, L. E.: Ventilation, perfusion, and gas exchange—the Va/Q concept. In Fenn, W. O., and Rahn, H., eds.: Handbook of Physiology. Sec. 3, Vol. 1. Baltimore, Williams & Wilkins, 1964, p. 125.
West, J. B.: Pulmonary gas exchange. Int Rev Physiol 14:83, 1977.

28

Transport of Oxygen and Carbon Dioxide Between the Alveoli and the Tissue Cells

PRESSURE DIFFERENCES OF OXYGEN AND CARBON DIOXIDE FROM THE LUNGS TO THE TISSUES

COMPOSITION OF ALVEOLAR AIR—ITS RELATION TO ATMOSPHERIC AIR

RATE AT WHICH ALVEOLAR AIR IS RENEWED BY ATMOSPHERIC AIR

OXYGEN CONCENTRATION AND PARTIAL PRESSURE IN THE ALVEOLI

CO_2 CONCENTRATION AND PARTIAL PRESSURE IN THE ALVEOLI

EXPIRED AIR

DIFFUSION OF GASES THROUGH THE RESPIRATORY MEMBRANE

DIFFUSING CAPACITY OF THE RESPIRATORY MEMBRANE

EFFECT OF THE VENTILATION-PERFUSION RATIO ON GAS EXCHANGE

TRANSPORT OF OXYGEN TO THE TISSUES

UPTAKE OF OXYGEN BY THE PULMONARY BLOOD

DIFFUSION OF OXYGEN FROM THE CAPILLARIES TO THE INTERSTITIAL FLUID

DIFFUSION OF OXYGEN FROM THE INTERSTITIAL FLUID INTO THE CELLS

TRANSPORT OF CARBON DIOXIDE TO THE LUNGS

DIFFUSION OF CARBON DIOXIDE FROM THE CELLS TO THE TISSUE CAPILLARIES

REMOVAL OF CARBON DIOXIDE FROM THE PULMONARY BLOOD

CHEMICAL AND PHYSICAL MEANS BY WHICH OXYGEN IS CARRIED IN THE BLOOD

THE REVERSIBLE COMBINATION OF OXYGEN WITH HEMOGLOBIN

METABOLIC USE OF OXYGEN BY THE CELLS—RELATIONSHIP TO CELLULAR PO_2

TRANSPORT OF OXYGEN IN THE DISSOLVED STATE

"POISONING" OF HEMOGLOBIN BY CARBON MONOXIDE

CHEMICAL AND PHYSICAL MEANS FOR CARRYING CARBON DIOXIDE IN THE BLOOD

CHEMICAL FORMS IN WHICH CARBON DIOXIDE IS CARRIED

THE CARBON DIOXIDE DISSOCIATION CURVE

THE RESPIRATORY EXCHANGE RATIO

PRESSURE DIFFERENCES OF OXYGEN AND CARBON DIOXIDE FROM THE LUNGS TO THE TISSUES

In the preceding chapter it was pointed out that gases can move from one point to another by diffusion and that the cause is always a pressure difference from the first point to the next. Thus, oxygen diffuses from the alveoli into the pulmonary capillary blood because of the pressure difference—that is, because the oxygen pressure (PO_2) in the alveoli is greater than it is in the pulmonary blood. The pulmonary blood is then transported by way of the circulation to the peripheral tissues. There the PO_2 is lower in the cells than in the arterial blood entering the capillaries. Here again, the much higher PO_2 in the capillary blood causes oxygen to diffuse out of the capillaries and through the interstitial fluid into the cells.

Then when oxygen is metabolized with the foods in the cells to form carbon dioxide, the carbon dioxide

305

pressure (PCO₂) rises to a high value in the cells, which causes carbon dioxide to diffuse from the cells into the tissue capillaries. Once in the blood, the carbon dioxide is transported to the pulmonary capillaries, where it diffuses out of the blood and into the alveoli, because the P_{CO_2} in the alveoli is lower than that in the blood.

Basically, then, the transport of oxygen and carbon dioxide to and from the tissues depends on both diffusion and the movement of blood. We now need to consider quantitatively the factors responsible for these effects and their significance in the overall physiology of respiration.

COMPOSITION OF ALVEOLAR AIR— ITS RELATIONSHIP TO ATMOSPHERIC AIR

Alveolar air does not have the same concentrations of gases as atmospheric air by any means. The differences can be readily seen by comparing the alveolar air composition in column 3 of Table 28–1 with the composition of atmospheric air in column 1. There are several reasons for the differences. First, the alveolar air is only partially replaced by atmospheric air with each breath. Second, oxygen is constantly being absorbed from the alveolar air. Third, carbon dioxide is constantly diffusing from the pulmonary blood into the alveoli. And, fourth, dry atmospheric air that enters the respiratory passages is humidified even before it reaches the alveoli.

Humidification of the Air as It Enters the Respiratory Passages. Column 1 of Table 28–1 shows that atmospheric air is composed almost entirely of nitrogen and oxygen; it normally contains almost no carbon dioxide and little water vapor. However, as soon as the atmospheric air enters the respiratory passages, it is exposed to the fluids covering the respiratory surfaces. Even before the air enters the alveoli, it becomes totally humidified.

The partial pressure of water vapor in humidified air at normal body temperature of 37°C is 47 mm Hg, which, therefore, is the partial pressure of water in the alveolar air. Since the total pressure in the alveoli cannot rise to more than the atmospheric pressure, this water vapor simply expands the volume of the air and thereby *dilutes* all the other gases in the inspired air. In column 2 of Table 28–1 it can be seen that humidification of the air has diluted the oxygen partial pressure at sea level from an average of 159 mm Hg in atmospheric air to 149 mm Hg in the humidified air, and it has diluted the nitrogen partial pressure from 597 to 563 mm Hg.

RATE AT WHICH ALVEOLAR AIR IS RENEWED BY ATMOSPHERIC AIR

In the preceding chapter it was pointed out that the *functional residual capacity* of the lungs, which is the amount of air remaining in the lungs at the end of normal expiration, measures approximately 2300 ml. Furthermore, only 350 ml of new air is brought into the alveoli with each normal respiration, and the same amount of old alveolar air is expired. Therefore, the amount of alveolar air replaced by new atmospheric air with each breath is only one seventh of the total, so that many breaths are required to exchange most of the alveolar air. Figure 28–1 illustrates this slow rate of renewal of the alveolar air. In the first alveolus of the figure an excess amount of a gas has been placed momentarily in all the alveoli. The second alveolus shows slight dilution of this gas with the first breath; the next alveolus shows still further dilution with the second breath, and so forth for the third, fourth, eighth, twelfth, and sixteenth breaths. Note that even at the end of 16 breaths the excess gas still has not been completely removed from the alveoli.

With normal alveolar ventilation, approximately half the gas is removed in 17 seconds. When a person's alveolar ventilation is only half the normal rate, half the gas is removed in 34 seconds, and, when ventilation is twice the normal rate, half is removed in about 8 seconds.

This slow replacement of alveolar air is of particular importance in preventing sudden changes in gaseous concentrations in the blood and helps to prevent excessive increases and decreases in tissue oxygenation, tissue carbon dioxide concentration, and tissue pH when respiration is temporarily interrupted.

OXYGEN CONCENTRATION AND PARTIAL PRESSURE IN THE ALVEOLI

Oxygen is continually being absorbed into the blood of the lungs, and new oxygen is continually entering the alveoli from the atmosphere. The more

Table 28–1. PARTIAL PRESSURES OF RESPIRATORY GASES AS THEY ENTER AND LEAVE THE LUNGS (AT SEA LEVEL)— PER CENT CONCENTRATIONS ARE GIVEN IN PARENTHESES

	Atmospheric Air* (mm Hg)		Humidified Air (mm Hg)		Alveolar Air (mm Hg)		Expired Air (mm Hg)	
N_2	597.0	(78.62%)	563.4	(74.09%)	569.0	(74.9%)	566.0	(74.5%)
O_2	159.0	(20.84%)	149.3	(19.67%)	104.0	(13.6%)	120.0	(15.7%)
CO_2	0.3	(0.04%)	0.3	(0.04%)	40.0	(5.3%)	27.0	(3.6%)
H_2O	3.7	(0.50%)	47.0	(6.20%)	47.0	(6.2%)	47.0	(6.2%)
TOTAL	760.0	(100.0%)	760.0	(100.0%)	760.0	(100.0%)	760.0	(100.0%)

*On an average cool, clear day.

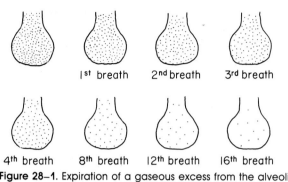

Figure 28-1. Expiration of a gaseous excess from the alveoli with successive breaths.

rapidly oxygen is absorbed, the lower becomes its concentration in the alveoli; on the other hand, the more rapidly new oxygen is brought into the alveoli from the atmosphere, the higher becomes its concentration. Therefore, oxygen concentration in the alveoli as well as its partial pressure is determined by the balance between the rate of absorption of oxygen into the blood and the rate of entry of new oxygen into the lungs by the ventilatory process. Its normal partial pressure in the alveoli is 104 mm Hg.

However, it must be noted that when a person is breathing air at normal sea-level pressure, even an extremely marked increase in alveolar ventilation can never increase the alveolar P_{O_2} above 149 mm Hg, for this is the maximum pressure of oxygen in humidified air.

CO_2 CONCENTRATION AND PARTIAL PRESSURE IN THE ALVEOLI

Carbon dioxide is continuously being formed in the body and then discharged into the alveoli, and it is continuously removed from the alveoli by the process of ventilation. Therefore, the two factors that determine carbon dioxide concentration and partial pressure (P_{CO_2}) in the lungs are (1) the rate of excretion of carbon dioxide from the blood into the alveoli and (2) the rate at which carbon dioxide is removed from the alveoli by alveolar ventilation. Quantitatively, one can easily understand that *the alveolar P_{CO_2} increases in direct proportion to the rate of carbon dioxide excretion, and it decreases in inverse proportion to alveolar ventilation.* The normal alveolar P_{CO_2} is 40 mm Hg.

EXPIRED AIR

Expired air is a combination of dead space air and alveolar air, and its overall composition is therefore determined by the proportion of the expired air that is dead space air and the proportion that is alveolar air. The initial portion of the expired air, the dead space air, is typical humidified air, as shown in column 2 of Table 28-1. Then progressively more alveolar air becomes mixed with the dead space air until all the dead space air has finally been washed out, and nothing but alveolar air is then expired. Thus, normal expired air, containing both dead space air and alveo-

lar air, has gaseous concentrations approximately as shown in column 4 of Table 28-1—that is, concentrations somewhere between those of humidified atmospheric air and alveolar air.

DIFFUSION OF GASES THROUGH THE RESPIRATORY MEMBRANE

The Respiratory Unit. The *respiratory unit* illustrated in Figure 28-2, is the terminal unit of the respiratory tree, where the gases exchange with those of the blood. Each respiratory unit is composed of a *respiratory bronchiole* and all of the other areas that it services, including *alveolar ducts, atria,* and *alveoli.* There are about 300 million alveoli in the two lungs, each alveolus having an average diameter of about 0.2 mm. The alveolar walls, as well as the walls of the other segments of the respiratory unit, are extremely thin, and within them is an almost solid network of interconnecting capillaries, as illustrated in Figure 28-3. Indeed, the flow of blood in the alveolar wall has been described as a "sheet" of flowing blood. Thus, it is obvious that the alveolar gases are in close proximity to the blood of the capillaries. Consequently, gaseous exchange between the alveolar air and the pulmonary blood occurs through the membranes of all these terminal portions of the lungs. These membranes are collectively known as the *respiratory membrane,* also called the *pulmonary membrane.*

The Respiratory Membrane. Figure 28-4 illustrates the ultrastructure of the respiratory membrane. It also shows the diffusion of oxygen from the alveolus into a red blood cell and diffusion of carbon dioxide in the opposite direction. Note the following different layers of the respiratory membrane:

1. A layer of fluid lining the alveolus and containing surfactant that reduces the surface tension of the alveolar fluid

2. The alveolar epithelium composed of very thin epithelial cells

3. An epithelial basement membrane

4. A very thin interstitial space between the alveolar epithelium and capillary membrane

5. A capillary basement membrane that in many places fuses with the epithelial basement membrane

6. The capillary endothelial membrane

Despite the large number of layers, the overall thickness of the respiratory membrane in some areas is as little as 0.2 micron and averages perhaps 0.6 micron.

From histologic studies it has been estimated that the total surface area of the respiratory membrane is approximately 160 square meters in the normal adult. This is equivalent to the floor area of a room 50 feet long by 30 feet wide. The total quantity of blood in the capillaries of the lung at any given instant is 60 to 140 ml. If this small amount of blood were spread over the entire surface of a 50 by 30-foot floor, one could readily understand the rapidity of respiratory exchange of gases.

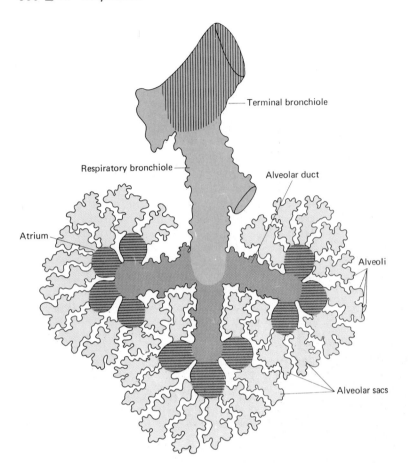

Terminal bronchiole

Respiratory bronchiole

Alveolar duct

Atrium

Alveoli

Alveolar sacs

Figure 28–2. The respiratory lobule. (From Miller: The Lung. Courtesy of Charles C Thomas, Publisher, Springfield, Illinois.)

Factors That Affect the Net Rate of Gas Diffusion Through the Respiratory Membrane

Referring to the discussion of diffusion of gases through water and tissues in the last chapter, one can apply the same principles and the same formula to diffusion of gases through the respiratory membrane. Thus, the factors that determine how rapidly a gas will pass through the membrane are (1) the *thickness of the membrane,* (2) the *surface area of the membrane, (3)* the *diffusion coefficient* of the gas in the substance of the membrane—that is, in water—and (4) the *pressure difference* between the two sides of the membrane.

The *thickness of the respiratory membrane* occasionally increases, often as a result of edema fluid in the interstitial spaces of the membrane and in the alveoli, so that the respiratory gases must diffuse not only through the membrane but also through this fluid. Because the rate of diffusion through the membrane is inversely proportional to the thickness of the membrane, any factor that increases the thickness to more than two to three times normal can interfere very significantly with normal respiratory exchange of gases.

The *surface area of the respiratory membrane* may be greatly decreased by many different conditions. For instance, removal of an entire lung decreases the surface area to half the normal amount. Also, in

emphysema many of the alveoli coalesce, with dissolution of many alveolar walls. When the total surface area is decreased to approximately one-third to one-fourth normal, exchange of gases through the membrane is impeded to a significant degree *even under resting conditions.* And during competitive sports and other strenuous exercise, even the slightest decrease in surface area of the lungs can be a serious detriment to respiratory exchange of gases.

The *diffusion coefficient* of each gas in the respiratory membrane is almost exactly the same as that in water, for reasons explained in the previous chapter. Therefore, for a given pressure difference, carbon dioxide diffuses through the membrane about 20 times as rapidly as oxygen. Oxygen in turn diffuses about two times as rapidly as nitrogen.

The *pressure difference* across the respiratory membrane is the difference between the partial pressure of the gas in the alveoli and the pressure of the gas in the blood. The partial pressure represents a measure of the total number of molecules of a particular gas striking a unit area of the alveolar surface of the membrane in unit time, and the pressure of the gas in the blood represents the number of molecules striking the same area of the membrane from the opposite side. Therefore, the difference between these two pressures is a measure of the *net tendency* for the gas to move through the membrane. Obviously, when the partial pressure of a gas in the alveoli is greater than the pressure of the gas in the

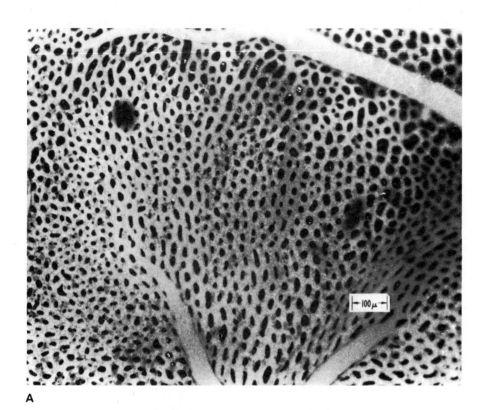

A

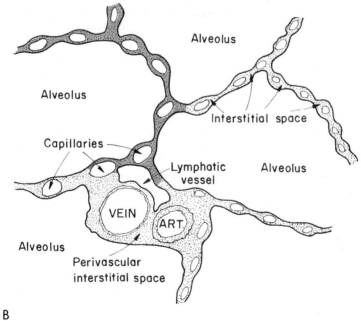

B

Figure 28–3. *A*, Surface view of capillaries in the alveolar wall. (From Maloney and Castle: Resp. Physiol., 7:150, 1969. Reproduced by permission of ASP Biological and Medical Press, North Holland Division.) *B*, Cross-sectional view of alveolar walls and their vascular supply.

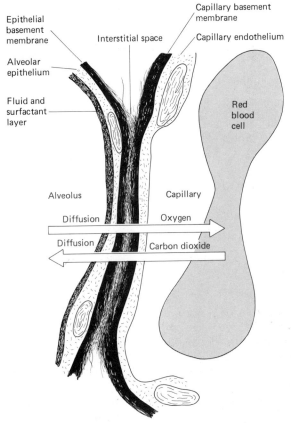

Epithelial
basement
membrane

Interstitial space

Capillary basement
membrane

Capillary endothelium

Alveolar
epithelium

Fluid and
surfactant
layer

Red
blood
cell

Alveolus

Capillary

Diffusion

Oxygen

Diffusion

Carbon dioxide

Figure 28–4. Ultrastructure of the respiratory membrane as shown in cross-section.

blood, as is true for oxygen, net diffusion from the alveoli into the blood occurs; but when the pressure of the gas in the blood is greater than in the alveoli, as is true for carbon dioxide, net diffusion from the blood into the alveoli occurs.

DIFFUSING CAPACITY OF THE RESPIRATORY MEMBRANE

The overall ability of the respiratory membrane to exchange a gas between the alveoli and the pulmonary blood can be expressed in terms of its *diffusing capacity,* which is defined as the *volume of a gas that diffuses through the membrane each minute for a pressure difference of 1 mm Hg.*

Obviously, all the factors discussed above that affect diffusion through the respiratory membrane can affect this diffusing capacity.

The Diffusing Capacity for Oxygen. In the young male adult the diffusing capacity for oxygen under resting conditions averages 21 ml per minute per mm Hg. The mean oxygen pressure difference across the respiratory membrane during normal, quiet breathing is approximately 11 mm Hg. Multiplying this pressure by the diffusing capacity (11×21) gives a total of about 230 ml of oxygen normally diffusing through the respiratory membrane each minute; this obviously is also equal to the rate at which the body uses oxygen.

Change in Oxygen-Diffusing Capacity During Exercise. During strenuous exercise, or during other conditions that greatly increase pulmonary activity, the diffusing capacity for oxygen increases about three-fold. This increase is caused by several different factors, among which are (1) opening of many previously dormant pulmonary capillaries, thereby increasing the surface area of the blood into which the oxygen can diffuse, and (2) dilatation of all the pulmonary capillaries that were already open. Therefore, during exercise the oxygenation of the blood is increased not only by increased alveolar ventilation but also by a greater capacity of the respiratory membrane for transmitting oxygen into the blood.

Diffusing Capacity for Carbon Dioxide. The diffusing capacity for carbon dioxide has never been measured because of the following technical difficulty: Carbon dioxide diffuses through the respiratory membrane so rapidly that the average P_{CO_2} in the pulmonary blood is not far different from the P_{CO_2} in the alveoli—the average difference is less than 1 mm Hg—and with the available techniques, this difference is too small to be measured.

Nevertheless, measurements of diffusion of other gases have shown that the diffusing capacity varies directly with the diffusion coefficient of the particular gas. Since the diffusion coefficient of carbon dioxide is 20 times that of oxygen, the diffusing capacity for carbon dioxide under resting conditions is about 400 to 450 ml and during exercise about 1200 to 1300 ml per minute per mm Hg.

The importance of these very large diffusing capacities for carbon dioxide is this: When the respiratory membrane becomes progressively damaged, its capacity for transmitting oxygen into the blood is often impaired enough to cause death of the person long before serious impairment of carbon dioxide diffusion occurs.

EFFECT OF THE VENTILATION-PERFUSION RATIO ON GAS EXCHANGE

Earlier in the chapter we discussed the importance of ventilation in determining both the P_{O_2} and P_{CO_2} in the alveoli. But we must also hasten to state that the rate of blood flow through the alveolar capillaries also is important in determining the effectiveness of gas exchange across the respiratory membrane—especially oxygen exchange but in some instances carbon dioxide exchange as well. Thus, the *ratio* of ventilation to pulmonary capillary blood flow, called the *ventilation-perfusion ratio,* is what is really important in determining gas exchange.

The Concept of Physiological Shunt (When the Ventilation-Perfusion Ratio Is Below Normal). Whenever the ventilation-perfusion ratio is below normal, there often is not ventilation enough to oxygenate the blood flowing through the alveolar capillaries. Therefore, a certain fraction of the venous blood passing through the pulmonary capillaries does not become oxygenated. This fraction is called *shunted blood*. The total quantitative amount of shunted blood per minute is called the *physiological shunt*.

Obviously, when the respiratory passageways to some lung areas are blocked—as occurs in emphysema, asthma, pneumonia, and many other diseases—this also causes a significant physiological shunt. That is, much blood passes through the lungs without being oxygenated.

The Concept of Physiological Dead Space (When the Ventilation-Perfusion Ratio is Above Normal). When the ventilation is great but blood flow is slow, there is then far more available oxygen in the alveoli than can be transported away from the alveoli by the flowing blood. Thus, a large portion of the ventilation is said to be *wasted*. The ventilation of the anatomical dead space areas of the lungs is also wasted. The sum of these two types of wasted ventilation is called the *physiological dead space*, a concept that was presented briefly in the previous chapter.

Obviously, also, when the blood flow to any part of the lungs is blocked for any reason, such as occurs in emphysema or lung cancer, all the ventilation to the affected area is wasted. This, too, adds to the physiological dead space.

When the physiological dead space is very great, much of the work of ventilation is wasted effort because so much of the ventilated air never reaches the blood.

In summary, for effective gas exchange to occur, it is very important that alveolar ventilation be appropriately balanced with pulmonary blood flow in each segment of the lungs.

TRANSPORT OF OXYGEN TO THE TISSUES

UPTAKE OF OXYGEN BY THE PULMONARY BLOOD

The top part of Figure 28–5 illustrates a pulmonary alveolus adjacent to a pulmonary capillary and shows diffusion of oxygen molecules between the alveolar air and the pulmonary blood. The P_{O_2} of the venous blood entering the capillary is only 40 mm Hg because a large amount of oxygen has been removed from this blood as it has passed through the tissue capillaries. The P_{O_2} in the alveolus is 104 mm Hg, giving an initial pressure difference for diffusion of oxygen into the pulmonary capillary of 104 − 40, or 64 mm Hg. Therefore, oxygen diffuses rapidly into the pulmonary capillary. The curve below the capillary shows the progressive rise in blood P_{O_2} as the blood passes through the capillary. This curve illustrates that the P_{O_2} rises almost to equal that of the alveolar air before reaching the midpoint of the capillary, becoming approximately 104 mm Hg. However, a small amount of pulmonary venous blood passes through

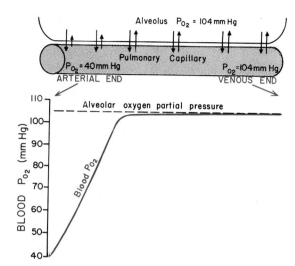

Figure 28–5. Uptake of oxygen by the pulmonary capillary blood.

poorly aerated alveoli and does not become oxygenated. When this blood mixes with the oxygenated blood in the left heart, the P_{O_2} in the aorta becomes about 95 mm Hg.

Uptake of Oxygen by the Pulmonary Blood During Exercise. During strenuous exercise, a person's body may require as much as 20 times the normal amount of oxygen. Yet because of the great *safety factor* for diffusion of still more oxygen through the pulmonary membrane and because the diffusing capacity for oxygen increases about threefold as discussed earlier, the blood is still within a mm Hg or so of being *completely saturated* with oxygen when it leaves the pulmonary capillaries.

DIFFUSION OF OXYGEN FROM THE CAPILLARIES TO THE INTERSTITIAL FLUID

At the tissue capillaries, oxygen diffuses into the tissues by a process essentially the same as that which takes place in the lung, as illustrated in Figure 28–6. That is, the P_{O_2} in the interstitial fluid immediately outside a capillary is low, averaging about 40 mm Hg, while that in the arterial blood is high, about 95 mm Hg. Therefore, at the arterial end of the capillary, a pressure difference of 55 mm Hg causes diffusion of oxygen. As illustrated in the figure, by the time the blood has passed through the capillary a large portion of the oxygen has diffused into the tissues, and the capillary P_{O_2} has now approached the 40 mm

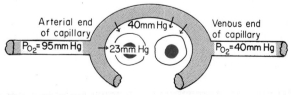

Figure 28–6. Diffusion of oxygen from a tissue capillary to the cells.

Hg oxygen pressure in the tissue fluids. Consequently, the venous blood leaving the tissue capillaries contains oxygen at essentially the same pressure as that immediately outside the tissue capillaries, 40 mm Hg.

DIFFUSION OF OXYGEN FROM THE INTERSTITIAL FLUID INTO THE CELLS

Since oxygen is always being used by the cells, the intracellular P_{O_2} remains lower than the interstitial fluid P_{O_2}. However, as was pointed out in Chapter 4, oxygen diffuses through cell membranes extremely rapidly. Therefore, the intracellular P_{O_2} is almost as great as that in the interstitial fluids.

Yet, in many instances, there is considerable distance between the capillaries and the cells. Therefore, the normal intracellular P_{O_2} ranges from as low as 5 mm Hg to as high as 60 mm Hg, averaging (by direct measurement in lower animals) 23 mm Hg, which is the value given for the cell in Figure 28–6. Since only 1 to 3 mm Hg oxygen pressure is required for full support of the metabolic processes of the cell, one can see that even this low cellular P_{O_2} is adequate and actually provides a considerable safety factor.

TRANSPORT OF CARBON DIOXIDE TO THE LUNGS

DIFFUSION OF CARBON DIOXIDE FROM THE CELLS TO THE TISSUE CAPILLARIES

Because of the continuous formation of large quantities of carbon dioxide in the cells, the intracellular P_{CO_2} tends to rise. However, carbon dioxide diffuses about 20 times as easily as oxygen, diffusing from the cells extremely rapidly into the interstitial fluids and thence into the capillary blood. Thus, in Figure 28–7 the intracellular P_{CO_2} is shown to be 46 mm Hg, while that in the interstitial fluid immediately adjacent to the capillaries is about 45 mm Hg, a pressure differential of only 1 mm Hg.

Arterial blood entering the tissue capillaries contains carbon dioxide at a pressure of approximately 40 mm Hg. As the blood passes through the capillaries, the blood P_{CO_2} rises to approach the 45 mm Hg P_{CO_2} of the interstitial fluid. Therefore, the P_{CO_2} of the blood leaving the capillaries and entering the veins is also about 45 mm Hg, within a fraction of a millimeter of reaching complete equilibrium with the P_{CO_2} of the interstitial fluid.

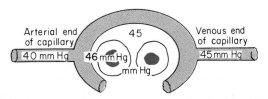

Figure 28–7. Uptake of carbon dioxide by the blood in the capillaries.

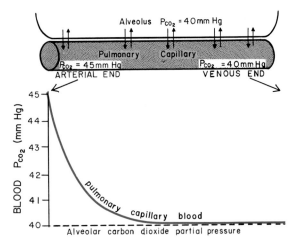

Figure 28–8. Diffusion of carbon dioxide from the pulmonary blood into the alveolus.

REMOVAL OF CARBON DIOXIDE FROM THE PULMONARY BLOOD

On arrival at the lungs, the P_{CO_2} of the venous blood is about 45 mm Hg while that in the alveoli is 40 mm Hg. Therefore, as illustrated in Figure 28–8, the initial pressure difference for diffusion is only 5 mm Hg, which is far less than that for diffusion of oxygen across the membrane. Yet even so, because of the 20 times as great diffusion coefficient for carbon dioxide as for oxygen, the excess carbon dioxide in the blood is rapidly transferred into the alveoli. Indeed, the figure shows that the P_{CO_2} of the pulmonary capillary blood becomes almost equal to that of the alveoli within the first four tenths of the blood's transit through the pulmonary capillary.

CHEMICAL AND PHYSICAL MEANS BY WHICH OXYGEN IS CARRIED IN THE BLOOD

Normally, about 97 per cent of the oxygen transported from the lungs to the tissues is carried in chemical combination with hemoglobin in the red blood cells, and the remaining 3 per cent is carried in the dissolved state in the water of the plasma and cells. Thus, *under normal conditions* the transport of oxygen in the dissolved state is negligible. However, when a person breathes oxygen at very high pressures, as much oxygen can sometimes be transported in the dissolved state as in chemical combination with hemoglobin. Therefore, the present discussion considers the transport of oxygen first in combination with hemoglobin and then in the dissolved state under special conditions.

THE REVERSIBLE COMBINATION OF OXYGEN WITH HEMOGLOBIN

The chemistry of hemoglobin was presented in Chapter 19, where it was pointed out that the oxygen

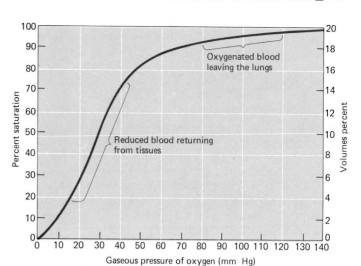

Figure 28–9. The oxygen-hemoglobin dissociation curve.

molecule combines loosely and reversibly with the heme portion of the hemoglobin. When the P_{O_2} is high, as in the pulmonary capillaries, oxygen binds with the hemoglobin, but when the P_{O_2} is low, as in the tissue capillaries, oxygen is released from the hemoglobin. This is the basis for transport of most of the oxygen from the lungs to the tissues.

The Oxygen-Hemoglobin Dissociation Curve

Figure 28–9 illustrates the oxygen-hemoglobin dissociation curve, which shows the progressive increase in the per cent of the hemoglobin that is bound with oxygen as the P_{O_2} increases. This is called the *per cent saturation of the hemoglobin*. Since the blood leaving the lungs usually has a P_{O_2} of about 100 mm Hg, one can see from the dissociation curve that the *usual oxygen saturation of arterial blood is about 97 per cent*. On the other hand, in normal venous blood the P_{O_2} is about 40 mm Hg and *the saturation of the hemoglobin is about 70 per cent*.

Maximum Amount of Oxygen That Can Combine with the Hemoglobin of the Blood. The blood of a normal person contains approximately 15 grams of hemoglobin in each 100 ml of blood, and each gram of hemoglobin binds with a maximum of about 1.34 ml of oxygen. Therefore, on the average the hemoglobin in 100 ml of blood can combine with a total of almost exactly 20 ml of oxygen when the hemoglobin is 100 per cent saturated. This is usually expressed as 20 *volumes per cent*. The oxygen-hemoglobin dissociation curve for the normal person, therefore, can also be expressed in terms of volume per cent of oxygen, as shown by the scale to the right in Figure 28–9 and also by Figure 28–10, rather than by per cent saturation of hemoglobin.

Amount of Oxygen Released from the Hemoglobin in the Tissues. The total quantity of oxygen *bound with hemoglobin* in normal arterial blood, which is normally 97 per cent saturated, is approximately 19.4 ml. This is illustrated in Figure 28–10 by the point at which the vertical line 95 mm Hg pressure crosses the

oxygen-hemoglobin dissociation curve. However, on passing through the tissue capillaries, this amount is reduced to 14.4 ml (P_{O_2} of 40 mm Hg, 72 per cent saturated), or a total loss of 5 ml of oxygen from each 100 ml of blood. Thus, *under normal conditions about 5 ml of oxygen is transported by each 100 ml of blood during each cycle through the tissues.*

However, during heavy exercise, tremendous amounts of oxygen are used by the muscles and the venous blood saturation then falls to as little as 20 per cent; therefore, the same blood now transports as much as 16 ml of oxygen in each 100 ml of blood instead of 5 ml, an increase of over threefold.

The Utilization Coefficient and the Effect of Exercise. The fraction of the blood that gives up its oxygen as it passes through the tissue capillaries is called the *utilization coefficient*. Normally, this is approximately 0.25, or 25 per cent, of the blood. That is, *the normal utilization coefficient is approximately one fourth*. During strenuous exercise, as much as 75 to 85 per cent of the blood can give up its oxygen; the utilization coefficient is then 0.75 to 0.85, which represents about three times as much oxygen delivery to the tissues as normal. These values are about the highest utilization coefficients that can be attained in the total body even when the tissues are in extreme need of oxygen. However, in local tissue areas where the blood flow is very slow or the

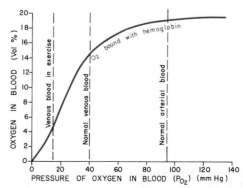

Figure 28–10. Effect of blood P_{O_2} on the quantity of oxygen bound with hemoglobin in each 100 ml of blood.

metabolic rate very high, utilization coefficients approaching 100 per cent have been recorded—that is, essentially all the oxygen is removed.

Total Rate of Oxygen Transport From the Lungs to the Tissues

If under resting conditions about 5 ml of oxygen is transported by each 100 ml of blood, and if the normal cardiac output is approximately 5000 ml per minute, the calculated total quantity of oxygen delivered to the tissues each minute is about 250 ml. This is also the amount measured by a respirometer.

This rate of oxygen transport to the tissues can be increased to about 15 times normal during heavy exercise or other instances of excessive need for oxygen (and very rarely to as high as 20 times normal in the best trained athletes). Oxygen transport can be increased to three times normal simply by an increase in the utilization coefficient, and it can be increased another fivefold as a result of increased cardiac output, thus accounting for the total 15-fold increase. Therefore, the maximum rate of oxygen transport to the tissues is about 15×250 ml, or 3750 ml per minute in the normal young adult. Special adaptations in athletic training, such as an increase in blood hemoglobin concentration and an increase in maximum cardiac output, can sometimes increase this value to as high as 4.5 to 6 liters per minute.

The Oxygen Buffer Function of Hemoglobin

Though hemoglobin is necessary for transport of oxygen to the tissues, it performs still another major function essential to life—its function as an oxygen buffer system. That is, it is the hemoglobin in the blood that mainly determines the oxygen pressure in the tissues and also keeps this pressure within a narrow controlled range. This can be explained as follows:

Under basal conditions the tissues require about 5 ml of oxygen from each 100 ml of blood passing through the tissue capillaries. Referring again to the oxygen-hemoglobin dissociation curve in Figure 28-10, one can see that for the 5 ml of oxygen to be released, the P_{O_2} must fall to about 40 mm Hg. Therefore, the tissue capillary P_{O_2} cannot rise above this 40 mm Hg level, for if that should occur, the oxygen needed by the tissues could not be released from the hemoglobin. In this way, the hemoglobin normally sets an upper limit on the gaseous pressure in the tissues at approximately 40 mm Hg.

On the other hand, in heavy exercise extra large amounts of oxygen must be delivered from the hemoglobin to the tissues. This can be achieved with very little further decrease in tissue P_{O_2} because of the steep slope of the dissociation curve—that is, a small fall in P_{O_2} causes extreme amounts of oxygen to be released from the hemoglobin. Therefore, the P_{O_2} rarely falls below 20 mm Hg.

It can be seen, then, that hemoglobin automatically delivers oxygen to the tissues at a pressure between approximately 20 and 40 mm Hg. This seems to be a wide range of P_{O_2} in the interstitial fluid, but when one considers how much the interstitial fluid P_{O_2} could theoretically change during exercise and other types of stress, this range of 20 to 40 mm Hg is relatively narrow.

This oxygen buffer function of hemoglobin is also very important when the alveolar P_{O_2} falls very low, as occurs at high altitudes, or rises very high, as occurs when one is breathing pure oxygen. Let us explain this:

It will be seen from the oxygen-hemoglobin dissociation curve in Figure 28–9 that when the alveolar P_{O_2} is decreased to as low as 60 mm Hg, which occurs at an altitude of about 2½ miles, the arterial hemoglobin is still 89 per cent saturated, only 8 per cent below the normal saturation of 97 per cent. Furthermore, the tissues still remove approximately 5 ml of oxygen from every 100 ml of blood that passes through the tissues; to remove this oxygen, the P_{O_2} of the venous blood falls to only slightly less than 40 mm Hg. Thus, a change in alveolar P_{O_2} from 104 to 60 mm Hg has almost no effect on tissue P_{O_2}.

On the other hand, when the alveolar P_{O_2} rises far above the normal value of 104 mm Hg, the maximum oxygen saturation of hemoglobin can never rise above 100 per cent. Therefore, even though the oxygen in the alveoli should rise to a partial pressure of 500 mm Hg or even more, the increase in the saturation of hemoglobin would be only 3 per cent, because even at 104 mm Hg P_{O_2}, 97 per cent of the hemoglobin is already combined with oxygen; and only a small amount of additional oxygen dissolves in the fluid of the blood, as will be discussed subsequently. Then, when the blood passes through the tissue capillaries, it still loses several milliliters of oxygen to the tissues, and this loss automatically reduces the P_{O_2} of the capillary blood to a value only a few millimeters greater than the normal 40 mm Hg.

Consequently, alveolar oxygen may vary greatly—from 60 to more than 500 mm Hg P_{O_2}—and still the P_{O_2} in the tissue does not vary more than a few millimeters from normal.

The specific properties of hemoglobin thus provide an essential role in buffering the tissue P_{O_2}, that is, keeping it always within a range that will not be lethal to the cells.

METABOLIC USE OF OXYGEN BY THE CELLS—RELATIONSHIP TO CELLULAR P_{O_2}

Only a minute level of oxygen pressure is required in the cells for normal intracellular chemical reactions to take place. The reason is that the respiratory enzyme systems of the cell, which are discussed in Chapter 45, are so geared that when the cellular P_{O_2} is more than 1 to 3 mm Hg, oxygen availability is no longer a limiting factor in the rates of the chemical reactions involving oxygen usage. Instead, a major

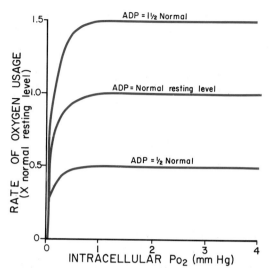

Figure 28–11. Effect of intracellular P_{O_2} on rate of oxygen usage by the cells. Note that increasing the intracellular concentration of adenosine diphosphate (ADP) increases the rate of oxygen usage.

limiting factor then is the *concentration of adenosine diphosphate* (ADP) in the cells, as was explained in Chapter 3. This effect is illustrated in Figure 28–11. Note that whenever the intracellular P_{O_2} is above 3 mm Hg, the rate of oxygen usage becomes constant for any given concentration of ADP in the cell. On the other hand, when the ADP increases, the rate of oxygen usage increases in proportion to the increase in ADP concentration.

It will be recalled from the discussion in Chapter 3 that when adenosine triphosphate (ATP) is utilized in the cells to provide energy, it is converted into ADP. The increasing concentration of ADP in turn increases the metabolic usage of oxygen and also of the various nutrients that combine with oxygen to release energy. This energy is used to re-form the ATP. Therefore, *under normal operating conditions, the rate of oxygen utilization by the cells is controlled by the rate of energy expenditure within the cells—that is, by the rate at which ADP is formed from ATP—and not by the degree of availability of oxygen to the cells.*

TRANSPORT OF OXYGEN IN THE DISSOLVED STATE

At the normal arterial P_{O_2} of 95 mm Hg, approximately 0.29 ml of oxygen is dissolved in every 100 ml of water in the blood. When the P_{O_2} of the blood falls to 40 mm Hg in the tissue capillaries, 0.12 ml of oxygen remains dissolved. In other words, 0.17 ml of oxygen is normally transported in the dissolved state to the tissues by each 100 ml of blood water. This compares with about 5.0 ml transported by the hemoglobin. Therefore, the amount of oxygen transported to the tissues in the dissolved state is normally slight, only about 3 per cent of the total as compared with the 97 per cent transported by the hemoglobin. During strenuous exercise, when hemoglobin transport of oxygen increases threefold, the relative quantity then

transported in the dissolved state falls to as little as 1.5 per cent. Yet if a person breathes oxygen at very high P_{O_2}s—at several thousand mm Hg P_{O_2}—the amount then transported in the dissolved state can become tremendous, so much so that serious excesses of oxygen occur in the tissues and "oxygen poisoning" ensues. This often leads to convulsions and even death; we discuss oxygen poisoning further in relation to high-pressure breathing in Chapter 30.

"POISONING" OF HEMOGLOBIN BY CARBON MONOXIDE

Carbon *mon*oxide combines with hemoglobin at the same point on the hemoglobin molecule as does oxygen. Furthermore, it binds with 230 times as much tenacity as oxygen. Therefore, a carbon monoxide pressure of only 0.4 mm Hg in the alveoli, 1/230 that of the alveolar oxygen, allows the carbon monoxide to compete equally with the oxygen for combination with the hemoglobin and causes half the hemoglobin in the blood to become bound to carbon monoxide instead of oxygen. And this carbon monoxide–bound hemoglobin becomes useless for transporting oxygen. A carbon monoxide pressure of 0.7 mm Hg (a concentration of about one part in a thousand in the air) can be lethal.

A person severely poisoned with carbon monoxide can be advantageously treated by the administration of pure oxygen, for oxygen at high alveolar pressures displaces carbon monoxide from combination with hemoglobin far more rapidly than can oxygen at the low pressure of atmospheric oxygen.

CHEMICAL AND PHYSICAL MEANS FOR CARRYING CARBON DIOXIDE IN THE BLOOD

Transport of carbon dioxide is not nearly so great a problem as transport of oxygen, because even in the most abnormal conditions carbon dioxide can usually be carried in the blood in far greater quantities than can oxygen. However, the amount of carbon dioxide in the blood does have much to do with the acid-base balance of the body fluids, which is discussed in detail in Chapter 26. Under normal resting conditions *an average of 4 ml of carbon dioxide is carried from the tissues to the lungs in each 100 ml of blood.*

CHEMICAL FORMS IN WHICH CARBON DIOXIDE IS CARRIED

To begin the process of carbon dioxide transport, carbon dioxide diffuses from the tissue cells to the capillaries. On entering the capillary, the chemical reactions illustrated in Figure 28–12 occur immediately. Most important, the dissolved carbon dioxide diffuses into the red blood cells, where it reacts with water to form carbonic acid. Inside the red cells an

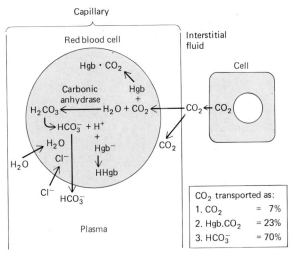

Figure 28-12. Transport of carbon dioxide in the blood.

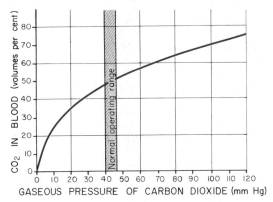

Figure 28-13. The carbon dioxide dissociation curve.

enzyme called *carbonic anhydrase* catalyzes this reaction between carbon dioxide and water, accelerating the rate of reaction about 5000-fold. Therefore, the reaction occurs almost instantaneously. The carbonic acid in turn dissociates into hydrogen ions and bicarbonate ions. The hydrogen ions combine mainly with the hemoglobin in the red cells, while many of the bicarbonate ions diffuse through the red cell membranes into the plasma. In the lungs, the exact reverse of these events occurs. About 70 per cent of the carbon dioxide is transported in this manner.

An additional one quarter of the carbon dioxide combines directly with hemoglobin to form a compound called *carbaminohemoglobin*. Since carbon dioxide dissociates from carbaminohemoglobin, this compound can release the carbon dioxide in the lungs for excretion.

Finally, a small amount of the carbon dioxide, about 7 per cent, is transported to the lungs in the dissolved form.

THE CARBON DIOXIDE DISSOCIATION CURVE

The total quantity of carbon dioxide combined with the blood in all its forms depends on the P_{CO_2}. The curve shown in Figure 28–13 depicts this dependence; this curve is called the *carbon dioxide dissociation curve*.

Note that the normal blood P_{CO_2} ranges between the limits of 40 mm Hg in arterial blood and 45 mm Hg in venous blood, which is a very narrow range. Note also that the normal concentration of carbon dioxide in the blood is about 50 ml/dl but that only 4 ml/dl of this is actually exchanged in the process of transporting carbon dioxide from the tissues to the lungs. That is, the concentration rises to about 52 ml/dl as the blood passes through the tissues, and falls to about 48 ml/dl as it passes through the lungs.

THE RESPIRATORY EXCHANGE RATIO

The discerning student will have noted that the normal amount of oxygen transported from the lungs to the tissues by each 100 ml of blood is about 5 ml, while the normal amount of carbon dioxide transported from the tissues to the lungs is about 4 ml. The ratio of carbon dioxide excretion to oxygen uptake is called the *respiratory exchange ratio* (R). That is,

$$R = \frac{\text{Rate of carbon dioxide excretion}}{\text{Rate of oxygen uptake}}$$

The value for R changes under different metabolic conditions. When a person is utilizing entirely carbohydrates for body metabolism, R rises to 1.00, because when oxygen is metabolized with carbohydrates, one molecule of carbon dioxide is formed for each molecule of oxygen consumed. But, when fats instead of carbohydrates are being metabolized, R falls to 0.7 because only 0.7 molecule of CO_2 is then formed for each molecule of O_2. This is discussed further in Chapter 47.

QUESTIONS

1. At normal respiration, approximately how long must a person breathe before half of the alveolar air is exchanged with atmospheric air?
2. What is the normal vapor pressure of the alveolar air at normal body temperature?
3. State the normal oxygen partial pressure in the alveoli. At maximum rate of breathing, how high can this rise when the person is breathing normal air at sea level?
4. What is the normal carbon dioxide concentration in the alveoli, and what are the factors that can increase or decrease this?
5. Describe the anatomy of the *respiratory unit*.

6. List the layers of the respiratory membrane. What is the average thickness of the respiratory membrane?
7. List and discuss the factors that determine how rapidly a gas will pass through the respiratory membrane.
8. Define the *diffusing capacity* of the respiratory membrane, and give approximate values for the diffusion capacity for oxygen and carbon dioxide at rest and during exercise.
9. Explain the concepts of *physiologic shunt* and *physiologic dead space*.
10. Give the approximate quantitative values for P_{O_2} in the alveoli, in the systemic arterial blood, in the interstitial fluid, and in the cells. Give the approximate quantitative values for P_{CO_2} in reverse order, from the cells back to the alveoli.
11. Draw the oxygen-hemoglobin dissociation curve, giving exact values for the scales on the abcissa and the ordinate.
12. What is meant by *utilization coefficient*? How does its value change during exercise?

13. Explain how hemoglobin buffers the interstitial fluid P_{O_2} during exercise, in conditions of low atmospheric oxygen and in conditions of high atmospheric oxygen.
14. What minimal intracellular concentration of oxygen is required to allow maximum rates of the oxygen-related metabolic reactions in the cell? When the oxygen P_{O_2} is above this minimal level, what determines the rate of oxygen utilization?
15. Explain why minute quantities of carbon monoxide can prevent the transport of oxygen to the tissues.
16. List the chemical forms in which carbon dioxide is transported from the cells to the lungs, and give the approximate proportions of the carbon dioxide transported in each form.
17. Draw the carbon dioxide dissociation curve for blood, and show the approximate normal range on this dissociation curve for transport of carbon dioxide.
18. Define the *respiratory exchange ratio*, and give its value when a person is metabolizing (1) carbohydrates and (2) fats.

References

Adamson, J. W., and Finch, C. A.: Hemoglobin function, oxygen affinity, and erythropoietin. Annu Rev Physiol 37:351, 1975.

Bartels, H., and Baumann, R.: Respiratory function of hemoglobin. Int Rev Physiol 14:107, 1977.

Bauer, C., et al., eds.: Biophysics and Physiology of Carbon Dioxide. New York, Springer-Verlag, 1980.

Cherniack, N. S., and Longobardo, G. S.: Oxygen and carbon dioxide gas stores of the body. Physiol Rev 50:196, 1970.

Forster, R. E.: CO₂: chemical, biochemical, and physiological aspects. Physiologist 13:398, 1970.

Grodins, F. S., and Yamashiro, S. M.: Optimization of the mammalian respiratory gas transport system. Annu Rev Biophys Bioeng 4:115, 1973.

Jöbsis, F. F.: Intracellular metabolism of oxygen. Am Rev Resp Dis 110:58, 1974.

Kessler, M., et al., eds.: Oxygen Supply. Baltimore, University Park Press, 1973.

Konigsberg, W.: Protein structure and molecular dysfunction: Hemoglobin. In Bondy, P. K., and Rosenberg, L. E., eds.: Metabolic Control and Disease, 8th ed. Philadelphia, W. B. Saunders Co., 1980, p. 27.

Michel, C. C.: The transport of oxygen and carbon dioxide by the blood. In MTP International Review of Science: Physiology. Vol. 2. Baltimore, University Park Press, 1974, p. 67.

Perutz, M. F.: Hemoglobin structure and respiratory transport. Sci Am 239(6):92, 1978.

Randall, D. J.: The Evolution of Air Breathing in Vertebrates. New York, Cambridge University Press, 1980.

Robin, E. D., and Simon, L. M.: Oxygen transport and cellular respiration. In Frohlich, E. D., ed.: Pathophysiology, 2nd ed. Philadelphia, J. B. Lippincott Co., 1976, p. 167.

West, J. B.: Pulmonary gas exchange. Int Rev Physiol 14:83, 1977.

Wittenberg, J. B.: Myoglobin-facilitated oxygen diffusion: Role of myoglobin in oxygen entry into muscle. Physiol Rev 50:559, 1970.

29

Regulation of Respiration and Respiratory Insufficiency

THE RESPIRATORY CENTER
   CONTROL OF OVERALL
     RESPIRATORY CENTER ACTIVITY
CHEMICAL CONTROL OF RESPIRATION
   DIRECT CHEMICAL CONTROL OF
     RESPIRATORY CENTER ACTIVITY BY
     CARBON DIOXIDE AND
     HYDROGEN IONS
THE PERIPHERAL CHEMORECEPTOR
  SYSTEM FOR CONTROL OF
  RESPIRATORY ACTIVITY—ROLE OF
  OXYGEN IN RESPIRATORY CONTROL
REGULATION OF RESPIRATION DURING
  EXERCISE
ABNORMALITIES OF RESPIRATORY
  CONTROL

RESPIRATORY CENTER DEPRESSION
PERIODIC BREATHING
PATHOPHYSIOLOGY OF RESPIRATORY
  INSUFFICIENCY IN COMMON
  RESPIRATORY DISEASES
  CHRONIC PULMONARY EMPHYSEMA
  PNEUMONIA
  ATELECATASIS
  ASTHMA
  TUBERCULOSIS
  CYANOSIS
  DYSPNEA
OXYGEN THERAPY IN DIFFERENT TYPES
  OF HYPOXIA

The nervous system adjusts the rate of alveolar ventilation almost exactly to the demands of the body so that the blood oxygen pressure (P_{O_2}) and carbon dioxide pressure (P_{CO_2}) are hardly altered even during strenuous exercise or other types of respiratory stress.

The first section of the present chapter describes the operation of this neurogenic system for regulation of respiration.

THE RESPIRATORY CENTER

The "respiratory center" is composed of several widely dispersed groups of neurons located *bilaterally* in the medulla oblongata and pons, as illustrated in Figure 29–1. It is divided into three major collections of neurons: (1) a *dorsal respiratory group*, located in the dorsal portion of the medulla, which mainly causes inspiration, (2) a *ventral respiratory group*, located in the ventrolateral part of the medulla, which can cause either expiration or inspiration depending upon which neurons in the group are stimulated, and (3) the *pneumotaxic center*, located in the superior portion of the pons, which helps control both the rate and pattern of breathing. The dorsal respiratory group of neurons plays the fundamental role in the control of respiration. Therefore, let us discuss its function first.

The Dorsal Respiratory Group of Neurons

The dorsal respiratory group of neurons extends approximately the entire length of the medulla. Either all or most of its neurons are located within the *tractus solitarius*, though additional neurons in the adjacent reticular substance of the medulla probably also play important roles in respiratory control. The nucleus of the tractus solitarius is also the sensory termination of both the vagal and glossopharyngeal

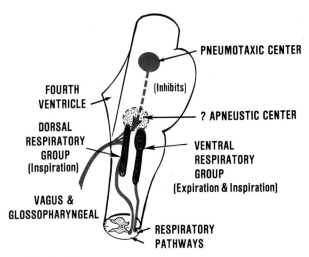

Figure 29–1. Organization of the respiratory center.

nerves, which transmit sensory signals into the respiratory center from the peripheral chemoreceptors, the baroreceptors, and several different types of receptors in the lung. All the signals from these peripheral areas help in the control of respiration.

The Inspiratory Function of the Dorsal Respiratory Group of Neurons. Stimulation of the neurons in the dorsal respiratory group always causes inspiration, never expiration. However, it will be recalled that normal quiet respiration is caused almost entirely, if not entirely, by contraction of the inspiratory muscles, especially the diaphragm. Then expiration is caused passively by elastic recoil of the distended chest and lungs.

Rhythmical Inspiratory Discharges from the Dorsal Respiratory Group. The basic rhythm of respiration is generated in the dorsal respiratory group of neurons. Unfortunately, though, the basic cause of the repetitive rhythmic discharges is still unknown. In primitive animals, neural networks have been found in which activity of one set of neurons excites a second set, which in turn inhibits the first. Then after a period of time the mechanism repeats itself, continuing throughout the life of the animal. Therefore, most respiratory physiologists believe that some similar network of neurons located within the medulla, probably involving not only the dorsal respiratory group but adjacent areas of the medulla as well, is responsible for the basic rhythm of respiration.

The Inspiratory Ramp Signal. The nervous signal that is transmitted to the inspiratory muscles is not an instantaneous burst of action potentials. Instead, in normal respiration, it increases steadily in a ramp (gradual) fashion for about 2 seconds. Then it abruptly ceases for approximately the next 3 seconds, then begins again for another cycle, repeating indefinitely. Thus, the inspiratory signal is said to be a *ramp signal*. The obvious advantage is that it causes a steady increase in the volume of the lungs during inspiration rather than inspiratory gasps.

There are two ways in which the inspiratory ramp is controlled:

(1) Control of the rate of increase of the ramp signal, so that during very active respiration the ramp increases rapidly and therefore fills the lungs rapidly as well.

(2) Control of the limiting point at which the ramp suddenly ceases. This is the usual method for controlling the rate of respiration; that is, the earlier the ramp ceases the shorter the duration of inspiration, and this also shortens the duration of expiration. Thus, the rate of respiration is increased.

The Pneumotaxic Center—Its Function in Limiting the Duration of Inspiration and Increasing Respiratory Rate

The pneumotaxic center, located in the *nucleus parabrachialis* of the upper pons, transmits impulses continuously to the inspiratory area. The effect of these is to control the "switch-off" point of the inspiratory ramp, thus controlling the duration of the filling phase of the lung cycle. When the pneumotaxic signals are strong, inspiration may last for as little as 0.5 second, but when weak, the inspiratory ramp may continue for perhaps as long as 5 to 10 seconds, thus filling the lungs with a great excess of air.

Therefore, the function of the pneumotaxic center is primarily to limit inspiration. However, this has a secondary effect on the rate of breathing because limitation of inspiration also shortens the entire period of respiration. Thus, a strong pneumotaxic signal can increase the rate of breathing up to 30 to 40 breaths per minute, whereas a weak pneumotaxic signal may reduce the rate to only a few breaths per minute.

Limitation of Inspiration by Lung Inflation Signals—The Hering-Breuer Inflation Reflex

Located in the walls of the bronchi and bronchioles throughout the lungs are *stretch receptors* that transmit signals through the *vagi* into the dorsal respiratory group of neurons when the lungs become overstretched. These signals affect inspiration in much the same way as signals from the pneumotaxic center; that is, they limit the duration of inspiration. Therefore, when the lungs begin to be overly inflated, the stretch receptors activate an appropriate feedback response that "switches-off" the inspiratory ramp and thus limits further inspiration. This is called the *Hering-Breuer inflation reflex*. This reflex also increases the rate of respiration because of the reduced period of inspiration, the same as is true for signals from the pneumotoxic center.

The Ventral Respiratory Group of Neurons—Its Function in Both Inspiration and Expiration

Located about 5 mm anterior and lateral to the dorsal respiratory group of neurons is still another group, the *ventral respiratory group,* that is important during more active breathing. These neurons, like the dorsal respiratory group, also are present in the entire length of the medulla. The function of this area differs from that of the dorsal respiratory group in several important ways:

(1) The neurons of the ventral respiratory group remain almost totally inactive during normal quiet respiration. Furthermore, there is no evidence that the ventral respiratory neurons participate in the basic rhythmic oscillation that controls respiration.

(2) When the respiratory drive for increased pulmonary ventilation becomes greater than normal, respiratory signals then spill over into the ventral respiratory neurons from the basic oscillating mechanism of the dorsal respiratory area. As a consequence, the ventral respiratory area then contributes its share to the respiratory drive as well.

(3) Electrical stimulation of some of the neurons in the ventral group causes inspiration whereas stimulation of others causes expiration. Therefore, these neurons contribute to both inspiration and expiration. However, they are especially important in providing the powerful expiratory forces during expiration. Thus, this area operates more or less as an overdrive mechanism when high levels of pulmonary ventilation are required.

An Apneustic Center in the Lower Pons

To add to the confusion of our knowledge about respiratory center function, there is another strange center in the lower part of the pons, called the *apneustic center.* Under certain conditions, the apneustic center sends signals to the dorsal respiratory group of neurons to prevent the "switch-off" of the inspiratory ramp signal. Therefore, the ramp continues for as long as 10 to 20 seconds, thus greatly overfilling the lungs. Consequently, the lungs become inflated near maximum, and only occasional short expiratory gasps occur.

The function of the apneustic center might be to provide extra drive to inspiration, but the pneumotaxic center and the stretch signals from the vagi normally override this excessive inspiratory drive and therefore allow normal respiration.

CONTROL OF OVERALL RESPIRATORY CENTER ACTIVITY

Up to this point we have discussed the basic mechanisms for causing inspiration and expiration, but it is also important to know how the respiratory center activity is controlled to match the ventilatory needs of the body. For example, during very heavy exercise, the rates of oxygen utilization and carbon dioxide formation are often increased to as much as 20 times normal, requiring commensurate increases in pulmonary ventilation. This is achieved in two different ways:

(1) By feedback excitation of respiratory center activity in response to changes in chemical composi-

tion of the blood, especially its concentrations of carbon dioxide, hydrogen ions, and oxygen.

(2) By excitatory signals from other parts of the nervous system; such signals are especially important during exercise.

The major purpose of the remainder of this chapter is to discuss this control of ventilation in response to the needs of the body.

CHEMICAL CONTROL OF RESPIRATION

The ultimate goal of respiration is to maintain proper concentrations of oxygen, carbon dioxide, and hydrogen ions in the body fluid. It is fortunate, therefore, that respiratory activity is highly responsive to changes in each one of these.

Excess carbon dioxide or hydrogen ions affect respiration mainly by excitatory effects on the respiratory center itself, causing greatly increased strength of both the inspiratory and expiratory signals to the respiratory muscles. The resulting increase in ventilation increases the elimination of carbon dioxide from the blood; this also removes hydrogen ions from the blood because decreased carbon dioxide decreases the blood carbonic acid.

Oxygen, on the other hand, does not have a significant *direct* effect on the respiratory center of the brain in controlling respiration. Instead, it acts either entirely or almost entirely on peripheral chemoreceptors located in the carotid and aortic bodies, and these in turn transmit appropriate nervous signals to the respiratory center for control of respiration.

Let us discuss first the stimulation of the respiratory center itself by carbon dioxide and hydrogen ions.

DIRECT CHEMICAL CONTROL OF RESPIRATORY CENTER ACTIVITY BY CARBON DIOXIDE AND HYDROGEN IONS

The Chemosensitive Area of the Respiratory Center. Thus far, we have discussed mainly three different areas of the respiratory center: the dorsal respiratory group of neurons, the ventral respiratory group, and the pneumotaxic center. However, it is believed that none of these are affected directly by changes in blood carbon dioxide concentration or hydrogen ion concentration. Instead, a very sensitive *chemosensitive* area, illustrated in Figure 29–2, is located bilaterally only a few microns beneath the surface of the medulla ventral to the entry of the glossopharyngeal and vagal nerves into the medulla. This area is highly sensitive to changes in either blood CO_2 or hydrogen ion concentration, and it in turn excites the other portions of the respiratory center. It has especially potent effects on increasing the degree of activity of the inspiratory center, increasing both the rate of rise of the inspiratory ramp signal and also the intensity of the signal. This in turn has an automatic secondary

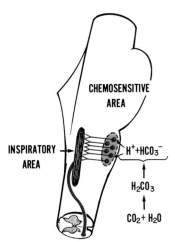

Figure 29–2. Stimulation of the inspiratory area by the *chemosensitive area* located bilaterally in the medulla, lying only a few microns beneath the ventral medullary surface. Note also that hydrogen ions stimulate the chemosensitive area, whereas mainly carbon dioxide in the fluid gives rise to the hydrogen ions.

effect of increasing the frequency of the respiratory rhythm.

Response of the Chemosensitive Neurons to Hydrogen Ions—The Primary Stimulus

The sensor neurons in the chemosensitive area are especially excited by hydrogen ions; in fact, it is believed that hydrogen ions are perhaps the only important direct stimulus for these neurons. Unfortunately, though, hydrogen ions do not easily cross either the blood-brain barrier or the blood–cerebrospinal fluid barrier. For this reason, changes in hydrogen ion concentration in the blood actually have considerably less effect in stimulating the chemosensitive neurons than do changes in carbon dioxide, even though carbon dioxide stimulates these neurons indirectly, as will be explained below.

Effect of Blood Carbon Dioxide on Stimulating the Chemosensitive Area

Though carbon dioxide has very little direct effect to stimulate the neurons in the chemosensitive area, it does have a very potent indirect effect. It does this by reacting with the water of the tissues to form carbonic acid. This in turn dissociates into hydrogen and bicarbonate ions; the hydrogen ions then have a potent direct stimulatory effect. These effects are illustrated in Figure 29–2.

But, why is it that blood CO_2 has a more potent effect to stimulate the chemosensitive neurons than do blood hydrogen ions? The answer is that hydrogen ions, as noted above, pass through both the blood-brain barrier and the blood-cerebrospinal fluid barrier only very poorly whereas carbon dioxide diffuses through both these barriers almost as if they did not exist. Consequently, whenever the blood carbon dioxide concentration increases, so also does the P_{CO_2} in

both the interstitial fluid of the medulla and also in the cerebrospinal fluid. And, in both of these fluids the carbon dioxide immediately reacts with the water to form hydrogen ions. Thus, paradoxically, more hydrogen ions appear in the neurons of the respiratory chemosensitive sensory area when the blood carbon dioxide concentration increases than when the blood hydrogen ion concentration increases. For this reason, respiratory center activity is affected considerably more by changes in blood carbon dioxide than by changes in blood hydrogen ions.

Quantitative Effects of Blood P_{CO_2} and Hydrogen Ion Concentration on Alveolar Ventilation

Figure 29–3 illustrates quantitatively the approximate effects of blood P_{CO_2} and blood pH (which is an inverse measure of hydrogen ion concentration) on alveolar ventilation. Note the marked increase in ventilation caused by the increase in P_{CO_2}. But note also the much smaller effect of decreased pH (that is, increased hydrogen ion concentration).

Finally, note that this *difference* in stimulation of ventilation is especially great in the normal P_{CO_2} and pH ranges: P_{CO_2}s between 30 and 50 mm Hg and pHs between 7.5 and 7.3. Therefore, from a practical point, changes in blood carbon dioxide play by far the greater role in the normal minute-by-minute control of pulmonary ventilation than do changes in pH.

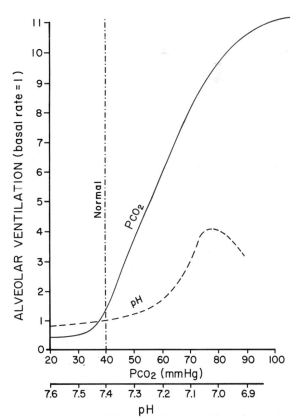

Figure 29–3. Effects of increased arterial P_{CO_2} and decreased arterial pH on the rate of alveolar ventilation.

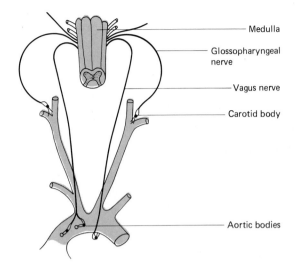

Figure 29–4. Respiratory control by the carotid and aortic bodies.

Value of Carbon Dioxide as a Regulator of Alveolar Ventilation. Since carbon dioxide is one of the end-products of metabolism, its concentration in the body fluids greatly affects the chemical reactions of all cells and also affects the tissue pH. For these reasons, the tissue fluid PCO_2 must be regulated exactly, and, as pointed out in the preceding chapter, the respiratory system is the only effective means that the body has to control the blood and tissue PCO_2. Therefore, stimulation of the respiratory center by carbon dioxide provides the necessary feedback mechanism for regulation of the concentration of carbon dioxide throughout the body.

THE PERIPHERAL CHEMORECEPTOR SYSTEM FOR CONTROL OF RESPIRATORY ACTIVITY—ROLE OF OXYGEN IN RESPIRATORY CONTROL

Aside from the direct sensitivity of the respiratory center itself to CO_2 and hydrogen ions, special chemical receptors called *chemoreceptors,* located outside the central nervous system, are also responsive to changes in oxygen, carbon dioxide, and hydrogen ion concentrations. These transmit signals to the respiratory center to help regulate respiratory activity.

The chemoreceptors are located in the *carotid* and *aortic bodies,* which are illustrated in Figure 29–4 along with their nerve connections to the respiratory center. The *carotid bodies* are located bilaterally in the bifurcations of the common carotid arteries, and their nerve fibers pass through *Hering's nerves* to the *glossopharyngeal nerves* and thence to the dorsal respiratory area of the medulla. The *aortic bodies* are located along the arch of the aorta; their nerve fibers pass through the *vagi* to the dorsal respiratory area. Each of these chemoreceptor bodies receives a special blood supply through a minute artery directly from the adjacent arterial trunk.

Stimulation of the Chemoreceptors by Decreased Arterial Oxygen. When the oxygen concentration in the arterial blood falls below normal, the chemoreceptors become strongly stimulated. This effect is illustrated in Figure 29–5, which shows the relationship between *arterial* PO_2 and rate of nerve impulse transmission from a carotid body. Note that the impulse rate is particularly sensitive to changes in arterial PO_2 in the range between 60 and 30 mm Hg, which is the range in which the arterial hemoglobin saturation with oxygen decreases rapidly.

Effect of Carbon Dioxide and Hydrogen Ion Concentration on Chemoreceptor Activity. An increase in either carbon dioxide concentration or hydrogen ion concentration also excites the chemoreceptors and in this way indirectly increases respiratory activity. However, the direct effects of both these factors in the respiratory center itself are so much more powerful than their effects mediated through the chemoreceptors that for most practical purposes the indirect effects through the chemoreceptors do not need to be considered. In the case of oxygen, on the other hand, this is not true because diminished oxygen in the arterial blood can affect the respiration significantly *only* by acting through the chemoreceptors.

Quantitative Effect of Low Blood PO_2 on Alveolar Ventilation

Low blood PO_2 normally will not increase alveolar ventilation significantly until the alveolar PO_2 falls almost to one half normal. This is illustrated in Figure 29–6. The lowermost curve of this figure shows that changing the alveolar arterial PO_2 from the normal value of slightly more than 100 mm Hg down to about 60 mm Hg has an imperceptible effect on ventilation. But, then, as the PO_2 falls from 60 mm Hg, down to 40 and then to 30 mm Hg, alveolar ventilation increases 1.5- to 1.7-fold. However, contrast this feeble increase in alveolar ventilation to the fourfold increase caused by decreasing blood pH or the elevenfold increase caused by increasing the PCO_2. Thus, it is clear that the effect of changes in blood PO_2 on respiratory activity is usually very slight, especially when compared with the effect of PCO_2.

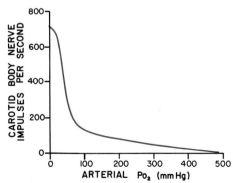

Figure 29–5. Effect of arterial PO_2 on impulse rate from the carotid body of a cat. (Curve drawn from data from several sources, but primarily from Von Euler.)

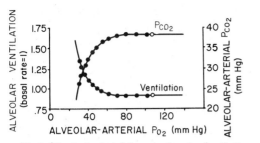

Figure 29–6. Effect of arterial P_{O_2} on alveolar ventilation and on the subsequent decrease in arterial P_{CO_2}. (From Gray: Pulmonary Ventilation and Its Physiological Regulation. Courtesy of Charles C Thomas, Publisher, Springfield, Illinois.)

Cause of the Poor Response of Respiration to Low P_{O_2}—The Opposing Effects of the P_{CO_2} and pH Regulatory Mechanisms. The cause of the poor effect of P_{O_2} changes on respiratory control is *opposition* caused by *both* the carbon dioxide and the hydrogen ion control mechanisms. This phenomenon can be explained by referring again to Figure 29–6. The increase in ventilation that does occur when the P_{O_2} falls blows off carbon dioxide from the blood and therefore decreases the P_{CO_2}, which is also illustrated in the figure; at the same time it also decreases the hydrogen ion concentration. Therefore, two powerful respiratory inhibitory effects are caused: (a) diminished carbon dioxide and (b) diminished hydrogen ions. These two exert inhibitory effects that oppose the excitatory effect of the diminished oxygen. As a result, they keep the decreased oxygen from causing a marked increase in ventilation until the P_{O_2} falls to 20 to 40 mm Hg, a range that is incompatible with life for more than a few minutes. Therefore, the maximum effect of decreased alveolar oxygen on alveolar ventilation, in the range compatible with life, is normally only about a 66 per cent (1.66-fold) increase.

Conditions Under Which Diminished Oxygen Does Play a Major Role in the Regulation of Respiration. In pneumonia, emphysema, and other lung ailments in which gases are not readily exchanged between the atmosphere and the pulmonary blood, the oxygen regulatory system *does* then play a major role in the regulation of respiration. Contrary to the normal effect, the increased ventilation then caused by oxygen lack is not followed by reduced arterial P_{CO_2} and hydrogen ion concentration, because the pulmonary disease also diminishes carbon dioxide exchange as well as oxygen exchange. Instead, the CO_2 either remains constant or builds up in the blood, and the hydrogen ion concentration behaves similarly. Therefore, the opposition effects of these other two control systems on the oxygen lack system are absent. As a result, the oxygen lack stimulation develops its full power and can increase alveolar ventilation as much as five- to sevenfold.

Effects of the Oxygen Lack Mechanism at High Altitudes. When a person first ascends to high altitudes (or in any other way is exposed to a rarefied atmosphere), the diminished oxygen in the air stimulates the oxygen lack control system of respiration. The respiration at first increases to a maximum of about 66 per cent above normal, which is a comparatively slight increase. Once again, the cause of this slight increase is the tremendous opposition effects of the carbon dioxide and hydrogen ion control mechanisms on the oxygen lack mechanism.

However, over several days, the respiratory center gradually becomes "adapted" to the diminished carbon dioxide, so that most of its opposition effect to the oxygen control is gradually lost, and alveolar ventilation then rises to as high as five to seven times normal. This is part of the acclimatization that occurs as a person slowly ascends a mountain, thus allowing the person to adjust respiration gradually to a level fitted for the higher altitude.

Why Oxygen Regulation of Respiration Is Not Normally Needed. On first thought, it seems strange that oxygen should play so small a role in the normal regulation of respiration, particularly since one of the primary functions of the respiratory center is to provide adequate intake of oxygen. However, oxygen control of respiration is not needed under most normal circumstances for the following reason:

The respiratory system ordinarily maintains an alveolar P_{O_2} actually *higher* than the level needed to saturate almost completely the hemoglobin of the arterial blood. It does not matter whether alveolar ventilation is normal or ten times normal, the blood will still be essentially fully saturated. Also, alveolar ventilation can decrease to as low as one half normal, and the blood still remains within 10 per cent of complete saturation. Therefore, one can see that alveolar ventilation can change tremendously without significantly affecting oxygen transport to the tissues.

On the other hand, changes in alveolar ventilation do have a tremendous effect on both blood and tissue carbon dioxide concentration, as was explained earlier in the chapter. Therefore, it is exceedingly important that carbon dioxide—not oxygen—be the major controller of respiration under normal conditions.

REGULATION OF RESPIRATION DURING EXERCISE

In strenuous exercise, oxygen utilization and carbon dioxide formation can increase as much as twentyfold, which is illustrated in Figure 29–7. Even so, alveolar ventilation ordinarily increases almost exactly in step with the increased level of metabolism as illustrated by Figure 29–8, which shows the increase in ventilation that occurs when oxygen consumption increases during exercise. Therefore, the blood P_{O_2}, P_{CO_2}, and pH all remain *almost exactly normal* despite the heavy exercise.

In trying to analyze the factors that cause increased ventilation during exercise, one is tempted immediately to ascribe this to chemical alterations in the

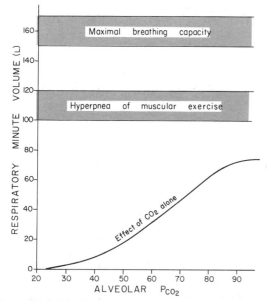

Figure 29–7. Relationship of hyperpnea caused by muscular exercise to that caused by increased alveolar P_{CO_2}. (Modified and reproduced from Comroe J. H., Jr.: THE LUNG: Clinical Physiology and Pulmonary Function Tests, 2nd edition. Copyright © 1962 by Year Book Medical Publishers, Inc., Chicago.)

body fluids during exercise. However, this is not valid, for measurements of arterial P_{CO_2}, pH, and P_{O_2} show that none of these usually changes significantly and certainly not enough to account for more than a small percentage of the increase in ventilation.

Therefore, the question must be asked: What is it during exercise that causes the intense increase in ventilation? This question has not been answered, but at least two different effects, illustrated in Figure 29–9, seem to be predominantly concerned:

1. The brain, on transmitting impulses to the contracting muscles, is believed to transmit collateral impulses into the brain stem to excite the respiratory center. This is analogous to the stimulatory effect of the higher centers of the brain on the vasomotor center of the brain stem during exercise, causing a rise in arterial pressure as well as an increase in ventilation.

2. During exercise, the body movements, especially of the limbs, are believed to increase pulmonary ventilation by exciting joint proprioceptors that then transmit excitatory impulses to the respiratory center. The reason for believing this is that even passive movements of the limbs often increase pulmonary ventilation severalfold.

It is possible that still other factors are also important in increasing pulmonary ventilation during exercise. For instance, some experiments even suggest that hypoxia developing in the muscles during exercise elicits afferent nerve signals to the respiratory center to excite respiration. However, since the increase in ventilation begins immediately upon the initiation of exercise, most of the increase in respiration probably results from the two neurogenic factors noted above, namely *stimulatory impulses from*

the higher centers of the brain and *proprioceptive stimulatory reflexes.*

When a person exercises, usually the nervous factors stimulate the respiratory center almost exactly the proper amount to supply the extra oxygen requirements for the exercise and to blow off the extra carbon dioxide. But, occasionally, the nervous signals are either too strong or too weak in their stimulation of the respiratory center. Only under these conditions do the chemical factors play a significant role in bringing about the final adjustment in respiration required to keep the carbon dioxide and hydrogen ion concentrations of the body fluids as nearly normal as possible.

ABNORMALITIES OF RESPIRATORY CONTROL

RESPIRATORY CENTER DEPRESSION

Cerebrovascular Disease. Probably the most common cause of long-term respiratory center depression is cerebrovascular disease in older-aged patients, especially following vascular occlusions or hemorrhages that damage the respiratory center areas. In such instances, a person may have chronically elevated arterial P_{CO_2}s and depressed P_{O_2}s.

Clinical Measurement of Respiratory Center Depression. In the clinical pulmonary function laboratory, the degree of respiratory center depression is frequently measured by the simple maneuver of having the patient breathe carbon dioxide at successively increasing concentrations. Then, from measurements of alveolar P_{CO_2} and alveolar ventilation, a *carbon dioxide–alveolar ventilation stimulation curve*, similar to that illustrated in Figure 29–3, is plotted. The degree of respiratory center depression is ascertained by comparing the slope of the carbon dioxide stimulation curve with that of the normal curve, assuming, of course, that all other aspects of pulmonary function are normal.

Acute Brain Edema. The activity of the respiratory center may be depressed or even totally inactivated

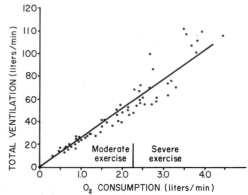

Figure 29–8. Effect of exercise on oxygen consumption and ventilatory rate. (From Gray: Pulmonary Ventilation and Its Physiological Regulation. Courtesy of Charles C Thomas, Publisher, Springfield, Illinois.)

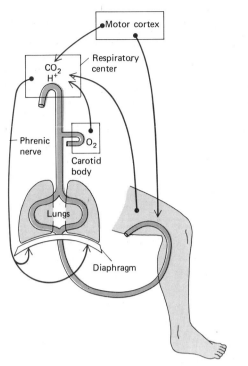

Figure 29–9. The different factors that enter into regulation of respiration during exercise.

by acute brain edema resulting from brain *concussion.* For instance, the head might be struck against some solid object, following which the damaged brain tissues swell, compressing the cerebral arteries against the cranial vault and thus totally or partially blocking the cerebral blood supply. As a result, the neurons of the respiratory center first become inactive and later die. In this manner brain edema may either depress or totally inactivate the respiratory center.

Occasionally, respiratory depression resulting from brain edema can be relieved temporarily by intravenous injection of hypertonic solutions such as highly concentrated mannitol solution. These solutions osmotically remove some of the intracellular fluids of the brain, thus relieving intracranial pressure and sometimes re-establishing respiration within a few minutes.

Anesthesia. Perhaps the most prevalent cause of respiratory depression and respiratory arrest is overdosage of anesthetics or narcotics. The best agent to be used for anesthesia is one that depresses the respiratory center the least while depressing the cerebral cortex the most. Ether is among the best of the anesthetics by these criteria, though halothane, cyclopropane, ethylene, nitrous oxide, and a few others have almost the same value. On the other hand, sodium pentobarbital is a poor anesthetic because it depresses the respiratory center considerably more than the above-mentioned agents. At one time, morphine was used as an anesthetic, but this drug is now used only as an adjunct to anesthetics because it greatly depresses the respiratory center.

PERIODIC BREATHING

An abnormality of respiration called *periodic breathing* occurs in a number of different disease conditions. The person breathes deeply for a short interval of time and then breathes slightly or not at all for an additional interval, the cycle repeating itself over and over again.

The most common type of periodic breathing, *Cheyne-Stokes breathing,* is characterized by slowly increasing and then decreasing respiration, occurring over and over again every 45 seconds to 3 minutes. The basic mechanism of this is the following:

Let us assume that the respiration becomes much more rapid and deeper than usual. This causes the P_{CO_2} in the pulmonary blood to *decrease.* A few seconds later the pulmonary blood reaches the brain, and the decreased P_{CO_2} inhibits respiration. As a result, the pulmonary blood P_{CO_2} now begins to *increase.* After another few seconds the blood carrying the increased CO_2 arrives at the respiratory center and stimulates respiration again, thus making the person overbreathe once again and initiating a new cycle of depressed respiration; and the cycles thus continue on and on, causing Cheyne-Stokes periodic breathing.

In the normal person, the respiratory control system is stable enough to prevent Cheyne-Stokes breathing, but a number of different abnormal conditions can overcome the stability of the feedback mechanisms and cause it to oscillate spontaneously. Two of these are (1) increased delay time in the flow of blood from the lungs to the brain, often caused by a weak heart and sluggish pumping of blood to the brain; and (2) abnormal feedback gain of the respiratory center mechanisms for control of respiration, usually caused by poor blood supply to portions of the respiratory center, which makes the center activity shut off entirely for short intervals of time until the buildup of CO_2 in the center periodically reactivates it.

PATHOPHYSIOLOGY OF RESPIRATORY INSUFFICIENCY IN COMMON RESPIRATORY DISEASES

CHRONIC PULMONARY EMPHYSEMA

The term *pulmonary emphysema* literally means excess air in the lungs. However, chronic pulmonary emphysema is a destructive process of the lungs, caused in all but a few of the patients by tobacco smoking. It results principally from *chronic infection* caused by inhaling smoke or other substances that irritate the bronchi and bronchioles. The principal reason for the chronic infection is that the irritant seriously deranges the normal protective mechanisms of the airways, including (a) partial paralysis of the cilia of the respiratory epithelium so that mucus cannot be moved easily out of the passageways, (b)

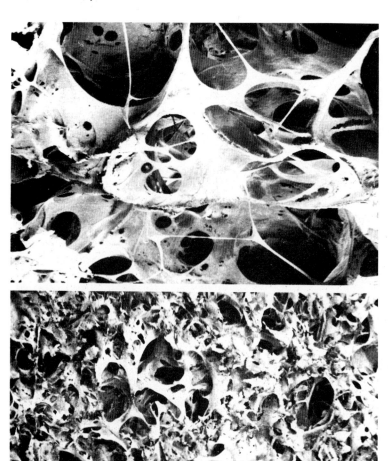

Figure 29–10. Contrast of the emphysematous lung (above) with the normal lung (below), showing extensive alveolar destruction. (Reproduced with permission of Patricia Delaney and the Department of Anatomy, The Medical College of Wisconsin.)

stimulation of excess mucus secretion, which further exacerbates the condition, and (c) inhibition of the alveolar macrophages so that they become less effective in combating infection.

The upper panel of Figure 29–10 illustrates an emphysematous lung compared with the normal lung in the lower panel. Note especially that as much as four fifths of the alveolar walls have been destroyed by the infection. In addition, many of the bronchioles have been partially or totally blocked by the infectious process.

The physiological effects of chronic emphysema are extremely varied, depending on the severity of the disease and on the relative degree of bronchiolar obstruction versus lung parenchymal destruction. However, among the different abnormalities are the following:

First, progressive bronchiolar obstruction greatly *increases airway resistance* and results in vastly increased work of breathing. It is especially difficult for the person to move air through the bronchioles during expiration because the compressive force on the outside of the lung not only compresses the alveoli but also compresses the bronchioles, which further increases their resistance during expiration.

Second, the marked loss of lung parenchyma greatly *decreases the diffusing capacity* of the lung, which reduces the ability of the lungs to oxygenate the blood and to remove carbon dioxide.

Third, the obstructive process is frequently much worse in some parts of the lungs than in other parts so that some portions of the lungs are well ventilated while other portions are poorly ventilated. This often causes *extremely abnormal ventilation-perfusion ratios*, with a *physiological shunt* in some parts resulting in poor aeration of the blood, and a *physiological dead space* in other parts resulting in wasted ventilation, both of these occurring in the same lungs. These effects greatly diminish the transport of gases between the alveoli and the blood, as discussed in the preceding chapter.

Fourth, loss of large portions of the lung parenchyma also decreases the number of pulmonary capillaries through which blood can pass. As a result, the pulmonary vascular resistance increases markedly, causing *pulmonary hypertension*. This in turn overloads the right heart and frequently causes right-heart failure.

Chronic emphysema usually progresses slowly over many years. The person develops hypoxia and hypercapnia (excess CO_2 in the body fluids) because of hypoventilation of many alveoli and because of loss of lung parenchyma. The net result of all of these effects is severe and prolonged air hunger that can last for years until the hypoxia and hypercapnia cause death—a very high penalty to pay for smoking.

PNEUMONIA

The term pneumonia describes any inflammatory condition of the lung in which the alveoli are usually filled with fluid and blood cells. A common type of pneumonia is *bacterial pneumonia,* caused most frequently by pneumococci. This disease begins with infection in the alveoli; the pulmonary membrane becomes inflamed and highly porous so that fluid and even red and white blood cells pass out of the blood into the alveoli. Thus, the infected alveoli become progressively filled with fluid and cells, and the infection spreads by extension of bacteria from alveolus to alveolus. Eventually, large areas of the lungs, sometimes whole lobes or even a whole lung, become "consolidated," which means that they are filled with fluid and cellular debris.

The pulmonary function of the lungs during pneumonia changes in different stages of the disease. In the early stages, the pneumonia process might well be localized to only one lung, and alveolar ventilation may be reduced even though blood flow through the lung continues normally. This results in two major pulmonary abnormalities: (1) reduction in the total available surface area of the respiratory membrane and (2) decreased ventilation-perfusion ratio. Both these effects cause reduced diffusing capacity, which results in hypoxemia (poor oxygenation of the blood).

ATELECTASIS

Atelectasis means collapse of the alveoli. It can occur in a localized area of a lung, in an entire lobe, or in an entire lung. Its most common causes are twofold: (1) obstruction of the airway, or (2) lack of surfactant in the fluids lining the alveoli.

Airway Obstruction. The airway obstruction type of atelectasis usually results from (a) blockage of many small bronchi with mucus or (b) obstruction of a major bronchus by either a large mucous plug or some solid object such as cancer. The air entrapped beyond the block is absorbed within minutes to hours by the blood flowing in the pulmonary capillaries. If the lung tissue is pliable enough, this will lead simply to collapse of the alveoli. However, if the lung tissue cannot collapse, absorption of air from the alveoli creates tremendously negative pressures within the alveoli and pulls fluid out of the pulmonary interstitium into the alveoli, thus causing the alveoli to fill completely with edema fluid. Collapse of the lung tissue not only occludes the alveoli but also increases the resistance to blood flow through the pulmonary vessels. This resistance increase occurs partially because of the collapse itself, which compresses and folds the vessels as the volume of the lung decreases. But, in addition, hypoxia in the collapsed alveoli causes additional vasoconstriction, as was explained in Chapter 12.

Because of the vascular constriction, blood flow through the atelectatic lung becomes slight. Most of the blood is routed through the ventilated lung and therefore becomes well aerated. As a result, the overall ventilation-perfusion ratio is only moderately compromised, so that the aortic blood has only mild oxygen desaturation.

Lack of Surfactant. In Chapter 27 it was pointed out that the substance surfactant is secreted by the alveolar epithelium into the fluids that line the alveoli. This substance decreases the surface tension in the alveoli two- to tenfold. In the normal lung this plays a major role in preventing alveolar collapse. However, in a number of different conditions the quantity of surfactant secreted by the alveoli is greatly decreased. Sometimes this is severe enough to cause atelectasis. For instance, in the condition called *hyaline membrane disease* or *respiratory distress syndrome,* which often occurs in newborn babies, the quantity of surfactant secreted by the alveoli is greatly depressed. This effect causes a serious tendency for the lungs of these babies to collapse, or to become filled with fluid as explained earlier; many of the infants die of suffocation as increasing portions of the lungs become atelectatic.

ASTHMA

Asthma is characterized by spastic contraction of the bronchioles, which causes extremely difficult breathing. It occurs in about 3 per cent of all persons at some time in life. The usual cause is hypersensitivity of the bronchioles to foreign substances in the air. In younger patients, under the age of 30 years, the asthma in about 70 per cent is caused by *allergic hypersensitivity,* especially sensitivity to plant pollens. In older persons, the cause in about 70 per cent is hypersensitivity to nonallergic types of irritants in the air, such as irritants in smog.

The allergic reaction that occurs in the allergic type of asthma is believed to occur in the following way: The typically allergic person has a tendency to form an abnormal type of antibody called IgE, and these antibodies cause allergic reactions when they react with their complementary antigens as was explained in Chapter 20. In asthma, these abnormal antibodies are mainly attached to mast cells that lie in the lung interstitium in close association with the bronchioles and small bronchi. Then when the person breathes a pollen to which he or she is sensitive (that is, to which the person has developed IgE antibodies), the pollen reacts with the mast cell–attached antibodies and causes these cells to release several different substances. Among them are *histamine, slow-reacting substance of anaphylaxis, eosinophilic chemotactic factor,* and *bradykinin.* The combined effects of all these factors, especially of the slow-reacting substance of anaphylaxis, are to produce (1) localized edema in the walls of the small bronchioles as well as secretion of thick mucus into the bronchiolar lumens, and (2) spasm of the bronchiolar smooth muscle. Obviously, therefore, the airway resistance increases greatly.

The bronchiolar diameter becomes more reduced during expiration than during inspiration in asthma. The reason for this is that the increased intrapulmonary pressure during expiratory effort not only compresses the air in the alveoli but compresses the outsides of the bronchioles as well. Therefore, the asthmatic person usually can inspire quite adequately but has great difficulty expiring.

The functional residual capacity and the residual volume of the lung become greatly increased during the asthmatic attack because of the difficulty in expiring air from the lungs. Over a long period of time the chest cage becomes permanently enlarged, causing a "barrel chest," and the functional residual capacity and residual volume also become permanently increased.

TUBERCULOSIS

In tuberculosis the tubercle bacilli cause a peculiar tissue reaction in the lungs including, first, invasion of the infected region by macrophages and, second, walling off of the lesion by fibrous tissue to form the so-called tubercle. This walling-off process helps to limit further transmission of the tubercle bacilli in the lungs and, therefore, is part of the protective process against the infection. However, in approximately 3 per cent of all persons who contract tuberculosis, the walling-off process fails, and tubercle bacilli spread throughout the lungs. Thus, tuberculosis in its late stages causes many areas of fibrosis throughout the lungs, and, secondly, it reduces the total amount of functional lung tissue. These effects cause (1) increased "work" on the part of the respiratory muscles to cause pulmonary ventilation and *reduced vital capacity and breathing capacity,* (2) *reduced total respiratory membrane surface area* and *increased thickness of the respiratory membrane,* these causing progressively diminished pulmonary diffusing capacity, and (3) *abnormal ventilation-perfusion ratio* in the lungs, further reducing the pulmonary diffusing capacity.

CYANOSIS

The term *cyanosis* means blueness of the skin, and its cause is excessive amounts of deoxygenated hemoglobin in the skin blood vessels, especially in the capillaries. This deoxygenated hemoglobin has an intense dark blue color that is transmitted through the skin. The presence of cyanosis is one of the most common clinical signs of different degrees of respiratory insufficiency.

DYSPNEA

Dyspnea means a desire for air or mental anguish associated with the act of ventilating enough to satisfy the air demand. A common synonym is *air hunger.*

At least three different factors often enter into the development of the sensation of dyspnea. These are: (1) abnormality of the respiratory gases in the body fluids, especially excess carbon dioxide and to a much less extent hypoxia, (2) the amount of work that must be performed by the respiratory muscles to provide adequate ventilation, and (3) the state of the mind.

At times, the levels of both carbon dioxide and oxygen in the body fluids are completely normal, but to attain this normality of the respiratory gases, the person has to breathe forcefully. In these instances the forceful activity of the respiratory muscles gives the person a sensation of air hunger.

Finally, the person's respiratory functions may be completely normal, and still dyspnea may be experienced because of an abnormal state of mind. This is called *neurogenic dyspnea* or, sometimes, *emotional dyspnea.* For instance, almost anyone momentarily thinking about the act of breathing may suddenly start taking breaths a little more deeply than ordinarily because of a feeling of mild dyspnea. This feeling is greatly enhanced in persons who have a fear of not being able to receive a sufficient quantity of air. For example, many persons on entering small or crowded rooms immediately experience emotional dyspnea, and patients with "cardiac neurosis" who have heard that dyspnea is associated with heart failure frequently experience severe psychic dyspnea even though the blood gases are completely normal. Neurogenic dyspnea has been known to be so intense that the person over-respires and causes alkalotic tetany.

OXYGEN THERAPY IN DIFFERENT TYPES OF HYPOXIA

Oxygen can be administered by (1) placing the patient's head in a tent that contains air fortified with oxygen, (2) allowing the patient to breathe either pure oxygen or high concentrations of oxygen from a mask, or (3) administering oxygen through a nasal tube.

Oxygen therapy is of great value in certain types of hypoxia but of almost no value at all in other types. However, recalling the basic physiological principles of the different types of hypoxia, one can readily decide when oxygen therapy is of value and, if so, how valuable. For instance:

In *atmospheric hypoxia,* that is, inadequate oxygen in the air, oxygen therapy can obviously completely correct the depressed oxygen level in the inspired gases and therefore provide 100 per cent effective therapy.

In *hypoventilation hypoxia* or *hypoxia caused by impaired diffusion,* a person breathing 100 per cent oxygen can move 5 times as much oxygen into the alveoli with each breath as when breathing normal air. Therefore, here again oxygen therapy can be extremely beneficial, increasing the available oxygen to as much as 400 per cent above normal.

In *hypoxia caused by anemia, carbon monoxide poisoning,* or *any other abnormality of hemoglobin transport,* oxygen therapy is of only slight value because the amount of oxygen transported by the hemoglobin is hardly altered. Yet, a small amount of extra oxygen can be transported in the dissolved state.

In the different types of *hypoxia caused by inadequate tissue use of oxygen,* such as when cyanide poisons the respiratory enzymes, there is no abnormality of oxygen pickup by the lungs or of transport to the tissues. Instead, the tissues simply cannot utilize the oxygen that is transported to them. Therefore, oxygen therapy is of essentially no benefit.

QUESTIONS

1. Describe the anatomical loci of the various portions of the so-called respiratory center.
2. What part of the respiratory center is responsible for the basic oscillating rhythm of respiration? What is meant by the inspiratory ramp signal?
3. How does the pneumotaxis center control the ramp?
4. What is the function of the Hering-Breuer inflation reflex?
5. What is the role of the ventral respiratory group of neurons in the respiratory center for controlling expiration?
6. How powerful is each of the following in directly controlling respiratory center activity: oxygen insufficiency, excess carbon dioxide, excess hydrogen ion concentration?
7. What is the relationship of the chemosensitive area of the respiratory center to the dorsal and ventral groups of respiratory neurons?
8. Approximately how much can excess carbon dioxide in the blood increase alveolar ventilation?
9. How much can excess hydrogen ion concentration in the blood increase ventilation?
10. Describe the relationship of the peripheral chemoreceptors to the respiratory center.
11. What is the importance of the peripheral chemoreceptors in the control of respiration by oxygen lack?
12. Why is oxygen regulation of respiration of minimal importance under normal conditions but very important in pneumonia and at high altitudes?
13. What special mechanisms cause powerful excitation of respiration during exercise?
14. What conditions frequently cause respiratory center depression?
15. Explain *periodic breathing,* especially of the *Cheyne-Stokes* type.
16. Describe the relationship of *pulmonary emphysema* to smoking, its pathological effects on the lungs, and its devastating effects on pulmonary function.
17. Describe the mechanism of *atelectasis* when there is either airway obstruction or lack of surfactant.
18. Why is it often much easier to inspire air than to expire air in asthma and in emphysema?
19. Define *cyanosis* and *dyspnea* and state their causes.
20. How valuble is oxygen therapy in each of the following types of hypoxia: *atmospheric hypoxia, hypoventilation hypoxia, hypoxia caused by carbon monoxide poisoning,* and *hypoxia caused by inadequate tissue use of oxygen?*

References

Regulation of Respiration

Cohen, M. I.: Central determinants of respiratory rhythm. Annu Rev Physiol 43:91, 1981.

Eldridge, F. L., and Millhorn, D. E.: Central regulation of respiration by endogenous neurotransmitters and neuromodulators. Annu Rev Physiol 43:121, 1981.

Eyzaguirre, C., et al.: Arterial chemoreceptors. In Shepherd, J. T., and Abboud, F. M., eds.: Handbook of Physiology. Sec. 2, Vol. 3. Bethesda, American Physiological Society, 1983, p. 557.

Flenley, D. C., and Warren, P. M.: Ventilatory Responses to O₂ and CO₂ during exercise. Annu Rev Physiol 45:415, 1983.

Guyton, A. C., et al.: Basic oscillating mechanism of Cheyne-Stokes breathing. Am. J. Physiol 187:395, 1956.

Haddad, G. G., and Mellins, R. B.: Hypoxia and respiratory control in early life. Annu Rev Physiol 46:629, 1984.

Jansen, A. H., and Chernick, V.: Development of respiratory control. Physiol Rev 63:437, 1983.

Kalia, M. P.: Anatomical organization of central respiratory neurons. Annu Rev Physiol 43:105, 1981.

Rigatto, H.: Control of ventilation in the newborn. Annu Rev Physiol 46:661, 1984.

Schlaefke, M. E., ed.: Central Neuron Environment and the Control Systems of Breathing and Circulation. New York, Springer-Verlag, 1983.

Von Euler, C., and Lagercrantz, H., eds.: Central Nervous Control Mechanisms in Breathing. New York, Pergamon Press, 1980.

Walker, D. W.: Peripheral and central chemoreceptors in the fetus and newborn. Annu Rev Physiol 46:687, 1984.

Whipp, B. J.: Ventilatory control during exercise in humans. Annu Rev Physiol 45:393, 1983.

Respiratory Abnormalities

Dawson, C. A.: Role of pulmonary vasomotion in physiology of the lung. Physiol Rev 64:544, 1984.

Dempsey, J. A., and Forster, H. V.: Mediation of ventilatory adaptations. Physiol Rev 62:262, 1982.

Fanta, C. H.: Calcium-channel blockers in prophylaxis and treatment of asthma. Am J Cardiol 55:202B, 1985.

Fisher, A. B., et al.: Oxygen toxicity of the lung: biochemical aspects. In Fishman, A. P., and Renkin, E. M., eds.: Pulmonary Edema. Baltimore, Waverly Press, 1979, p. 207.

Fishman, A. P., and Pietra, G. G.: Primary pulmonary hypertension. Annu Rev Med 31:421, 1980.

Hodgkin, J. E.. ed.: Chronic Obstructive Pulmonary Disease: Current Concepts in Diagnosis and Comprehensive Care. Park Ridge, Ill., American College of Chest Physicians, 1979.

Killian, K. J., and Campbell, E. J. M.: Dyspnea and exercise. Annu Rev Physiol 45:465, 1983.

Malik, A. B.: Pulmonary microembolism. Physiol Rev 63:1114, 1983.

McFadden, E. R., Jr., and Ingram, R. H., Jr.: Exercise-induced airway obstruction. Annu Rev Physiol 45:453, 1983.

Spector, S. L.: The use of corticosteroids in the treatment of asthma. Chest 87:73S, 1985.

Wolfe, W. G., and Sabiston, D. C.: Pulmonary Embolism. Philadelphia, W. B. Saunders Co., 1980.

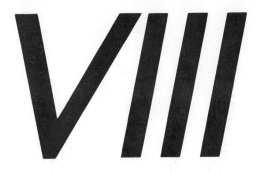

AVIATION, SPACE, AND DEEP SEA DIVING PHYSIOLOGY

30 ■ Aviation, Space, and Deep Sea Diving Physiology

30

Aviation, Space, and Deep Sea Diving Physiology

EFFECTS OF LOW OXYGEN PRESSURE
  ON THE BODY
  ALVEOLAR Po₂ AT DIFFERENT
    ELEVATIONS
  EFFECTS OF BREATHING PURE
    OXYGEN ON THE ALVEOLAR Po₂
    AT DIFFERENT ALTITUDES
  EFFECTS OF HYPOXIA
  ACCLIMATIZATION TO LOW Po₂
  NATURAL ACCLIMATIZATION OF
    PERSONS LIVING AT HIGH
    ALTITUDES
EFFECTS OF ACCELERATORY FORCES
  ON THE BODY IN AVIATION AND
  SPACE PHYSIOLOGY
  CENTRIFUGAL ACCELERATORY
    FORCES
  EFFECTS OF LINEAR ACCELERATORY
    FORCES ON THE BODY

RADIATION HAZARDS IN SPACE
ARTIFICIAL CLIMATE IN THE SEALED
  SPACECRAFT
WEIGHTLESSNESS IN SPACE
PHYSIOLOGY OF DEEP SEA DIVING
  AND OTHER HIGH PRESSURE
  OPERATIONS
  EFFECTS OF HIGH PARTIAL
    PRESSURES OF GASES ON THE
    BODY
  DECOMPRESSION OF DIVERS AFTER
    EXPOSURE TO HIGH PRESSURES
SCUBA (SELF-CONTAINED
  UNDERWATER BREATHING
  APPARATUS) DIVING
SPECIAL PHYSIOLOGICAL PROBLEMS
  OF SUBMARINES
HYPERBARIC OXYGEN THERAPY

As people have ascended to higher and higher altitudes in aviation, in mountain climbing, and in space vehicles, it has become progressively more important to understand the effects of altitude and low gas pressures on the human body. And as divers have gone deeper in the sea, it has become necessary to understand the effects of high gas pressures as well.

The present chapter deals with these problems: first, hypoxia at high altitudes; second, the other physical factors affecting the body at high altitudes; third, the tremendous acceleratory forces that occur in both aviation and space physiology; and, finally, the effects of high-pressure gases at the depths of the sea.

EFFECTS OF LOW OXYGEN PRESSURE ON THE BODY

Barometric Pressures at Different Altitudes. Table 30–1 gives the barometric pressures at different alti-

tudes, showing that at sea level the pressure is 760 mm Hg, while at 10,000 feet it is only 523 mm Hg, and at 50,000 feet, 87 mm Hg. The decrease in barometric pressure is the basic cause of all the hypoxia problems in high altitude physiology, for as the barometric pressure decreases, the oxygen pressure decreases proportionately, remaining at all times slightly less than 21 per cent of the total barometric pressure.

Oxygen Partial Pressures in the Atmosphere at Different Elevations. Table 30–1 also shows that the partial pressure of oxygen (Po_2) in dry air at sea level is approximately 159 mm Hg, though this can be decreased as much as 10 mm when large amounts of water vapor exist in the air. The Po_2 at 10,000 feet is approximately 110 mm Hg, at 20,000 feet 73 mm Hg, and at 50,000 feet 18 mm Hg.

ALVEOLAR Po₂ AT DIFFERENT ELEVATIONS

Obviously, when the Po_2 in the atmosphere decreases at higher elevations, a decrease in alveolar

Table 30-1. EFFECTS OF ACUTE EXPOSURE TO LOW ATMOSPHERIC PRESSURES ON ALVEOLAR GAS CONCENTRATIONS AND ON ARTERIAL OXYGEN SATURATION

Altitude (ft)	Barometric Pressure (mm Hg)	P_{O_2} in Air (mm Hg)	Breathing Air			Breathing Pure Oxygen		
			P_{CO_2} in Alveoli (mm Hg)	P_{O_2} in Alveoli (mm Hg)	Arterial Oxygen Saturation (%)	P_{CO_2} in Alveoli (mm Hg)	P_{O_2} in Alveoli (mm Hg)	Arterial Oxygen Saturation (%)
0	760	159	40	104	97	40	673	100
10,000	523	110	36	67	90	40	436	100
20,000	349	73	24	40	73	40	262	100
30,000	226	47	24	21	30	40	139	99
40,000	141	29	24	12	15	36	58	87
50,000	87	18	24	2	2	24	16	22

P_{O_2} is also to be expected. At low altitudes the alveolar P_{O_2} does not decrease quite so much as the atmospheric P_{O_2} because increased pulmonary ventilation helps to compensate for the diminished atmospheric oxygen. But at higher altitudes the alveolar P_{O_2} decreases even more than atmospheric P_{O_2} for peculiar reasons that are explained as follows:

Carbon Dioxide and Water Vapor Decrease the Alveolar Oxygen. Carbon dioxide is continually excreted from the pulmonary blood into the alveoli. Also, water vaporizes into the alveolar space from the respiratory surfaces. These two gases therefore dilute the oxygen and nitrogen already in the alveoli, thus reducing the oxygen concentration.

The presence of carbon dioxide and water vapor in the alveoli becomes exceedingly important at high altitudes, because the total barometric pressure falls to low levels while the pressures of carbon dioxide and water vapor do not fall comparably. Water vapor pressure remains at 47 mm Hg as long as the body temperature is normal, regardless of altitude; and the pressure of carbon dioxide falls from about 40 mm Hg at sea level only to about 24 mm Hg because of its continued excretion from the blood into the alveoli.

Now let us see how the pressures of these two gases affect the available space for oxygen. Let us assume that the total barometric pressure falls to 100 mm Hg; 47 mm Hg of this must be water vapor, leaving only 53 mm Hg for all the other gases; 24 mm Hg of the 53 mm Hg must be carbon dioxide, leaving a remaining space of only 29 mm Hg. If there were no uptake of oxygen from the alveoli by the blood, one fifth of this 29 mm Hg would be oxygen and four fifths would be nitrogen; or, the P_{O_2} in the alveoli would be 6 mm Hg. However, most of this last remaining alveolar oxygen is absorbed into the blood, leaving only about 3 mm Hg oxygen pressure in the alveoli. Therefore, at a barometric pressure of 100 mm Hg (an altitude of about 47,000 feet), the person could not possibly survive when breathing air. But the effect is very much different if the person is breathing pure oxygen, as we shall see later.

The fifth column in Table 30-1 shows the P_{O_2}'s in the alveoli at different altitudes when one is breathing air. The P_{O_2} is 104 mm Hg at sea level; it falls to approximately 67 mm Hg at 10,000 feet, and to only 2 mm Hg at 50,000 feet.

Saturation of Hemoglobin With Oxygen at Different Altitudes When Breathing Air. The lower curve of Figure 30-1 illustrates arterial oxygen saturation at different altitudes when one is breathing air, and the actual percentage of saturation at each 10,000 foot level is given in the sixth column of Table 30-1. Up to an altitude of approximately 10,000 feet, the arterial oxygen saturation remains at least as high as 90 per cent. However, above 10,000 feet the saturation falls progressively until it is only 73 per cent at 20,000 feet altitude and still less at higher altitudes. At these altitudes above 20,000 feet, the delivery of oxygen to the tissues begins to be seriously compromised.

EFFECTS OF BREATHING PURE OXYGEN ON THE ALVEOLAR P_{O_2} AT DIFFERENT ALTITUDES

Referring once again to Table 30-1, note that when a person breathes air at 30,000 feet, the alveolar P_{O_2} is only 21 mm Hg, even though the barometric pressure is 226 mm Hg. Much of this difference is caused by the fact that a considerable proportion of the alveolar air is nitrogen. But if a person breathes

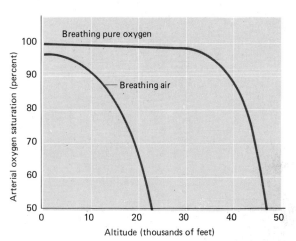

Figure 30-1. Effect of low atmospheric pressure on arterial oxygen saturation when breathing air and when breathing pure oxygen.

pure oxygen instead of air, most of the space in the alveoli formerly occupied by nitrogen is now occupied by oxygen instead. Theoretically, at this altitude the flier breathing pure oxygen could have an alveolar P_{O_2} of 139 mm Hg instead of the 21 mm Hg when breathing air.

The upper curve of Figure 30–1 illustrates the arterial oxygen saturation at different altitudes when breathing pure oxygen. Note that the saturation remains above 90 per cent until the flier ascends to approximately 39,000 feet, about three times the altitude for the same saturation when breathing air. Then the saturation falls rapidly to approximately 50 per cent at about 47,000 feet. This is about the lowest limit that the flier can tolerate for a long time, so that this altitude is called the ceiling.

EFFECTS OF HYPOXIA

The rate of pulmonary ventilation ordinarily does not increase significantly until one has ascended to about 8000 feet. At this height, the arterial oxygen saturation has fallen to approximately 93 per cent, at which level the chemoreceptors begin to respond significantly. Above 8000 feet, the chemoreceptor stimulatory mechanism progressively increases the ventilation until approximately 16,000 to 20,000 feet, at which altitude the ventilation has reached a maximum of approximately 65 per cent above normal. Further increase in altitude does not further activate the chemoreceptors.

Other effects of hypoxia, beginning at an altitude of about 12,000 feet, are drowsiness, lassitude, mental fatigue, sometimes headache, occasionally nausea, and sometimes euphoria. Most of these symptoms increase in intensity at still higher altitudes, the headache often becoming especially prominent and the cerebral symptoms sometimes progressing to the stage of twitchings or convulsions and, above 23,000 feet in the unacclimatized person, to coma.

One of the most important effects of hypoxia is decreased mental proficiency, which decreases judgment, memory, and the performance of discrete motor movements. Ordinarily these abilities remain absolutely normal up to approximately 9000 feet, and they may be completely normal for a short time up to elevations of 15,000 feet. But, during exposure to hypoxia for a long time, mental proficiency, as measured by reaction times, handwriting, and other psychological tests, may decrease to 80 per cent of normal even at altitudes as low as 11,000. If a person stays at 15,000 feet for one hour without supplemental oxygen, mental proficiency ordinarily will have fallen to approximately 50 per cent of normal, and after 18 hours at this level, to approximately 20 per cent of normal.

ACCLIMATIZATION TO LOW P_{O_2}

A person remaining at high altitudes for days, weeks, or years gradually becomes acclimatized to the low P_{O_2}, so that it causes fewer and fewer deleterious effects to the body and also so that it becomes possible to work harder or to ascend to still higher altitudes. Several means by which acclimatization comes about are (1) further increase in pulmonary ventilation, (2) increased hemoglobin in the blood, and (3) increased vascularity of the tissues.

Further Increase in Pulmonary Ventilation. On immediate exposure to low P_{O_2}, the hypoxic stimulation of the chemoreceptors increases alveolar ventilation to a maximum of about 65 per cent. This increase is an immediate compensation for the high altitude, and even this small increase in breathing allows the person to rise several thousand feet higher than would be possible without the increased ventilation. But, if a person remains at a very high altitude for several days, ventilation gradually increases to as much as five to seven times normal. The basic cause of this gradual increase is the following:

The immediate 65 per cent increase in pulmonary ventilation on rising to a high altitude blows off large quantities of carbon dioxide, which reduces the P_{CO_2} and increases the pH of the body fluids. Both of these changes *inhibit* the respiratory center and thereby *oppose the stimulation by the hypoxia*. However, during the next two to five days, most of this inhibition fades away, allowing the respiratory center now to respond with full force to the chemoreceptor stimuli resulting from hypoxia, and the ventilation increases to about five to seven times normal.

Increase in Hemoglobin During Acclimatization. It will be recalled from Chapter 19 that hypoxia is the principal stimulus for an increase in red blood cell production. Ordinarily, in full acclimatization to low oxygen the hematocrit rises from a normal value of 40 to 45 to an average of 60 to 65, with an average increase in hemoglobin concentration from the normal of 15 gm per cent to about 22 gm per cent.

In addition, the blood volume also increases, often by as much as 20 to 30 per cent, resulting in a total increase in circulating hemoglobin of as much as 50 to 90 per cent.

Unfortunately, this increase in hemoglobin and blood volume is slow in occurring, having almost no effect until after two to three weeks, reaching half development in a month or so, and becoming fully developed only after many months.

Increased Vascularity. Histological studies of animals that normally live at high altitudes show *increased vascularity* (increased numbers and sizes of capillaries) of the hypoxic tissues. This helps to explain what happens to the 20 to 30 per cent increase in blood volume, and it means that the blood comes into much closer contact with the tissue cells than normally.

NATURAL ACCLIMATIZATION OF PERSONS LIVING AT HIGH ALTITUDES

Many natives of the Andes and the Himalayas live at altitudes above 13,000 feet; one group in the

Peruvian Andes actually lives at an altitude of 17,500 feet and works a mine at an altitude of 19,000 feet. Many of these persons are born at these altitudes and live there all their lives. In all of the aspects of acclimatization listed earlier, the natives are superior to even the best acclimatized lowlanders, even though the lowlanders may also have lived at high altitudes for ten or more years. The process of acclimatization of the natives begins in infancy. The chest size, especially, is greatly increased, whereas the body size is somewhat decreased, giving a high ratio of ventilatory capacity to body mass. In addition, the heart, particularly the right heart, which provides a high pulmonary arterial pressure to pump blood through a greatly expanded pulmonary capillary system, is considerably larger than the heart of a lowlander.

The following table gives an idea of the importance of acclimatization. At an altitude of 17,000 feet, the work capacities by percentage of the sea level maximum for a normal person are

	Per cent
Unacclimatized	50
Acclimatized for two months	68
Native living at 13,200 feet but working at 17,000 feet	87

Thus, naturally acclimatized natives can achieve a daily work output even at these high altitudes almost equal to that of a normal person at sea level, but even well-acclimatized lowlanders almost never can achieve this result.

EFFECTS OF ACCELERATORY FORCES ON THE BODY IN AVIATION AND SPACE PHYSIOLOGY

Because of rapid changes in velocity and direction of motion in airplanes and space ships, several types of acceleratory forces often affect the body during flight. At the beginning of flight, simple linear acceleration occurs; at the end of flight, deceleration; and every time the airplane turns, angular and centrifugal acceleration occur. In aviation physiology it is usually centrifugal acceleration that demands greatest consideration, because the structure of the airplane is capable of withstanding much greater centrifugal acceleration than is the human body.

CENTRIFUGAL ACCELERATORY FORCES

When an airplane makes a turn, the force of centrifugal acceleration is determined by the following relationship:

$$f = \frac{mv^2}{r}$$

in which f is the centrifugal acceleratory force, m is the mass of the object, v is the velocity of travel, and r is the radius of curvature of the turn. From this formula it is obvious that as the velocity increases, the force increases in proportion to the square of the velocity. It is also obvious that the force of acceleration is directly proportional to the sharpness of the turn, that is, as the radius of the turn decreases.

Measurement of the Acceleratory Force—G. When a person is simply sitting in his seat, the force with which he is pressing against the seat results from the pull of gravity, and it is equal to his weight. The intensity of this force is 1 G because it is equal to one times the pull of gravity. If the force with which he presses against his seat becomes five times his normal weight during a pullout from a dive because of extra force caused by centrifugation, the force acting upon the seat is 5 G.

If the airplane goes through an outside loop, so that the pilot is held down by his seat belt, *negative G* is applied to his body, and if the force with which he is thrown against his belt is equal to the weight of his body, the negative force is said to be −1 G.

Effects of Centrifugal Acceleratory Force on the Body

Effects on the Circulatory System. The most important effect of centrifugal acceleration is on the circulatory system, because blood is mobile and can be translocated within the blood vessels by centrifugal force. Centrifugal force also tends to displace the tissues, but because of their more solid structure, they only sag—ordinarily not enough to cause abnormal function.

When the flier is subject to *positive G,* his blood is centrifuged toward the lower part of his body. Thus, if the centrifugal acceleratory force is 5 G and the person is in a standing position, the hydrostatic pressure in the veins of the feet is five times normal, or approximately 450 mm Hg, and even in the sitting position this pressure is nearly 300 mm Hg. As the pressure in the vessels of the lower part of the body increases, the vessels passively dilate, and a major proportion of the blood from the upper part of the body is translocated into these lower vessels. Because the heart cannot pump unless blood returns to it, the greater the quantity of blood pooled in the lower body, the less the cardiac output.

When the acceleration rises to 4 G and the flier is in the seated position, the systemic arterial pressure at the level of the heart falls approximately 40 mm Hg, and blood flow to the brain almost ceases. Acceleration greater than 4 to 6 G ordinarily causes "black-out" of vision within a few seconds and then unconsciousness shortly thereafter.

EFFECTS OF LINEAR ACCELERATORY FORCES ON THE BODY

Acceleratory Forces in Space Travel. In contrast with aircraft, a spacecraft cannot make rapid turns; therefore, centrifugal acceleration is of little importance except when the spacecraft goes into abnormal gyrations. On the other hand, blast-off acceleration

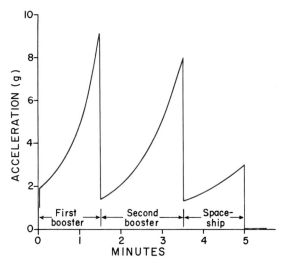

Figure 30–2. Acceleratory forces during the takeoff of a spacecraft.

and landing deceleration can be tremendous; both of these are types of linear acceleration.

Figure 30–2 illustrates a typical profile of the acceleration during blast-off in a three-stage spacecraft, showing that the first-stage booster causes acceleration as high as 9 G and the second-stage booster as high as 8 G. In the standing position, the human body could not endure this much acceleration, but in a reclining position *transverse to the axis of acceleration,* this amount of acceleration can be withstood with ease despite the fact that the acceleratory forces continue for as long as five minutes at a time. We therefore see the reason for the reclining seats used by the astronauts.

Problems also occur during deceleration when the spacecraft re-enters the atmosphere. A person traveling at Mach 1 (the speed of sound and of fast airplanes) can be safely decelerated in a distance of approximately 0.12 mile, whereas a person traveling at a speed of Mach 100 (a speed possible in interplanetary space travel) requires a distance of about 10,000 miles for safe deceleration. The principal reason for this difference is that the total amount of energy that must be dispelled during deceleration is proportional to the *square* of the velocity, which alone increases the distance 10,000-fold. But, in addition, a human being can withstand far less deceleration if it lasts for a long time than for a short time. Therefore, deceleration must be accomplished much more slowly from the very high velocities than is necessary at the lower velocities.

RADIATION HAZARDS IN SPACE

Large quantities of cosmic particles are continually bombarding the earth's upper atmosphere, some originating from the sun and some from outer space. The magnetic field of the earth traps many of these cosmic particles in two major belts around the earth called *Van Allen radiation belts.* The inner belt begins at an altitude of about 300 miles and extends to about 3000 miles. The outer belt begins at about 6000 miles and extends to 20,000 miles. Even with the best possible shielding, a person traversing these two belts in an interplanetary space trip can receive as much as 1.0 rad of radiation, which is about one four hundredth the lethal dose; and a person in a spacecraft orbiting the earth within one of these two belts can receive enough radiation to cause death.

Thus, it is important to orbit spacecraft below an altitude of 200 to 300 miles, an altitude at which the radiation hazard is slight.

ARTIFICIAL CLIMATE IN THE SEALED SPACECRAFT

Since there is no atmosphere in outer space, a special atmosphere and other conditions of climate must be provided artificially in the spacecraft cabin. The ability of a person to survive in this artificial climate depends entirely on appropriate engineering design.

Most important of all, the oxygen concentration must remain high enough and the carbon dioxide concentration low enough. In some space missions, a capsule atmosphere containing pure oxygen at about 260 mm Hg pressure has been used. In others, normal air at 760 mm Hg pressure has been used. The presence of nitrogen in the mixture greatly diminishes the likelihood of fire and explosion.

For space travel lasting several years, it will be impractical to carry along an adequate oxygen supply and enough carbon dioxide absorbent. For this reason, recycling techniques are being developed for use of the same oxygen over and over again. These techniques also frequently include reuse of the same food and water. Basically, they involve (1) a method for resynthesizing oxygen from carbon dioxide, (2) a method for removing water from the human excreta so that the water can be reused, and (3) use of the human excreta for resynthesizing or growing an adequate food supply.

Large amounts of energy are required for these processes, and the real problem at present is to derive enough energy from the sun's radiation to energize the necessary chemical reactions. Some recycling processes depend on purely physical procedures, such as distillation, electrolysis of water, and capture of the sun's energy by solar batteries, whereas others depend on biological methods, such as use of algae, with its large store of chlorophyll, to generate foodstuffs by photosynthesis. Unfortunately, a completely practical system for recycling is yet to be achieved. The problem is the weight of the equipment that must be carried.

WEIGHTLESSNESS IN SPACE

A person in an orbiting satellite or in any nonpropelled spacecraft experiences weightlessness (and therefore is not drawn toward the bottom, sides, or top of the spacecraft but simply floats inside its chamber). The cause is not failure of gravity to pull on the body, because gravity from any nearby heavenly body is still active. However, the gravity acts on both the spacecraft and the person at the same time, and since there is no resistance to movement in space, both are pulled with exactly the same forces and in the same direction.

Weightlessness causes engineering problems such as the necessity for providing special techniques for eating and drinking (food and water will not stay in open plates or glasses), special waste disposal systems (the excreta will float in the cabin atmosphere—a problem that has actually occurred), and adequate hand holds or other means for stabilizing the astronauts so that they adequately control the operation of the ship.

Physiological Problems of Weightlessness. Fortunately, the physiological problems of weightlessness have not proved to be severe. Most of the problems that do occur appear to be related to two effects of the weightlessness: (1) translocation of fluids within the body because of failure of gravity to cause hydrostatic pressures, and (2) diminishment of physical activity because no strength of muscle contraction is required to oppose the force of gravity.

The observed effects of prolonged stay in space are the following: (1) decrease in blood volume, (2) decrease in red cell mass, (3) decreased work capacity, (4) decrease in maximum cardiac output, and (5) loss of calcium from the bones. Because of the circulatory changes, astronauts frequently faint when they first return to earth and stand up against gravity. Essentially, these same effects also occur in persons lying in bed for an extended period of time. For this reason, an extensive exercise program is carried out when it is practical, and all of the above effects are greatly reduced.

PHYSIOLOGY OF DEEP SEA DIVING AND OTHER HIGH PRESSURE OPERATIONS

When human beings descend into the sea, the pressure around them increases tremendously. To keep their lungs from collapsing, air must be supplied at an equally high pressure, which exposes the blood in the lungs to extremely high alveolar gas pressures. Beyond certain limits, these high pressures can cause tremendous alterations in the physiology of the body.

Also exposed to high atmospheric pressures are caisson workers who, in digging tunnels beneath rivers or elsewhere, often must work in a pressurized area to keep the tunnel from caving in. Here again, the same problems of excessively high gas pressures in the alveoli occur.

Before explaining the effects of high alveolar gas pressures on the body, it is necessary to review some physical principles of pressure and volume changes at different depths beneath the sea.

TABLE 30–2. EFFECT OF DEPTH ON PRESSURE

Depth (Feet)	Atmosphere(s)
Sea level	1
33	2
66	3
100	4
133	5
166	6
200	7
300	10
400	13
500	16

Relationship of Sea Depth to Pressure. A column of sea water 33 feet deep exerts the same pressure at its bottom as all the atmosphere above the earth. Therefore, a person 33 feet beneath the ocean surface is exposed to a pressure of 2 atmospheres, 1 atmosphere of pressure caused by the air above the water and the second atmosphere by the weight of the water itself. At 66 feet the pressure is 3 atmospheres, and so forth, in accord with Table 30–2.

Effect of Depth on the Volume of Gases. Another important effect of depth is the compression of gases to smaller and smaller volumes. At 33 feet beneath the surface of the sea, where the pressure is 2 atmospheres, a one-liter volume at sea level is compressed to only one-half liter. At 100 feet, where the pressure is 4 atmospheres, the volume is compressed to one-fourth liter, and at 8 atmospheres (233 feet) to one-eighth liter. This is an extremely important effect in diving, because it can cause the air chambers of the diver's body, including the lungs, to become so small in some instances that serious damage results.

EFFECTS OF HIGH PARTIAL PRESSURES OF GASES ON THE BODY

The three gases to which a diver breathing air is normally exposed are nitrogen, oxygen, and carbon dioxide.

Nitrogen Narcosis at High Nitrogen Pressures. Approximately four fifths of the air is nitrogen. At sea level pressure it has no known effect on bodily function, but at high pressures, nitrogen can cause varying degrees of narcosis. When a diver remains in the sea for an hour or more and is breathing compressed air, the depth at which the first symptoms of mild narcosis appear is approximately 120 feet, at which level the diver begins to exhibit joviality and to lose many cares. At 150 to 200 feet, drowsiness occurs. At 200 to 250 feet, the diver's strength wanes considerably, and he or she often becomes too clumsy to perform the work required. Beyond 250 feet (8.5 atmospheres pressure), the diver usually becomes almost useless as a result of nitrogen narcosis caused by remaining at these depths too long.

Nitrogen narcosis has characteristics similar to those of alcohol intoxication, and for this reason it has frequently been called rapture of the depths.

The mechanism of the narcotic effect is believed to

be the same as that of essentially all the gas anesthetics. That is, nitrogen dissolves freely in the fats of the body. Presumably, like most other anesthetic gases, it then dissolves in the membranes or other lipid structures of the brain neurons and, because of its *physical* effect on altering electrical charge transfer through the membranes, reduces the excitability.

Oxygen Toxicity at High Pressures. Breathing oxygen under very high partial pressure can be detrimental to the central nervous system, sometimes causing epileptic convulsions followed by coma. Indeed, exposure to 3 atmospheres pressure of oxygen (P_{O_2} = 2280 mm Hg) will cause convulsions and coma in most persons after about one hour. These convulsions often occur without any warning, and they obviously are likely to be lethal to a diver submerged in the sea.

The cause or causes of oxygen toxicity are yet unknown, but experiments have shown that excess oxygen in the tissues causes the development of large concentrations of oxidizing free radicals such as superoxide (O_2^-), which can cause oxidative destruction of many essential elements of the cells, thereby damaging the metabolic systems of the cells.

Carbon Dioxide Toxicity at Great Depths. If the diving gear is properly designed and functions as it should, a diver has no problem with carbon dioxide toxicity, for depth alone does not increase the carbon dioxide partial pressure in the alveoli. This is true because carbon dioxide is manufactured in the body, and as long as a diver continues to breathe a normal tidal volume, the carbon dioxide is expired as it is formed, maintaining the alveolar carbon dioxide partial pressure at a normal value.

Unfortunately, though, in certain types of diving gear, such as the diving helmet and different types of rebreathing apparatuses, carbon dioxide can frequently build up in the dead space air of the apparatus and be rebreathed by the diver. Up to a carbon dioxide pressure (P_{CO_2}) of about 80 mm Hg, two times that of normal alveoli, the diver tolerates this buildup, the minute respiratory volume increasing up to a maximum of 6- to 10-fold to compensate for the increased carbon dioxide. However, beyond the 80 mm Hg level, the situation becomes intolerable, and eventually the respiratory center begins to be depressed rather than excited; the diver's respiration then actually begins to fail rather than to compensate. In addition, severe respiratory acidosis develops, and varying degrees of lethargy and finally coma ensue.

DECOMPRESSION OF DIVERS AFTER EXPOSURE TO HIGH PRESSURES

When a person breathes air under high pressure for a long time, the amount of nitrogen dissolved in his body fluids becomes very large. The reason is the following: The blood flowing through the pulmonary capillaries becomes saturated with nitrogen at the same pressure as that in the breathing mixture. Over several hours, enough nitrogen is carried to all the tissues of the body to saturate them also with dissolved nitrogen. And, since nitrogen is not metabolized by the body, it remains dissolved until the nitrogen pressure in the lung decreases, at which time the nitrogen is then removed by the reverse respiratory process.

Volume of Nitrogen Dissolved in the Body Fluids at Different Depths. At sea level almost 1 liter of nitrogen is dissolved in the entire body. After the diver has become totally saturated with nitrogen, the *sea level volume of nitrogen* dissolved in his body fluids at the different depths is

Feet	Liters
33	2
100	4
200	7
300	10

However, several hours are required for the body to become saturated with nitrogen at each new depth, simply because the blood does not flow rapidly enough and the nitrogen does not diffuse rapidly enough to cause instantaneous saturation. For this reason, if a person remains at deep levels for only a few minutes, not much nitrogen dissolves in his fluids and tissues, whereas if he remains at a deep level for several hours, his fluids and tissues become almost completely saturated with nitrogen.

Decompression Sickness (Synonyms: Compressed Air Sickness, Bends, Caisson Disease, Diver's Paralysis, Dysbarism). If a diver has been in the sea so long that large amounts of nitrogen have dissolved in his body and then suddenly comes back to the surface of the sea, significant quantities of nitrogen bubbles can develop in both the intracellular and extracellular body fluids, and these can cause minor or serious damage in almost any area of the body, depending on the number of bubbles formed. The cause of these bubbles is as follows:

As long as a diver remains deep in the sea, the pressure against the outside of his body compresses all the body tissues sufficiently to keep the dissolved gases in solution. Then, with a sudden rise to sea level, the pressure on the outside of the body becomes only 1 atmosphere (760 mm Hg), while the pressure of dissolved gases inside the body fluids is usually several thousand mm Hg, a value far greater than the pressure on the outside of the body. Therefore, the gases can now escape from the dissolved state and actually form bubbles inside the tissues.

Symptoms of Decompression Sickness. In persons who have developed decompression sickness, symptoms have occurred with the following frequencies:

	Per cent
Local pain in the legs or arms	89
Dizziness	5.3
Paralysis	2.3
Shortness of breath ("the chokes")	1.6
Extreme fatigue and pain	1.3
Collapse with unconsciousness	0.5

From the above list of symptoms of decompression sickness, it can be seen that the most serious problems are usually related to bubble formation in the nervous system. Bubbles sometimes actually disrupt important pathways in the brain or spinal cord, and bubbles in the peripheral nerves can cause severe pain. Unfortunately, large bubbles in the central nervous system occasionally lead to permanent paralysis or permanent mental disturbance.

But the nervous system is not the only locus of damage in decompression sickness, for bubbles can also form in the blood and can become caught in the capillaries of the lungs; these bubbles block pulmonary blood flow and cause "the chokes," characterized by serious shortness of breath. This is often followed by severe pulmonary edema, which further aggravates the condition and can cause death.

The symptoms of decompression sickness usually appear within a few minutes to an hour after sudden decompression. However, occasional symptoms of decompression sickness develop as long as six hours or more after decompression.

Rate of Nitrogen Elimination from the Body—Decompression Tables. Fortunately, if a diver is brought to the surface slowly, the dissolved nitrogen is eliminated through his lungs rapidly enough to prevent decompression sickness. Approximately two thirds of the total nitrogen is liberated in one hour and about 90 per cent in six hours. However, some excess nitrogen is still present in the body fluids for many more hours, and the diver is not completely safe for as long as 9 to 12 hours. Therefore, a diver must be "decompressed" sometimes for many hours if he has been deep in the sea for a long time.

The rate at which a diver can be brought to the surface depends, first, on the *depth* to which he has descended and, second, on the *amount of time* he has been there. Therefore, *decompression tables* have been established to designate safe procedures for decompression. Only 20 minutes at a depth of 300 feet requires over two and a half hours decompression time (45 minutes at 300 feet requires over five hours). On the other hand, a person can remain at 50 feet for as long as three hours and yet be decompressed in only 12 minutes.

Use of Helium-Oxygen Mixtures in Deep Dives. In deep dives, helium has advantages over nitrogen, including (1) decreased decompression time, (2) lack of narcotic effect, and (3) decreased airway resistance in the lungs. The decreased decompression time results from two properties of helium: (a) Only 40 per cent as much helium dissolves in the body as does nitrogen; (b) because of its small atomic size, it diffuses through the tissues about two and a half times as quickly as nitrogen and therefore can be transported to the blood and expired much more rapidly than can nitrogen.

SCUBA (SELF-CONTAINED UNDERWATER BREATHING APPARATUS) DIVING

Prior to the 1940s, almost all diving was done using a diving helmet connected to a hose through which

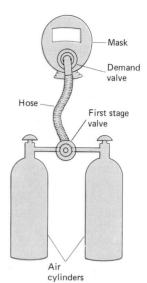

Figure 30–3. The open circuit demand type of SCUBA apparatus.

air was pumped to the diver from the surface. Then, in 1943, Jacques Cousteau developed and popularized the *self-contained underwater breathing apparatus* which is popularly known simply as the SCUBA diving equipment. Figure 30–3 illustrates one type of SCUBA diving gear showing the following components: (1) one or more tanks of compressed air or of some other breathing mixture, (2) a first-stage reducing valve for reducing the pressure from the tanks to a constant low-pressure level, (3) a combination inhalation "demand" valve and exhalation valve, which allows air to be pulled into the lungs with very slight negative pressure and then to be exhausted into the sea, and (4) a mask and tube system with little "dead space."

Basically, the demand system operates as follows: The first-stage reducing valve reduces the pressure from the tanks to about 140 lb per square inch. However, the breathing mixture does not flow continually into the mask. Instead, with each inspiration, slight negative pressure in the mask pulls the diaphragm of the demand valve inward, and this automatically releases air from the hose into the mask and lungs. In this way, only the amount of air needed for inhalation enters the system. Then, on expiration, the air cannot go back into the tank but instead is expired through the expiration valve.

The most important problem in use of the self-contained underwater breathing apparatus is the time limit that one can remain beneath the surface; only a few minutes are possible at great depths because tremendous airflow from the tanks is required to wash carbon dioxide out of the lungs—the greater the depth, the greater the airflow required, because all the gases are compressed to smaller volumes at the deeper levels.

SPECIAL PHYSIOLOGICAL PROBLEMS OF SUBMARINES

Escape from Submarines. Essentially the same problems as those of deep sea diving are often met in submarines, especially when it is necessary to escape from a submerged submarine. Escape is possible from as deep as 300 feet even without the use of any special type of apparatus. Proper use of rebreathing devices using helium or hydrogen can theoretically allow escape from as deep as 600 feet or perhaps more.

One of the major problems of escape is prevention of air embolism. As the person ascends, the air in his lungs expands and sometimes ruptures a major pulmonary vessel, allowing the alveolar air to enter into the pulmonary vascular system and cause embolism of the circulation. Therefore, the person must exhale continually during ascent to prevent this.

Expansion and exhalation of gases from the lungs during ascent, even without breathing, is often rapid enough to blow off the accumulating carbon dioxide in the lungs. This keeps the concentration of carbon dioxide from building up in the blood and reduces the desire to breath. Therefore, a person can hold his breath for an extremely long time during ascent.

Health Problems in the Submarine Internal Environment. Except for escape submarine medicine generally centers on several engineering problems to keep hazards out of the internal environment of the submarine. In nuclear submarines there exists the problem of radiation hazards, but with appropriate shielding, the amount of radiation received by the submerged crew has actually been less than the normal radiation received above the surface of the sea from cosmic rays. Therefore, no essential hazard results from this unless some failure in the apparatus causes unexpected release of radioactive materials.

Also, poisonous gases on occasion escape into the atmosphere of the submarine and must be controlled. For instance, during several weeks' submergence, cigarette smoking by the crew can liberate sufficient amounts of carbon monoxide, if not removed from the air, to cause carbon monoxide poisoning, and on occasion even Freon gas has been found to diffuse through the tubes in refrigeration systems in sufficient quantity to cause toxicity.

HYPERBARIC OXYGEN THERAPY

In recent years it has been learned that the intense oxidizing properties of high-pressure oxygen (*hyperbaric oxygen*) can have very valuable therapeutic effects in several important clinical conditions. Therefore, large pressure tanks are now available in many medical centers into which patients can be placed and treated with hyperbaric oxygen. The oxygen is usually administered at PO_2s of 2 to 3 atmospheres of pressure. It is believed that the same oxidizing free radicals responsible for oxygen toxicity are also responsible for the therapeutic benefits.

Probably the most successful use of hyperbaric oxygen has been in the treatment of *gas gangrene*. The bacteria that cause this condition, the *clostridial organisms*, grow best under anaerobic conditions and actually stop growing at oxygen pressures greater than about 70 mm Hg. Therefore, hyperbaric oxygenation of the tissues can frequently stop the infectious process entirely and thus convert a condition that formerly was almost 100 per cent fatal into one that is cured in most instances.

Recent results also suggest that hyperbaric oxygenation might have almost as dramatic an effect in curing *leprosy* as in curing gas gangrene—also because of the susceptibility of the leprosy bacillus to destruction by high oxygen pressures.

Other conditions in which hyperbaric oxygen therapy has been valuable include decompression sickness, arterial gas embolism, carbon monoxide poisoning, osteomyelitis, and possibly myocardial infarction.

QUESTIONS

1. Approximately how much is the atmospheric PO_2 decreased from normal at an altitude of 20,000 feet?
2. Why does water vapor pressure remain approximately constant in the alveoli at 47 mm Hg regardless of the altitude?
3. Why does the PCO_2 not decrease nearly so much in the alveoli at high altitudes as does the PO_2?
4. At what altitude does the saturation of arterial blood with hemoglobin fall below approximately 50 per cent, which is the approximate ceiling at which a person can survive?
5. How does breathing pure oxygen change the PO_2 in the alveoli at 20,000 feet and at 50,000 feet, and what is the approximate ceiling at which a person can survive when breathing pure oxygen?
6. What are the effects of hypoxia on the body, especially the brain?
7. Discuss the different physiological changes that allow a person to become acclimatized to high altitudes.
8. What is the relationship of centrifugal acceleratory force to the velocity of movement and the sharpness of a turn?
9. What is meant by G force?
10. Why are linear acceleratory forces important in space travel?
11. Discuss the problems of artificial climate and weightlessness in space.
12. How deep below sea level must one go for the pressure of gases in the lungs to reach 4 atmospheres?
13. Explain the phenomenon of *nitrogen narcosis*, which occurs at deep levels below the sea surface when breathing air.
14. What are the effects of *oxygen toxicity* at great depths below the sea surface?

15. Explain the cause and the effects of *decompression sickness*.
16. In SCUBA diving, why is the compressed air mixture that the diver breathes used up far more rapidly at 200 feet than at 50 feet below the sea surface? What is the relationship of carbon dioxide to this difference?

17. Discuss the physiology of escape from a submarine and also some of the special physiological problems of the submarine internal environment.
18. How is *hyperbaric oxygen therapy* used in various clinical conditions?

References

Aviation and Space Physiology

American Physiological Society: High Altitude and Man. Washington, D.C., American Physiological Society, 1984.

Blomqvist, C. G., and Stone, H. L.: Cardiovascular adjustments to gravitational stress. In Shepherd, J. T., and Abboud, F. M., eds.: Handbook of Physiology. Sec. 2, Vol. 3, Bethesda, American Physiological Society, 1983, p. 1025.

Brendel, W. ed.: High Altitude Physiology and Medicine. I. Physiology of Adaptation. New York, Springer-Verlag, 1982.

Bullard, R. W.: Physiological problems of space travel. Annu Rev Physiol 34:205, 1972.

Ciba Foundation Symposia: High Altitude Physiology. New York, Churchill Livingstone, 1971.

Hochachka, P. W.: Living Without Oxygen: Closed and Open Systems of Hypoxia Tolerance. Cambridge, Mass., Harvard University Press, 1980.

Kellogg, R. H.: Altitude acclimatization, a historical introduction emphasizing the regulation of breathing. Physiologist 11:37, 1968.

Lahiri, S.: Physiological responses and adaptations to high altitude. In MTP International Review of Science: Physiology. Vol. 7. Baltimore, University Park Press, 1974, p. 271.

Sloan, A. W.: Man in Extreme Environments. Springfield, Ill., Charles C Thomas, 1979.

Sutton, J. R., et al.: Exercise at altitude. Annu Rev Physiol 45:427, 1983.

Diving Physiology

Behnke, A. R., Jr., and Lanphier, E. H.: Underwater physiology. In Fenn, W. O., and Rahn, H., eds.: Handbook of Physiology. Sec. 3, Vol. 2. Baltimore, Williams & Wilkins, 1965, p. 1159.

Bennett, P. B., and Elliott, D. H.: The Physiology and Medicine of Diving and Compressed Air Work, 2nd ed. Baltimore, Williams & Wilkins, 1975.

Burakovsky, V. I.: Hyperbaric Oxygenation and Its Value in Cardiovascular Surgery. Chicago, Imported Publications, 1981.

Fridovich, I.: Superoxide radical: An endogenous toxicant. Ann Rev Pharmacol Toxicol 23:239, 1983.

Gamarra, J. A.: Decompression Sickness. Hagerstown, Md., Harper & Row, 1974.

Halsey, M. J.: Effects of high pressure on the central nervous system. Physiol Rev 62:1341, 1982.

Oxygen Free Radicals and Tissue Damage. Ciba Foundation Symposium. New York, Excerpta Medica, 1979.

Shilling, C. W., and Beckett, M. W., eds.: Underwater Physiology IV. Bethesda, Md., Federation of American Societies for Experimental Biology, 1978.

Vail, E. G.: Hyperbaric respiratory mechanics. Aerospace Med 42:536, 1971.

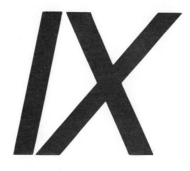

THE CENTRAL NERVOUS SYSTEM

31 ■ Organization of the Nervous System; Basic Functions of Synapses and Neuronal Circuits

32 ■ Sensory Receptors and Mechanoreceptive Somatic Sensations

33 ■ Somatic Sensations: Pain, Visceral Pain, Headache, and Thermal Sensations

34 ■ The Spinal Cord and Brain Stem Reflexes; Function of the Vestibular Apparatus

35 ■ Motor Control by the Motor Cortex, the Basal Ganglia, and the Cerebellum

36 ■ The Cerebral Cortex and Intellectual Functions of the Brain

37 ■ Activation of the Brain; Wakefulness and Sleep; Behavioral Function of the Brain

38 ■ The Autonomic Nervous System; the Adrenal Medulla

31

Organization of the Nervous System; Basic Functions of Synapses and Neuronal Circuits

GENERAL DESIGN OF THE NERVOUS SYSTEM
THE SENSORY DIVISION—SENSORY RECEPTORS
THE MOTOR DIVISION—THE EFFECTORS
PROCESSING OF INFORMATION—THE INTEGRATIVE FUNCTION OF THE NERVOUS SYSTEM
STORAGE OF INFORMATION—MEMORY
THE THREE MAJOR LEVELS OF CENTRAL NERVOUS SYSTEM FUNCTION
THE CENTRAL NERVOUS SYSTEM SYNAPSES
PHYSIOLOGICAL ANATOMY OF THE SYNAPSE
ELECTRICAL EVENTS DURING NEURONAL EXCITATION
ELECTRICAL EVENTS DURING NEURONAL INHIBITION
SUMMATION OF POSTSYNAPTIC POTENTIALS

SPECIAL FUNCTIONS OF DENDRITES IN EXCITING NEURONS
RELATION OF STATE OF EXCITATION OF THE NEURON TO RATE OF FIRING
SOME SPECIAL CHARACTERISTICS OF SYNAPTIC TRANSMISSION
TRANSMISSION AND PROCESSING OF SIGNALS IN NEURONAL POOLS
RELAYING OF SIGNALS THROUGH NEURONAL POOLS
TRANSMISSION OF SPATIAL PATTERNS THROUGH SUCCESSIVE NEURONAL POOLS
PROLONGATION OF A SIGNAL BY A NEURONAL POOL—AFTER-DISCHARGE
RHYTHMIC SIGNAL OUTPUT
INSTABILITY AND STABILITY OF NEURONAL CIRCUITS

The nervous system, along with the endocrine system, provides most of the control functions for the body. In general, the nervous system controls the rapid activities of the body, such as muscular contractions, rapidly changing visceral events, and even the rate of secretion of some endocrine glands. The endocrine system, by contrast, regulates principally the metabolic functions of the body.

The nervous system is unique in the vast complexity of the control actions that it can perform. It receives literally millions of bits of information from the different sensory organs and then integrates all these to determine the response to be made by the body. The purpose of this chapter is to present a general outline of the overall mechanisms by which the nervous system performs such functions and then to discuss the basic functions of synapses and neuronal circuits. Before beginning this discussion, however, the reader should refer to Chapters 5 and 7, which present the principles of membrane potentials and the transmission of signals through neuromuscular junctions, respectively.

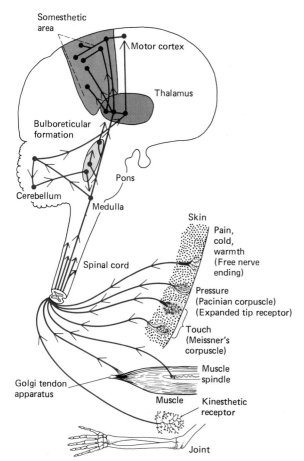

Figure 31-1. The somatic sensory axis of the nervous system.

GENERAL DESIGN OF THE NERVOUS SYSTEM

THE SENSORY DIVISION— SENSORY RECEPTORS

Most activities of the nervous system are initiated by sensory experience emanating from *sensory receptors*—visual, auditory, tactile (on the surface of the body), or other kinds of receptors. This sensory experience can cause an immediate reaction, or its memory can be stored in the brain for minutes, weeks, or years and then can help to determine the bodily reactions at some future date.

Figure 31-1 illustrates the *somatic* portion of the sensory system, which transmits sensory information from the receptors of the entire surface of the body and deep structures. This information enters the nervous system through the spinal nerves and is conducted to essentially all segments of the central nervous system.

THE MOTOR DIVISION— THE EFFECTORS

The most important ultimate role of the nervous system is to control the bodily activities. This is achieved by controlling (1) contractions of skeletal

muscles throughout the body, (2) contractions of smooth muscle in the internal organs, and (3) the secretions of both exocrine and endocrine glands in many parts of the body. These activities are collectively called *motor functions* of the nervous system, and the muscles and glands are called *effectors* because they perform the functions dictated by the nerve signals.

Figure 31-2 illustrates the *motor axis* of the nervous system for controlling skeletal muscle contraction. Operating parallel with this axis is another similar system for control of the smooth muscles and glands; it is the *autonomic nervous system*, which is described in detail in Chapter 38. Note in Figure 31-2 that the skeletal muscles can be controlled from many different levels of the central nervous system. Each of these different areas plays its own specific role in the control of body movements, the lower regions of the central nervous system being concerned primarily with automatic, instantaneous responses of the body to sensory stimuli and the higher regions with deliberate movements controlled by the thought processes of the cerebrum.

PROCESSING OF INFORMATION—THE INTEGRATIVE FUNCTION OF THE NERVOUS SYSTEM

The nervous system would not be at all effective in controlling bodily functions if each bit of sensory information caused some motor reaction. Therefore, one of the major functions of the nervous system is to process incoming information in such a way that

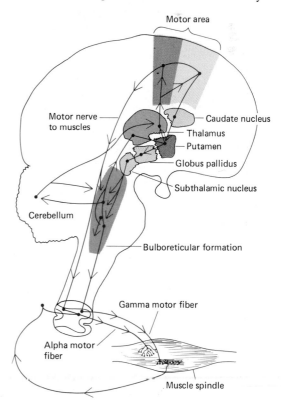

Figure 31-2. The motor axis of the nervous system.

appropriate motor responses occur. Indeed, more than 99 per cent of all sensory information is discarded by the brain as irrelevant and unimportant. For instance, one is ordinarily totally unaware of the parts of the body that are in contact with clothing and is also unaware of the seat pressure when sitting. Likewise, attention is drawn only to an occasional object in one's field of vision, and even the perpetual noise of our surroundings is usually relegated to the background.

After the important sensory information has been selected, it is then channeled into proper motor regions of the brain to cause the desired responses, which is called the *integrative function* of the nervous system. Thus, if a person places a hand on a hot stove, the desired response is to lift the hand, plus other associated responses such as moving the entire body away from the stove and perhaps even shouting with pain. Yet even these responses represent activity by only a small fraction of the total motor system of the body.

Role of Synapses in Processing Information. The synapse is the junction point from one neuron to the next and, therefore, is an advantageous site for control of signal transmission. The synapses determine the directions that the nervous signals spread in the nervous system. Some synapses transmit signals from one neuron to the next with ease, while others transmit signals only with difficulty. Also, facilitatory and inhibitory signals from other areas in the nervous system can control synaptic activity, sometimes opening the synapses for transmission and other times closing them. In addition, some postsynaptic neurons respond with large numbers of impulses, while others respond with only a few.

Thus, the synapses perform a selective action, often blocking the weak signals while allowing the strong signals to pass, often selecting and amplifying certain weak signals, and often channeling the signal in many different directions rather than simply in one direction.

STORAGE OF INFORMATION—MEMORY

Only a small fraction of the important sensory information causes an immediate motor response. Much of the remainder is stored for future control of motor activities and for use in the thinking processes. Most of this storage occurs in the *cerebral cortex,* but not all, for even the basal regions of the brain and perhaps even the spinal cord can store small amounts of information.

The storage of information is the process we call *memory,* and this too is a function of the synapses. That is, each time certain types of sensory signals pass through sequences of synapses, these synapses become more capable of transmitting the same signals the next time, which process is called *facilitation.* After the sensory signals have passed through the synapses a large number of times, the synapses become so facilitated that signals generated within the brain itself can also cause transmission of impulses through the same sequences of synapses even though the sensory input has not been excited. This gives the person a perception of experiencing the original sensations, though in effect they are only memories of the sensations.

Unfortunately, we do not know the precise mechanism by which facilitation of synapses occurs in the memory process, but what is known about this and other details of the memory process is discussed in Chapter 36.

Once memories have been stored in the nervous system, they become part of the processing mechanism. The thought processes of the brain compare new sensory experiences with the stored memories; the memories help to select the important new sensory information and to channel this into appropriate storage areas for future use or into motor areas to cause bodily responses.

THE THREE MAJOR LEVELS OF CENTRAL NERVOUS SYSTEM FUNCTION

The human nervous system has inherited specific characteristics from each stage of evolutionary development. From this heritage, three major levels of the central nervous system have specific functional attributes: (1) the *spinal cord level,* (2) the *lower brain level,* and (3) the *higher brain* or *cortical level.*

The Spinal Cord Level

We often think of the spinal cord as being only a conduit for signals from the periphery of the body to the brain or in the opposite direction from the brain back to the body. However, this is far from the truth. Even after the spinal cord has been cut in the high neck region, many spinal cord functions still occur. For instance, neuronal circuits in the cord can cause
 (1) walking movements
 (2) reflexes that withdraw portions of the body from objects
 (3) reflexes that stiffen the legs to support the body against gravity
 (4) reflexes that control local blood vessels, gastrointestinal movements, and so forth
 (5) and many other functions.
In fact, the upper levels of the nervous system often operate, not by sending signals directly to the periphery of the body, but instead by sending signals to the control centers of the cord, simply "commanding" the cord centers to perform their functions.

The Lower Brain Level

Many, if not most, of what we call subconscious activities of the body are controlled in the lower areas of the brain—in the medulla, pons, mesencephalon, hypothalamus, thalamus, cerebellum, and basal ganglia. Subconscious control of arterial pressure and respiration is achieved mainly in the medulla and pons. Control of equilibrium is a combined function of the older portions of the cerebellum and the reticular substance of the medulla, pons, and mesencephalon. Feeding reflexes, such as salivation in response to the taste of food and the licking of the lips, are controlled by areas in the medulla, pons, mesencephalon, amygdala, and hypothalamus; and many emotional patterns, such as anger, excitement, sexual activities, reaction to pain, or reaction of pleasure, can occur in animals without a cerebral cortex.

The Higher Brain or Cortical Level

After recounting all the nervous system functions that can occur at the cord and lower brain levels, what is left for the cerebral cortex to do? The answer to this is a complex one, but it begins with the fact that the cerebral cortex is an *extremely large memory storehouse.* The cortex never functions alone but always in association with the lower centers of the nervous system.

Without the cerebral cortex, the functions of the lower brain centers are often very imprecise. The vast storehouse of cortical information usually converts these functions to very determinative and precise operations.

Finally, the cerebral cortex is essential for most of our thought processes even though it also cannot function alone in this. In fact, it is the lower centers that cause *wakefulness* in the cerebral cortex, thus opening its bank of memories to the thinking machinery of the brain.

Hence, each portion of the nervous system performs specific functions. Many integrative functions are well developed in the spinal cord, and many of the subconscious functions of the brain are originated and executed entirely in the lower regions of the brain. But it is the cortex that opens the world for one's mind.

THE CENTRAL NERVOUS SYSTEM SYNAPSES

Almost every student is aware that information is transmitted in the central nervous system mainly in the form of nerve impulses through a succession of neurons, one after another. However, it is not immediately apparent that each impulse (a) may be blocked in its transmission from one neuron to the next, (b) may be changed from a single impulse into repetitive impulses, or (c) may be integrated with impulses from other neurons to cause highly intricate patterns of impulses in successive neurons. All these functions are called the *synaptic functions of neurons.*

Virtually all the synapses utilized for signal transmission in the central nervous system are *chemical synapses.* In them, the first neuron secretes a chemical substance called a *neurotransmitter* at the synapse, and this transmitter in turn acts on receptor proteins in the membrane of the next neuron to excite the neuron, to inhibit it, or to modify its sensitivity in some other way. Over 30 different transmitter substances have been discovered thus far.

One-Way Conduction Through the Chemical Synapses. Chemical synapses have one exceedingly important characteristic that makes them highly desirable as the form of transmission of nervous system signals: they always transmit the signals in one direction—that is, from the neuron that secretes the transmitter, called the *presynaptic neuron,* to the neuron on which the transmitter acts, called the *postsynaptic neuron.* This is the principle of *one-way conduction.*

Think for a moment about the extreme importance of the one-way conduction mechanism. It allows signals to be directed toward specific goals. Indeed, it is this specific transmission of signals to discrete and highly focused areas in the nervous system that allows the nervous system to perform its myriad functions of sensation, motor control, memory, and many others.

PHYSIOLOGICAL ANATOMY OF THE SYNAPSE

Figure 31–3 illustrates a typical *motor neuron* in the anterior horn of the spinal cord. It is composed of three major parts: the *soma,* which is the main body of the neuron; a single *axon,* which extends from the soma into the peripheral nerve; and the *dendrites,* which are thin projections of the soma that

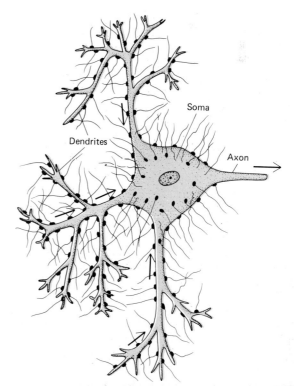

Figure 31–3. A typical motor neuron, showing presynaptic terminals on the neuronal soma and dendrites. Note also the single axon.

extend up to 1 mm into the surrounding areas of the cord.

An average of about 6000 small knobs called *presynaptic terminals* lie on the surfaces of the dendrites and soma of the motor neuron, approximately 80 to 90 per cent of them on the dendrites and only 10 to 20 per cent on the soma. These terminals are the ends of nerve fibrils that originate in many other neurons. Later it will become evident that many of these presynaptic terminals are *excitatory* and secrete a substance that excites the postsynaptic neuron, whereas others are *inhibitory* and secrete a substance that inhibits the neuron.

Neurons in other parts of the cord and brain differ markedly from the motor neuron in (1) the size of the cell body, (2) the length, size, and number of dendrites, ranging in length from almost none at all up to as long as many centimeters, (3) the length and size of the axon, and (4) the number of presynaptic terminals, which may range from only a few to more than a hundred thousand. These differences make neurons in different parts of the nervous system react differently to incoming signals and therefore perform different functions.

The Presynaptic Terminals. Electron microscopic studies of the presynaptic terminals show that they have varied anatomical forms, but most resemble small round or oval knobs and therefore are frequently called *terminal knobs, boutons, end-feet,* or *synaptic knobs.*

Figure 31–4 illustrates the basic structure of the presynaptic terminal. It is separated from the neuronal soma by a *synaptic cleft* having a width usually of 200 to 300 Angstroms. The terminal has two internal structures important to the excitatory or inhibitory functions of the synapse: the *synaptic vesicles* and the *mitochondria.* The synaptic vesicles contain a *transmitter substance* which, when released into the synaptic cleft, either *excites* or *inhibits* the neurons—excites if the neuronal membrane contains *excitatory receptors,* inhibits if it contains *inhibitory receptors.* The mitochondria provide ATP, which is required to synthesize new transmitter substance. The transmitter must be synthesized extremely rapidly because the amount stored in the vesicles is sufficient to last for only a few seconds to a few minutes of maximum activity.

When an action potential spreads over a presynaptic terminal, the membrane depolarization causes emptying of a small number of vesicles into the cleft; the released transmitter in turn causes an immediate change in the permeability characteristics of the postsynaptic neuronal membrane, which leads to excitation or inhibition of the neuron, depending on its receptor characteristics.

Mechanism by Which Action Potentials Cause Transmitter Release at the Presynaptic Terminals—Role of Calcium Ions. The synaptic membrane of the presynaptic terminals contains a large number of *voltage-gated calcium channels.* For this reason, when the action potential depolarizes the terminal, large numbers of calcium ions, along with the sodium ions that cause the action potential, flow into the terminal. And the quantity of transmitter substance that is released into the synaptic cleft is directly related to the number of calcium ions that enter the terminal. The precise mechanism by which the calcium ions cause this release is not known, but it is believed that the calcium ions bind with protein receptors on the inside surfaces of the synaptic membrane called *release sites.* This in turn causes the transmitter vesicles in the local vicinity to bind with the membrane and actually to fuse with it and, finally, to open to the exterior by the process called *exocytosis* that was described in Chapter 2. Often several hundred vesicles release their transmitter into the cleft following a single action potential.

One transmitter substance that occurs in certain parts of the nervous system is acetylcholine, as is discussed later. It has been calculated that about 3000 molecules of acetylcholine are present in each vesicle, and enough vesicles are present in the presynaptic terminal on a neuron to transmit a few thousand impulses.

Synthesis of New Transmitter Substance. Fortunately, the presynaptic terminals have the capability of continually synthesizing new transmitter substance. Were it not for this, synaptic transmission would become completely ineffective within a few minutes. The synthesis occurs either partially or totally in the cytoplasm of the presynaptic terminals, and then the newly synthesized transmitter is immediately absorbed into the vesicles and stored until needed.

As an example, acetylcholine is synthesized from acetyl-CoA and choline in the presence of the enzyme *choline acetyltransferase,* an enzyme that is present in abundance in the cytoplasm of the cholinergic type of presynaptic terminal. When acetylcholine is released from the terminal into the synaptic cleft, it is rapidly split again to acetate and choline by the enzyme *cholinesterase* that is adherent to the proteoglycan reticulum that fills the space of the synaptic cleft. Then the choline is actively transported back

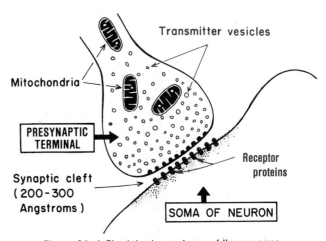

Figure 31–4. Physiologic anatomy of the synapse.

into the terminal to be used once more for synthesis of new acetylcholine.

Action of the Transmitter Substance on the Postsynaptic Neuron—The Function of Receptors. At the synapse, the membrane of the postsynaptic neuron contains large numbers of *receptor proteins,* illustrated in Figure 31–4. These receptors have two important components: (1) a *binding component* that protrudes outward from the membrane into the synaptic cleft—it binds with the neurotransmitter from the presynaptic terminal and activates the receptor, and (2) an *ionophore component* that protrudes through the membrane to the interior of the postsynaptic neuron and opens an ion channel when the receptor is activated.

The ion channels are mainly of three types: (a) *sodium channels* that allow mainly sodium ions (but some potassium ions as well) to pass through, (b) *potassium channels* that allow mainly potassium ions to pass, and (c) *chloride channels* that allow chloride and a few other anions to pass. We shall learn later that opening the sodium channels excites the postsynaptic neuron. Therefore, a transmitter substance that opens the sodium channels is called an *excitatory transmitter.* On the other hand, opening of potassium and chloride channels inhibits the neuron, and transmitters that open either or both of these are called *inhibitory transmitters.*

Duration of Action of the Transmitter, and Removal of the Transmitter from the Synapse. When either an excitatory or an inhibitory transmitter is released into the synaptic cleft, it binds almost instantly with its specific receptor-activated ion channels and opens these either to the flow of sodium ions in the case of the excitatory transmitter or the flow of potassium or chloride ions in the case of the inhibitory transmitter. However, after these channels have remained open for only 1 to 2 milliseconds, in most instances they close equally as rapidly. The reason for this is that the transmitter agent itself is rapidly removed from the synaptic cleft. This is achieved in three different ways:

(1) By *diffusion* of the transmitter out of the cleft into the surrounding fluids.

(2) By *enzymatic destruction* within the cleft itself. For instance, in the case of acetylcholine, the enzyme *cholinesterase* is present in the cleft, bound in the proteoglycan matrix that fills the space. Each molecule of this enzyme can split as many as ten molecules of acetylcholine each millisecond, thus inactivating this transmitter substance. Similar effects occur for other transmitters.

(3) Many of the transmitters are *actively transported back into the presynaptic terminal itself* and are then reused again and again. This is called *transmitter re-uptake.* It occurs especially prominently at the presynaptic terminals of the sympathetic nervous system for the re-uptake of norepinephrine, as we shall discuss in Chapter 38.

The degree to which each of these methods of removal is utilized is different for each type of transmitter.

Excitation and Inhibition. Whether a transmitter will cause excitation or inhibition is determined not only by the nature of the transmitter but also by the nature of the receptor in the postsynaptic membrane. To give an example, the same neuron might be excited at one synapse that releases acetylcholine but at the same time be inhibited at still another synapse that releases glycine. Thus, the neuronal membrane at the first synapse contains an *excitatory receptor* for acetylcholine and at the second synapse an *inhibitory receptor* for glycine. To give another example, norepinephrine released at some synapses in the central nervous system causes inhibition, whereas at other synapses it causes excitation. In the first case, the postsynaptic neuronal membranes contain an inhibitory receptor for norepinephrine while the others contain an excitatory receptor for the same transmitter.

Chemical Substances That Function As Neurotransmitters

More than 30 different chemical substances have either been proved or postulated to be synaptic transmitters; most are listed in Table 31–1. Some of the more important of the transmitters are the following:

Acetylcholine is secreted by neurons in many areas of the brain, but specifically by the large pyramidal

---

Table 31–1. NEUROTRANSMITTERS

Class I:
    Acetylcholine

Class II: The Amines
    Norepinephrine
    Epinephrine
    Dopamine
    Serotonin

Class III: Amino Acids
    γ-Aminobutyric acid (GABA)
    Glycine
    Glutamate

Class IV: Peptides
    A. Hypothalamic-releasing hormones
        Thyrotropin-releasing hormone
        Luteinizing hormone–releasing hormone
        Somatostatin (growth hormone–inhibitory factor)
    B. Pituitary peptides
        ACTH
        β-Endorphin
        α-Melanocyte-stimulating hormone
        Vasopressin
        Oxytocin
    C. Peptides that act on gut and brain
        Leucine enkephalin
        Methionine enkephalin
        Substance P
        Cholecystokinin
        Vasoactive intestinal polypeptide (VIP)
        Neurotensin
        Insulin
        Glucagon
    D. From other tissues
        Angiotensin II
        Bradykinin
        Carnosine
        Bombesin

cells of the motor cortex, by many different neurons in the basal ganglia, by the motor neurons that innervate the skeletal muscles, by the preganglionic neurons of the autonomic nervous system, by the postganglionic neurons of the parasympathetic nervous system, and by some of the postganglionic neurons of the sympathetic nervous system. In most instances acetylcholine has an excitatory effect; however, it is known to have inhibitory effects at some of the peripheral parasympathetic nerve endings, such as inhibition of the heart by the vagus nerves.

Norepinephrine is secreted by many neurons whose cell bodies are located in the brain stem and hypothalamus. Specifically, norepinephrine-secreting neurons located in the *locus ceruleus* in the pons send nerve fibers to widespread areas of the brain and help control the overall activity and mood of the mind. In many of these areas it probably causes excitation, but in others inhibition. Norepinephrine is also secreted by most of the postganglionic neurons of the sympathetic nervous system, where it excites some organs but inhibits others.

Dopamine is secreted by neurons that originate in the substantia nigra. The terminations of these neurons are mainly in the striatal region of the basal ganglia. The effect of dopamine is usually inhibition.

Glycine is secreted mainly at synapses in the spinal cord. It probably always acts as an inhibitory transmitter.

Gamma-aminobutyric acid (GABA) is secreted by nerve terminals in the spinal cord, the cerebellum, the basal ganglia, and many areas of the cortex. It is believed always to cause inhibition.

Glutamate is probably secreted by the presynaptic terminals in many of the sensory pathways as well as in many areas of the cortex. It probably always causes excitation.

Substance P is probably released by pain fiber terminals in the dorsal horns of the spinal cord. And it is also found in the basal ganglia and hypothalamus. In general, it causes excitation.

Enkephalins are probably secreted by nerve terminals in the spinal cord, in the brain stem, in the thalamus, and in the hypothalamus. These probably act as excitatory transmitters to excite other systems that inhibit the transmission of pain.

Serotonin is secreted by nuclei that originate in the median raphe of the brain stem and project to many brain areas, especially to the dorsal horns of the spinal cord and to the hypothalamus. Serotonin acts as an inhibitor of pain pathways in the cord, and its effect in the brain is believed to help control the mood of the person, perhaps even to cause sleep.

Release of Only a Single Type of Transmitter Substance by Each Neuron. Except in special cases, it is believed that each neuron releases only one type of transmitter, and it releases this same transmitter at all of its separate terminals. This is frequently called the *Dale principle*, in honor of the physiologist most instrumental in developing the concept.

ELECTRICAL EVENTS DURING NEURONAL EXCITATION

The electrical events in neuronal excitation have been studied in the large motor neurons of the anterior horn of the spinal cord. Therefore, the events to be described in the following few sections pertain essentially to these neurons. However, except for some quantitative differences, they apply to most other neurons of the nervous system as well.

The Resting Membrane Potential of the Neuronal Soma. Figure 31–5 illustrates the soma of a motor neuron, showing the resting membrane potential to be about −65 millivolts. This is somewhat less than the −80 to −90 millivolts found in large peripheral nerve fibers and in skeletal muscle fibers; the lower voltage is important, however, because it allows both positive and negative control of the degree of excitability of the neuron. That is, decreasing the voltage to a less negative value makes the membrane of the neuron more excitable, whereas increasing this voltage to a more negative value makes the neuron less excitable. This is the basis of the two modes of function of the neuron—either excitation or inhibition—as we will explain in detail in the following sections.

Concentration Differences of Ions Across the Neuronal Somal Membrane. Figure 31–5 also illustrates the concentration differences across the neuronal somal membrane of the three ions that are most important for neuronal function: sodium ions, potassium ions, and chloride ions.

At the top, the sodium ion concentration is shown to be very great in the extracellular fluid but low inside the neuron. This sodium concentration gradient is caused by a strong sodium pump that continually pumps sodium out of the neuron.

The figure also shows that the potassium ion concentration is large inside the neuronal soma but very low in the extracellular fluid. It illustrates that there is also a potassium pump (the other half of the Na^+-K^+ pump, as described in Chapter 4) that tends to pump potassium to the interior. However, because

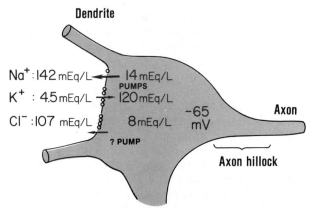

Figure 31–5. Distribution of sodium, potassium, and chloride ions across the neuronal somal membrane; origin of the intrasomal membrane potential.

there is a very high degree of permeability to potassium, the potassium ions leak through the neuronal somal pores so readily that this nullifies most but not all of the effectiveness of the pump.

Figure 31–5 shows the chloride ion to be of high concentration in the extracellular fluid but low concentration inside the neuron. It also shows that the membrane is highly permeable to chloride ions and that there may be a weak chloride pump. But whether there is or is not a chloride pump, most of the reason for the low concentration of chloride ions inside the neuron is the −65 millivolts in the neuron. This negative voltage repels the negatively charged chloride ions, forcing them outward through the pores until the concentration difference is much greater outside the membrane than on the inside.

Let us recall at this point what we learned in Chapters 4 and 5 about the relationship of ionic concentration differences to membrane potentials. It will be recalled that an electrical potential across the membrane can exactly oppose the movement of ions through a membrane despite concentration differences if the potential is of the proper polarity and magnitude. A potential that exactly opposes movement of each type of ion is called the Nernst potential for that ion, the equation for which is the following:

$$EMF(mV) = \pm 61 \times \log \left(\frac{\text{Concentration outside}}{\text{Concentration inside}} \right)$$

in which EMF is the Nernst potential in millivolts on the *inside of the membrane*. The potential will be positive (+) for a positive ion and negative (−) for a negative ion.

Now, let us calculate the Nernst potential that will exactly oppose the movement of each of the three separate ions: sodium, potassium, and chloride.

For the sodium concentration difference shown in Figure 31–5, 142 mEq/liter on the exterior and 14 mEq/liter on the interior, the membrane potential that would exactly oppose sodium ion movement through the sodium channels would be + 61 millivolts. However, the actual membrane potential is − 65 millivolts, not + 61 millivolts. Therefore, sodium ions normally diffuse inward through the sodium channels when they are open; however, not many sodium ions will diffuse because most of the sodium channels are normally closed. Furthermore, those sodium ions that do diffuse to the interior are normally pumped immediately back to the exterior by the sodium pump.

For potassium ions, the concentration gradient is 140 mEq/liter inside the neuron and 4.5 mEq/liter outside. This gives a Nernst potential of − 86 millivolts inside the neuron, which is more negative than the − 65 that actually exists. Therefore, there is a tendency for potassium ions to diffuse to the outside of the neuron, but this is partly opposed by the continual pumping of these potassium ions back to the interior.

Finally, the chloride ion gradient, 107 mEq/liter

outside and 8 mEq/liter inside, yields a Nernst potential of − 70 millivolts inside the neuron, which is slightly more negative than the actual value measured. Therefore, chloride ions tend normally to leak to the interior of the neuron, but those that do leak are moved back to the exterior, perhaps by an active chloride pump.

Keep these three Nernst potentials in mind and also remember the direction in which the different ions tend to diffuse, for this information will be important in understanding both excitation and inhibition of the neuron by synaptic transmission.

Origin of the Resting Membrane Potential of the Neuronal Soma. The basic cause of the − 65 millivolt resting membrane potential of the neuronal soma is the sodium-potassium pump. This pump causes the extrusion of more positively charged sodium ions to the exterior than potassium to the interior—3 sodium ions for each 2 potassium ions. Since there are large numbers of negatively charged ions inside the soma that cannot diffuse through the membrane—protein ions, phosphate ions, and many others—extrusion of the excess positive ions to the exterior leaves all these nondiffusible negative ions inside the cell unbalanced by positive ions. Therefore, the interior of the neuron becomes negatively charged as the result of the sodium-potassium pump. This principle is discussed in more detail in Chapter 5 in relation to the resting membrane potential of nerve fibers.

Uniform Distribution of the Potential Inside the Soma. The interior of the neuronal soma contains a very highly conductive electrolytic solution, the intracellular fluid of the neuron. Furthermore, the diameter of the neuronal soma is very large (from 10 to 80 microns in diameter); as a result there is almost no resistance to conduction of electrical current from one part of the somal interior to another part. Therefore, any change in potential in any part of the intrasomal fluid causes an almost exactly equal change in potential at all other points inside the soma. This is an important principle because it plays a major role in the summation of signals entering the neuron from multiple sources, as we shall see in subsequent sections of this chapter.

Effect of Synaptic Excitation on the Postsynaptic Membrane—The Excitatory Postsynaptic Potential. Figure 31–6A illustrates the resting neuron with an unexcited presynaptic terminal resting upon its surface. The resting membrane potential everywhere in the soma is − 65 millivolts.

Figure 31–6B illustrates a presynaptic terminal that has secreted a transmitter into the cleft between the terminal and the neuronal somal membrane. This transmitter acts on a membrane excitatory receptor *to increase the membrane's permeability to Na^+*. Because of the large electrochemical gradient that tends to move sodium inward, this large opening of the membrane pores mainly allows sodium ions to rush to the inside of the membrane. And, because the sodium ions are positively charged, this influx immediately neutralizes part of the negativity of the resting

A

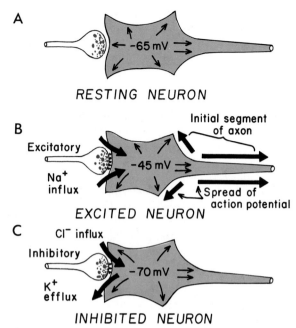

RESTING NEURON

B

Initial segment
of axon

Excitatory

Na⁺
influx

−45 mV

Spread of
action potential

EXCITED NEURON

C

Cl⁻ influx

Inhibitory

K⁺
efflux

−70 mV

INHIBITED NEURON

Figure 31–6. Three states of a neuron. *A*, A resting neuron. *B*, A neuron in an excited state, with increased intraneuronal potential caused by sodium influx. *C*, A neuron in an inhibited state, with decreased intraneuronal membrane potential caused by potassium ion efflux and chloride ion influx.

membrane potential. Thus, in Figure 31–6B the resting membrane potential has been increased from −65 millivolts to −45 millivolts. This +20 millivolt *increase* in voltage above the normal resting neuronal potential—that is, to a less negative value—is called the *excitatory postsynaptic potential* (or EPSP), because when this potential rises high enough it will elicit an action potential in the neuron, thus exciting it.

However, we must issue a word of warning at this point. Discharge of a single presynaptic terminal can never increase the neuronal potential from −65 millivolts up to −45 millivolts. Instead, an increase of this magnitude requires the simultaneous discharge of many terminals—about 70 for the usual anterior motor neuron—at the same time or in rapid succession, which occurs by a process called *summation,* discussed in following sections.

Generation of Action Potentials at the Axon Hillock of the Neuron—Threshold for Excitation. When the membrane potential inside the neuron rises high enough, there comes a point at which this initiates an action potential in the neuron. However, the action potential does not begin on the somal membrane adjacent to the excitatory synapses. Instead, it begins in the *axon hillock,* which is the point of origin of the axon from the neuronal soma. The main reason for this point of origin of the action potential is that the soma has relatively few voltage-gated sodium channels in its membrane, which makes it difficult to open the required number of channels in the somal membrane to elicit an action potential. On the other hand, the membrane of the axon hillock has seven times as

great a concentration of voltage-gated sodium channels and therefore can generate an action potential with much greater ease than can the soma. The excitatory postsynaptic potential that will elicit an action potential at the axon hillock is between +15 and +20 millivolts, in contrast to approximately +30 millivolts required on the soma.

Once the action potential begins, it travels both peripherally along the axon and also backward over the soma. In many instances, it travels backward into the dendrites, too, but not into all of them because they, like the neuronal soma, also have very few voltage-gated sodium channels.

Thus, in Figure 31–6B, it is shown that under normal conditions the *threshold* for excitation of the neuron is about −45 millivolts, which represents an excitatory postsynaptic potential of +20 millivolts—that is, 20 millivolts more positive than the normal resting neuronal potential of −65 millivolts.

ELECTRICAL EVENTS DURING NEURONAL INHIBITION

Effect of Inhibitory Synapses on the Postsynaptic Membrane—The Inhibitory Postsynaptic Potential. It was pointed out earlier that the excitatory synapses open "sodium" channels in the postsynaptic membrane, and these allow easy passage mainly of sodium ions. And, because of the very large difference between the resting membrane potential (−65 mV) and the Nernst potential for sodium (+61 mV), especially large numbers of sodium ions move into the neuron and cause the excitatory postsynaptic potential. The inhibitory synapses, by contrast, open the *potassium* and *chloride channels,* allowing easy passage of both these ions. Now, to understand how the inhibitory synapses inhibit the postsynaptic neuron, we must recall what we learned about the Nernst potentials for both the potassium ions and the chloride ions. We calculated this potential for potassium ions to be about −86 millivolts; for chloride ions, about −70 millivolts. Both these potentials are more negative than the −65 millivolts normally present inside the resting neuronal membrane. Therefore, opening the potassium channels will allow potassium ions to move to the exterior, which will make the membrane potential more negative than normal and opening the chloride channels will allow the chloride ions to move to the interior, which *also* will make the membrane potential more negative than usual. Hence, the degree of intracellular negativity is increased, which is called *hyperpolarization.* This increase obviously inhibits the neuron, because the membrane potential is now farther away than ever from the threshold for excitation. Therefore, the increase in negativity beyond the normal resting membrane potential level is called the *inhibitory postsynaptic potential* (IPSP).

Thus Figure 31–6C illustrates the effect on the membrane potential caused by excitation of inhibitory synapses, allowing chloride influx into the cell and potassium efflux from the cell, with the membrane potential decreasing from its normal value of -65 millivolts to the more negative value of -70 millivolts. By this means, an inhibitory postsynaptic potential of -5 millivolts occurs.

Inhibition of Neurons Without Causing an Inhibitory Postsynaptic Potential—Short Circuiting of the Membrane. Sometimes activation of the inhibitory synapses causes little or no inhibitory postsynaptic potential but nevertheless still inhibits the neuron.

The reason that the potential often does not change is that in some neurons the concentration differences across the membrane for the potassium and chloride ions are only able to cause a diffusion potential equal to the normal resting potential. Therefore, when the inhibitory pores open, there is no net flow of ions to cause an inhibitory postsynaptic potential. Yet, both the potassium and the chloride ions do diffuse bidirectionally through the wide-open pores many times as rapidly as normally, and this high flux of these two ions inhibits the neuron in the following way: When excitatory synapses fire and sodium ions flow into the neuron, this now causes far less excitatory postsynaptic potential than usual because any tendency for the membrane potential to change away from the resting potential is immediately opposed by rapid flux of potassium and chloride ions through the inhibitory pores. That is, the rapid flux of these other ions tends to bring the potential back to the negative equilibrium potential for these two ions. Therefore, the influx of sodium ions now required to cause excitation may be as much as 5 to 20 times normal.

This tendency for the potassium and chloride ions to maintain the membrane potential near the resting value when the inhibitory pores are wide open is called short circuiting of the membrane, thus making the sodium current flow caused by excitatory synapses ineffective in exciting the cell.

Presynaptic Inhibition

In addition to the inhibition caused by inhibitory synapses operating at the neuronal membrane, called *postsynaptic inhibition,* another type of inhibition often occurs before the signal reaches the synapse. This type of inhibition, called *presynaptic inhibition,* is believed to occur in the following way:

In presynaptic inhibition, the inhibition is caused by "presynaptic" synapses that lie on the terminal nerve fibrils before they themselves terminate on the following neuron. It is believed that these presynaptic synapses secrete a transmitter substance that in some way not yet understood depresses the voltage of the action potential that occurs at the synaptic membrane of the presynaptic terminal. This greatly decreases the amount of calcium ions that enter the terminal and therefore also decreases the amount of transmitter released by the terminal. Therefore, the degree of excitation of the neuron is also greatly suppressed, or inhibited.

Presynaptic inhibition occurs in many of the sensory pathways in the nervous system. That is, the adjacent nerve fibers inhibit each other, which minimizes the spread of signals from one fiber to the next. We will discuss this phenomenon more fully in the following chapter.

SUMMATION OF POSTSYNAPTIC POTENTIALS

Time Course of Postsynaptic Potentials. When a synapse excites the anterior motor neuron the neuronal membrane becomes highly permeable for only 1 to 2 milliseconds. During this time sodium ions diffuse rapidly to the interior of the cell to increase the intraneuronal potential, thus creating the *excitatory postsynaptic potential.* This potential then persists for about 15 milliseconds, because this is the time required for potassium ions to leak out or chloride ions to leak in to re-establish the normal resting membrane potential.

Precisely the opposite effect occurs for the inhibitory postsynaptic potential. That is, the inhibitory synapse increases the permeability of the membrane to potassium and chloride ions for 1 to 2 milliseconds, which usually decreases the intraneuronal potential to a more negative value than normal, thereby creating the *inhibitory postsynaptic potential.* This potential also persists for about 15 milliseconds.

However, other types of transmitter substances acting on other neurons can perhaps excite or inhibit for hundreds of milliseconds or even for seconds, minutes, or hours.

Spatial Summation of the Postsynaptic Potentials. It has already been pointed out that excitation of a single presynaptic terminal on the surface of a neuron will almost never excite the neuron. The reason for this is that sufficient transmitter substance is released by a single terminal to cause an excitatory postsynaptic potential of usually no more than a millivolt at most, instead of the required 15 to 20 millivolts to reach the usual threshold for excitation. However, during excitation in a neuronal pool of the nervous system, many presynaptic terminals are usually stimulated at the same time, and even though these terminals are spread over wide areas of the neuron, their effects can still summate. The reason for this summation is the following: It has already been pointed out that a change in the potential at any single point within the soma will cause the potential to change everywhere in the soma almost exactly equally. Therefore, for each excitatory synapse that discharges simultaneously, the intrasomal potential becomes more positive by as much as a small fraction of a millivolt up to about 1 millivolt. When the excitatory postsynaptic potential becomes great enough, the threshold for firing will be reached, and an action potential will generate at the axon hillock. This effect of summing simultaneous postsynaptic potentials by excitation of multiple terminals on widely spaced areas of the membrane is called *spatial summation.*

Temporal Summation. Most presynaptic terminals can fire repetitively in rapid succession only a few milliseconds apart. Each time a terminal fires, the released transmitter substance opens the membrane channels for a millisecond or so. Since the postsynaptic potential lasts up to 15 milliseconds, a second opening of the same channel can increase the postsynaptic potential to a still greater level. Therefore, the more rapid the rate of terminal stimulation, the greater the effective postsynaptic potential. Thus, successive postsynaptic potentials of individual presynaptic terminals, if they occur rapidly enough, can summate in the same way as postsynaptic potentials from widely distributed terminals over the surface of the neuron. This event is called *temporal summation.*

Simultaneous Summation of Inhibitory and Excitatory Postsynaptic Potentials. Obviously, if an inhibitory postsynaptic potential is tending to decrease the membrane potential to a more negative value while an excitatory postsynaptic potential is tending to increase the potential at the same time, these two effects can either completely or partially nullify each other. Also, inhibitory short circuiting of the membrane potential can nullify much of an excitatory potential. Thus, if a neuron is currently being excited by an excitatory postsynaptic potential, then an inhibitory signal from another source can easily reduce the postsynaptic potential to less than the threshold value for excitation, turning off the activity of the neuron.

Facilitation of Neurons. Often the summated postsynaptic potential is excitatory in nature but has not risen high enough to reach the threshold for excitation. When this happens, the neuron is said to be *facilitated.* That is, its membrane potential is nearer the threshold for firing than normally but not yet to the firing level. Consequently, a signal entering the neuron from some other source can then excite the neuron very easily. Diffuse signals in the nervous system often facilitate large groups of neurons so that they can respond quickly and easily to signals arriving from second sources.

SPECIAL FUNCTIONS OF DENDRITES IN EXCITING NEURONS

The Large Spatial Field of Excitation of the Dendrites. The dendrites of the anterior motor neurons extend for 0.5 to 1 millimeter in all directions from the neuronal soma. Therefore, these dendrites can receive signals from a large spatial area around the motor neuron. This circumstance provides vast opportunity for summation of signals from many separate presynaptic neurons.

It is also important that between 80 and 90 per cent of all the presynaptic terminals terminate on the dendrites of the anterior motor neuron in contrast to only 10 to 20 per cent terminating on the neuronal soma. Therefore, the preponderant share of the excitation of the neuron is provided by signals transmitted over the dendrites. However, a large share of the excitatory postsynaptic potential is lost before it reaches the soma. The reason for this is that the dendrites are long and thin, and their membranes are

also leaky to electrical current. Therefore, before the excitatory potentials can reach the soma, a large share of the potential is lost by leakage through the membrane. This decrease in membrane potential as it spreads electrotonically along dendrites toward the soma is called *decremental conduction.*

It is therefore obvious that the nearer the excitatory synapse is to the soma of the neuron, the smaller will be the decrement of conduction. Consequently, those synapses that lie near the soma have far more excitatory effect than those that lie far away from the soma.

Rapid Re-Excitation of the Neuron by the Dendrites After the Neuron Fires. When an action potential is generated in a neuron, this action potential spreads back over the soma but not always over the dendrites. Therefore, the excitatory postsynaptic potentials in the dendrites often are only partially disturbed by the action potential, so that just as soon as the action potential is over, the potentials still existing in the dendrites are ready and waiting to excite the neuron again. Thus, the dendrites have a "holding capacity" for the excitatory signal from presynaptic sources.

RELATION OF STATE OF EXCITATION OF THE NEURON TO RATE OF FIRING

The Excitatory State. The *excitatory state* of a neuron is defined as the degree of excitatory drive to the neuron. If there is a higher degree of excitation than inhibition of the neuron at any given instant, it is said that there is an *excitatory state.* On the other hand, if there is more inhibition than excitation, then it is said that there is an *inhibitory state.*

When the excitatory state of a neuron rises above the threshold for excitation, then the neuron will fire repetitively as long as the excitatory state remains at this level. Furthermore, and for obvious reasons, *the rate at which it will fire is determined by how much the excitatory state is above threshold.*

Response Characteristics of Different Neurons to Increasing Levels of Excitatory State. Histological study of the nervous system immediately convinces one of the widely varying types of neurons in different parts of the nervous system. And, physiologically, the different types of neurons perform different functions. Therefore, as would be expected, the ability to respond to stimulation by the synapses varies from one type of neuron to another.

Figure 31-7 illustrates theoretical responses of three different types of neurons to varying levels of excitatory state. Note that neuron #1 has a low threshold for excitation, while neuron #3 has a high threshold. But note also that neuron #2 has the lowest maximum frequency of discharge, while neuron #3 has the highest maximum frequency.

Some neurons in the central nervous system fire continuously because even the normal excitatory state is above the threshold level. Their frequency of firing can usually be increased still more by further increas-

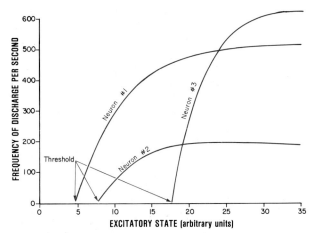

Figure 31-7. Response characteristics of different types of neurons to progressively increasing levels of excitatory state.

ing their excitatory state. Or the frequency may be decreased, or firing even be stopped, by superimposing an inhibitory state on the neuron.

Thus, different neurons respond differently, have different thresholds for excitation, and have widely differing maximal frequencies of discharge. With a little imagination, one can readily understand the importance of having neurons with many different types of response characteristics to perform the widely varying functions of the nervous system.

SOME SPECIAL CHARACTERISTICS OF SYNAPTIC TRANSMISSION

Fatigue of Synaptic Transmission. When excitatory synapses are repetitively stimulated at a rapid rate, the number of discharges in the post-synaptic neuron is at first very great, but it becomes progressively less in succeeding milliseconds or seconds. This is called *fatigue* of synaptic transmission.

Fatigue is an exceedingly important characteristic of synaptic function, for when areas of the nervous system become overexcited, fatigue causes them to lose this excess excitability after a while. For example, fatigue is probably the most important means by which the excess excitability of the brain during an epileptic convulsion is finally subdued so that the convulsion ceases. Thus, the development of fatigue is a protective mechanism against excess neuronal activity. This will be discussed further in the description of reverberating neuronal circuits later in the chapter.

The mechanism of fatigue is mainly exhaustion of the stores of transmitter substance in the synaptic terminals, particularly since it has been calculated that the excitatory terminals can store enough excitatory transmitter for only 10,000 normal synaptic transmissions, an amount that can be exhausted in only a few seconds to a few minutes. However, part of the fatigue process probably also results from two other factors as well: (1) progressive inactivation of many of the postsynaptic membrane receptors and

(2) slow buildup of calcium ions inside the neuronal cell, caused by the successive action potentials—these calcium ions in turn open calcium-activated potassium channels, which cause an inhibitory effect on the postsynaptic neuron.

Effects of Acidosis and Alkalosis on Synaptic Transmission. The neurons are highly responsive to changes in pH of the surrounding interstitial fluids. *Alkalosis greatly increases neuronal excitability.* For instance, a rise in arterial pH from the normal of 7.4 to about 7.8 often causes cerebral convulsions because of increased excitability of the neurons. This effect can be demonstrated especially well by having a person who is predisposed to epileptic convulsions overbreathe. The overbreathing elevates the pH of the blood only momentarily, but even this short interval can often precipitate an epileptic attack.

On the other hand, *acidosis greatly depresses neuronal activity;* a fall in pH from 7.4 to below 7.0 usually causes a comatose state. For instance, in very severe diabetic or uremic acidosis, coma always develops.

Effect of Hypoxia on Synaptic Transmission. Neuronal excitability is also highly dependent on an adequate supply of oxygen. Cessation of oxygen supply for only a few seconds can cause complete inexcitability of the neurons. This occurrence is often seen when the cerebral circulation is temporarily interrupted, for within 3 to 5 seconds the person becomes unconscious.

Effects of Drugs on Synaptic Transmission. Many different drugs are known to increase the excitability of neurons, and others are known to decrease the excitability. For instance, caffeine, theophylline, and theobromine, which are found in coffee, tea, and cocoa, respectively, all increase neuronal excitability, presumably by reducing the threshold for excitation of the neurons. However, strychnine, which is one of the best known of all the agents that increase the excitability of neurons, does not reduce the threshold for excitation of the neurons at all but, instead, *inhibits the action of at least some of the inhibitory transmitters* on the neurons, probably especially the inhibitory effect of glycine in the spinal cord. In consequence, the effects of the excitatory transmitters become overwhelming, and the neurons become so excited that they go into rapidly repetitive discharge, causing severe convulsions.

Most anesthetics increase the membrane threshold for excitation and thereby decrease synaptic transmission at many points in the nervous system. Because most of the anesthetics are lipid-soluble, it has been reasoned that they might change the physical characteristics of the neuronal membranes, making them less responsive to excitatory agents.

TRANSMISSION AND PROCESSING OF SIGNALS IN NEURONAL POOLS

The central nervous system is made up of literally hundreds or even thousands of separate *neuronal pools*, some of which contain very few neurons while others hold vast numbers. For instance, the entire cerebral cortex could be considered to be a single large neuronal pool. It has many separate fiber tracts coming to it (afferent fibers) and others leaving it (efferent fibers). Furthermore it maintains the same quality of spatial orientation as that found in the nerve bundles, individual points of the cortex connecting with specific points elsewhere in the nervous system or connecting through the peripheral nerves with specific points in the body. However, within this pool of neurons are large numbers of short nerve fibers whereby signals spread horizontally from neuron to neuron within the pool itself.

Other neuronal pools include the different basal ganglia, the specific nuclei in the thalamus, cerebellum, mesencephalon, pons, and medulla. Also, the entire dorsal gray matter of the spinal cord could be considered to be one long pool of neurons, and the entire anterior gray matter another long neuronal pool. Each pool has its own special characteristics of organization which cause it to process signals in its own special way, thus allowing these special characteristics to determine the multitude of functions of the nervous system. Yet, despite their differences in function, the pools also have many similarities that are described in the following pages.

RELAYING OF SIGNALS
THROUGH NEURONAL POOLS

Signals. In the transmission of information, it is frequently not desirable to speak in terms of the individual impulses but instead to refer to the overall pattern of impulses; this pattern is called a *signal*. As an example, when pressure is applied to a large area of skin, impulses are transmitted by large numbers of parallel nerve fibers, and the total pattern of impulses transmitted by all these fibers is a signal. Thus, we can speak of visual signals, auditory signals, somesthetic sensory signals, motor signals, and so forth.

Organization of Neurons for Relaying Signals. Figure 31–8 is a schematic diagram of several neurons in a neuronal pool, showing "input" fibers to the left and "output" fibers to the right. Each input fiber divides hundreds to thousands of times, providing an average of a thousand or more terminal fibrils that spread over a large area in the pool to synapse with the dendrites or cell bodies of the neurons in the pool. The dendrites of some of the neurons also arborize and spread in the pool. The neuronal area stimulated by each incoming nerve fiber is called its *stimulatory field*. Note that each input fiber arborizes so that large numbers of its terminals lie on the centermost neurons in its "field," but progressively fewer terminals lie on the neurons farther from the center of the field.

Threshold and Subthreshold Stimuli—Facilitation. From the discussion of synaptic function earlier in the chapter, it will be recalled that discharge of a

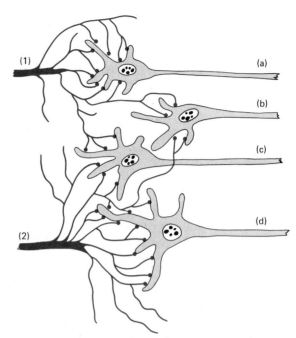

Figure 31–8. Basic organization of a neuronal pool.

single excitatory presynaptic terminal almost never stimulates the postsynaptic neuron. Instead, large numbers of terminals must discharge on the same neuron either simultaneously or in rapid succession to cause excitation. For instance, in Figure 31–8, let us assume that six separate terminals must discharge simultaneously to excite any one of the neurons. If the student will count the number of terminals on each one of the neurons from each input fiber, it can be seen that input fiber (1) has more than enough terminals to cause neuron (a) to discharge. Therefore, the stimulus from input fiber (1) to this neuron is said to be an *excitatory stimulus*, or it is also called a *threshold stimulus* because it is above the threshold required for excitation.

Input fiber (1) also contributes terminals to neurons (b) and (c) but not enough to cause excitation. Nevertheless, discharge of these terminals makes both these neurons more excitable to signals arriving through other incoming nerve fibers. Therefore, the stimulus to these neurons is said to be *subthreshold*, and the neurons are said to be *facilitated*.

Similarly, for input fiber (2), the stimulus to neuron (d) is a threshold stimulus and to neurons (b) and (c), a subthreshold but facilitating stimulus.

It must be recognized that Figure 31–8 represents a highly condensed version of a neuronal pool, for each input nerve fiber usually provides terminals to hundreds or thousands of separate neurons in its distribution field.

Inhibition of a Neuronal Pool. We must also remember that some incoming fibers inhibit neurons rather than excite them. This is exactly the opposite of facilitation, and the entire field of the inhibitory branches is called the *inhibitory zone*. The degree of inhibition in the center of this zone is very great

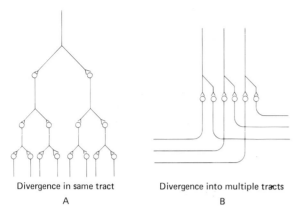

Divergence in same tract

A

Divergence into multiple tracts

B

Figure 31–9. "Divergence" in neuronal pathways. A, Divergence within a pathway to cause "amplification" of the signal. B, Divergence into multiple tracts to transmit the signal to separate areas.

because of large numbers of endings in the center, while the inhibition becomes progressively less toward its edges.

Divergence of Signals Passing Through Neuronal Pools

Often it is important for signals entering a neuronal pool to excite far greater numbers of nerve fibers leaving the pool. This phenomenon is called *divergence*. Two major types of divergence occur and have entirely different purposes. These are illustrated in Figure 31–9 and may be described as follows:

An *amplifying* type of divergence often occurs, illustrated in Figure 31–9A. This means simply that an input signal spreads to an increasing number of neurons as it passes through successive pools of a nervous pathway. This type of divergence is characteristic of the corticospinal pathway in its control of skeletal muscles, as follows: Stimulation of a single large pyramidal cell in the motor cortex transmits a single impulse into the spinal cord. Yet, under appropriate conditions of very strong cord facilitation, this impulse can stimulate perhaps several hundred interneurons and anterior motor neurons. Each of the motor neurons then stimulates as many as 100 or more muscle fibers. Thus, there is a total divergence, or amplification, of as much as 10,000-fold.

The second type of divergence, illustrated in Figure 31–9B, is *divergence into multiple tracts*. In this case, the signal is transmitted in two separate directions from the pool, to different parts of the nervous system where it is needed. For instance, information transmitted in the dorsal columns of the spinal cord takes two courses in the lower part of the brain: (1) into the cerebellum, and (2) on through the lower regions of the brain to the thalamus and cerebral cortex.

Convergence of Signals

Often it is important for signals from multiple incoming neurons to excite the same neuron. That is, these incoming fibers *converge* on this same neuron.

Like divergence, there are also two basic types of convergence, illustrated in Figure 31–10.

Section A of this figure shows *convergence from a single source*. That is, multiple terminals from an incoming fiber tract terminate on the same neuron. The importance of this fact is that neurons are almost never excited by an action potential from a single input terminal. But action potentials from multiple input terminals will provide enough summation to bring the neuron to the threshold required for discharge.

However, *convergence can also result from input signals* (excitatory or inhibitory) *from several different sources*, which is illustrated in Figure 31–10B. For instance, the interneurons of the spinal cord receive converging signals from (a) peripheral nerve fibers entering the cord, (b) propriospinal fibers passing from one segment of the cord to another, (c) corticospinal fibers from the cerebral cortex, and (d) several other long pathways descending from the brain into the spinal cord. Then the signals from the interneurons converge on the anterior motor neurons to control muscle function.

Such convergence allows summation of information from different sources, and the resulting response is a summated effect of all the different types of information. Obviously, therefore, convergence is one of the important means by which the central nervous system correlates, summates, and sorts different types of information.

Neuronal Circuit Causing Both Excitatory and Inhibitory Output Signals

Sometimes an incoming signal to a neuronal pool causes an output excitatory signal going in one direction and, at the same time, an inhibitory signal going elsewhere. For instance, at the same time that an excitatory signal is transmitted by one set of neurons in the spinal cord to cause forward movement of a leg, an inhibitory signal is transmitted simultaneously through a separate set of neurons to inhibit the muscles on the back of the leg so that they will not oppose the forward movement. This type of circuit is

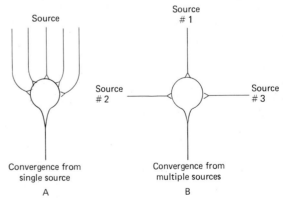

Source

Source
1

Source
2

Source
3

Convergence from
single source

A

Convergence from
multiple sources

B

Figure 31–10. "Convergence" of multiple input fibers on a single neuron. A, Input fibers from a single source. B, Input fibers from multiple sources.

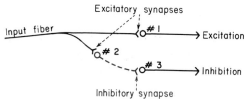

Figure 31-11. Inhibitory circuit. Neuron 2 is an inhibitory neuron.

characteristic of control of all antagonistic pairs of muscles, and it is called the *reciprocal inhibition circuit*.

Figure 31–11 illustrates the means by which the inhibition is achieved. The input fiber directly excites the excitatory output pathway, but it stimulates an intermediate *inhibitory neuron* (neuron 2), which then inhibits the second output pathway from the pool.

TRANSMISSION OF SPATIAL PATTERNS THROUGH SUCCESSIVE NEURONAL POOLS

Most information is transmitted from one part of the nervous system to another through several successive neuronal pools. For instance, sensory information from the skin passes first through the peripheral nerve fibers, then through second order neurons that originate either in the spinal cord or in the cuneate and gracile nuclei of the medulla, and finally through third order neurons originating in the thalamus to the cerebral cortex. Such a pathway is illustrated at the top of Figure 31-12. Note that the sensory nerve endings in the skin overlap each other tremendously; and the terminal fibrils of each nerve fiber, on entering each neuronal pool, spread to many adjacent neurons, innervating perhaps 100 or more separate neurons. On first thought, one would expect signals from the skin to become completely mixed up by this haphazard arrangement of terminal fibrils in each neuronal pool. For statistical reasons, however, this does not occur, which can be explained as follows:

First, if a single point is stimulated in the skin, the nerve fiber with the most nerve endings in that particular spot becomes stimulated to the strongest extent, while the immediately adjacent nerve fibers become stimulated less strongly, and the nerve fibers still farther away become stimulated only weakly. When this signal arrives at the first neuronal pool, the stimulus spreads in many directions in the terminal fibrils of the neuronal pool. Yet the *greatest number* of *excited presynaptic terminals* lies very near the point of entry of the most excited input nerve fiber. Therefore, the neuron closest to this central point is the one that becomes stimulated to the greatest extent. Exactly the same effect occurs in the second neuronal pool in the thalamus and again when the signal reaches the cerebral cortex.

Yet it is true that a signal passing through *highly facilitated neuronal pools* could diverge so much that the spatial pattern at the terminus of the pathway would be completely obscured. This effect is illustrated in Figure 31–12A, which shows successively

expanding spatial patterns of neuron stimulation in such a facilitated, diverging pathway.

However, the degree of facilitation of the different neuronal pools varies from time to time. Under some conditions, the degree of facilitation is so low that the pathway becomes converging, as illustrated in Figure 31-12B. In this case, a broad area of the skin is stimulated, but the signal loses part of its fringe stimuli as it passes through each successive pool until the breadth of the stimulus becomes contracted at the opposite end. One can achieve this type of stimulation by pressing ever so lightly with a flat object on the skin. The signal converges to give the person a sensation of almost a point contact.

In Figure 31-12C, four separate points are simultaneously stimulated on the skin, and the degree of excitability in each neuronal pool is exactly that amount required to prevent either divergence or convergence. Therefore, a reasonably true spatial pattern of each of the four points of stimulation is transmitted through the entire pathway.

Lateral Inhibition to Provide Contrast in the Spatial Pattern. When a single point of the skin or other sensory area is stimulated, not only is a single fiber excited but a number of "fringe" fibers are excited less strongly at the same time, as already explained. Therefore, the spatial pattern is blurred even before the signal begins to be transmitted through the pathway. However, in almost all pathways that transmit very exact information, such as the critical sensory pathways, lateral *inhibitory circuits* inhibit the fringe neurons and re-establish a truer spatial pattern.

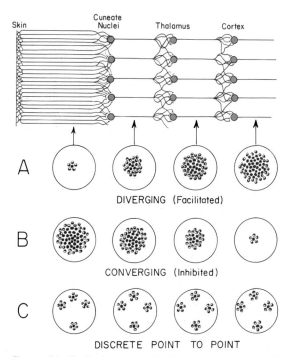

Figure 31-12. Typical organization of a sensory pathway from the skin to the cerebral cortex. *Below:* The patterns of fiber stimulation at different points in the pathway following stimulation by a pinprick when the pathway is *A*, facilitated; *B*, inhibited; and *C*, normally excitable.

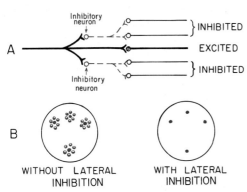

Figure 31–13. *A,* One type of lateral inhibitory circuit by which an excited fiber of a neuronal pool can cause inhibition of adjacent fibers. *B,* Increase in contrast of the stimulus pattern caused by the inhibitory circuit.

Figure 31–13A illustrates one type of lateral inhibitory circuit, showing that the nerve fibers of a pathway give off collateral fibers that excite inhibitory neurons. These inhibitory neurons in turn inhibit the less excited fringe neurons in the signal pathway. The effect on transmission of the spatial pattern is illustrated in Figure 31–13B, which shows the same point-to-point transmission pattern that was illustrated in Figure 31–12C. The left-hand pattern illustrates four strongly excited fibers (the solid fibers) with penumbras of fringe excitation surrounding each of these. In the illustration to the right, the penumbras have been removed by the lateral inhibitory circuits; obviously, this removal increases the *contrast* in the signal and helps in the *faithfulness* of transmission of the spatial pattern.

PROLONGATION OF A SIGNAL BY A NEURONAL POOL—AFTER-DISCHARGE

Thus far, we have considered signals that are merely relayed through neuronal pools. However, in many instances, a signal entering a pool causes a prolonged output discharge, called *after-discharge,* even after the incoming signal is over, and lasting from a few milliseconds to as long as many minutes. The three basic mechanisms by which after-discharge occurs are the following:

Synaptic After-Discharge. When excitatory synapses discharge on the surfaces of dendrites or the soma of a neuron, a postsynaptic potential develops in the neuron and lasts for many milliseconds—in the anterior motor neuron for up to 15 milliseconds, though perhaps much longer in other neurons, especially so when some of the long-acting synaptic transmitter substances are involved. As long as this potential lasts, it can continue to excite the neuron, causing it to transmit a continuous train of output impulses. Thus it is possible for a single instantaneous input to cause a sustained signal output (a series of repetitive discharges) lasting as long as 15 or more milliseconds.

The Parallel Circuit Type of After-Discharge. Figure 31–14 illustrates a second type of neuronal circuit that can cause intermediate periods of after-discharge. In this case, the input signal spreads through a series of neurons in the neuronal pool, and from each of these neurons, impulses then converge onto an output neuron. Because a signal is delayed at each synapse for about 0.5 millisecond, called the *synaptic delay,* signals passing through a succession of intermediate neurons reach the output neuron one by one after varying periods. Therefore, the output neuron continues to be stimulated for many milliseconds.

It is doubtful whether more than a few dozen successive neurons ordinarily enter into a parallel after-discharge circuit. Therefore, one would suspect that this type of after-discharge circuit could cause after-discharges that last for no more than perhaps 25 to 50 milliseconds. Yet this circuit does represent a means by which a single input signal, lasting less than 1 millisecond, can be converted into a sustained output signal lasting for a rather precise period of time.

The Reverberatory (Oscillatory) Circuit as a Cause of After-Discharge. Many neurophysiologists believe that one of the most important of all circuits in the entire nervous system is the *reverberatory,* or *oscillatory, circuit.* Such circuits are caused by positive feedback within the neuronal pool. That is, the output of a neuronal circuit feeds back to re-excite the same circuit. Consequently, once stimulated, the circuit discharges repetitively for a long time.

Several different postulated varieties of reverberatory circuits are illustrated in Figure 31–15, the simplest—in Figure 31–15A—involving only a single neuron. In this case, the output neuron simply sends a collateral nerve fiber back to its own dendrites or soma to restimulate itself; therefore, once the neuron discharges, the feedback stimuli could theoretically help keep the neuron discharging for a long time thereafter.

Figure 31–15B illustrates a few additional neurons in the feedback circuit, which would give a longer period of time between the initial discharge and the feedback signal. Figure 31–15C illustrates a still more complex system in which both facilitatory and inhibitory fibers impinge on the reverberating pool. A facilitatory signal increases the ease with which reverberation takes place, whereas an inhibitory signal decreases the ease of reverberation.

Figure 31–15D illustrates that most reverberating pathways are constituted of many parallel fibers, and

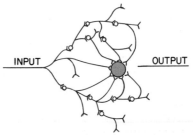

Figure 31–14. The parallel after-discharge circuit.

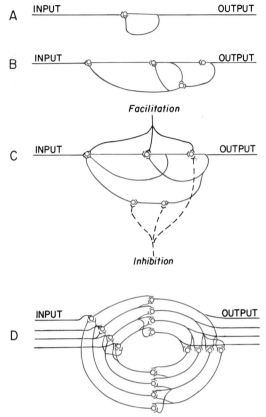

Figure 31–15. Reverberatory circuits of increasing complexity.

at each cell station the terminal fibrils diffuse widely. In such a system, the total reverberating signal can be either weak or strong, depending on how many parallel nerve fibers are momentarily involved in the reverberation.

Finally, reverberation need not occur only in a single neuronal pool; it can occur through a circuit involving two or more successive pools in the positive feedback pathway.

Characteristics of After-Discharge from a Reverberatory Circuit. The input stimulus need last only 1 millisecond or so, and yet the output can last for many milliseconds or even minutes. Furthermore, the duration of the after-discharge is determined by the degree of inhibition or facilitation of the neuronal pool. In this way, signals from other parts of the brain can control the reaction of the pool to the input stimulus.

One of the most important factors that determines the duration of the reverberatory type of after-discharge is the rapidity with which the involved synapses fatigue. Rapid fatigue obviously tends to shorten the period of after-discharge. On the other hand, the greater the number of successive stages of neurons in the reverberatory pathway and the greater the number of collateral feedback fibrils, the easier it would be to keep the reverberation going.

Some Reverberatory Systems of the Nervous System and Their Durations of Reverberation. Even though neurophysiologists are not certain which functions of the nervous system can rightfully be ascribed to reverberatory circuits, some of those that have been postulated have reverberatory durations from as short as 10 milliseconds up to as long as several minutes or perhaps even hours. Some examples include: (1) In an animal whose spinal cord is transected in the neck, a sudden painful stimulus to the animal's paw will cause the flexor muscles to contract and remain contracted from a fraction of a second to as much as several seconds after the stimulus ends. (2) During respiration the inspiratory neuronal pool in the medulla becomes excited for about 2 seconds during each respiratory cycle. One theory suggests that this excitation is caused by reverberation within the inspiratory neuronal pool. And (3) one theory of wakefulness is that continual reverberation occurs somewhere within the brain stem to keep a wakefulness area excited during the waking hours. If this be true, then this would represent a 14- to 18-hour period of reverberation.

RHYTHMIC SIGNAL OUTPUT

Many neuronal circuits emit rhythmic output signals—for instance, the rhythmic respiratory signal originating in the medulla and pons. This repetitive rhythmic signal continues throughout life, while other rhythmic signals, such as those that cause walking movements, require input stimuli into the respective circuits to initiate the signals.

Many rhythmic signals are postulated to result from reverberating circuits or successive reverberating circuits that feed excitatory or inhibitory signals from one neuronal pool to the next. Obviously, facilitatory or inhibitory inputs can affect rhythmic signal output in the same way that they can affect any other neuronal function. For instance, when the carotid body is stimulated by arterial oxygen deficiency, the frequency and amplitude of the rhythmic respiratory signal pattern increase progressively.

INSTABILITY AND STABILITY OF NEURONAL CIRCUITS

Almost every part of the brain connects either directly or indirectly with every other part, and this creates a serious problem. If the first part excites the second, the second the third, and so on until finally the signal re-excites the first part, it is clear that an excitatory signal entering any part of the brain would set off a continuous cycle of re-excitation of all parts. If this circumstance should occur, the brain would be inundated by a mass of uncontrolled reverberating signals—signals that would be transmitting no information but would nevertheless be consuming the circuits of the brain so that none of the informational signals could be transmitted. Such an effect actually occurs in widespread areas of the brain during *epileptic convulsions*.

How does the central nervous system prevent this from happening all the time? Part of the answer seems to lie in the phenomenon of synaptic fatigue, described in the following paragraphs.

Synaptic Fatigue as a Means for Stabilizing the Nervous System. Synaptic fatigue means simply that the signal transmission through the synapses becomes progressively weaker the more prolonged the period of excitation. Let us apply this phenomenon of fatigue to multiple pathways in the brain. Those pathways that are overused become fatigued, so that their sensitivities will be reduced. On the other hand, those that are underused become rested and their sensitivities increase. Thus, fatigue and recovery from fatigue constitute an important means for moderating the sensitivities of the different nervous system circuits, helping to keep them operating in a range of sensitivity that allows effective function.

Long-Term Changes in Synaptic Sensitivity Caused by Automatic Downgrading or Upgrading of Synaptic Receptors. Recently, it has been learned that the long-term sensitivities of synapses can change tremendously as a result of downgrading the number of receptor proteins at the synaptic sites when there is overactivity and upgrading the receptors when there is underactivity. The mechanism for this is believed to be the following: Receptor proteins are constantly formed by the endoplasmic reticulum–Golgi apparatus system and are constantly inserted into the synaptic membrane. However, when the synapses are overused, excesses of transmitter substance combine with the receptor proteins and cause many of these proteins to be inactivated permanently. Therefore overusage of a circuit will lead to gradually decreasing sensitivity of the synapses because of decreased receptor proteins, while underusage will cause prolonged increase in sensitivity. These opposite reactions represent still another mechanism for continually adjusting the sensitivities of the respective neuronal circuits.

It is indeed fortunate that fatigue and downgrading or upgrading of receptors, as well as other control mechanisms of the nervous system, continually adjust the sensitivity in each circuit to almost the exact level required for proper function. Think for a moment how serious it would be if the sensitivities of only a few of these circuits should be abnormally high; one might then expect almost continual muscle cramps, convulsions, psychotic disturbances, hallucinations, tension, or many other nervous disorders. But the automatic controls normally readjust the sensitivities of the circuits back to a controllable range of reactivity any time the circuits begin to be too active.

QUESTIONS

1. Discuss in general the *sensory and motor divisions* and the *integrative function* of the nervous system.
2. What are the general functions at the three major levels of the central nervous system: the *spinal cord*, the *lower brain*, and the *higher brain*, or *cortical*, *levels*?
3. Describe the structure of the typical *synapse*.
4. What is the role of calcium ions in the release of *transmitter substance* at a synapse?
5. How is transmitter substance synthesized in the presynaptic terminals?
6. Explain the action of the transmitter substance on the postsynaptic neuron membrane.
7. What determines whether a transmitter substance will be excitatory or inhibitory? Name the specific characteristics of several of the more important neurotransmitter substances.
8. Give the concentrations of the important ions for neuronal function on the two sides of the neuronal cell membrane.
9. Explain what is meant by the *Nernst potential* and what is the mechanism for developing the resting membrane potential of the neuronal cell membrane.
10. Explain the sequence of events and changes in membrane potential that occur when an excitatory transmitter is released at a synapse.
11. Explain also the events that occur when an inhibitory transmitter is released.
12. Why do the action potentials in the postsynaptic neuron originate in the axon hillock?
13. Explain the mechanism of inhibition called short-circuiting.
14. What is the difference between presynaptic and postsynaptic inhibition?
15. Explain *spatial* and *temporal summation* of postsynaptic potentials; also explain the phenomenon of *facilitation*.
16. What are the special functions of *dendrites* in synaptic transmission?
17. What is the relationship between the excitatory state of a neuron and its rate of firing?
18. What is the mechanism of *synaptic fatigue*?
19. Describe the mechanisms of *divergence* and *convergence* in neuronal pools.
20. What is the function of the *reciprocal inhibition* circuit?
21. What is the function of *lateral inhibition* in the transmission of nervous signals through neuronal pools?
22. What are the differences between *synaptic after-discharge*, after-discharge caused by the *parallel circuit*, and after-discharge caused by a *reverberatory circuit*?
23. Explain the functions of several specific reverberatory neuronal circuits.
24. What is the mechanism of rhythmic signal outputs from neuronal pools?
25. Why is the nervous system likely to be unstable, and what are the roles of synaptic fatigue and synaptic receptor changes in stabilizing the nervous system?

References

Barde, Y. A., et al.: New neurotrophic factors. Annu Rev Physiol 45:601, 1983.

Buchtel, H. A.: The Conceptual Nervous System. New York, Pergamon Press, 1982.

Changeux, J. P., et al.: Acetylcholine receptor: An allosteric protein. Science 225:1335, 1984.

Eyzaguirre, C.: Physiology of the Nervous System. Chicago, Year Book Medical Publishers, 1985.

Hanin, I., ed.: Dynamics of Neurotransmitter Function. New York, Raven Press, 1984.

Kehoe, J., and Marty, A.: Certain slow synaptic responses: their properties and possible underlying mechanisms. Annu Rev Biophys Bioeng 9:437, 1980.

Kostyuk, P. G.: Intracellular perfusion of nerve cells and its effects on membrane currents. Physiol Rev 64:435, 1984.

Krnjevic, K.: Transmitters in motor systems. In Brooks, V. B., ed.: Handbook of Physiology, Sec. 1, Vol. 2. Bethesda, American Physiological Society, 1981, p. 107.

Landis, S. C.: Neuronal growth cones. Annu Rev Physiol 45:567, 1983.

McKay, R. D. G.: Molecular approach to the nervous system. Annu Rev Neurosci 6:527, 1983.

McKerns, K. W., ed.: Hormonally Active Brain Peptides. Structure and Function. New York, Plenum Publishing Corp., 1982.

Purves, D., and Lichtman, J. W.: Specific connections between nerve cells. Annu Rev Physiol 45:553, 1983.

Schubert, D.: Developmental Biology of Cultured Nerve, Muscle and Glia. New York, John Wiley & Sons, 1984.

Stein, J. F.: Introduction to Neurophysiology. St. Louis, C. V. Mosby, 1982.

Tucek, S.: Regulation of acetylcholine synthesis in the brain. J Neurochem 44:11, 1985.

Wright, E. M.: Electrophysiology of plasma membrane vesicles. Am J Physiol 246:F363, 1984.

32

Sensory Receptors and Mechanoreceptive Somatic Sensations

TYPES OF SENSORY RECEPTORS AND
   THE SENSORY STIMULI THEY DETECT
   *DIFFERENTIAL SENSITIVITY OF
      RECEPTORS*
TRANSDUCTION OF SENSORY STIMULI
   INTO NERVE IMPULSES
   *LOCAL CURRENTS AT NERVE
      ENDINGS—RECEPTOR POTENTIALS*
   ADAPTATION OF RECEPTORS
PSYCHIC INTERPRETATION OF
   STIMULUS STRENGTH
PHYSIOLOGICAL CLASSIFICATION OF
   NERVE FIBERS
THE SOMATIC SENSES
DETECTION AND TRANSMISSION OF
   TACTILE SENSATIONS
   DETECTION OF VIBRATION
THE DUAL SYSTEM FOR TRANSMISSION
   OF MECHANORECEPTIVE SOMATIC
   SENSORY SIGNALS INTO THE
   CENTRAL NERVOUS SYSTEM
FUNCTION OF THE SPINAL CORD
   NEURONS IN TRANSMITTING
   SENSORY SIGNALS

TRANSMISSION IN THE DORSAL
   COLUMN–LEMNISCAL SYSTEM
   *ANATOMY OF THE DORSAL
      COLUMN–LEMNISCAL SYSTEM*
   THE SOMATIC SENSORY CORTEX
   *FUNCTIONS OF SOMATIC SENSORY
      AREA I*
   *SOMATIC SENSORY ASSOCIATION
      AREA*
   *CHARACTERISTICS OF
      TRANSMISSION IN THE DORSAL
      COLUMN–LEMNISCAL SYSTEM*
   THE POSITION SENSE
TRANSMISSION IN THE ANTEROLATERAL
   SYSTEM
   *ANATOMY OF THE ANTEROLATERAL
      PATHWAY*
SOME SPECIAL ASPECTS OF SENSORY
   FUNCTION

Input to the nervous system is provided by the sensory receptors that detect such sensory stimuli as touch, sound, light, cold, and warmth. The purposes of the present chapter are to discuss the basic mechanisms by which these receptors change sensory stimuli into nerve signals and also how both the type of sensory stimulus and its strength are detected by the brain.

TYPES OF SENSORY RECEPTORS AND THE SENSORY STIMULI THEY DETECT

Table 32–1 gives a list and classification of most of the body's sensory receptors. This table shows that there are basically five different types of sensory receptors: (1) *mechanoreceptors,* which detect mechanical deformation of the receptor itself or of cells adjacent to the receptor; (2) *thermoreceptors,* which detect changes in temperature, some receptors detecting cold and others warmth; (3) *nociceptors,* which detect pain, usually caused by physical or chemical damage to the tissues; (4) *electromagnetic receptors*, which detect light on the retina of the eye; and (5) *chemoreceptors*, which detect taste in the mouth, smell in the nose, oxygen level in the arterial blood, osmolality of the body fluids, carbon dioxide concentration, and perhaps other factors that make up the chemistry of the body.

This chapter especially discusses the function of

Table 32–1. CLASSIFICATION OF SENSORY RECEPTORS

Mechanoreceptors
Skin tactile sensibilities (epidermis and dermis)
  Free nerve endings
  Expanded tip endings
    Merkel's disks
    Plus several other variants
  Spray endings
    Ruffini's endings
  Encapsulated endings
    Meissner's corpuscles
    Krause's corpuscles
  Hair end-organs
Deep tissue sensibilities
  Free nerve endings
  Expanded tip endings
    Plus a few other variants
  Spray endings
    Ruffini's endings
  Encapsulated endings
    Pacinian corpuscles
    Plus a few other variants
  Muscle endings
    Muscle spindles
    Golgi tendon receptors
Hearing
  Sound receptors of cochlea
Equilibrium
  Vestibular receptors
Arterial pressure
  Baroreceptors of carotid sinuses and aorta

Thermoreceptors
Cold
  Cold receptors
Warmth
  Possibly free nerve endings

Nociceptors
Pain
  Free nerve endings

Electromagnetic Receptors
Vision
  Rods
  Cones

Chemoreceptors
Taste
  Receptors of taste buds
Smell
  Receptors of olfactory epithelium
Arterial oxygen
  Receptors of aortic and carotid bodies
Osmolality
  Probably neurons of supraoptic nuclei
Blood CO_2
  Receptors in or on surface of medulla and in aortic and
    carotid bodies
Blood glucose, amino acids, fatty acids
  Receptors in hypothalamus

certain receptors, primarily peripheral mechanoreceptors, to illustrate some of the basic principles by which receptors in general operate. Other receptors are discussed in relation to the sensory systems that they subserve. Figure 32–1 illustrates some of the different types of mechanoreceptors found in the skin or in the deep structures of the body, and Table 32–1 gives their respective sensory functions. The functions of some of these are described briefly, as follows:

Free nerve endings are found in all parts of the

body. A very large proportion of these detect pain. However, other free nerve endings detect crude touch, pressure, tickle, and itch sensations and possibly warmth and cold.

Several of the more complex receptors listed in Table 32–1 detect tissue deformation. These include the *Merkel's disks*, the *tactile hairs, Pacini's corpuscles, Meissner's corpuscles, Krause's corpuscles,* and *Ruffini's end-organs.* In the skin, it is these receptors that detect the tactile sensations of touch and pressure. In the deep tissues, they detect stretch, deep pressure, or any other type of tissue deformation—even the stretch of joint capsules and ligaments to determine the movements of joints.

Golgi tendon apparatus detects tension in tendons, and the *muscle spindle* detects relative changes in muscle length. These two receptors will be discussed in Chapter 34 in relation to the muscle and tendon reflexes.

DIFFERENTIAL SENSITIVITY OF RECEPTORS

The first question that must be answered is, How do two types of sensory receptors detect different types of sensory stimuli? The answer is, By virtue of differential sensitivities. That is, each type of receptor is very highly sensitive to the one type of stimulus for which it is designed and yet is almost nonresponsive to normal intensities of the other types of sensory stimuli. Thus, the rods and cones are highly responsive to light but are almost completely nonresponsive to heat, cold, pressure on the eyeballs, or chemical changes in the blood. The osmoreceptors of the supraoptic nuclei in the hypothalamus detect minute changes in the osmolality of the body fluids but have

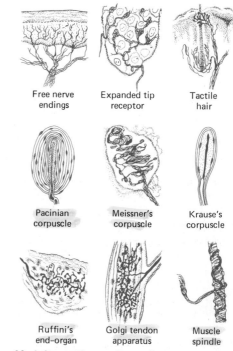

Free nerve endings	Expanded tip receptor	Tactile hair
Pacinian corpuscle	Meissner's corpuscle	Krause's corpuscle
Ruffini's end-organ	Golgi tendon apparatus	Muscle spindle

Figure 32–1. Several types of somatic sensory nerve endings.

never been known to respond to sound. Finally, pain receptors in the skin are almost never stimulated by usual touch or pressure stimuli but do become highly active the moment tactile stimuli become severe enough to damage the tissues.

Modality of Sensation— The Labeled Line Principle

Each of the principal types of sensation that we can experience—pain, touch, sight, sound, and so forth—is called a *modality* of sensation. Yet, despite the fact that we experience these different modalities of sensation, nerve fibers transmit only impulses. Therefore, how is it that different nerve fibers transmit different modalities of sensation?

The answer to this is that each nerve tract terminates at a specific point in the central nervous system, and the type of sensation felt when a nerve fiber is stimulated is determined by this point in the nervous system to which the fiber leads. For instance, if a pain fiber is stimulated, the person perceives pain regardless of what type of stimulus excites the fiber. The stimulus can be electricity, heat, crushing, or stimulation of the pain nerve ending by damage to the tissue cells. Yet, whatever the means of stimulation, the person still perceives pain. Likewise, if a touch fiber is stimulated by exciting a touch receptor electrically or in any other way, the person perceives touch because touch fibers lead to specific touch areas in the brain. Similarly, fibers from the retina of the eye terminate in the vision areas of the brain, fibers from the ear terminate in the auditory areas of the brain, and temperature fibers terminate in the temperature areas.

This specificity of nerve fibers for transmitting only one modality of sensation is called the *labeled line principle*.

TRANSDUCTION OF SENSORY STIMULI INTO NERVE IMPULSES

LOCAL CURRENTS AT NERVE ENDINGS— RECEPTOR POTENTIALS

All sensory receptors have one feature in common. Whatever the type of stimulus that excites the receptor, its immediate effect is to change the potential across the receptor membrane. This change in potential is called a *receptor potential,* and it in turn excites action potentials in the attached nerve fiber.

Different receptors can be excited in several different ways to cause receptor potentials: (1) by mechanical deformation of the receptor, which stretches the membrane and opens ion channels; (2) by application of a chemical to the membrane, which also opens ion channels; (3) by change of the temperature of the membrane, which alters the permeability of the membrane; or (4) by the effects of electromagnetic radiation such as light on the receptor, which either directly

or indirectly changes the membrane characteristics and allows ions to flow through membrane channels. In all these instances, the basic cause of the change in membrane potential is a change in receptor membrane permeability, which allows ions to diffuse more or less readily through the membrane and thereby change the transmembrane potential.

The Receptor Potential of the Pacinian Corpuscle. The pacinian corpuscle is a very large and easily dissected sensory receptor. For this reason, one can study in detail the mechanism by which tactile stimuli excite it and by which it causes action potentials in the sensory nerve fiber leading from it. Note in Figure 32–1 that the pacinian corpuscle has a central nonmyelinated tip of a nerve fiber extending through its core. Surrounding this fiber are many concentric capsule layers so that compression on the outside of the corpuscle tends to elongate, indent, or otherwise deform the central core of the fiber, depending on how the compression is applied, as illustrated in Figure 32–2. This deformation causes the sudden opening of ion channels that mainly carry positively charged sodium ions to the interior of the fiber. This in turn creates more positivity in the fiber, which is the receptor potential. The receptor potential in turn induces a local circuit of current flow that spreads along the nerve fiber. At the first node of Ranvier, which itself lies inside the capsule of the pacinian corpuscle, the local current flow initiates action potentials in the fiber. That is, the current flow through the node depolarizes it, and this then sets off a typical action potential that is transmitted along the nerve fiber toward the central nervous system.

ADAPTATION OF RECEPTORS

A special characteristic of all sensory receptors is that they *adapt* either partially or completely to their stimuli after a period of time. That is, when a continuous sensory stimulus is applied, the receptors respond at first with a very high impulse rate, then at a progressively lower rate until finally many of them no longer respond at all.

Figure 32–3 illustrates typical adaptation of certain types of receptors. Note that the pacinian corpuscle adapts extremely rapidly and the hair receptor within

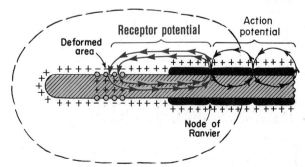

Figure 32–2. Excitation of a sensory nerve fiber by a receptor potential produced in a pacinian corpuscle. (Modified from Loëwenstein: Ann NY Acad Sci 94:510, 1961.)

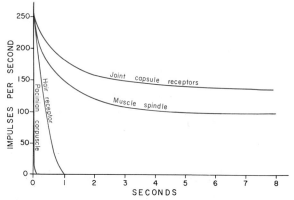

Figure 32–3. Adaptation of different types of receptors, showing rapid adaptation of some receptors and slow adaptation of others.

a second or so, while joint capsule and muscle spindle receptors adapt very slowly.

Furthermore, some sensory receptors adapt to a far greater extent than others. For example, the pacinian corpuscles adapt to "extinction" within a few thousandths to a few hundredths of a second, and the hair base receptors within a second or more. It is probable that all other mechanoreceptors also completely adapt eventually, but some require hours or days to do so, for which reason they are frequently called nonadapting receptors.

Some of the other types of receptors, the chemoreceptors and pain receptors, for instance, probably never adapt completely.

Mechanisms by Which Receptors Adapt. Adaptation of receptors is an individual property of each type of receptor in much the same way that development of a receptor potential is an indivdual property. For instance, in the eye, the rods and cones adapt by changing their chemical compositions (which is discussed in Chapter 39). In the case of the mechanoreceptors, the receptor that has been studied for adaptation in greatest detail is the pacinian corpuscle. Adaptation occurs in this receptor mainly by the corpuscular structure itself very rapidly adapting to the deformation of the tissue. That is, within a few thousandths to a few hundredths of a second after compression, the fluid within the corpuscle redistributes so that the pressure becomes essentially equal again all through the corpuscle. Thus, a receptor potential appears at the onset of compression but then disappears within a small fraction of a second even though the compression continues.

Then, when the distorting force is removed from the corpuscle, essentially the reverse events occur. The sudden removal of the distortion from one side of the corpuscle allows rapid expansion on that side, and a corresponding distortion of the central core occurs once more. This signals the offset of compression in the same manner that the onset of compression had been signaled.

Function of the Slowly Adapting and Nonadapting Receptors to Detect Continuous Stimulus Strength—

The Tonic Receptors. The slowly adapting receptors continue to transmit impulses to the brain for many minutes or hours. Therefore, they keep the brain constantly apprised of the status of the body and its relation to its surroundings. For instance, impulses from the slowly adapting joint capsule receptors allow the person to "know" at all times the degree of bending of the joints and therefore the positions of the different parts of the body. And impulses from muscle spindles and Golgi's tendon apparatuses allow the central nervous system to know, respectively, the status of muscle contraction and the load on the muscle tendon at each instant.

Other types of slowly adapting receptors include the receptors of the macula in the vestibular apparatus, the pain receptors, the baroreceptors of the arterial tree, the chemoreceptors of the carotid and aortic bodies, and some of the tactile receptors, such as Ruffini's endings and Merkel's disks.

Because the slowly adapting receptors can continue to transmit information for many hours, they are called *tonic* receptors. Many of these slowly adapting receptors will adapt to extinction if the intensity of the stimulus remains absolutely constant for several hours or days. Fortunately, because of our continually changing bodily state, these receptors almost never reach a state of complete adaptation.

Function of the Rapidly Adapting Receptors to Detect Change in Stimulus Strength—The Rate Receptors (Movement, or Phasic, Receptors). Obviously, receptors that adapt rapidly cannot be used to transmit a continuous signal because these receptors are stimulated only when the stimulus strength changes. Yet they react strongly *while a change is actually taking place.* Furthermore, the number of impulses transmitted is directly related to the *rate at which the change takes place.* Therefore, these receptors are called *rate* receptors, *movement* receptors, or *phasic* receptors. Thus, in the case of the pacinian corpuscle, sudden pressure applied to the skin excites this receptor for a few milliseconds, and then its excitation is over even though the pressure continues. But then it transmits a signal again when the pressure is released. In other words, the pacinian corpuscle is exceedingly important for transmitting information about rapid changes in pressure against the body, but it is useless for transmitting information about constant pressure applied to the body.

Importance of the Rate Receptors—Their Predictive Function. If one knows the rate at which some change in bodily status is taking place, one can predict the state of the body a few seconds or even a few minutes later. For instance, the receptors of the semicircular canals in the vestibular apparatus of the ear detect the rate at which the head begins to turn when one runs around a curve. Using this information, a person can predict a turn of 10, 30, or some other number of degrees within the next 10 seconds and can adjust the motion of the limbs *ahead of time* to keep from losing balance. Likewise, pacinian corpuscles and other receptors located in or near the joint capsules help detect the rates of movement of the different parts of the body. Therefore, when one is running, information from these receptors allows the nervous system to predict ahead of time where the feet will be during any precise fraction of a second, and appropriate motor signals can be transmitted to the muscles of the legs to make any necessary anticipatory corrections in limb position so that one will not fall. Loss of this predictive function makes it impossible for a person to run.

PSYCHIC INTERPRETATION OF STIMULUS STRENGTH

The ultimate goal of most sensory stimulation is to apprise the psyche of the state of the body and its surroundings. Therefore, it is important that we discuss briefly some of the principles related to the transmission of sensory stimulus strength to the higher levels of the nervous system.

The first question that comes to mind is: How is it possible for the sensory system to transmit sensory experiences of tremendously varying intensities? For instance, the auditory system can detect the weakest possible whisper but can also discern the meanings of an explosive sound only a few feet away, even though the sound intensities of these two experiences can vary more than ten billionfold; the eyes can see visual images with light intensities that vary as much as a half millionfold; or the skin can detect pressure differences of ten thousand- to one hundred thousand-fold.

As a partial explanation of these effects, many receptors are capable of accurately measuring extremely minute changes in stimulus strength at low-intensity levels, but at high-intensity levels the change in stimulus strength must be much greater to cause the same amount of change in receptor potential.

The Weber-Fechner Principle—Detection of Stimulus Strength. In the mid-1800s, Weber first and Fechner later proposed the principle that *gradations of stimulus strength are discriminated approximately in proportion to the logarithm of stimulus strength.* That is, a person can barely detect a 1-gram increase in weight when holding 30 grams, or a 10-gram increase when holding 300 grams. Thus, the *ratio* of the change in stimulus strength required for detection of a *change* remains essentially constant, about 1 to 30, which is what the logarithmic principle means. Because the Weber-Fechner principle offers a ready explanation for the tremendous range of stimulus strength that our nervous system can discern, it unfortunately became widely accepted for all types of sensory experience and for all levels of background sensory intensity. More recently it has become evident that this principle applies mainly to higher intensities of visual, auditory, and cutaneous sensory experience and applies only poorly to most other types of sensory experience.

PHYSIOLOGICAL CLASSIFICATION OF NERVE FIBERS

Some sensory signals need to be transmitted to the central nervous system extremely rapidly; otherwise the information would be useless. An example of this is the sensory signals that apprise the brain of the momentary positions of the limbs at each fraction of a second during running. At the other extreme, some types of sensory information, such as that depicting prolonged, aching pain, do not need to be transmitted rapidly at all so that very slowly conducting fibers will suffice. Fortunately, nerve fibers come in all sizes between 0.2 and 20 microns in diameter—the larger the diameter, the greater the conducting velocity. The range of conducting velocities is between 0.5 and 120 meters per second.

Figure 32–4 gives two different classifications of nerve fibers that are in general use. One of these is a general classification that encompasses both sensory and motor fibers, including the autonomic nerve fibers. The other is a classification of sensory nerve fibers that is used primarily by sensory neurophysiologists.

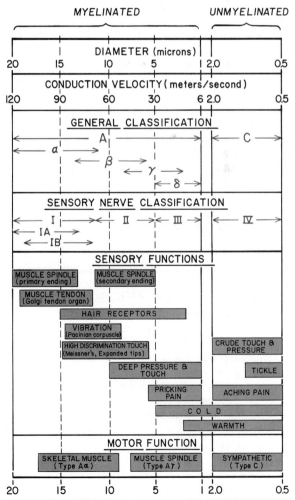

Figure 32–4. Physiological classifications and functions of nerve fibers.

In the *general classification,* the fibers are divided into types A and C, and the type A fibers are further subdivided into α, β, γ, and δ fibers.

Type A fibers are the typical myelinated fibers of spinal nerves. Type C fibers are the very small, unmyelinated nerve fibers that conduct impulses at low velocities. These constitute more than half the sensory fibers in most peripheral nerves and also all of the post-ganglionic autonomic fibers.

In the *sensory fiber classification,* the fibers are divided into Groups Ia, Ib, II, III, and IV. The group I fibers are the largest, and the group IV fibers, the very smallest, are the unmyelinated fibers that are the same as the type C fibers in the general classification.

THE SOMATIC SENSES

The *somatic senses* are the nervous mechanisms that collect sensory information from the body. These senses are contradistinguished from the *special senses,* which mean specifically sight, hearing, smell, taste, and equilibrium.

The somatic senses can be classified into three different physiologic types: (1) the *mechanoreceptive somatic senses,* stimulated by mechanical displacement of some tissues of the body; (2) the *thermoreceptive senses*, which detect heat and cold; and (3) the *pain sense,* which is activated mainly by factors that damage the tissues. This section deals with the mechanoreceptive somatic senses; the following chapter deals with the thermoreceptive and pain senses.

The mechanoreceptive senses include *touch, pressure*, and *position senses*, the last of which determines the relative positions and rates of movement of the different parts of the body.

Somatic sensations are also grouped together in special classes that are not necessarily mutually exclusive, as follows:

Exteroceptive sensations are from the surface of the body.

Proprioceptive sensations are those having to do with the physical state of the body, including position and tendon and muscle sensations, pressure sensations from the bottom of the feet, and even the sensation of equilibrium, which is generally considered to be a "special" sensation rather than a somatic sensation.

Visceral sensations are those from the viscera of the body; this term usually refers specifically to sensations from the internal organs.

The *deep sensations* are those that come from the deep tissues, such as bone and fascia. These include mainly "deep" pressure, pain, and vibration.

DETECTION AND TRANSMISSION OF TACTILE SENSATIONS

Interrelationships Among the Tactile Sensations of Touch, Pressure, and Vibration. Though touch, pres-sure, and vibration are frequently classified as separate sensations, they are all detected by the same types of receptors. The only differences among these three are (1) touch sensation, which generally results from stimulation of tactile receptors in the skin or in tissues immediately beneath the skin; (2) pressure sensation, which generally results from deformation of deeper tissues; and (3) vibration sensation, which results from rapidly repetitive sensory signals, but for this last sensation, the receptors for both touch and pressure are utilized—specifically, the rapidly adapting receptors.

The Tactile Receptors. At least six entirely different types of tactile receptors are known; in addition, there are many more similar to these types. Some of these receptors are illustrated in Figure 32–1; their special characteristics are as follows:

First, some of the *free nerve endings*, which are found everywhere in the skin and in many other tissues, can detect touch and pressure. For instance, even light contact with the cornea of the eye, which contains only free nerve endings, can nevertheless elicit touch and pressure sensations.

Second, a touch receptor of special sensitivity is *Meissner's corpuscle,* an encapsulated nerve ending that excites a large myelinated sensory nerve fiber. Inside the capsulation are many whorls of terminal nerve filaments. These receptors are particularly abundant in the fingertips, lips, and other areas of the skin in which the ability to discern spatial characteristics of touch sensations is highly developed. They (along with the expanded tip receptors described subsequently) are mainly responsible for one's ability to recognize exactly what point of the body is touched and to recognize the texture of objects touched. Meissner's corpuscles adapt within a second after they are stimulated, which means that they are particularly sensitive to movement of very light objects over the surface of the skin and also to low-frequency vibration.

Third, the fingertips and other areas that contain large numbers of Meissner's corpuscles also contain *expanded tip tactile receptors*, one type of which is *Merkel's disks.* These receptors differ from Meissner's corpuscles in that they transmit an initial strong but partially adapting signal followed by a continuing weaker signal that adapts only slowly. For this reason, they are responsible for giving steady state signals that allow one to distinguish the continuous pressure of objects against the skin. The hairy parts of the body contain almost no Meissner's corpuscles but do contain a few expanded tip receptors.

Fourth, slight movement of any hair on the body stimulates the nerve fiber entwining its base. Thus, each hair and its basal nerve fiber, called the *hair end-organ,* is also a type of touch receptor. This receptor adapts readily and therefore, like Meissner's corpuscles, detects mainly movement of objects on the surface of the body.

Fifth, located in the deeper layers of the skin and also in deeper tissues of the body are many *Ruffini's end-organs,* which are multibranched endings as illustrated in Figure 32–1. These endings adapt very little and therefore are important for signaling continuous states of deformation of the skin and deeper tissues, such as heavy and continuous touch and pressure signals. They are also found in joint capsules and signal the degree of joint rotation.

Sixth, many *pacinian corpuscles*, which were discussed in detail earlier in the chapter, lie both beneath the skin and deep in the tissues of the body. These are stimulated only by very rapid movement of the tissues because these receptors adapt in a small fraction of a second. Therefore, they are particularly important for detecting tissue vibration or other extremely rapid changes in the mechanical state of the tissues.

Transmission of Tactile Sensations in Peripheral Nerve Fibers. The specialized sensory receptors such as Meissner's corpuscles, expanded tip endings, pacinian corpuscles, and Ruffini's endings all transmit their signals in beta type A nerve fibers that have transmission velocities of 30 to 70 meters per second. On the other hand, most free nerve ending tactile receptors transmit signals mainly via the small delta type A nerve fibers that conduct at velocities from 5 to 30 meters per second, but a few transmit via type C fibers at velocities of about 1 meter per second, probably subserving the sensations of tickling and itching.

Thus, the more critical types of sensory signals—those that help to determine precise localization on the skin, minute gradations of intensity, or rapid changes in sensory signal intensity—are all transmitted in the rapidly conducting types of sensory nerve fibers. On the other hand, the cruder types of signals, such as crude touch and tickling and itching, are transmitted via such slower nerve fibers, fibers that are very small and therefore require much less space in the nerves.

DETECTION OF VIBRATION

All the tactile receptors are involved in detection of vibration, though different receptors detect different frequencies of vibration. Pacinian corpuscles can signal vibrations between 60 and 500 cycles per second because they respond extremely rapidly to minute and rapid deformations of the tissues and because they transmit their signals over beta type A nerve fibers, which can transmit more than 1000 impulses per second.

Low-frequency vibrations up to 80 cycles per second, on the other hand, stimulate other tactile receptors—especially Meissner's corpuscles, which adapt less rapidly than pacinian corpuscles.

THE DUAL SYSTEM FOR TRANSMISSION OF MECHANORECEPTIVE SOMATIC SENSORY SIGNALS INTO THE CENTRAL NERVOUS SYSTEM

Either all or almost all sensory information from the somatic segments of the body enters the spinal cord through the dorsal roots of the spinal nerves. However, from this point to the brain, the sensory signals are carried through one of two alternate sensory pathways: (1) the *dorsal column—leminiscal system* or (2) the *anterolateral system*. These two systems come together again at the level of the thalamus.

Comparison of the Dorsal Column–Lemniscal System with the Anterolateral System. The distinguishing difference between the dorsal column–lemniscal system and the anterolateral system is that the dorsal column–lemniscal system is constituted mainly of large myelinated nerve fibers that transmit signals to the brain at velocities of 30 to 110 meters per second, while the anterolateral system consists of much smaller myelinated fibers that transmit impulses at velocities ranging between 10 to 60 meters per second.

Another difference between the two systems is that the dorsal system has a very high degree of spatial orientation of the nerve fibers with respect to their origin on the surface of the body, while the anterolateral system has a much smaller degree of spatial orientation.

These differences in the two systems immediately characterize the types of sensory information that can be conveyed by the two systems. First, sensory information that must be sent rapidly and with temporal fidelity is transmitted in the dorsal column–lemniscal system, while information that does not need to be communicated rapidly is transmitted mainly in the anterolateral system. Second, those sensations that detect fine gradations of intensity are signaled in the dorsal system, while those that lack the fine gradations are handled in the anterolateral system. And, third, sensations that are discretely localized to exact points in the body are transmitted in the dorsal system, while those conveyed in the anterolateral system can be localized much less exactly. On the other hand, the anterolateral system has a special capability that the dorsal system does not have: the ability to transmit a broad spectrum of sensory modalities—pain, warmth, cold, and crude tactile sensations; the dorsal system is limited to mechanoreceptive sensations alone. With this differentiation in mind we can now list the types of sensations transmitted in the two systems.

The Dorsal Column–Lemniscal System

1. Touch sensations requiring a high degree of localization of the stimulus
2. Touch sensations requiring transmission of fine gradations of intensity
3. Phasic (such as vibratory) sensations
4. Sensations that signal movement against the skin
5. Positional sensations
6. Pressure sensations with fine degrees of pressure intensity

The Anterolateral System

1. Pain
2. Thermal sensations, including both warmth and cold

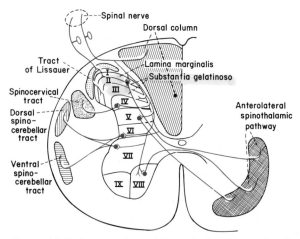

Figure 32–5. Cross-section of the spinal cord showing the anatomical laminae I through IX of the cord gray matter and the ascending sensory tracts in the white columns of the spinal cord.

3. Crude touch and pressure that can be only crudely localized on the surface of the body and requires little intensity discrimination
4. Tickling and itching
5. Sexual sensations

FUNCTION OF THE SPINAL CORD NEURONS IN TRANSMITTING SENSORY SIGNALS

Relay of Sensory Signals in the Spinal Cord. Upon first entering the spinal cord through the dorsal roots, as illustrated in Figure 32–5, most of the large sensory nerve fibers, mainly type Aβ fibers, turn medially toward the dorsal columns. Then they usually divide into two branches. One ascends upward through the dorsal white columns to the brain, and the other enters the anterior portion of the dorsal horn of the spinal cord gray matter.

In the dorsal horn gray matter, the terminals of the *large* fibers synapse with second order neurons of two types: (1) local neurons that play an intricate role in the control of spinal cord reflexes and (2) relay neurons that give rise to long, ascending fiber tracts that transmit sensory information to the brain. Most of the fibers from these relay neurons ascend in the *spinocervical tract* located in the dorsal part of the lateral column, also shown in Figure 32–5.

The smaller fibers entering the spinal cord from the dorsal roots take a more lateral pathway than the larger fibers; either they enter the gray matter of the dorsal horn immediately or they ascend or descend a few segments and then enter the dorsal horn. Most of these fibers terminate on small neurons in the posterior portions of the dorsal horns, and these often give rise to short fibers that terminate somewhere else in the gray matter before the sensory information is finally relayed to other areas of the cord or to the long ascending pathways. Essentially all the sensory

information from the smaller fibers eventually enters the *anterolateral tract* that crosses to the opposite side of the cord in the anterior commissure and then ascends to the brain.

TRANSMISSION IN THE DORSAL COLUMN–LEMNISCAL SYSTEM

ANATOMY OF THE DORSAL COLUMN–LEMNISCAL SYSTEM

Sensory signals are transmitted to the brain by way of two major pathways in the dorsal lemniscal system: (1) the *dorsal column pathway* and (2) the *spinocervical pathway*. The routes that these take to the brain are illustrated in Figure 32–6.

Anatomy of the Dorsal Column Pathway. Note in Figure 32–6 that the nerve fibers entering the dorsal columns pass up these columns to the medulla, where they synapse in the *dorsal column nuclei* (the *cuneate* and *gracile nuclei*). From here, *second order neurons* decussate immediately to the opposite side and then pass upward to the thalamus through bilateral path-

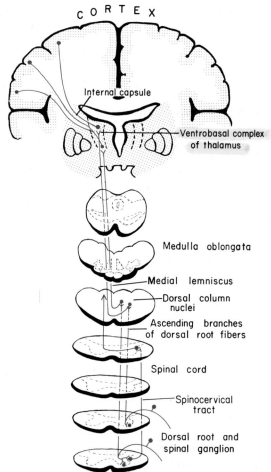

Figure 32–6. The dorsal column and spinocervical pathways for transmitting critical types of tactile signals. (Modified from Ranson and Clark: Anatomy of the Nervous System. Philadelphia, W. B. Saunders Company, 1959.)

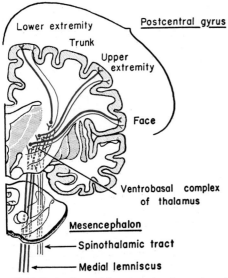

Figure 32–7. Projection of the dorsal column–lemniscal system from the thalamus to the somatic sensory cortex. (Modified from Brodal: Neurological Anatomy in Relation to Clinical Medicine. New York, Oxford University Press, 1969.)

ways called the *medial lemnisci*. Each medial lemniscus then terminates in the *ventrobasal complex*, located mainly in the ventral posterolateral nucleus of the *thalamus*.

From the ventrobasal complex, *third order neurons* project, as shown in Figure 32–7, mainly to the *postcentral gyrus* of the *cerebral cortex*, called the *somatic sensory area I*.

Anatomy of the Spinocervical Pathway. The anatomy of the spinocervical pathway is much less well known than that of the dorsal column pathway. However, many of the large sensory fibers that enter the cord in the dorsal roots soon synapse, mainly in lamina IV of the cord gray matter, as shown in Figure 32–5, giving rise to second order fibers that enter the *dorsolateral white columns* and ascend in the *spinocervical tract* to the cervical region of the cord or even to the medulla. At these points the fibers again synapse, and third order neurons decussate to the opposite side and pass along with the nerve fibers of the dorsal column pathway upward to the thalamus through the *medial lemnisci*. The pathway within the brain thus parallels that of the dorsal column pathway.

Separation of Sensory Modalities Between the Dorsal Column Pathway and the Spinocervical Pathway

The dorsal column pathway mainly transmits signals from rapidly adapting sensory receptors. For instance, it is through the dorsal column pathway that signals are transmitted from the extremely rapidly adapting pacinian corpuscles. Also, most of the signals from the Meissner's corpuscles and from the hair receptors, both of which are rapidly adapting receptors, are transmitted through this pathway.

On the other hand, some of the more slowly adapting signals from the Merkel's disks, from the deep-tissue Ruffini's end-organs, and from the slowly adapting Ruffini's position sense receptors of the joint capsules seem to be transmitted through the spinocervical pathway.

Spatial Orientation of the Nerve Fibers in the Dorsal Column–Lemniscal System

One of the distinguishing features of the dorsal column–lemniscal system is also a distinct spatial orientation of nerve fibers from the individual parts of the body that is maintained throughout. For instance, in the dorsal columns, the fibers from the lower parts of the body lie toward the center, while those that enter the spinal cord at progressively higher segmental levels form successive layers laterally.

The spatial orientation in the spinocervical pathway is less well known. However, stimulation experiments of single fibers within this pathway have shown that the sensory signals diverge very little, indicating a high degree of spatial orientation in this pathway as well.

THE SOMATIC SENSORY CORTEX

The area of the cerebral cortex to which the sensory signals are projected is called the *somatic sensory cortex*. In the human being, this area lies mainly in the anterior portions of the parietal lobes. Two distinct and separate areas are known to receive direct afferent nerve fibers from the relay nuclei of the thalamus; these, called *somatic sensory area I* and *somatic sensory area II*, are illustrated in Figure 32–8. However, somatic sensory area I is extremely important to the sensory functions of the body, while the functions of somatic sensory area II are mainly unknown. Therefore, in popular usage, the term *somatic sensory cortex* is almost always used to mean area I alone.

Projection of the Body in Somatic Sensory Area I. Somatic sensory area I lies in the postcentral gyrus of the parietal lobe of the cerebral cortex. A distinct spatial orientation exists in this area for reception of

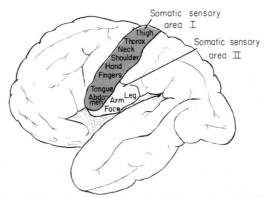

Figure 32–8. The two somatic sensory cortical areas, somatic sensory areas I and II.

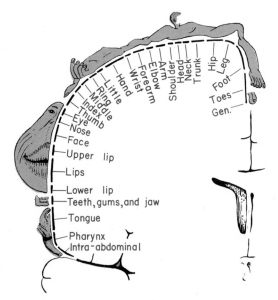

Figure 32–9. Representation of the different areas of the body in the somatic sensory area I of the cortex. (From THE CEREBRAL CORTEX OF MAN by Wilder Penfield and Theodore Rasmussen. Copyright 1950 by Macrnillan Publishing Company, renewed 1978 by Theodore Rasmussen. Reprinted with permission of the publisher.)

nerve signals from the different regions of the body. Figure 32–9 illustrates a cross section through the brain at the level of the postcentral gyrus, showing the representations of the different parts of the body in separate areas of somatic sensory area I. Note, however, that each side of the cortex receives its sensory information from the opposite side of the body, not from the same side.

Some areas of the body are represented by large areas in the somatic cortex—the lips by far the greatest of all, followed by the face and thumb—while the entire trunk and lower part of the body are represented by relatively small areas. The sizes of these areas are directly proportional to the number of specialized sensory receptors in each respective peripheral area of the body. For instance, a great number of specialized nerve endings are found in the lips and thumb, while only a few are present in the skin of the trunk.

Note also that the head is represented in the lower, lateral portion of the postcentral gyrus, while the lower part of the body is represented in the medial, upper portion of the postcentral gyrus.

Excitation of Vertical Columns of Neurons in the Somatic Sensory Cortex

The cerebral cortex contains *six* separate layers of neurons, and, as would be expected, the neurons in each layer perform functions different from those in other layers. Also, the neurons are arranged functionally in *vertical columns* extending all the way through the six layers of the cortex, each column having a diameter of about 0.33 to 1 millimeter and

containing about 100,000 neuronal cell bodies. Unfortunately, we still know relatively little about the functions of these columns of cells but we are certain about the following facts:

1. The incoming sensory signal mainly excites neuronal layer IV first (the fourth layer from the surface of the brain); then the signal spreads toward the surface of the cortex and also toward the deeper layers.

2. Layers I and II (the two layers nearest the surface) receive a diffuse, nonspecific input from lower brain centers called the reticular activating system, which can activate the whole or portions of the brain at once; this system is described in Chapter 37.

3. The neurons in layers V and VI send axons to other parts of the nervous system—some to other areas of the cortex, some to deeper structures of the brain, such as the thalamus or brain stem, and some even to the spinal cord.

Similar vertical columns of neurons exist in all other areas of the cortex as they do in the somatic sensory cortex.

Each vertical column of neurons seems to be able to decipher a specific quality of information from the sensory signal. Presumably, in the somatic cortex each column detects a separate quality of signal (angles of orientation of lengths of edges, perhaps roundness of objects, perhaps sharpness of objects, and so forth) from specific surface areas of the body.

FUNCTIONS OF SOMATIC SENSORY AREA I

Destruction of somatic sensory area I causes loss of the following types of sensory judgment:

1. The person is unable to localize discretely sensations in the different parts of the body. However, he or she can still localize these sensations crudely, for example, to a particular hand, which indicates that the thalamus or parts of the cerebral cortex not normally considered to be concerned with somatic sensations can perform some degree of localization.

2. Such a person is unable to distinguish critical degrees of pressure.

3. He or she is unable to discriminate among the weights of objects.

4. He or she is unable to determine what are the shapes or forms of objects. This is called *astereognosis*.

5. The injured person is unable to evaluate texture of materials, for this type of judgment depends on highly critical sensations caused by movement of the skin over the surface.

Note in the above list that nothing has been said about loss of pain and temperature senses. However, in the absence of somatic sensory area I, the appreciation of these sensory modalities may be altered either in quality or in intensity. But more important, the pain or temperature sensations that do occur are poorly localized, indicating that pain and temperature localization probably depend mainly upon simultaneous stimulation of tactile sensors that use the topographical map of the body in somatic sensory area I to locate the source.

SOMATIC SENSORY ASSOCIATION AREA

The parietal cortex immediately behind somatic sensory area I plays important roles in deciphering the sensory information that enters the somatic sensory areas. Therefore, this area is called the *somatic sensory association area*.

Electrical stimulation in the somatic association area can occasionally cause a person to experience a complex somatic sensation, sometimes even the "feeling" of an object such as a knife or a ball. Therefore, it seems clear that the somatic association area combines information from multiple points in the somatic sensory area to decipher its meaning. This assumption also fits with the anatomical arrangement of the neuronal tracts that enter the somatic sensory association area, for it receives signals directly from (a) somatic sensory area I, (b) the ventrobasal complex of the thalamus, (c) other areas of the thalamus which themselves receive input from the ventrobasal complex, (d) the visual cortex, and (e) the auditory cortex.

Effect of Removing the Somatic Sensory Association Area—Amorphosynthesis. When the somatic sensory association area is removed, the person especially loses the ability to recognize by touch complex objects and complex forms. In addition, the person loses most of the sense of form of his or her own body. An especially interesting fact is that loss of the somatic sensory association area on one side of the brain causes the person sometimes to be oblivious of the opposite side of the body—that is, to forget that it is there. Likewise, when handling an object, the person tends to feel only one side of the object and to forget that the other side even exists. This complex sensory deficit is called *amorphosynthesis*.

CHARACTERISTICS OF TRANSMISSION IN THE DORSAL COLUMN–LEMNISCAL SYSTEM

Basic Neuronal Circuit and Discharge Pattern in the Dorsal Column–Lemniscal System. The lower part of Figure 32–10 illustrates the basic organization of the neuronal circuit of the dorsal column pathway, showing that at each synaptic stage divergence occurs. However, the upper part of the figure shows that a single receptor stimulus on the skin does not cause all the cortical neurons with which that receptor connects to discharge at the same rate. Instead, the cortical neurons that discharge to the greatest extent are those in a central part of the cortical "field" for each respective skin receptor. Thus, a weak stimulus causes only the centermost neurons to fire. A stronger stimulus causes still more neurons to fire, but those in the center still discharge at a considerably more rapid rate than those farther away from the center.

Two-Point Discrimination. A method frequently used to test tactile capabilities is to determine a person's so-called two-point discriminatory ability. In this test, two needles are pressed against the skin, and the person determines whether two points of stimulus are felt or one point. On the tips of the fingers a person can distinguish two separate points when the needles are as close together as 1 to 2 mm because of the many specialized nerve endings in the finger tips. However, on the person's back, the needles must usually be as far apart as 30 to 70 mm before two separate points can be detected.

Figure 32–11 illustrates the mechanism by which the dorsal column pathway transmits two-point discriminatory information. This figure shows two adjacent points on the skin that are strongly stimulated, and it also shows the small area of the somatic sensory cortex (greatly enlarged) that is excited by signals from the two stimulated points. The solid black curve shows the spatial pattern of cortical excitation when both skin points are stimulated simultaneously. Note that the resultant zone of excitation has two separate peaks. It is these two peaks separated by a valley that allow the sensory cortex to detect the presence of two stimulatory points rather than a single point. However, the capability of the sensorium to distinguish between two points of stimulation is strongly influenced by another mechanism, the mechanism of lateral inhibition, as explained in the following section.

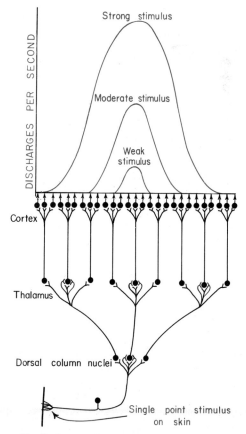

Figure 32–10. Transmission of pinpoint stimulus signal to the cortex.

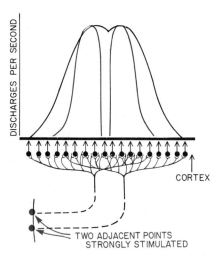

Figure 32–11. Transmission of signals to the cortex from two adjacent pinpoint stimuli. The solid black curve represents the pattern of cortical stimulation without "surround" inhibition, and the two colored curves represent the pattern with "surround" inhibition.

Increase in Contrast in the Perceived Spatial Pattern Caused by Lateral Inhibition. In Chapter 31 it was pointed out that contrast in sensory patterns is increased by inhibitory signals transmitted laterally in the sensory pathway. In the case of the dorsal column–lemniscal system, an excited receptor in the skin transmits not only excitatory signals to the somesthetic cortex but also inhibitory signals laterally to adjacent fiber pathways. These inhibitory signals help to block lateral spread of the excitatory signal, a process called *lateral inhibition*, or *surround inhibition*. As a result, the peak of excitation stands out, and much of the surrounding diffuse stimulation is blocked. This effect is illustrated by the two colored curves in Figure 32–11, showing complete separation of the peaks when the surround inhibition is very great. Obviously, this mechanism accentuates the contrast between the areas of peak stimulation and the surrounding areas, thus greatly increasing the contrast or sharpness of the perceived spatial pattern.

THE POSITION SENSE

The position sense can be divided into two subtypes: (1) *static position,* which means conscious recognition of the orientation of the different parts of the body with respect to each other, and (2) *kinesthesia,* which means conscious recognition of rates of movement of the different parts of the body. The position sensations are transmitted to the sensorium through the dorsal column–lemniscal system.

The Position Sense Receptors. Sensory information from many different types of receptors is used to determine both static position and kinesthesia. These include especially the extensive sensory endings in the joint capsules and ligaments but also receptors in the skin and deep tissues near the joints.

Three major types of nerve endings have been described in the joint capsules and the ligaments

about the joints: (1) By far the most abundant of these are spray-type *Ruffini's endings,* one of which was illustrated in Figure 32–1. These endings are stimulated strongly when the joint is suddenly moved; they adapt slightly at first but transmit a steady signal thereafter. (2) A second type of ending resembling the stretch receptors found in muscle tendons (called *Golgi's receptors*) is found particularly in the ligaments about the joints. Though far less numerous than the Ruffini's endings, they have essentially the same response properties. (3) A few *pacinian corpuscles* are also found in the tissues around the joints. These adapt extremely rapidly and presumably help to detect *rate of rotation* at the joint.

Detection of Static Position by the Joint Receptors. Figure 32–12 illustrates the excitation of seven different nerve fibers leading from separate joint receptors in the capsule of a cat's knee joint. Note that at 180 degrees of joint rotation one of the receptors is stimulated; then at 150 degrees still another is stimulated; at 140 degrees two are stimulated, and so forth. The information from these joint receptors continually apprises the central nervous system of the momentary rotation of the joint. That is, the rotation determines *which* receptor is stimulated and how much it is stimulated, and from this information, the brain knows how far the joint is bent.

Detection of Rate of Movement (Kinesthesia) at the Joint. Rate of movement at the joint is probably detected mainly in the following way: The Ruffini's and Golgi's endings in the joint tissues are stimulated very strongly at first by joint movement, but within a fraction of a second, this strong level of stimulation fades to a lower, steady state rate of firing. This early overshoot in receptor stimulation is directly proportional to the rate of joint movement and is believed to be the signal mainly used by the brain to discern the rate of movement. However, it is likely that the few pacinian corpuscles also play at least some role in this process.

TRANSMISSION IN THE ANTEROLATERAL SYSTEM

It was pointed out earlier in the chapter that the anterolateral system transmits sensory signals that do

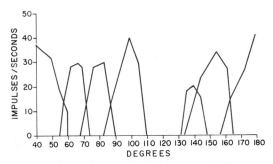

Figure 32–12. Responses of seven different nerve fibers from knee joint receptors in a cat at different degrees of rotation. (Modified from Skoglund: Acta Physiol Scand [Suppl 124] 36:1, 1956.)

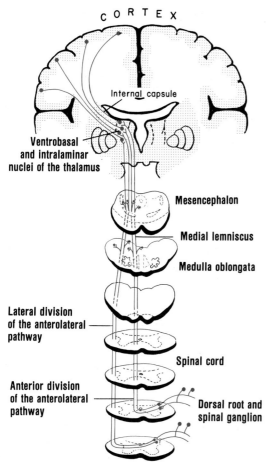

Figure 32–13. The anterior and lateral divisions of the anterolateral pathway.

mainly twofold: (1) throughout the *reticular nuclei of the brain stem* and (2) in two different nuclear complexes of the thalamus, the *ventrobasal complex* and the *intralaminar nuclei.* In general, the tactile signals are transmitted mainly into the ventrobasal complex, which is probably also true for the temperature signals. From here the tactile signals are relayed to the somatic sensory cortex along with the signals from the dorsal columns. On the other hand, only part of the pain signals project to this complex. Instead, most of these enter the reticular nuclei of the brain stem and intralaminal nuclei of the thalamus, as is discussed in greater detail in the following chapter.

Characteristics of Transmission in the Anterolateral Pathway. In general, the same principles apply to transmission in the anterolateral pathway as in the dorsal column–lemniscal system except for the following differences: (a) the velocities of transmission in the anterolaterol pathway are only one third to one half those in the dorsal system; (b) the degree of spatial localization of signals is poor, especially in the pain pathways; (c) the gradations of intensities are also far less acute, most of the sensations being recognized in 10 to 20 gradations of strength rather than as many as 100 gradations for the dorsal system; and (d) the ability to transmit repetitive sensations is poor.

Thus, it is evident that the anterolateral system is a cruder type of transmission system than the dorsal column–lemniscal system. Even so, certain modalities of sensation are transmitted in this system only and not at all in the dorsal column–lemniscal system. These are pain, thermal, tickling and itching, and sexual sensations.

SOME SPECIAL ASPECTS OF SENSORY FUNCTION

Function of the Thalamus in Somatic Sensation. When the somatic sensory cortex of a human being is destroyed, he loses most critical tactile sensibilities, but a slight degree of crude tactile sensibility does return. Therefore, it must be assumed that the thalamus has a slight ability to discriminate tactile sensation but functions mainly to relay this type of information to the cortex.

On the other hand, loss of the somatic sensory cortex has little effect on one's perception of pain sensation and only a moderate effect on the perception of temperature. Therefore, there is much reason to believe that the thalamus and other associated basal regions of the brain perhaps play the dominant role in discrimination of these sensibilities; it is interesting that these sensibilities appeared very early in the phylogenetic development of animalhood, while the critical tactile sensibilities were a late development.

Cortical Control of Sensory Sensitivity. The conscious brain is capable of directing its attention to

not provide highly discrete localization of the signal source and that do not discriminate fine gradations of intensity. These include pain; heat; cold; and the crude tactile, tickling and itching and sexual sensations. In the following chapter, pain and temperature sensations are discussed, while the present section is concerned principally with transmission of the tactile sensations.

ANATOMY OF THE ANTEROLATERAL PATHWAY

The anterolateral fibers originate mainly in laminae I, IV, V, and VI in the dorsal horns, where the small, peripheral, sensory nerve fibers terminate after entering the cord (see Figure 32–5). Then, as illustrated in Figure 32–13, the fibers immediately cross in the anterior commissure of the cord to the opposite anterolateral white column, where they turn upward toward the brain. These fibers ascend rather diffusely throughout the anterolateral columns. However, most anatomists still separate this pathway into an *anterior spinothalamic tract* and a *lateral spinothalamic tract* as illustrated in Figure 32–13, even though physiologically it has been difficult to make this differentiation using electrical recording techniques.

The upper terminus of the anterolateral pathway is

different segments of the sensory system. One of the mechanisms for doing so is the following:

"Corticofugal" signals can be transmitted from the cortex to the lower relay stations of the sensory pathways to *inhibit* transmission in the thalamus, in the brain stem reticular nuclei, in the dorsal column nuclei, and especially in the dorsal horn relay station of the anterolateral system. Also, similar inhibitory mechanisms are known for the visual, auditory, and olfactory systems, which are discussed in later chap-

ters. Each corticofugal pathway begins in the part of the cortex in which the sensory pathway that it controls terminates. Thus, a feedback control loop exists for each sensory pathway.

Obviously, corticofugal control of sensory input could allow the cerebral cortex to alter the threshold for different sensory signals. Also, it might help the brain to focus its attention on specific types of information, which is an important and necessary quality of nervous system function.

QUESTIONS

1. What are the functions of the following types of sensory receptors: *free nerve endings, Merkel's disks, pacinian corpuscles, Meissner's corpuscles, Ruffini's end-organs,* and *muscle spindles?*
2. Explain the labeled line principle.
3. What causes receptor potentials in sensory receptors?
4. Which receptors adapt rapidly and which slowly? Why is it important to have some receptors adapt very rapidly?
5. Explain the principal mechanism by which pacinian corpuscles adapt.
6. Explain the Weber-Fechner principle.
7. Explain the differences between A and C types of nerve fibers.
8. Name the characteristics of the types of sensations that are transmitted in the *dorsal column–lemniscal system.*
9. Give the characteristics of the types of sensations that are transmitted in the *anterolateral system.*
10. Describe the anatomy for signal transmission in the dorsal column–lemniscal system.
11. What is the general difference between the sensations transmitted in the *dorsal columns* and those transmitted in the *spinocervical pathway?*
12. Describe the localization of somatic sensation within *somatic sensory area I.*
13. What are the functions of *somatic sensory area I?*
14. What is the function of the *somatic sensory association area?*
15. Explain the mechanism for two-point discrimination by the sensory nervous system. What is the importance of lateral inhibition in this process?
16. Explain how one determines the degrees of rotation of the joints.
17. Explain how the nervous system determines the rate of movement (called kinesthesia) at a joint.
18. Describe the anatomy of the anterolateral sensory pathway.
19. What are the roles of the thalamus in somatic sensation?
20. Explain the mechanisms for cortical control of sensory sensitivity.

References

American Physiological Society: Sensory Processes. Washington, D.C., American Physiological Society, 1984.

Anderson, D. J., et al.: Sensory mechanisms in mammalian teeth and their supporting structures. Physiol Rev 50:171, 1970.

Bate, C. M., et al.: Development of Sensory System, New York, Springer-Verlag, 1978.

Bennett, T. L.: The Sensory World: An Introduction to Sensation and Perception. Monterey, Cal., Brooks/Cole Publishing Co., 1978.

Catton, W. T.: Mechanoreceptor function. Physiol Rev 50:297, 1970.

Darian-Smith, I.: The sense of touch: Performance and peripheral neural processes. In Darian-Smith I., ed.: Handbook of Physiology. Sec. 1, Vol. III. Bethesda, American Physiological Society, 1984, p. 739.

Friedhoff, A. J., and Miller, J. C.: Clinical implications of receptor sensitivity modification. Annu Rev Neurosci 6:121, 1983.

Goldstein, E. B.: Sensation and Perception. Belmont. Cal., Wadsworth Publishing Co., 1980.

Hochberg, J.: Perception. In Darian-Smith, I., ed.: Handbook of Physiology. Sec. 1, Vol. III. Bethesda, American Physiological Society, 1984, p. 75.

Jung, R.: Sensory research in historical perceptive: Some philosophical foundations of perception. In Darian-Smith, I., ed.: Handbook of Physiology. Sec. 1, Vol. III. Bethesda, American Physiological Society, 1984, p. 1.

McCloskey, D. I.: Kinesthetic sensibility. Physiol Rev 58:763, 1978.

Neff, W. D., ed.: Contributions to Sensory Physiology. New York, Academic Press, 1982.

Porter, R., ed.: Studies in Neurophysiology. New York, Cambridge University Press, 1978.

Schmidt, R. F., ed.: Fundamentals of Sensory Physiology. New York, Springer-Verlag, 1978.

Somjen, G.: Sensory Coding in the Mammalian Nervous System. New York, Appleton-Century-Crofts, 1972.

Weiss, T. F.: Relation of receptor potentials of cochlear hair cells to spike discharges of cochlear neurons. Annu Rev Physiol 46:247, 1984.

Wiersma, C. A. G., and Roach, J. L. M.: Principles in the organization of invertebrate sensory systems. In Brookhart, J. M., and Mountcastle, V. B., eds.: Handbook of Physiology. Sec. 1, Vol. 1. Baltimore, Williams & Wilkins, 1977, p. 1089.

33

Somatic Sensations: Pain, Visceral Pain, Headache, and Thermal Sensations

THE TWO TYPES OF PAIN—ACUTE AND
  SLOW—AND THEIR QUALITIES
  *METHODS FOR MEASURING THE
    PERCEPTION OF PAIN*
THE PAIN RECEPTORS AND THEIR
  STIMULATION
  *RATE OF TISSUE DAMAGE AS THE
    CAUSE OF PAIN*
THE DUAL PATHWAY FOR
  TRANSMISSION OF PAIN SIGNALS
  INTO THE CENTRAL NERVOUS
  SYSTEM
A PAIN-CONTROL (ANALGESIC)

SYSTEM IN THE BRAIN AND THE
  SPINAL CORD
  *INHIBITION OF PAIN TRANSMISSION
    AT THE CORD LEVEL BY TACTILE
    SIGNALS*
REFERRED PAIN
VISCERAL PAIN
  SPECIFIC EXAMPLES
HEADACHE
TICKLING AND ITCHING SENSATIONS
THERMAL SENSATIONS
  *TRANSMISSION OF THE THERMAL
    SIGNALS IN THE NERVOUS SYSTEM*

Many, if not most, ailments of the body cause pain. Furthermore, the ability to diagnose different diseases depends to a great extent on a doctor's knowledge of the different qualities of pain. For these reasons, the present chapter is devoted mainly to pain and to the physiologic basis of some of the associated clinical phenomena.

The Purpose of Pain. Pain is a protective mechanism for the body; it occurs whenever any tissues are being damaged, and it causes the individual to react to remove the pain stimulus. Even such simple activities as sitting for a long time on the ischia can cause tissue destruction because of lack of blood flow to the skin where the skin is compressed by the weight of the body. When the skin becomes painful as a result of the ischemia, the person shifts weight unconsciously. A person who has lost the pain sense, such as after spinal cord injury, fails to feel the pain and therefore fails to shift weight. This eventually results in ulceration at the areas of pressure unless special measures are taken to move the person from time to time.

THE TWO TYPES OF PAIN—ACUTE AND SLOW—AND THEIR QUALITIES

Pain has been classified into two major types: *acute* and *slow*. Acute pain occurs within about 0.1 second when a pain stimulus is applied, whereas slow pain begins only after a second or more and then increases slowly over a period of many seconds and sometimes even minutes. During the course of this chapter we shall see that the conduction pathways for these two types of pain are different and that each of them has specific qualities.

Acute pain is also described by many alternate names, such as *sharp, pricking, fast, and electric,* among others. This type of pain is felt when a needle is stuck into the skin or when the skin is cut with a knife and is also felt when the skin is subjected to electric shock. Acute, sharp pain is not felt in most of the deeper tissues of the body.

Slow pain goes by multiple additional names, including *burning, aching, throbbing, nauseous, and chronic pain.* This type of pain is usually associated

377

with *tissue destruction*. It can become excruciating and can lead to prolonged, unbearable suffering. It can occur both in the skin and in almost any internal tissue or organ.

We will learn later that the acute type of pain is transmitted through type Aδ pain fibers, whereas the slow type results from stimulation of the more primitive type C fibers.

METHODS FOR MEASURING THE PERCEPTION OF PAIN

The intensity of a stimulus necessary to cause pain can be measured in many different ways, but the most used methods have been pricking the skin with a pin at measured pressures, pressing a solid object against a protruding bone with measured force, or heating the skin with measured amounts of heat. The last of these methods has proved to be especially accurate from a quantitative point of view.

Strength-Duration Curve for Expressing Pain Threshold. Figure 33–1 illustrates a typical strength-duration curve obtained by using a heat procedure for measuring pain threshold. Note that a very intense stimulus applied for only a second elicits a sensation of pain, while a stimulus of much less intensity may require many seconds. The lowest intensity of stimulus that will excite the sensation of pain when the stimulus is applied for a prolonged period of time is called the *pain threshold*.

Uniformity of Pain Threshold in Different People. Figure 33–2 shows graphically the lowest skin temperature at which pain is perceived by different persons. By far the greatest number of subjects barely begin to perceive pain when the skin temperature rises to 45°C, and almost everyone perceives pain before the temperature reaches 47°C. In other words, it is almost never true that some persons are unusually sensitive or insensitive to pain. Indeed, measurements in people as widely diverse as Eskimos, American Indians, and whites have shown no significant differences in their *thresholds for pain*. However, different people do *react* very differently to pain, as is discussed in subsequent sections of this chapter.

THE PAIN RECEPTORS AND THEIR STIMULATION

Free Nerve Endings as Pain Receptors. The pain receptors in the skin and other tissues are all free nerve endings. They are widespread in the superficial layers of the *skin* and also in certain internal tissues, such as the *periosteum*, the *arterial walls*, the *joints*, and the *falx* and *tentorium* of the cranial vault. Most of the other deep tissues are not extensively supplied with pain endings but are weakly supplied; nevertheless, any widespread tissue damage can still summate to cause the slow—chronic—aching type of pain even in these areas.

Types of Stimuli That Excite Pain Receptors— Mechanical, Thermal, and Chemical. Some pain fi-

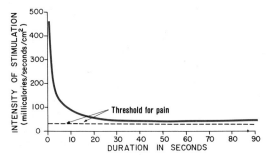

Figure 33–1. Strength-duration curve for depicting pain threshold. (Reprinted with permission from J Chronic Dis, Vol. 4, J. D. Hardy, Copyright 1956, Pergamon Press.)

bers are excited almost entirely by excessive mechanical stress or mechanical damage to the tissues; these are called *mechanosensitive pain receptors*. Others are sensitive to extremes of heat or cold and therefore are called *thermosensitive pain receptors*. And still others, called *chemosensitive pain receptors*, are sensitive to various chemical substances. Some of the chemicals that excite the chemosensitive receptors include *bradykinin, serotonin, histamine, potassium ions, acids, prostaglandins, acetylcholine,* and *proteolytic enzymes*.

Though some pain receptors are mainly sensitive to only one of the above types of stimuli, most are sensitive to more than one.

RATE OF TISSUE DAMAGE AS THE CAUSE OF PAIN

The average critical temperature of 45°C at which a person first begins to perceive pain is also the temperature at which the tissues begin to be damaged by heat; indeed, the tissues are eventually completely destroyed if the temperature remains at this level indefinitely. Therefore, it is immediately apparent

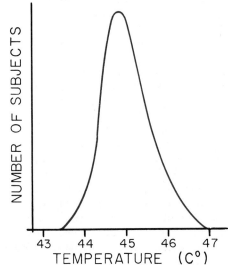

Figure 33–2. Distribution curve obtained from a large number of subjects of the minimal skin temperature that causes pain. (Modified and reprinted with permission from J Chronic Dis, Vol. 4, J. D. Hardy, Copyright 1956, Pergamon Press.)

that pain resulting from heat is closely correlated with the ability of heat to damage the tissues.

Furthermore, in studying soldiers who had been severely wounded in World War II, it was found that the majority of them felt little or no pain except for a short time after the severe wound had been sustained. This, too, indicates that *pain generally is not felt after damage has been done* but only *while damage is being done.*

Special Importance of Chemical Pain Stimuli During Tissue Damage. Extracts from damaged tissues cause intense pain when injected beneath the normal skin. Among the substances that are especially painful in such extracts are *bradykinin, histamine, prostaglandins, acids, excesses of potassium ions, serotonin,* and *proteolytic enzymes,* which are the same substances that are known from electrophysiological data to excite the pain nerve endings. Obviously, many of these substances, especially the proteolytic enzymes, could cause direct damage to the pain nerve endings. But some of the other substances, such as bradykinin and some of the prostaglandins, can cause direct, extreme stimulation of pain nerve fibers without necessarily damaging them.

Release of the various substances listed above not only stimulates the chemosensitive pain endings but also greatly decreases the threshold for stimulation of the mechanosensitive and thermosensitive pain receptors as well. A widely known example of this is the extreme pain caused by slight mechanical or heat stimuli following tissue damage by sunburn.

THE DUAL PATHWAY FOR TRANSMISSION OF PAIN SIGNALS INTO THE CENTRAL NERVOUS SYSTEM

Even though all pain endings are free nerve endings, they utilize two separate pathways for transmitting pain signals into the central nervous system. The two pathways correspond to the two types of pain, an *acute-sharp pain pathway,* and a *slow-chronic pain pathway.*

The Peripheral Pain Fibers—"Fast" and "Slow" Fibers. The acute–sharp pain signals are transmitted in the peripheral nerves to the spinal cord by small type Aδ fibers at velocities of between 6 and 30 meters per second. On the other hand, the slow-chronic type of pain is transmitted by type C fibers at velocities of between 0.5 and 2 meters per second. When the type Aδ fibers are blocked by moderate compression of the nerve trunk without blocking the C fibers, the acute-sharp pain disappears. On the other hand, when the type C fibers are blocked by low concentrations of local anesthetic without blocking the delta fibers, the slow-chronic-aching type of pain disappears.

Because of this double system of pain innervation, a sudden onset of painful stimulus gives a "double" pain sensation: a fast, sharp pain followed a second or so later by a slow, burning pain. The sharp pain

apprises a person very rapidly of a damaging influence and therefore plays an important role in making the person react immediately to remove himself or herself from the stimulus. On the other hand, the slow, burning sensation tends to become more and more painful over a period of time. This sensation gives one the almost intolerable suffering of long-continued pain.

Transmission in the Anterolateral Sensory Pathway. Pain fibers enter the cord through the dorsal roots, ascend or descend one to two segments, and then terminate on neurons in the dorsal horns of the cord gray matter, the type Aδ fibers in laminae I and V and the type C fibers in laminae II and III, an area also called the substantia gelatinosa. Most of the signals then pass through one or more additional short-fibered neurons, finally giving rise to long fibers that cross to the opposite side of the cord and pass upward to the brain via the anterolateral sensory pathway, which is described in the previous chapter.

As the pain pathways pass into the brain they separate into the (1) *fast–acute pain pathway,* composed almost entirely of type A delta fibers, and (2) the *slow–chronic pain pathway,* composed almost entirely of the slow type C fibers.

Termination of the Fast–Acute Pain Pathway in the Brain Stem and Thalamus. Figure 33–3 illustrates the pain pathways entering the brain stem from the spinal cord. About three quarters to nine tenths of all pain fibers terminate in the reticular formation of the medulla, pons, and mesencephalon. However, a small proportion of the pain fibers, especially those that transmit the fast-acute type of pain, pass directly to the thalamus and terminate in the *ventrobasal complex of the thalamus,* along with the sensory fibers from the dorsal column–lemniscal pathway. From

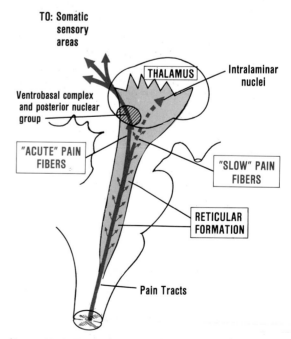

Figure 33–3. Transmission of pain signals into the hindbrain, thalamus, and cortex via the "pricking pain" pathway and the "burning pain" pathway.

here signals are transmitted into other areas of the thalamus and also to the somatic sensory cortex. The signals to the cortex are probably important mainly for localizing the pain, not for interpreting it.

Termination of the Slow–Chronic Pain Fibers in the Brain Stem and Thalamus. In contrast with the fibers of the acute-fast pain pathway, those of the slow-chronic pathway terminate almost entirely in the reticular formation of the medulla, pons, and mesencephalon. However, great numbers of signals are relayed upward through this formation via short nerve fibers and finally into the intralaminar nuclei of the thalamus, which are themselves an upward extension of the reticular formation protruding among the specific thalamic nuclei. The reticular area of the brain stem transmits activating signals into essentially all parts of the brain, especially upward through the thalamus to all areas of the cerebral cortex.

Thus, the slow–burning–aching pain fibers, because they do excite the reticular activating system, have a very potent effect in activating essentially the entire nervous system—that is, arousing one from sleep, creating a state of excitement, a sense of urgency, and promoting defense and aversion reactions designed to rid the person or animal of the painful stimulus.

The signals that are transmitted through the slow–burning–aching pain pathway can be localized only to very gross areas of the body. Therefore, these signals are designed almost entirely for the single purpose of calling one's attention to injurious processes in the body. They create suffering that is sometimes intolerable. Their gradation of intensity is poor; instead, even weak pain signals can, over a period of time by a process of temporal summation, create an unbearable feeling even though the same pain for short periods of time may be relatively mild.

Function of the Reticular Formation, Thalamus, and Cerebral Cortex in the Appreciation of Pain. Complete removal of the somatic sensory areas of the cerebral cortex does not destroy one's ability to perceive pain. Therefore, it is believed that pain impulses entering only the reticular formation, thalamus, and other lower centers can cause conscious perception of pain. However, this does not mean that the cerebral cortex has nothing to do with normal pain appreciation; indeed, electrical stimulation of the cortical somatic sensory areas causes a person to perceive mild pain in approximately 3 per cent of the stimulations. It is believed that the cortex plays an important role in interpreting the quality of pain and localizing the pain even though pain perception might be a function of lower centers.

A PAIN-CONTROL (ANALGESIC) SYSTEM IN THE BRAIN AND THE SPINAL CORD

The degree to which each person reacts to pain varies tremendously. This results partly from the capability of the brain itself to control the degree of input of pain signals to the nervous system by activation of a pain control system, called an *analgesic system.*

The analgesic system is illustrated in Figure 33–4. It consists of three major components (plus other accessory components):

(1) The *periaqueductal gray area* of the mesencephalon and the upper pons surrounding the aqueduct of Sylvius. Neurons from this area send their signals to

(2) The *raphe magnus nucleus,* a thin midline nucleus located in the lower pons and upper medulla. From here the signals are transmitted down the spinal cord to

(3) A *pain-inhibitory complex located in the dorsal horns of the spinal cord.* At this point the pain signals can be blocked before they are relayed on to the brain.

Electrical stimulation in either the periaqueductal gray area or in the raphe magnus nucleus can almost completely suppress many very strong pain signals entering by way of the dorsal spinal roots. Stimulation of areas at still higher levels of the brain that in turn excite the periaqueductal gray can also suppress pain.

Several different transmitter substances are involved in the analgesic system; especially involved are *enkephalin* and *serotonin.* Many of the nerve fibers derived from both the periventricular nuclei and the periaqueductal gray area secrete enkephalin at their endings. For instance, as shown in Figure 33–4, the endings of many of the fibers in the raphe magnus nucleus release enkephalin. On the other hand, the fibers originating in this nucleus but ter-

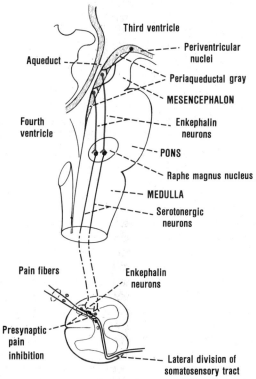

Figure 33–4. The analgesia system of the brain stem and spinal cord, showing inhibition of incoming pain signals at the cord level.

minating in the dorsal horns of the spinal cord secrete serotonin at their endings. The serotonin in turn acts on still another set of local cord neurons that are believed to secrete enkephalin. The enkephalin, in some way not presently understood, is believed to cause presynaptic inhibition of the incoming pain fibers in laminae I through V in the dorsal horns.

Thus, the analgesic system can block pain signals at the initial entry point to the spinal cord. In fact, it can also block many of the local cord reflexes that result from pain signals, especially the withdrawal reflexes that are described in the following chapter.

It is probable that this analgesic system can also inhibit pain transmission at other points in the pain pathway, especially in the reticular nuclei in the brain stem and in the intralaminar nuclei of the thalamus.

Most important, it must be noted that this pain analgesic system is capable of blocking both the fast-sharp and the slow-burning-aching types of pain.

The Brain's Opiate System— The Endorphins and Enkephalins

More than 20 years ago, it was discovered that injection of extremely minute quantities of morphine into either the periventricular nucleus around the third ventricle of the diencephalon or into the peri-aqueductal gray area of the brain stem will cause an extreme degree of analgesia. In subsequent studies, it has been found that morphine acts at many other points in the analgesic system, including both the raphe magnus nucleus and the dorsal horns of the spinal cord. Because most drugs that alter the excitability of neurons do so by acting on synaptic receptors, it was assumed that the "morphine receptors" of the analgesic system must in fact be receptors for some morphine-like neurotransmitter that is naturally secreted in the brain. Therefore, an extensive search was set in motion for a natural opiate of the brain. At least nine such opiate-like substances have now been found at different points in the nervous system. Furthermore, multiple areas of the brain have been shown to have opiate receptors, especially areas in the analgesic system. Among the more important of the opiate substances are

(1) β-endorphin,
(2) met-enkephalin,
(3) leu-enkephalin, and
(4) dynorphin.

The two enkephalins are found in the portions of the analgesic system described earlier, and β-endorphin is present both in the hypothalamus and in the pituitary gland. Dynorphin, though found only in minute quantities in nervous tissue, is important because it is an extremely powerful opiate, having 200 times as much pain-killing effect as morphine when injected directly into the analgesic system.

Thus, although all the fine details of the brain's opiate system are not yet entirely understood, nevertheless activation of the analgesic system either by nervous signals entering the periaqueductal gray area or by morphine-like drugs can totally or almost totally suppress many pain signals entering through the peripheral nerves.

INHIBITION OF PAIN TRANSMISSION AT THE CORD LEVEL BY TACTILE SIGNALS

Another important landmark in the saga of pain control was the discovery that stimulation of large sensory fibers from the peripheral tactile receptors depresses the transmission of pain signals either from the same area of the body or even from areas sometimes located many segments away. This explains why such simple maneuvers as rubbing the skin near painful areas is often very effective in relieving pain. And it probably also explains why *liniments* are often useful in the relief of pain. This mechanism and simultaneous psychogenic excitation of the central analgesic system are probably also the basis of pain relief by *acupuncture*.

Treatment of Pain by Electrical Stimulation. Several clinical procedures have been developed recently for suppressing pain by stimulating large sensory nerve fibers. The stimulating electrodes are placed on selected areas of the skin, or on occasion they have been implanted over the spinal cord to stimulate the dorsal sensory columns. And, in a few patients, electrodes have even been placed stereotaxically in the periventricular, periaqueductal, or other areas of the diencephalon. The patient can then personally control the degree of stimulation. Dramatic relief has been reported in some instances.

REFERRED PAIN

Often a person feels pain in a part of his or her body that is considerably removed from the tissues causing the pain. This pain is called *referred pain.* Usually the pain is initiated in one of the visceral organs and referred to an area on the body surface. Also, pain may be referred to another deep area of the body not coincident with the location of the viscus producing the pain. A knowledge of these different types of referred pain is extremely important in clinical diagnosis because many visceral ailments produce no other signs except referred pain.

Mechanism of Referred Pain. Figure 33–5 illustrates the most likely mechanism by which most pain is referred. In the figure, branches of visceral pain fibers are shown to synapse in the spinal cord with some of the same second-order neurons that receive pain fibers from the skin. When the visceral pain fibers are stimulated, pain signals from the viscera are then conducted through at least some of the same neurons that conduct pain signals from the skin, and the person has the feeling that the sensations actually originate in the skin itself.

VISCERAL PAIN

In clinical diagnosis, pain from the different viscera of the abdomen and chest is one of the few criteria

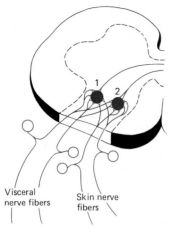

Figure 33–5. Mechanism of referred pain and referred hyperalgesia.

that can be used for diagnosing visceral inflammation, disease, and other ailments. In general, the viscera have receptors for no other types of sensation besides pain. Also, visceral pain differs from surface pain in several important aspects.

One of the most important differences between surface pain and visceral pain is that some highly localized types of damage to the viscera may not cause severe pain. For instance, a surgeon can cut the gut entirely in two in a patient who is awake without causing significant pain. On the other hand, any stimulus that causes *diffuse stimulation of pain nerve endings* throughout a viscus causes pain that can be extremely severe. For instance, ischemia caused by occluding the blood supply to a large area of the gut causes severe tissue damage and stimulates many diffuse pain fibers, resulting in extreme pain.

The Pathway for Transmission of Visceral Pain. Most of the internal organs of the body are supplied by type C pain fibers that pass along the visceral sympathetic nerves into the spinal cord and thence up the lateral division of the anterolateral sensory pathway along with the pain fibers from the body's surface.

Localization of Referred Pain Transmitted by the Visceral Pathways. The position in the cord to which visceral afferent fibers pass from each organ depends on the segment of the body from which the organ developed embryologically. For instance, the heart originated in the neck and upper thorax. Consequently, the heart's visceral pain fibers enter the cord all the way from segment C-3 down to T-5. The stomach had its origin in the lower thoracic segments of the embryo, and consequently the visceral afferents from the stomach enter the spinal cord at these levels. The gallbladder had its origin almost entirely in the ninth thoracic segment, so that the visceral afferents from the gallbladder enter the spinal cord at T-9.

Because the visceral afferent pain fibers are responsible for transmitting referred pain from the viscera, the location of the referred pain on the surface of the body is in the skin area of the segment from which the visceral organ was originally derived

in the embryo. Some of the areas of referred pain on the surface of the body are shown in Figure 33–6.

SPECIFIC EXAMPLES

Cardiac Pain. Almost all pain that originates in the heart results from ischemia secondary to coronary sclerosis. This pain is referred mainly to the base of the neck, over the shoulders, over the pectoral muscles, and down the arms. Most frequently, the referred pain is on the left side rather than on the right—probably because the left side of the heart is much more frequently involved in coronary disease than is the right side—but occasionally mild referred pain occurs on the right side of the body as well as on the left.

When coronary ischemia is extremely severe, such as immediately after a coronary thrombosis, intense cardiac pain often occurs directly underneath the sternum simultaneously with pain referred to other areas. This direct pain from underneath the sternum is difficult to explain on the basis of the visceral nerve connections. Therefore, it is highly probable that sensory nerve endings passing from the heart through the pericardial reflections around the great vessels conduct this pain directly into the spinal nerves at this level of the chest.

Gastric Pain. Pain arising in the stomach—usually caused by gastritis—is referred to the anterior surface of the chest or upper abdomen from slightly below the heart to an inch or so below the xyphoid process. This pain is frequently characterized as burning pain; and it, or pain from the lower esophagus, causes the condition known as heartburn.

Most *peptic ulcers* occur within 1 to 2 inches on either side of the pylorus in the stomach or in the duodenum, and pain from such ulcers is usually referred to a surface point approximately midway

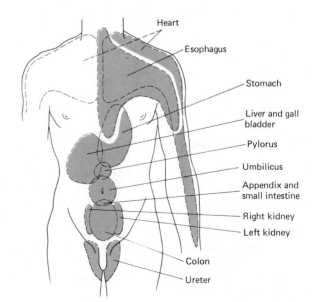

Figure 33–6. Surface areas of referred pain from different visceral organs.

between the umbilicus and the xyphoid process. The origin of ulcer pain is almost undoubtedly chemical because when the acid juices of the stomach are not allowed to reach the pain fibers in the ulcer crater, the pain does not exist. Characteristically, this pain is intensely burning.

Biliary and Gallbladder Pain. Pain from the bile ducts and gallbladder is localized in the midepigastrium almost at the same point as pain caused by peptic ulcers. Also, biliary and gallbladder pain is sometimes burning, like that from ulcers, though cramps usually occur because of intermittent spastic contractions of the gallbladder wall.

Biliary disease, in addition to causing pain on the abdominal surface, frequently refers pain to a small area at the tip of the right scapula. This pain is transmitted through sympathetic afferent fibers that enter the ninth thoracic segment of the spinal cord.

Uterine Pain. Both direct and visceral afferent pain may be transmitted from the uterus. The low abdominal cramping pains at the time of menstruation are visceral pains mediated through the sympathetic afferents, and an operation to cut the sympathetic hypogastric nerves to the uterus will in many instances relieve this pain. On the other hand, lesions of the uterus that spread into the surroundings of the uterus, or lesions of the fallopian tubes and broad ligaments, usually cause pain in the lower back or side. This pain is conducted over direct nerve fibers to the surface areas of the body and is usually sharp rather than resembling the diffuse cramping pain of true dysmenorrhea.

HEADACHE

Headaches are actually pain referred to the surface of the head from the deep structures. The brain itself is almost totally insensitive to pain. Even cutting or electrically stimulating the sensory centers of the cortex when a person is awake only occasionally causes pain; instead, it causes tactile paresthesia on the area of the body represented by the portion of the cortex stimulated. Therefore, most of the pain of headache probably is not caused by damage within the brain itself.

On the other hand, *tugging on the venous sinuses* or *damage to the membranes covering the brain* can cause intense pain that is recognized as headache.

Headache of Meningitis. One of the most severe headaches of all is that resulting from meningitis, which causes inflammation of all the meninges, including the sensitive areas of the dura and the sensitive areas around the venous sinuses. Such intense damage as this can cause extreme headache pain referred over the entire head.

Migraine Headache. Migraine headache is a special type of headache that is thought to result from abnormal vascular phenomena, though the exact mechanism is unknown.

Migraine headaches often begin with various prodromal sensations, such as nausea, loss of vision in parts of the fields of vision, visual aura, or other types of sensory hallucinations. Ordinarily, the prodromal symptoms begin half an hour to an hour prior to the beginning of the headache itself. Therefore, any theory that explains migraine headache must also explain these prodromal symptoms.

One of the theories of the cause of migraine headaches is that prolonged emotion or tension causes reflex vasospasm of some of the arteries of the head, including arteries that supply the brain itself. The vasospasm theoretically produces ischemia (poor nourishment) of portions of the brain, which is responsible for the prodromal symptoms. Then, as a result of the intense ischemia, something happens to the vascular wall to allow it to become flaccid and incapable of maintaining vascular tone for the next 24 to 48 hours. The blood pressure in the vessels causes them to dilate and pulsate intensely, and it is supposedly the excessive stretching of the walls of the arteries—including the extracranial arteries such as the temporal artery—that causes the actual pain of migraine headaches. However, it is possible that diffuse aftereffects of ischemia in the brain itself are at least partially responsible for this type of headache.

Alcoholic Headache. As many people have experienced, a headache usually follows an alcoholic binge. It is most likely that alcohol, because it is toxic to tissues, directly damages the meninges and causes the cerebral pain.

Headache Caused by Constipation. Constipation causes headache in many persons. This probably results from absorbed toxic products that affect the brain and surrounding tissues, or the headache could result from changes in the circulatory system. Indeed, constipation sometimes causes temporary loss of plasma into the wall of the gut, and a resulting poor flow of blood to the head could be the cause of the headache.

Headache Caused by Irritation of the Nasal Structures and Their Accessories. The mucous membranes of the nose and also of all the nasal sinuses are sensitive to pain. As a consequence, infection or other irritative processes in widespread areas of the nasal structures usually cause headache that is referred behind the eyes or, in the case of frontal sinus infection, to the frontal surfaces of the forehead and scalp.

Headache Caused by Eye Disorders. Difficulty in focusing one's eyes clearly may cause excessive contraction of the muscles of the eye in an attempt to gain clear vision. Even though these muscles are extremely small, tonic contraction of them could be the cause of retro-orbital headache.

TICKLING AND ITCHING SENSATIONS

The phenomena of tickling and itching have often been stated to be caused by very mild stimulation of pain nerve endings, because whenever pain is blocked by anesthesia of a nerve or by compressing the nerve, the phenomena of tickling and itching also disappear.

However, recent neurophysiological studies have demonstrated the existence of very sensitive free nerve endings that elicit only the itching sensation. Furthermore, these endings are found almost exclusively in the superficial layers of the skin, which is also the only tissue from which the itching sensation can be elicited. Also, exciting itch receptors in animals initiates scratch reflexes, contrasting with the effect of exciting pain nerve endings, which always causes withdrawal reflexes instead.

Therefore, it seems clear that itching and tickling sensations are transmitted by very small type C fibers similar to those that transmit burning type of pain; these fibers, however, are distinctly separate from pain fibers.

The purpose of the itching sensation is presumably to call attention to mild surface stimuli such as a flea crawling on the skin or a fly about to bite, and the elicited signals then lead to scratching or other maneuvers that rid the host of the irritant.

The relief of itching by the process of scratching occurs only when the irritant is removed or when the scratch is strong enough to elicit pain (or other overriding sensations). The pain signals are believed to suppress the itch signals in the cord by a process of inhibition that is described earlier in the chapter.

THERMAL SENSATIONS

Thermal Receptors and Their Excitation

The human being can perceive gradations of cold and heat, progressing from *freezing cold* to *cold* to *cool* to *neutral* to *warm* to *hot* to *burning hot*.

Thermal gradations are discriminated by at least three different types of sensory receptors: the cold receptors, the warmth receptors, and pain receptors. The pain receptors are stimulated only by extreme degrees of heat or cold and therefore are responsible, along with the cold and warmth receptors, for "freezing cold" and "burning hot" sensations.

The cold and warmth receptors are located immediately under the skin at discrete points, each having a stimulatory diameter of about 1 mm. In most areas of the body there are three to ten times as many cold receptors as warmth receptors, and the number in different areas of the body varies from as great as 15 to 25 cold points per square centimeter in the lips, to 3 to 5 cold points per square centimeter in the finger, to less than 1 cold point per square centimeter in some broad surface areas of the trunk. There are correspondingly fewer numbers of warmth points. A definitive cold receptor has been identified. It is a special, small, type Aδ myelinated nerve ending with a number of branches, the tips of which protrude into the bottom surfaces of basal epidermal cells.

On the other hand, a definitive warmth receptor has not been found. This receptor is believed to be one variety of free nerve ending.

Stimulation of Thermal Receptors—Sensations of Cold, Cool, Neutral, Warm, and Hot. Figure 33–7

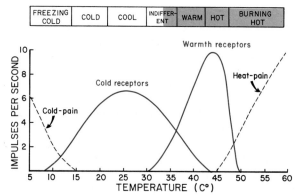

Figure 33–7. Frequencies of discharge of (1) a cold-pain fiber, (2) a cold fiber, (3) a warmth fiber, and (4) a heat-pain fiber. (The responses of these fibers are drawn from original data collected in separate experiments by Zotterman, Hensel, and Kenshalo.)

illustrates the effects of different temperatures on the responses of four different nerve fibers: (1) a pain fiber stimulated by cold, (2) a cold fiber, (3) a warmth fiber, and (4) a pain fiber stimulated by heat. Note especially that these fibers respond differently at different levels of temperature. For instance, in the *very* cold region only the pain fibers are stimulated (if the skin becomes even colder so that it nearly freezes or actually does freeze, even these fibers cannot be stimulated). As the temperature rises to 10 to 15° C, pain impulses cease, but the cold receptors begin to be stimulated. Then above about 30° C, the warmth receptors become stimulated, while the cold receptors fade out at about 43° C. Finally, at around 45° C, pain fibers begin to be stimulated by heat.

One can understand from Figure 33-7, therefore, that a person determines the different gradations of thermal sensations by the relative degrees of stimulation of the different types of endings. One can understand also from this figure why extreme degrees of cold or heat can both be painful and why both these sensations, when intense enough, may give almost exactly the same quality of sensation—that is, freezing cold and burning hot sensations feel almost alike; they are both very painful.

Stimulatory Effects of Rising and Falling Temperatures—Adaptation of Thermal Receptors. When a thermal receptor is suddenly subjected to an abrupt change in temperature, it becomes strongly stimulated at first, but this stimulation fades rapidly during the first few seconds and progressively more slowly during the next half hour or more. In other words, the receptor adapts to a great extent but not entirely.

Thus, it is evident that the thermal senses respond markedly to *changes in temperature* in addition to being able to respond to steady states of temperature. This means that when the temperature of the skin is actively falling, a person feels much colder than when the temperature remains at the same level. Conversely, if the temperature is actively rising, the person feels much warmer than at the same temperature when it is not rising.

Mechanism of Stimulation of the Thermal Receptors. It is believed that the thermal receptors are stimulated by changes in their metabolic rates, these changes resulting from the fact that temperature alters the rates of intracellular chemical reactions more than twofold for each 10° C change. In other words, thermal detection probably results not from direct physical stimulation but instead from chemical stimulation of the endings as modified by the temperature.

Spatial Summation of Thermal Sensations. The number of cold or warmth endings in any small surface area of the body is very small, so that it is difficult to judge gradations of temperature when small areas are stimulated. However, when a large area of the body is stimulated, the thermal signals from the entire area summate. Indeed, one reaches his maximum ability to discern minute temperature variations when his entire body is subjected to a temperature change all at once. For instance, rapid changes in temperature of as little as 0.01° C can be detected if this change affects the entire surface of the body simultaneously. On the other hand, temperature changes 100 times this great might not be detected when the skin surface affected is only a square centimeter or so in size.

TRANSMISSION OF THE THERMAL SIGNALS IN THE NERVOUS SYSTEM

In general, thermal signals are transmitted in pathways that closely parallel the pathways for pain signals. On entering the spinal cord, the signals travel for a few segments upward or downward, then are processed by one or more cord neurons, and finally enter long, ascending thermal fibers that cross to the opposite lateral division of the anterolateral tract and terminate in (a) the reticular areas of the brain stem and (b) the ventrobasal complex of the thalamus. A few thermal signals are also relayed to the somatic sensory cortex from the ventrobasal complex. Occasionally, a neuron in somatic sensory area I has been found by microelectrode studies to be directly responsive to either cold or warm stimuli in specific areas of the skin. Furthermore, it is known that removal of the postcentral gyrus in the human being reduces his ability to distinguish different gradations of temperature.

QUESTIONS

1. Discuss the differences between *acute pain* and *slow pain*.
2. Explain what is meant by the uniformity of *pain thresholds* in different people.
3. What are the different types of pain receptor endings, and what is the relationship between tissue damage and pain?
4. Describe the two separate pathways for transmission of pain signals into the central nervous system and their functional differences.
5. Describe the functions of the reticular formation, the thalamus, and the cerebral cortex in the appreciation of pain.
6. Describe the pain-control (analgesic) system of the brain and spinal cord.
7. What is meant by the brain's *opiate system*?
8. Explain the mechanism of *referred pain*. Why is referred pain from the viscera often localized far from the organ causing the pain?
9. Describe briefly the characteristics of cardiac, gastric, biliary and gall bladder, and uterine pains.
10. What pain receptor regions within the head are responsible for headache?
11. What is the theoretical mechanism for *migraine headache*?
12. Explain the mechanism by which a person determines the temperature of objects touched by the skin.
13. Explain the mechanism of spatial summation of thermal sensations. How important is this mechanism in the appreciation of changes in temperature?

References

Akil, H., et al.: Endogenous opioids: etiology and function. Annu Rev Neurosci 7:223, 1984.

Basbaum, A. I., and Fields, H. L.: Endogenous pain control systems: brainstem spinal pathways and endorphin circuitry. Annu Rev Neurosci 7:309, 1984.

Bond, M. R.: Pain—Its Nature, Analysis, and Treatment. New York, Churchill Livingstone, 1984.

Darian-Smith, I.: Thermal sensibility. In Darian-Smith, I., ed.: Handbook of Physiology. Sec. 1, Vol. 3. Bethesda, American Physiological Society, 1984, p. 879.

Dubner, R., and Bennett, G. J.: Spinal and trigeminal mechanisms of nociception. Annu Rev Neurosci 6:381, 1983.

Friedhoff, A. J., and Miller, J. C.: Clinical implications of receptor sensitivity modification. Annu Rev Neurosci 6:121, 1983.

Gelmers, H. J.: Calcium-channel blockers in the treatment of migraine. Am J Cardiol 55:139B, 1985.

Guyton, A. C., and Reeder, R. C.: Pain and contracture in poliomyelitis. Arch Neurol Psychiatr 63:954, 1950.

Haft, J. I., ed.: Differential Diagnosis of Chest Pain and Other Cardiac Symptoms. Mt. Kisco, N.Y., Futura Publishing Co., 1983.

Hyvarinen, J.: Posterior parietal lobe of the primate brain. Physiol Rev 62:1060, 1982.

Kaas, J. H.: What, if anything, is SI? Organization of first somatosensory area of cortex. Physiol Rev 63:206, 1983.

Kaas, J. J., et al.: The reorganization of the somatosensory cortex following peripheral nerve damage in adult and developing mammals. Annu Rev Neurosci 6:325, 1983.

Kruger, L., ed.: Neural Mechanisms of Pain. New York, Raven Press, 1984.

Neff, W. D., ed.: Contributions to Sensory Physiology. New York, Academic Press, 1982.

Perl, E. R.: Pain and nociception. In Darian-Smith, I., ed.: Handbook of Physiology. Sec. 1, Vol. 3. Bethesda, American Physiological Society, 1984, p. 915.

Raskin, N. H.: Chemical headaches. Annu Rev Med 32:63, 1981.

Raskin, N. H., and Appenzeller, O.: Headache. Philadelphia, W. B. Saunders Co., 1980.

Stimmel, B.: Pain, Analgesia, and Addiction. The Pharmacologic Treatment of Pain. New York, Raven Press, 1983.

34

The Spinal Cord and Brain Stem Reflexes and Function of the Vestibular Apparatus

ORGANIZATION OF THE SPINAL
CORD FOR MOTOR FUNCTIONS
THE MUSCLE RECEPTORS—MUSCLE
SPINDLES AND GOLGI'S TENDON
ORGANS—AND THEIR ROLES IN
MUSCLE CONTROL
RECEPTOR FUNCTION OF THE
MUSCLE SPINDLE
THE STRETCH REFLEX (ALSO CALLED
THE MYOTATIC REFLEX)
ROLE OF THE MUSCLE SPINDLE IN
VOLUNTARY MOTOR ACTIVITY
CLINICAL APPLICATION OF THE
STRETCH REFLEX—THE KNEE JERK
AND OTHER MUSCLE JERKS
THE TENDON REFLEX
THE FLEXOR REFLEX
THE CROSSED EXTENSOR REFLEX
RECIPROCAL INHIBITION (RECIPROCAL
INNERVATION)
THE REFLEXES OF POSTURE AND
LOCOMOTION
SPINAL CORD REFLEXES THAT CAUSE
MUSCLE SPASM

SPINAL CORD TRANSECTION AND
SPINAL SHOCK
THE BRAIN STEM
THE RETICULAR FORMATION AND
SUPPORT OF THE BODY AGAINST
GRAVITY
VESTIBULAR SENSATIONS AND THE
MAINTENANCE OF EQUILIBRIUM
THE VESTIBULAR APPARATUS
FUNCTION OF THE UTRICLE AND THE
SACCULE IN THE MAINTENANCE
OF STATIC EQUILIBRIUM
THE SEMICIRCULAR CANALS AND
THEIR DETECTION OF ANGULAR
ACCELERATION
OTHER FACTORS CONCERNED WITH
EQUILIBRIUM
FUNCTIONS OF THE RETICULAR
FORMATION AND SPECIFIC BRAIN
STEM NUCLEI IN CONTROLLING
SUBCONSCIOUS, STEREOTYPED
MOVEMENTS
SUMMARY OF THE FUNCTIONS OF THE
CORD AND BRAIN STEM IN POSTURE
AND LOCOMOTION

In the discussion of the nervous system thus far, we have considered principally the input of sensory information. In the following chapters we discuss the origin and output of motor signals, the signals that cause muscle contraction and other motor effects throughout the body. Sensory information is integrated at all levels of the nervous system and causes appropriate motor responses, beginning in the spinal cord with relatively simple reflexes, extending into the brain stem with more complicated responses, and finally into the cerebrum where the most complicated responses are controlled. The present chapter discusses the control of motor function at the spinal cord and lower brain stem level.

ORGANIZATION OF THE SPINAL CORD FOR MOTOR FUNCTIONS

The cord gray matter is the integrative area for the cord reflexes and other motor functions. Figure 34–1 shows the typical organization of the cord gray matter in a single cord segment. Sensory signals enter the cord through the sensory roots. After entering the cord, every sensory signal travels to two separate

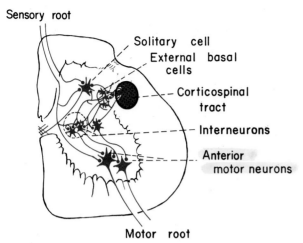

Sensory root

Solitary cell
External basal cells

Corticospinal tract

Interneurons

Anterior motor neurons

Motor root

Figure 34–1. Connections of the sensory fibers and cortico-spinal fibers with the interneurons and anterior motor neurons of the spinal cord.

destinations. First, either in the same segment of the cord or in nearby segments, the sensory nerve or its collaterals terminate in the gray matter of the cord and elicit local segmental responses—local excitatory or facilitory effects, reflexes, or others. Second, the signals travel to higher levels of the nervous system—to higher levels in the cord itself, to the brain stem, or even to the cerebral cortex. It is these sensory signals that cause the sensory effects described in the past few chapters.

Each segment of the spinal cord has several million neurons in its gray matter. Aside from the sensory relay neurons already discussed, the remainder of these neurons are divided into two separate types, the *anterior motor neurons* and the *interneurons*.

The Anterior Motor Neurons. Located in each segment of the anterior horns of the cord gray matter are several thousand neurons that are 50 to 100 per cent larger than most of the others and called anterior motor neurons. These neurons give rise to the nerve fibers that leave the cord via the anterior roots and then proceed to the muscles to innervate the skeletal muscle fibers. They can be divided into two major types, the *alpha motor neurons* and the *gamma motor neurons*.

The Alpha Motor Neurons. The alpha motor neurons give rise to large, type A alpha nerve fibers, ranging from 9 to 20 microns in diameter, that pass through the spinal nerves to innervate the skeletal muscle fibers. Stimulation of a single nerve fiber excites from three to several hundred skeletal muscle fibers that are collectively called the *motor unit*. Transmission of nerve impulses into skeletal muscles and their stimulation of the muscle fibers was discussed in Chapters 5 through 7.

The Gamma Motor Neurons. In addition to the alpha motor neurons that excite contraction of the skeletal muscle fibers, about one half as many much smaller gamma motor neurons are located along with the alpha motor neurons in the anterior horns. These transmit impulses through type A gamma (Aγ) fibers, averaging 5 microns in diameter, to very small, special skeletal muscle fibers called *intrafusal fibers*. These are part of the *muscle spindle*, which is discussed later in the chapter.

The Interneurons. The interneurons are present in all areas of the cord gray matter—in the dorsal horns, in the anterior horns, and in the intermediate areas between these two. These cells are numerous—approximately 30 times as numerous as the anterior motor neurons. They are small and highly excitable, often exhibiting spontaneous activity and capable of firing as rapidly as 1500 times per second. The interneurons have many interconnections, and many of them directly innervate the anterior motor neurons as illustrated in Figure 34–1. The interconnections among the interneurons and anterior motor neurons are responsible for many of the integrative functions of the spinal cord that are discussed in the remainder of this chapter.

Essentially all the different types of neuronal circuits described in Chapter 31 are found in the interneuron pool of cells of the spinal cord, including the *diverging, converging,* and *repetitive-discharge* circuits. In this chapter we will see many applications of these different circuits to the performance of specific reflex acts by the spinal cord.

Only a few incoming sensory signals from the spinal nerves or signals from the brain terminate directly on the anterior motor neurons. Instead, most of them are transmitted first through interneurons, where they are appropriately processed. Thus, in Figure 34–1, it is shown that the corticospinal tract terminates almost entirely on interneurons, and it is only after the signals from this tract have been integrated in the interneuron pool with signals from other spinal tracts or from the spinal nerves that they finally impinge on the anterior motor neurons to control muscular function.

THE MUSCLE RECEPTORS—MUSCLE SPINDLES AND GOLGI'S TENDON ORGANS—AND THEIR ROLES IN MUSCLE CONTROL

Proper control of muscle function requires not only excitation of the muscle by the anterior motor neurons but also continuous feedback of information from each muscle to the nervous system, giving the status of the muscle at each instant. To provide this function, the muscles and their tendons are supplied abundantly with two special types of sensory receptors: (1) *muscle spindles,* which are distributed throughout the belly of the muscle and which send information to the nervous system about either the muscle length or rate of change of its length, and (2) *Golgi's tendon organs,* which transmit information about tension or rate of change of tension.

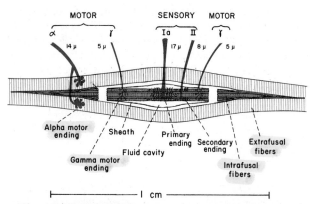

Figure 34–2. The muscle spindle, showing its relationship to the large extrafusal skeletal muscle fibers. Note also both the motor and the sensory innervation of the muscle spindle.

RECEPTOR FUNCTION OF THE MUSCLE SPINDLE

Structure and Innervation of the Muscle Spindle. The physiologic organization of the muscle spindle is illustrated in Figure 34–2. Each spindle is built around 3 to 12 small *intrafusal muscle fibers* that are pointed at their ends and are attached to the surrounding *extrafusal* skeletal muscle fibers. Each intrafusal fiber is a very small skeletal muscle fiber. However, the central region of each of these fibers—that is, the area midway between its two ends—has either no or few actin and myosin filaments. Therefore, this central portion does not contract when the ends do. Instead, it functions as a sensory receptor. The end portions are excited by the small *gamma motor nerve fibers* originating from the gamma motor neurons described earlier. These fibers are also called *gamma efferent fibers*, in contradistinction to the *alpha efferent fibers* that innervate the extrafusal skeletal muscle.

The receptor area of the spindle has two types of sensory nerve endings, the *primary ending* and the *secondary ending*, which have slightly different functions.

The Primary Ending. A very large type Ia sensory fiber innervates the very center of the spindle receptor. This fiber spirals around the intrafusal fibers, forming the so-called *primary ending*, also called the *annulospiral ending*. When the receptor portion of the spindle is stretched, this ending is stimulated. And, because the innervating fiber is so large, signals are transmitted to the spinal cord at a velocity approaching 100 meters per second, a velocity as great as that in almost any part of the nervous system.

The Secondary Ending. A type II nerve fiber innervates the receptor to one side of the primary ending. This fiber, like the Ia fiber, also spirals around the intrafusal fibers, and when the receptor portion of the intrafusal fibers is stretched, this nerve ending also is stimulated. It is called the *secondary ending*.

Static Response of Both the Primary and the Secondary Endings. When the receptor portion of the muscle spindle is stretched *slowly,* the number of impulses transmitted from both types of endings increases almost directly in proportion to the degree of stretch, and the endings continue to transmit these impulses for many minutes. This effect is called the *static response* of the spindle receptor, meaning simply that the receptor responds to a change in length of the spindle and also continues to transmit its signal for a prolonged period of time.

Dynamic Response of the Primary Ending. In addition to its static response, the primary, but not the secondary, ending also exhibits a very strong *dynamic response,* which means that it responds extremely strongly to sudden *changes* in length. When the length of the spindle receptor area increases only a fraction of a micron, if this increase occurs rapidly, the primary receptor transmits tremendous numbers of impulses into the Ia fiber, but only *while the length is actually increasing.* As soon as the length has stopped increasing, the rate of impulse discharge returns to the much weaker static response level that is still present in the signal.

Conversely, when the spindle receptor area shortens, this change momentarily decreases the impulse output from the primary ending; as soon as the receptor area has reached its new shortened length, the static response impulses reappear in the Ia fiber within a fraction of a second. Thus, the primary ending sends extremely strong signals to the central nervous system to apprise it of any change in length of the spindle receptor area.

Function of the Muscle Spindle in Comparing Intrafusal and Extrafusal Muscle Lengths

From the foregoing description of the muscle spindle, one can see that there are two different ways in which the spindle can be stimulated: (1) *By stretching the whole muscle.* This lengthens the entire spindle and therefore stretches the spindle receptor. (2) *By contracting the intrafusal muscle fibers* while the extrafusal fibers remain at their normal length. Since the intrafusal fibers only contract near their two ends, this stretches the central receptor portion of the intrafusal fibers, obviously exciting the spindle nerve endings.

In effect, the muscle spindle acts as a *comparator* of the lengths of the two types of muscle fibers, the extrafusal and the intrafusal. When the length of the extrafusal fibers is greater than that of the intrafusal fibers, the spindle becomes excited. On the other hand, when the length of the extrafusal fiber is shorter than that of the intrafusal fiber, the spindle is inhibited.

Continuous Discharge of the Muscle Spindles Under Normal Conditions. Normally, particularly when there is a slight amount of intrafusal fiber contraction caused by gamma efferent excitation, the muscle spindles emit sensory nerve impulses all of the time. Stretching the muscle spindles increases the rate of firing, whereas shortening the spindle decreases this rate of firing. Thus, the spindles can operate in both directions; that is, their normal signal output can be either increased or decreased from normal.

THE STRETCH REFLEX (ALSO CALLED THE MYOTATIC REFLEX)

Sudden stretch of a muscle excites the muscle spindle, and this in turn sends strong signals to the spinal cord, which then transmits signals through the alpha efferent nerve fibers to the extrafusal muscle fibers, causing reflex contraction of the *same* muscle. For obvious reasons, this reflex is frequently simply called a muscle *stretch reflex*. This reflex has a dynamic component and a static component.

The Dynamic Stretch Reflex. The dynamic stretch reflex is caused by the potent dynamic signal from the muscle spindles. That is, when the muscle is suddenly stretched, a very strong signal is transmitted to the spinal cord from the primary endings, but this signal is potent *only while the length of the muscle is increasing.* On entering the spinal cord, most of the signal goes directly to the anterior motor neurons without passing through interneurons, as shown in Figure 34–3, and it causes reflex contraction of the same muscle from which the muscle spindle signals originated. Thus, a sudden stretch of a muscle causes reflex contraction of the same muscle, and *this opposes further stretch of the muscle.*

The Static Stretch Reflex. Though the dynamic stretch reflex is over within a fraction of a second after the muscle has been stretched to its new length, a weaker static stretch reflex continues for a prolonged period of time thereafter. This reflex is elicited by continuous static receptor signals transmitted from both the primary and secondary endings of the muscle spindles. The importance of the static stretch reflex is that is continues to cause muscle contraction as long as the muscle is maintained at an excessive length (for as long as several hours, but not for days). Thus, the muscle contraction opposes the force that is causing the excess length.

The Negative Stretch Reflex. When a muscle is suddenly shortened, exactly opposite effects occur.

That is, extrafusal fibers of the muscle lose their stimulation, and the muscle relaxes. Thus, *this negative stretch reflex* opposes the shortening of the muscle in the same way that the positive stretch reflex opposes lengthening of the muscle. Therefore, one can begin to see that the muscle spindle reflex tends to maintain the status quo for the length of a muscle.

Function of the Static Stretch Reflex to Nullify the Effects of Changes in Load During Muscle Contraction

Let us assume that a person's biceps is contracted so that the forearm is horizontal to the earth. Then assume that a five-pound weight is put in the hand. The hand will immediately drop. However, the amount that the hand will drop is determined to a great extent by the degree of activity of the static muscle spindle reflex. If the static reflex is very active, even slight lengthening of the biceps, and therefore also of the muscle spindles in the biceps, will cause a strong feedback contraction of the extrafusal skeletal muscle fibers of the biceps. This contraction in turn will limit the degree of fall of the hand, thus automatically maintaining the forearm in a nearly horizontal position despite the increased load. This response is called a *load reflex.*

The Damping Function of the Stretch Reflex. Another extremely important function of the reflex—indeed, probably more important than the load reflex—is the ability of the muscle spindle reflex to prevent oscillation and jerkiness of the body movements. This is a damping, or smoothing, function. An example is the following:

Use of the Damping Mechanism in Smoothing Muscle Contraction. Occasionally, signals from other parts of the nervous system are transmitted to a muscle in an uneven fashion, first increasing in intensity for a few milliseconds, then decreasing in intensity, then changing to another intensity level, and so forth. When the muscle spindle apparatus is not functioning satisfactorily, the muscle contraction can be jerky during the course of such a signal. This effect is illustrated in Figure 34–4, which shows an experiment in which a sensory nerve signal entering one side of the cord is transmitted to a motor nerve on the other side of the cord to excite a muscle. In curve A the muscle spindle reflex of the excited muscle is intact. Note that the contraction is relatively smooth even though the sensory nerve is excited at a slow frequency of 8 per second. Curve B, on the other hand, shows the same experiment in an animal whose muscle spindle sensory nerves had been sectioned three months earlier. Note the spasmodic muscle contraction. Thus, curve A illustrates graphically the ability of the damping mechanism of the muscle spindle to make muscle contractions smooth even though the input signals to the muscle motor system are jerky. This effect can also be called a *signal averaging* function of the muscle spindle.

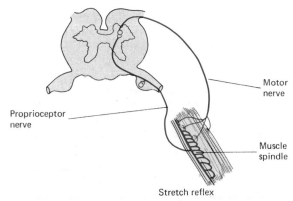

Motor nerve

Proprioceptor nerve

Muscle spindle

Stretch reflex

Figure 34–3. Neuronal circuit of the stretch reflex.

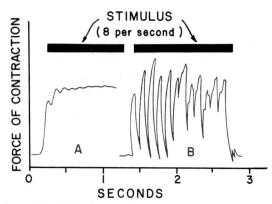

Figure 34–4. Muscle contraction caused by a spinal cord signal under two different conditions: A, in a normal muscle, and B, in a muscle whose muscle spindles had been denervated by section of the posterior roots of the cord 82 days previously. Note the smoothing effect of the muscle spindle reflex in A. (Modified from Creed et al.)

Function of the Gamma Efferent System in Controlling the Intensity of the Stretch Reflex

The gamma efferent system plays a potent role in determining the effectivenesss of the load reflex and also the degree of damping. For instance, there are times when a person wishes his limbs to move extremely rapidly in response to rapidly changing input signals. Under such conditions, one would wish less damping and less load reflex. On the other hand, at other times it is important that the muscle contractions be very smooth. Under these conditions one would like a potent stretch reflex. This is achieved by gamma efferent stimulation of the spindle intrafusal muscle fibers, a condition that tenses the intrafusal fibers and therefore greatly enhances the excitability of the muscle spindles.

ROLE OF THE MUSCLE SPINDLE IN VOLUNTARY MOTOR ACTIVITY

To emphasize the importance of the muscle spindles and the gamma efferent system, one needs only to recognize that 31 per cent of all the motor nerve fibers to the muscles are gamma efferent fibers to the intrafusal muscle fibers of the spindles rather than large type A alpha motor fibers to the extrafusal muscle. Whenever signals are transmitted from the motor cortex or from any other area of the brain to the alpha motor neurons, almost invariably the gamma motor neurons are stimulated simultaneously, a principle called *gamma efferent coactivation*. This dual stimulation causes the intrafusal muscle fibers to contract at the same time that the whole muscle contracts.

The purpose of contracting the muscle spindle fibers at the same time that the large skeletal muscle fibers contract is twofold: First, it keeps the muscle spindle from opposing the muscle contraction. Second, it also maintains proper damping of the muscle

regardless of change in muscle strength. For instance, if the muscle spindle did not contract and relax along with the large muscle fibers, the receptor portion of the spindle would sometimes be flail and at other times be overstretched, in neither instance operating under optimal conditions for spindle function.

CLINICAL APPLICATION OF THE STRETCH REFLEX—THE KNEE JERK AND OTHER MUSCLE JERKS

Clinically, a method used to determine the functional integrity of the stretch reflexes is to elicit the knee jerk and other muscle jerks. The knee jerk can be elicited by simply striking the patellar tendon with a reflex hammer; this stretches the quadriceps muscle and initiates a *dynamic stretch reflex* that causes the lower leg to jerk forward.

Similar reflexes can be obtained from almost any muscle of the body either by striking the tendon of the muscle or by striking the belly of the muscle itself. In other words, sudden stretch of muscle spindles is all that is required to elicit a stretch reflex.

The muscle jerks are used by neurologists to assess the degree of facilitation of spinal cord centers. When large numbers of facilitatory impulses are being transmitted from the upper regions of the central nervous system into the cord, the muscle jerks are greatly exacerbated. On the other hand, if the facilitatory impulses are depressed or abrogated, the muscle jerks are considerably weakened or completely absent. These reflexes are used most frequently to determine the presence or absence of muscle spasticity following lesions in the motor areas of the brain. Ordinarily, diffuse lesions in the motor areas of the opposite side of the cerebral cortex cause greatly exacerbated muscle jerks. This often occurs in patients who have had a stroke, which is damage to the brain resulting from loss of its blood supply.

THE TENDON REFLEX

The Golgi's Tendon Organ and Its Excitation. Golgi's tendon organs, one of which is illustrated in Figure 34–5, lie within muscle tendons immediately beyond their attachments to the muscle fibers. An average of 10 to 15 muscle fibers are usually connected in series with each Golgi's tendon organ, and

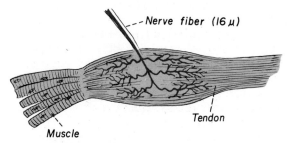

Figure 34–5. Golgi tendon organ.

the organ is stimulated by the tension in the tendon produced by this small bundle of muscle fibers. Thus, the major difference between the function of the Golgi's tendon apparatus and the muscle spindle is that the spindle detects relative extrafusal-intrafusal muscle length, and the tendon organ detects muscle *tension.*

Inhibitory Nature of the Tendon Reflex. Signals from the Golgi's tendon organ, when it is stretched, are transmitted into the spinal cord to cause reflex effects in the same muscle. However, this reflex *inhibits* the muscle instead of exciting it, the exact opposite of the muscle spindle reflex. The signal from the tendon organ is believed to excite inhibitory interneurons, and these in turn to inhibit the alpha motor neurons to the muscle.

When tension on the muscle and therefore on the tendon becomes extreme, the inhibitory effect from the tendon organ can be so great that this inhibition causes sudden relaxation of the entire muscle. This effect is called the *lengthening reaction;* it is probably a protective mechanism to prevent tearing of the muscle or avulsion of the tendon from its attachments to the bone.

Possibly as important as this protective reaction is the function of the tendon reflex as a part of the overall control of muscle contraction, which occurs in the following manner:

The Tendon Reflex as a Control Mechanism for Muscle Tension. In the same way that the stretch reflex operates as a feedback mechanism to control the length of a muscle, the tendon reflex theoretically can operate as a feedback mechanism to control muscle tension. That is, if the tension on the muscle becomes too great, inhibition from the tendon organ decreases this tension back to a lower value. On the other hand, if the tension becomes too slack, impulses from the tendon organ cease and the resulting loss of inhibition allows the alpha motor neurons to become active again, thus increasing muscle tension to a higher level.

Little is known at present about the function of or control of this tension feedback mechanism, but it is thought to operate in the following basic manner: Signals from the brain are presumably transmitted to the cord centers to set the sensitivity of the tendon feedback system. This can be done by changing the degree of facilitation of the neurons in the feedback loop. If the neuron excitability is high, then this system will be extremely sensitive to signals coming from the tendon organs; on the other hand, lack of excitatory signals from the brain could make the system very insensitive to the signals from the tendon organ. In this way, control signals from higher nervous centers could automatically set the level of tension at which the muscle would be maintained.

An obvious value of a mechanism for setting the degree of muscle tension would be to allow a muscle to apply a desired amount of force (that is, maintain constant tension on the tendon) irrespective of the length of the muscle.

THE FLEXOR REFLEX

In the spinal or decerebrate animal, almost any type of sensory stimulus to a limb is likely to cause the flexor muscles of the limb to contract strongly, thereby withdrawing the limb from the stimulus. This is called the flexor reflex.

In this classic form, the flexor reflex is elicited most frequently by stimulation of pain endings by pinprick, heat, or some other painful stimulus, for which reason it is also frequently called a *nociceptive reflex*, or simply, a *pain reflex*. However, even stimulation of the touch receptors can also occasionally elicit a weaker and less prolonged flexor reflex.

If some part of the body besides one of the limbs is painfully stimulated, this part will be withdrawn from the stimulus in a similar manner, but the reflex may not be confined entirely to flexor muscles even though it is basically the same type of reflex. Therefore, the reflex is frequently called a *withdrawal reflex,* too.

Neuronal Mechanism of the Flexor Reflex. The left-hand portion of Figure 34-6 illustrates the neuronal pathways for the flexor reflex. In this instance, a painful stimulus is applied to the hand; as a result, the flexor muscles of the upper arm become excited by reflex thus withdrawing the hand from the painful stimulus.

The nervous pathways for eliciting the flexor reflex do not pass directly to the anterior motor neurons but instead pass first into the interneuron pool of neurons and then to the motor neurons.

Within a few milliseconds after a pain nerve is first stimulated, the flexor response appears. Then, during the next few seconds, the reflex begins to *fatigue,* even though the pain nerve endings continue to be stimulated; this is characteristic of essentially all of the more complex integrative reflexes of the spinal cord. After the pain stimulus is over, the contraction

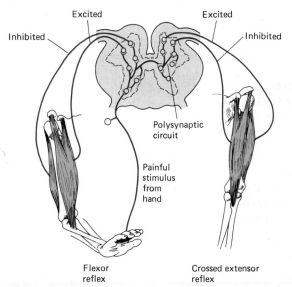

Figure 34-6. The flexor reflex, the crossed extensor reflex, and reciprocal inhibition.

of the muscle begins to return toward the baseline, but because of *after-discharge* in the interneurons of the cord, it will not return all the way for many milliseconds. The duration of the after-discharge depends on the intensity of the sensory stimulus that elicited the reflex; a weak stimulus causes almost no after-discharge; in contrast an after-discharge lasting for several seconds follows a very strong stimulus.

The after-discharge that occurs in the flexor reflex almost certainly involves *reverberating circuits* in the interneurons, which transmit impulses to the anterior motor neurons, sometimes for several seconds after the incoming sensory signal is completely over.

Thus, the flexor reflex is appropriately organized to withdraw a pained or otherwise irritated part of the body from the stimulus. Furthermore, because of the after-discharge it will continue to hold the irritated part away from the stimulus for up to one to three seconds after the irritation ceases. During this time, other reflexes as well as actions of the central nervous system can move the entire body away from the painful stimulus.

The Pattern of Withdrawal. The pattern of withdrawal that results when a flexor (withdrawal) reflex is elicited depends on the sensory nerve that is stimulated. Thus, a painful stimulus on the inside of the arm not only elicits a flexor reflex in the arm but also contracts the abductor muscles to pull the arm outward. In other words, the integrative centers of the cord cause those muscles to contract that can most effectively remove the pained part of the body from the object that causes pain. This same principle applies to any part of the body but especially to the limbs, because they have highly developed flexor reflexes.

THE CROSSED EXTENSOR REFLEX

Approximately 0.2 to 0.5 second after a stimulus elicits a flexor reflex in one limb, the opposite limb begins to extend. This is called the *crossed extensor reflex.* Extension of the opposite limb obviously can push the entire body away from the object causing the painful stimulus.

Neuronal Mechanism of the Cross Extensor Reflex. The right-hand portion of Figure 34–6 illustrates the neuronal circuit responsible for the crossed extensor reflex, showing that signals from the sensory nerves cross to the opposite side of the cord to cause exactly opposite reactions to those of the flexor reflex, namely, to extend the limb. Because the crossed extensor reflex usually does not begin until 200 to 500 milliseconds following the initial pain stimulus, it is certain that many internuncial neurons are in the circuit between the incoming sensory neuron and the motor neurons of the opposite side of the cord responsible for the crossed extension. Furthermore, after the painful stimulus is removed, the crossed extensor reflex has an even longer period of *after-discharge* than that of the flexor reflex. Again, it is

almost certain that this prolonged after-discharge results from *reverberatory circuits* among the internuncial cells.

RECIPROCAL INHIBITION (RECIPROCAL INNERVATION)

In the foregoing paragraphs we have pointed out several times that excitation of one group of muscles is often associated with inhibition of another group. For instance, when a stretch reflex excites one muscle, it simultaneously inhibits the antagonist muscles. This is the phenomenon of *reciprocal inhibition,* and the neuronal mechanism that causes this reciprocal relationship is simply the presence of an inhibitory neuron somewhere in the circuit. Likewise, reciprocal relationships exist between the two sides of the cord as exemplified by the flexor and extensor reflexes as described above.

We will see below that the principle of reciprocal innervation is also important in most of the cord reflexes that subserve locomotion, for it helps to cause forward movement of one limb and simultaneous backward movement of the opposite limb. It also causes alternate movements between the forelimbs and the hindlimbs.

THE REFLEXES OF POSTURE AND LOCOMOTION

The Positive Supportive Reaction. Pressure on the footpad of a decerebrate animal causes the limb to extend against the pressure that is being applied to the foot. Indeed, this reflex can sometimes be so strong that an animal whose spinal cord was transected several months previously can often be placed on its feet, and the pressure on the footpads will reflexly stiffen the limbs sufficiently to support the weight of the body. This reflex is called the *positive supportive reaction.*

The positive supportive reaction involves a complex circuit in the interneurons similar to those responsible for the flexor and the crossed extensor reflexes. Furthermore, the locus of the pressure on the pad of the foot determines the position to which the limb is extended.

The Rhythmic Stepping Reflex. Rhythmic stepping movements are frequently observed in the limbs of spinal animals. Indeed, even when the lower portion is separated from the remainder of the spinal cord and a longitudinal section is made down the center of the cord to block neuronal connections between the two limbs, each hind limb can still perform stepping functions. Forward flexion of the limb is followed a second or so later by backward extension. Then flexion occurs again, and the cycle is repeated over and over.

If the lumbar spinal cord is not sectioned down its center, every time stepping occurs in the forward

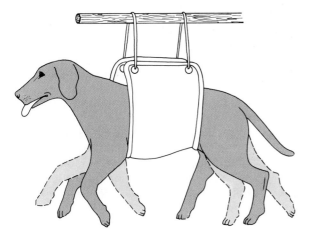

Figure 34–7. Diagonal stepping movements exhibited by a spinal animal.

direction in one limb, the opposite limb ordinarily steps backward. This effect results from reciprocal innervation between the two limbs.

Diagonal Stepping of All Four Limbs—the Mark Time Reflex. Stepping reflexes that involve all four limbs can also be demonstrated in a spinal animal. In general, stepping occurs diagonally between the fore- and hindlimbs. That is, the right hindlimb and the left forelimb move backward together while the right forelimb and left hindlimb move forward. This diagonal response is another manifestation of reciprocal innervation, this time occurring the entire distance up and down the cord between the fore- and hindlimbs. Such a walking pattern, illustrated in a spinal dog hanging in a sling in Figure 34–7, is often called a *mark time reflex.*

The Galloping Reflex. Another type of reflex that occasionally develops in the spinal animal is the galloping reflex, in which both forelimbs move backward in unison while both hindlimbs move forward. If stretch or pressure stimuli are applied almost exactly equally to opposite limbs at the same time, a galloping reflex is likely to result, whereas unequal stimulation of one side versus the other elicits the diagonal walking reflex. This is in keeping with the normal patterns of walking and galloping, for in walking only one limb at a time is stimulated, which would predispose to continued walking. Conversely, when the animal strikes the ground during galloping, the limbs on both sides are stimulated approximately equally, which obviously would predispose to further galloping and continuation of this pattern of motion in contradistinction to the walking pattern.

SPINAL CORD REFLEXES THAT CAUSE MUSCLE SPASM

In human beings, local muscle spasm is often observed. The mechanism of this has not been elucidated to complete satisfaction even in experimental animals, but it is known that pain stimuli can cause reflex spasm of local muscles, which presumably is the cause of much if not most of the muscle spasm observed in localized regions of the human body.

Abdominal Spasm in Peritonitis. A type of local muscle spasm caused by a cord reflex is the abdominal spasm resulting from irritation of the parietal peritoneum by peritonitis. Relief of the pain caused by the peritonitis allows the spastic muscles to relax. Almost the same type of spasm often occurs during surgical operations; pain impulses from the parietal peritoneum cause the abdominal muscles to contract extensively and sometimes actually to squeeze the abdomen and to extrude the intestines through the surgical wound. For this reason deep surgical anesthesia is usually required for intrabdominal operations.

Muscle Cramps. Another type of local spasm is the typical muscle cramp. Any local irritating factor or metabolic abnormality of a muscle—such as severe cold, lack of blood flow to the muscle, or overexercise of the muscle—can elicit pain or other types of sensory impulses that are transmitted from the muscle to the spinal cord, thus causing reflex muscle contraction. The contraction in turn stimulates the same sensory receptors still more, which causes the spinal cord to increase the intensity of contraction still further. Thus, a positive feedback mechanism occurs, so that a small amount of initial irritation causes more and more contraction until a full-blown muscle cramp ensues.

SPINAL CORD TRANSECTION AND SPINAL SHOCK

When the spinal cord is suddenly transected in the neck, essentially all cord functions, including the cord reflexes, immediately become almost completely blocked, a response called *spinal shock.* The reason for this shock is that normal activity of the cord neurons depends to a great extent on continual *faciatory signals* from higher centers, particularly signals transmitted through the vestibulospinal tract, the reticulospinal tracts, and the corticospinal tracts.

Some of the spinal functions specifically affected during spinal shock are these: (1) The arterial blood pressure falls immediately—sometimes to as low as 40 mm Hg—thus illustrating that sympathetic activity becomes blocked almost to extinction. However, the pressure ordinarily returns to normal within a few hours in lower animals and within a few days in the human being. (2) All skeletal muscle reflexes integrated in the spinal cord are completely blocked during the initial stages of spinal shock. In lower animals, a few hours to a week or so are required for these reflexes to return to normal, and in human beings several weeks are often required. (3) The sacral reflexes for control of bladder and colon evacuation are completely suppressed in humans for the first few weeks following cord transection, but they eventually return. These effects are discussed in Chapters 26 and 42.

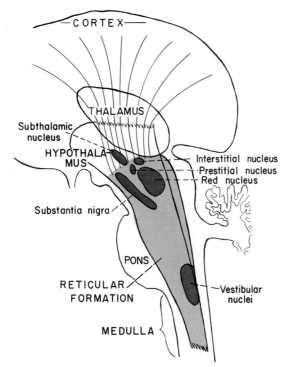

Figure 34–8. The reticular formation and associated nuclei.

THE BRAIN STEM

The brain stem is a complex extension of the spinal cord, including in it the *medulla, pons, and mesencephalon.* Collected in it are numerous neuronal circuits to control respiration, cardiovascular function, gastrointestinal function, eye movement, equilibrium, support of the body against gravity, and many special stereotyped movements of the body. Some of these functions—such as control of respiration and cardiovascular functions—are described in special sections of this text. The present discussion deals primarily with the control of whole body movement and equilibrium.

THE RETICULAR FORMATION AND SUPPORT OF THE BODY AGAINST GRAVITY

Throughout the entire extent of the brain stem—in the medulla, pons, and mesencephalon—are areas of diffuse neurons collectively known as the *reticular formation.* Figure 34–8 illustrates the extent of the reticular formation, showing it to begin at the upper end of the spinal cord and to extend upward through the medulla, pons, and mesencephalon. Many of the ascending and descending fiber tracts between the brain and spinal cord pass through the reticular formation, and as they do so they also provide collateral nerve endings to all reticular areas. In turn, the reticular formation provides multiple afferent fibers that pass both upward and downward in the axis of the nervous system.

Interspersed throughout the reticular formation are both motor and sensory neurons; these vary in size from very small to very large. The small neurons, which constitute the greater number, make multiple connections within the reticular formation itself. The large neurons are mainly motor in function, and their axons often bifurcate almost immediately, with one division extending downward to the spinal cord and the other extending upward to the thalamus or other basal regions of the diencephalon or cerebrum. The axons passing into the spinal cord help control the axial and girdle movements—that is, the trunk, neck, shoulder, hip, and proximal limb movements. On the other hand, the nerve fibers extending into the diencephalon and cerebrum play important roles in controlling the overall activity of the brain. These especially play prominent roles in the control of wakefulness and sleep, as we shall discuss in Chapter 37.

The input signals to the reticular formation are derived from multiple sources, including: (1) multiple tracts from the spinal cord, (2) the vestibular nuclei, (3) the cerebellum, (4) the basal ganglia, (5) the cerebral cortex, from both the sensory and the motor regions, and (6) the hypothalamus and other nearby areas.

Some of the neurons in the reticular formation are collected into *specific nuclei,* which are labeled in Figure 34–8. In general, these specific nuclei are the loci of "preprogrammed" control of stereotyped movements such as bending the body, turning the head, and so forth. Note especially in Figure 34–8 the location of the *vestibular nuclei* in the posterior portion of the lower pons and upper medulla. These nuclei provide preprogrammed attitudinal contractions of appropriate muscles for maintaining equilibrium.

The Motor Pathways from the Brain Stem to the Spinal Cord. Figure 34–9 illustrates the principal motor pathways from the brain stem to the spinal cord. These include two *vestibulospinal tracts* and two *reticulospinal tracts.* All of these eventually terminate on anterior motor neurons in the spinal cord or on interneurons that in turn terminate on the anterior motor neurons.

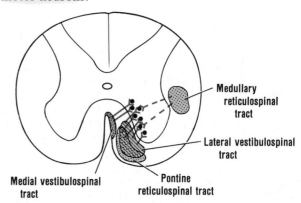

Figure 34–9. The vestibulospinal and reticulospinal tracts descending in the spinal cord to excite (solid lines) or inhibit (dashed lines) the anterior motor neurons that control the body's axial musculature.

Excitation of the Antigravity Muscles by the Brain Stem—The Decerebrate Animal

Both the vestibular nuclei and the pontine portion of the reticular formation, the two of which function in very close association with each other, are intrinsically excitable. However, this excitability is usually held in check by inhibitory signals that originate mainly in the basal ganglia but to a lesser extent in the cerebral cortex and cerebellum. When the brain stem is sectioned *above the vestibular nuclei* at the midpontine level, the intrinsic activity of these nuclei immediately takes over and causes a considerable degree of rigidity of all the antigravity muscles in the body. If this section is made still higher in the brain stem, for instance at the midlevel of the mesencephalon, then the intrinsic activity of the pontine and lower mesencephalic portion of the reticular formation adds still more to the rigidity of the antigravity muscles, and the animal can usually stand on its feet. This is called the *decerebrate animal.* Finally, if the cerebellum is removed at the same time to remove its inhibitory influences, the rigidity becomes still further enchanced.

Thus, the principal role of the brain stem in the control of motor function is to provide *background contractions of the trunk and neck musculature and proximal portions of the limbs;* and the most important function of these contractions is to provide support of the body against gravity.

The relative degree of contraction of the individual antigravity muscles is determined by the equilibrium mechanisms. Thus, if an animal begins to fall to one side, the extensor muscles on that side stiffen while those on the opposite side relax. In turn, the equilibrium mechanisms are controlled by signals mainly from the *vestibular apparatuses,* which are the sensory organs for equilibrium that will be discussed fully in subsequent sections of this chapter.

VESTIBULAR SENSATIONS AND THE MAINTENANCE OF EQUILIBRIUM

THE VESTIBULAR APPARATUS

The vestibular apparatus is the organ that detects sensations concerned with equilibrium. It is composed of a system of bony tubes and chambers in the petrous portion of the temporal bone called the *bony labyrinth* and within this a system of membranous tubes and chambers called the *membranous labyrinth,* which is the functional part of the apparatus. The top of Figure 34–10 illustrates the membranous labyrinth; it is composed mainly of the *cochlear duct,* three *semicircular canals,* and two large chambers known as the *utricle* and the *saccule.* The cochlear duct is the major sensory area for hearing and has nothing to do with equilibrium. However, the *utricle,* the *semicircular canals,* and probably the *saccule* are all integral parts of the equilibrium mechanism.

The Maculae—The Sensory Organs of the Utricle and the Saccule for Detecting the Orientation of the Head with Respect to Gravity. Located on the inside surface of each utricle and saccule is a small sensory area slightly over 2 mm in diameter called a *macula.* The macula of the utricle lies in the horizontal plane on the inferior surface of the utricle and plays an important role in determining the normal orientation of the head with respect to the direction of gravitational or acceleratory forces. On the other hand, the macula of the saccule is located in a vertical plane on the medial wall of the saccule. It probably operates as an equilibrium apparatus when the head is *not* in a vertical position.

Each macula is covered by a gelatinous layer in which many small calcium carbonate crystals called *statoconia* (or *otoliths*) are embedded. Also, in the macula are thousands of *hair cells,* which project *cilia* up into the gelatinous layer. The bases and sides of the hair cells synapse with sensory axons of the vestibular nerve.

Even under resting conditions, most of the nerve fibers leading from the hair cells transmit a continuous

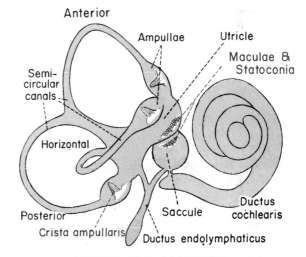

MEMBRANOUS LABYRINTH

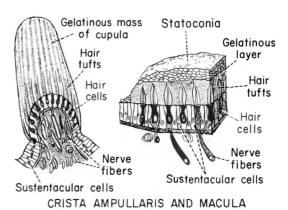

CRISTA AMPULLARIS AND MACULA

Figure 34–10. The membranous labyrinth, and organization of the crista ampullaris and the macula. (Modified from Clemente, C. D. (Ed.): Gray's Anatomy. Philadelphia, Lea & Febiger, 1985.)

series of nerve impulses. Bending the cilia of a hair cell to one side causes the impulse traffic in its nerve fibers to increase markedly; bending the cilia to the opposite side decreases the impulse traffic, often turning it off completely. Therefore, as the orientation of the head in space changes and the weight of the statoconia (whose specific gravity is about 3 times that of the surrounding tissues) bends the cilia, appropriate signals are transmitted to the brain to control equilibrium.

In each macula the different hair cells are oriented in different directions so that some of them are stimulated when the head bends forward, some when it bends backward, others when it bends to one side, and so forth. Therefore, a different pattern of excitation occurs in the macula for each position of the head; it is this "pattern" that apprises the brain of the head's orientation.

The Semicircular Canals. The three semicircular canals in each vestibular apparatus, known respectively as the *anterior, posterior,* and *horizontal semicircular canals,* are arranged at right angles to each other so that they represent all three planes in space.

Each semicircular canal has an enlargement at one of its ends called the *ampulla,* and the canals are filled with a viscous fluid called *endolymph.* Flow of this fluid in the canals excites a sensory organ in the ampulla. As illustrated in Figure 34–10, located in each ampulla is a small crest called a *crista ampullaris,* and on top of the crista is a gelatinous mass, similar to that in the utricle, known as the *cupula.* Into the cupula are projected cilia from hair cells located along the ampullary crest, and these hair cells in turn are connected to sensory nerve fibers that pass into the *vestibular nerve.* Bending the cupula to one side, caused by flow of fluid in the canal, stimulates the hair cells, while bending in the opposite direction inhibits them. Thus, appropriate signals are sent through the vestibular nerve to apprise the central nervous system of fluid movement in the respective canal.

Directional Sensitivity of the Hair Cells—The Kinocilium. As illustrated in Figure 34–11, each hair cell, whether in a macula or a cupula, has an average of about 50 small cilia, called *stereocilia,* plus one very large cilium called the *kinocilium.* This kinocilium is located to one side of the hair cell, always on the same side of the cell with respect to its orientation on the ampullary crest. This is the cause of the directional sensitivity of the hair cells: namely, stimulation when the cilia are bent toward the side of the kinocilium and inhibition when bent in the opposite direction.

Neuronal Connections of the Vestibular Apparatus with the Central Nervous System. Figure 34–12 illustrates the central connections of the vestibular nerve. Most of the vestibular nerve fibers end in the *vestibular nuclei,* which are located approximately at the junction of the medulla and the pons, but some fibers pass without synapsing into the cerebellum. The fibers that end in the vestibular nuclei synapse with second

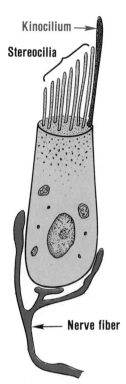

Figure 34–11. A hair cell of the membranous labyrinth of the equilibrium apparatus.

order neurons that in turn send fibers into the cerebellum, into the spinal cord, and especially into the brain stem reticular nuclei.

Note especially the very close association between the vestibular apparatus, the vestibular nuclei, and the cerebellum. The primary pathway for the reflexes of equilibrium begins in the vestibular nerves and passes next to both the vestibular nuclei and the cerebellum. Then, along with two-way traffic of impulses between these two, signals are also sent into the reticular nuclei of the brain stem and down the spinal cord via the vestibulospinal and reticulospinal tracts. In turn, the signals to the cord control the

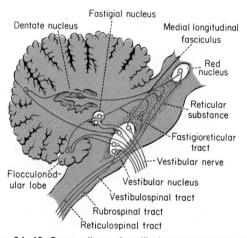

Figure 34–12. Connections of vestibular nerves in the central nervous system.

interplay between facilitation and inhibition of the antigravity muscles, thus controlling equilibrium.

FUNCTION OF THE UTRICLE AND THE SACCULE IN THE MAINTENANCE OF STATIC EQUILIBRIUM

It is especially important that the different hair cells are oriented in all different directions in the maculae of the utricles and saccules so that at different positions of the head, different hair cells become stimulated. The "patterns" of stimulation of the different hair cells apprise the nervous system of the position of the head with respect to the pull of gravity. In turn, the vestibular, cerebellar, and reticular motor systems reflexly excite the appropriate muscles to maintain proper equilibrium.

Detection of Linear Acceleration by the Utricle and Saccule. When the body is suddenly thrust forward, which is called linear acceleration, the statoconia, which have greater inertia than the surrounding fluids, fall backward on the hair cells. Therefore, information of malequilibrium is sent into the nervous centers, causing the person to feel as if he or she were falling backward. This automatically causes the body to lean forward until the anterior shift of the statoconia caused by the forward leaning exactly equals the tendency for the statoconia to fall backward because of the linear acceleration. At this point, the nervous system detects a state of proper equilibrium and therefore stops the body from leaning farther forward. As long as the degree of linear acceleration remains constant and the body is maintained in this forward leaning position, the person falls neither forward nor backward. Thus, the statoconia operate to maintain equilibrium during linear acceleration in exactly the same manner as they operate in static equilibrium.

The statoconia *do not* operate for the detection of linear *motion*. When a runner first begins to run, leaning far forward keeps the body from falling over backward because of acceleration, but once running speed has been achieved a runner in a vacuum would not have to lean forward at all. In air a runner leans forward to maintain equilibrium only because of the air resistance against the body, and in this instance it is not the statoconia but the pressure of the air acting on pressure end-organs in the skin, which initiate the appropriate equilibrium adjustments.

THE SEMICIRCULAR CANALS AND THEIR DETECTION OF ANGULAR ACCELERATION

When the head suddenly *begins* to rotate in any direction, the endolymph in the membranous semicircular canals, because of its inertia, tends to remain stationary while the semicircular canals themselves turn. This causes relative fluid flow in the canals in a direction opposite to the rotation of the head; this relative flow lasts for a few seconds, thus activating the semicular canal receptors; and the person perceives this onset of rotation, which is called *angular acceleration*.

When the rotation suddenly stops, exactly the opposite effects take place: That is, the endolymph continues to rotate while the semicircular canal stops, and the canal receptors are activated in the opposite direction; the person perceives the termination of rotation.

Predictive Function of the Semicircular Canals in the Maintenance of Equilibrium. Since the semicircular canals do not detect that the body is off balance in the forward direction, in the side direction, or in the backward direction, one might ask, What is the function of the semicircular canals in the maintenance of equilibrium? All they detect is that the person's head is beginning to rotate or is stopping rotation in one direction or another. Therefore, the function of the semicircular canals is not likely to be the maintenance of static equilibrium nor of equilibrium during linear acceleration. Yet loss of function of the semicircular canals causes a person to have very poor equilibrium when he attempts to perform *rapid* and *intricate* body movements.

We can explain the function of the semicircular canals best by the following illustrations. If a person is running forward rapidly and then suddenly begins to turn to one side, he falls off balance a second or so later unless appropriate corrections are made *ahead of time*. Unfortunately, the utricle and saccule cannot detect that he is off balance until *after* this has occurred. On the other hand, the semicircular canals will have already detected that the person is beginning to turn, and this information can easily apprise the central nervous system that malequilibrium will occur within the next second or so unless some correction is made. In other words, the semicircular canal mechanism *predicts* that malequilibrium is going to occur when the person begins to turn and thereby causes the equilibrium centers to make appropriate preventive adjustments.

OTHER FACTORS CONCERNED WITH EQUILIBRIUM

The Neck Proprioceptors. The vestibular apparatus detects the orientation and movements *only of the head*. Therefore, it is essential that the nervous centers also receive appropriate information depicting the orientation of the head with respect to the body as well as the orientation of the different parts of the body with respect to each other.

By far the most important proprioceptive information needed for the maintenance of equilibrium is that derived from the *joint receptors of the neck*, for this apprises the nervous system of the orientation of the head with respect to the body. When the head is bent in one direction an appropriate signal from the vestibular apparatuses says that the head is leaning. However, at the same time, signals from the neck receptors keep the vestibular apparatuses from giving the person a sense of malequilibrium. They do this by transmitting signals that exactly oppose the signals transmitted from the vestibular apparatuses. However, *when the entire body* is changed to a new position with respect to gravity, the signals from the vestibular apparatuses *are not opposed* by the neck proprioceptors because the neck is not then bent; therefore, the person in this instance does perceive a change in equilibrium status.

Importance of Visual Information in the Maintenance of Equilibrium. After complete destruction of the vestibular apparatuses, and even after loss of most proprioceptive information from the body, a person can still use his visual mechanisms effectively for maintaining equilibrium. Visual images help the person maintain equilibrium simply by visual detection of the upright stance. Many persons with complete destruction of the vestibular apparatus have almost normal equilibrium as long as their eyes are open and as long as they perform all motions slowly. But when they move rapidly or close their eyes, equilibrium is immediately lost.

FUNCTIONS OF THE RETICULAR FORMATION AND SPECIFIC BRAIN STEM NUCLEI IN CONTROLLING SUBCONSCIOUS, STEREOTYPED MOVEMENTS

Rarely, an anencephalic monster—a child without brain structures above the mesencephalic region—is born. Some of these children have been kept alive for many months. Such a child is able to perform essentially all the functions of feeding, such as suckling, extrusion of unpleasant food from the mouth, and moving its hands to its mouth to suck its fingers. In addition, it can yawn and stretch. It can cry and follow objects with its eyes and by movements of its head. Also, placing pressure on the upper anterior parts of its legs will cause it to pull to the sitting position.

Therefore, it is obvious that many of the stereotyped motor functions of the human being are integrated in the brain stem. Unfortunately, the loci of most of these different motor control systems have not been found except for the following:

Stereotyped Body Movements. Most movements of the trunk and head can be classified into several simple movements such as forward flexion, extension, rotation, and turning movements of the entire body. These types of movements are controlled by special nuclei located mainly in the mesencephalic and lower diencephalic region. For instance, *rotational movements* of the head and eyes are controlled by the *interstitial nucleus*, which is illustrated in Figure 34–8. The *raising movements* of the head and body are controlled by the *prestitial nucleus*. The flexing movements of the head and body are controlled by the *nucleus precommissuralis* located at the level of the posterior commissure. The *turning movements* of the body involve both the pontile and mesencephalic reticular formation. And *backward extension of the head and upper trunk* is accomplished by a portion of the *red nucleus*.

SUMMARY OF THE FUNCTIONS OF THE CORD AND BRAIN STEM IN POSTURE AND LOCOMOTION

From the discussions in this chapter, we see that almost all of the discrete "patterns" of muscle movements required for posture and locomotion can be elicited by the spinal cord alone. However, coordination of these patterns to provide equilibrium, progression, and purposefulness of movement requires neuronal function at progressively higher levels of the central nervous system. Centers in the brain stem provide most of the nervous energy required to maintain the postural tone for support of the body against gravity. In addition, brain stem centers provide especially the equilibrium adjustments of the body and the control of most stereotyped movements of body as well.

In the following chapter we will discuss the functions of still higher centers in the brain to provide the voluntary movements of the body.

QUESTIONS

1. Describe the organization of the typical segment of the spinal cord for motor control.
2. Explain the roles of the *alpha motor neurons*, the *gamma motor neurons*, and the *interneurons* in the control of muscle contraction.
3. Describe the *muscle spindle*, its innervation, and the anatomy of its receptor region.
4. What are the functional differences between the *primary* and *secondary sensory endings* of the muscle spindle?
5. Explain the manner in which the spindle receptor is stimulated by (a) stretching the whole muscle or (b) contracting the intrafusal muscle fibers of the spindle.
   What is meant by the comparator function of the muscle spindle?
6. Explain the difference between the *dynamic stretch reflex* and the *static stretch reflex*.
7. Describe the neuronal circuit of the stretch reflex.
8. How does the stretch reflex help to damp jerky muscle movements?
9. How does the stretch reflex prevent large changes in muscle length when different levels of load are applied to the muscle?
10. Describe the *Golgi's tendon organ* and the means by which it is excited.
11. Describe the neuronal circuit of the *tendon reflex*.

12. How does the tendon reflex function as a means for controlling muscle tension?
13. Explain the neuronal circuit of the *flexor reflex* and the function of the flexor reflex. Why is the flexor sometimes called a *withdrawal reflex*?
14. Explain the phenomenon of *reciprocal inhibition* as it applies to the *crossed extensor reflex*.
15. Describe the following reflexes of posture and locomotion: the *positive supportive reaction*, the *rhythmic stepping reflex*, and the *galloping reflex*.
16. Why does peritonitis cause *abdominal spasm*?
17. Describe the *reticular formation* of the brain stem and its role in the support of the body against gravity.
18. What are the characteristics of the *decerebrate animal*?

19. Describe the *macula* of the *utricle* or the *saccule*, including the orientation of hair cells within the macula and function of the macula for detection of equilibrium.
20. Why are the maculae in the utricle and saccule the principal equilibrium sensory receptors organs for both static equilibrium and detection of linear acceleration?
21. Explain the detection of angular acceleration by the *semicircular canals* and the importance of detecting this for the maintenance of balance during rapid movements.
22. Why are the *neck reflexes* of importance in the maintenance of equilibrium?
23. What are some of the stereotyped movements that are controlled by specific nuclei in the brain stem?

References

Spinal Cord

Austin, G.: The Spinal Cord, New York, Igaku Shoin Medical Publishers, 1981.

Baldissera, F., Hultborn, H., and Illert, M.: Integration in spinal neuronal systems. *In* Brooks, V. B., ed.: Handbook of Physiology. Sec I, Vol. 2. Bethesda, American Physiological Society, 1981, p. 509.

Burke, R. E.: Motor units: Anatomy, physiology, and functional organization. In Brooks, V. B., ed.: Handbook of Physiology. Sec. 1, Vol. 2. Bethesda, American Physiological Society, 1981, p. 345.

Creed, R. S., et al.: Reflex Activity of the Spinal Cord. New York, Oxford University Press, 1932.

Freund, H-J.: Motor unit and muscle activity in voluntary motor control. Physiol Rev 63:387, 1983.

Grillner, S.: Neurobiological bases of rhythmic motor acts in vertebrates. Science 228:143, 1985.

Henneman, E., and Mendell, L. M.: Functional organization of motoneuron pool and its inputs. In Brooks, V. B., ed.: Handbook of Physiology. Sec. 1, Vol. 2. Bethesda, American Physiological Society, 1981, p. 423.

Houk, J. C., and Rymer, W. Z.: Neural control of muscle length and tension. In Brooks, V. B., ed.: Handbook of Physiology. Sec. 1, Vol. 2. Bethesda, American Physiological Society, 1981, p. 257.

Matthews, P. B. C.: Muscle spindles: their messages and their fusimotor supply. In Brooks, V. B., ed.: Handbook of Physiology, Sec. 1, Vol. 2, Bethesda, American Physiological Society, 1981, p. 189.

Mendell, L. M.: Modifiability of spinal synapses. Physiol Rev 64:260, 1984.

Pearson, K.: The control of walking. Sci Am 235(6):72, 1976.

Stein, R. B.: Peripheral control of movement. Physiol Rev 54:215, 1974.

Brain Stem and Vestibular Apparatus

Dampney, R. A., et al.: Identification of cardiovascular cell groups in the brain stem. Clin Exp Hypertens 6:205, 1984.

Dublin, W. B.: Fundamentals of Vestibular Pathology. St. Louis, Warren H. Green, Inc., 1985.

Elder, H. Y., and Trueman, E. R., eds.: Aspects of Animal Movement. New York, Cambridge University Press, 1980.

Goldberg, J. M., and Fernandez, C.: The vestibular system. In Darian-Smith, I., ed.: Handbook of Physiology. Sec. 1, Vol. 3. Bethesda, American Physiological Society, 1984, p. 977.

Granit, R., and Pompeiano, O., eds.: Reflex Control of Posture and Movement. New York, Elsevier Scientific Publishing Co., 1979.

Grillner, S.: Control of locomotion in bipeds, tetrapods, and fish. In Brooks, V. B., ed.: Handbook of Physiology. Sec. 1, Vol. 2. Bethesda, American Physiological Society, 1981, p. 1179.

Hobson, J. A., and Brazier, M. A. B., eds.: The Reticular Formation Revisited: Specifying Function for a Nonspecific System. New York, Raven Press, 1980.

Silverman, A. J.: Magnocellular neurosecretory system. Annu Rev Neurosci 6:357, 1983.

Stein, R. B., and Lee, R. G.: Tremor and clonus. In Brooks, V. B. ed.: Handbook of Physiology. Sec. 1, Vol. 2. Bethesda, American Physiological Society, 1981, p. 325.

Valentinuzzi, M.: The Organs of Equilibrium and Orientation as a Control System. New York, Harwood Academic Publishers, 1980.

Wilson, V. J., and Peterson, B. W.: Vestibulospinal and reticulospinal systems. In Brooks, V. B., ed.: Handbook of Physiology, Sec. 1, Vol. 2. Bethesda, American Physiological Society, 1981, p. 667.

35

Motor Control by the Motor Cortex, the Basal Ganglia, and the Cerebellum

PHYSIOLOGICAL ANATOMY OF THE
   MOTOR AREAS OF THE CORTEX AND
   THEIR PATHWAYS TO THE CORD
   THE PRIMARY MOTOR CORTEX OF
      THE HUMAN BEING
   COMPLEX MOVEMENTS ELICITED BY
      STIMULATING THE CORTEX
      ANTERIOR TO THE PRIMARY
      MOTOR CORTEX—THE PREMOTOR
      CORTEX
   EFFECTS OF LESIONS IN THE MOTOR
      AND THE PREMOTOR CORTEX
STIMULATION OF THE SPINAL MOTOR
   NEURONS BY MOTOR SIGNALS
   FROM THE BRAIN
MOTOR FUNCTIONS OF THE BASAL
   GANGLIA
   FUNCTIONS OF THE DIFFERENT
      BASAL GANGLIA
   CLINICAL SYNDROMES RESULTING
      FROM DAMAGE TO THE BASAL
      GANGLIA

THE CEREBELLUM AND ITS MOTOR
   FUNCTIONS
   THE INPUT SYSTEM OF THE
      CEREBELLUM
   OUTPUT SIGNALS FROM THE
      CEREBELLUM
   THE NEURONAL CIRCUIT OF THE
      CEREBELLUM
   FUNCTION OF THE CEREBELLUM IN
      VOLUNTARY MOVEMENTS
SENSORY FEEDBACK CONTROL OF
   MOTOR FUNCTIONS
   THE SENSORY ENGRAM FOR MOTOR
      MOVEMENTS
   ESTABLISHMENT OF RAPID "SKILLED"
      MOTOR PATTERNS
INITIATION OF VOLUNTARY MOTOR
   ACTIVITY

In preceding chapters we have been concerned with the subconscious motor activities integrated in the spinal cord and brain stem, especially those responsible for locomotion. In the present chapter we will discuss the control of motor function by the cerebral cortex, the basal ganglia, and the cerebellum, much of which is "voluntary" control in contradistinction to the "involuntary" control effected by the lower centers.

PHYSIOLOGICAL ANATOMY OF THE MOTOR AREAS OF THE CORTEX AND THEIR PATHWAYS TO THE CORD

Electrical stimulation anywhere within a large area of the cerebral cortex can at times cause muscle

contraction. This area, illustrated in Figure 35–1, is called the *motor cortex*. The area immediately in front of the central sulcus, designated in the figure by the darkest shading, contains large numbers of *giant Betz cells*, or *pyramidal cells* that send nerve fibers directly to the spinal cord to control the muscles. This area causes motor movements following the least amount of electrical excitation and is therefore also called the *primary motor cortex*.

The Pyramidal Tract (Corticospinal Tract). One of the major pathways by which motor signals are transmitted from the motor areas of the cortex to the anterior motor neurons of the spinal cord is the *pyramidal tract* or *corticospinal tract*, which is illustrated in Figure 35–2. This tract originates in all the shaded areas in Figure 35–1, including both the motor and the somatic sensory areas, about four fifths from

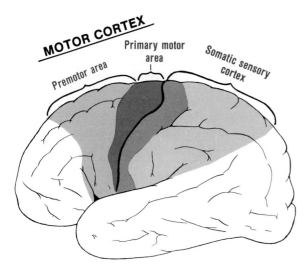

Figure 35–1. Relationship of the motor cortex to the somatic sensory cortex.

the motor area and about one fifth from the sensory regions posterior to the central sulcus. The function of the fibers from the sensory cortex is probably not motor, but instead is to cause feedback control of sensory input to the nervous system.

The most impressive fibers in the pyramidal tract are the large myelinated fibers that originate in the giant Betz cells of the motor area. These account for approximately 34,000 large fibers (mean diameter of about 16 microns) in the pyramidal tract from *each* side of the cortex.

The pyramidal tract passes downward through the *brain stem*; then the tract from each side crosses to the opposite side. The fibers then descend in the *lateral corticospinal tracts* of the cord and terminate principally on interneurons at the bases of the dorsal horns of the cord gray matter.

The Extrapyramidal Tracts. The extrapyramidal tracts are additional tracts besides the pyramidal tract itself that transmit motor signals from the cortex and subcortical motor areas. For instance, large numbers of signals are transmitted from the motor cortex into the *caudate nucleus* and then through the *putamen, globus pallidus, subthalamic nucleus, substantia nigra,* and *reticular nuclei of the brain stem* before passing into the spinal cord. And many other signals pass from the cortex to the red nucleus and thence to the cord. The multiplicity of connections within these intermediate nuclei will be presented later in the chapter.

The final pathways for transmission of extrapyramidal signals into the cord are the *reticulospinal tracts,* which lie in both the ventral and lateral columns of the cord, the *rubrospinal tract,* the *vestibulospinal tracts,* and the *tectospinal tract.*

THE PRIMARY MOTOR CORTEX OF THE HUMAN BEING

Figure 35–3 gives an approximate map of the human brain showing the points in the primary motor

cortex that, when stimulated, cause muscle contractions in different parts of the body.

Note in the figure that stimulation of the most lateral portions of the motor cortex causes muscular contractions related to swallowing, chewing, and facial movements, while stimulation of the midline portion of the motor cortex where it bends over into the longitudinal fissure causes contraction of the legs, feet, or toes. The spatial organization is similar to that of the somatic sensory cortex I, which is shown in Chapter 32.

Degree of Representation of Different Muscle Groups in the Primary Motor Cortex. The different muscle groups of the body are not represented equally in the motor cortex. In general, the degree of representation is proportional to the discreteness of movement required of the respective part of the body. Thus, the thumb and fingers have large representations, as is true also of the lips, tongue, and vocal cords. The relative degrees of representation of the different parts of the body are illustrated in Figure 35–4, a figure constructed on the basis of stimulatory

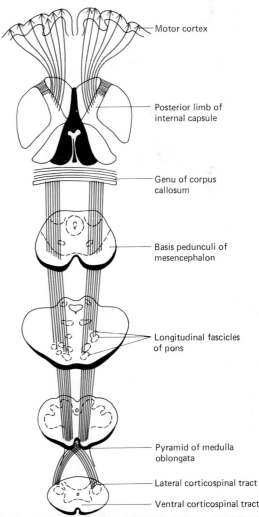

Motor cortex

Posterior limb of internal capsule

Genu of corpus callosum

Basis pedunculi of mesencephalon

Longitudinal fascicles of pons

Pyramid of medulla oblongata

Lateral corticospinal tract

Ventral corticospinal tract

Figure 35–2. The pyramidal tract. (From Ranson and Clark: Anatomy of the Nervous System. Philadelphia, W. B. Saunders Company, 1959.)

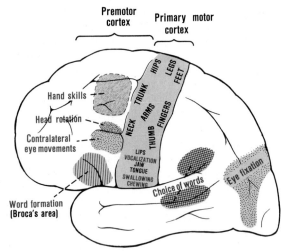

Figure 35–3. Representation of the different muscles of the body in the motor cortex and location of other cortical areas responsible for certain types of motor movements.

charts made of the human motor cortex during hundreds of brain operations.

When very weak electrical stimuli are used, only small segments of the peripheral musculature ordinarily contract at a time. In the "finger" and "thumb" regions, which have tremendous representation in the cerebral cortex, weak stimuli can sometimes cause single muscles or, at times, even single fasciculi of muscles to contract, thus illustrating that a high degree of control is exercised by this portion of the motor cortex over discrete muscular movement.

On the other hand, weak stimuli in the trunk region of the body might cause as many as 30 to 50 small back muscles to contract simultaneously, thus illustrating that the motor cortex does not control discrete trunk muscles but instead controls *groups* of muscles. Similarly, weak stimuli in the lip, tongue, and vocal cord regions of the motor cortex cause contraction of minute muscular areas, whereas stimulation in the leg region ordinarily excites several synergistic muscles at a time, causing some gross movement of the leg.

COMPLEX MOVEMENTS ELICITED BY STIMULATING THE CORTEX ANTERIOR TO THE PRIMARY MOTOR CORTEX— THE PREMOTOR CORTEX

Electrical stimulation of the cerebral cortex for distances 1 to 3 centimeters in front of the primary motor cortex will often elicit complex contractions of groups of muscles. Occasionally, vocalization occurs, or rhythmic movements such as alternate thrusting of a leg forward and backward, coordinate moving of the eyes, chewing, swallowing, or contortion of parts of the body into different postural positions.

Some neurophysiologists have called this area the *premotor cortex* and have ascribed to it special capabilities to control coordinated movements involving many muscles simultaneously. One might also call

the premotor cortex a *motor association area*. It is peculiarly organized to control coordinated muscle contractions for the following reasons: (1) The premotor cortex has long subcortical neuronal connections with the sensory association areas of the parietal lobe. (2) It has direct subcortical connections with the primary motor cortex. (3) It connects with areas in the thalamus contiguous with the thalamic areas that connect with the primary motor cortex. (4) The premotor area has abundant direct connections with the basal ganglia.

Still another reason for the belief that the premotor cortex controls coordinate muscle contractions is that damage to this area causes loss of certain coordinate skills, as follows:

Broca's Area and Speech. Referring again to Figure 35–3, note that immediately anterior to the primary motor cortex and immediately above the sylvian fissure is an area labeled "word formation." This region is called *Broca's area*. Damage to it does not prevent a person from vocalizing, but it does make it impossible for the person to speak whole words other than simple utterances such as no or yes. A cortical area located immediately above Broca's area causes appropriate respiratory function, so that the vocal cords can be activated simultaneously with the movements of the mouth and tongue during speech. Thus, the coordinate muscle contractions that are related to Broca's area are highly complex.

The Voluntary Eye Movement Field. Above Broca's area is a locus for controlling eye movements. Damage to this area prevents a person from voluntarily moving his or her eyes toward different objects. Instead, the eyes tend to lock on specific objects, an effect controlled by signals from the occipital region,

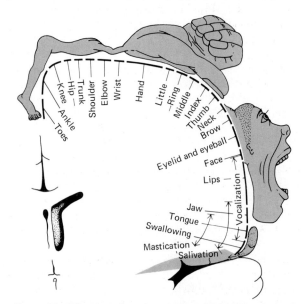

Figure 35–4. Degree of representation of the different muscles of the body in the motor cortex. (From THE CEREBRAL CORTEX OF MAN by Wilder Penfield and Theodore Rasmussen. Copyright 1950 by Macmillan Publishing Company, renewed 1978 by Theodore Rasmussen. Reprinted with permission of the publisher.)

as explained in Chapter 40. This frontal area also controls eyelid movements such as blinking.

Head Rotation Area. Still slightly higher in the "premotor region," electrical stimulation will elicit head rotation. This area is closely associated with the eye movement field and is presumably related to directing the head toward different objects.

Area for Hand Skills. In the frontal area immediately anterior to the primary motor cortex for the hands and fingers is a region neurosurgeons have observed to be an area for hand skills. That is, when tumors or other lesions cause destruction in this area, the hand movements become incoordinate and nonpurposeful, a condition called *motor apraxia.*

Summary of Functions of the Premotor Areas. It is clear that the area anterior to the primary motor cortex, the premotor area, can cause complex coordinate movements, such as speech movements, eye movements, head movements, and even hand skills. However, it should be remembered that all of these areas are closely connected with corresponding areas in the primary motor cortex, the thalamus, and the basal ganglia. Therefore, the complex coordinate movements almost certainly result from a cooperative effort of all these structures.

EFFECTS OF LESIONS IN THE MOTOR AND THE PREMOTOR CORTEX

The motor cortex is frequently damaged, especially by the common abnormality called a stroke, which is caused by loss of blood supply to the cortex resulting from blood vessel rupture or occlusion. Also, experiments have been performed in animals to remove selectively different parts of the motor cortex.

Ablation of the Primary Motor Cortex. Removal of a very small portion of the primary motor cortex in a monkey causes loss of much of the control of the represented muscles. If the sublying caudate nucleus is not damaged, gross postural and limb "fixation" movements can still be performed, but the animal loses voluntary control of discrete movements of the distal segments of the limbs—of the hands and fingers, especially. This does not mean that the muscles themselves cannot contract, but that the animal's ability to control the fine movements is gone.

From these results one can conclude that the primary motor cortex is concerned mainly with voluntary initiation of finely controlled movements. On the other hand, the deeper motor areas, particularly the basal ganglia and lower brain stem, are responsible mainly for the involuntary and postural body movements.

Muscle Spasticity Caused by Ablation of Large Areas of the Motor and the Premotor Cortex— Extrapyramidal Lesions as the Basis of Spasticity. It should be recalled that the motor cortex gives rise to tracts that descend to the spinal cord through both the pyramidal tract and the extrapyramidal tracts. These two tracts have opposing effects on the tone of the body muscles. The pyramidal tract causes continuous facilitation and therefore a tendency to increased muscle tone throughout the body. On the other hand, the extrapyramidal system transmits signals through the basal ganglia to inhibit the reticular formation of the brain stem, with resultant inhibition of muscle action. When the motor cortex is destroyed, the balance between these two opposing effects may be altered. If the lesion is located discretely in the primary motor cortex where the large Betz cells lie, very little change in muscle tone results because both pyramidal and extrapyramidal elements are affected about equally. On the other hand, the usual lesion caused by a stroke is very large, involving large portions of the cortex both anterior and posterior to the primary motor area, and these regions normally transmit inhibitory signals through the extrapyramidal tracts. Therefore, loss of extrapyramidal inhibition is the dominant feature, thus leading to muscle spasm.

If the lesion involves the basal ganglia as well as the motor cortex, the spasm is even more intense because the basal ganglia normally provide additional strong inhibition of the postural control system of the reticular formation, and loss of this inhibition further exacerbates the reticular excitation of the muscles. In patients with strokes, the lesion almost invariably affects both the motor cortex itself and the sublying basal ganglia, so that very intense spasm normally occurs in the muscles of the opposite side of the body.

STIMULATION OF THE SPINAL MOTOR NEURONS BY MOTOR SIGNALS FROM THE BRAIN

Figure 35–5 shows several different motor tracts entering a segment of the spinal cord from the brain. The corticospinal tract (pyramidal tract) terminates mainly on small *interneurons* in the base of the dorsal horns, although a few tracts also terminate directly on the anterior motor neurons themselves. From the

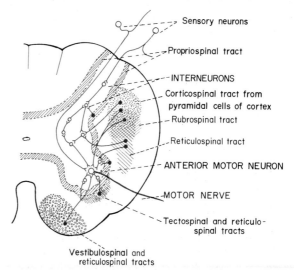

Figure 35–5. Convergence of all the different motor pathways on the anterior motor neurons.

primary interneurons, most of the motor signals are transmitted through still other interneurons before finally exciting the anterior motor neurons.

Figure 35–5 shows several other descending tracts from the brain, collectively called the *extrapyramidal tracts*, as explained earlier, which also carry signals to the anterior motor neurons: (1) the *rubrospinal tract*, (2) the *reticulospinal tracts*, (3) the *tectospinal tract*, and (4) the *vestibulospinal tract*. In addition, sensory signals arriving through the dorsal sensory roots, as well as signals transmitted from segment to segment of the spinal cord, stimulate the anterior motor neurons.

The corticospinal tract causes specific muscle contractions. On the other hand, the extrapyramidal tracts provide less specific muscle contractions. Instead, they provide such effects as general facilitation, general inhibition, or gross postural signals, all of which provide the background against which the corticospinal system operates.

Patterns of Movement Elicited by Spinal Cord Centers. From Chapter 34, recall that the spinal cord can provide specific reflex patterns of movement in response to sensory nerve stimulation. Many of these same patterns are also activated when the anterior motor neurons are excited by signals from the brain. For instance, the stretch reflex is functional at all times, helping to damp the motor movements initiated from the brain. Also, when a brain signal excites an agonist muscle, it is not necessary to transmit an inverse signal to the antagonist at the same time; this transmission will be achieved by the reciprocal innervation circuit that is always present in the cord for coordinating the functions of antagonistic pairs of muscles.

Finally, parts or all of the other reflex patterns— withdrawal, walking, postural mechanisms, and so forth—are at times activated by signals from the brain. Very simple signals from the brain can lead to many of our normal motor activities, particularly such functions as walking and the attainment of different postural attitudes of the body.

On the other hand, at times it is important to suppress the cord mechanisms to prevent their interference with the performance of patterns of motor activity generated within the brain itself. This suppression is believed to be one of the functions of the inhibitory signals transmitted through some of the reticulospinal tracts.

MOTOR FUNCTIONS OF THE BASAL GANGLIA

Physiologic Anatomy of the Basal Ganglia. The anatomy of the basal ganglia is so complex and so poorly known in its details that it would be pointless to attempt a complete description at this time. However, Figure 35–6 illustrates the principal structures of the basal ganglia and their neural connections with other parts of the nervous system. Anatomically, the

basal ganglia include the *caudate nucleus, putamen, globus pallidus, amygdaloid nucleus*, and *claustrum*. The amygdaloid nucleus, which will be discussed in Chapter 37, and the claustrum are not concerned directly with motor functions of the central nervous system. On the other hand, the *thalamus, subthalamus*, and *substantia nigra* all operate in close association with the caudate nucleus, putamen, and globus pallidus and are considered to be part of the basal ganglia system for motor control.

Some important features of the different neuronal circuits among the basal ganglia are the following:

1. Pathway from Cortex to Basal Ganglia and Back to Cortex. Figure 35–7 illustrates the pathway that involves the greatest number of nerve fibers in the basal ganglia system. The pathway begins in all areas of the cerebral cortex and passes through the following four stages: (a) from the *cortex* to the *caudate nucleus* and *putamen* (which together are called the *neostriatum*), (b) from the neostriatum to the *globus pallidus*, (c) from the globus pallidus to the *thalamus*, and (d) from the ventroanterior and the ventrolateral nuclei of the thalamus *back to all areas of the cortex*.

Essentially all the nerve fibers from the neostriatum to the globus pallidus (stage b in the above circuit) are inhibitory pathways, secreting the inhibitory transmitter GABA at their nerve endings. Because of this inhibitory step, the circular pathway beginning in the cortex and returning once again to the cortex is a *negative feedback loop* that provides stability to many aspects of the motor control interactions.

2. Mutual Inhibitory Pathways Between the Neostriatum and the Substantia Nigra. Figure 35–8 illustrates a pathway from the *caudate nucleus* and *putamen* (the neostriatum) to the *substantia nigra* that secretes the inhibitory transmitter *GABA* at its ter-

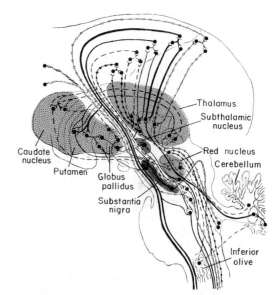

Figure 35–6. Pathways through the basal ganglia and related structures of the brain stem, thalamus, and cerebral cortex. (From Jung and Hassler: Handbook of Physiology, Vol. 2, Sec. 1. Baltimore, Williams & Wilkins Company, 1960.)

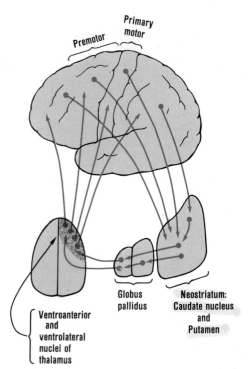

Figure 35–7. Feedback circuit from the cerebral cortex to the basal ganglia, then through the thalamus back to the cortex.

minus in the substantia nigra. In turn, a group of dark-staining cells in the substantia nigra sends axons back to the caudate nucleus and putamen, secreting the inhibitory transmitter *dopamine* at their terminals. This mutual inhibitory pathway normally maintains a certain degree of inhibition of the two separate areas. Lesions in these pathways are the basis of a number of different clinical syndromes involving the basal ganglia, including the important syndrome called Parkinson's disease that we shall discuss later.

3. Outflow Tracts from the Basal Ganglia Toward the Lower Brain Stem. Even though it is known that the basal ganglia can have important effects on the motor control functions of the brain stem, there are surprisingly few direct nerve fiber projections from the basal ganglia to the lower brain stem. Nevertheless, several small pathways pass mainly from the globus pallidus through either the subthalamic nucleus or the substantia nigra before entering the reticular formation.

FUNCTIONS OF THE DIFFERENT BASAL GANGLIA

Before attempting to discuss the functions of the basal ganglia in humans, we should speak briefly of the better known functions of these ganglia in lower animals. In birds, for instance, the cerebral cortex is poorly developed, while the basal ganglia are highly developed. These ganglia perform essentially all the motor functions, even controlling the voluntary movements in much the same manner as does the motor cortex of the human being. Furthermore, in the cat,

and to a lesser extent in the dog, decortication removes only the discrete types of motor functions and does not interfere with the animal's ability to walk, eat, fight, develop rage, have periodic sleep and wakefulness, and even participate naturally in sexual activities. However, if a major portion of the basal ganglia is destroyed, only gross stereotyped body movements, which were discussed in the previous chapter in relation to the lower brain stem animal, remain.

Finally, in the human being, cortical lesions in very young persons destroy the discrete movements of the body, particularly of the hands and distal portions of the lower limbs, but do not destroy the person's ability to walk crudely, to control his or her equilibrium, or to perform many other subconscious types of movements. However, simultaneous destruction of a major portion of the caudate nuclei almost totally paralyzes the opposite side of the body except for a few stereotyped reflexes integrated in the cord and brain stem.

With this brief background of the overall function of the basal ganglia, we can attempt to describe the functions of the individual portions of the basal ganglia system, realizing that the system actually operates as a total unit and that individual functions cannot be ascribed completely to the different parts of the basal ganglia.

Inhibition of Motor Tone by the Basal Ganglia. Though it is wrong to ascribe a single function to all the basal ganglia, nevertheless one of the general effects of diffuse basal ganglia excitation is to inhibit muscle tone throughout the body. This effect results from inhibitory signals transmitted from the basal ganglia to the brain stem reticular formation. Therefore, whenever widespread destruction of the basal

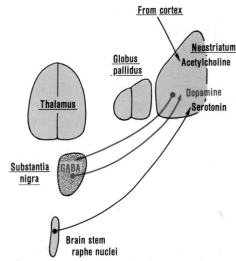

Figure 35–8. Interrelationships between the neostriatum (caudate nucleus and putamen) and the substantia nigra and raphe nuclei in the brain stem. This figure also shows several different transmitter substances involved in nerve transmission, especially secretion of GABA in the substantia nigra and dopamine in the neostriatum, both of which function as inhibitory transmitters.

ganglia occurs, the *loss* of inhibition of the postural control system of the reticular formation causes muscle rigidity throughout the body. For instance, when the brain stem is transected at the mesencephalic level, which removes the inhibitory effects of the basal ganglia, the phenomenon called *decerebrate rigidity*, discussed in the previous chapter, occurs.

Yet, despite this general inhibitory effect of the basal ganglia, stimulation of specific areas within the basal ganglia can at times elicit positive muscle contractions and at times even complex patterns of movements.

Function of the Caudate Nucleus and Putamen—The Neostriatum. The caudate nucleus and putamen together, called the neostriatum, function together to initiate and regulate *gross intentional movements of the body*, such as changing the position of the body, bending the body, and moving the arms. To perform this function they transmit impulses through two different pathways: (1) into the *globus pallidus*, thence by way of the *thalamus* to the *cerebral cortex*, and finally downward into the spinal cord through the *corticospinal pathway*; (2) downward through the *globus pallidus* and the *substantia nigra* by way of short axons into the *reticular formation*, and finally into the spinal cord mainly through the *reticulospinal tracts*.

In summary, the neostriatum helps to control gross intentional movements that we normally perform subconsciously. However, this control also involves the motor cortex, with which the neostriatum is very closely connected.

Function of the Globus Pallidus. It is already clear that almost all the outflow of signals from the basal ganglia are channelled through the globus pallidus en route either back to the cortex or on their way to lower brain centers. However, in addition to this motor relay function, the globus pallidus seems to have still another function that operates in close association with the subthalamus and brain stem to help control the axial and girdle movements of the body. These movements provide the background positioning of the body and proximal limbs so that the more discrete motor functions of the hands and feet can then be performed. That is, a person wishing to perform an exact function with a hand first positions the body, next positions the legs and arms, and finally tenses all the axial and girdle muscles to provide background stability of all the proximal portions of the body. These associated tonic contractions are supposedly initiated by circuits that strongly involve the globus pallidus but also operate through the axial and girdle motor control areas of the reticular formation. Lesions of the globus pallidus seriously interfere with the attitudinal movements that are necessary to position the hand and therefore make it difficult or impossible for one to use the hand for discrete activities.

Electrical stimulation of the globus pallidus while an animal is performing a gross body movement often will stop the movement in a static position, the animal holding that position for many seconds while the stimulation continues. This fits with the concept that the globus pallidus is involved in some type of servofeedback motor control system that is capable of locking the different parts of the body into specific positions.

CLINICAL SYNDROMES RESULTING FROM DAMAGE TO THE BASAL GANGLIA

Much of what we know about the function of the basal ganglia comes from study of patients with basal ganglia lesions whose brains have undergone pathologic studies after death. Among the different clinical syndromes are these:

Athetosis. In this disease, slow, writhing movements of a hand, the neck, the face, the tongue, or some other part of the body occur continually. The movements are likely to be wormlike, first with overextension of the hands and fingers, then flexion, then rotary twisting to the side—all these continuing in a slow, rhythmic, writhing pattern. The contracting muscles exhibit a high degree of spasm, and the movements are enhanced by emotions or by excessive signals from the sensory organs. Furthermore, voluntary movements in the affected area are greatly impaired or sometimes even impossible.

The damage in athetosis is usually found in the *lateral portion of the globus pallidus* or in this area and the neostriatum. Athetosis is usually attributed to the interruption of feedback circuits among the basal ganglia, thalamus, and cerebral cortex. The normal feedback circuits presumably allow a constant and rapid interplay between antagonistic muscle groups so that finely controlled movements can take place. However, if the feedback circuits are blocked, it is supposed that the detouring impulses may take devious routes through the basal ganglia, thalamus, and motor cortex, causing a succession of abnormal movements.

Parkinson's Disease. Parkinson's disease, which is also known as *paralysis agitans*, results almost invariably from *widespread destruction of the substantia nigra*, often associated with lesions of the subthalamus and other related areas. The disease is characterized by (1) *rigidity* of the musculature, either in widespread areas of the body or in isolated areas, (2) *tremor at rest* of the involved areas in most but not all instances, and (3) a *serious inability to initiate movement*, called *akinesia*.

These abnormal motor activities are almost certainly related to *loss of dopamine secretion* in the caudate nucleus and putamen by the nerve endings of the *nigrostriatal tract*. Destruction of the substantia nigra causes this tract to degenerate, and the *inhibitory* transmitter dopamine normally secreted in the caudate nucleus and putamen is no longer present. But still present are large numbers of neurons that secrete acetylcholine, an *excitatory* transmitter. It is believed that the dopamine from the nigrostriatal pathway normally acts to inhibit these acetylcholine-producing neurons or in some other way to counter their activity. But, in the absence of dopamine secretion, the acetylcholine pathways become overly active, which presumably is the basis for the rigidity and other motor symptoms in Parkinson's disease.

Tremor usually, though not always, occurs in Parkinson's disease. The frequency of the tremor is four to six cycles per second. When the person performs voluntary movements, weak tremors become temporarily blocked, but not strong tremors. The mechanism of the tremor is probably the lack of dopamine in the basal ganglia to inhibit the multiple feedbacks in the striatum-globus pallidus-thalamus-cortex circuit, which allows overactivity of many of these ganglia and causes them to oscillate.

Though the muscle rigidity and the tremor are both distressing to the parkinsonian patient, often even more serious is the *akinesia* that occurs in the final stages of the disease. To perform even the simplest of movements, the patient must exert the highest degree of concentration, mental effort, and even mental anguish to cause voluntary muscle contractions—that is, to overcome "motor stiffness" of his musculature. Thus, the person with Parkinson's disease has a masklike face, showing almost no automatic emotional facial expressions; he is usually bent forward because of his muscle rigidity; and all his movements of necessity are highly deliberate rather than characterized by the many casual subconscious movements that are normally a part of our everyday life.

The cause of the akinesia in Parkinson's disease is not known, and again we must resort to theory. It is presumed that *loss of dopamine secretion in the caudate nucleus and putamen by the nigrostriatal fibers* allows excessive excitation caused by the acetylcholine-producing neurons. But normal operation of the basal ganglia requires a balance between both excitatory and inhibitory activities, and loss of this balance, in effect, leads to a functionless basal ganglia system. We have already pointed out that the basal ganglia are responsible for many of the subconscious movements of the body and even for the background movements of the trunk, legs, neck, and upper arms that are a required preliminary to performing the more discrete movements of the hands. If the subconscious and the background movements cannot occur, then other neural mechanisms must be substituted, especially those of the motor cortex and cerebellum. Unfortunately, though, these cannot reduplicate the movements normally controlled by the basal ganglia and certainly cannot function at a subconscious level.

Treatment with L-Dopa. Administration of the drug L-dopa to patients with Parkinson's disease ameliorates most of the symptoms, especially the rigidity and the akinesia, in about two thirds of the patients. The reason for this seems to be the following: The dopamine secreted in the caudate nucleus and putamen by the nigrostriatal fibers is a derivative of L-dopa. When the substantia nigra is destroyed and a person develops Parkinson's disease, the administration of L-dopa is believed to substitute for the dopamine no longer secreted by the destroyed neurons. This causes more or less normal inhibition of the basal ganglia and relieves much or most of the akinesia and rigidity.

THE CEREBELLUM AND ITS MOTOR FUNCTIONS

The cerebellum has long been called a *silent area* of the brain principally because electrical excitation of this structure causes no sensation and rarely causes any motor movement. However, as we shall see, removal of the cerebellum does cause the motor movements to become highly abnormal. The cerebellum is especially vital to the control of very rapid muscular activities such as running, typing, playing the piano, and even talking. Loss of this area of the brain can cause almost total incoordination of these activities even though it does not cause paralysis of muscles.

But how is it that the cerebellum can be so important when it has no direct control over muscle contraction? The answer is that it *monitors and makes corrective adjustments in the motor activities elicited by other parts of the brain.* It receives continuously updated information from the peripheral parts of the body to determine instantaneously the status of each part of the body—its position, its rate of movement, forces acting on it, and so forth. And it is believed that the cerebellum *compares* the actual physical status of each part of the body, as depicted by the sensory signals, with the status that is intended by the motor system. If the two do not compare favorably, then appropriate corrective signals are instantaneously transmitted into the motor system to increase or decrease the levels of activation of the specific muscles.

Since the cerebellum must make major motor corrections extremely rapidly, *while the motor movements are actually occurring,* a very extensive and rapidly acting cerebellar input system is required both from the peripheral parts of the body and from the cerebral motor areas. Also, an extensive output system feeding equally rapidly into the motor system is necessary to provide the necessary corrections of the motor signals.

THE INPUT SYSTEM OF THE CEREBELLUM

The Afferent Pathways. The basic afferent pathways to the cerebellum are illustrated in Figure 35–9. An extensive and important afferent pathway is the *corticocerebellar pathway,* which originates in the *motor cortex* and then passes by way of the *pontile nuclei* and *pontocerebellar tracts* to the cortex of the cerebellum.

The cerebellum also receives important sensory

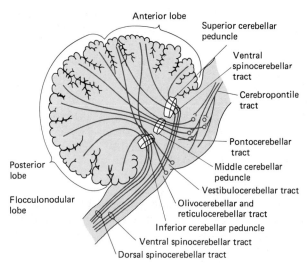

Figure 35–9. The principal afferent tracts to the cerebellum.

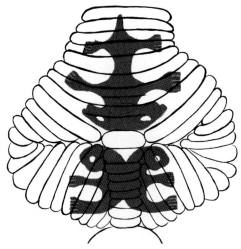

Figure 35–10. The sensory projection areas, called "homunculi," on the cortex of the cerebellum. (From Snider, R. S.: SCIENTIFIC AMERICAN, August, 1958. © 1958, by Scientific American, Inc. All rights reserved.)

signals directly from the peripheral parts of the body, which reach the cerebellum by way of the *ventral* and *dorsal spinocerebellar* tracts. The signals transmitted in these tracts originate in the muscle spindles, the Golgi's tendon organs, and the large tactile receptors of the skin and joints; they apprise the cerebellum of the momentary status of muscle contraction, degree of tension on the muscle tendons, positions of the parts of the body, and forces acting on the surfaces of the body. All of this information keeps the cerebellum constantly apprised of the physical status of the body at every instant.

In addition to the signals in the spinocerebellar tracts, other signals are transmitted up the cord through the *spinoreticular pathway* to the reticular substance of the brain stem and through the *spinoolivary pathway* to the inferior olivary nucleus and then relayed to the cerebellum. Thus, the cerebellum collects continual information about all parts of the body even though it is operating at a subconscious level.

Spatial Localization of Sensory Input to the Cerebellum. Afferent fibers entering the cerebellum terminate in distinct spatially oriented areas of the cerebellar cortex. Figure 35–10 illustrates the cerebellum, showing the approximate sensory terminations.

It is also important to note that the joints in the cerebellum representing specific muscles also receive information from the points in the motor cortex that excite the same muscles. Thus, the cerebellum receives information directly from the motor cortex concerning the motor signals that activate the muscle and also from the muscle concerning the effect actually produced. Then it projects corrective signals back into the motor pathway to the same part of this system.

The Longitudinal Functional Divisions of the Cerebellum. From a functional point of view, the cerebellum is organized into longitudinal sections, as illustrated in Figure 35–11. Note down the center of

the cerebellum a narrow band separated from the remainder of the cerebellum by shallow grooves. This band is called the *vermis*. In this area most cerebellar control functions for the muscle movements of the axial body, the neck, and the shoulders and hips are located.

To each side of the vermis is a large, laterally protruding *cerebellar hemisphere*, and each of these hemispheres is divided into an *intermediate zone* and a *lateral zone*. The intermediate zone of the hemisphere is concerned with the control of muscular contractions in the distal portions of both the upper and lower limbs, especially of the hands and fingers and feet and toes. The lateral zone of the hemisphere, which is called the *neocerebellum*, operates at a much more remote level, for this area seems to join into the overall planning of sequential motor movements. Without this lateral zone, most discrete motor activ-

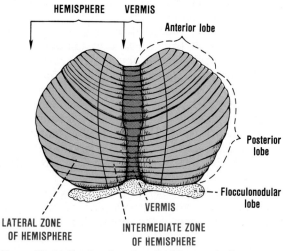

Figure 35–11. The functional parts of the cerebellum as seen from the posteroinferior view, with the inferiormost portion of the cerebellum rolled outward to flatten the surface.

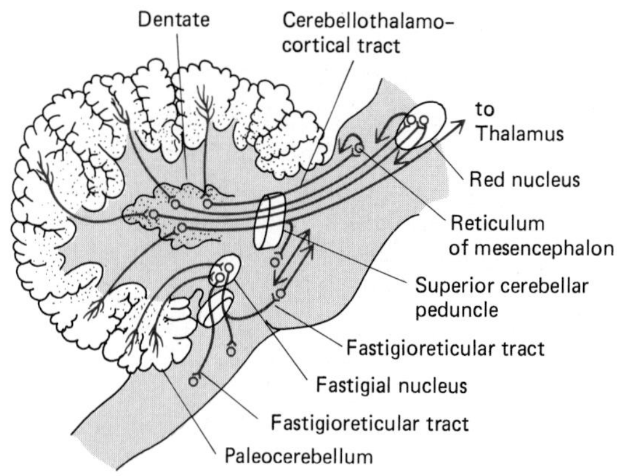

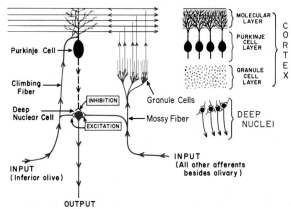

Figure 35–12. Principal efferent tracts from the cerebellum.

ities of the body would lose their appropriate timing and therefore become highly incoordinate, as we shall discuss more fully later.

OUTPUT SIGNALS FROM THE CEREBELLUM

The Deep Cerebellar Nuclei and the Efferent Pathways. Located deep in the cerebellar mass are three *deep cerebellar nuclei:* the *dentate, interpositus,* and *fastigial nuclei.* All of the output tracts from the cerebellum arise in the deep nuclei—that is, the cerebellar cortex always transmits its output signals only through the deep nuclei. The output signals are transmitted to many portions of the motor system, including (1) the motor cortex, (2) the basal ganglia, (3) the red nucleus, (4) the reticular formation of the brain stem, and (5) the vestibular nuclei. The important tracts are illustrated in Figure 35–12.

THE NEURONAL CIRCUIT OF THE CEREBELLUM

The structure of the cerebellar cortex is entirely different from that of the cerebral cortex. Furthermore, each minute part of the cerebellar cortex has a neuronal organization almost precisely the same as that in all other parts.

The human cerebellum is actually a large folded sheet, approximately 17 cm wide by 120 cm long, the folds lying crosswise, as illustrated in Figure 35–11.

The Functional Unit of the Cerebellar Cortex—the Purkinje Cells. The cerebellum has approximately 30 million nearly identical functional units, one of which is illustrated in Figure 35–13. This functional unit centers around the Purkinje cell, of which there are also 30 million in the cerebellar cortex.

Note to the far right in Figure 35–13 the three major layers of the cerebellar cortex: the *molecular layer,* the *Purkinje cell layer,* and the *granular cell layer.* Beneath these cortical layers are *deep nuclei* located in the center of the cerebellar mass.

The Neuronal Circuit of the Functional Unit

Figure 35–13 illustrates the neuronal circuit of the cerebellar functional unit. The output of this unit is

from a *deep nuclear cell* that sends a nervous signal back to the motor cortex or to the brain stem. Each of these deep nuclear cells is continually under the influence of both excitatory and inhibitory signals. The excitatory signals come from the incoming nerve fibers immediately after they enter the cerebellum. Each incoming fiber sends excitatory branches to the deep nuclear cells. The inhibitory signals arise entirely from the *Purkinje cells* in the cortex of the cerebellum, because the nerve endings from the Purkinje cells secrete an inhibitory transmitter.

The incoming fibers are of two types, called the *climbing fiber type* and the *mossy fiber type.* Each sends its branches to the deep nuclear cells and continues on to the cerebellar cortex. The climbing fibers synapse directly with the Purkinje cells and provide strong excitatory signals to these cells. On the other hand, the mossy fibers terminate, not directly on the Purkinje cells, but on literally millions of minute neuronal cells called *granule cells.* These cells in turn send millions of extremely tiny axons in both horizontal directions in the cerebellum, and very large numbers of these fibers synapse with each Purkinje cell. Because of the small size of these fibers and their slow transmission, the signal reaches the Purkinje cells after a short delay period, which is undoubtedly important for cerebellar function.

After the Purkinje cell has been excited by both the climbing and the mossy fiber circuits, it in turn sends a signal that, because its axon secretes an inhibitory transmitter substance, inhibits rather than excites the deep nuclear cell. Note, also, that this inhibitory signal arrives at the deep nuclear cell after a short delay time. That is, at the beginning of a motor action, there is, first, excitation of the deep nuclear cell by the direct incoming signals to the cerebellum, followed a few milliseconds later by inhibition from the Purkinje cells.

Keep in mind this dual stimulation of the deep nuclear cell with a slight delay between excitation and inhibition, for this sequence is believed to be of great significance in cerebellar function. That is, after initial excitation by a motor signal, a negative feedback signal from the cerebellum occurs a short time

Figure 35–13. Basic neuronal circuit of the cerebellum, showing excitatory pathways in color. At right are the three major layers of the cerebellar cortex and also the deep nuclei.

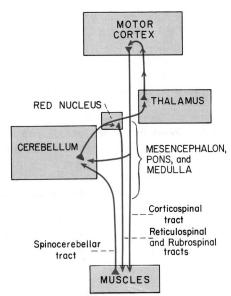

Figure 35-14. Pathways for cerebellar control of voluntary movements.

later to stop the muscle movement from overshooting its mark, a cardinal feature of cerebellar function.

FUNCTION OF THE CEREBELLUM IN VOLUNTARY MOVEMENTS

The cerebellum functions only in association with activities initiated elsewhere in the central nervous system. These activities may originate in the spinal cord, in the reticular formation, in the basal ganglia, or in the motor areas of the cerebral cortex.

Figure 35-14 illustrates the basic cerebellar pathways involved in cerebellar control of voluntary movements. When motor signals are transmitted from the cerebral cortex downward through the pyramidal and extrapyramidal tracts to excite the muscles, collateral signals are transmitted simultaneously into the cerebellum through the pontocerebellar and olivocerebellar tracts. Therefore, for every motor movement that is performed, not only do the muscles receive activating signals, but the cerebellum receives similar signals at the same time.

When the muscles contract, the muscle spindles, Golgi's tendon apparatuses, joint receptors, and other peripheral receptors transmit signals upward mainly through the spinocerebellar and spino-olivary pathways to terminate in the cerebellum.

After the signals from the periphery and those from the motor cortex are integrated in the cerebellum, efferent impulses are transmitted from the cerebellar deep nuclei upward through the ventrolateral nuclei of the thalamus back to the motor cortex.

"Error Control" by the Cerebellum. One will readily recognize that the circuit described above represents a complicated feedback circuit beginning in the cerebral part of the motor control system and then returning also to this area. Ordinarily, the motor cortex transmits far more impulses than are needed

to perform each intended movement, and the cerebellum therefore must act to inhibit the motor cortex at the appropriate time after the muscle has begun to move. The cerebellum seems to assess the rate of movement and to calculate the time that will be required to reach the point of intention. Then appropriate inhibitory impulses are transmitted to the motor cortex to inhibit the agonist muscles and to excite the antagonist muscles. In this way, appropriate "brakes" are applied to stop the movement at the precise point of intention.

Since all these events transpire much too rapidly for the motor cortex to reverse the excitation "voluntarily," it is evident that the excitation of the antagonist muscle toward the end of a movement is an entirely automatic and subconscious function and is not a "willed" contraction of the same nature as the original contraction of the agonist muscle. We shall see below that in patients with serious cerebellar damage, excitation of the antagonist muscles occurs not at the appropriate time but instead always too late. Therefore, it is almost certain that one of the major functions of the cerebellum is automatic excitation of antagonist muscles at the end of a movement and, at the same time, inhibition of agonist muscles that started the movement.

The "Damping" Function of the Cerebellum— Intension Tremor. One of the by-products of the cerebellar feedback mechanism is its ability to "damp" muscular movements. To explain the meaning of "damping" we must first point out that essentially all movements of the body are "pendular." For instance, when an arm is moved, momentum develops, and the momentum must be overcome before the movement can be stopped. And, because of the momentum, the arm has a tendency to overshoot. If overshooting does occur in a person whose cerebellum has been destroyed, the conscious centers of the cerebrum eventually recognize this and initiate a movement in the opposite direction to bring the arm toward its intended position. But again the arm, by virtue of its momentum now in the opposite direction, again overshoots, and appropriate corrective signals must again be instituted. Thus, the arm oscillates back and forth past its intended point for several cycles before it finally fixes on its mark. This effect is called an *action tremor*, or *intention tremor*.

However, if the cerebellum is intact, appropriate subconscious signals stop the movement precisely at the intended point, thereby preventing the overshoot and also the tremor. This is the basic characteristic of a damping system. All control systems regulating pendular elements that have inertia must have damping circuits built into the mechanisms. In the motor control system of our central nervous system, the cerebellum provides much of this damping function.

Function of the Cerebellum in Prediction—Dysmetria. Another important by-product of the cerebellar feedback mechanism seems to be an ability to help the central nervous system predict future positions of moving parts of the body. Without the cerebellum a person "loses" his limbs *when they move rapidly*, indicating that feedback information from the periphery probably must be analyzed by the cerebellum if the brain is to keep up with the motor movements. Thus, the cerebellum detects from the incoming sensory signals the rate at which the limb is moving and then predicts from this the projected time course of movement. This allows the cerebellum, operating through the cerebellar output circuits, to inhibit the agonist muscles and to excite the antagonist muscles when the movement approaches the point of intention.

Without the cerebellum this predictive function is so deficient that moving parts of the body move much farther than the point of intention. This failure to control the distance that the parts of the body move is called *dysmetria*, which means simply poor control of the distance of movement.

Function of the Large Lateral Zone of the Cerebellar Hemisphere in Planning Sequential Movements

In human beings, the lateral zones of the two cerebellar hemispheres have become very highly developed and greatly enlarged, along with the human ability to perform intricate movements with the hands and fingers and to speak. Yet, strangely enough, these large lateral portions of the cerebellar hemispheres have no direct informational input from the peripheral parts of the body. Also, almost all the communication between these lateral cerebellar areas and the cortex is not with the primary motor cortex but with the premotor and the sensory areas of the cortex. Even so, destruction of the lateral portions of the cerebellar hemispheres along with their deep nuclei, the dentate nuclei, can lead to extreme incoordination of the purposeful movements of the hands, fingers, feet, and speech apparatus. This has been hard to understand because of lack of direct communication between this part of the cerebellum and the primary motor cortex. However, recent experimental studies suggest that these portions of the cerebellum are concerned with the planning of sequential movements.

The Planning Function. The planning of sequential movements is believed to be related to the fact that the lateral hemispheres communicate with the premotor and sensory portions of the cerebral cortex. It seems that the plan of the sequential movements is transmitted from the sensory and premotor areas of the cortex to the lateral zones of the cerebellar hemispheres, and two-way traffic between the cerebellum and the cortex is necessary to provide appropriate transition from one movement to the next. An exceedingly interesting observation that supports this view is that many of the neurons in the dentate nuclei display the activity pattern of the next movement at the same time that the present movement is occurring. Thus, the lateral hemispheres appear to be involved not with what is happening at a given moment but

instead with *what will be happening during the next sequential movement*.

To summarize, one of the most important features of normal motor function is one's ability to progress smoothly from one movement to the next in orderly succession. In the absence of the cerebellar hemispheres this capability is seriously disturbed, especially for rapid movements.

Extramotor Predictive Functions of the Cerebellum. The cerebellum also plays a role in predicting other events besides simply movements of the body. For instance, the rates of progression of both auditory and visual phenomena can be predicted. As an example, a person can predict from the changing visual scene how rapidly he is approaching an object. A striking experiment that demonstrates the importance of the cerebellum in this ability is the effect of removing the visual portion of the cerebellum in monkeys. A monkey so treated occasionally charges the wall of a corridor and literally bashes its brains out because it is unable to predict when it will reach the wall.

SENSORY FEEDBACK CONTROL OF MOTOR FUNCTIONS

THE SENSORY ENGRAM FOR MOTOR MOVEMENTS

It is primarily in the sensory and sensory association areas that a person records memories of the different patterns of motor movements. These are called *sensory engrams*. When one wishes to achieve some purposeful act, the engram automatically sets the motor system of the brain into action to reproduce the sensory pattern of the engram.

The Proprioceptor Feedback Servomechanism for Reproducing the Sensory Engram. From the discussion of cerebellar function earlier in the chapter, it is clear how proprioceptor signals from the periphery can affect motor activity. However, in addition to looping through the cerebellum, feedback pathways pass from the muscles, joints, and other parts of the body directly back to the cerebral cortex. Each of these pathways is capable of modifying the motor response. For instance, if a person learns to cut with scissors, the movements involved in this process cause a particular sequential pattern of proprioceptive impulses to pass to the somatic sensory area. Once this pattern has been "learned" by the sensory cortex, the memory engram of the pattern can activate the motor system to perform the same sequential pattern whenever it is required.

To do this, the proprioceptor signals from the fingers, hands, and arms are compared with the engram, and if the two do not match each other, the difference, called the error, initiates additional motor signals that automatically activate appropriate muscles to bring the fingers, hands, and arms into the necessary sequential attitudes for performance of the task. Each successive portion of the engram is projected according to a time sequence, and the motor control system automatically follows from one point to the next so that the fingers go through the precise motions necessary to duplicate exactly the sensory engram of the motor activity.

Thus, one can see that the motor system in this case actually acts as a servomechanism; that is, it is not the motor cortex itself that controls the pattern of activity to be accomplished. Instead, the pattern is located in the sensory part of the brain, and the motor system merely follows the pattern, which is the definition of a servomechanism. If ever the motor system fails to follow the pattern, signals are fed back to the cerebral cortex to apprise the sensorium of this failure and appropriate corrective signals are transmitted to the muscles.

Besides somatic sensory signals, other sensory signals, particularly visual ones are involved in motor control. However, these other sensory systems are often slower to recognize error than is the somatic proprioceptor system. Therefore, when the sensory engram depends on visual feedback for control purposes, the motor movements are usually considerably slowed in comparison with those that depend on somatic feedback.

An experiment that demonstrates the importance of the sensory engram for control of motor movements is one in which a monkey has been trained to perform some complex task and then various portions of its cortex removed. Removal of small portions of the motor cortex that control the muscles normally used for the task does not prevent the monkey from performing it. Instead, the monkey automatically uses other muscles in place of the paralyzed ones to perform the same task. On the other hand, if the corresponding somatic sensory cortex is removed but the motor cortex is left intact, the monkey then loses all ability to perform the task. This experiment demonstrates that the motor system acts automatically as a servomechanism to use whatever muscles are available to follow the pattern of the sensory engram, and if some muscles are missing, other muscles are substituted automatically. The experiment also demonstrates forcefully that the somatic sensory cortex is essential to at least some types of "learned" motor performance, especially the complex patterns.

ESTABLISHMENT OF RAPID "SKILLED" MOTOR PATTERNS

Many motor activities are performed so rapidly that there is insufficient time for sensory feedback signals to control them. For instance, the movements of the fingers during typing occur much too rapidly for feedback signals to be transmitted either to the somatic sensory cortex or even directly to the motor cortex. It is believed that the patterns for control of these rapid coordinate muscular movements are es-

tablished in the motor system itself, probably involving complex circuitry in the primary motor cortex, in the premotor area of the cortex, in the basal ganglia, and even in the cerebellum. Indeed, lesions in any of these areas can destroy or at least greatly alter one's ability to peform rapid coordinated muscular contractions, such as those required during the act of typing, talking, or writing by hand.

Role of Sensory Feedback During Establishment of the Rapid Motor Patterns. Even a highly skilled motor activity can be performed the very first time, provided that it is performed extremely slowly—slowly enough for sensory feedback to guide the movements through each step. However, to be really useful, many skilled motor activities must be performed rapidly. This probably is achieved by successive performances of the same skilled activity, at first very slowly, then progressively more rapidly, until finally an engram of the skilled activity is laid down in the motor system as well as in the sensory system. This motor engram causes a precise set of muscles to go through a specific sequence of movements required to perform the skilled activity. Such an engram is called *a pattern of skilled motor function*, and the motor areas of the brain are primarily concerned with this.

After a person has performed a skilled activity many times, the motor pattern of this activity can thereafter cause the hand or arm or other part of the body to go through the same pattern of activity again and again, now entirely *without* sensory feedback control. However, even though sensory feedback control is no longer present, the sensory system still determines in retrospect whether or not the act has been performed correctly. If it has not, information from the sensory system supposedly can help to correct the pattern the next time it is performed.

Thus, eventually, hundreds of patterns of coordinate movements are laid down in the motor system, and these can be called upon one at a time in different sequential orders to perform literally thousands of still more complex motor activities.

An interesting experiment that demonstrates the applicability of these theoretical methods of muscular control is one in which the eyes are made to follow an object that moves around and around in a circle. At first, the eyes can follow the object around the circle only when it moves slowly, and even then the eye movements are extremely jerky. Thus, sensory feedback is being utilized to control the eye movements for following the object. However, after a few seconds, the eyes begin to follow the moving object rather faithfully, and the rapidity of movement around the circle can be increased to many times per second, and still the eyes continue to follow the object. Sensory feedback control of each stage of the eye movements at these rapid rates would be completely impossible. Therefore, by this time, the eyes have developed a pattern of movement that is not dependent upon step-by-step sensory feedback.

Nevertheless, if the eyes should fail to follow the object around the circle, the sensory system would immediately become aware of this and presumably could make corrections in the pattern of movement.

INITIATION OF VOLUNTARY MOTOR ACTIVITY

Because of the spectacular properties of the primary motor cortex (the area pyramidalis) and of the instantaneous muscle contractions that can be achieved by electrically stimulating this area, it has been customary to think that the initial brain signals eliciting voluntary muscle contractions begin in the primary motor cortex. However, this almost certainly is far from the truth. Indeed, experiments have shown that the cerebellum and the basal ganglia are activated at almost exactly the same time or even before the motor cortex is activated. Furthermore, there is no known mechanism by which the motor cortex can conceive the entire sequential pattern that is to be achieved by the motor movements.

Therefore, we are left with an unanswered question: What is the locus of the initiation of involuntary motor activity? A partial answer comes from the fact that neuronal activity begins in the sensory areas of the brain as long as a second before voluntary motor activity occurs. Also, neuronal activity begins in the premotor areas of the cortex and in some areas of the basal ganglia many milliseconds before motor activity occurs in the motor cortex. Therefore, it is currently thought that *cerebration* occurring in these "integrative" portions of the brain, operating in association with the cerebellum, conceives and plans the complex sequence of movements that is to be executed. Only after the plan has been established is the primary motor system set into action to cause the sequential events. In the following chapter, we shall discuss the planning and execution of speech, which is an excellent illustration of these principles of voluntary motor control.

QUESTIONS

1. Describe the *primary motor cortex* and the *pyramidal tract*.
2. What is meant by the term *extrapyramidal tracts?*
3. What is the difference between the functions of the *premotor cortex* and the primary motor cortex?
4. Describe *Broca's area* for control of speech.
5. What are the functions of the following premotor areas: the voluntary eye movement field, the head rotation area, and the area for hand skills?
6. What type of muscle activity is affected to the greatest extent by ablation of the primary motor cortex?
7. Explain why lesions of the premotor cortex and of the basal ganglia cause spasticity, while lesions limited to the primary motor cortex fail to do so.
8. Describe the neuronal circuit from the cortex to the basal ganglia and then back to the cortex. What are some possible functions of this neuronal circuit?
9. Describe the neuronal circuit between the neostriatum and the substantia nigra. What are some of the possible functions of this pathway?
10. In lower animals in which the cerebral cortex has been removed, what are some of the remaining functions of the basal ganglia?
11. What is a possible cause of the clinical condition called *athetosis?*
12. Give possible physiological explanations for the following three abnormalities found in *Parkinson's disease*: (a) rigidity, (b) tremor at rest, and (c) akinesia.
13. How does the drug L-dopa function in the treatment of Parkinson's disease?
14. Describe both the afferent and efferent nerve tracts of the cerebellum.
15. Describe the spatial localization of signals from the body in the cerebellum.
16. Explain the balance between excitation and inhibition that controls the output from the deep nuclear cells of the cerebellum.
17. How does the cerebellum delay the onset of the inhibitory output signal that occurs at the end of a motor movement?
18. Discuss the principle of error control by the cerebellum.
19. Explain the function of the cerebellum in *prediction* and the phenomena of *dysmetria* and *intention tremor*.
20. Explain the function of the *lateral zone of the cerebellar hemispheres* in planning sequential movements.
21. What is the role of the *sensory engram for motor movements* in the learning of and control of learned motor activities?
22. Explain how one establishes rapid skilled motor patterns in the motor portions of the cerebral cortex.
23. What is the probable mechanism for the initiation of voluntary motor activity?

References

Allen, G. I., and Tsukahara, N.: Cerebrocerebellar communication systems. Physiol Rev 54:957, 1974.

Asanuma, H.: The pyramidal tract. In Brooks, V. B., ed.: Handbook of Physiology. Sec. 1, Vol. 2. Bethesda, American Physiological Society, 1981, p. 703.

Bloedel, J. R., and Courville, J.: Cerebellar afferent systems. In Brooks,

V. B., ed.: Handbook of Physiology. Sec. 1. Vol. 2. Bethesda, American Physiological Society, 1981, p. 735.

Brooks, V. B., and Thach, W. T.: Cerebellar control of posture and movement. In Brooks, V. B., ed.: Handbook of Physiology. Sec. 1, Vol. 2. Bethesda, American Physiological Society, 1981, p. 877.

Desmedt, J. E. ed.: Cerebral Motor Control in Man: Long Loop Mechanisms. New York, S. Karger, 1978.

Evarts, E. V.: Role of motor cortex in voluntary movements in primates. In Brooks, V. B., ed.: Handbook of Physiology. Sec. 1. Vol. 2. Bethesda, American Physiological Society, 1981, p. 1083.

Fuster, J. M.: Prefrontal cortex in motor control. In Brooks, V. B., ed.: Handbook of Physiology. Sec. 1, Vol. 2. Bethesda, American Physiological Society, 1981, p. 1149.

Keele, S. W.: Behavioral analysis of movements. In Brooks, V. B., ed.: Handbook of Physiology. Sec. 1, Vol. 2. Bethesda, American Physiological Society, 1981, p. 1391.

Llinas, R.: Eighteenth Bowditch lecture. Motor aspects of cerebellar control. Physiologist 17:19, 1974.

Orlovsky, G. N., and Shik, M. L.: Control of locomotion: a neurophysiological analysis of the cat locomotor system. Int Rev Physiol 10:281, 1976.

Pearson, K.: The control of walking. Sci Am 235(6):72, 1976.

Porter, R.: Internal organization of the motor cortex for input-output arrangements. In Brooks, V. B., ed.: Handbook of Physiology. Sec. 1, Vol. 2. Bethesda, American Physiological Society, 1981, p. 1063.

Shik, M. L., and Orlovsky, G. N.: Neurophysiology of locomotor automatism. Physiol Rev 56:465, 1976.

Stein, P. S. G.: Motor systems with specific reference to the control of locomotion. Annu Rev Neurosci 1:61, 1978.

Wiesendanger, M., and Miles, T. S.: Ascending pathway of low-threshold muscle afferents to the cerebral cortex and its possible role in motor control. Physiol Rev 62:1234, 1982.

36

The Cerebral Cortex and Intellectual Functions of the Brain

PHYSIOLOGICAL ANATOMY OF THE
CEREBRAL CORTEX
**FUNCTIONS OF CERTAIN SPECIFIC
CORTICAL AREAS**
SPECIFIC FUNCTIONS OF THE
PRIMARY SENSORY AREAS
THE SENSORY ASSOCIATION AREAS
INTERPRETATIVE FUNCTION OF THE
POSTERIOR PART OF THE

SUPERIOR TEMPORAL
LOBE—WERNICKE'S AREA
THE PREFRONTAL AREAS
**THOUGHTS, CONSCIOUSNESS, AND
MEMORY**
MEMORY AND TYPES OF MEMORY
PHYSIOLOGICAL BASIS OF MEMORY
**FUNCTION OF THE BRAIN IN
COMMUNICATION**

It is ironic that of all parts of the brain, we know least about the mechanisms of the cerebral cortex, even though it is by far the largest portion of the nervous system. Yet, we do know the effects of destruction or of stimulation of various portions of the cortex, and still more has been learned from electrical recordings from the cortex. In the early part of the present chapter the known facts about cortical functions are discussed, and then basic theories of the neuronal mechanisms involved in thought processes, memory, analysis of sensory information, and so forth are presented briefly.

PHYSIOLOGICAL ANATOMY OF THE CEREBRAL CORTEX

The functional portion of the cerebral cortex is composed mainly of a thin layer of neurons 2 to 5 mm thick, covering the surface of all the convolutions of the cerebrum and having a total area of about one-quarter of a square meter. The total cerebral cortex contains approximately 100 billion neurons.

Figure 36–1 illustrates the typical structure of the cerebral cortex, showing successive layers of different groups of cells. Most of the cells are of three types; *granular, fusiform,* and *pyramidal,* the latter named for their characteristic pyramidal shape.

To the right in Figure 36–1 is illustrated the typical organization of nerve fibers within the different layers of the cortex. Note particularly the large number of horizontal fibers extending between adjacent areas of the cortex, but note also the vertical fibers that extend to and from the cortex to lower areas of the brain stem or to distant regions of the cerebral cortex, or even all the way to the spinal cord, through long bundles of fibers.

Anatomical Relationship of the Cerebral Cortex to the Thalamus and Other Lower Centers. All areas of the cerebral cortex have both direct afferent and efferent connections with the thalamus. Figure 36–2 shows the areas of the cerebral cortex connected with specific parts of the thalamus. These connections are in *two* directions, both from the thalamus to the cortex and then from the cortex back to essentially the same area of the thalamus. Furthermore, when the thalamic connections are cut, the functions of the corresponding cortical areas become either entirely or almost entirely abrogated. The cortex therefore operates in close association with the thalamus and can almost be considered, both anatomically and functionally, a large outgrowth of the thalamus; for this reason the thalamus and the cortex together are called the *thalamocortical system,* as is discussed in the following chapter. Also, all pathways from the

415

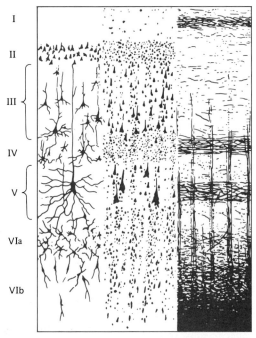

Figure 36–1. Structure of the cerebral cortex, illustrating *I*, molecular layer; *II*, external granular layer; *III*, layer of pyramidal cells; *IV*, internal granular layer; *V*, large pyramidal cell layer; *VI*, layer of fusiform or polymorphic cells. (From Ranson and Clark [after Brodmann]: Anatomy of the Nervous System. Philadelphia, W. B. Saunders Company, 1959.)

sensory nerve endings to the cortex pass through the thalamus, with the single exception of the sensory pathways of the olfactory tract.

FUNCTIONS OF CERTAIN SPECIFIC CORTICAL AREAS

Studies in human beings by neurosurgeons have shown that some specific functions are localized to certain localized areas of the cerebral cortex. Figure 36–3 gives a map of some of these areas as determined by Penfield and Rasmussen from electrical stimulation of the cortex or neurological examination of patients

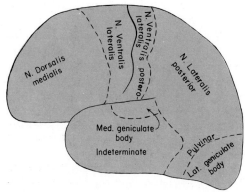

Figure 36–2. Areas of the cerebral cortex that connect with specific portions of the thalamus. (Modified from Elliott: Textbook of the Nervous System. Philadelphia, J. B. Lippincott Co.)

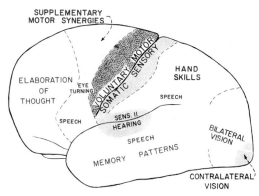

Figure 36–3. Functional areas of the human cerebral cortex as determined by electrical stimulation of the cortex during neurosurgical operations and by neurologic examinations of patients with destroyed cortical regions. (From THE CEREBRAL CORTEX OF MAN by Wilder Penfield and Theodore Rasmussen. Copyright 1950 by Macmillan Publishing Company, renewed 1978 by Theodore Rasmussen. Reprinted with permission of the publisher.)

after portions of the cortex had been removed. The lightly shaded areas are *primary sensory areas,* while the darkly shaded area is the *voluntary motor area* (also called *primary motor area*) from which muscular movements can be elicited with relatively weak electrical stimuli. These primary sensory and motor areas have highly specific functions, while other areas of the cortex perform more general functions that we call association or cerebration.

SPECIFIC FUNCTIONS OF THE PRIMARY SENSORY AREAS

The primary sensory areas all have certain functions in common. For instance, somatic, visual, and auditory sensory areas all have spatial localizations of signals from the peripheral receptors (which are discussed in detail in Chapters 32, 40, and 41).

Electrical stimulation of the primary sensory areas in the parietal lobes in patients who are awake gives relatively uncomplicated sensations. For instance, in the somatic sensory area, the patient experiences a tingling in the skin, numbness, mild "electric" or, rarely, mild degrees of temperature sensations. And these sensations are localized to discrete areas of the body in accordance with the spatial representation in the somatic sensory cortex, as described in Chapter 32. Therefore, it is believed that the primary somatic sensory cortex analyzes only the simple aspects of sensations and that analysis of intricate patterns of sensory experience requires adjacent parts of the parietal lobe called *sensory association areas.*

Electrical stimulation of the primary visual cortex in the occipital lobes causes a person to see flashes of light, bright lines, colors, or other simple visions. Here again, the visual images are localized to specific regions of the visual fields in accordance with the portion of the primary visual cortex stimulated, as described in Chapter 40. But the visual cortex alone is not capable of complete analysis of complicated visual patterns; for this, the visual cortex must operate in association with adjacent regions of the occipital cortex, the *visual association areas.*

Electrical stimulation of the auditory cortex in the temporal lobes causes a person to hear a simple sound that may be weak or loud, of low or high frequency, or may have other uncomplicated characteristics, such as a squeak or even an undulation. But never are words or any other fully intelligible sound heard. Thus, the primary auditory cortex, like the other primary sensory areas, can detect the individual elements of auditory experience but cannot analyze complicated sounds. Therefore, the primary auditory cortex alone is not sufficient for even the usual auditory experiences; these can be achieved, however, when the primary area operates together with the *auditory association areas* located in adjacent regions of the temporal lobes.

Despite the inability of the primary sensory areas to analyze fully the incoming sensations, when these areas are destroyed, the ability of the person to utilize the sensations usually suffers drastically. For instance, loss of the primary visual cortex in one occipital lobe causes a person to become blind in the ipsilateral halves of both retinae, and loss of the primary visual cortices in both hemispheres causes total blindness. Likewise, loss of both primary auditory cortices causes almost total deafness.

THE SENSORY ASSOCIATION AREAS

Around the borders of the primary sensory areas are regions called *sensory association areas* or *secondary sensory areas.* In general, these areas extend 1 to 5 centimeters in one or more directions from the primary sensory areas; each time a primary area receives a sensory signal, secondary signals spread after a delay of a few milliseconds into the respective association area. Part of this spread occurs in the cortex itself, but a major part also occurs in the thalamus, beginning in the thalamic sensory relay nuclei, passing next to corresponding *thalamic* association areas, and then traveling to the association cortex.

The general function of the sensory association areas is to provide a higher level of interpretation of the sensory experiences. The general areas for the interpretative functions for somatic, visual, and auditory experiences are illustrated in Figure 36–4.

Destruction of the sensory association areas greatly reduces the capability of the brain to analyze different characteristics of sensory experiences. For instances, damage in the temporal lobe below and behind the primary auditory area in the dominant hemisphere of the brain often causes a person to be unable to understand the meaning of words though he hears the words and can even repeat them.

Likewise, destruction of the visual association areas of the occipital lobe in the dominant hemisphere does not cause blindness or prevent normal activation of the primary visual cortex but does greatly reduce the person's ability to interpret what he sees. Such a person often loses his ability to recognize the mean-

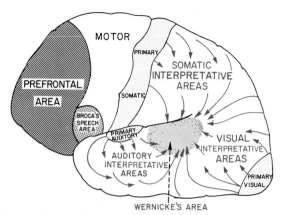

Figure 36–4. Organization of the somatic, auditory, and visual association areas into a general mechanism for interpretation of sensory experience. All these feed also into *Wernicke's* area located in the posterosuperior portion of the temporal lobe. Note also the prefrontal area, and Broca's speech area.

ings of words that he reads, a condition that is called *word blindness* or *dyslexia.*

Finally, destruction of the somatic sensory association area in the parietal cortex posterior to primary somatic area I causes the person to lose his spatial perception for location of the different parts of his body. In the case of the hand that has been "lost," the skills of the hand are greatly reduced. Thus, this area of the cortex seems to be necessary for interpretation of somatic sensory experiences.

The functions of the association areas are described in more detail in Chapter 32 for somatic, in Chapter 40 for visual, and in Chapter 41 for auditory experiences.

INTERPRETATIVE FUNCTION OF THE POSTERIOR PART OF THE SUPERIOR TEMPORAL LOBE—WERNICKE'S AREA

The somatic, visual, and auditory association areas, which can actually be called interpretative areas, all meet in the posterior part of the superior temporal lobe where the temporal, parietal, and occipital lobes all come together, as shown in Figure 36–4. This area of confluence of the sensory interpretative areas is especially highly developed in the dominant side of the brain—the *left side* in right-handed persons—and it plays the greatest single role of any part of the cerebral cortex in the higher levels of brain function that we call *cerebration.* Therefore, this region has frequently been called by different names suggestive of the area having almost global importance: the *general interpretative area,* the *gnostic area,* the *knowing area,* the *tertiary association area,* and so forth. However, it is best known as *Wernicke's area* in honor of the neurologist who first described its special significance in intellectual processes.

Following severe damage in Wernicke's area, a person may hear perfectly well and even recognize different words but still may be unable to arrange these words into a coherent thought. Likewise, the person may be able to read words from the printed page but be unable to recognize the thought that is conveyed.

Electrical stimulation in Wernicke's area of the conscious patient occasionally causes a highly complex thought. This is particularly true when the stimulatory electrode is passed deep enough into the brain to approach the corresponding connecting areas of the thalamus. The types of thoughts that might be experienced include memories of complicated visual scenes that one might remember from childhood, auditory hallucinations such as a specific musical piece, or even a discourse by a specific person. For this reason it is believed that complicated memory patterns involving more than one sensory modality are stored at least partially in this area, or that activation of Wernicke's area can call forth the memories even if they may be stored elsewhere. This belief is in accord with the importance of Wernicke's area in interpretation of the complicated meanings of different sensory experiences.

The Angular Gyrus—Interpretation of Visual Information. The angular gyrus is the most inferior portion of the posterior parietal lobe, lying immediately behind Wernicke's area and fusing posteriorly into the visual areas of the occipital lobe as well. If this region is destroyed while Wernicke's area in the temporal lobe is still intact, the person can still interpret auditory experiences as usual, but the stream of visual experiences passing into Wernicke's area from the visual cortex is mainly blocked. Therefore, the person may be able to see words and may even know they are words but, nevertheless, is not able to interpret their meanings. This is the condition called *dyslexia,* or *word blindness.*

Let us again emphasize the global importance of Wernicke's area for most intellectual functions of the brain. Loss of this area in an adult usually leads thereafter to a lifetime of almost demented existence.

The Concept of the Dominant Hemisphere

The general interpretative functions of Wernicke's area and of the angular gyrus, and also the functions of the speech and motor control areas, are usually much more highly developed in one cerebral hemisphere than in the other. Therefore, this hemisphere is called the *dominant hemisphere.* In about 95 per cent of all persons, the left hemisphere is the dominant one. Even at birth, Wernicke's area of the brain is already as much as 50 per cent larger in the left hemisphere than in the right in more than one half of newborn babies. Therefore, it is easy to understand why the left side of the brain might become dominant over the right side. However, if for some reason the dominant Wernicke's area is removed in early childhood, the opposite side of the brain can develop fully dominant characteristics.

Usually associated with the dominant temporal lobe also is dominance of certain other cortical functions. For instance, as discussed later in the chapter, the premotor speech area (Broca's area) is almost always also dominant on the left side of the brain. And the motor area for controlling the hand on the opposite side of the body is dominant on the left side of the brain in about nine of ten persons, thus causing right-handedness in most people.

Though Wernicke's area is highly developed in only a single hemisphere, it receives sensory information from both hemispheres and also is capable of controlling motor activities in both hemispheres, utilizing mainly fiber pathways in the *corpus callosum* for communication between the two hemispheres. This unitary, cross-feeding organization prevents interference between the functions of the two sides of the brain; such interference, obviously, could create havoc with both thoughts and motor responses.

Role of Language in Function of Wernicke's Area and in Intellectual Functions

A major share of our sensory experience is converted into its language equivalent before being stored in the memory areas of the brain and before being processed for other intellectual purposes. For instance, when we read a book, we do not store the visual images of the printed words but instead store the words themselves in language form. Also, the information conveyed by the words is usually converted to language form before its meaning is discerned.

The sensory area of the dominant hemisphere for interpretation of language is Wernicke's area, which is very closely associated with both the primary hearing area and the auditory association areas of the temporal lobe. This close relationship probably results from the fact that the first introduction to language is by way of hearing. Later in life, when visual perception of language through the medium of reading develops, the visual information is then presumably channeled into the already developed language regions of the dominant temporal lobe.

Wernicke's Area in the Nondominant Hemisphere. When Wernicke's area in the dominant hemisphere is destroyed, the person normally loses almost all intellectual functions associated with language or verbal symbolism, such as the ability to read, the ability to perform mathematical operations, and even the ability to think through logical problems. However, many other types of interpretative capabilities utilize the temporal lobe and angular gyrus regions of the opposite hemisphere, and these capabilities are retained. Psychological studies in patients with damage to their nondominant hemispheres have suggested that this hemisphere may be especially important for understanding and interpreting music, nonverbal visual experiences such as visual patterns, spatial relationships between the person and the surroundings, and probably also for interpreting many somatic experiences related to use of the limbs and the hands. Thus, even though we speak of the dominant hemisphere, this dominance is primarily for language- or verbal symbolism–related intellectual functions; the opposite hemisphere is actually dominant for some other types of intelligence.

THE PREFRONTAL AREAS

The prefrontal areas are those portions of the frontal lobes that lie anterior to the motor regions, as shown in Figure 36-4. For years, this part of the cortex has been considered to be the locus of the higher intellect of the human being, principally because the main difference between the brains of monkeys and those of human beings is the great prominence of the human prefrontal areas. Yet efforts to show that the prefrontal cortex is more important in higher intellectual functions than other portions of the cortex have not been successful. Indeed, destruction of the posterior temporal lobe (Wernicke's area) and the angular gyrus region in the dominant hemisphere causes infinitely more harm to the intellect than does destruction of both prefrontal areas.

Yet, the prefrontal areas do have some specific functions that are all their own. One of these has to do with control of some types of behavior, especially choice of behavioral options for each social or physical situation. Some of the other possible functions of the prefrontal lobes include:

Prevention of Distractibility—Importance for Sequencing Thoughts. One of the outstanding characteristics of a person who has lost the prefrontal areas is the ease with which he or she can be *distracted* from a sequence of thoughts. Likewise, the ability to concentrate on psychological tests is almost completely lost. The human being without prefrontal areas is still capable of performing many intellectual tasks, such as answering short questions and performing simple arithmetic computations (such as $9 \times 6 = 54$), thus illustrating that the basic intellectual activities of the cerebral cortex are still intact without the prefrontal areas. Yet if concerted *sequences* of cerebral functions are required, the person becomes completely disorganized. Therefore, the prefrontal areas seem to be important in keeping the mental functions directed toward goals.

Elaboration of Thought, Prognostication, and Performance of Higher Intellectual Functions by the Prefrontal Areas. Another function that has been ascribed to the prefrontal areas by psychologists and neurologists is *elaboration of thought*. This means simply an increase in depth and abstractness of the thoughts. Psychological tests have shown that prefrontal lobectomized lower animals presented with successive bits of sensory information fail to store these bits even in temporary memory—probably because the animals are distracted so easily that they cannot hold thoughts long enough for storage to take place. This ability of the prefrontal areas to cause storage—even though it be temporary—of many bits of information simultaneously, and then to cause recall of this information bit by bit as it is needed for subsequent thoughts, could well explain the many functions of the brain that we associate with higher intelligence, such as the abilities to (1) prognosticate, (2) plan for the future, (3) delay action in response to incoming sensory signals so that the sensory infor-

mation can be weighed and the best course of response decided, (4) consider the consequences of motor actions even before these are performed, (5) solve complicated mathematical, legal, or philosophical problems, (6) correlate all avenues of information in diagnosing rare diseases, and (7) control one's activities in accord with moral laws.

Effects of Destruction of the Prefrontal Areas

Human beings without prefrontal areas ordinarily act precipitously in response to incoming sensory signals, such as reacting angrily to slight provocations, but also forgetting the event equally as rapidly. In addition, they are likely to lose many or most of their morals; they have little embarrassment in relation to excretory, sexual, and social activities; and they are prone to quickly changing moods of hate, joy, sadness, exhilaration, and rage. And they lose both ambition and drive toward goals. In short, they are highly *distractible* persons with lack of ability to pursue long and complicated thoughts.

THOUGHTS, CONSCIOUSNESS, AND MEMORY

Our most difficult problem in discussing consciousness, thoughts, memory, and learning is that we do not know the neural mechanism of a thought. We know that destruction of large portions of the cerebral cortex does not prevent a person from having thoughts, but it usually does reduce the *degree* of awareness of the surroundings.

Each thought almost certainly involves simultaneous signals in many portions of the cerebral cortex, thalamus, limbic system, and reticular formation of the brain stem. Some crude thoughts probably depend almost entirely on lower centers; the thought of pain is probably a good example, for electrical stimulation of the human cortex rarely elicits anything more than the mildest degrees of pain, whereas stimulation of certain areas of the hypothalamus and mesencephalon in animals appears to cause excruciating pain. On the other hand, a type of thought pattern that requires mainly the cerebral cortex is that involving vision, because loss of the visual cortex causes complete inability to perceive visual form or color.

Therefore, we might formulate a definition of a thought in terms of neural activity as follows: A thought probably results from the momentary "pattern" of stimulation of many different parts of the nervous system all at the same time, probably involving most importantly the cerebral cortex, the thalamus, the limbic system, and the upper reticular formation of the brain stem. This is called the *holistic theory* of thoughts. The stimulated areas of the limbic system, thalamus, and reticular formation perhaps determine the general nature of the thought, giving it such qualities as pleasure, displeasure, pain, comfort, crude modalities of sensation, localization to gross areas of the body, and other general characteristics. On the other hand, the stimulated areas of the cerebral cortex probably determine the discrete characteristics of the thought such as specific localization of sensations on the body and of objects in the fields of vision, discrete patterns of sensation such as the rectangular pattern of a concrete block wall or the texture of a rug, and other individual characteristics that enter into the overall awareness of a particular instant.

And consciousness can perhaps be described as our continuing stream of awareness of either our surroundings or our sequential thoughts.

MEMORY AND TYPES OF MEMORY

If we accept the above approximation of what constitutes a thought, we can see immediately that the mechanism of memory must be equally as complex as the mechanism of a thought, for, to provide memory, the nervous system must recreate the same spatial and temporal pattern (the "holistic" pattern) of stimulation in the central nervous system at some future date. Though we cannot explain in detail what a memory is, we do know some of the basic psychological and neuronal processes that probably lead to the process of memory.

All of us know that all degrees of memory occur, some memories lasting a few seconds and others lasting hours, days, months, or years. Possibly all these types of memory are caused by the same mechanism operating to different degrees of fulfillment. Yet, it is also possible that different mechanisms of memory do exist. Indeed, most physiologists classify memory into from two to four different types. For the purpose of the present discussion, we will use the following classification:

(1) sensory memory, (2) primary memory, and (3) secondary memory.

The basic characteristics of these types of memory are the following:

Sensory Memory. Sensory memory means the ability to retain sensory signals in the sensory areas of the brain for a very short interval of time following the actual sensory experience. Usually these signals remain available for analysis for several hundred milliseconds but are replaced by new sensory signals in less than one second. Nevertheless, during the short interval of time that the instantaneous sensory information remains in the brain it can continue to be used for further processing; most important, it can be "scanned" to pick out the important points. Thus, this is the initial stage of the memory process.

Primary Memory. Primary memory is the ability to recall facts, words, numbers, letters, or other information for a few seconds to a few minutes at a time. This is typified by a person's memory of the digits in a telephone number for a short period of time after he has looked up the number in the telephone directory. It is also typified by the ability of a person to look at a visual scene, then to turn the head away

and still be able to recall for seconds or a minute or more many features of the scene.

Secondary Memory. Secondary memory is the storage in the brain of information that can be recalled hours, days, months, or years later. This type of memory has been called long-term memory, fixed memory, permanent memory, and several other names. One of its characteristics is that, except when the memory is very deeply engrained, one must "search" through the memory stores for seconds to minutes before it is possible to recall the memory.

PHYSIOLOGICAL BASIS OF MEMORY

Despite the many advances in neurophysiology during the past half century, we still cannot explain what is perhaps the most important function of the brain: its capacity for memory. Yet physiological experiments are beginning to generate conceptual theories of the means by which memory could occur. Some of these are discussed in the following few sections.

Possible Mechanisms for Primary Memory. Primary memory requires a neuronal mechanism that can hold specific information signals for a few seconds to at most a minute or more. Several such mechanisms are the following:

Reverberating Circuit Theory of Primary Memory. When an appropriate tetanizing electrical stimulus is applied directly to the surface of the cerebral cortex and then is removed after a second or more, the local area excited by this stimulus often continues to emit rhythmic action potentials for short periods of time. This effect is believed to result from local reverberating circuits, the signals passing through a multistage circuit of neurons in the local area of the cortex itself or perhaps even back and forth between the cortex and the thalamus.

It is postulated that sensory signals reaching the cerebral cortex can set up similar reverberating oscillations and that these could be the basis for primary memory. Then, as the reverberating circuit fatigues, or as new signals interfere with the reverberations, the primary memory fades away.

One of the principal observations in support of this theory is that any factor that suddenly blocks brain function, such as a blow on the head that causes temporary coma or such as anesthesia, erases the primary memory. The memory cannot be recalled when the disturbance is over unless a portion of this memory had already been placed into the secondary memory store, as discussed in subsequent sections.

Post-Tetanic Potentiation Theory of Primary Memory. In most parts of the nervous system, including even the anterior motor neurons of the spinal cord, tetanic stimulation of a synapse for a few seconds causes a short period of synaptic fatigue for the next few seconds but then increased excitability of the synapse for still another few seconds to a few hours. If during this time of increased excitability the synapse is stimulated again, the neuron responds much more vigorously than normally, a phenomenon called *post-tetanic potentiation*. This obviously is a type of memory that depends on change in the excitability of the synapse, and it could be the basis for primary memory. Recent experiments have shown that post-tetanic potentiation is caused by excessive accumulation of calcium ions in the presynaptic terminals, these ions in turn increasing the release of transmitter substance by the terminals.

Presynaptic Facilitation and Inhibition as Possible Causes of Primary Memory. Many presynaptic terminals of the central nervous system lie on the surfaces of other presynaptic terminals or even on terminal nerve fibrils. When such terminals are stimulated, they can cause either inhibition or facilitation of the secondary terminals, depending on the type of transmitter released. Furthermore, this inhibition or facilitation can last at times for many minutes and perhaps even for an hour or more. Such events are a type of memory, though it still is not known whether this is one of the mechanisms of primary memory.

Mechanism of Secondary Memory— Enhancement of Synaptic Transmission Facility

Secondary memory is the ability of the nervous system to recall thoughts long after initial elicitation of the thoughts is over. We know that secondary memory does not depend on continued activity of the nervous system, because the brain can be totally inactivated by cooling, by general anesthesia, by hypoxia, by ischemia, or by any other method, and yet secondary memories that have been previously stored are still retained when the brain becomes active once again. Therefore, secondary memory must result from some actual alterations of the synapses, either physical or chemical.

Many different theories have been offered to explain the synaptic changes that cause long-term memory. Among the most important of these are:

1. Anatomical Changes in the Synapses. Cajal, almost a century ago, discovered that the number of terminal fibrils ending on neuronal cells and dendrites in the cerebral cortex increases with age. Conversely, physiologists have shown that inactivity of regions of the cortex causes thinning of the cortex: for instance, thinning of the primary visual cortex in animals that have lost their eyesight. Also, intense activity of a particular part of the cortex can cause excessive thickening of the cortical shell in that area alone. Finally, some neuroanatomists have observed electron micrographic changes in presynaptic terminals that have been subjected to intense and prolonged activity.

All these observations have led to a theory that fixation of memories in the brain may result from anatomical changes in the synapses themselves: perhaps changes in numbers of presynaptic terminals, in sizes of the terminals, or in the sizes and conductivities of the dendrites. Such anatomical changes could

cause permanent or semipermanent increase in the degree of facilitation of specific neuronal circuits, thus allowing signals to pass through the circuits with greater ease the more often the memory trace is used.

2. Physical or Chemical Changes in the Presynaptic Terminal or the Postsynaptic Membrane. Recent studies by Kandel and others in the large snail *Aplysia* have uncovered several mechanisms of memory that result from either physical or chemical changes in the presynaptic terminal or possibly even in the entire presynaptic neuron. One such mechanism, illustrated in Figure 36–5, functions in the following way: In this figure there are two separate presynaptic terminals, one of which is from a primary input sensory neuron and terminates on the surface of a secondary neuron that is to be stimulated; this is called the *sensory terminal*. The other presynaptic terminal lies on the surface of the sensory terminal and is called the *facilitator terminal*. When the sensory terminal is stimulated repeatedly but without stimulating the facilitator terminal, signal transmission to the postsynaptic neuron is at first very great, but becomes less and less intense with repeated stimulation until transmission almost ceases. This phenomenon is called *habituation*. It is a type of memory that causes the neuronal circuit to lose its response to repeated events that are insignificant.

On the other hand, if a noxious stimulus excites the facilitator terminal at the same time that the sensory terminal is stimulated, then, instead of the transmitted signal becoming progressively weaker, the ease of transmission becomes much stronger and will remain strong for hours, days, or perhaps weeks even without further stimulation of the facilitator terminal. Thus, the noxious stimulus causes the memory pathway to become facilitated for days or weeks thereafter. It is especially interesting that only a few repeated action potentials are required to cause either habituation or facilitation. However, once habituation has occurred, the synapses can become facilitated very rapidly with only a few noxious stimuli.

At the molecular level, the habituation effect in the sensory terminal results from progressive closure of calcium channels of the terminal membrane, though the cause of this is not fully known. As a result, much less transmitter is released because cal-

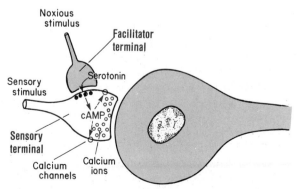

Figure 36–5. A memory system that has been discovered in the snail *Aplysia*.

cium entry at the time of the action potential is the stimulus for transmitter release (as was discussed in Chapter 31).

In the case of facilitation, the molecular mechanism is believed to be the following: Stimulation of the facilitator neuron causes serotonin release at the facilitator synapse on the sensory presynaptic terminal. This in turn, through a series of intermediate effects, eventually blocks the potassium channels, leading to great prolongation of the action potential and consequently to much greater release of synaptic transmitter.

Thus, in an indirect way the associative effect of stimulating the facilitator neuron at the same time that the sensory neuron is stimulated causes a prolonged change in the sensory terminal that produces a long-term memory trace.

Summary. The theory that at present seems most likely to explain secondary memory is that some actual anatomical, physical, or chemical change occurs in the presynaptic terminals or perhaps in whole neurons that permanently facilitate the transmission of impulses at the synapses. If all the synapses are thus facilitated in a thought circuit, this circuit can be re-excited by any one of many diverse signals at later dates, thereby causing memory. The overall facilitated circuit is called a *memory engram,* or a *memory trace.*

Consolidation of Memory

For a primary memory to be converted into a secondary memory that can be recalled days later, it must become "consolidated"—that is, the synapses must become permanently facilitated. This process requires 5 to 10 minutes for minimal consolidation and an hour or more for maximal consolidation. For instance, if a strong sensory impression is made on the brain but is then followed within a minute or so by an electrically induced brain convulsion, the sensory experience will not be remembered at all. Likewise, brain concussion, sudden application of deep general anesthesia, and other effects that temporarily block the dynamic function of the brain can prevent consolidation.

The process of consolidation and the time required for consolidation can probably be explained by the phenomenon of *rehearsal* of the primary memory as follows:

Role of Rehearsal in Transference of Primary Memory into Secondary Memory. Psychological studies have shown that rehearsal of the same information again and again accelerates and potentiates the degree of transfer of primary memory into secondary memory, and therefore also accelerates and potentiates the process of consolidation. The brain has a natural tendency to rehearse newfound information, and especially information that catches the mind's attention. Therefore, over a period of time the important features of sensory experiences become progressively more and more fixed in the secondary memory stores. This explains why a person can remember small amounts of information studied in depth far better than large amounts of information studied only superficially. And it also explains why a person who is wide-awake will consolidate memories far better than will a person who is in a state of mental fatigue.

Codifying of Memories During the Process of Consolidation. One of the most important features of the process of consolidation is that memories to be placed permanently into the secondary memory storehouse are first codified into different classes of information. During this process similar previously stored information is recalled from the secondary storage bins and is used to help process the new information. The new and old are compared for similarities and for differences, and part of the storage process is to store the information about these similarities and differences rather than simply to store the unprocessed information. Thus, during the process of consolidation, the new memories are not stored randomly in the brain but instead are stored in direct association with other memories of the same type. This is obviously necessary if one is to be able to "search" the memory store at a later date to find the required information.

Role of Specific Parts of the Brain in the Memory Process

Role of the Hippocampus for Rehearsal, Codification, and Consolidation of Memories—Anterograde Amnesia Following Hippocampal Lesions. The hippocampus is the most medial portion of the inferior temporal lobe cortex where it folds underneath the brain and then upward into the lower surface of the lateral ventricle. The two hippocampi have been removed for the treatment of epilepsy in a number of patients. This procedure hardly affects the person's memory for information stored in the brain prior to removal of the hippocampi. However, after removal, these persons have very little capability for transferring *verbal and symbolic types* of primary memories into secondary memories. That is, they do not have the ability to separate out the important information, to codify it, to rehearse it, and to consolidate it in the secondary memory store. Therefore, these persons are unable to establish new long-term memories of those types of information that are the basis of intelligence. This is called *anterograde amnesia.*

Retrograde Amnesia. *Retrograde amnesia* means inability to recall memories from the past—that is, from the secondary memory storage bins—even though the memories are known to be still there. When retrograde amnesia occurs, the degree of amnesia for recent events is likely to be much greater than for events of the distant past. The reason for this difference is probably that the distant memories have been rehearsed so many times that elements of these memories are stored in widespread areas of the brain.

In some persons who have hippocampal lesions, some degree of retrograde amnesia usually occurs along with the anterograde amnesia just discussed, which suggests that these two types of amnesia are at least partially related and that hippocampal lesions can cause both. However, it has also been claimed that damage in some thalamic areas can lead specifically to retrograde amnesia without causing significant anterograde amnesia.

FUNCTION OF THE BRAIN IN COMMUNICATION

One of the most important differences between human beings and lower animals is the facility with which human beings can communicate with one another. Therefore, we will review rapidly the function of the cortex in communication; from the review, one can see immediately how the principles of sensory analysis and motor control apply to this art.

There are two aspects to communication: first, the *sensory aspect,* involving the ears and eyes, and, second, the *motor aspect,* involving vocalization and its control.

Sensory Aspects of Communication. We noted earlier in the chapter that destruction of portions of the *auditory* or *visual association areas* of the cortex can result in inability to understand the spoken or the written word. These effects are called, respectively, *auditory receptive aphasia* and *visual receptive aphasia* or, more commonly, *word deafness* and *word blindness* (or *dyslexia*).

Wernicke's Aphasia (Sensory Aphasia). Some persons are perfectly capable of understanding either the spoken word or the written word but are *unable to interpret the thought* that is expressed. This results most frequently when *Wernicke's area* in the *posterior portion of the dominant hemisphere superior temporal gyrus* is damaged or destroyed. Therefore, this type of aphasia is generally called *Wernicke's aphasia,* or frequently, simply sensory aphasia.

When the lesion in Wernicke's area is widespread and extends (a) backward into the angular gyrus region, (b) inferiorly into the lower areas of the temporal lobe, and (c) superiorly into the superior border of the sylvian fissure, the person is said to have *global aphasia,* meaning that he or she is almost totally demented.

Motor Aspects of Communication. The process of speech involves two principal stages of mentation: (1) formation in the mind of thoughts to be expressed and choice of words to be used, then (2) motor control of vocalization and the actual act of vocalization itself. The formation of thoughts and choice of words is the function of the sensory areas of the brain. Again, it is Wernicke's area in the posterior part of the superior temporal gyrus that is most important for this ability. Therefore, persons with either Wernicke's aphasia or global aphasia are unable to formulate the thoughts that are to be communicated. Or, if the lesion is less severe, the person may be able to formulate thoughts but yet be unable to put together the appropriate words to express the thought. Often, a person may be very fluent in speech but the words that are spoken may present a jumbled mass of confusion.

Motor Aphasia. Often a person is perfectly capable of deciding what he wishes to say and is capable of vocalizing but simply cannot make his or her vocal system emit words instead of noises. This effect, called *motor aphasia,* often results from damage to *Broca's speech area,* which lies in the *premotor* facial region of the cortex—about 95 per cent of the time in the left hemisphere, as illustrated in Figures 36–3 and 36–4. Therefore, we assume that the *skilled motor patterns* for control of the larynx, lips, mouth, respiratory system, and other accessory muscles of articulation are all controlled in this area.

Articulation. Finally, we have the act of articulation itself, which means the muscular movements of the mouth, tongue, larynx, and so forth that are responsible for the actual emission of sound. The *facial and laryngeal regions of the motor cortex* activate these muscles, and the *cerebellum, basal ganglia,* and *sensory cortex* all help control the muscle contractions by feedback mechanisms described in Chapter 35. Destruction of these regions can cause either total or partial inability to speak distinctly.

QUESTIONS

1. Describe briefly the physiological anatomy of the cerebral cortex.
2. Review the different areas of the cerebral cortex for which specific functions are known.
3. Draw a map of the cerebral cortex showing the *primary sensory areas* and the *sensory association areas*.
4. On the above map, exactly place *Wernicke's area*. Also show the locus of the *angular gyrus*. What are the functions of Wernicke's area and the angular gyrus?
5. Explain what is meant by the *dominant hemisphere* and explain why it is important to have a single dominant hemisphere.
6. What is the role of language in the function of Wernicke's area?
7. What are some of the important functions of Wernicke's area in the nondominant hemisphere?
8. What are the functions of the *prefrontal areas* of the cerebral cortex, and what happens to a person whose prefrontal areas have been destroyed?
9. Explain the *holistic theory* of thoughts.
10. Explain the characteristics of *sensory memory, primary memory,* and *secondary memory*.
11. Describe the theories for establishment of secondary memory, especially the theory involving the presynaptic terminals.
12. What is meant by *consolidation of memories* and by *codification of memories?*
13. What is the role of the *hippocampus* in the consolidation of memories? How does this relate to *anterograde amnesia?*
14. Explain the differences between *sensory aphasia* and *motor aphasia*.

References

Bindman, L.: The Neurophysiology of the Cerebral Cortex. Austin, University of Texas Press, 1981.

Buchtel, H. A.: The Conceptual Nervous System. New York, Pergamon Press, 1982.

Damasio, A. R., and Geschwind, N.: The neural basis of language. Annu Rev Neurosci 7:127, 1984.

Daniloff, R., et al.: The Physiological Bases of Verbal Communication. Englewood Cliffs, N.J., Prentice-Hall, 1980.

Hixon, T. J., et al., eds.: Introduction to Communicative Disorders. Englewood Cliffs, N.J., Prentice-Hall, 1980.

Klopf, A. H.: The Hedonistic Neuron. A Theory of Memory, Learning, and Intelligence. Washington, D.C., Hemisphere Publishers, 1982.

McCloskey, D. I.: Corollary discharges: motor commands and perception. In Brooks, V. B., ed.: Handbook of Physiology. Sec. 1, Vol. 2. Bethesda, American Physiological Society, 1981, p. 1415.

Mitzdorf, U.: Current source-density method and application in cat cerebral cortex: investigation of evoked potentials and EEG phenomena. Physiol Rev 65:37, 1985.

Moskowitz, B. A.: The acquisition of language. Sci Am 239(5):92, 1978.

Rosenbek, J. C., ed.: Apraxia of Speech. Physiology, Acoustics, Linguistics, Management. San Diego, College-Hill Press, 1984.

Thompson, R. F., et al.: Cellular processes of learning and memory in the mammalian CNS. Annu Rev Neurosci 6:447, 1983.

Trevarthen, C.: Hemispheric specialization. In Darian-Smith, I., ed.: Handbook of Physiology. Sec. 1, Vol. 3. Bethesda, American Physiological Society, 1984, p. 1129.

Truman, J. W.: Cell death in invertebrate nervous systems. Annu Rev Neurosci 7:171, 1984.

Walters, E. T., and Byrne, J. H.: Associative conditioning of single sensory neurons suggests a cellular mechanism for learning. Science 219:405, 1983.

Wong, R. K., et al.: Local circuit interactions in synchronization of cortical neurones. J Exp Biol 112:169, 1984.

37

Activation of the Brain; Wakefulness and Sleep; Behavioral Functions of the Brain

THE RETICULAR ACTIVATING SYSTEM
AND ITS ROLE IN WAKEFULNESS
SPECIFIC NEURONAL SYSTEMS
ASSOCIATED WITH THE RETICULAR
FORMATION
THE GENERALIZED
THALAMOCORTICAL SYSTEM—ITS
POSSIBLE FUNCTION IN ATTENTION
AND IN SEARCHING THE MEMORY
STORE
BRAIN WAVES AND LEVEL OF BRAIN
ACTIVITY
SLEEP
SLOW-WAVE SLEEP
REM SLEEP (PARADOXICAL SLEEP,
DESYNCHRONIZED SLEEP)
BASIC THEORIES OF SLEEP
PHYSIOLOGICAL EFFECTS OF SLEEP
COMA
EPILEPSY

BEHAVIORAL FUNCTIONS OF THE
BRAIN: THE LIMBIC SYSTEM AND THE
ROLE OF THE HYPOTHALAMUS
THE LIMBIC SYSTEM
THE HYPOTHALAMUS, A MAJOR
OUTPUT PATHWAY OF THE LIMBIC
SYSTEM
BEHAVIORAL FUNCTIONS OF THE
LIMBIC SYSTEM
TRANSMISSION OF PSYCHOSOMATIC
EFFECTS THROUGH THE
AUTONOMIC NERVOUS SYSTEM
BEHAVIORAL FUNCTIONS OF THE
AMYGDALA
FUNCTIONS OF THE HIPPOCAMPUS
FUNCTION OF THE LIMBIC CORTEX
FUNCTIONS OF SPECIFIC CHEMICAL
TRANSMITTER SYSTEMS FOR
BEHAVIOR CONTROL

One of the remaining great mysteries of the brain is how the brain controls itself. For instance, what sets the overall level of activity? Also, why do we go to sleep or wake up? And perhaps even more mysterious is how behavior is controlled.

Though the answers to these questions are mainly unknown, glimmers of information are beginning to appear that will at least let us construct plausible, even though questionable, theories about activation of the brain, wakefulness, sleep, and behavior.

THE RETICULAR ACTIVATING SYSTEM AND ITS ROLE IN WAKEFULNESS

Diffuse electrical stimulation in the *mesencephalic and pontile portions of the reticular formation*—an area discussed in Chapter 34 in relation to the motor functions of the nervous system—causes immediate and marked activation of the cerebral cortex and will even cause a sleeping animal to awaken instantaneously. This area is represented in Figure 37–1 by the bold arrow directed upward through the brain stem. Extending upward into the cerebrum from the mesencephalic reticular formation are multiple diffuse pathways that terminate in almost all areas of both the diencephalon and the cerebrum. This entire system is called the *reticular activating system.*

Certain regions of the reticular formation as well as portions of the upward radiating distribution system have discrete anatomical organizations, discrete distribution pathways, and different effects on different parts of the brain—sometimes causing increased

425

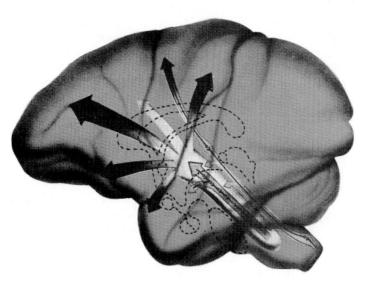

Figure 37–1. The reticular activating system schematically projected on a monkey brain. (From Lindsley: Reticular Formation of the Brain. Little, Brown and Co.)

activity and other times decreased activity. We shall discuss these more specific systems later, but for now let us address the more general functions.

Function of the Mesencephalic Portion of the Reticular Activating System to Cause Wakefulness. Cutting the brain stem in the midpontile region, leaving the mesencephalon and upper pons attached to the cerebrum, causes the cerebrum to become active and to remain active indefinitely as if it remains continuously awake. Therefore, the reticular formation of the mesencephalon and upper pons seems to provide intrinsic activation of the brain. However, as we shall see later, areas in the brain stem below the midlevel of the pons can inhibit this activating system and cause sleep.

Function of the Thalamic Portion of the Activating System. Electrical stimulation in different areas of the thalamic portion of the activating system activates specific regions of the cerebral cortex more than others. This result is distinctly different from stimulation in the mesencephalic portion, which activates large areas of the brain at the same time. Therefore, it is postulated that selective stimulation of portions of the thalamus by the internal signals of the brain might be the cause of specific activation of certain areas of the cerebral cortex in distinction to other areas.

Stimulation of the Reticular Activating System by Nerve Signals from Elsewhere

The reticular activating system itself is subject to stimulation and therefore to increased levels of activation. Also, it is subject to inhibition, which can lead to sleep, as we shall discuss in detail later in the chapter.

Two basic types of stimuli are especially likely to increase the activity of the activating system. These are (1) sensory stimuli from almost any part of the body and (2) retrograde stimuli from the cerebrum,

feeding mainly into the mesencephalic portion of the reticular formation.

Almost any sensory signal entering the nervous system will cause at least some degree of activation of the reticular activating system. However, some signals are much more stimulatory than others, especially pain and proprioceptive somatic impulses, both of which are likely to require some immediate action by the brain. When an animal is asleep and appropriate sensory signals suddenly enter the reticular activating system, this can cause the animal to awaken immediately. This is called the *arousal reaction.*

Stimulation of the reticular activating system by the cerebrum, especially by the cerebral cortex, is mediated through direct fiber pathways into the reticular formation from almost all parts of the cerebrum. An especially large number of nerve fibers pass from the motor regions of the cerebral cortex to the reticular formation; therefore, motor activity in particular is associated with a high degree of reticular activation, which partially explains the importance of moving around when one wishes to remain awake.

SPECIFIC NEURONAL SYSTEMS ASSOCIATED WITH THE RETICULAR FORMATION

As more has been learned about the reticular formation, specific anatomically distinct neuronal systems have been discovered. Four of these have special importance in controlling specific activities of the diencephalon and cerebrum. Illustrated in Figure 37–2, these are

1. *The gigantocellular nucleus of the reticular formation.* This area lies in the medial portions of the reticular formation in the mesencephalon and upper pons. The neurons of this nucleus are very large and their fibers divide immediately into two branches, one passing upward into the higher levels of the brain and the other passing downward through the reticulo-

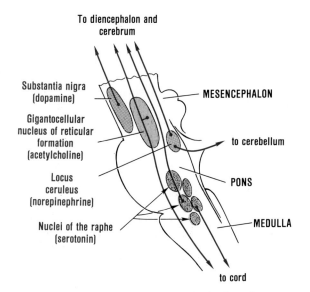

Figure 37–2. Multiple centers in the brain stem, the neurons of which secrete different transmitter substances. These neurons send control signals upward into the diencephalon and cerebrum and downward into the spinal cord.

spinal tracts into the spinal cord. This is a principal activator portion of the reticular activating system.

The neurons of this nucleus release *acetylcholine* at their terminals, and this normally functions as an excitatory transmitter.

2. *The substantia nigra.* This nucleus is discussed in Chapter 35 in relation to the basal ganglia. It lies in the anterior portion of the mesencephalon and contains neuronal cell bodies that secrete *dopamine* at their nerve endings. Fibers from this area pass to the the striatum, the hypothalamus, the cerebral cortex, and the limbic system. The dopamine released at the nerve endings functions in the striatum (the upper part of the basal ganglia) as an inhibitory transmitter, which is perhaps also true in other areas of the brain.

It will be recalled from Chapter 35 that destruction of the dopaminergic neurons in the substantia nigra eliminates their normal inhibitory effect on the striatum, and that is the basic cause of Parkinson's disease.

3. *The locus ceruleus.* This is a small area located bilaterally and posteriorly at the junction point between the mesencephalon and the pons. Nerve fibers from this area secrete norepinephrine. They spread very widely through the diencephalon and the cerebrum, as well as into the cerebellum and lower regions of the brain stem. The norepinephrine released by the endings of these neurons may have either excitatory or inhibitory effects on different structures, depending on the character of the receptors in the postsynaptic neurons. Later in the chapter we shall see that the locus ceruleus probably plays a role in one type of sleep called REM sleep.

4. *The raphe nuclei.* In the midline of the lower pons and medulla are several very thin nuclei called the raphe nuclei. Many of the neurons in these nuclei secrete serotonin, and they send fibers to widespread areas in the diencephalon and also to the spinal cord.

The cord fibers have the capability of suppressing pain, which was discussed in Chapter 33. The serotonin released in the diencephalon and cerebrum almost certainly plays an essential role in causing normal sleep, as we shall discuss later in the chapter.

THE GENERALIZED THALAMOCORTICAL SYSTEM—ITS POSSIBLE FUNCTION IN ATTENTION AND IN SEARCHING THE MEMORY STORE

The thalamus is the entryway for all sensory nervous signals to the cerebral cortex, with the single exception of signals from the olfactory system. Those thalamic nuclei that relay these sensory signals to the cerebral cortex are called the *specific* thalamic nuclei, and this sensory input system to the cerebral cortex is known as the *specific thalamocortical system.*

In addition to the *specific* thalamocortical system, there is a second, separate system called the *generalized thalamocortical system.* This latter system is principally composed of the reticular activating nerve pathway discussed earlier that feeds upward from the thalamus to the cortex. The signals of this pathway are relayed in the thalamus by multiple small diffuse neurons that lie mainly between the specific thalamic nuclei or on the outer surface of the thalamus. Many of these neurons make multiple connections with the specific thalamic nuclei, but especially they project very small fibers to all parts of the cerebral cortex.

Mechanism of Cortical Activation by the Generalized Thalamocortical System. The way in which the generalized thalamocortical system activates the cerebral cortex is entirely different from activation by the specific sensory systems. Some of the differences are the following:

1. Stimulation of a specific thalamic nucleus—such as the ventrobasal complex that transmits somatic signals to the somatic sensory cortex—activates the cortex within 1 to 2 milliseconds, whereas stimulation of the generalized system causes no activation for approximately the first 25 milliseconds. The activation level builds up over a period of many milliseconds.

2. At the end of stimulation, the activation of the cortex by the specific nuclei dies away within another few milliseconds, whereas the activation by the generalized system often continues as an after-discharge for as long as 30 seconds.

3. Signals from the specific nuclei to the cortex activate mainly layer IV of the cortex, whereas activation of the generalized thalamic system activates mainly layers I and II of the cortex. Since this latter activation is prolonged and because layers I and II are the loci of many of the dendrites of the deeper cortical neurons, these circumstances in turn cause a generalized increase in the degree of facilitation of the cortex. When the cortex is thus facilitated, specific signals that enter the cortex from other sources are exuberantly received.

4. Stimulation in the generalized thalamic system *facilitates* an *area* of several square centimeters in the

cortex, while stimulation at a point in a specific thalamic nucleus *excites* a specific point in the cortex.

In summary, the generalized thalamocortical system controls the overall degree of activity of the cortex. It can at times facilitate activity in regional areas of the cortex distinct from the remainder of the cortex.

Possible Mechanisms for Attention and for Searching the Memory Store

We are all aware that we can direct our attention toward certain of our mental activities individually and can also search through our memory store for specific memories. Because of the capability of the generalized thalamocortical system to activate small areas of the cerebral cortex at a time, it is tempting to believe that specific activation of regional portions of the cortex may be the way in which we do indeed direct our attention and may also be the basis for searching through memory stores.

One other bit of information also suggests that the generalized thalamocortical system might be important in searching for memories: It has been reported that specific lesions in the thalamus are sometimes associated with retrograde amnesia—that is, inability to recall memories that are known to be stored within the brain.

BRAIN WAVES AND LEVEL OF BRAIN ACTIVITY

When the brain becomes activated, the neurons exhibit intense electrical activity, and electrical recordings from the surface of the brain or even from the surface of the scalp demonstrate this circumstance. Both the intensity and the patterns of this electrical activity are determined to a great extent by the overall level of excitation of the brain resulting from stimulation by the reticular activating system. The undulations in the recorded electrical potentials shown in Figure 37–3 are called *brain waves,* and the entire record is called an *electroencephalogram* (EEG).

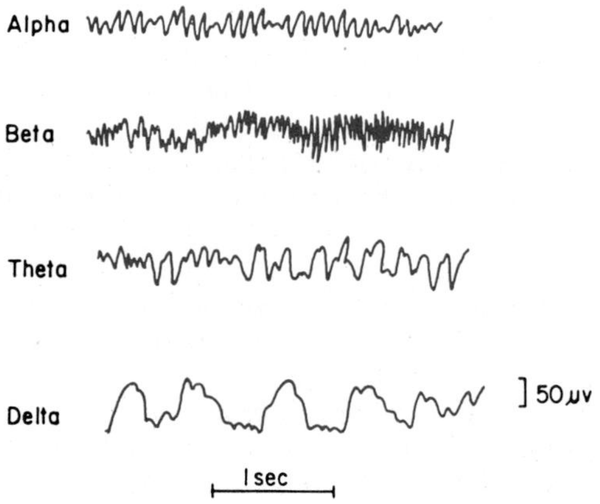

The intensities of the brain waves on the surface of the scalp range from zero to 300 microvolts, and their frequencies range from once every few seconds to 50 or more per second. The character of the waves is highly dependent on the degree of activity of the cerebral cortex, and the waves change markedly among the states of wakefulness, sleep, and coma.

Much of the time, the brain waves are irregular, and no general pattern can be discerned in the EEG. However, at other times, distinct patterns do appear. Some of these are characteristic of specific abnormalities of the brain such as epilepsy, which is discussed later. Others occur even in normal persons and can be classified into *alpha, beta, theta,* and *delta waves,* which are all illustrated in Figure 37–3.

Alpha waves are rhythmic waves occurring at a frequency between 8 and 13 per second and are found in the EEGs of almost all normal persons when they are awake in a quiet, resting state of cerebration. During sleep the alpha waves disappear entirely, and when the awake person's attention is directed to some specific type of mental activity, the alpha waves are replaced by asynchronous, higher frequency but lower voltage waves of the beta type.

Beta waves occur at frequencies of more than 14 cycles per second and as high as 25 and, rarely, 50 cycles per second. Most beta waves appear during *intense* activation of the central nervous system or during tension.

Theta waves have frequencies between 4 and 7 cycles per second. They occur mainly in the parietal and temporal regions in children, and they occur during emotional stress in some adults, particularly during disappointment and frustration. They can often be brought out in the EEG of a frustrated person by allowing him to enjoy some pleasant experience and then suddenly removing this element of pleasure; this often causes approximately 20 seconds of theta waves. These same waves also occur in many brain disorders.

Delta waves include all waves of the EEG below 3½ cycles per second and are sometimes as low as 1 cycle every 2 to 3 seconds. These waves occur in deep sleep, in infancy, and in very serious organic brain disease. And they occur in the cortex of animals that have had subcortical transections separating the cerebral cortex from the thalamus. Therefore, delta waves can occur locally in the cortex independently of activities in lower regions of the brain.

Effects of Varying Degrees of Cerebral Activity on the Basic Rhythm of the Electroencephalogram. There is a general relationship between the degree of cerebral activity and the average frequency of the electroencephalographic rhythm, the frequency increasing progressively with higher degrees of activity. Delta waves, in general, occur in stupor, in surgical anesthesia, and in sleep; theta waves, in psychomotor states and in infants; alpha waves, during relaxed states; and beta waves, during periods of intense mental activity.

Figure 37–3. Different types of normal electroencephalographic waves.

SLEEP

Sleep is defined as a state of unconsciousness from which a person can be aroused by appropriate sensory or other stimuli.

Two Types of Sleep—(1) Slow Wave Sleep and (2) REM Sleep. During each night a person goes through stages of two types of sleep that alternate with each other. These are called (1) *slow wave sleep,* because in this type of sleep the brain waves are very slow, and (2) *REM sleep,* which stands for *rapid eye movement* sleep, because in this type of sleep the eyes undergo rapid movements.

Most of the sleep during each night is of the slow wave variety; this is the deep, restful type of sleep that the person experiences during the first hour of sleep after having been kept awake for many hours. Episodes of REM sleep occur periodically during sleep and occupy about 25 per cent of the sleep time of the young adult; they normally recur about every 90 minutes. This type of sleep is not so restful, and it is usually associated with dreaming, as we shall discuss later.

Electroencephalographic Changes in the Different Stages of Wakefulness and Sleep

Figure 37–4 illustrates the electroencephalogram from a typical person in different stages of wakefulness and sleep. Alert wakefulness is characterized by high frequency *beta waves,* whereas quiet wakefulness is usually associated with *alpha waves,* as illustrated in the figure.

Slow wave sleep is generally divided into four stages. In the first stage, a stage of very light sleep, the voltage of the electroencephalographic waves becomes very low but this is broken by *sleep spindles,* that is, short spindle-shaped bursts of alpha waves that occur periodically. In stages 2, 3, and 4 of slow

Alert wakefulness (beta waves)

Quiet wakefulness (alpha waves)

Stage 1 (low voltage and spindles)

] 50 uv

Stages 2 and 3 (theta waves)

Stage 4 slow wave sleep (delta waves)

REM sleep (beta waves)

|— 1 sec —|

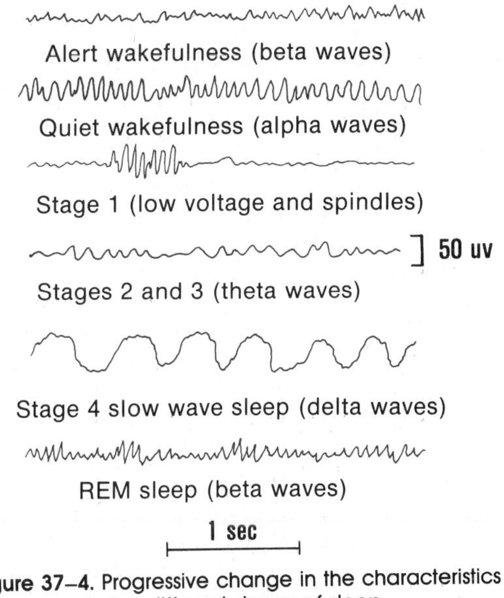

Figure 37–4. Progressive change in the characteristics of the brain waves during different stages of sleep.

wave sleep the frequency of the electroencephalogram becomes progressively slower until it reaches, in stage 4, a frequency of only two to three waves per second; these are typical *delta waves.*

In REM sleep, the electroencephalogram suddenly changes to the characteristics of the early stages of wakefulness, indicating a high level of activity in the brain during this period of sleep.

SLOW WAVE SLEEP

Most of us can understand the characteristics of deep slow wave sleep by remembering the last time that we were kept awake for more than 24 hours and the deep sleep that occurred within 30 minutes to an hour after going to sleep. This sleep is exceedingly restful and is associated with a 10 to 30 per cent decrease in blood pressure, respiratory rate, and basal metabolic rate.

Though slow wave sleep is frequently called dreamless sleep, dreams actually occur very often during slow wave sleep, and nightmares even occur during this type of sleep. However, the difference between the dreams occurring in slow wave sleep and those in REM sleep is that those of REM sleep are remembered whereas those of slow wave sleep usually are not. That is, during slow wave sleep the process of consolidation of the dreams in memory does not occur.

REM SLEEP (PARADOXICAL SLEEP, DESYNCHRONIZED SLEEP)

In a normal night of sleep, bouts of REM sleep lasting 5 to 30 minutes usually appear on an average of every 90 minutes, the first such period occurring 80 to 100 minutes after the person falls asleep. When a person is extremely tired, the duration of each bout of REM sleep is very short, and it may even be absent. On the other hand, as a person becomes more rested through the night, the duration of the REM bouts greatly increases.

There are several important characteristics of REM sleep:

1. It is usually associated with active dreaming.

2. The muscle tone throughout the body is exceedingly depressed, indicating strong inhibition of the spinal projections from the reticular formation of the brain stem.

3. The heart rate and respiration usually become irregular, which is characteristic of the dream state.

4. Despite the extreme inhibition of the peripheral muscles, a few irregular muscle movements occur. These include, in particular, rapid movements of the eyes; this is the origin of the acronym REM, for "rapid eye movements."

5. The electroencephalogram shows a desynchronized pattern of beta waves similar to those that occur during wakefulness. Therefore, this type of sleep is also frequently called *desynchronized sleep,* meaning desynchronized brain waves; it is also called *paradox-*

ical sleep because it is a paradox that a person can still be asleep despite marked activity in the brain.

In summary, REM sleep is a type of sleep in which the brain is quite active. However, the brain activity is not directed toward awareness of one's surroundings.

BASIC THEORIES OF SLEEP

The Active Theory of Sleep. An earlier theory of sleep was that the reticular activating system and other parts of the brain simply fatigued over the period of a waking day and therefore became inactive as a result. This was called the *passive theory of sleep*. However, an important effect quoted earlier in this chapter changed this view to the current belief that sleep most likely is caused by an active inhibitory process. That is, it was discovered that transecting the brain stem in the midpontile region leads to a brain that never goes to sleep. In other words, there seems to be some center or centers located below the midpontile level of the brain stem that actively causes sleep by inhibiting other parts of the brain. This is called the *active theory* of sleep.

Neuronal Centers, Transmitters, and Mechanisms That Can Cause Sleep

The most conspicuous stimulation area for causing almost natural sleep is the *raphe nuclei* in the lower half of the pons and in the medulla. These are a thin sheet of nuclei located in the midline. Nerve fibers from these nuclei spread widely in the reticular formation and also upward into the thalamus and the neocortex, the hypothalamus, and most areas of the limbic cortex. In addition, they extend downward into the spinal cord, terminating in the posterior horns, where they can inhibit incoming pain signals, as was discussed in Chapter 33. It is also known that the endings of fibers from these raphe neurons secrete *serotonin*. Therefore, it is assumed that serotonin is the major transmitter substance associated with production of sleep.

Stimulation of several other regions in the diencephalon can also help promote sleep. These areas include (a) the rostral part of the hypothalamus, mainly in the suprachiasmal area, and (b) an occasional area in the diffuse nuclei of the thalamus.

Effect of Lesions in the Sleep-Promoting Centers. Discrete lesions in the raphe nuclei lead to a high state of wakefulness. This is also true of bilateral lesions in the mediorostral suprachiasmal portion of the anterior hypothalamus. In both instances, the reticular activating system seems to be released from inhibition. Indeed, the lesions of the anterior hypothalamus can sometimes cause such intense wakefulness that the animal actually dies of exhaustion.

Other Possible Transmitter Substances Related to Sleep. Experiments have shown that both the cerebrospinal fluid and the blood of animals that have been kept awake for several days contain a substance or substances that cause sleep when injected into the ventricular system of another animal. One of these substances is a small polypeptide with a molecular weight of less than 500. When cerebrospinal fluid containing this sleep-producing substance or substances is injected into the third ventricle, almost natural sleep occurs within a few minutes, and the animal may then stay asleep for several hours. Therefore, it is possible that prolonged wakefulness causes progressive accumulation of a sleep factor in the brain stem or in the cerebrospinal fluid that leads to sleep.

Possible Causes of REM Sleep

Why slow wave sleep is broken periodically by REM sleep is not understood. However, a lesion in the *locus ceruleus* on each side of the brain stem can reduce REM sleep, and if the lesion includes other contiguous areas of the brain stem, REM sleep can be prevented altogether. Therefore, it has been postulated that when stimulated, the norepinephrine-secreting nerve fibers that originate in the locus ceruleus can activate many portions of the brain. This stimulation theoretically causes the excess activity that occurs in certain regions of the brain in REM sleep, but the signals are not channeled appropriately to cause the normal conscious awareness that is characteristic of the wakefulness state.

The Cycle Between Sleep and Wakefulness

The preceding discussions have merely identified neuronal areas, transmitters, and mechanisms that are related to sleep. However, they have not explained the alternating, reciprocal operation of the sleep-wakefulness cycle. It is quite possible that this is caused by a free-running intrinsic oscillator within the brain stem that cycles back and forth between the sleep centers and areas in the reticular activating system that cause wakefulness.

However, there is much reason to believe that feedback signals from the cerebral cortex and from the peripheral nerve receptors might also play an important role in helping control the sleep-wakefulness rhythm. One reason for this belief is that sensory signals feeding into the reticular activating system will often arouse a person from deep sleep. Also, as explained earlier, stimulation of the cerebral cortex will powerfully stimulate the reticular activating system.

Therefore, a very likely mechanism for the rhythmicity of the sleep-wakefulness cycle is the following:

When the sleep centers are quiescent, the reticular activating system then presumably begins spontaneous activity. This in turn excites both the cerebral cortex and the peripheral nervous system. Next, positive feedback signals return from both these areas to the reticular activating system to arouse it still further. Thus, once the wakefulness state begins, it has a natural tendency to sustain itself.

However, after the brain remains active for many hours, even the neurons within the activating system presumably will fatigue to some extent, and other factors presumably activate the sleep centers. Consequently, the positive feedback cycle between the reticular activating system and the cortex and between the reticular activating system and the periphery will fade, and the inhibitory effects of the sleep centers as well as possible sleep-producing chemical transmitter substances will take over, leading to rapid transition from the wakefulness state to the sleep state.

Then one could postulate that during sleep the excitatory neurons of the reticular activating system gradually become more and more excitable because of the prolonged rest, while the inhibitory neurons of the sleep centers become less excitable, thus leading to a new cycle of wakefulness.

This theory obviously can explain the rapid transitions from sleep to wakefulness and from wakefulness to sleep. It can also explain arousal, the insomnia that occurs when a person's mind becomes preoccupied with a thought, the wakefulness that is produced by bodily activity, and many other conditions that affect a person's state of sleep or wakefulness.

PHYSIOLOGICAL EFFECTS OF SLEEP

Prolonged wakefulness is often associated with progressive malfunction of the mind and also causes abnormal behavioral activities of the nervous system. We are all familiar with the increased sluggishness of thought that occurs toward the end of a prolonged wakeful period, but in addition, a person can become irritable or even psychotic following forced wakefulness for prolonged periods of time.

Therefore, one can assume that sleep in some way not presently understood restores normal sensitivities of and "balance" among the different parts of the central nervous system. This might be likened to the "rezeroing" of electronic analog computers after prolonged use, for all computers of this type gradually lose their base line of operation; it is reasonable to assume that the same effect occurs in the central nervous system, because overuse of some neurons during wakefulness could easily throw all these out of balance with the remainder of the nervous system. Therefore, in the absence of any definitely demonstrated functional value of sleep, we might postulate that the principal value of sleep is to restore the natural balance among the neuronal centers.

Wakefulness and sleep also have moderate effects on the peripheral body. For instance, there is enhanced sympathetic activity during wakefulness and enhanced numbers of impulses to the skeletal musculature to increase muscle tone. Conversely, during sleep, sympathetic activity decreases while parasympathetic activity increases. Therefore, arterial blood pressure falls, pulse rate decreases, skin vessels dilate, activity of the gastrointestinal tract sometimes increases, muscles fall into a mainly relaxed state, and the overall basal metabolic rate of the body falls by 10 to 30 per cent.

COMA

Coma is distinct from sleep in that a person cannot be aroused from coma. In some coma patients all parts of the brain, not just the reticular activating system, are inactivated. In this case, all electrical activity of the brain ceases—that is, the brain waves are said to be "flat." This is the condition called *brain death,* and the person can then remain alive only by being sustained on artificial respiration, administration of nutrition by stomach tube or intravenously, and use of various supportive drugs and fluids to maintain appropriate blood circulation.

Coma can result from any factor that diminishes or stops activity in the mesencephalic portion of the reticular activating system. Such factors can include brain tumors, vascular lesions, infections, pressure on the brain, and so forth.

EPILEPSY

Epilepsy is characterized by uncontrolled excessive activity of either all or a part of the central nervous system. A person who is predisposed to epilepsy has attacks when the basal level of excitability of the nervous system (or of the part that is susceptible to the epileptic state) rises above a certain critical threshold. But as long as the degree of excitability is held below this threshold, no attack occurs.

Two important types of epilepsy are grand mal epilepsy and petit mal epilepsy.

Grand Mal Epilepsy. Grand mal epilepsy is characterized by extreme neuronal discharges originating in the mesencephalic portion of the reticular activating system. These spread throughout the entire central nervous system to the cortex, to the deeper parts of the brain, and even into the spinal cord to cause generalized *convulsions* of the entire body. The grand mal seizure lasts from a few seconds to as a long as three to four minutes and is characterized by post seizure depression of the entire nervous system; the person remains in stupor for one to many minutes after the attack is over and then often remains severely fatigued for many hours thereafter.

The top recording of Figure 37–5 illustrates a typical electroencephalogram from almost any region of the cortex during a grand mal attack. This illustrates that high voltage discharges occur over the entire cortex and have almost the same periodicity as the normal alpha waves. Furthermore, the same type of discharge occurs on both sides of the brain at the same time, illustrating that the origin of the abnormality is in the lower centers of the brain that control the overall activity of the cerebral cortex and not in the cerebral cortex itself.

In experimental animals or even in human beings, grand mal attacks can be initiated by administering neuronal stimulants such as the drug Metrazol, or they can be caused by insulin hypoglycemia or by the passage of alternating electrical currents directly through the brain.

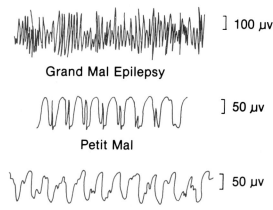

Grand Mal Epilepsy

Petit Mal

Psychomotor

Figure 37–5. Electroencephalograms in different types of epilepsy.

Presumably, a grand mal attack is caused by intrinsic overexcitability of the neurons that make up the mesencephalic portion of the reticular activating system or by some abnormality of the local neuronal circuitry. The discharges from this region could result from local reverberating circuits.

One might ask What stops the grand mal attack after a given time? Cessation is believed to result from (1) *fatigue of the neurons* throughout the brain and (2) *active inhibition* by certain structures of the brain. The stupor and fatigue that occur after a grand mal seizure is over are believed to result from the extreme fatigue of the neurons following their intensive activity during the grand mal attack.

Petit Mal Epilepsy. Petit mal epilepsy is closely allied to grand mal epilepsy in that it too almost certainly originates in the reticular activating system. It is characterized by 3 to 30 seconds of unconsciousness during which the person has several twitchlike contractions of the muscles, usually in the head region—especially blinking of the eyes; this period is followed by return of consciousness and resumption of previous activities. The patient may have one such attack in many months or in rare instances he may have a rapid series of attacks, one following the other. However, the usual course is for the petit mal attacks to appear in late childhood and then to disappear entirely by the age of 30.

The brain wave pattern in petit mal epilepsy is illustrated by the middle record of Figure 37–5, which is typified by a *spike and dome pattern*. The spike portion of this recording is almost identical with the spikes that occur in grand mal epilepsy, but the dome portion is distinctly different. The spike and dome can be recorded over the entire cerebral cortex, illustrating that the seizure originates in the reticular activating system of the brain.

BEHAVIORAL FUNCTIONS OF THE BRAIN: THE LIMBIC SYSTEM AND THE ROLE OF THE HYPOTHALAMUS

Behavior is a function of the entire nervous system, not of any particular portion. Even the discrete cord reflexes are an element of behavior, and the wakefulness and sleep cycle discussed earlier in this chapter is certainly one of the most important of our behavioral patterns. However, in this section we will deal with those special types of behavior associated with emotions, subconscious motor and sensory drives, and the intrinsic feelings of pain and pleasure. These functions of the nervous system are performed mainly by structures located in the basal regions of the brain. This overall group of brain structures is frequently called the *limbic system*.

THE LIMBIC SYSTEM

Figure 37–6 illustrates the anatomical structures of the limbic system, showing them to be an interconnected complex of basal brain elements. Located in the midst of them is the *hypothalamus*, which is considered by many anatomists to be a separate structure from the remainder of the limbic system but which, from a physiological point of view, is one of the central elements of the system. Figure 37–7 illustrates schematically this key position of the hypothalamus in the limbic system and, surrounding it, the other subcortical structures of the limbic system. Notice that surrounding the subcortical structures is the *limbic cortex* composed of a ring of cerebral cortex (1) beginning in the *orbitofrontal area* on the ventral surface of the frontal lobes, (2) extending upward in front of and over the corpus callosum, onto the medial aspect of the cerebral hemisphere to the *cingulate gyrus*, and finally (3) passing posterior to the corpus callosum and downward onto the ventromedial surface of the temporal lobe, to the *hippocampal gyrus, pyriform area*, and *uncus*. Thus, on the medial and ventral surfaces of each cerebral hemisphere is a ring of paleocortex that surrounds a group of deep structures intimately associated with overall behavior and with emotions.

THE HYPOTHALAMUS, A MAJOR OUTPUT PATHWAY OF THE LIMBIC SYSTEM

Note in Figure 37–7 that the hypothalamus lies in the very middle of the limbic system. It also has communicating pathways with all levels of this system. In turn, the hypothalamus and its closely allied structures send output signals in three directions: (1) downward through the brain stem, mainly into the reticular formation of the mesencephalon, pons, and medulla; (2) upward toward many higher areas of the diencephalon and cerebrum, especially the anterior thalamus and the limbic cortex; and (3) into the infundibulum to control most of the secretory functions of both the posterior and anterior pituitary glands.

In summary, the hypothalamus, which represents less than 1 per cent of the brain mass, nevertheless is the most important of all the motor output pathways of the limbic system. It controls most of the vegetative and endocrine functions of the body as well as many aspects of emotional behavior. Let us discuss first the

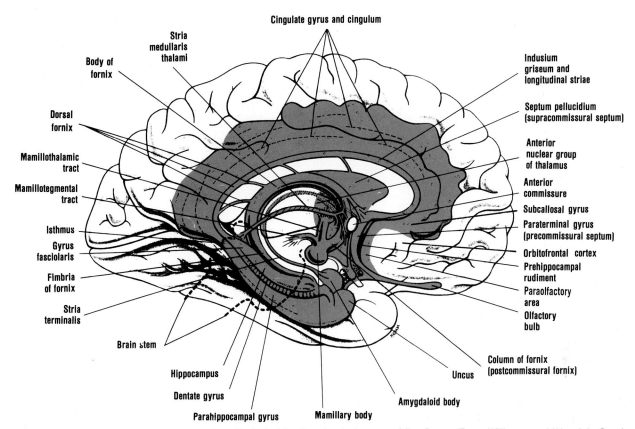

Figure 37–6. Anatomy of the limbic system illustrated by the shaded areas of the figure. (From Williams and Warwick: Gray's Anatomy. 36th Br. ed. London, Longman Group, Ltd., 1980.)

vegetative and endocrine control functions of the hypothalamus and then return to its behavioral functions to see how all these operate together.

Figure 37–8 shows an enlargement of the hypothalamus, which represented only a small area in Figure 37–6. Please take a few minutes to study this diagram, especially to read the multiple functions that are excited or inhibited when respective hypothalamic nuclei are stimulated. Some of these functions include regulation of (1) heart rate and arterial pressure, (2) body temperature, (3) body fluid osmolarity, (4) food

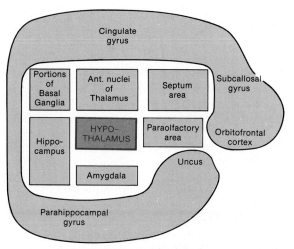

Figure 37–7. The limbic system.

intake, and (5) secretion of the pituitary hormones. Each of these functions is discussed elsewhere in this text in relation to the physiological system it affects.

BEHAVIORAL FUNCTIONS OF THE LIMBIC SYSTEM

Pleasure and Pain: Reward and Punishment

In recent years, it has been learned that many hypothalamic and other limbic structures are particularly concerned with the affective nature of sensory sensations—that is, with whether the sensations are *pleasant* or *painful*. These affective qualities are also called *reward* and *punishment* or *satisfaction* and *aversion*. Electrical stimulation of certain regions pleases or satisfies the animal, whereas electrical stimulation of other regions causes extreme pain, fear, defense, escape reactions, and all the other elements of punishment. Obviously, these two oppositely responding systems greatly affect the behavior of the animal.

Reward Centers. Figure 37–9 illustrates a technique that has been used for localizing the specific reward and punishment areas of the brain. In this technique a lever is placed at the side of the cage and is arranged so that depressing the lever makes electrical contact with a stimulator. Electrodes are placed successively in different areas in the brain so that the animal can stimulate the area by pressing the lever.

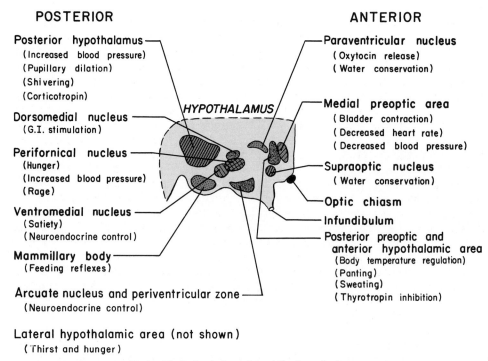

POSTERIOR   ANTERIOR

Posterior hypothalamus
(Increased blood pressure)
(Pupillary dilation)
(Shivering)
(Corticotropin)

Dorsomedial nucleus
(G.I. stimulation)

Perifornical nucleus
(Hunger)
(Increased blood pressure)
(Rage)

Ventromedial nucleus
(Satiety)
(Neuroendocrine control)

Mammillary body
(Feeding reflexes)

Arcuate nucleus and periventricular zone
(Neuroendocrine control)

HYPOTHALAMUS

Paraventricular nucleus
(Oxytocin release)
(Water conservation)

Medial preoptic area
(Bladder contraction)
(Decreased heart rate)
(Decreased blood pressure)

Supraoptic nucleus
(Water conservation)

Optic chiasm

Infundibulum

Posterior preoptic and
anterior hypothalamic area
(Body temperature regulation)
(Panting)
(Sweating)
(Thyrotropin inhibition)

Lateral hypothalamic area (not shown)
(Thirst and hunger)

Figure 37–8. Control centers of the hypothalamus.

If stimulating the particular area gives the animal a sense of reward, then the animal will quickly learn to press the lever again and again, sometimes as much as 10,000 times per hour. Furthermore, when offered the choice of eating some delectable food or stimulating the reward center, the animal often chooses the electrical stimulation.

By use of this procedure, the major reward centers have been found to be located *along the course of the medial forebrain bundle*, especially *in the lateral* and *ventromedial nuclei of the hypothalamus*. Less potent reward centers, which are probably secondary to the major ones in the hypothalamus, are found in the septum, the amygdala, certain areas of the thalamus and basal ganglia, and, finally, extending downward into the basal tegmentum of the mesencephalon.

Punishment Centers. The apparatus illustrated in Figure 37–9 can also be connected so that pressing the lever *turns off* rather than turns on the electrical stimulus. In this case, the animal will not turn the stimulus off when the electrode is in one of the reward areas, but when it is in certain other areas he immediately learns to turn it off. Stimulation in these areas causes the animal to show all the signs of displeasure, fear, terror, and punishment. Furthermore, prolonged stimulation for 24 hours or more can cause the animal to become severely sick and can actually lead to death.

By means of this technique, the principal centers for punishment and escape tendencies have been found in the *central gray area surrounding the aqueduct of Sylvius in the mesencephalon* and extending upward into the *periventricular structures of the hypothalamus and thalamus*.

It is particularly interesting that stimulation in the punishment centers can frequently inhibit the reward and pleasure centers completely, illustrating that pain can take precedence over pleasure and reward.

Importance of Reward and Punishment in Behavior. Almost everything that we do depends on reward or punishment. If we are doing something that is rewarding, we continue to do it; if it is punishing, we cease to do it. Therefore, the reward and punishment centers undoubtedly constitute one of the most important of all the controllers of our bodily activities, our motivations, and so forth.

Importance of Reward and Punishment in Learning and Memory—Habituation or Reinforcement. Ani-

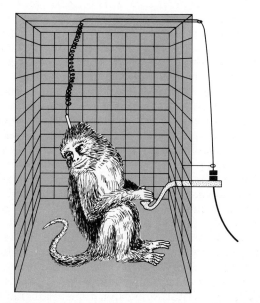

Figure 37–9. Technique for localizing reward and punishment centers in the brain of a monkey.

mal experiments have shown that a sensory experience causing neither reward nor punishment is remembered hardly at all. Electrical recordings have shown that new and novel sensory stimuli always excite the cerebral cortex. But repetition of the stimulus over and over leads to almost complete extinction of the cortical response if the sensory experience does not elicit either a sense of reward or punishment. Thus, the animal or human being becomes *habituated* to the sensory stimulus, and thereafter ignores it.

However, if the stimulus causes either reward or punishment rather than indifference, the cortical response becomes progressively more intense with repetitive stimulation instead of fading away, and the response is said to be *reinforced*. Thus, an animal builds up strong memory traces for sensations and thoughts that are either rewarding or punishing but, on the other hand, develops complete habituation to indifferent sensory stimuli. Therefore, it is evident that the reward and punishment centers of the limbic system have much to do with selecting the information that we learn.

Effect of Tranquilizers on the Reward and Punishment Centers. Administration of a tranquilizer, such as chlorpromazine, inhibits both the reward and punishment centers, thereby greatly decreasing the affective reactivity of the animal. Therefore, it is presumed that tranquilizers function in psychotic states by suppressing many of the important behavioral areas of the hypothalamus and its associated regions of the brain.

Rage

An emotional pattern that involves the hypothalamus and has been well characterized is the *rage pattern*. This can be described as follows:

Stimulation of the punishment centers of the brain, especially the *periventricular areas of the hypothalamus*, which are also the hypothalamic regions that give the most intense sensation of punishment, causes the animal to (1) develop a defense posture, (2) extend its claws, (3) lift its tail, (4) hiss, (5) spit, (6) growl, and (7) develop piloerection, wide-open eyes, and dilated pupils. Furthermore, even the slightest provocation causes an immediate, savage attack. This is approximately the behavior that one would expect from an animal being severely punished, and it is the pattern of behavior called *rage*.

Placidity and Tameness. Exactly the opposite emotional behavioral pattern—placidity and tameness—occurs when the reward centers are stimulated.

TRANSMISSION OF PSYCHOSOMATIC EFFECTS THROUGH THE AUTONOMIC NERVOUS SYSTEM

Many psychosomatic abnormalities result from stimulation of either the sympathetic or parasympathetic system by the hypothalamus and other portions of the limbic system. The usual effects of sympathetic hyperactivity are (1) increased heart rate—sometimes with palpitation of the heart, (2) increased arterial pressure, (3) constipation, and (4) increased metabolic rate. On the other hand, parasympathetic signals are likely to be much more focal. For instance, signals transmitted to specific areas in the dorsal motor nuclei of the vagus nerves can cause more or less specifically (1) increased or decreased heart rate and palpitation of the heart, (2) esophageal spasm, (3) increased peristalsis in the upper gastrointestinal tract, or (4) increased hyperacidity of the stomach with resultant development of peptic ulcer. Stimulation of the sacral region of the parasympathetic system, on the other hand, is likely to cause extreme colonic glandular secretion and peristalsis with resulting diarrhea. One can readily see, then, that emotional patterns controlling the sympathetic and parasympathetic centers of the hypothalamus can cause wide varieties of peripheral psychosomatic effects.

BEHAVIORAL FUNCTIONS OF THE AMYGDALA

The amygdala is a complex of nuclei located in the pole of each temporal lobe of the cerebral cortex. It receives impulses from all portions of the limbic cortex—from the orbital surfaces of the frontal lobes, from the cingulate gyrus, and from the hippocampal gyrus. In turn, the amygdala transmits signals (1) back into these same cortical areas, (2) into the hippocampus, (3) into the septum, (4) into the thalamus, and especially (5) into the hypothalamus.

Effects of Stimulating the Amygdala. In general, stimulation of the amygdala can cause almost all the same effects as those elicited by stimulation of the hypothalamus, plus still other effects, including (1) tonic movements, such as raising the head or bending the body, (2) circling movements, (3) occasionally, clonic, rhythmic movements, and (4) different types of movements associated with olfaction and eating, such as licking, chewing, and swallowing. And stimulation can alter respiration or at other times stop all movements of an animal, freezing the animal in its present postural state, a phenomenon called the *arrest reaction*.

In addition, stimulation of certain amygdaloid nuclei can rarely cause a pattern of rage, of escape, of being punished, and of pain similar to the rage pattern elicited from the hypothalamus as described above. And stimulation of other nuclei can give reactions of reward and pleasure.

Finally, excitation of still other portions of the amygdala can cause sexual activities that include erection, copulatory movements, ejaculation, ovulation, uterine activity, and premature labor.

In short, stimulation of appropriate portions of the amygdaloid nuclei can produce almost any pattern of behavior. It is believed that the normal function of the amygdaloid nuclei is to help control the overall pattern of behavior demanded for each social or environmental occasion.

FUNCTIONS OF THE HIPPOCAMPUS

The hippocampus is an elongated structure composed of a modified type of cerebral cortex. It folds inward from the basomedial surface of the temporal lobe to form the ventral surface of the inferior horn of the lateral ventricle. One end of the hippocampus abuts against the amygdaloid nuclei, and it also fuses along one of its borders with the hippocampal gyrus, which is the cortex of the ventromedial surface of the temporal lobe. The hippocampus has numerous connections with almost all parts of the limbic system, including especially the amygdala, the hippocampal gyrus, the cingulate gyrus, the hypothalamus, and other areas closely related to the hypothalamus.

One of the most remarkable effects of hippocampal stimulation in the conscious human being is immediate *loss of contact* with any person with whom he might be talking, indicating that the hippocampus can play a role in determining a person's attention.

A special feature of the hippocampus is that weak electrical stimuli can cause local epileptic seizures in this region. These seizures cause various psychomotor effects including olfactory, visual, auditory, tactile, and other types of hallucinations that are uncontrollable even though the person has not lost consciousness and knows the hallucinations to be unreal.

Theoretical Function of the Hippocampus in Learning. The hippocampus originated as part of the olfactory cortex. In the very lowest animals, it plays essential roles in such decisions as whether the animal will eat a particular food, whether the smell of a particular object suggests danger, whether the odor is sexually inviting, and in other decisions that are of life and death importance. Thus, very early in the development of the brain, the hippocampus presumably became a critical decision-making neuronal mechanism, determining the importance and type of incoming sensory signals. Presumably, as the remainder of the brain developed, the connections from the other sensory areas into the hypothalamus continued to utilize this decision-making capability.

Earlier in the chapter, it was pointed out that reward and punishment play a major role in determining whether or not the information will be stored in memory. A person rapidly becomes habituated to indifferent stimuli but learns assiduously any sensory experience that causes either pleasure or punishment. Yet what is the mechanism by which this occurs? It has been suggested that the hippocampus acts as the area responsible for causing the translation of primary memory into long-term, secondary memory—that is, it transmits an additional signal to the long-term memory storage area directing that storage take place.

Whatever the mechanism, without the hippocampi *consolidation* of most long-term memories does not take place. This is especially true for verbal information, perhaps because the temporal lobes, in which the hippocampi are located, are particularly concerned with verbal information.

FUNCTION OF THE LIMBIC CORTEX

Probably the most poorly understood portion of the entire limbic system is the ring of cerebral cortex, called the *limbic cortex*, that surrounds the subcortical limbic structures. The limbic cortex is among the oldest of all parts of the cerebral cortex. In lower animals it plays a major role in various olfactory, gustatory, and feeding phenomena. However, in the human being, these functions of the limbic cortex are of minor importance. Instead, the limbic cortex of the human being is believed to be the cerebral association cortex for control of the lower centers that have to do primarily with behavior.

Yet we find ourselves still perplexed regarding the function of the cortical regions of the limbic system. The probable reason is that these regions correlate information from many sources but cause no direct, overt effects that can be observed objectively. Thus, in the insular and anterior temporal cortex we find gustatory and olfactory associations that affect behavior. In the hippocampal gyrus, there is a tendency for auditory associations with behavior. In the cingulate cortex, there is some reason to believe that sensorimotor control of behavior occurs. And, finally, the orbitofrontal cortex presumably acts as a bridge between behavior and the analytical functions of the prefrontal lobes.

Therefore, until further information is available, it is perhaps best to state that the cortical regions of the limbic system occupy intermediate associative positions between the functions of the remainder of the cerebral cortex and the functions of the lower centers for control of behavioral patterns. Thus, thoughts or other stimuli that spill over into portions of the limbic cortex can probably elicit almost any type of behavior that is appropriate for the occasion.

FUNCTIONS OF SPECIFIC CHEMICAL TRANSMITTER SYSTEMS FOR BEHAVIOR CONTROL

In several chapters it has already been pointed out that certain special collections of neurons in the brain stem radiate to multiple areas of the forebrain, each releasing a specific chemical transmitter substance. Three of these special chemical transmitter systems have received particular attention as behavior modifiers; these are the norepinephrine system, the serotonin system, and the dopamine system.

The Norepinephrine and Serotonin Systems and Their Relationship to Depression and to Manic-Depressive Psychoses. Earlier in the chapter it was pointed out that large numbers of *norepinephrine-secreting neurons* are located in the reticular formation, especially in the *locus ceruleus*, and that these send fibers upward to most parts of the limbic system, the thalamus, and cerebral cortex. Also, many *serotonin-producing neurons* are located in the *midline* *raphe nuclei* of the lower pons and medulla and also project fibers to many areas of the limbic system and to some other areas of the brain as well.

In the past few years, much evidence has accumulated to show that the psychosis called *depression*, which afflicts about 8 million people in the United States at any one time, might be caused by diminished formation of either norepinephrine or serotonin or both. These patients experience symptoms of grief, unhappiness, despair, and misery. In addition, they lose their appetite and sex drive and also have severe insomnia. And associated with all these is a state of psychomotor agitation despite the depression.

A principal reason for believing that depression is caused by diminished activity of the norepinephrine and serotonin systems is that drugs that block the secretion of norepinephrine and serotonin, such as the drug *reserpine*, frequently cause depression. Conversely, about 70 per cent of depressive patients can be treated very effectively with one of two types of drugs that increase norepinephrine and serotonin at the nerve endings: (1) *monoamine oxidase inhibitors* that block destruction of norepinephrine and serotonin once they are formed, and (2) *tricyclic antidepressants* that block re-uptake of norepinephrine and serotonin by the nerve endings so that these transmitters remain active for longer periods of time after secretion.

Some patients with depression alternate between depression and mania, which is called the *manic-depressive psychosis*, and a few persons exhibit only mania without the depressive episodes. Drugs that block the formation or action of norepinephrine and serotonin, such as lithium compounds, can be effective in treating the manic condition.

Therefore, it is presumed that the norepinephrine and serotonin systems normally function to provide motor drive to the limbic system to increase a person's sense of well being, to create happiness, contentment, good appetite, appropriate sex drive, and psychomotor balance, though too much of a good thing can cause mania.

The Dopamine System and Its Relationship to Schizophrenia. There are many reasons to believe that schizophrenia might be caused by excess secretion of dopamine in the brain. In Chapter 35 we discussed the dopaminergic neurons that project from the substantia nigra to the basal ganglia and exert an important inhibitory restraint on basal ganglial activity. In addition to the dopaminergic neurons in the substantia nigra, still other dopaminergic neurons are located in the ventral tegmentum of the mesencephalon medial and superior to the substantia nigra. These neurons give rise to the so-called *mesolimbic dopaminergic system* that projects nerve fibers mainly into the medial and anterior portions of the limbic system, especially into the amygdala, the anterior caudate nucleus, and the anterior cingulate gyrus of the cortex, all of which are powerful behavioral control centers.

Some of the reasons for believing the mesolimbic dopaminergic system to be related to schizophrenia are the following: When Parkinson's disease patients are treated with L-dopa, which releases dopamine in the brain, the parkinsonian patient sometimes develops schizophrenic symptoms, indicating that excess dopaminergic activity can cause dissociation of a person's drives and thought patterns. However, an even more compelling reason for believing that schizophrenia might be caused by excess production of dopamine is that those drugs that are effective in treating schizophrenia, such as *chlorpromazine* and *haloperidol*, all decrease the secretion of dopamine by the dopaminergic nerve endings or decrease the effect of dopamine on the subsequent neurons.

Almost certainly there are other factors in schizophrenia besides excess secretion of dopamine, but the symptoms of schizophrenia are nevertheless believed to be similar to the behavioral effects of excessive dopamine, as follows: (1) a sense of persecution from outside sources, (2) hearing voices, (3) incoherent speech, (4) dissociation of ideas and abnormal sequences of thought, and (5) sometimes abnormal postures or rigidities.

QUESTIONS

1. Describe the reticular activating system and tell how it causes wakefulness.
2. How does function of the *mesencephalic portion* of the *reticular activating system* differ from function of the *thalamic portion*?
3. Explain the *arousal reaction*.
4. What is the difference between the function of the *generalized* thalamocortical system and the *specific* thalamocortical system?
5. Explain how the thalamic portion of the reticular activating system may function in the phenomenon of attention and in searching the memory store.
6. What are the four major types of brain waves, and what are the characteristics of each?
7. Describe the successive changes in the brain waves as one passes through all stages of wakefulness and sleep.
8. Characterize *slow wave sleep*.
9. How does *REM sleep* differ from slow wave sleep?
10. Describe the function of the *serotonin-secreting neurons* of the raphe nuclei and their role in causing sleep.
11. What is the role of the *locus ceruleus* and its norepinephrine-secreting nerve fibers in causing REM sleep?
12. Explain, theoretically, the cycling process between wakefulness and sleep.

13. What are the physiological effects of sleep?
14. How does *coma* differ from sleep?
15. Characterize *grand mal epilepsy*, and explain what stops an epileptic attack.
16. Characterize *petit mal epilepsy*.
17. Explain what is meant by the *limbic system*, and describe, in general, its anatomy.
18. List the control functions of the various hypothalamic nuclei that have to do with behavior.
19. Explain the principle of *reward* and *punishment centers* in the hypothalamus and other portions of the limbic system.
20. What are the roles of reward and punishment in learning and memory? How does the *hippocampus* fit into this scheme?
21. How does the *amygdala* help to control the pattern of behavior demanded for each social occasion?
22. Explain the association function of the *limbic cortex* in behavioral control.
23. What are the relationships of the norepinephrine and serotonin systems to *depression* and *manic-depressive psychoses*?
24. What is the relationship of the dopamine system to *schizophrenia*?

References

Activation of the Brain; Wakefulness and Sleep

Block, G. D., and Page,T. L.: Circadian pacemakers in the nervous system. Annu Rev Neurosci 1:19, 1978.
Enright, J. T.: The Timing of Sleep and Wakefulness: on the Substructure and Dynamics of the Circadian Pacemakers Underlying the Wake-Sleep Cycle. New York, Springer-Verlag, 1979.
Fuller, R. W.: Pharmacology of central serotonin neurons. Annu Rev Pharmacol Toxicol 20:111, 1980.
Hobson, J. A., and Brazier, M. A. B., eds.: The Reticular Formation Revisited: Specifying Function for a Nonspecific System. New York, Raven Press, 1980.
Jones, E. G.: Organization of the thalamocortical complex and its relation to sensory processes. In Darian-Smith, I., ed.: Handbook of Physiology. Sec. 1, Vol. 3. Bethesda, American Physiological Society, 1984, p. 149.
Klee, M., ed.: Physiology and Pharmacology of Epileptogenic Phenomena. New York, Raven Press, 1982.
Mitzdorf, U.: Current source-density method and application in cat cerebral cortex; investigation of evoked potentials and EEG phenomena. Physiol Rev 65:37, 1985.
Plum, F., and Posner, J. B.: The Diagnosis of Stupor and Coma, 3rd ed. Philadelphia, F. A. Davis, 1980.
Tucek, S.: Regulation of acetylcholine synthesis in the brain. J Neurochem 44:11, 1985.

Behavioral Functions

Berger, P. A., et al.: Behavioral pharmacology of the endorphins. Annu Rev Med 33:397, 1982.
Burchfield, S. R., ed.: Stress, Physiological and Psychological Interactions. Washington, D.C., Hemisphere Publishing Corp., 1985.
Buzsaki, G.: Feed-forward inhibition in the hippocampal formation. Prog Neurobiol 22:131, 1984.
Cohen, D. H., and Randall, D. C.: Classical conditioning of cardiovascular responses. Annu Rev Physiol 46:187, 1984.
Engel, B. T., and Schneiderman, N.: Operant conditioning and the modulation of cardiovascular function. Annu Rev Physiol 46:199, 1984.
Foote, S. L., et. al.: Nucleus locus ceruleus: new evidence of anatomical and physiological specificity. Physiol Rev 63:844, 1983.
Fuller, R. W.: Pharmacology of brain epinephrine neurons. Annu Rev Pharmacol Toxicol 22:31, 1982.
Givens, J. R.: The Hypothalamus in Health and Disease. Chicago, Year Book Medical Publishers, 1984.
Iversen, L. L.: Nonopioid neuropeptides in mammalian CNS. Annu Rev Pharmacol Toxicol 230:1, 1984.
Lechtenberg, R.: Psychiatrist's Guide to Diseases of the Nervous System. New York, John Wiley & Sons, 1982.
McFadden, D., ed.: Neural Mechanisms in Behavior. New York, Springer-Verlag, 1980.
Russell, R. W.: Cholinergic system in behavior: the search for mechanisms of action. Annu Rev Pharmacol Toxicol 22:435, 1982.
Smith, O. A., and DeVito, J. L.: Central neural integration for the control of autonomic responses associated with emotion. Annu Rev Neurosci 7:43, 1984.
Stephenson, R. B.: Modification of reflex regulation of blood pressure by behavior. Annu Rev Physiol 46:133, 1984.
Swanson, L. W., and Sawchenko, P. E.: Hypothalamic integration: organization of the paraventricular and supraoptic nuclei. Annu Rev Neurosci 6:269, 1983.
Usdin, E.: Stress, The Role of Catecholamines and Other Neurotransmitters, New York, Gordon Press Publishers, 1984.
Verrier, R. L., and Lown, B.: Behavioral stress and cardiac arrhythmias. Annu Rev Physiol 46:155, 1984.

38

The Autonomic Nervous System; The Adrenal Medulla

GENERAL ORGANIZATION OF THE
AUTONOMIC NERVOUS SYSTEM
*PHYSIOLOGICAL ANATOMY OF THE
SYMPATHETIC NERVOUS SYSTEM*
*PHYSIOLOGICAL ANATOMY OF THE
PARASYMPATHETIC NERVOUS
SYSTEM*
BASIC CHARACTERISTICS OF
SYMPATHETIC AND
PARASYMPATHETIC FUNCTIONS
*CHOLINERGIC AND ADRENERGIC
FIBERS—SECRETION OF
ACETYLCHOLINE OR
NOREPINEPHRINE AT THE
POSTGANGLIONIC NERVE
ENDINGS*
*RECEPTORS OF THE EFFECTOR
ORGANS*
*EXCITATORY AND INHIBITORY
ACTIONS OF SYMPATHETIC AND*

PARASYMPATHETIC STIMULATION
*EFFECTS OF SYMPATHETIC AND
PARASYMPATHETIC STIMULATION
ON SPECIFIC ORGANS*
*FUNCTION OF THE ADRENAL
MEDULLAE*
*SYMPATHETIC AND
PARASYMPATHETIC TONE*
STIMULATION BY THE SYMPATHETIC
AND PARASYMPATHETIC SYSTEMS OF
DISCRETE ORGANS IN SOME
INSTANCES, MASS STIMULATION IN
OTHER INSTANCES
*ALARM OR STRESS FUNCTION OF
THE SYMPATHETIC NERVOUS
SYSTEM*
*MEDULLARY, PONTINE, AND
MESENCEPHALIC CONTROL OF
THE AUTONOMIC NERVOUS
SYSTEM*

The portion of the nervous system that controls the visceral functions of the body is called the *autonomic nervous system*. This system helps to control arterial pressure, gastrointestinal motility and secretion, sweating, body temperature, and many other activities, some of which are controlled almost entirely by the autonomic nervous system and some only partially.

GENERAL ORGANIZATION OF THE AUTONOMIC NERVOUS SYSTEM

The autonomic nervous system is activated mainly by centers located in the *spinal cord, brain stem,* and *hypothalamus*. Also, all of the limbic system can transmit signals to the lower brain centers and in this way influence autonomic control. Often the auto-

nomic nervous system operates by means of *autonomic reflexes*. That is, sensory signals from peripheral nerve receptors send signals into the centers of the cord, brain stem, or hypothalamus, and these in turn transmit appropriate reflex responses back to the peripheral organs or tissues to control their activities.

The autonomic signals are transmitted to the body through two major subdivisions, called the *sympathetic* and *parasympathetic systems,* the characteristics and functions of which follow.

PHYSIOLOGICAL ANATOMY OF THE SYMPATHETIC NERVOUS SYSTEM

Figure 38–1 illustrates the general organization of the sympathetic nervous system, showing one of the two *sympathetic chains* found respectively on each side of the spinal column, with nerves extending to

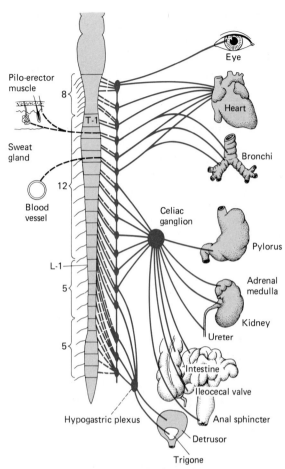

Figure 38–1. The sympathetic nervous system. Dashed lines represent postganglionic fibers in the gray rami leading into the spinal nerves for distribution to blood vessels, sweat glands, and piloerector muscles.

the different internal organs. The sympathetic nerves originate in the spinal cord between the segments T-1 and L-2.

Preganglionic and Postganglionic Sympathetic Neurons. The sympathetic nerves are different from skeletal motor nerves in the following way: Each skeletal motor pathway to a skeletal muscle is composed of a single fiber originating in the cord. In contrast, each sympathetic pathway is composed of two successive fibers, a *preganglionic fiber* and a *postganglionic fiber.* The cell body of the preganglionic fiber lies in the intermediolateral horn of the spinal cord and then passes through an *anterior root* of the cord into a *spinal nerve.* After traveling for a few centimeters with the spinal nerve, the preganglionic fiber leaves the nerve and passes to a *ganglion* of the *sympathetic chain,* illustrated in red to the right of the spinal cord in Figure 38–1. Here the fiber either synapses immediately with postganglionic neurons or, often, passes on through the chain into one of its radiating nerves to synapse with postganglionic neurons in an outlying sympathetic ganglion. The postganglionic neuron then gives rise to a nerve fiber that travels to its destination in one of the organs.

Many of the postganglionic fibers in the sympathetic chain pass back into the spinal nerves at all levels of the cord. These fibers extend to all parts of the body in the spinal nerves. They control the blood vessels, sweat glands, and piloerector muscles of the hairs.

Segmental Distribution of Sympathetic Nerves. The sympathetic fibers originating in the different segments of the spinal cord are not necessarily distributed to that same local area of the body. Instead, the *sympathetic fibers from T-1 generally pass up the sympathetic chain into the head; from T-2 into the neck; from T-3, T-4, T-5, and T-6 into the thorax; from T-7, T-8, T-9, T-10, and T-11 into the abdomen; from T-12, L-1 and L-2, into the legs.*

The distribution of sympathetic nerves to each organ is determined partly by the position in the embryo at which the organ originates. For instance, the heart receives many sympathetic nerves from the neck portion of the sympathetic chain because the heart originates in the neck of the embryo. Likewise, the abdominal organs receive their sympathetic innervation from the lower thoracic segments because the primitive gut originates in the lower thoracic area.

Special Nature of the Sympathetic Nerve Endings in the Adrenal Medullae. Preganglionic sympathetic nerve fibers pass without synapsing all the way from the intermediolateral horn cells of the spinal cord, through the sympathetic chains, through the splanchnic nerves, and finally into the adrenal medullae. There they end directly on special cells that *secrete epinephrine* and *norepinephrine.* These secretory cells are embryologically derived from nervous tissue and are analogous to postganglionic neurons; indeed, they even sprout rudimentary nerve fibers.

PHYSIOLOGICAL ANATOMY OF THE PARASYMPATHETIC NERVOUS SYSTEM

The parasympathetic nervous system is illustrated in Figure 38–2, which shows that parasympathetic fibers leave the central nervous system through several of the cranial nerves as well as through the second and third sacral spinal nerves, and occasionally through the first and fourth sacral nerves as well. About 75 per cent of all parasympathetic nerve fibers are in the *vagus nerves* (also called the *tenth cranial nerves*), passing to the entire thoracic and abdominal regions of the body. The vagus nerves supply parasympathetic nerves to the heart, the lungs, the esophagus, the stomach, the small intestine, the proximal half of the colon, the liver, the gallbladder, the pancreas, and the upper portions of the ureters.

Parasympathetic fibers in the *third cranial nerve* flow to the pupillary sphincters and ciliary muscles of the eye. Fibers from the *seventh cranial nerve* pass to the lacrimal, nasal, and submandibular glands, and fibers from the *ninth cranial nerve* pass to the parotid gland.

The sacral parasympathetic fibers combine to form the *nervi erigentes,* which leave the sacral plexus on

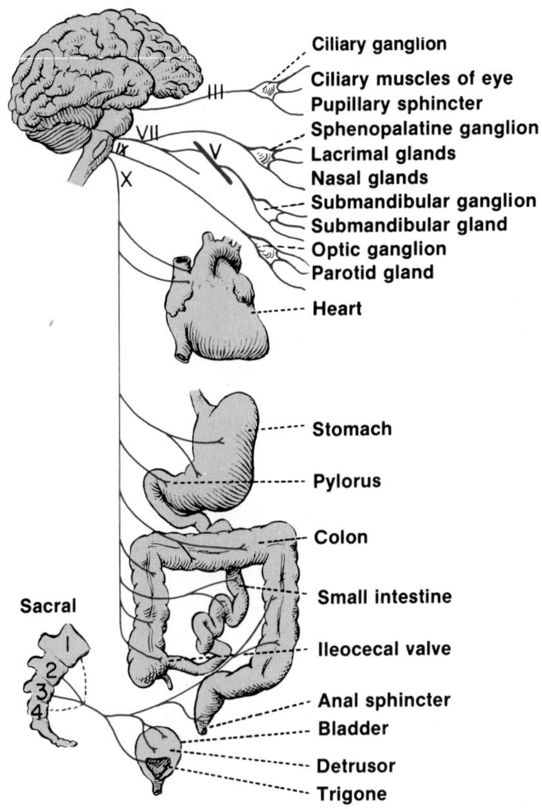

Figure 38–2. The parasympathetic nervous system.

each side of the cord and distribute their peripheral fibers to the descending colon, rectum, bladder and lower portions of the ureters. Also, this sacral group of parasympathetics supplies fibers to the external genitalia to cause various sexual reactions.

Preganglionic and Postganglionic Parasympathetic Fibers. The parasympathetic system, like the sympathetic, has both preganglionic and postganglionic fibers, but the preganglionic fibers usually pass uninterrupted to the organ that is to be excited by parasympathetic signals. Then, in the wall of the organ are located the *parasympathetic postganglionic neurons.* The preganglionic fibers synapse with these; and then short postganglionic fibers, 1 millimeter to several centimeters in length, leave the neuronal cell bodies to spread in the substance of the organ.

BASIC CHARACTERISTICS OF SYMPATHETIC AND PARASYMPATHETIC FUNCTIONS

CHOLINERGIC AND ADRENERGIC FIBERS—SECRETION OF ACETYLCHOLINE OR NOREPINEPHRINE AT THE POSTGANGLIONIC NERVE ENDINGS

It will be recalled from Chapter 7 that skeletal nerve endings secrete acetylcholine. This is also true of the *preganglionic fibers* of both the sympathetic

and parasympathetic system, and it is true, too, of the *parasympathetic postganglionic fibers.* Therefore, all these fibers are said to be *cholinergic because they secrete acetylcholine at their nerve endings.*

A few of the postganglionic endings of the sympathetic nervous system also secrete acetylcholine; these fibers, too, are cholinergic; but by far the majority of the sympathetic postganglionic endings secrete *norepinephrine.* These fibers are said to be *adrenergic,* a term derived from *noradrenalin,* which is the English name for norepinephrine. Thus, there is a basic functional difference between the postganglionic fibers of the parasympathetic and sympathetic systems, one secreting acetylcholine and the other principally norepinephrine. The chemical structures of these substances are the following:

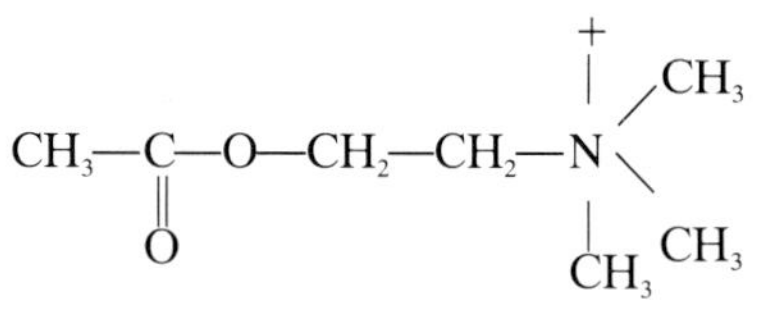

$$CH_3-C-O-CH_2-CH_2-\overset{+}{N}\diagdown \begin{matrix} CH_3 \\ CH_3 \\ CH_3 \end{matrix}$$
$$\underset{O}{|}$$

Acetylcholine

$$HO-\underset{HO}{\bigcirc}-CH-CH_2-NH_2$$
$$\underset{OH}{|}$$

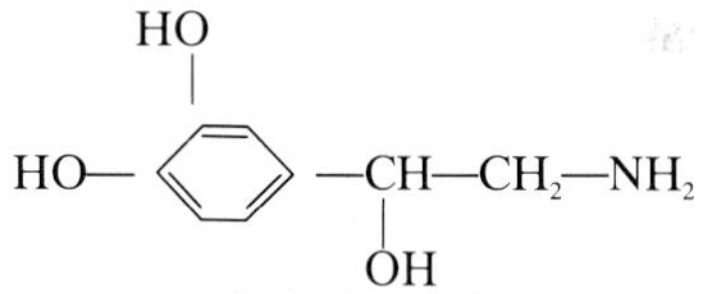

Norepinephrine

The acetylcholine and norepinephrine secreted by the postganglionic fibers act on the different organs to cause the respective parasympathetic or sympathetic effects. Therefore, these substances are called *parasympathetic* and *sympathetic mediators,* respectively, or sometimes *cholinergic* and *adrenergic mediators.*

Once *acetylcholine* has been secreted by the cholinergic nerve ending, it is split into acetate ion and choline by the enzyme *acetylcholinesterase* that is present both in the synapse and in the tissues of the receptor organ. Therefore, the action of acetylcholine lasts for a few seconds at most and usually for only a fraction of a second. Much of the choline derived from the acetylcholine is then transported back into the nerve terminal to be used in the formation of new acetylcholine.

Following secretion of *norepinephrine* by the adrenergic nerve endings, it is removed from the secretory site mainly in two different ways: (1) re-uptake into the adrenergic nerve endings themselves by an active transport process—accounting for removal of 50 to 80 per cent of the secreted norepinephrine; and (2) diffusion away from the nerve endings into the surrounding body fluids and thence into the blood—accounting for removal of most of the remainder of the norepinephrine, after which it is destroyed by enzymes in about one minute.

Ordinarily, the norepinephrine secreted directly in a tissue by adrenergic nerve endings remains active for only a few seconds, illustrating that its re-uptake and diffusion away from the tissue is rapid. However, the norepinephrine and epinephrine secreted into the blood by the adrenal medullae remain active until they diffuse into some tissue where they are destroyed by enzymes; this occurs mainly in the liver. Therefore, when secreted into the blood, both norepinephrine and epinephrine remain active for 10 to 30 seconds, followed by decreasing activity thereafter for one to several minutes.

RECEPTORS OF THE EFFECTOR ORGANS

The acetylcholine, norepinephrine, and epinephrine secreted by the autonomic nervous system all stimulate the effector organs by binding with *receptors* of the effector cells. The receptor in most instances is in the cell membrane and is a glycoprotein molecule. The usual mechanism for function of the receptor is that when the transmitter binds with the receptor, this causes a basic change in the structure of the protein molecule. Because the receptor is an integral part of the cell membrane, this structural change often opens or closes *ion channels*, thus altering the permeability of the cell membrane to various ions—for instance, to allow rapid influx or to diminish influx of sodium or calcium ions into the cell or to alter the efflux of potassium ions out of the cell.

These ionic changes then usually alter the membrane potential, which in turn alters the organ function. Or at other times, the ions themselves have direct effects within the receptor cells, such as calcium ions' promotion of smooth muscle contraction.

Another way that the receptor can function, besides changing the membrane permeability, is to activate an enzyme in the cell membrane; this enzyme in turn promotes chemical reactions within the cell. For instance, epinephrine increases the activity of *adenyl cyclase* in some cell membranes, and this then causes the formation of cyclic AMP at the inner surfaces of the membranes; the cyclic AMP then initiates many intracellular activities.

The effect that occurs in each instance is determined by the nature of the receptors in each organ.

The Acetylcholine Receptors—Muscarinic and Nicotinic Receptors. Acetylcholine activates two different types of receptors. These are called *muscarinic* and *nicotinic* receptors. The reason for these names is that muscarine, a poison from toadstools, also activates the muscarinic receptors but not the nicotinic receptors, whereas nicotine will activate only the other receptors; acetylcholine activates both of them.

The muscarinic receptors are found in all the effector cells stimulated by the postganglionic neurons of the parasympathetic nervous system, as well as those stimulated by the postganglionic cholinergic neurons of the sympathetic system.

The nicotinic receptors are found in the synapses between the pre- and postganglionic neurons of both the sympathetic and parasympathetic systems and also in the membranes of skeletal muscle fibers at the neuromuscular junction (discussed in Chapter 7).

Table 38–1. ADRENERGIC RECEPTORS AND THEIR FUNCTIONS

Alpha Receptor	Beta Receptor
Vasoconstriction	Vasodilatation (β_2)
Iris dilatation	Cardioacceleration (β_1)
Intestinal relaxation	Increased myocardial strength (β_1)
Intestinal sphincter contraction	Intestinal relaxation (β_2)
	Uterus relaxation (β_2)
Pilomotor contraction	Bronchodilatation (β_2)
	Calorigenesis (β_2)
Bladder sphincter contraction	Glycogenolysis (β_2)
	Lipolysis (β_1)
	Bladder relaxation (β_2)

An understanding of the two different types of receptors is especially important because specific drugs are frequently used to stimulate or to block one or the other of the two types of receptors.

The Adrenergic Receptors—Alpha and Beta Receptors. Research experiments using drugs (called *sympathomimetic drugs*) that mimic the action of norepinephrine on sympathetic effector organs have shown that there are two major types of adrenergic receptors, called *alpha receptors* and *beta receptors*. (The beta receptors in turn are divided into *beta₁* and *beta₂* receptors because certain drugs affect some beta receptors but not all of them.)

Norepinephrine and epinephrine, both of which are secreted by the adrenal medulla, have somewhat different effects in exciting the alpha and beta receptors. Norepinephrine excites mainly alpha receptors but excites the beta receptors to a slight extent as well. On the other hand, epinephrine excites both types of receptors approximately equally. Therefore, the relative effects of norepinephrine and epinephrine on different effector organs is determined by the types of receptors in the organs. Obviously, if they are all beta receptors, epinephrine will be the more effective excitant.

Table 38–1 gives the distribution of alpha and beta receptors in some of the organs and systems controlled by the sympathetic nerves. Note that certain alpha functions are excitatory while others are inhibitory. Likewise, certain beta functions are excitatory and others are inhibitory. Therefore, alpha and beta receptors are not necessarily associated with excitation or inhibition but simply with the affinity of the hormone for the receptors in a given effector organ.

EXCITATORY AND INHIBITORY ACTIONS OF SYMPATHETIC AND PARASYMPATHETIC STIMULATION

Table 38–2 gives the effects on different visceral functions of the body caused by stimulation of the parasympathetic and sympathetic nerves. From this table it can be seen that *sympathetic stimulation causes excitatory effects in some organs but inhibitory effects in others. Likewise, parasympathetic stimulation causes excitation in some organs but inhibition in others.* Also, when sympathetic stimulation excites a particular organ, parasympathetic stimulation often

Table 38–2. AUTONOMIC EFFECTS ON VARIOUS ORGANS OF THE BODY

Organ	Effect of Sympathetic Stimulation	Effect of Parasympathetic Stimulation
Eye: Pupil	Dilated	Constricted
Ciliary muscle	Slight relaxation	Constricted
Glands: Nasal	Vasoconstriction and slight secretion	Stimulation of copious (except
Lacrimal		pancreas) secretion (containing
Parotid		many enzymes for enzyme-
Submandibular		secreting glands)
Gastric		
Pancreatic		
Sweat glands	Copious sweating (cholinergic)	None
Apocrine glands	Thick, odoriferous secretion	None
Heart: Muscle	Increased rate	Slowed rate
	Increased force of contraction	Decreased force of contraction
		(especially of atrium)
Coronaries	Dilated (β_2); constricted (α)	Dilated
Lungs: Bronchi	Dilated	Constricted
Blood vessels	Mildly constricted	? Dilated
Gut: Lumen	Decreased peristalsis and tone	Increased peristalsis and tone
Sphincter	Increased tone (most times)	Relaxed (most times)
Liver	Glucose released	Slight glycogen synthesis
Gallbladder and bile ducts	Relaxed	Contracted
Kidney	Decreased output and renin	None
	secretion	
Bladder: Detrusor	Relaxed (slight)	Excited
Trigone	Excited	Relaxed
Penis	Ejaculation	Erection
Systemic arterioles:		
Abdominal	Constricted	None
Muscle	Constricted (adrenergic α)	None
	Dilated (adrenergic β_2)	
	Dilated (cholinergic)	
Skin	Constricted	None
Blood: Coagulation	Increased	None
Glucose	Increased	None
Basal metabolism	Increased up to 100%	None
Adrenal medullary secretion	Increased	None
Mental activity	Increased	None
Piloerector muscles	Excited	None
Skeletal muscle	Increased glycogenolysis	None
	Increased strength	

inhibits it, illustrating that the two systems occasionally act reciprocally to each other. However, most organs are dominantly controlled by one or the other of the two systems, so that, except in a few instances, the two systems do not actively oppose each other.

There is no generalization to explain whether sympathetic or parasympathetic stimulation will cause excitation or inhibition of a particular organ. Therefore, to understand sympathetic and parasympathetic functions, one must learn the functions of these two nervous systems as listed in Table 38–2. Some of these functions need to be clarified in still greater detail, as follows:

EFFECTS OF SYMPATHETIC AND PARASYMPATHETIC STIMULATION ON SPECIFIC ORGANS

The Eye. Two functions of the eye are controlled by the autonomic nervous system: the pupillary opening and the focus of the lens. Sympathetic stimulation dilates the pupil, while parasympathetic stimulation constricts the pupil. The parasympathetics that control the pupil are reflexly stimulated when excess light enters the eyes; this reflex reduces the pupillary opening and decreases the amount of light that strikes the retina. On the other hand, the sympathetics become stimulated during periods of excitement and therefore increase the pupillary opening at these times.

Focusing of the lens is controlled almost entirely by the parasympathetic nervous system. The lens is normally held in a flattened state by tension on its radial ligaments. Parasympathetic excitation contracts the *ciliary muscle,* which loosens this tension and allows the lens to become more convex, causing the eye to focus on objects near at hand. The focusing mechanism is discussed in Chapters 39 and 40 in relation to function of the eyes.

The Gastrointestinal System. The gastrointestinal system has its own intrinsic set of nerves, known as the *gastrointestinal intramural plexus.* However, both parasympathetic and sympathetic stimulation can affect gastrointestinal activity. Parasympathetic stimulation, in general, increases the overall activity of the gastrointestinal tract by promoting peristalsis, thus allowing rapid propulsion of the intraluminal contents along the tract. This propulsive effect is associated with simultaneous increase in rate of secretion by many of the gastrointestinal glands.

Normal function of the gastrointestinal tract is not very dependent on sympathetic stimulation. However, in some diseases, strong sympathetic stimulation inhibits peristalsis and increases the tone of the sphincters. The net result is greatly slowed propulsion of food through the tract.

The Heart. In general, sympathetic stimulation increases the overall activity of the heart. This is accomplished by increasing both the rate and force of the heartbeat. Parasympathetic stimulation causes mainly the opposite effects, decreasing the overall activity of the heart. To express these effects in another way, sympathetic stimulation increases the effectiveness of the heart as a pump, whereas parasympathetic stimulation decreases its effectiveness.

Systemic Control of the Blood Vessels. Most blood vessels are constricted by sympathetic stimulation. Parasympathetic stimulation generally has almost no effects on most blood vessels but does dilate vessels in certain restricted areas such as the blush area of the face.

Effect of Sympathetic and Parasympathetic Stimulation on Arterial Pressure. The arterial pressure in the circulatory system is caused by propulsion of blood by the heart and by resistance to flow of this blood through the vascular system. In general, sympathetic stimulation increases both propulsion by the heart and resistance to flow, which can cause the pressure to increase greatly.

On the other hand, parasympathetic stimulation decreases the pumping effectiveness of the heart, which can lower the pressure on occasion. However, this reduction occurs only rarely.

Effects of Sympathetic and Parasympathetic Stimulation on Other Functions of the Body. Because of the great importance of the sympathetic and parasympathetic control systems, these systems are discussed many times in this text in relation to a myriad of body functions that are not considered in detail here. In general, most of the entodermal structures, such as the ducts of the liver, the gallbladder, the ureter, and the urinary bladder, are inhibited by sympathetic stimulation but excited by parasympathetic stimulation.

Sympathetic stimulation also has metabolic effects, causing release of glucose from the liver, and increase in blood glucose concentration, in glycogenolysis in muscle, in muscle strength, in basal metabolic rate, and in mental activity.

Finally, the sympathetic and parasympathetic nerves are involved in regulating the male and female sexual acts, as will be explained in Chapters 54 and 55.

FUNCTION OF THE ADRENAL MEDULLAE

Stimulation of the sympathetic nerves to the adrenal medullae causes large quantities of epinephrine and norepinephrine to be released into the circulating blood, and these two hormones in turn are carried in the blood to all tissues of the body.

The circulating hormones have almost the same effects on the different organs as those caused by direct sympathetic stimulation, except that *the effects last about ten times as long* because norepinephrine and epinephrine are only slowly removed from the blood. For instance, they cause constriction of essentially all the blood vessels of the body; they cause increased activity of the heart, inhibition of the gastrointestinal tract, dilation of the pupil of the eye, and so forth.

In summary, stimulation of the adrenal medullae causes the release of hormones that have almost the same effects throughout the body as direct sympathetic stimulation, except that the effects are greatly prolonged.

Value of the Adrenal Medullae to the Function of the Sympathetic Nervous System. Often, when the sympathetic nervous system is stimulated, major portions of the entire system are stimulated. At the same time, norepinephrine and epinephrine are almost always released by the adrenal medullae. Therefore, the body's organs are actually stimulated in two different ways simultaneously, directly by the sympathetic nerves and indirectly by the medullary hormones. The two means of stimulation support each other, and either can usually substitute for the other. For instance, destruction of the direct sympathetic pathways to the organs does not abrogate excitation of the organs, because norepinephrine and epinephrine are still released into the circulating fluids and indirectly cause stimulation. Likewise, total loss of the two adrenal medullae usually has little effect on the operation of the sympathetic nervous system because the direct pathways can still perform almost all the necessary duties.

Another important value of the adrenal medullae is the capability of epinephrine and norepinephrine to stimulate structures of the body that are not innervated by direct sympathetic fibers. For instance, the metabolic rate of every cell of the body is increased by these hormones, especially by epinephrine, even though only a small proportion of all the cells in the body are innervated by sympathetic fibers.

SYMPATHETIC AND PARASYMPATHETIC TONE

The sympathetic and parasympathetic systems are continually active, and the basal rates of stimulation are known, respectively, as *sympathetic tone* and *parasympathetic tone.*

The value of tone is that it allows a single nervous system either to increase or to decrease the activity of an organ. For instance, sympathetic tone normally keeps almost all the blood vessels of the body constricted to approximately half their maximum diameter. By increasing the degree of sympathetic stimulation, the vessels can be constricted even more, but, on the other hand, by decreasing the level of sympathetic stimulation the vessels can be dilated. If it were not for normal sympathetic tone, the sympathetic system could only be used to cause vasoconstriction, never vasodilatation.

Another interesting example of tone is parasympathetic tone in the gastrointestinal tract. Surgical removal of the parasympathetic nerves to the gut by cutting the vagi can cause serious and prolonged gastric and intestinal "atony," thus illustrating that in normal function the parasympathetic tone to the gut is necessary to maintain normal gastrointestinal activity. This tone can be decreased by the brain, thereby inhibiting gastrointestinal activity, or on the other hand, it can be increased, thereby promoting increased gastrointestinal activity.

STIMULATION BY THE SYMPATHETIC AND PARASYMPATHETIC SYSTEMS OF DISCRETE ORGANS IN SOME INSTANCES, MASS STIMULATION IN OTHER INSTANCES

The Sympathetic System. In many instances, the sympathetic nervous system discharges almost as a complete unit, a phenomenon called *mass discharge.* This frequently occurs when the hypothalamus becomes activated by fright or fear or severe pain. The result is a widespread reaction throughout the body called the *alarm* or *stress response,* which we shall discuss shortly.

However, at other times sympathetic activation occurs in isolated portions of the system. The most important of these are (1) in the process of heat regulation, the sympathetics control sweating and blood flow in the skin without affecting other organs innervated by the sympathetics; (2) during muscular activity in some animals, sympathetic cholinergic vasodilator fibers of the skeletal muscles are stimulated independently of all the remainder of the sympathetic system; and (3) many "local reflexes" involving the spinal cord but usually not the higher nervous centers affect local areas. For instance, many sympathetic reflexes that control gastrointestinal functions are discrete, operating sometimes by way of nerve pathways that do not even enter the spinal cord, merely passing from the gut to the sympathetic ganglia and then back to the gut through the sympathetic nerves to control motor or secretory activity.

The Parasympathetic System. In contrast to the sympathetic system, most control functions of the parasympathetic system are very specific. For instance, parasympathetic cardiovascular reflexes usually act only on the heart to increase or decrease its rate of beating. Likewise, parasympathetic reflexes frequently cause secretion mainly in the mouth or, in other instances, secretion mainly by the stomach glands. Finally, the rectal emptying reflex does not affect other parts of the bowel to a major extent.

Yet there is often association between closely allied parasympathetic functions. For instance, though salivary secretion can occur independently of gastric secretion, these two also often occur together, and pancreatic secretion frequently occurs at the same time. Also, the rectal emptying reflex often initiates a bladder emptying reflex, resulting in simultaneous emptying of both the bladder and rectum. Conversely, the bladder emptying reflex can help initiate rectal emptying.

ALARM OR STRESS FUNCTION OF THE SYMPATHETIC NERVOUS SYSTEM

From the above discussions of the sympathetic nervous system, one can already see that mass sympathetic discharge increases in many ways the capability of the body to perform vigorous muscle activity. Let us quickly summarize these ways:
  1. Increased arterial pressure
  2. Increased blood flow to active muscles concurrent with decreased blood flow to organs that are not needed for rapid activity
  3. Increased rates of cellular metabolism throughout the body
  4. Increased blood glucose concentration
  5. Increased glycolysis in muscle
  6. Increased muscle strength
  7. Increased mental activity

The sum of these effects permits the person to perform far more strenuous physical activity than would otherwise be possible. Since it is physical *stress* that usually excites the sympathetic system, it is frequently said that the purpose of the sympathetic system is to provide extra activation of the body in states of stress; this is often called the *sympathetic stress response.*

The sympathetic system is also strongly activated in many emotional states. For instance, in the state of *rage,* which is elicited mainly by stimulating the hypothalamus, signals are transmitted downward through the reticular formation and spinal cord to cause massive sympathetic discharge, and all the sympathetic events listed above ensue immediately. This is called the sympathetic *alarm reaction.* It is also frequently called the *fight or flight reaction* because an animal in this state decides almost instantly whether to stand and fight or to run. In either event, the sympathetic alarm reaction makes the animal's subsequent activities extremely vigorous.

MEDULLARY, PONTINE, AND MESENCEPHALIC CONTROL OF THE AUTONOMIC NERVOUS SYSTEM

Many areas in the reticular substance of the medulla, pons, and mesencephalon, as well as many special nuclei (Fig. 38–3), control autonomic functions, such as arterial pressure, heart rate, glandular secretion in the upper part of the gastrointestinal tract, gastrointestinal peristalsis, the degree of contraction of the urinary bladder, and many others. The control of each of these is discussed at appropriate points in this text. Suffice it to point out here that the most important factors controlled in the lower

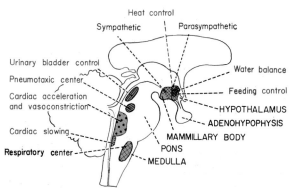

Figure 38–3. Autonomic control centers of the brain stem.

brain stem are arterial pressure, heart rate, and respiration. Indeed, transection of the brain stem at the midpontile level allows normal basal control of arterial pressure to continue as before but prevents its modulation by higher nervous centers, particularly the hypothalamus. On the other hand, transection immediately below the medulla causes the arterial pressure to fall to about one-half normal. Closely associated with the cardiovascular regulatory centers in the medulla is the medullary center for regulation of respiration, discussed in detail in Chapter 29. Though this is not considered to be an autonomic function, it is one of the *involuntary* functions of the body.

In the previous chapter it was pointed out that many of the behavioral responses of an animal are mediated through the hypothalamus, the reticular formation, and the autonomic nervous system. Indeed, the higher areas of the brain can alter the function of the whole autonomic nervous system or of portions of it strongly enough to cause severe autonomic-induced disease, such as peptic ulcer, constipation, heart palpitation, and even heart attacks.

QUESTIONS

1. Describe the anatomy of the *sympathetic nervous system*, including the pathways of the *preganglionic* neurons into the sympathetic chain and of the *postganglionic neurons* to the organs that are to be controlled.
2. Describe the *parasympathetic nervous system* as well as its preganglionic and postganglionic neurons.
3. At what points in the sympathetic and parasympathetic nervous systems are *acetylcholine* and *norepinephrine* secreted?
4. What determines whether or not an organ will be excited or inhibited by sympathetic or parasympathetic stimulation?
5. What is meant by *muscarinic* and *nicotinic receptors*, and by *alpha* and *beta adrenergic receptors*?
6. Describe briefly the effects of sympathetic and parasympathetic stimulation on (1) the eye, (2) the gastrointestinal system, (3) the heart, (4) the blood vessels, and (5) arterial pressure.
7. Explain the function of the *adrenal medullae* and why this function is important.
8. Explain how sympathetic and parasympathetic tone can allow the sympathetic and parasympathetic systems to cause both excitation and inhibition of an organ.
9. Explain the *mass discharge* response of the sympathetic system and its role in *alarm* and *stress reactions*.
10. How do the alarm and stress reactions prepare an animal for increased activity?

References

Abboud, F. M., ed.: Disturbances in Neurogenic Control of the Circulation. Baltimore, Williams and Wilkins, 1981.

Burattini, R., and Borgdorff, P.: Closed-loop baroreflex control of total peripheral resistance in the cat: identification of gains by aid of a model. Cardiovasc Res 18:715, 1984.

Burchfield, S. R., ed.: Stress. Physiological and Psychological Interactions. Washington, D.C., Hemisphere Publishing Corp., 1985.

Christensen, N. J., and Galbo, H.: Sympathetic nervous activity during exercise. Annu Rev Physiol 45:139, 1983.

Davies, A. O., and Lefkowitz, R. J.: Regulation of β-adrenergic receptors by steroid hormones. Annu Rev Physiol 46:119, 1984.

Donald, D. E., and Shepherd, J. T.: Autonomic regulation of the peripheral circulation. Annu Rev Physiol 42:429, 1980.

Givens, J. R.: The Hypothalamus in Health and Disease. Chicago, Year Book Medical Publishers, 1984.

Landsberg, L., and Young, J. B.: Catecholamines and the adrenal medulla. In Bondy, P. K., and Rosenberg, L. E., eds.: Metabolic Control and Disease, 8th ed. Philadelphia, W. B. Saunders Co., 1980, p. 1621.

Livett, B. G.: Adrenal medullary chromaffin cells in vitro. Physiol Rev 64:1103, 1984.

Robinson, R.: Tumours That Secrete Catecholamines: A Study of Their Natural History and Their Diagnosis. New York, John Wiley & Sons, 1980.

Rowell, L. B.: Reflex control of regional circulations in humans. J Auton Nerv Syst 11:101, 1984.

Stiles, G. L., et al.: β-Adrenergic receptors: biochemical mechanisms of physiological regulation. Physiol Rev 64:661, 1984.

Tauc, L.: Nonvesicular release of neurotransmitter. Physiol Rev 62:857, 1982.

Ungar, A., and Phillips, J. H.: Regulation of the adrenal medulla. Physiol Rev 63:787, 1983.

Usdin, E.: Stress. The Role of Catecholamines and Other Neurotransmitters. New York, Gordon Press Publishers, 1984.

Westfall, T. C.: Local regulations of adrenergic neurotransmission. Physiol Rev 57:659, 1977.

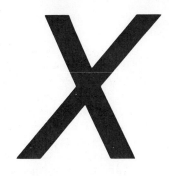

THE SPECIAL SENSES

39 ■ The Eye: I. Optics of Vision and Function of the Retina

40 ■ The Eye: II. Neurophysiology of Vision

41 ■ The Sense of Hearing and the Chemical Senses of Taste and Smell

39

The Eye: I. Optics of Vision and Function of the Retina

THE OPTICS OF THE EYE
   THE EYE AS A CAMERA
   THE MECHANISM OF
      ACCOMMODATION
   THE PUPILLARY APERTURE
   ERRORS OF REFRACTION
   CATARACTS
   SIZE OF THE IMAGE ON THE RETINA
      AND VISUAL ACUITY
   DETERIMINATION OF DISTANCE OF
      AN OBJECT FROM THE
      EYE—DEPTH PERCEPTION
THE RETINA
PHOTOCHEMISTRY OF VISION

   THE RHODOPSIN-RETINAL VISUAL
      CYCLE AND EXCITATION OF THE
      RODS
   PHOTOCHEMISTRY OF COLOR
      VISION BY THE CONES
   AUTOMATIC REGULATION OF
      RETINAL SENSITIVITY—DARK AND
      LIGHT ADAPTATION
   FUSION OF FLICKERING LIGHT BY
      THE RETINA
COLOR VISION
   THE TRICOLOR MECHANISM OF
      COLOR PERCEPTION
   COLOR BLINDNESS

THE OPTICS OF THE EYE

THE EYE AS A CAMERA

The eye, as illustrated in Figure 39–1, is optically equivalent to the usual photographic camera, for it has a lens system, a variable aperture system, and a retina that corresponds to the film. The refractive surfaces of the eye's lens system are (1) the interface between air and the anterior surface of the cornea, (2) the interface between the posterior surface of the cornea and the aqueous humor, (3) the interface between the aqueous humor and the anterior surface of the lens, and (4) the interface between the posterior surface of the lens and the vitreous humor. The *difference* between the refractive indices on the two sides of each surface is one of the factors that determine the focusing strength of each surface. Another factor is the curvature of the surface.

The Reduced Eye. If all the refractive surfaces of the eye are algebraically added together and then considered to be one single lens, the optics of the normal eye may be simplified and represented schematically as a "reduced eye." This is useful in simple calculations. In the reduced eye, a single lens is considered to exist with its central point 17 mm in front of the retina and to have a total refractive power of approximately 59 diopters when the lens is accommodated for distant vision. (A lens that will focus parallel light rays at a distance of 1 meter beyond the lens has a strength of 1 diopter. A 59-diopter lens is 59 times as strong and will focus the same parallel rays at a distance of 1/59 meter beyond the lens.)

The anterior surface of the cornea provides about 48 diopters of the eye's total dioptric strength mainly because the refractive index of the cornea is markedly different from that of air, as shown by the numbers in Figure 39–1.

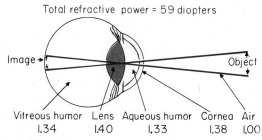

Figure 39–1. The eye as a camera. The numbers are the refractive indices.

The posterior surface of the cornea is concave and actually acts as a concave lens, which has *negative* focusing power, but because the difference in refractive index of the cornea and the aqueous humor is slight, this posterior surface of the cornea has a refractive power of only about −4 diopters, which neutralizes only a small part of the refractive power of the other refractive surfaces of the eye.

The total refractive power of the crystalline lens of the eye when it is surrounded by fluid on each side is only 15 diopters of the total refractive power of the eye's lens system. If this lens were removed from the eye and then surrounded by air, its refractive power would be about 100 diopters. Thus, it can be seen that the lens inside the eye is not nearly so powerful as it is outside the eye. The reason is that the fluids surrounding the lens have refractive indices not greatly different from the refractive index of the lens itself, the smallness of the differences greatly decreasing the amount of light refraction at the lens interfaces. But the importance of the crystalline lens is that its curvature, and therefore its strength as well, can change to provide accommodation, which will be discussed later in the chapter.

Formation of an Image on the Retina. In exactly the same manner that a glass lens can focus an image on a sheet of paper, the lens system of the eye can also focus an image on the retina. The image is inverted, and reversed with respect to the object. However, the mind perceives objects in the upright position despite the upside-down orientation of the retinal image because the brain is trained to consider an inverted image as the normal.

THE MECHANISM OF ACCOMMODATION

The refractive power of the crystalline lens of the eye can voluntarily be increased from 15 diopters to approximately 29 diopters in young children; this is a total accommodation of 14 diopters. To do this, the shape of the lens is changed from that of a moderately convex lens to that of a very convex lens. The mechanism of this shift is as follows:

Normally, the lens is composed of a strong elastic capsule filled with viscous proteinaceous but transparent fibers. When the lens is in a relaxed state, with no tension on its capsule, it assumes a spherical shape, owing entirely to the elasticity of the lens capsule. However, as illustrated in Figure 39–2, approximately 70 ligaments attach radially around the lens, pulling the lens edges toward the edge of the choroid. These ligaments are constantly tensed by the elastic pull of their attachments to the choroid, and the tension on the ligaments causes the lens to remain relatively flat under normal resting conditions of the eye. At the insertions of the ligaments in the choroid is the ciliary muscle, which has two sets of smooth muscle fibers, the *meridional fibers* and the *circular fibers*. The meridional fibers extend from the corneoscleral junction to the insertions of the ligaments in the choroid, approximately 2 to 3 mm behind the

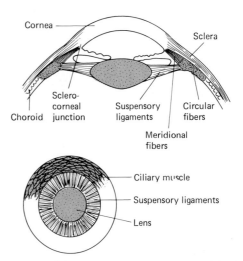

Figure 39–2. Mechanism of accommodation (focusing).

junction. When these muscle fibers contract, the ligaments are pulled forward, thereby releasing a certain amount of tension on the crystalline lens. The circular fibers are arranged circularly all the way around the eye so that when they contract a sphincterlike action occurs, decreasing the diameter of the circle of ligament attachments and allowing the ligaments to pull less on the lens capsule.

Thus, contraction of both sets of smooth muscle fibers in the ciliary muscle relaxes the ligaments to the lens capsule, and the lens assumes a more spherical shape, like that of a balloon, because of elasticity of its capsule. Therefore, when the ciliary muscle is completely relaxed, the ligaments are tensed and the dioptric strength of the lens is as weak as it can become. On the other hand, when the ciliary muscle contracts as strongly as possible, the ligaments become relaxed and the dioptric strength of the lens then becomes maximal.

Autonomic Control of Accommodation. The ciliary muscle is controlled almost entirely by parasympathetic nerve fibers from the third cranial nerve. Stimulation of these fibers contracts the ciliary muscle, which in turn relaxes the ligaments of the lens and increases its refractive power. With an increased refractive power, the eye is more capable of focusing on objects that are nearer to it than is an eye with less refractive power. Consequently, as a distant object moves toward the eye, the number of parasympathetic impulses impinging on the ciliary muscle must be progressively increased for the eye to keep the object constantly in focus.

Presbyopia. As a person grows older, his lens loses its elastic nature and becomes a relatively solid mass, probably because of progressive denaturation of the proteins. Therefore, the ability of the lens to assume a spherical shape progressively decreases, and the power of accommodation (the amount that the lens strength can change in response to contraction of the ciliary muscle) decreases from approximately 14 diopters shortly after birth to approximately 2 diopters at the age of 45 to 50. Thereafter, the lens of the eye may be considered to be almost totally nonaccommodating, a condition known as presbyopia.

Once a person has reached the state of presbyopia, each eye remains focused permanently at an almost constant distance; this distance depends on the physical characteristics of each individual's eyes. Obviously, the eyes can no longer accommodate for both near and far vision. Therefore, for an older person to see clearly both in the distance and nearby, he must wear bifocal glasses with the upper segment focused for distant vision and the lower segment focused for near vision.

THE PUPILLARY APERTURE

A major function of the iris is to increase the amount of light that enters the eye during darkness and to decrease the light that enters the eye in bright light. The reflexes for controlling this mechanism are considered in the discussion of the neurology of the eye in Chapter 40. The amount of light that enters the eye through the pupil is *proportional to the area of the pupil or to the square of the diameter* of the pupil. The pupil of the human eye can become as small as approximately 1.5 mm and as large as 8 mm in diameter. Therefore, the quantity of light entering the eye may vary approximately 30 times as a result of changes in pupillary aperture size.

Depth of Focus of the Lens System of the Eye. Figure 39–3 illustrates two separate eyes that are exactly alike except that the diameters of the pupillary apertures are different. In the upper eye the pupillary aperture is small, and in the lower eye the aperture is large. In front of each of these two eyes are two small point sources of light, and light from each passes through the pupillary aperture and focuses on the retina. Consequently, in both eyes the retina sees two spots of light in perfect focus. It is evident from the diagrams, however, that if the retina is moved forward or backward to an out-of-focus position, the size of each spot will not change much in the upper eye, but in the lower eye the size of each spot will

increase greatly at any distance from the lens except at the exact focus point, and the spot becomes a blurred circle. In other words, the upper lens system has far greater *depth of focus* than the bottom lens system. When the lens system of the eye has great depth of focus—that is, a smaller aperture diameter—the retina can be considerably displaced from the focal plane and still discern the various features of an image rather distinctly; whereas, when a lens system has a shallow depth of focus, moving the retina only slightly away from the focal plane causes extreme blurring of the image. This explains why a person with poor focus of his lens system can see much more clearly in bright light when the pupil is small.

ERRORS OF REFRACTION

Emmetropia. As shown in Figure 39–4, the eye is considered to be normal, or emmetropic, if, when the ciliary muscle is completely relaxed, parallel light rays from distant objects are in sharp focus on the retina. This means that the emmetropic eye can, with its ciliary muscle completely relaxed, see all distant objects clearly, but to focus objects at close range it must contract its ciliary muscle and thereby provide various degrees of accommodation.

Hypermetropia (Hyperopia). Hypermetropia, also known as "far-sightedness," usually results from an eyeball that is too short. In this condition, parallel light rays are not bent sufficiently by the lens system to come to a focus by the time they reach the retina. In order to overcome this abnormality, the ciliary muscle must contract to increase the strength of the lens. Unfortunately, in old age, when the lens becomes presbyopic, the far-sighted person often is not able to accommodate the lens sufficiently to focus

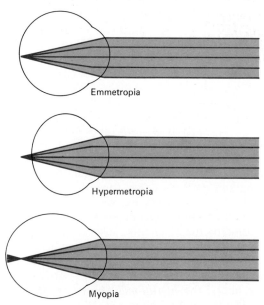

Figure 39–4. Parallel light rays focus on the retina in emmetropia, behind the retina in hypermetropia, and in front of the retina in myopia.

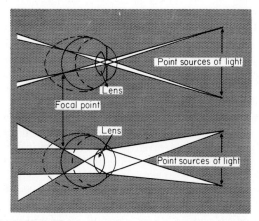

Figure 39–3. Effect of small and large pupillary apertures on the depth of focus.

even on distant objects, much less to focus on near objects.

Myopia. Myopia, or "near-sightedness," usually results from an eyeball that is too long. Therefore, the lens system focuses the light rays in front of the retina.

No mechanism exists by which the eye can decrease the strength of its lens below that which exists when the ciliary muscle is completely relaxed. Therefore, the myopic person has no mechanism by which he can ever focus distant objects sharply on his retina. However, as an object comes nearer and nearer to his eye, it finally comes near enough that its image is focused on the retina. Then, when the object comes still closer to the eye, the person can use his mechanism for accommodation to keep the image focused clearly. Therefore, a myopic person has a definite limiting "far point" for sharp vision.

Correction of Myopia and Hypermetropia by Use of Lenses. It will be recalled that light rays passing through a concave lens diverge. Therefore, if the refractive surfaces of the eye have too much refractive power in relation to the length of the eyeball, as in myopia, some of this excessive refractive power can be neutralized by placing in front of the eye a concave spherical lens, which will diverge the incoming rays. On the other hand, in a person who has hypermetropia—that is, one who has too weak a lens for the distance of the retina away from the lens—the abnormal vision can be corrected by adding refractive power with a convex lens in front of the eye. These corrections are illustrated in Figure 39–5. One usually determines the strength of the concave or convex lens needed for clear vision by trial and error—that is, by trying first a strong lens and then a stronger or a weaker lens until the one that gives the best visual acuity is found.

Astigmatism. Astigmatism is a refractive error of the lens system of the eye usually caused by an oblong shape of the cornea or, rarely, by an oblong shape of the lens. A lens surface like the side of an egg lying edgewise to the incoming light would be an example of an astigmatic lens. The degree of curvature in the

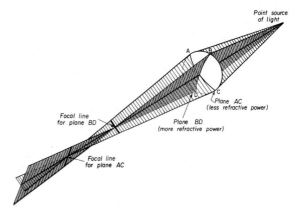

Figure 39–6. Astigmatism, illustrating that light rays focus at one focal distance in one focal plane and at another focal distance in the plane at right angles.

plane through the long axis of the egg is not nearly so great as the degree of curvature in the plane through the short axis. The same is true of an astigmatic lens of the eye. Because the curvature of the astigmatic lens along one plane is less than the curvature along the other plane, light rays striking the peripheral portions of the lens in one plane are not bent nearly so much as are rays striking the peripheral portions of the other plane.

This circumstance is illustrated in Figure 39–6, which shows what happens to rays of light emanating from a point source of passing through on oblong astigmatic lens. The light rays in the vertical plane, which is indicated by plane BD, are refracted greatly by the astigmatic lens because of the greater curvature in the vertical direction than in the horizontal direction. However, the light rays in the horizontal plane, indicated by plane AC, are bent not nearly so much as the light rays in the vertical plane. It is obvious, therefore, that the light rays passing through an astigmatic lens do not all come to a common focal point because the light rays passing through one plane of the lens focus far in front of those passing through the other plane.

Placing an appropriate *spherical* lens in front of an astigmatic eye can bring the light rays that pass through *one plane* of the lens into focus on the retina, but spherical lenses can never bring *all* the light rays into complete focus at the same time. For this reason astigmatism is a very undesirable refractive error of the eyes. Furthermore, the accommodative power of the eye cannot compensate for astigmatism for the reason that a spherical lens in front of the eye cannot correct the condition.

Correction of Astigmatism with a Cylindrical Lens. In correcting astigmatism with lenses, one can consider the astigmatic eye lens to be a spherical lens with a superimposed cylindrical lens (a lens that is curved in only one plane and not at all in the other plane). To correct the focusing of this system, it is necessary to determine both the *strength* of the cylindrical lens needed to neutralize the excess cylindrical power of the eye lens and the *axis* of this abnormal cylindrical lens.

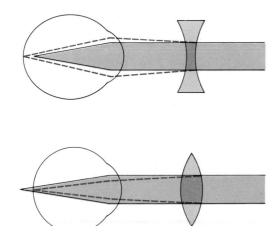

Figure 39–5. Correction of myopia with a concave lens, and correction of hypermetropia with a convex lens.

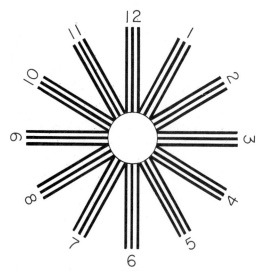

Figure 39–7. Chart composed of parallel black bars for determining the axis of astigmatism.

There are several methods for determining the axis of the abnormal cylindrical component of the lens system of the eye. One of these methods is based on the use of parallel black bars, as shown in Figure 39–7. Some of these parallel bars are vertical, some are horizontal, and some are at various angles to the vertical and horizontal axes. After placing, by trial and error, various spherical lenses in front of the astigmatic eye, a strength of lens will usually be found that will cause sharp focus of one set of these parallel bars on the retina of the astigmatic eye.

It can be shown from the physical principles of optics that the axis of the *out-of-focus* cylindrical component of the optical system is parallel to the black bars that are fuzziest in appearance. Once this axis is found, the examiner tries progressively stronger positive or negative cylindrical lenses, the axes of which are placed parallel to the out-of-focus bars, until the person sees all the cross bars with equal clarity. When this has been accomplished, the examiner directs the optician to grind a special lens having both the spherical correction plus the cylindrical correction at the appropriate axis.

CATARACTS

Cataracts are an especially common lens abnormality that occurs in older people. A cataract is a cloudy or an opaque area in the lens. In the early stage of cataract formation, the proteins in the lens fibers become denatured. Later, these same proteins coagulate to form opaque areas in place of the normal transparent protein fibers of the lens. Finally, in still later stages, calcium is often deposited in the coagulated proteins, thus further increasing the opacity.

When a cataract has obscured light transmission so greatly that it seriously impairs vision, the condition can be corrected by surgical removal of the entire lens. When this is done, however, the eye loses a large portion of its refractive power, which must be replaced by a powerful convex lens (about +15 diopters) in front of the eye or by putting an artificial plastic lens inside the eye in place of the natural lens that is removed.

SIZE OF THE IMAGE ON THE RETINA AND VISUAL ACUITY

If the distance from an object to the eye lens is 17 meters and the distance from the center of the lens to the retina is 17 millimeters, the ratio of the object size to image size is 1000 to 1. Therefore, an object 17 meters in front of the eye and 1 meter in size produces an image on the retina 1 millimeter in size.

Theoretically, a point of light from a distant point source, when focused on the retina, should be infinitely small. However, since the lens system of the eye is not perfect, such a retinal spot ordinarily has a total diameter of about 11 microns even with maximum resolution of the optical system. However, it is brightest in its very center and shades off gradually toward the edges.

The average diameter of cones *in the fovea* of the retina, the central part of the retina in which vision is most highly developed, is approximately 1.5 microns, which is one seventh the diameter of the spot of light. Nevertheless, since the spot of light has a bright center point and shaded edges, a person can distinguish two separate points if their centers lie approximately 2 microns apart on the retina, which is slightly greater than the width of a foveal cone. This means that a person with maximal visual acuity looking at two bright pinpoint spots of light 10 meters away can barely distinguish the spots as separate spots when they are 1 millimeter apart.

The foveal portion of the retina is only about half a millimeter in diameter, which means that maximum visual acuity occurs only in a small area in the very center of the visual field. Outside this foveal area, the visual acuity is reduced five- to tenfold, and it becomes progressively poorer as the periphery is approached.

Clinical Method for Stating Visual Acuity. Usually the test chart for testing eyes is placed 20 feet away from the tested person, and if the person can see the letters of the size that he should be able to see at 20 feet, he is said to have 20/20 vision—that is, normal vision. If he can only see letters that he should be able to see at 200 feet, he is said to have 20/200 vision. On the other hand, if he can see at 20 feet letters he should be able to see at only 15 feet, he is said to have 20/15 vision. In other words, the clinical method for expressing visual acuity is to use a mathematical fraction that expresses the ratio of two distances, which is also the ratio of one's visual acuity to normal vision.

DETERMINATION OF DISTANCE OF AN OBJECT FROM THE EYE—DEPTH PERCEPTION

There are three major means by which the visual apparatus normally perceives distance, a phenome-

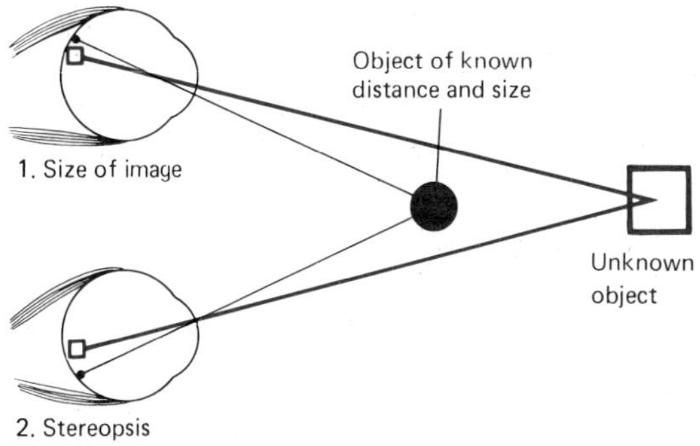

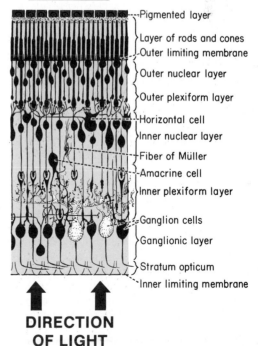

Figure 39–8. Perception of distance (1) by the size of the image on the retina, and (2) as a result of stereopsis.

non that is known as *depth perception*. They are (1) relative sizes of objects, (2) moving parallax, and (3) stereopsis.

Determination of Distance by Relative Sizes. If one knows that a man is 6 feet tall and then sees this man even with only one eye, how far away the man is can be determined simply by the size of the image on the retina. Without consciously thinking about it, the brain has learned to determine automatically from the image size the distance of an object from the eye when the dimensions of the object already are known.

Determination of Distance by Moving Parallax. Another important means by which the eyes determine distance is that of moving parallax. If a person looks off into the distance with the eyes completely still, he or she perceives no moving parallax, but when moving the head to one side or another, the images of objects close by move rapidly across the retinae while the images of distant objects remain rather stationary. For instance, if an object is only 1 inch in front of the eye, by moving the head 1 inch then the image moves almost all the way across the retinae, whereas the image of an object 200 feet away does not move perceptibly. Thus, by this mechanism of moving parallax, one can tell the *relative distances* of different objects even though only one eye is used.

Determination of Distance by Stereopsis. Another method by which one perceives parallax is that of binocular vision. Because the eyes are a little more than 2 inches apart, the images on the two retinae are different—that is, an object that is 1 inch in front of the bridge of the nose forms an image on the temporal portion of the retina of each eye, whereas the image of a small object 20 feet in front of the nose is nearly in the middle of each eye. This type of parallax is illustrated in Figure 39–8, which shows the images of a black spot and a square actually reversed on the two retinae because they are at different distances in front of the eyes. This difference gives a type of parallax that is present at all times when both eyes are used. It is almost entirely this binocular parallax (called stereopsis) that gives a person with two eyes far greater ability to judge relative distances (*when objects are nearby*) than a person who has only one eye. However, stereopsis is virtually useless for depth perception at distances beyond 200 feet.

THE RETINA

The retina is the light-sensitive portion of the eye containing the *cones*, which are mainly responsible for color vision, and the *rods*, which are mainly responsible for vision in the dark. When the rods and cones are excited, signals are transmitted through successive neurons in the retina itself and finally into the optic nerve fibers and cerebral cortex. The purpose of the present discussion is to explain specifically the mechanisms by which the rods and cones detect both white and colored light.

The Layers of the Retina. Figure 39–9 shows the functional components of the retina arranged in layers from the outside to the inside as follows: (1) pigment layer, (2) layer of rods and cones projecting into the pigment, (3) outer limiting membrane, (4) outer nuclear layer containing the cell bodies of the rods and cones, (5) outer plexiform layer, (6) inner nuclear layer, (7) inner plexiform layer, (8) ganglionic layer, (9) layer of optic nerve fibers, and (10) inner limiting membrane.

After light passes through the lens system of the eye and then through the vitreous humor, it enters the retina at the point designated at the bottom of Figure 39–9; that is, it passes through the ganglion cells, the plexiform layer, the nuclear layers, and the limiting membranes before it finally reaches the rods and cones located all the way on the opposite side of the retina. This distance is a thickness of several hundred microns; visual acuity is obviously decreased by this passage through such nonhomogeneous tissue. However, in the central region of the retina, as will

OUTSIDE

Pigmented layer
Layer of rods and cones
Outer limiting membrane
Outer nuclear layer
Outer plexiform layer
Horizontal cell
Inner nuclear layer
Fiber of Müller
Amacrine cell
Inner plexiform layer
Ganglion cells
Ganglionic layer
Stratum opticum
Inner limiting membrane

DIRECTION OF LIGHT

Figure 39–9. Plan of the retinal neurons. (Modified from Polyak, S. L.: The Retina. Chicago, University of Chicago Press, 1941.)

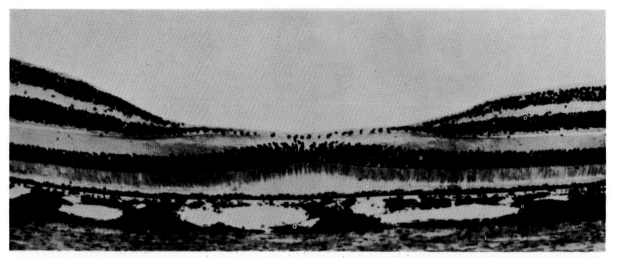

Figure 39–10. Photomicrograph of the macula and of the fovea in its center. Note that the inner layers of the retina are pulled to the side to decrease the interference with light transmission. (From Bloom and Fawcett: A Textbook of Histology. 10th ed. Philadelphia, W. B. Saunders Company, 1975; courtesy of H. Mizoguchi.)

be discussed below, the initial layers are pulled aside to prevent this loss of acuity.

The Foveal Region of the Retina and Its Importance in Acute Vision. A minute area in the center of the retina (illustrated in Figure 39–10) called the *macula*, which occupies a total area of less than 1 square millimeter, is especially capable of acute and detailed vision. This area is composed entirely of cones, but the cones are very much elongated and have a diameter of only 1.5 microns in contradistinction to the very large cones located farther peripherally in the retina. The central portion of the macula, only 0.4 mm in diameter, is called the *fovea*; in this region the blood vessels, the ganglion cells, the inner nuclear layer of cells, and the plexiform layers are all displaced to one side rather than resting directly on top of the cones. This arrangement allows light to pass unimpeded to the cones rather than through several layers of retina, which aids immensely in the acuity of visual perception by this foveal region of the retina.

The Rods and Cones. Figure 39–11 is a diagrammatic representation of a photoreceptor (either a rod or a cone), though the cones are distinguished by having a conical upper end as shown in Figure 39–12. In general, the rods are narrower and longer than the cones, but this is not always the case. In the peripheral portions of the retina, the rods are 2 to 5 microns in diameter whereas the cones are 5 to 8 microns in diameter; in the central part of the retina, in the fovea, the cones have a diameter of only 1.5 microns.

To the right in Figure 39–11, the four major functional segments of either a rod or a cone are labeled: (1) the *outer segment*, (2) the *inner segment*, (3) the *nucleus*, and (4) the *synaptic body*. In the outer segment, the light-sensitive photochemical is found. In the case of the rods, this is *rhodopsin*, and in the cones it is one of several photochemicals collectively called *iodopsin*, which is almost exactly

the same as rhodopsin except for a difference in spectral sensitivity.

Note in both Figures 39–11 and 39–12 the large numbers of discs in both the rods and the cones. Each of the discs is actually an infolded shelf of cell membrane. There are as many as 1000 discs in each rod or cone. At the tips of the rods, the discs are continually degenerating, but new ones are also being formed at a rate of about 50 to 100 per day at the base of the outer segment. In the cones, similar degeneration and replacement occurs, but it occurs along the entire extent of the outer segment.

Both rhodopsin and iodopsin are proteins incor-

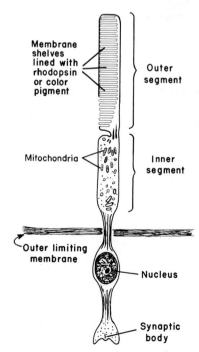

Figure 39–11. Schematic drawing of the functional parts of the rods and cones.

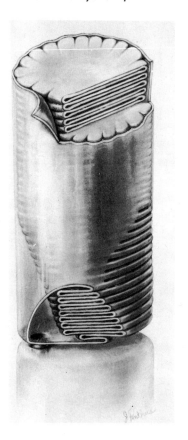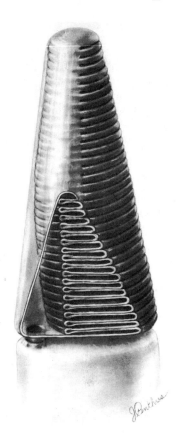

Figure 39-12. Membranous structures of the outer segments of a rod (left) and a cone (right). (Courtesy of Dr. Richard Young.)

porated into the membranes of the discs in the form of transmembrane proteins. The concentrations of these photosensitive pigments are so great that they constitute approximately 40 per cent of the entire mass of the outer segment.

The inner segment contains the usual cytoplasm of the cell with the usual cytoplasmic organelles. Particularly important are the mitochondria, for we shall see later that the mitochondria in this segment play an important role in providing most of the energy for function of the photoreceptors.

The synaptic body is the portion of the rod and cone that connects with the subsequent neuronal cells, the horizontal and bipolar cells, that represent the next stages in the vision chain.

The Pigment Layer of the Retina. The black pigment *melanin* in the pigment layer, together with still more melanin in the choroid, prevents light reflection throughout the globe of the eyeball; this is extremely important for acute vision. The pigment performs the same function in the eye as black paint inside the bellows of a camera. Without it, light rays would be reflected in all directions within the eyeball and would cause diffuse lighting of the retina rather than the contrasts between dark and light spots required for formation of precise images.

The importance of melanin in the pigment layer and choroid is well illustrated by its absence in *albino* persons who hereditarily lack melanin pigment in all parts of their bodies. When an albino enters a bright area, light that impinges on the retina is reflected in all directions by the white surface of the unpigmented choroid, so that a single discrete spot of light that would normally excite only a few rods or cones is reflected everywhere and excites many of the receptors. As a result, the visual acuity of albinos, even with the best of optical correction, is rarely better than 20/100 to 20/200.

The pigment layer also stores large quantities of *vitamin A*. This vitamin is exchanged back and forth through the membranes of the outer segments of the rods and cones, which themselves penetrate into the pigment layer. We shall see later that vitamin A is an important precursor of the photosensitive pigments and that this interchange of vitamin A is very important for adjustment of the light sensitivity of the receptors.

PHOTOCHEMISTRY OF VISION

Both the rods and cones contain chemicals that decompose on exposure to light and, in the process, excite the nerve fibers leading from the eye. The chemical in the *rods* is called *rhodopsin*; the light-sensitive chemicals in the *cones* have compositions only slightly different from that of rhodopsin and are collectively called *iodopsin*.

In the present section we will discuss principally the photochemistry of rhodopsin, but we can apply almost exactly the same principles to the photochemistry of the iodopsin of the cones.

THE RHODOPSIN-RETINAL VISUAL CYCLE AND EXCITATION OF THE RODS

Rhodopsin and Its Decomposition by Light Energy. The outer segment of the rod that projects into the pigment layer of the retina has a concentration of about 40 per cent of the light-sensitive pigment called *rhodopsin*, or *visual purple*. This substance is a combination of the protein *scotopsin* and the carotenoid pigment *retinal* (also called retinene). Furthermore, the retinal is a particular type called 11-*cis* retinal. This *cis* form of the retinal is important because only this form can combine with scotopsin to synthesize rhodopsin.

When light energy is absorbed by rhodopsin, the rhodopsin immediately begins to decompose, as shown at the top of Figure 39–13. The cause of this decomposition is photoactivation of electrons in the retinal portion of the rhodopsin, which leads to an instantaneous change (in the order of trillionths of a second) of the *cis* form of retinal into an all-*trans* form, which still has the same chemical structure as the *cis* form but has a different physical structure—a straight rather than a curved molecule. Because the three-dimensional orientation of the reactive sites of the all-*trans* retinal no longer fits with that of the reactive sites on the protein scotopsin, it begins to pull away from the scotopsin. The immedite product is *prelumirhodopsin*, which is a partially split combination of the all-*trans* retinal and scotopsin. However, prelumirhodopsin is an extremely unstable compound and decays in billionths of a second to *lumirhodopsin*. This decays in microseconds to *metarhodopsin I*, then in about a millisecond to *metarhodopsin II*, and, finally, much more slowly (in seconds) into the completely split products *scotopsin* and *all-trans retinal*.

During the first stages of splitting, the rods are excited and signals are transmitted into the central nervous system, as we shall discuss later.

Reformation of Rhodopsin. The first stage in the reformation of rhodopsin, as shown in Figure 39–13, is to reconvert the all-*trans* retinal into 11-*cis* retinal. This process is catalyzed by the enzyme *retinal isomerase*. Once the 11-*cis* retinal is formed, it automatically recombines with the scotopsin to reform rhodopsin. The product, rhodopsin, is a stable compound until its decomposition is again triggered by absorption of light energy.

The Role of Vitamin A in the Formation of Rhodopsin. Note in Figure 39–13 that there is a second chemical route by which all-*trans* retinal can be converted into 11-*cis* retinal. This is by conversion of the all-*trans* retinal first into all-*trans retinol*, which is one form of vitamin A. Then, the all-*trans* retinol is converted into 11-*cis* retinol under the influence of the enzyme isomerase. And, finally the 11-*cis* retinol is converted into 11-*cis* retinal.

Vitamin A is present both in the cytoplasm of the rods and in the pigment layer of the retina as well. Therefore, vitamin A is normally always available to form new retinal when needed. On the other hand, when there is excess retinal in the retina, the excess is converted back into vitamin A, thus reducing the amount of light-sensitive pigment in the retina. We shall see later that this interconversion between retinal and vitamin A is especially important in long-term adaptation of the retina to different light intensities.

Night Blindness. Night blindness occurs in severe vitamin A deficiency. The simple reason is that not enough vitamin A is then available to form adequate quantities of retinal. Therefore, the amounts of rhodopsin that can be formed in the rods, as well as the amounts of iodopsin in the cones, are all depressed. This condition is called *night blindness* because the amount of light available at night is then too little to permit adequate vision, though in daylight the rods and cones can still be excited despite their reduction in photochemical substances.

For night blindness to occur, a person usually must remain on a vitamin A–deficient diet for months, mainly because large quantities of vitamin A are normally stored in the liver. However, once night blindness does develop, it can sometimes be completely cured in less than an hour by intravenous injection of vitamin A.

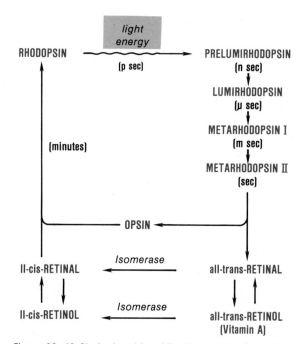

Figure 39–13. Photochemistry of the rhodopsin-retinal-vitamin A visual cycle.

Excitation of the Rod When Rhodopsin Decomposes

Generation of the Rod Receptor Potential. Generation of the rod receptor potential is entirely different from the generation of receptor potentials in almost all other sensory receptors. That is, excitation of the rod causes *increased negativity* of the membrane potential, which is a state of *hyperpolarization*, rather than decreased negativity, which is the process of depolarization that is characteristic of almost all other sensory receptors.

But, how does the breakdown of rhodopsin cause hyperpolarization? The answer is that *when rhodopsin decomposes, it decreases the membrane conductance for sodium ions in the outer segment of the rod.* And this causes hyperpolarization of the entire rod membrane in the following way:

Figure 39–14 illustrates movement of sodium ions in a complete electrical circuit through the inner and outer segments of the rod. The inner segment continually pumps sodium from inside the rod to the outside, thereby creating a negative potential on the inside of the cell. However, the membrane of the outer segment, in the *dark* state, is very leaky to sodium. Therefore, sodium continually leaks back to the inside of the rod and thereby neutralizes much of the negativity on the inside of the entire cell. Thus, under normal conditions when the rod is not excited, there is a reduced amount of electronegativity inside the membrane of the rod, normally about -30 millivolts.

When the rhodopsin in the outer segment of the rod is exposed to light and begins to decompose, however, this *decreases* the conductance of sodium to the interior of the rod even though sodium ions continue to be pumped out. Thus, more sodium ions now leave the rod than leak back in. Because these are positive ions, their loss from inside the rod creates increased negativity inside the membrane; and the greater the amount of light energy striking the rod, the greater the electronegativity—that is, the greater the degree of *hyperpolarization*. At maximum light intensity, the membrane potential approaches -90 millivolts, which is the equilibrium potential for potassium ions across the membrane.

Duration of the Receptor Potential and Logarithmic Relationship of the Receptor Potential to Light Intensity. When a sudden pulse of light strikes the retina, the transient hyperpolarization—that is, the receptor potential that occurs—lasts about one twentieth to one half of a second, depending on the intensity of the light and other factors. Therefore, a visual image impinged on the retina for only a millionth of a second nevertheless can cause the sensation of seeing the image, sometimes for up to half a second.

Another characteristic of the receptor potential is that it is approximately proportional to the logarithm of the light intensity. This feature is exceedingly important, because it allows the eye to discriminate light intensities through a range many thousand times as great as would be possible otherwise.

PHOTOCHEMISTRY OF COLOR VISION BY THE CONES

It was pointed out at the outset of this discussion that the photochemicals, collectively called iodopsin, in the cones have almost exactly the same chemical composition as that of rhodopsin in the rods. The only difference is that the protein portions in the cones, the opsins, called *photopsins,* are different from the scotopsin of the rods. The retinal portions are exactly the same in the cones as in the rods. The color-sensitive pigments of the cones therefore are combinations of retinal and photopsins.

In the discussion of color vision later in the chapter, it will become evident that three different types of photochemicals are present in different cones, thus making these cones selectively sensitive to the colors of blue, green, and red. These photochemicals are called respectively *blue-sensitive pigment, green-sensitive pigment,* and *red-sensitive pigment.* These pigments show peak light absorbencies at light wavelengths of 445, 535, and 570 millimicrons, respectively. These are also the wavelengths for peak light sensitivity for each type of cone, which begins to explain how the retina differentiates the colors. The approximate absorption curves for these three pigments are shown in Figure 39–15. Also shown is the absorption curve for the rhodopsin of the rods, which has a peak at 505 millimicrons.

AUTOMATIC REGULATION OF RETINAL SENSITIVITY— DARK AND LIGHT ADAPTATION

Relationship of Sensitivity to Photochemical Concentration. The sensitivity of rods is approximately proportional to the antilogarithm of the rhodopsin concentration, and it is assumed that this relationship also holds true in the cones. Therefore, the sensitivity of the rods and cones can be tremendously altered

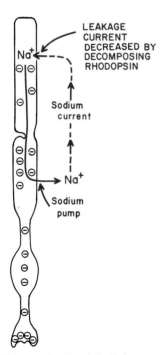

Figure 39–14. Theoretical basis for the generation of a hyperpolarization receptor potential caused by rhodopsin decomposition.

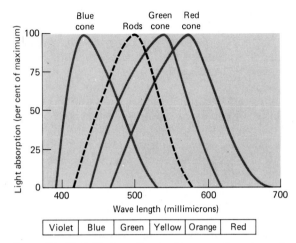

Figure 39–15. Light absorption by the respective pigments of the three color-receptive cones of the human retina. (Drawn from curves recorded by Marks et al.: Science 143:1181, 1964, and by Brown and Wald: Science 144:45, 1964.)

up or down by only slight changes in concentrations of the photosensitive chemicals.

Light and Dark Adaptations. If a person has been in bright light for a long time, large proportions of the photochemicals in both the rods and cones will have been reduced to retinal and opsins. Furthermore, most of the retinal of both the rods and cones will have been converted into vitamin A. Because of these two effects, the concentrations of the photosensitive chemicals are considerably reduced, and the sensitivity of the eye to light is even more reduced. This is called *light adaptation.*

On the other hand, if the person remains in darkness for a long time, essentially all the retinal and opsins in the rods and cones become converted into light-sensitive pigments. Furthermore, large amounts of vitamin A are converted into retinal, which is then changed into additional light-sensitive pigments, the final limit being determined by the amount of opsins in the rods and cones. Because of these two effects, the visual receptors gradually become so sensitive that even the most minute amount of light causes excitation. This is called *dark adaptation.*

Value of Light and Dark Adaptation in Vision. Between the limits of maximal dark adaptation and maximal light adaptation, the eye can change its sensitivity to light by as much as 500,000 to 1,000,000 times, the sensitivity automatically adjusting to changes in illumination.

Since the registration of images by the retina requires detection of both dark and light spots in the image, it is essential that the sensitivity of the retina always be adjusted so that the receptors respond to the lighter areas but not to the darker areas. An example of maladjustment of the retina occurs when a person leaves a movie theater and enters the bright sunlight; even the dark spots in the images then seem exceedingly bright, and as a consequence, the entire visual image is bleached, having little contrast between its different parts. Obviously, this is poor

vision, and it remains poor until the retina has adapted sufficiently that the dark spots of the image no longer stimulate the receptors excessively.

FUSION OF FLICKERING LIGHT BY THE RETINA

A flickering light is one in which intensity alternately increases and decreases rapidly. An instantaneous flash of light excites the visual receptors for as long as 1/5 to 1/10 second, and because of this *persistence* of excitation, rapidly successive flashes of light become *fused* together to give the appearance of being continuous. This well-known effect is demonstrated when one observes motion pictures or television. The images on the motion picture screen are flashed at a rate of 24 frames per second, while those of the television screen are flashed at a rate of 60 frames per second. As a result, the images fuse together, and continuous motion is observed.

The frequency at which flicker fusion occurs, called the *critical frequency for fusion,* varies with the light intensity. At a very low intensity, fusion results even when the rate of flicker is as low as 2 to 6 per second. However, in very bright illumination, the critical frequency for fusion rises to as great as 60 flashes per second. This difference results at least partly from the fact that the cones, which operate mainly at high levels of illumination, can detect much more rapid alterations in illumination than can the rods.

COLOR VISION

From the preceding sections, we know that different cones are sensitive to different colors of light. The present section is a discussion of the mechanisms by which the retina detects the different gradations of color in the visual spectrum.

THE TRICOLOR MECHANISM OF COLOR PERCEPTION

Many different theories have been proposed to explain the phenomenon of color vision, but they are all based on the well-known observation that the human eye can detect almost all gradations of colors when red, green, and blue monochromatic lights are appropriately mixed in different combinations.

The first important theory of color vision, that of Young, was later expanded and given a more experimental basis by Helmholz. Therefore, the theory is known as the *Young-Helmholz theory.* According to this theory, there are three different types of cones, each of which responds maximally to a different color.

As time has gone by, the Young-Helmholz theory has been further expanded, and more details have been worked out. It now is generally accepted as *the* mechanism of color vision.

Spectral Sensitivities of the Three Types of Cones. On the basis of psychological tests, the spectral sen-

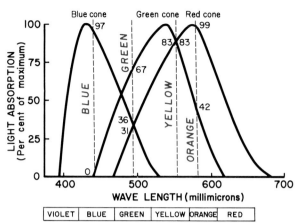

Figure 39-16. Demonstration of the degree of stimulation of the different color-sensitive cones by monochromatic lights of four separate colors: blue green, yellow, and orange.

sitivities of the three different types of cones in human beings are essentially the same as the light absorption curves for the three types of pigment found in the respective cones. These were illustrated in Figure 39-15 and are also shown in Figure 39-16. These curves can readily explain all the phenomena of color vision.

Interpretation of Color in the Nervous System. Referring to Figure 39-16, one can see that an orange monochromatic light with a wavelength of 580 millimicrons stimulates the red cones to a stimulus value of approximately 99 (99 per cent of the peak stimulation at optimum wavelength), while it stimulates the green cones to a value of approximately 42 and the blue cones not at all. Thus, the ratios of stimulation of the three different types of cones in this instance are 99:42:0. The nervous system interprets this set of ratios as the sensation of orange. On the other hand, a monochromatic blue light with a wavelength of 450 millimicrons stimulates the red cones to a stimulus value of 0, the green cones to a value of 0, and the blue cones to a value of 97. This set of ratios—0:0:97—is interpreted by the nervous system as blue. Likewise, ratios of 83:83:0 are interpreted as yellow and 31:67:36 as green.

This scheme also shows how it is possible for a person to perceive a sensation of yellow when a red light and a green light are shined into the eye at the same time, for this stimulates the red and green cones approximately equally, which gives a sensation of yellow even though no wavelength of light corresponding to yellow is present.

Perception of White Light. Approximately equal stimulation of all the red, green, and blue cones give one the sensation of seeing white. Yet there is no wavelength of light corresponding to white; instead, white is a combination of all the wavelengths of the spectrum. Furthermore, the sensation of white can be achieved by stimulating the retina with a proper combination of only three chosen colors that stimulate the respective types of cones equally.

COLOR BLINDNESS

Red-Green Color Blindness. When a single group of color receptive cones is missing from the eye, the person is unable to distinguish some colors from others. As can be observed by studying Figures 39-15 and 39-16, if the red cones are missing, light of 525 to 625 millimicrons wavelength can stimulate only the green-sensitive cones, so that the *ratio* of stimulation of the different cones does not change as the color shifts from green all the way through the red spectrum. Therefore, within this wavelength range, all colors appear to be the same to this color blind person.

On the other hand, if the green-sensitive cones are missing, the colors in the range from green to red can stimulate only the red-sensitive cones, and the person also perceives only one color within these limits. Therefore, when a person lacks either the red or green types of cones, he is said to be red-green color blind.

Blue Weakness. Occasionally, a person has blue weakness, which results from diminished blue receptors.

Stilling and Ishihara Test Charts. A rapid method for determining color blindness is based on the use of spot-charts such as those illustrated in Figure 39-17, some of which were developed by Stilling and others by Ishihara. These charts are arranged with a confusion of spots of several different colors. In the top chart, the normal person reads "74," while the red or green color blind person reads "21." In the bottom chart, the normal person reads "42," while the red blind person reads "2," and the green blind person reads "4."

If one studies these charts while at the same time observing the spectral sensitivity curves of the different cones in Figure 39-16, he can readily understand why excessive emphasis can be placed on spots of certain colors by color blind persons in comparison with normal persons.

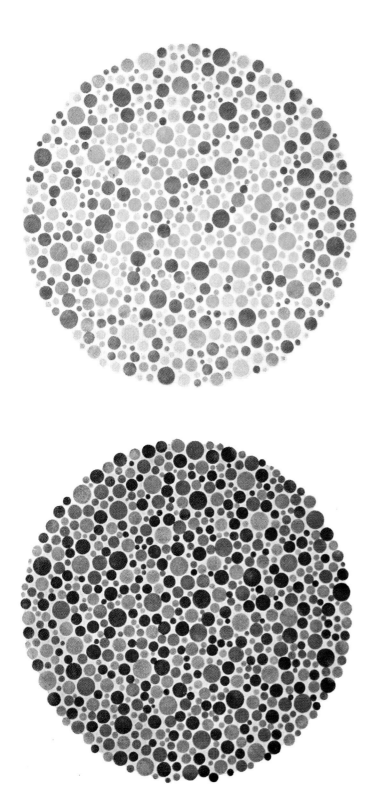

Figure 39–17. Two Ishihara charts. *Upper*: In this chart, the normal person reads "74," whereas the red-green color blind person reads "21." *Lower*: In this chart, the red-blind person (protanope) reads "2," while the green-blind person (deuteranope) reads "4." The normal person reads "42." (The charts have been reproduced from Ishihara: Tests for Colour-Blindness. Tokyo, Kanehara and Co., Ltd., Tokyo, Japan, but tests for color blindness cannot be conducted with this material. For accurate testing the original plate should be used.)

QUESTIONS

1. Why is the anterior surface of the cornea the major refractive surface of the eye's lens system?
2. When the ciliary muscle of the eye is completely relaxed, what happens to the tension on the *radial ligaments of the lens*? What happens to the shape of the lens and its focusing strength?
3. What happens to the range of accommodation of the lens as a person becomes older? What is meant by *presbyopia*?
4. What is meant by *depth of focus*? What happens to the depth of focus of the eye's focusing system when the pupillary aperture becomes very small?
5. What are the causes of *hypermetropia, myopia,* and *astigmatism*?
6. What type of lens is necessary to correct each of the above abnormalities of vision?
7. How far apart on the retina must two separate points of light be separated in order for a person to distinguish that there are two points rather than a single point?
8. If a person is said to have 20/50 vision, what is meant?
9. Explain how the visual system determines distance of an object from the eyes by the mechanisms of *moving parallax* and *stereopsis*.
10. Give the structure of a typical *rod*. How do *cones* differ from the rods?
11. Describe the *fovea* and its function in high acuity vision.
12. List the major functional segments of a rod or cone. Also describe the *discs* and their relationship to *rhodopsin* or *iodopsin*.
13. What is the relationship of the pigment layer of the retina to the rods and cones, and what is the importance of this relationship?
14. Describe the physical and chemical events that take place after rhodopsin is exposed to an instantaneous bright light.
15. Describe the reformation of rhodopsin after it has been decomposed in bright light.
16. What is the relationship between vitamin A and the visual pigments of the rods and cones?
17. How does generation of the receptor potential in the rods differ from the generation of a receptor potential in most sensory receptors of the body? Explain the mechanism for generating this potential.
18. What are the respective wavelengths for peak absorption by the different types of cones?
19. Why are light and dark adaptation very important in vision?
20. Explain how the brain interprets color by the visual signals received from the retina.
21. What is the cause of color blindness? What types of color blindness are common?

References

Optics

Allen, E. W.: Essentials of Ophthalmic Optics. New York, Oxford University Press, 1979.

Davson, H., and Graham, L. T., Jr.: The Eye. Vols. 1–6. New York, Academic Press, 1969–1974.

Fischbarg, J., and Lim, J. J.: Fluid and electrolyte transports across corneal endothelium. Curr Top Eye Res 4:201, 1984.

Hartstein, J.: Basics of Contact Lenses, 3rd ed. San Francisco, American Academy of Ophthalmology, 1979.

Kavner, R. S., and Dusky, L.: Total Vision. New York, A & W Publishers, 1980.

Kuszak, J. R., et al.: Sutures of the crystalline lens: a review. Scan Electron Microsc (Pt. 3):1369, 1984.

Lesperace: Ophthalmic Lasers. Photocoagulation, Photoradiation and Surgery. St. Louis, C. V. Mosby, 1983.

Miller, D.: Ophthalmology: The Essentials. Boston, Houghton Mifflin, 1979.

Morgan, M. W.: The Optics of Ophthalmic Lenses. Chicago, Professional Press, 1978.

Moses, R. A.: Adler's Physiology of the Eye: Clinical Application. 7th Ed. St. Louis, C. V. Mosby, 1981.

Records, R. E.: Physiology of the Human Eye and Visual System. Hagerstown, Md., Harper & Row, 1979.

Roth, H. W., and Roth-Wittig, M.: Contact Lenses. Hagerstown, Md., Harper & Row, 1980.

Safir, A., ed.: Refraction and Clinical Optics. Hagerstown, Md., Harper & Row, 1980.

Sloane, A. E., ed.: Manual of Refraction. Boston, Little, Brown, 1979.

The Retina

Allansmith, M. R.: The Eye and Immunology. St. Louis, C. V. Mosby, 1983.

Cunha-Vaz, J. G., ed.: The Blood-Retinal Barriers. New York, Plenum Press, 1980.

DeValois, R. L., and Jacobs, G. H.: Neural mechanisms of color vision. In Darian-Smith, I., ed.: Handbook of Physiology. Sec. 1, Vol. 3. Bethesda, American Physiological Society, 1984, p. 525.

Dowling, J. E., and Dubin, M. W.: The vertebrate retina. In Darian-Smith, I. ed.: Handbook of Physiology. Sec. 1, Vol. 3. Bethesda, American Physiological Society, 1984, p. 317.

Hillman, P., et al.: Transduction in invertebrate photoreceptors: role of pigment bistability. Physiol Rev 63:668, 1983.

Kanski, J. J., ed.: BIMR Ophthalmology. Vol. 1. Disorders of the Vitreous, Retina, and Choroid. Woburn, Mass, Butterworths, 1983.

MacNichol, E. F., Jr.: Three-pigment color vision. Sci Am 211:48, 1964.

Marks, W. B., et al.: Visual pigments of single primate cones. Science 143:1181, 1964.

Michaelson, I. C.: Textbook of the Fundus of The Eye. New York, Churchill Livingstone, 1980.

Schepens, C. L.: Retinal Detachment and Allied Diseases. Philadelphia, W. B. Saunders Co., 1983.

Wolf, G.: Multiple functions of vitamin A. Physiol Rev 64:873, 1984.

40

The Eye: II. Neurophysiology of Vision

THE VISUAL PATHWAY
NEURAL FUNCTION OF THE RETINA
NEURAL ORGANIZATION OF THE
RETINA
STIMULATION OF THE RODS AND
CONES
STIMULATION OF THE BIPOLAR CELLS
STIMULATION AND FUNCTION OF
THE HORIZONTAL CELLS
STIMULATION AND FUNCTION OF
THE AMACRINE CELLS
EXCITATION OF THE GANGLION
CELLS
DIFFERENT TYPES OF SIGNALS
TRANSMITTED BY THE GANGLION
CELLS THROUGH THE OPTIC NERVE
**FUNCTION OF THE LATERAL
GENICULATE BODY**
**FUNCTION OF THE PRIMARY VISUAL
CORTEX**

DETECTION OF LINES AND BORDERS
BY THE PRIMARY VISUAL CORTEX
ANALYSIS OF COLOR BY THE VISUAL
CORTEX
PERCEPTION OF LUMINOSITY
TRANSMISSION OF VISUAL
INFORMATION INTO OTHER
REGIONS OF THE CEREBRAL
CORTEX
THE FIELDS OF VISION; PERIMETRY
EYE MOVEMENTS AND THEIR CONTROL
FIXATION MOVEMENTS OF THE EYES
FUSION OF THE VISUAL IMAGES
**AUTONOMIC CONTROL OF
ACCOMMODATION AND PUPILLARY
APERTURE**
CONTROL OF ACCOMMODATION
CONTROL OF THE PUPILLARY
APERTURE

THE VISUAL PATHWAY

Figure 40–1 illustrates the visual pathway from the two retinae back to the *visual cortex*. After impulses leave the retinae they pass backward through the *optic nerves*. At the *optic chiasm* all the fibers from the nasal halves of the opposite retinae cross and join the fibers from the temporal retinae to form the *optic tracts*. The fibers of each optic tract synapse in the *lateral geniculate body*, and from here the *geniculocalcarine fibers* pass through the *optic radiation*, or *geniculocalcarine tract*, to the *optic*, or *visual*, *cortex* in the calcarine area of the occipital lobe.

In addition, visual fibers pass to lower areas of the brain, into the lateral thalamus, the superior colliculi, and the pretectal nuclei.

NEURAL FUNCTION OF THE RETINA

NEURAL ORGANIZATION OF THE RETINA

The detailed anatomy of the retina was illustrated in Figure 39–9 of the preceding chapter; Figure 40–2

illustrates the essentials of the retina's neural connections: to the left is the general organization of the neural elements in a peripheral retinal area, and to the right the organization in the foveal area. Note that in the peripheral region both rods and cones converge on *bipolar cells*, which in turn converge on *ganglion cells*. In the fovea, where only cones exist, there is little convergence; instead, the cones are represented by approximately equal numbers of bipolar and ganglion cells.

In addition, two other special types of cells are present in the retina, (1) the *horizontal cells* and (2) the *amacrine cells*. These will be discussed later.

Each retina contains about 125 million rods and 5.5 million cones; yet, as counted with the light microscope, only one million optic nerve fibers lead from the retina to the brain. Thus, an average of 125 rods and 6 cones converge on each optic nerve fiber. However, there are major differences between the peripheral retina and the central retina, for nearer the fovea increasingly fewer rods and cones converge on each optic fiber, and the rods and cones both

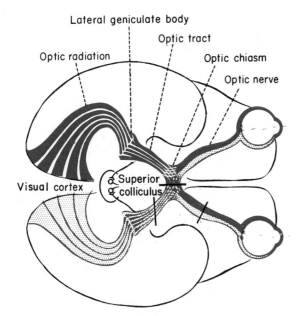

Figure 40–1. The visual pathways from the eyes to the visual cortex. (Modified from Polyak, S. L.: The Retina. University of Chicago Press, 1941.)

become more slender. These two effects progressively increase the acuity of vision toward the central retina. In the very central portion, in the fovea, there are no rods at all. Also, the number of optic nerve fibers leading from this part of the retina is almost equal to the number of cones in the fovea, as shown to the right in Figure 40–2. This circumstance mainly explains the high degree of visual acuity in the central portion of the retina in comparison with the very poor acuity in the peripheral portions.

Another difference between the peripheral and central portions of the retina is that there is consid-

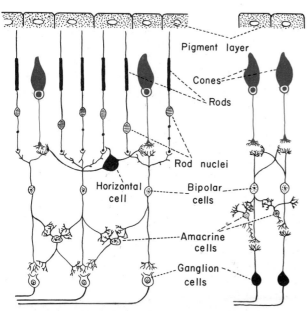

Figure 40–2. Neural organization of the retina: peripheral area to the left, foveal area to the right.

erably greater sensitivity of the peripheral retina to weak light. This increase in sensitivity results partly from the fact that as many as 300 rods converge on the same optic nerve fiber in the most peripheral portions of the retina, but the rods are also more sensitive to weak light than are the cones.

STIMULATION OF THE RODS AND CONES

Neither the rods nor the cones generate action potentials. Instead, the hyperpolarization receptor potentials generated in the outer segments of the rods and cones, which were discussed in the previous chapter, are transmitted through the bodies of these receptors to the *synaptic bodies* at their other ends. This transmission is by direct conduction of the electrical voltage itself, which is called *electrotonic conduction*. Then, at the synaptic body, the receptor potential controls the release of a transmitter substance the chemical nature of which is still not known. The transmitter in turn induces signals in the successive neurons, the *bipolar* and the *horizontal cells*. The signals in both these cells are also transmitted by electrotonic conduction, not by action potentials.

STIMULATION OF THE BIPOLAR CELLS

The most direct pathway from the rods and cones to the ganglion cells is through the bipolar cells. However, there are two different types of bipolar cells, the *depolarizing bipolar cell* and the *hyperpolarizing bipolar cell*.

The depolarizing bipolar cell is stimulated by the rods and cones when they are exposed to light. However, the hyperpolarizing cell becomes inhibited.

Because of this difference between the two types of bipolar cells, both positive signals and negative signals can be transmitted through different bipolar cells from the rods and cones to the amacrine and ganglion cells.

STIMULATION AND FUNCTION OF THE HORIZONTAL CELLS

The horizontal cells, illustrated to the left in Figure 40–2, connect laterally in the retina. The input to these cells is principally from the rods and cones; in turn, the cells excite the dendrites of bipolar cells located many microns laterally.

The horizontal cells respond to the rods and cones in the same manner as do the depolarizing bipolar cells. That is, they are excited by light. However, they in turn release an *inhibitory* transmitter that inhibits the laterally displaced bipolar cells with which they connect. Therefore, the horizontal cells represent a *lateral inhibitory pathway* in the retina.

STIMULATION AND FUNCTION OF THE AMACRINE CELLS

The amacrine cells are excited by the bipolar cells and in turn excite the ganglion cells. Many of the fiber pathways of the amacrine cells travel laterally in the inner plexiform layer of the retina, so this represents another pathway by which lateral signals can be transmitted, though this time the signals are excitatory in contrast to the inhibitory signals of the horizontal cells.

Perhaps the most important characteristic of the amacrine cells is that when they are stimulated by the bipolar cells, they at first respond very strongly, but the signal dies away to almost nothing in a fraction of a second. Therefore, it is believed that the amacrine cells send strong signals to the brain to indicate sudden changes in light intensity.

EXCITATION OF THE GANGLION CELLS

Spontaneous, Continuous Discharge of the Ganglion Cells. The ganglion cells transmit their signals through the optic nerve fibers to the brain in the form of action potentials. These cells, even when unstimulated, transmit continuous nerve impulses at an average rate of about 5 per second. The visual signal is superimposed on this basic level of ganglion cell stimulation. The signal can be either excitatory, with the number of impulses increasing to greater than 5 per second, or inhibitory, with the number of nerve impulses decreasing to below 5 per second—often all the way to zero.

Summation at the Ganglion Cells of Signals from the Bipolar, the Horizontal, and the Amacrine Cells. The depolarizing bipolar cells transmit the main direct *excitatory* information from the rods and the cones to the ganglion cells; the hyperpolarizing bipolar cells and the horizontal cells transmit *inhibitory* information from laterally displaced rods and cones to surrounding bipolar cells and then to the ganglion cells; the amacrine cells seem to transmit direct but short-lived transient signals indicating a *change* in the level of illumination of the retina. Thus, each of these types of cells performs a separate function in stimulating the ganglion cells.

DIFFERENT TYPES OF SIGNALS TRANSMITTED BY THE GANGLION CELLS THROUGH THE OPTIC NERVE

Transmission of Signals Depicting Contrasts in the Visual Scene— The Role of Lateral Inhibition

Most of the ganglion cells do not respond to the actual level of illumination of the scene; instead they respond only to the contrast borders. Since it seems that this response is the major means by which the form of the scene is transmitted to the brain, let us explain how the process occurs.

When flat light is applied to the entire retina—that is, when all the photoreceptors are stimulated equally by the incident light—the ganglion cell is neither stimulated nor inhibited. The reason is that the signals transmitted *directly* from the photoreceptors through

the depolarizing bipolar cells are excitatory, whereas the signals transmitted *laterally* through the hyperpolarizing bipolar cells and horizontal cells are inhibitory. Thus, the direct excitatory signal through one pathway is likely to be completely neutralized by the inhibitory signals through the lateral pathways. One such circuit is illustrated in Figure 40–3, which shows three photoreceptors; the central receptor excites a depolarizing bipolar cell. At the same time, the two receptors on either side are connected to this same bipolar cell through inhibitory horizontal cells that neutralize the direct excitatory signal.

Now, let us examine what happens when a contrast border occurs in the visual scene. Referring again to Figure 40–3, let us assume that the central photoreceptor is stimulated by a bright spot of light while the two lateral receptors are in the dark. The bright spot of light will excite the direct pathway through the bipolar cell. In addition, the fact that the two lateral photoreceptors are in the dark causes the two horizontal cells to be inhibited, and these cells lose their inhibitory effect, thus allowing still more excitation of the bipolar cell. Therefore, when light is everywhere, the excitatory and inhibitory signals to the bipolar cells mainly neutralize each other, but when contrasts occur, the signals through the direct and lateral pathways actually accentuate each other.

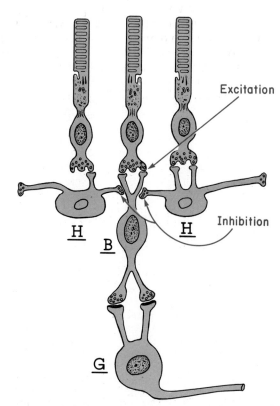

Figure 40–3. Typical arrangement of rods, horizontal cells (H), a bipolar cell (B), and a ganglion cell (G) in the retina, showing excitation at the synapses between the rods and the horizontal cells but inhibition between the horizontal cells and the bipolar cells.

Thus, the mechanism of lateral inhibition functions in the eye in the same way that it functions in most other sensory systems that is, to provide contrast detection and enhancement.

Detection of Instantaneous Changes in Light Intensity—The On-Off Response. Many of the ganglion cells are especially excited by *change* in light intensity. This ability to detect and transmit signals related to *change* in light intensity is caused by a rapid phase of "adaptation" of neurons in the visual chain. Since adaptation is known to be rapid in the amacrine cells, it has been suggested that the amacrine cells may be peculiarly adapted to detecting light intensity changes.

This capability to detect change in light intensity is especially well developed in the peripheral retina. For instance, a minute gnat flying across the peripheral field of vision is instantaneously detected. On the other hand, the same gnat sitting quietly in the peripheral field of vision remains entirely below the threshold of visual detection.

Transmission of Color Signals by the Ganglion Cells. A single ganglion cell may be stimulated by many cones or by a very few. When all three types of cones—the red, blue, and green stimulate the same ganglion cell, the signal transmitted through the ganglion cell is the same for any color of the spectrum. Therefore this signal plays no role in the detection of the different colors. Instead, it is a "white" signal.

On the other hand, many of the ganglion cells are excited by only one type of color cone but are inhibited by a second type. For instance, this is a frequent occurrence with the red and green cones, red causing excitation and green causing inhibition—or vice versa—green causing excitation and red, inhibition. The same type of reciprocal effect also occurs between blue cones on the one hand and a combination of red and green cones on the other hand, giving a reciprocal excitation-inhibition relationship between the blue and yellow colors.

The mechanism of this opposing effect of colors is as follows: One color-type cone excites the ganglion cell by the direct excitatory route through a depolarizing bipolar cell, while the other color type inhibits the ganglion cell by the indirect inhibitory route through a horizontal cell or a hyperpolarizing bipolar cell.

The importance of these color-contrast mechanisms is that they represent a method by which the retina itself begins to differentiate colors. Thus each color-contrast type of ganglion cell is excited by one color but inhibited by the opposing color. Therefore, the process of color analysis begins in the retina and is not entirely a function of the brain.

Thus, specific features of visual information begin to be dissected from other features before the visual signals leave the retina; then the different types of information are transmitted through the optic nerves and optic tracts mainly to the lateral geniculate body.

FUNCTION OF THE LATERAL GENICULATE BODY

Each lateral geniculate body is composed of six nuclear layers. Layers 2, 3, and 5 (from the surface inward) receive optic nerve fibers from the temporal portion of the ipsilateral retina, while layers 1, 4, and 6 receive fibers from the nasal retina of the opposite eye.

All layers of the lateral geniculate body relay visual information to the *visual cortex* through the *geniculocalcarine tract*.

The pairing of layers from the two eyes probably plays a major role in *fusion of vision*, because corresponding retinal fields in the two eyes connect with respective neurons that are approximately superimposed over each other in the successive layers. Also, with a little imagination, one can postulate that interaction between the successive layers could be part of the mechanism by which stereoscopic depth perception occurs, because this also depends on comparing the visual images of the two eyes and determining their slight differences, as was discussed in Chapter 39.

The signals recorded in the relay neurons of the lateral geniculate body are similar to those recorded in the ganglion cells of the retina. A few of the neurons transmit luminosity signals, while the majority transmit signals depicting only contrast borders in the visual image; also, many of the neurons are particularly responsive to movement of objects across the visual scene. However, the signals of the geniculate neurons are different from those in the ganglion cells in that a greater number of the complex interactions are found. That is, a much higher percentage of the neurons respond to contrast in the visual scene or to movement. These more complex reactions presumably result from convergence of signals from two or more ganglion cells on the relay neurons of the lateral geniculate body.

FUNCTION OF THE PRIMARY VISUAL CORTEX

The ability of the visual system to detect spatial organization of the visual scene—that is, to detect the forms of objects, brightness of the individual parts of the objects, shading, and so forth—is dependent on the function of the *primary visual cortex*, the anatomy of which is illustrated in Figure 40–4. This area lies mainly in the *calcarine fissure*, located bilaterally on the medial aspect of each occipital cortex. Specific points of the retina connect with specific points of the visual cortex, the right halves of the two respective retinae connecting with the right visual cortex and the left halves with the left visual cortex. The macula is represented at the occipital pole of the

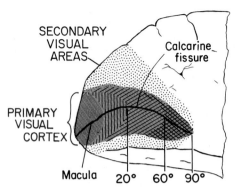

Figure 40–4. The visual cortex.

visual cortex and the peripheral regions of the retina are represented in concentric arcs progressively farther forward from the occipital pole. The upper portion of the retina is represented superiorly in the visual cortex and the lower portion inferiorly. Note the large area of cortex receiving signals from the macular region of the retina. It is in this region that the fovea, which gives the highest degree of visual acuity, is represented.

DETECTION OF LINES AND BORDERS BY THE PRIMARY VISUAL CORTEX

If a person looks at a blank wall, only a few neurons of the primary visual cortex will be stimulated, whether the illumination of the wall is bright or dark. Therefore, the question must be asked, What does the visual cortex do? To answer this question, let us now place on the wall a large cross such as that shown to the left in Figure 40–5. To the right is illustrated the spatial pattern of the greater majority of the excited neurons that one finds in the visual cortex. *Note that the areas of excitation occur along the sharp borders of the visual pattern.* Thus, by the time the visual signal is recorded in the primary visual cortex, it is concerned mainly with the *contrasts* in the visual scene rather than with the flat areas. At each point in the visual scene where there is a change from dark to light or light to dark, the corresponding area of the primary visual cortex becomes stimulated. The intensity of stimulation is determined by the *gradient of contrast*. That is, the greater the sharpness in the contrast border and the greater the difference in

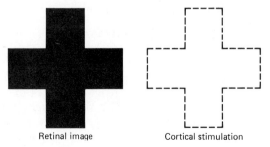

Retinal image   Cortical stimulation

Figure 40–5. Pattern of excitation occurring in the visual cortex in response to a retinal image of a dark cross.

intensities between the light and dark areas, the greater is the degree of stimulation.

Thus, the *pattern of contrasts* in the visual scene is impressed upon the neurons of the visual cortex, and this pattern has a spatial orientation roughly the same as that of the retinal image.

Not only does the visual cortex detect the *existence* of lines and borders in the different areas of the retinal image, but it also detects the *orientation* of each line or border as well as its length. This discernment is achieved by excitation of specific secondary neurons by lines of one orientation and length and other secondary neurons by lines of other orientations and lengths.

ANALYSIS OF COLOR BY THE VISUAL CORTEX

Some of the neurons in the visual cortex respond specifically to colors rather than simply to lines. However, as is true in the retina and also in the lateral geniculate body, stimulation of these neurons usually requires contrasting colors, especially the red-green and the blue-yellow opponent colors. The deciphering of color information is believed also to become more complex at successive levels of neuronal organization. In fact, full appreciation of color probably does not occur in the primary visual cortex alone, for it has recently been found in human beings that lesions on the ventral surface of the occipital lobe can cause lack of color reception. It is suggested, therefore, that this ventral surface area may be a final region for color signal processing.

PERCEPTION OF LUMINOSITY

Very little is known about the way in which the brain detects the level of luminosity. However, it is believed that this detection results at least partly from the effects of luminosity in increasing the intensity of the visual contrasts caused by lines, borders, moving objects, and opponent colors in the visual scene. That is, the greater the light intensity, the greater are the degrees of contrast and therefore the more strongly the visual cortex is stimulated.

In addition, some of the ganglion cells of the retina do respond to luminosity, especially some of the very small ganglion cells. These transmit luminosity signals into the pretectal region of the brain stem to control the size of the pupil. It is possible that this same information is used to help a person appreciate the level of illumination.

TRANSMISSION OF VISUAL INFORMATION INTO OTHER REGIONS OF THE CEREBRAL CORTEX

Signals from the primary visual cortex project laterally in the occipital cortex into *visual association areas* (also called *secondary visual areas*), which are loci for additional processing of visual information.

Here the neurons respond to more complex patterns than do those in the primary visual cortex. For instance, some cells are stimulated by simple geometric patterns such as curving borders or angles. It presumably is these progressively more complex interpretations that eventually decode the visual information, giving a person the overall impression of the visual scene that is observed.

Human beings who have destructive lesions of the visual association areas have difficulty with certain types of visual perception and visual learning. For instance, a lesion in the angular gyrus of the occipital lobe, one of the visual association areas, can cause the abnormality known as *dyslexia* or *word blindness*, meaning difficulty in understanding the meanings of words that are seen.

THE FIELDS OF VISION; PERIMETRY

The *field of vision* is the area seen by an eye at a given instant. The area to the nasal side is called the *nasal field of vision*, and the area to the lateral side, the *temporal field of vision*.

To diagnose blindness in specific portions of the retinas, one charts the field of vision for each eye by a process known as *perimetry*. This is done by having the subject look with one eye toward a central spot directly in front of the eye. Then a small dot of light or a small object is moved back and forth in all areas of the field of vision, laterally and nasally, upward and downward, and the person indicates when the spot of light or object can be seen and when it cannot. At the same time, a chart (Fig. 40–6) is made for the eye, showing the areas in which the subject can and cannot see the spot. Thus the field of vision is plotted.

In all perimetry charts, a *blind spot* caused by lack of rods and cones in the retina over the *optic disc* (where the optic nerve leaves the eyeball) is found

approximately 15 degrees lateral to the central point of vision, as illustrated in the figure. Other blind spots frequently occur where there are retinal lesions such as those found in diabetes and, frequently, in persons who smoke too much.

EYE MOVEMENTS AND THEIR CONTROL

To make use of the abilities of the eyes, almost as important as the system for interpretation of the visual signals from the eyes is the cerebral control system for directing the eyes toward the object to be viewed.

Muscular Control of Eye Movements. The eye movements are controlled by three separate pairs of muscles, shown in Figure 40–7: (1) the medial and lateral recti, (2) the superior and inferior recti, and (3) the superior and inferior obliques. The medial and lateral recti contract reciprocally to move the eyes from side to side. The superior and inferior recti contract reciprocally to move the eyes upward or downward. And the oblique muscles function mainly to rotate the eyeballs to keep the visual fields in the upright position.

Neural Pathways for Control of Eye Movements. Figure 40–7 also illustrates the nuclei of the third, fourth, and sixth cranial nerves and their innervation of the ocular muscles. Shown, too, are the interconnections between these three nuclei through the *medial longitudinal fasciculus*. Either by way of this fasciculus or by way of other closely associated pathways, each of the three sets of muscles to each eye is *reciprocally* innervated, so that one muscle of the pair relaxes while the other contracts.

Figure 40–8 illustrates cortical control of the oculomotor apparatus, showing spread of signals from the occipital visual areas through occipitotectal and occipitocollicular tracts into the pretectal and superior collicular areas of the brain stem. In addition, a frontotectal tract passes from the frontal cortex into the pretectal area. From both the pretectal and the

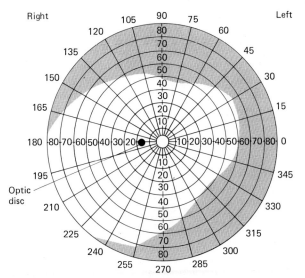

Figure 40–6. A perimetry chart, showing the field of vision for the left eye.

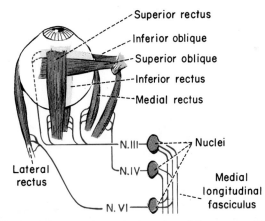

Figure 40–7. The extraocular muscles of the eye and their innervation.

superior collicular areas, the oculomotor control signals then pass to the nuclei of the oculomotor nerves. Finally, strong signals are also transmitted into the oculomotor system from the vestibular nuclei by way of the medial longitudinal fasciculus.

FIXATION MOVEMENTS OF THE EYES

Perhaps the most important movements of the eyes are those that cause the eyes to "fix" on a discrete portion of the field of vision.

Fixation movements are controlled by two entirely different neuronal mechanisms. The first of these allows a person to move his or her eyes voluntarily to find the object upon which to fix his or her vision; this is called the *voluntary fixation mechanism.* The second is an involuntary mechanism that holds the eyes firmly on the object once it has been found; this is called the *involuntary fixation mechanism.*

The voluntary fixation movements are controlled by a small cortical area located bilaterally in the premotor cortical regions of the frontal lobes, as illustrated in Figure 40–8. Bilateral dysfunction or destruction of these areas makes it difficult or almost impossible to "unlock" the eyes from one point of fixation and then move them to another point. It is usually necessary to blink the eyes or put a hand over them for a short time, which then allows movement of the eyes.

On the other hand, the fixation mechanism that causes the eyes to "lock" on the object of attention once it is found is controlled by an *involuntary fixation area of the occipital cortex,* which is also illustrated in Figure 40–8. When this area is destroyed bilaterally, the person has difficulty or becomes completely unable to keep his or her eyes directed toward a given fixation point.

Mechanism of Involuntary Fixation. Visual fixation results from a negative feedback mechanism that prevents the object of attention from leaving the foveal portion of the retina. Once a spot of light has become fixed on the foveal region of the retina, each time the spot drifts as far as the edge of the fovea, a sudden *flicking movement* of the eyes occurs to move the spot away from the edge back toward the center, which is an automatic response to keep the image from drifting off the fovea. These drifting and flicking motions are illustrated in Figure 40–9, which shows by dashed lines the slow drifting across the retina and by solid lines the flicks that keep the image from leaving the foveal region.

Saccadic Movement of the Eyes

When the visual scene is moving continuously before the eyes, as when one is riding in a car or turning around, the eyes fix on one highlight after another in the visual field, jumping from one to the next at a rate of two to three times per second. These jumps are called *saccades.* The saccades occur so rapidly that not more than 10 per cent of the total time is spent in moving the eyes, 90 per cent of the time

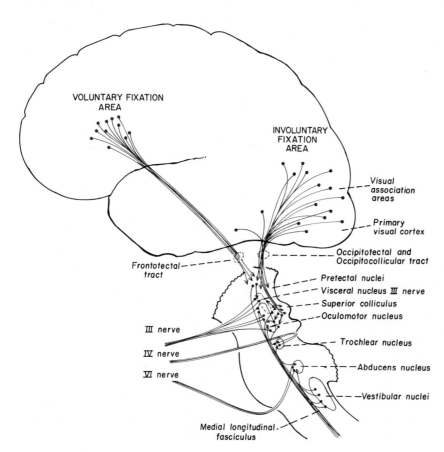

Figure 40–8. Neural pathways for control of conjugate movement of the eyes.

VOLUNTARY FIXATION AREA

INVOLUNTARY FIXATION AREA

Visual association areas

Primary visual cortex

Occipitotectal and Occipitocollicular tract

Frontotectal tract

Pretectal nuclei

Visceral nucleus III nerve

Superior colliculus

Oculomotor nucleus

III nerve

Trochlear nucleus

IV nerve

Abducens nucleus

VI nerve

Vestibular nuclei

Medial longitudinal fasciculus

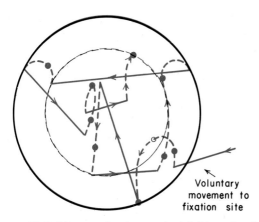

Figure 40–9. Movements of a spot of light on the fovea, showing sudden "flicking" movements to move the spot back toward the center of the fovea whenever it drifts to the foveal edge. (The dashed lines represent slow drifting movements, and the solid lines represent sudden flicking movements.)

Voluntary movement to fixation site

being allocated to the fixation sites. Also, the brain suppresses the visual image during the saccades so that one is completely unconscious of the movements from point to point.

Saccadic Movements During Reading. During the process of reading, a person usually makes several saccadic movements of the eyes for each line. In this case, the visual scene is not moving past the eyes, but the eyes are trained to scan in saccadic jumps across the visual scene to extract the important information. Similar saccades occur when, for example, a person observes a painting or examines someone of the opposite sex, except that the saccades occur in one direction after another, from one highlight to another, then another, and so forth.

FUSION OF THE VISUAL IMAGES

To make the visual perceptions more meaningful and also to aid in depth perception by the mechanism of stereopsis, discussed in Chapter 39, the visual images in the two eyes normally *fuse* with each other on corresponding points of the two retinas.

The visual cortex plays a very important role in fusion. It was pointed out earlier in the chapter that corresponding points of the two retinas transmit visual signals to different neuronal layers of the lateral geniculate body; these signals in turn are relayed to adjacent parallel stripes of neurons in the visual cortex. Interactions occur between the stripes of cortical neurons; these cause *interference patterns of excitation* in some of the local neuronal cells when the two visual images are not precisely "in register"—that is, not precisely fused. This excitation presumably provides the signal that is transmitted to the oculomotor apparatus to cause convergence or divergence or rotation of the eyes so that fusion can be reestablished. Once the corresponding points of the retinas are precisely in register, the excitation of the specific cells in the visual cortex disappears.

AUTONOMIC CONTROL OF ACCOMMODATION AND PUPILLARY APERTURE

The Autonomic Nerves to the Eyes. The eye is innervated by both parasympathetic and sympathetic fibers, as illustrated in Figure 40–10. The parasympathetic fibers arise in the *Edinger-Westphal nucleus* (also called the *visceral nucleus of the third nerve*) and then pass in the *third nerve* to the *ciliary ganglion*, which lies about 1 cm behind the eye. Here the fibers synapse with postganglionic parasympathetic neurons that pass through the *ciliary nerves* into the eyeball. These nerves excite the ciliary muscle and the sphincter of the iris.

The sympathetic innervation of the eye originates in the *intermediolateral horn cells* of the first thoracic segment of the spinal cord. From here, presynaptic fibers enter the sympathetic chain and pass upward to the *superior cervical ganglion*, where they synapse with postganglionic neurons. Fibers from these neurons spread along the carotid artery and along successively smaller arteries until they reach the eyeball. There the sympathetic fibers innervate the radial fibers of the iris as well as several extraocular structures around the eye. They also supply very weak inhibitory innervation to the ciliary muscle.

CONTROL OF ACCOMMODATION

Continuous nervous control of the accommodation mechanism—the mechanism that focuses the lens

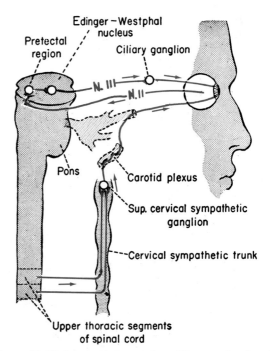

Figure 40–10. Autonomic innervation of the eye, showing also the reflex arc of the light reflex. (Modified from Ranson and Clark: Anatomy of the Nervous System. Philadelphia, W. B. Saunders Company, 1959.)

system of the eye—is essential to achieve a high degree of visual acuity. Accommodation results from contraction or relaxation of the ciliary muscle— contraction causing increased strength of the lens systems as explained in Chapter 39 and relaxation causing decreased strength. The question that must be answered now is, How does one adjust this accommodation to keep the eyes in focus all the time?

Accommodation of the lens is regulated by a negative feedback mechanism that automatically adjusts the focal power of the lens to attain the highest degree of visual acuity. When the eyes have been looking at some far object and then suddenly look at a near object, the lens accommodates for maximum acuity of vision usually within one second; the precise control mechanism that causes this rapid and accurate focusing of the eye is still unclear. However, some of the different types of clues that can help the lens change its strength in the proper direction include the following: (1) *Chromatic aberration* appears to be important. That is, the red light rays focus on the retina slightly posteriorly to the blue light rays. The eyes appear to be able to detect which of these two types of rays is in better focus, and this clue relays the information to the accommodating mechanism to make the lens stronger or weaker. (2) When the eyes fixate on a near object they also converge toward each other. The neural mechanisms for *convergence cause a simultaneous signal to strengthen the lens of the eye.* (3) *Since the fovea is a depressed area, the clarity of focus in the depth of the fovea compared with the clarity of focus on the edges will be different.* It has been suggested that this circumstance also gives clues as to which way the strength of the lens needs to be changed. (4) It has been found that *the degree of accommodation of the lens oscillates slightly* all of the time at a frequency of as much as two times per second. It has been suggested that the visual image becomes clearer when the lens strength oscillates in the appropriate direction and poorer when the lens strength oscillates in the wrong direction. This difference could give a rapid clue as to which way the strength of the lens needs to change to provide the appropriate focus.

CONTROL OF THE PUPILLARY APERTURE

Stimulation of the parasympathetic nerves excites the pupillary sphincter, thereby decreasing the pupillary aperture; this is called *miosis*. On the other hand, stimulation of the sympathetic nerves excites the radial fibers of the iris and causes pupillary dilatation, which is called *mydriasis*.

The Pupillary Light Reflex. When light shines into the eyes, the pupils constrict, a reaction called the pupillary light reflex. The neuronal pathway for this reflex is illustrated in Figure 40–10. When light impinges on the retina, the resulting impulses pass through the optic nerves and optic tracts and thence into nerve branches that terminate in the *pretectal nuclei* of the brain stem, near the oculomotor nuclei. From here, impulses pass to the *Edinger-Westphal nucleus* and finally pass back through the *parasympathetic nerves* to constrict the sphincter of the iris. In darkness, the Edinger-Westphal nucleus becomes inhibited, which results in dilatation of the pupil.

The function of the light reflex is to help the eye adapt extremely rapidly to changing light conditions, the importance of which was explained in the previous chapter. The limits of pupillary diameter are about 1.5 mm on the small side and 8 mm on the large side. Therefore, the range of light adaptation that can be effected by the pupillary reflex is about 30 to 1.

QUESTIONS

1. Describe the visual pathway.
2. Describe in sequence the stimulation and the functions of the *rods* and *cones*, the *bipolar cells*, the *horizontal cells*, the *amacrine cells*, and the *ganglion cells*.
3. Explain the function of *lateral inhibition* in the retina as a means for highlighting contrasts in the visual scene.
4. Explain the transmission of color signals by ganglion cells. What is meant by *opponent colors*, and how do they stimulate the ganglion cells?
5. Discuss the relaying of visual signals through the *lateral geniculate body*.
6. Where is the *primary visual cortex* located in the brain?
7. Describe the localization of signals from different parts of the retina in the primary visual cortex.
8. Explain why the visual cortex detects mainly lines and borders rather than flat areas in the visual scene.
9. How does the visual cortex function in the analysis of color and in the perception of luminosity?
10. What is meant by the *fields of vision*? Explain how one finds blind spots in the field of vision of an eye by the method of *perimetry*.
11. What are the three separate pairs of *extraoccular muscles* that control eye movements? Also, give the nervous pathways for control of the eye movements.
12. What is the difference between the *voluntary* and the *involuntary fixation* mechanisms?
13. Explain the feedback mechanism, from the eye to the brain and back to the extraocular muscles, that causes involuntary fixation.
14. What is meant by *saccadic movements* of the eyes, and how do these function during reading?
15. What is the neural mechanism that causes *fusion* of the visual images from the two eyes?
16. Explain the neural mechanism for control of *accommodation*. What are some of the clues in the visual signals that help to control accommodation?
17. Describe the neural circuitry for control of the diameter of the pupil.

References

Anderson, D. R.: Testing the Field of Vision. St. Louis, C. V. Mosby, 1983.

Bishop, P. O.: Processing of visual information within the retinostriate system. In Darian-Smith, I., ed.: Handbook of Physiology. Sec. 1, Vol. 3. Bethesda, American Physiological Society, 1984, p. 341.

Buttner, E. J. ed.: Neuroanatomy of the Oculomotor System. New York, Elsevier Science Publishing Co., 1984.

DeValois, R. L., and Jacobs, G. H.: Neural mechanisms of color vision. In Darian-Smith, I., ed.: Handbook of Physiology. Sec. 1, Vol. 3. Bethesda, American Physiological Society, 1984, p. 525.

Fregnac, Y., and Imbert, M.: Development of neuronal selectivity in primary visual cortex of cat. Physiol Rev 64:325, 1984.

Gilbert, C. D.: Microcircuitry of the visual cortex. Annu Rev Neurosci 6:217, 1983.

Hubel, D. H., and Wiesel, T. N.: Receptive fields of cells in striate cortex of very young, visually inexperienced kittens. J Neurophysiol 26:994, 1963.

Hubel, D. H., and Wiesel, T. N.: Brain mechanisms of vision. Sci Am 241(3):150, 1979.

Poggio, G. F., and Poggio, T.: The analysis of stereopsis. Annu Rev Neurosci 7:379, 1984.

Robinson, D. A.: Control of eye movements. In Brooks, V. B., ed.: Handbook of Physiology. Sec. 1, Vol. 2. Bethesda, American Physiological Society, 1981, p. 1275.

Schiller, P. H.: The superior colliculus and visual function. In Darian-Smith, I., ed.: Handbook of Physiology. Sec. 1, Vol. 3. Bethesda, American Physiological Society, 1984, p. 457.

Sherman, S. M., and Spear, P. D.: Organization of visual pathways in normal and visually deprived cats. Physiol Rev 62:738, 1982.

Simpson, J. I.: The accessory optic system. Annu Rev Neurosci 7:13, 1984.

Woolsey, C. N., ed.: Cortical Sensory Organization. Multiple Visual Areas. Clifton, NJ Humana Press, 1981.

Wurtz, R. H., and Albano, J. E.: Visual-motor function of the primate superior colliculus. Annu Rev Neurosci 3:189, 1980.

41

The Sense of Hearing and the Chemical Senses of Taste and Smell

HEARING
    THE TYMPANIC MEMBRANE AND THE
       OSSICULAR SYSTEM
    THE COCHLEA
    FUNCTION OF THE ORGAN OF
       CORTI
    DETERMINATION OF PITCH—THE
       PLACE PRINCIPLE
    DETERMINATION OF LOUDNESS
    FREQUENCY RANGE OF HEARING
    CENTRAL AUDITORY MECHANISMS
    FUNCTION OF THE CEREBRAL
       CORTEX IN HEARING
    DISCRIMINATION OF DIRECTION
       FROM WHICH SOUND EMANATES
    DEAFNESS

THE SENSE OF TASTE
    THE PRIMARY SENSATIONS OF TASTE
    THE TASTE BUD AND ITS FUNCTION
    TRANSMISSION OF TASTE SIGNALS
       INTO THE CENTRAL NERVOUS
       SYSTEM
    SPECIAL ATTRIBUTES OF THE TASTE
       SENSE
THE SENSE OF SMELL
    THE OLFACTORY MEMBRANE
    STIMULATION OF THE OLFACTORY
       CELLS
    TRANSMISSION OF SMELL
       SENSATIONS INTO THE CENTRAL
       NERVOUS SYSTEM

HEARING

The purpose of the first half of this chapter is to describe and to explain the mechanism by which the ear receives sound waves, discriminates their frequencies, and finally transmits auditory information into the central nervous system.

THE TYMPANIC MEMBRANE AND THE OSSICULAR SYSTEM

Figure 41–1 illustrates the *tympanic membrane* (commonly called the *eardrum*) and the *ossicular system,* which transmits sound through the middle ear. The tympanic membrane is cone-shaped, with its concavity facing downward toward the auditory canal. Attached to the very center of the tympanic membrane is the *handle* of the *malleus*. At its other end, the malleus is tightly bound to the *incus* by ligaments, so that whenever the malleus moves, the incus moves in unison with it. The opposite end of the incus in

turn articulates with the stem of the *stapes*, and the *faceplate* of the stapes lies against the membranous labyrinth in the opening of the oval window where sound waves are transmitted into the inner ear, the *cochlea*.

The ossicles of the middle ear are suspended by ligaments in such a way that the combined malleus

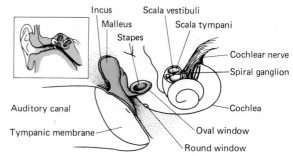

Figure 41–1. The tympanic membrane, the ossicular system of the middle ear, and the inner ear.

and incus act as a single lever having its fulcrum approximately at the border of the tympanic membrane. The large *head* of the malleus, which is on the opposite side of the fulcrum from the handle, almost exactly balances the other end of the lever, so that changes in position of the body will not increase or decrease the tension on the tympanic membrane.

The handle of the malleus is constantly pulled inward by ligaments and by the *tensor tympani muscle*, which keeps the tympanic membrane tensed. This arrangement allows sound vibrations on *any* portion of the tympanic membrane to be transmitted to the malleus, which would not be true if the membrane were lax.

Impedance Matching by the Ossicular System. The amplitude of movement of the stapes faceplate with each sound vibration is only three fourths as much as the movement of the handle of the malleus. Therefore, the ossicular lever system does not amplify the distance of movement as is commonly believed, but instead the system increases the *force* of movement about 1.3 times. Also, the surface area of the tympanic membrane is approximately 55 sq mm, whereas the surface area of the stapes averages 3.2 sq mm. This 17-fold difference times the 1.3-fold ratio of the lever system allows all the energy of a sound wave impinging on the tympanic membrane to be applied to the small faceplate of the stapes, causing approximately 22 times as much *pressure* on the fluid of the cochlea as is exerted by the sound wave against the tympanic membrane. Since fluid has far greater inertia than air, it is easily understood that increased amounts of pressure are needed to cause vibration in the fluid. Therefore, the tympanic membrane and ossicular system provide *impedance matching* between the sound waves in air and the sound vibrations in the fluid of the cochlea.

In the absence of the ossicular system and tympanum, sound waves can travel directly through the air of the middle ear and can even enter the cochlea at the oval window. However, the sensitivity for hearing is then 20 decibels less than for ossicular transmission—equivalent to a decrease from loud shouting to a barely audible voice level.

Attenuation of Sound by Contraction of the Stapedius and the Tensor Tympani Muscles. When loud sounds are transmitted through the ossicular system into the central nervous system, a reflex occurs after a latent period of 40 to 80 milliseconds to cause contraction of both the *stapedius* and *tensor tympani muscles*. The tensor tympani muscle pulls the handle of the malleus inward, while the stapedius muscle pulls the stapes outward. These two forces oppose each other and thereby cause the entire ossicular system to develop a high degree of rigidity, thus greatly reducing the ossicular conduction of low-frequency sound, mainly frequencies below 1000 cycles per second.

This *attenuation reflex* can reduce the intensity of sound transmission by as much as 30 to 40 decibels, which is about the same difference as that between a whisper and the sound emitted by a loud voice. The function of this mechanism is twofold: (1) To *protect* the cochlea from damaging vibrations caused by excessively loud sound. (2) To *mask* low-frequency sounds in loud environments. This usually removes a major share of the background noise and allows a person to concentrate on sounds above 1000 cycles per second frequency. It is in this upper-frequency range that most of the pertinent information in voice communication is achieved.

Another function of the tensor tympani and stapedius muscles is to decrease the person's hearing sensitivity to his own speech. This effect is activated by collateral signals transmitted to these muscles at the same time that his brain activates his voice mechanism.

THE COCHLEA

The cochlea is a system of coiled tubes, shown in Figure 41–1 and in cross-section in Figures 41–2 and 41–3 with three different tubes coiled side by side: the *scala vestibuli*, the *scala media*, and the *scala tympani*. The scala vestibuli and scala media are separated from each other by *Reissner's membrane* (also called the *vestibular membrane*), and the scala tympani and scala media are separated from each other by the *basilar membrane*. On the surface of the basilar membrane lies a structure, the *organ of Corti*, which contains a series of mechanically sensitive cells, the *hair cells*. These are the receptive end-organs that generate nerve impulses in response to sound vibrations.

Figure 41–4 illustrates schematically the functional parts of the uncoiled cochlea for transmission of sound vibrations. First, note that Reissner's membrane is missing from this figure. This membrane is so thin and so easily moved that it does not obstruct the passage of sound vibrations from the scala vestibuli into the scala media at all. Therefore, so far as the transmission of sound is concerned, the scala

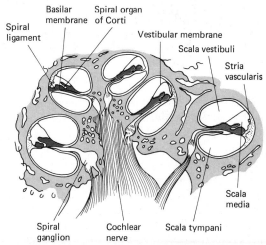

Figure 41–2. The cochlea. (From Clemente, C. O. (Ed.): *Gray's Anatomy*, Lea & Febiger, Philadelphia, 1985.)

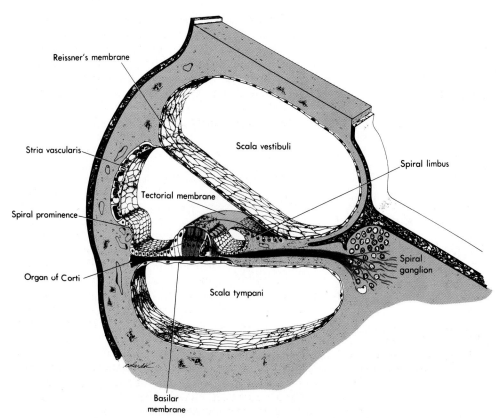

Figure 41–3. A section through one of the turns of the cochlea. (Drawn by Sylvia Colard Keene. From Bloom and Fawcett: A Textbook of Histology. Philadelphia, W. B. Saunders Company, 1975.)

vestibuli and scala media are considered to be a single chamber. The importance of Reissner's membrane is to maintain a special fluid in the scala media that is required for optimal function of the sound-receptive hair cells.

Sound vibrations enter the scala vestibuli from the faceplate of the stapes at the oval window. The faceplate is connected with the edges of the window by a relatively loose annular ligament, so that it can move inward and outward with the sound vibrations. Inward movement causes forward movement of the fluid in the scala vestibuli and scala media.

Note from Figure 41–4 that the distal end of the scala vestibuli and scala tympani open directly into each other by way of the *helicotrema*. If the stapes moves inward *very slowly*, fluid from the scala vestibuli is pushed through the helicotrema into the scala tympani, and this causes the round window to bulge outward. However, if the stapes vibrates inward and outward rapidly, the fluid simply does not have time to pass all the way to the helicotrema and the round window and then back again to the oval window between successive vibrations. Instead, the fluid wave takes a short-cut through the basilar membrane, causing this membrane to bulge back and forth with each sound vibration. We shall see later that each frequency of sound causes a different pattern of vibration in the basilar membrane and that this is the important means by which the sound frequencies are discriminated.

The Basilar Membrane and Resonance in the Cochlea. The basilar membrane contains about 25,000 *basilar fibers* that project from the bony center of the cochlea, the *modiolus*, toward the outer wall. These fibers are stiff, elastic, reedlike structures that are not solidly fixed at their distal ends though they are embedded in the basilar membrane. Because they are stiff and free at one end, they can vibrate like the reeds of a harmonica.

The lengths of the basilar fibers increase progressively from the base of the cochlea to the helicotrema, from approximately 0.04 mm near the oval window to 0.5 mm at the helicotrema, a 12-fold increase in length.

The diameters of the fibers, on the other hand, decrease from the base to the helicotrema, so that their overall stiffness decreases more than 100-fold. As a result, the stiff, short fibers near the base of the

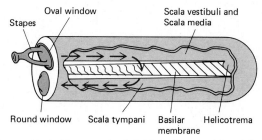

Figure 41–4. Movement of fluid in the cochlea following forward thrust of the stapes.

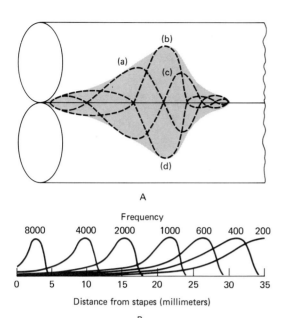

Figure 41–5. *A,* Amplitude pattern of vibration of the basilar membrane for a medium frequency sound. *B,* Amplitude patterns for sounds of all frequencies between 200 and 8000 per second, showing the points of maximum amplitude (the resonance points) on the basilar membrane for the different frequencies.

cochlea tend to vibrate at a high frequency, while the long, limber fibers near the helicotrema tend to vibrate at a low frequency.

In addition to the differences in stiffness of the basilar fibers, they are also differently "loaded" by the fluid mass of the cochlea. That is, when an area of the basilar membrane vibrates back and forth, all the fluid between the vibrating membrane and the oval and round windows must also move back and forth at the same time. For a basilar fiber vibrating near the base of the cochlea, the total mass of moving fluid is slight in comparison with that for a fiber vibrating near the helicotrema. This difference, too, favors high-frequency vibration near the windows and low-frequency vibration near the tip of the cochlea.

Thus, high-frequency resonance of the basilar membrane occurs near the base and low-frequency resonance occurs near the apex because of (1) difference in stiffness of the basilar fibers and (2) difference in "loading."

Pattern of Vibration of the Basilar Membrane. The dashed curves of Figure 41–5A show the position of a sound wave of a particular sound frequency on the basilar membrane when the stapes (*a*) is all the way inward, (*b*) has moved back to the neutral point, (*c*) is all the way outward, and (*d*) has moved back again to the neutral point but is moving inward. The shaded area around these different waves shows the complete pattern of vibration of the basilar membrane during a complete vibratory cycle for this particular sound frequency.

Figure 41–5B shows the amplitude patterns of vibration for different frequencies, showing that the

maximum amplitude for 8000 cycles occurs near the base of the cochlea, while that for frequencies less than 200 cycles per second occurs at the helicotrema. The principal method by which sound frequencies are distinguished from each other is based on the "place" of maximum stimulation of the nerve fibers from the organ of Corti, which rests on the basilar membrane, as will be explained in the following section.

FUNCTION OF THE ORGAN OF CORTI

The organ of Corti, illustrated in Figures 41–2, 41–3, and 41–6, is the receptor organ that generates nerve impulses in response to vibration of the basilar membrane. Note that the organ of Corti lies on the surface of the basilar fibers and basilar membrane. The actual sensory receptors in the organ of Corti are two types of *hair cells*—a single row of *internal hair cells*, numbering about 3500, and three to four rows of *external hair cells*, numbering about 20,000. The bases and sides of the hair cells are enmeshed by a network of cochlear nerve endings. These lead to the *spiral ganglion of Corti*, which lies in the modiolus (the center) of the cochlea. The spiral ganglion in turn sends axons into the *cochlear nerve* and thence into the central nervous system at the level of the upper medulla. The relationship of the organ of Corti to the spiral ganglion and to the cochlear nerve is illustrated in Figure 41–2.

Excitation of the Hair Cells. Note in Figure 41–6 that minute hairs, or cilia, project upward from the hair cells and either touch or are embedded in the surface gel coating of the *tectorial membrane*, which lies above the cilia in the scala media. These hair cells are similar to the hair cells found in the maculae and cristae ampullaris of the vestibular apparatus, which were discussed in Chapter 34. Bending of the hairs excites the hair cells, and this in turn excites the nerve fibers synapsing with their bases.

Upward movement of the basilar fiber rocks the hair cells upward and *inward*. Then, when the basilar membrane moves downward, the cells rock downward and *outward*. The inward and outward motion causes the hairs to shear back and forth against the tectorial membrane, thus exciting the cochlear nerve fibers whenever the basilar membrane vibrates.

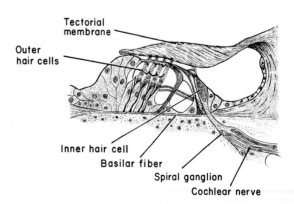

Figure 41–6. The organ of Corti, showing especially the hair cells and the tectorial membrane against the projecting hairs.

Mechanism by Which the Hair Cells Excite the Nerve Fibers—Receptor Potential. Back and forth bending of the hairs causes alternate changes in the electrical potential across the hair cell membrane. This alternating potential is the *receptor potential* of the hair cell; it in turn stimulates the cochlear nerve endings that terminate on the hair cells. Some physiologists believe that the receptor potential stimulates the endings by direct electrical excitation, but others believe that a transmitter substance may be released by the hair cells to excite the nerves.

DETERMINATION OF PITCH—THE PLACE PRINCIPLE

From earlier discussions in this chapter it is already apparent that low-pitched (or low-frequency) sounds cause maximal activation of the basilar membrane near the apex of the cochlea; high-pitched (or high-frequency) sounds activate the basilar membrane near the base of the cochlea; intermediate frequencies activate the membrane at intermediate distances between these two extremes. Furthermore, there is a spatial organization of the cochlear nerve fibers from the cochlea to the cochlear nuclei in the brain stem, with the fibers from each respective area of the basilar membrane terminating in a corresponding area in the cochlear nuclei. We shall see later that this spatial organization also continues all the way up to the cerebral cortex. The recording of signals from the auditory tracts in the brain stem and from the auditory receptive fields in the cerebral cortex shows that specific neurons are activated by specific pitches. Therefore, the method used by the nervous system to detect different pitches is to determine the position along the basilar membrane that is most stimulated. This is called the *place principle* for determination of pitch.

DETERMINATION OF LOUDNESS

Loudness is determined by the amplitude of vibration of the basilar membrane and hair cells. Increasing the amplitude excites the nerve endings at more rapid rates and also causes more and more of the hair cells on the fingers of the vibrating portion of the basilar membrane to become stimulated, thus causing *spatial summation* of impulses—that is, transmission through many nerve fibers rather than through a few.

The interpreted sensation of sound changes approximately in proportion to the cube root of the actual sound intensity. To express this another way, the ear can discriminate changes in sound intensity from the softest whisper to the loudest possible noise—nearly *one trillion times* as much sound energy. Yet the ear interprets this much difference in sound level as approximately a 10,000-fold change. Thus, the scale of intensity is greatly "compressed" by the sound perception mechanisms of the auditory system. This obviously allows a person to interpret differences in sound intensities over an extremely wide range, a far broader range than would be possible were it not for compression of the scale.

The Decibel Unit. Because of the extreme changes in sound intensities that the ear can detect and discriminate, sound intensities are usually expressed in terms of the logarithm of their actual intensities. A 10-fold increase in sound energy is called 1 *bel*, and one-tenth bel is called 1 *decibel*. One decibel represents an actual increase in intensity of 1.26 times.

Another reason for using the decibel system in expressing changes in loudness is that, in the usual sound intensity range for communication, the ears can detect approximately a 1-decibel change in sound intensity.

FREQUENCY RANGE OF HEARING

The frequencies of sound that a young person can hear, before aging has affected the ears, are generally said to be between 20 and 20,000 cycles per second. However, the sound range depends to a great extent on intensity. If the intensity is only −60 decibels, the sound range is 500 to 5000 cycles per second, but if the sound intensity is −20 decibels, the frequency range is about 70 to 15,000 cycles per second, and only with very loud sounds can the complete range of 20 to 20,000 cycles be achieved. In old age, the frequency range falls to 50 to 8000 cycles per second or less.

CENTRAL AUDITORY MECHANISMS

Figure 41–7 illustrates the major auditory pathways. It shows that nerve fibers from the *spiral*

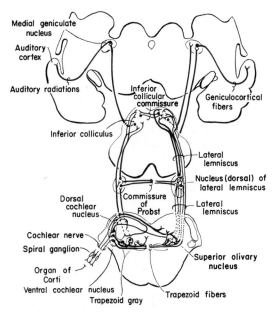

Figure 41–7. The auditory pathway. (Reprinted with permission of Macmillan Publishing Company from Correlative Anatomy of the Nervous System, by Crosby, Humphrey, and Lauer. © 1962 by Macmillan Publishing Company.)

ganglion of the organ of Corti enter the *cochlear nuclei,* located in the upper part of the medulla. At this point, all the fibers synapse. Part of the signal then travels up the same side of the brain stem, but most of it passes to the opposite side and is transmitted upward through successive neurons in the *superior olivary nucleus,* the *inferior colliculus,* and the *medial geniculate nucleus,* finally terminating in the *auditory cortex,* located in the superior gyrus of the temporal lobe.

Several points of importance in relation to the auditory pathway should be noted. First, impulses from either ear are transmitted through the auditory pathways of both sides of the brain stem with only slight preponderance of transmission in the contralateral pathway.

Second, many collateral fibers from the auditory tracts pass directly into the reticular activating system of the brain stem. Therefore, sound can activate the whole brain.

Third, a high degree of spatial orientation is maintained in the fiber tracts, from the cochlea all the way to the cortex. In fact, there are three different spatial representations of sound frequencies in the cochlear nuclei, two representations in the inferior colliculi, a precise representation of discrete sound frequencies in the auditory cortex, and as many as five less precise representations.

FUNCTION OF THE CEREBRAL CORTEX IN HEARING

The projection of the auditory pathway onto the cerebral cortex is illustrated in Figure 41–8, which shows that the auditory cortex lies principally on the *supratemporal plane of the superior temporal gyrus* but also extends over the *lateral border of the temporal lobe,* over much of the *insular cortex,* and even into the most lateral portion of the *parietal lobe.*

Two separate areas are shown in Figure 41–8: the *primary auditory cortex* and the *auditory association cortex.* The primary auditory cortex is directly excited by projections from the nucleus of the medial geniculate body, while the auditory association areas are usually excited secondarily by signals both from the primary auditory cortex and from the thalamic association areas adjacent to the medial geniculate body.

Locus of Sound Frequency Perception in the Primary Auditory Cortex. At least six different *tonotopic maps* have been found in the primary auditory cortex and auditory association areas. In each of these maps, high-frequency sounds excite neurons at one end of the map while low-frequency sounds excite the neurons at the opposite end. In most, the low-frequency sounds are located anteriorly, as shown in Figure 41–8, and the high-freqency sounds posteriorly. However, this is not true for all the maps. The question that one must ask is why does the auditory cortex have so many different *tonotopic* maps? The answer presumably is that each of the separate areas dissects out some specific feature of the sounds. For instance, one of the large maps in the primary auditory cortex almost certainly discriminates the sound frequencies themselves and gives a person the psychic sensation of sound pitches. Another one of the maps probably is used to detect the direction from which the sound comes.

A large share of the neurons in the auditory cortex, especially in the auditory association cortex, do not respond to specific sound frequencies in the ear. It is believed that these neurons associate different sound frequencies with each other or associate sound information with information from other sensory areas of the cortex. Indeed, the parietal portion of the auditory association cortex partly overlaps somatic sensory area II, which could provide easy opportunity for association of auditory information with somatic sensory information.

Discrimination of Sound Patterns by the Auditory Cortex. Complete bilateral removal of the auditory cortex does not prevent an animal from detecting sounds or reacting in a crude manner to the sounds. However, it does greatly reduce or sometimes even abolish the animal's ability to discriminate different sound pitches and especially *patterns of sound.* For instance, an animal that has been trained to recognize a combination or sequence of tones, one following the other in a particular pattern, loses this ability when the auditory cortex is destroyed, and furthermore, it cannot relearn this type of response. Therefore, the auditory cortex is important in the discrimination of *tonal* and *sequential sound patterns.*

In the human being, lesions affecting the auditory association areas but not the primary auditory cortex allow the person full capability to hear and to differentiate sound tones as well as to interpret at least a few sample patterns of sound. However, the person will often be completely unable to interpret the *meaning* of the sounds. For instance, lesions in the poste-

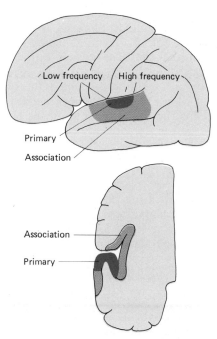

Figure 41–8. The auditory cortex.

rior portion of the superior temporal gyrus, either in or near Wernicke's area, often make it impossible to interpret the meanings of words even though the person hears them perfectly well and often can even repeat them. These functions of the auditory association areas and their relationship to the overall intellectual functions of the brain were discussed in detail in Chapter 36.

DISCRIMINATION OF DIRECTION FROM WHICH SOUND EMANATES

A person determines the direction from which sound emanates by two principal mechanisms: (1) the time lag between the entry of sound into one ear and into the opposite ear and (2) the difference between the intensities of the sounds in the two ears. The first mechanism functions best for frequencies below 3000 cycles per second, and the intensity mechanism operates best at higher frequencies because the head acts as a sound barrier at these frequencies. The time lag mechanism discriminates direction much more exactly than the intensity mechanism, for the time lag mechanism does not depend on extraneous factors but only on an exact interval of time between two acoustical signals. If a person is looking straight toward the sound, the sound reaches both ears at exactly the same instant, while if the right ear is closer to the sound than the left ear, the sound signals from the right ear are perceived ahead of those from the left ear.

Neural Mechanisms for Detecting Sound Direction. Destruction of the auditory cortex on both sides of the brain, in either man or lower mammals, causes loss of almost all ability to detect the direction from which sound comes. Yet the mechanism for this detection process begins in the superior olivary nuclei, even though it requires the neural pathways all the way from these nuclei to the cortex for interpretation of the signals. The mechanism is believed to function as follows.

First, the superior olivary nucleus is divided into two sections, (a) the *medial superior olivary nucleus* and (b) the *lateral superior olivary nucleus*. The lateral nucleus is concerned with detecting the direction from which the sound is coming by the *difference in intensities of the sound* reaching the two ears, presumably by simply comparing the two intensities and sending an appropriate signal to the auditory cortex to estimate the direction.

The *medial superior olivary nucleus*, on the other hand, has a very specific mechanism for *detecting the time-lag between acoustic signals entering the two ears*. This nucleus contains large numbers of neurons that have two major dendrites, one projecting to the right and the other to the left. The acoustical signal from the right ear impinges on the right dendrite, the signal from the left ear on the left dendrite. The degree of excitation of each of these neurons is highly sensitive to a specific time-lag between the two acoustical signals from the two ears. The neurons near one border of the nucleus respond maximally to a short time-lag; whereas those near the opposite border respond to a very long time-lag; and those between, to intermediate time-lags. Thus, a spatial pattern of neuronal stimulation develops in the medial superior olivary nucleus, with sound from directly in front of the head stimulating one set of olivary neurons maximally and sounds from different side angles stimulating other sets of neurons maximally. This spatial orientation of signals is then transmitted all the way to the auditory cortex, where sound direction is determined by the locus in the cortex that is stimulated maximally. It is believed that the signals for determining sound direction are transmitted through a different pathway and that this pathway terminates in the cerebral cortex in a different locus from the transmission pathway and the termination locus for tonal patterns of sound.

This mechanism for detection of sound direction indicates again how the information in sensory signals is dissected out as the signals pass through different levels of neuronal activity. In this case, the quality of sound direction is separated from the quality of sound tones at the level of the superior olivary nuclei.

DEAFNESS

Deafness is usually divided into two types; first, that caused by impairment of the cochlea or auditory nerve, which is usually classified as nerve deafness and, second, that caused by impairment of the middle ear mechanisms for transmitting sound into the cochlea, which is usually called conduction deafness. Obviously, if either the cochlea or the auditory nerve is completely destroyed, the person is completely deaf. However, if the cochlea and nerve are still intact but the ossicular system has been destroyed or ankylosed ("frozen" in place by fibrous tissue or calcification), sound waves can still be conducted into the cochlea by means of bone conduction (such as conduction of sound from the butt of a vibrating tuning fork applied directly to the skull). The person with conduction deafness can often be made to hear again almost normally by an operation to remove the stapes and replacing it with a minute Teflon or metal prosthesis that transmits the sound from the incus to the oval window.

THE SENSE OF TASTE

Taste is mainly a function of the *taste buds* in the mouth, and its importance lies in the fact that it allows a person to select food in accord with his or her desires and perhaps also in accord with the needs of the tissues for specific nutritive substances.

On the basis of psychological studies, there are considered to be four *primary* sensations of taste: *sour, salty, sweet,* and *bitter*. Yet we know that a person can perceive literally hundreds of different tastes. These are all supposedly combinations of the four primary sensations in the same manner that all the colors of the spectrum are combinations of three primary color sensations, as described in Chapter 39.

THE PRIMARY SENSATIONS OF TASTE

The Sour Taste. The sour taste is caused by acids, and the intensity of the taste sensation is approximately proportional to the logarithm of the *hydrogen ion concentration*. That is, the more acidic the substance, the stronger becomes the sensation.

The Salty Taste. The salty taste is elicited by ionized salts. The quality of the taste varies somewhat from one salt to another because the salts also elicit other taste sensations besides saltiness.

The Sweet Taste. The sweet taste is not caused by any single class of chemicals. A list of some of the types of chemicals that cause this taste includes sugars, glycols, alcohols, aldehydes, ketones, amides, esters, amino acids, sulfonic acids, halogenated acids, and inorganic salts of lead and beryllium. Note specifically that most substances with a sweet taste are organic chemicals; the only inorganic substances that elicit the sweet taste are certain salts of lead and beryllium.

Saccharin is a substance more than 600 times as sweet as common table sugar and is an important noncalorigenic sweetening agent.

The Bitter Taste. The bitter taste, like the sweet taste, is not caused by any single type of chemical agent, but here again, the substances that give the bitter taste are almost entirely organic substances. Two particular classes of substances are especially likely to cause bitter taste sensations: (1) long-chain organic substances and (2) alkaloids. The alkaloids include many of the drugs used in medicines, such as quinine, caffeine, strychnine, and nicotine.

The bitter taste, when it occurs in high intensity, usually causes the person or animal to reject the food. This is undoubtedly an important purposive function of the bitter taste sensation, because many of the deadly toxins found in poisonous plants are alkaloids, and these all have an intensely bitter taste.

Threshold for Taste

The threshold for stimulation of the sour taste by hydrochloric acid averages 0.0009 moles/liter; for stimulation of the salty taste by sodium chloride: 0.01 moles/liter; for the sweet taste by sucrose (table sugar): 0.01 moles/liter; and for the bitter taste by quinine: 0.000008 moles/liter. Note especially how much more sensitive is the bitter taste sense to stimuli than all the others, which would be expected since this sensation provides an important protective function.

THE TASTE BUD AND ITS FUNCTION

Figure 41–9 illustrates a taste bud, which has a diameter of about 1/30 millimeter and a length of about 1/16 millimeter. The taste bud is composed of about 40 modified epithelial cells called *taste cells*.

The outer tips of the taste cells are arranged around a minute *taste pore*, shown in Figure 41–9. From the tip of each cell, several *microvilli*, or *taste hairs*, about 2 to 3 microns in length and 0.2 micron in width, protrude outward through the taste pore to approach the cavity of the mouth. These microvilli are believed to provide the receptor surface for taste.

Interwoven among the taste cells is a branching terminal network of several *taste nerve fibers* that are stimulated by the taste cells. These fibers invaginate deeply into folds of the taste cell membranes, so that there is extremely intimate contact between the taste cells and the nerves.

Location of the Taste Buds. The taste buds are found on three out of four different types of papillae of the tongue, as follows: (1) A large number of taste buds are on the walls of the troughs surrounding the circumvallate papillae, which form a V line toward the posterior of the tongue. (2) Moderate numbers of taste buds are on the fungiform papillae over the front surface of the tongue. (3) Moderate numbers are on the foliate papillae located in the folds along the posterolateral surfaces of the tongue.

Additional taste buds are located on the palate, a few on the tonsillar pillars and at other points around the nasopharynx. Adults have approximately 10,000 taste buds, and children a few more. Beyond the age of 45 many taste buds rapidly degenerate, causing the taste sensation to become progressively less critical.

Specificity of Taste Buds for the Primary Taste Stimuli. Psychological tests using different types of taste stimuli carefully applied to individual taste buds, one at a time, have suggested that we have four distinctly different varieties of taste buds, each sensitive for only one type of taste. Yet microelectrode studies from single taste buds while they are stimulated successively by the four different primary taste stimuli have shown that most of them can be excited by two, three, or even four of the primary taste stimuli, though usually with one or two of these predominating. Thus, at present, there are conflicting beliefs about the degree of specificity of taste buds,

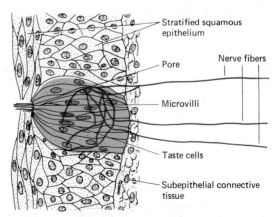

Figure 41–9. The taste bud.

some physiologists believing them always to be highly specific for only one primary taste stimulus and other physiologists believing this specificity to be true only in a statistical sense because of dominance of one taste perception over the others.

Regardless of which theory is correct, one can well understand that the hundreds of different types of tastes that we experience result from different quantitative degrees of stimulation of the four primary sensations of tastes (as well as simultaneous stimulation of smell in the nose and tactile and pain nerve endings in the mouth).

TRANSMISSION OF TASTE SIGNALS INTO THE CENTRAL NERVOUS SYSTEM

Figure 41–10 illustrates the neuronal pathways for transmission of taste sensations from the tongue and pharyngeal region into the central nervous system. Taste impulses pass through the fifth, seventh, ninth, and tenth nerves into the brain stem, where they terminate in the *tractus solitarius*. From here, signals pass first to the *thalamus* and thence to the *parietal opercular-insular area* of the cerebral cortex. This lies at the very most lateral margin of the postcentral gyrus of the parietal lobe in the sylvian fissure, in close association with, or even superimposed on, the tongue area of somatic sensory area I.

From this description of the taste pathways, it immediately becomes evident that they parallel closely the somatic sensory pathways from the tongue as described in Chapter 32.

SPECIAL ATTRIBUTES OF THE TASTE SENSE

Importance of the Sense of Smell in Taste. Persons with severe colds frequently state that they have lost their sense of taste. However, on testing the taste sensations, these are found to be completely normal. This illustrates that much of what we call taste is

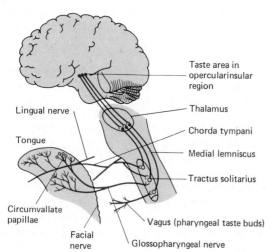

Figure 41–10. Transmission of taste impulses into the central nervous system.

actually smell. Odors from the food can pass upward into the nose, often stimulating the olfactory system thousands of times as strongly as the taste system. For instance, if the olfactory system is intact, alcohol can be "tasted" in 1/25,000 the concentration required when the olfactory system is not intact.

Taste Preference and Control of the Diet. Taste preferences mean simply that an animal will choose certain types of food in preference to others, and it automatically uses this to help control the type of diet it eats. Furthermore, its taste preferences often change in accordance with the needs of the body for certain specific substances. The following experimental studies illustrate this ability of an animal to choose food in accordance with bodily need: First, adrenalectomized animals, which lose excessive amounts of sodium chloride in the urine, automatically select drinking water with a high concentration of sodium chloride in preference to pure water, and this choice in many instances is sufficient to supply the needs of the body and to prevent death as a result of salt depletion. Second, an animal injected with excessive amounts of insulin develops a depleted blood sugar, and it automatically chooses the sweetest food from among many samples. Third, parathyroidectomized animals, which have depleted calcium ions in the blood, automatically choose drinking water with a high concentration of calcium chloride.

These same phenomena are also observed in many instances of everyday life. For instance, the salt licks of the desert region are known to attract animals from far and wide, and even the human being rejects any food that has an unpleasant sensation, which certainly in many instances protects our bodies from undesirable substances.

THE SENSE OF SMELL

Smell is the least understood sense. This lack of knowledge results partly from the location of the olfactory membrane high in the nose, where it is difficult to study, and partly from the fact that the sense of smell is a subjective phenomenon that cannot be studied with ease in lower animals. Still another complication is the fact that the sense of smell is almost rudimentary in the human being in comparison with some lower animals.

THE OLFACTORY MEMBRANE

The olfactory membrane lies in the superior part of each nostril, as illustrated in Figure 41–11. Medially, it folds downward over the surface of the septum, and laterally, it folds over the superior concha and even over a small portion of the upper surface of the middle concha. In each nostril the olfactory membrane has a surface area of approximately 2.4 square centimeters.

The Olfactory Cells. The receptor cells for the smell sensation are the *olfactory cells*, which are actually bipolar nerve cells derived originally from

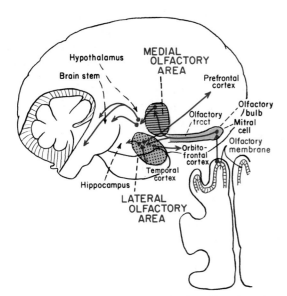

Figure 41–11. Neural connections of the olfactory system.

the central nervous system itself. There are about 100 million of these cells in the olfactory epithelium, interspersed among *sustentacular cells,* as shown in Figure 41–12. The mucosal end of the olfactory cell forms a knob from which 6 to 12 *olfactory hairs,* or *cilia,* 0.3 micron in diameter and 50 to 80 microns in length, project into the mucus that coats the inner surface of the nasal cavity. These projecting cilia form a dense mat in the mucus, and it is these cilia that react to odors in the air and then stimulate the olfactory cells, as discussed below. Spaced among the olfactory cells in the olfactory membrane are many small *glands of Bowman* that secrete mucus onto the surface of the olfactory membrane.

STIMULATION OF THE OLFACTORY CELLS

The Necessary Stimulus for Smell. We do not know what it takes chemically to stimulate the olfactory cells. Yet we do know the physical characteristics of

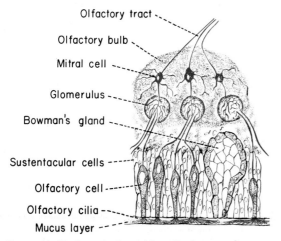

Figure 41–12. Organization of the olfactory membrane.

the substances that cause olfactory stimulation: First, the substance must be volatile so that it can be breathed into the nostrils. Second, it must be at least slightly water soluble so that it can pass through the mucus to the cilia. And, third, it must also be lipid soluble, presumably because the olfactory cilia are principally composed of lipid materials.

Regardless of the basic mechanism by which the olfactory cells are stimulated, it is known that they become stimulated only when air blasts upward into the superior region of the nose. Therefore, smell occurs in cycles along with the inspirations, which indicates that the olfactory receptors respond in milliseconds to volatile agents. Because smell intensity is enhanced by blasting air through the upper reaches of the nose, a person can greatly enhance the sense of smell by the well-known sniffing technique.

Search for the Primary Sensations of Smell. Most physiologists are convinced that the many smell sensations are subserved by a few rather discrete primary sensations in the same way that taste is subserved by sour, sweet, bitter, and salty sensations. But thus far only minor success has been achieved in classifying the primary sensations of smell. Yet on the basis of psychological tests and action potential studies from various points in the olfactory nerve pathways, it has been postulated that about seven different primary classes of olfactory stimulants preferentially excite separate olfactory cells. These classes of olfactory stimulants may be characterized as follows:
1. Camphoraceous
2. Musky
3. Floral
4. Pepperminty
5. Ethereal
6. Pungent
7. Putrid

However, it is unlikely that this list actually represents the true primary sensations of smell even though it does illustrate the results of one of the many attempts to classify them. Indeed, several clues in recent years have indicated that there may be as many as *50* or more primary sensations of smell—a marked contrast to only *three* primary sensations of color detected by the eyes and only *four* primary sensations of taste detected by the tongue. For instance, individual persons have been found who are specifically *odor-blind* for a single substance; and such discrete odor blindness has been identified for more than 50 different substances. Since it is presumed that odor-blindness for each substance represents a lack of the appropriate receptor for that substance, it is postulated that the sense of smell might be subserved by 50 or more primary smell sensations.

Mechanism for Excitation of the Olfactory Cells. The basic mechanism by which the olfactory cells are stimulated is not known, but two principal theories have been proposed. One of these is a *physical theory*, which suggests that it is the physical shapes of the odor molecules that determine which olfactory cells will be stimulated, but the evidence for this theory is weak. The second theory, a *chemical theory*, is much more likely to be correct. It assumes that the odor molecules bind chemically to protein *receptors* in the membranes of the olfactory cilia. The type of receptor in each olfactory cell determines the type of stimulant that will excite the cell. The reaction between the stimulant and the receptor supposedly increases the permeability of the olfactory ciliary membrane, and this in turn creates the receptor potential in the olfactory cell that generates impulses in the olfactory nerve fibers.

Threshold for Smell. One of the principal characteristics of smell is the minute concentration of the stimulating agent in the air required to effect a smell sensation. For instance, the substance *methyl mercaptan* can be smelled when only 1/25,000,000,000 mg is present in each milliliter of air. Because of the low threshold, this substance is mixed with natural gas to give it an odor that can be detected when it leaks from a gas pipe.

TRANSMISSION OF SMELL SENSATIONS INTO THE CENTRAL NERVOUS SYSTEM

The function of the central nervous system in olfaction is almost as vague as the function of the peripheral receptors. However, Figures 41–11 and 41–12 illustrate the general plan for transmission of olfactory sensations into the central nervous system. Figure 41–11 shows a number of separate *olfactory cells* sending axons into the *olfactory bulb* to end on *dendrites from mitral cells* in a structure called the *glomerulus*. Approximately 25,000 axons from olfactory cells enter each glomerulus and synapse with about 25 mitral cells that in turn send signals into the brain. There is a total of about 5000 glomeruli.

Figure 41–12 shows the major pathways for transmission of olfactory signals from the mitral cells into the brain. The fibers from the cells travel through the *olfactory tract* and terminate either primarily or after relay neurons in two principal areas of the brain called the *medial olfactory area* and the *lateral olfactory area*, respectively. The medial olfactory area is composed of a group of nuclei located in the midportion of the brain anterior to the hypothalamus. This group includes the *olfactory nucleus,* the *olfactory tubercle,* parts of the *hypothalamus,* and other adjacent areas.

The lateral olfactory area is composed mainly of the *prepyriform* and *pyriform cortex* and part of the *amygdaloid nuclei.*

Secondary olfactory tracts pass from both the medial and lateral olfactory areas into many other portions of the *limbic system* and into associated regions of the *thalamus* and *brain stem nuclei.*

The lateral olfactory area, especially parts of the *amygdala* and the overlying cortex, the *pyriform* and *prepyriform* areas, is believed to be responsible for the more complex aspects of olfaction, such as association of olfactory sensations with somatic, visual, tactile, and other types of sensation. These regions of the brain, operating in association with other areas of the cortex located more anteriorly in the *uncus, orbitofrontal cortex,* and *frontal cortex,* are probably responsible for a person's specific appetites for certain types of foods. For instance, it might be in these areas that one develops special likes or dislikes for certain foods, depending upon previous experience with the foods.

The *pyriform area* of the temporal cortex is frequently considered to be the *primary olfactory cortex.* It is particularly interesting that this is the only part of the entire cerebral cortex that receives primary sensory signals that are not relayed through the thalamus.

Complete removal of the lateral olfactory area hardly affects the primitive responses to olfaction, such as licking lips, salivation, and other feeding responses caused by the smell of food or such as the various emotions associated with smell. On the other hand, its removal does abolish the more complicated conditioned reflexes that depend on olfactory stimuli.

QUESTIONS

1. Describe the *tympanic membrane* and the *ossicular system* and their roles in the transmission of sound to the oval window. Explain what is meant by *impedance matching* in this system.
2. Explain how the *attenuation reflex* protects the ear from damaging noises.
3. Trace the movement of fluid in the *cochlear* chambers during each phase of a complete sound wave.
4. Explain the role of each of the following in the *resonance* process that occurs in the cochlea: the length of the basilar fibers, the stiffness of the basilar fibers, and the loading effect of the fluid in the scala vestibuli, scala media, and scala tympani.
5. Draw a diagram showing the respective points in the cochlea where the greatest amplitude of vibration occurs on the basilar membrane for the different sound frequencies.
6. Describe the anatomy of the *organ of Corti* and the mechanism by which the *hair cells* are excited when sound waves cause them to move.
7. What is meant by the place principle for the determination of pitch?
8. Explain how the cochlea determines loudness of a sound and how the ear can operate in a tremendous range of sound intensity.
9. Describe the neural pathway for transmission of sound signals to the cerebral cortex.
10. Describe the function of the *auditory cortex*, including (a) what is meant by *tonotopic maps* in the auditory cortex and (b) the discrimination of sound patterns.

11. How does a person determine the direction from which a sound is coming?
12. Explain the differences between *nerve deafness* and *conduction deafness,* as well as the surgical treatment of conduction deafness.
13. Give the four primary sensations of taste and the types of chemical substances that excite each of these sensations.
14. Describe the *taste bud*, its stimulation, and its specificity for specific types of taste stimuli.
15. Trace the neural circuit for transmission of taste signals into the central nervous system.
16. What role does taste play in the control of the diet?
17. Describe the *olfactory membrane*, the *olfactory cells*, and the sensory portions of the olfactory cells.
18. What are the characteristics of substances that cause smell?
19. What do we know about the primary sensations of smell?
20. Give the *chemical theory* for detection of the different types of smell.
21. Trace the neural pathway for transmission of olfactory signals from the olfactory cells to the brain.
22. What are the differences between the functions of the *medial olfactory area* and the *lateral olfactory area* of the brain?

References

Hearing

Aitkin, L. M., et al.: Central neural mechanisms of hearing. In Darian-Smith, I., ed.: Handbook of Physiology. Sec 1, Vol 3. Bethesda, American Physiological Society, 1984, p. 675.
Ballenger, J. J., ed.: Diseases of the Nose, Throat, Ear, Head, and Neck. Philadelphia, Lea & Febiger, 1985.
Dallos, P.: Peripheral mechanisms of hearing. In Darian-Smith, I., ed. Handbook of Physiology. Sec 1, Vol 3. Bethesda, American Physiological Society, 1984, p. 595.
Green, D. M., and Wier, C. C.: Auditory perception. In Darian-Smith, I., ed.: Handbook of Physiology. Sec 1, Vol 3. Bethesda, American Physiological Society, 1984, p. 557.
Guth, P. S., and Melamed, B.: Neurotransmission in the auditory system: a primer for pharmacologists. Annu Rev Pharmacol. Toxicol 22:383, 1982.
Hudspeth, A. J.: Mechanoelectrical transduction by hair cells in the acousticolateralis sensory system. Annu Rev Neurosci 6:187, 1983.
Imig, T. J., and Morel, A.: Organization of the thalamocortical auditory system in the cat. Annu Rev Neurosci 6:95, 1983.
Kay, R. H.: Hearing of modulation in sounds. Physiol Rev 62:894, 1982.
Masterton, R. B., and Imig, T. J.: Neural mechanisms of sound localization. Annu Rev Physiol 46:275, 1984.
Rhode, W. S.: Cochlear mechanics. Annu Rev Physiol 46:231, 1984.
Sachs, M. B.: Neural coding of complex sounds: Speech. Annu Rev Physiol 46:261, 1984.
Schneiderman, C. R.: Basic Anatomy and Physiology in Speech and Hearing. San Diego, College-Hill Press, 1984.
Stevens, S. S.: Hearing. Its Psychology and Physiology. New York, Acoustical Society of America, 1983.
Weiss, T. F.: Relation of receptor potentials of cochlear hair cells to spike discharges of cochlear neurons. Annu Rev Physiol 46:247, 1984.
Woolsey, D. N., ed.: Cortical Sensory Organization. Multiple Auditory Areas. Clifton, NJ, Humana Press, 1982.

Taste and Smell

Douek, E.: The Sense of Smell and Its Abnormalities. New York, Churchill Livingstone, 1974.
Kashara, Y., ed.: Proceedings of the Seventeenth Japanese Symposium on Taste and Smell. Arlington, VA, IRL Press, 1984.
McBurney, D. H.: Taste and olfaction: Sensory discrimination. In Darian-Smith, I., ed.: Handbook of Physiology. Sec 1, Vol 3. Bethesda, American Physiological Society, 1984, p. 1067.
Norgren, R.: Central neural mechanisms of taste. In Darian-Smith, I., ed.: Handbook of Physiology. Sec 1, Vol 3. Bethesda, American Physiological Society, 1984, p. 1087.
Ohloff, G., and Thomas, A. F., eds.: Gustation and Olfaction. New York, Academic Press, 1971.
Shepherd, G. M.: The olfactory bulb: a simple system in the mammalian brain. In Brookhart, J. M., and Mountcastle, V. B., eds.: Handbook of Physiology. Sec 1, Vol 1. Baltimore, Williams & Wilkins, 1977, p. 945.
Takagi, S. F.: The olfactory nervous system of the Old World monkey. Jpn J Physiol 34:561, 1984.

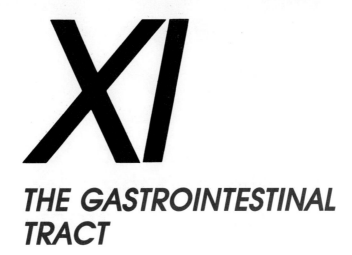

THE GASTROINTESTINAL TRACT

42 ■ Movement of Food Through the Alimentary Tract

43 ■ Secretory Functions of the Alimentary Tract

44 ■ Digestion and Absorption in the Gastrointestinal Tract; Gastrointestinal Disorders

42

Movement of Food Through the Alimentary Tract

GENERAL PRINCIPLES OF INTESTINAL MOTILITY
CHARACTERISTICS OF THE INTESTINAL WALL
CHARACTERISTICS OF INTESTINAL SMOOTH MUSCLE
INNERVATION OF THE GUT—THE ENTERIC NERVOUS SYSTEM
FUNCTIONAL TYPES OF MOVEMENTS IN THE GASTROINTESTINAL TRACT
THE MIXING MOVEMENTS
THE PROPULSIVE MOVEMENTS—PERISTALSIS
INGESTION OF FOOD
MASTICATION (CHEWING)
SWALLOWING (DEGLUTITION)

FUNCTION OF THE LOWER ESOPHAGEAL SPHINCTER
MOTOR FUNCTIONS OF THE STOMACH
STORAGE FUNCTION OF THE STOMACH
MIXING IN THE STOMACH
EMPTYING OF THE STOMACH
REGULATION OF STOMACH EMPTYING
MOVEMENTS OF THE SMALL INTESTINE
MIXING CONTRACTIONS (SEGMENTATION CONTRACTIONS)
PROPULSIVE MOVEMENTS
FUNCTION OF THE ILEOCECAL VALVE
MOVEMENTS OF THE COLON
DEFECATION

The primary function of the alimentary tract is to provide the body with a continuous supply of water, electrolytes, and nutrients, but before this can be achieved, food must be moved along the alimentary tract at an appropriate rate for the digestive and absorptive functions to take place. Therefore, discussion of the alimentary system is presented in three different phases in this and the next two chapters: (1) movement of food through the alimentary tract, (2) secretion of the digestive juices, and (3) absorption of the digested foods, water, and the various electrolytes.

Figure 42–1 illustrates the entire alimentary tract, showing major anatomical differences between its parts. Each part is adapted for specific functions, such as (1) simple passage of food from one point to another, as in the esophagus, (2) storage of food in the body of the stomach or fecal matter in the descending colon, (3) digestion of food in the stomach, duodenum, jejunum, and ileum, and (4) absorption of the digestive end-products in the entire small intestine and proximal half of the colon. One of the most important features of the gastrointestinal tract that is discussed in the present chapter, is the myriad of autoregulatory processes in the gut that keep the food moving at an appropriate pace—slow enough for digestion and absorption to take place but fast enough to provide the nutrients needed by the body.

GENERAL PRINCIPLES OF INTESTINAL MOTILITY

CHARACTERISTICS OF THE INTESTINAL WALL

Figure 42–2 illustrates a typical section of the intestinal wall, showing the following layers from the outside inward: (1) the *serosa*, (2) a *longitudinal muscle layer*, (3) a *circular muscle layer*, (4) the *submucosa*, and (5) the *mucosa*. In addition, a sparse layer of smooth muscle fibers, the *muscularis mucosae*, lies in the deeper layers of the mucosa. The motor functions of the gut are performed by the different layers of smooth muscle.

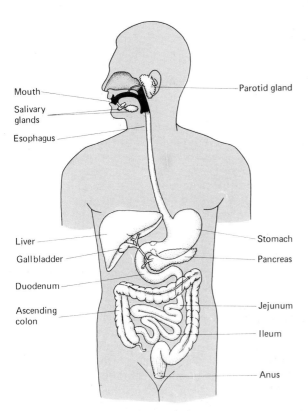

Figure 42–1. The alimentary tract.

CHARACTERISTICS OF INTESTINAL SMOOTH MUSCLE

The general characteristics of smooth muscle and its function were discussed in Chapter 7. However, some specific characteristics of smooth muscle in the gut are the following:

The Functioning Syncytium. The individual smooth muscle fibers in the gastrointestinal tract are arranged in bundles of as many as a thousand parallel fibers. In the longitudinal muscle layer, these bundles extend longitudinally down the intestinal tract; in the circular muscle layer they extend around the gut. Within each

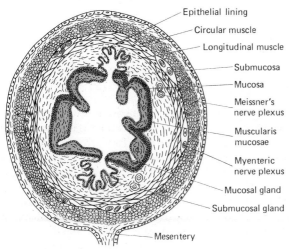

Figure 42–2. Typical cross-section of the gut.

bundle the muscle fibers are electrically connected with each other through large numbers of *gap junctions* that allow low resistance movement of ions from one cell to the next. Therefore, electrical signals can travel readily from one fiber to the next.

Each bundle of smooth muscle fibers is separated from the next by loose connective tissue, but the bundles fuse with each other at many points, so that in reality each muscle layer represents a branching latticework of smooth muscle bundles. Therefore, each muscle layer functions as a *syncytium*—that is, when an action potential is elicited anywhere within the muscle mass, it generally travels in all directions in the muscle and causes widespread contraction. However, the distance that the action potential travels depends upon the excitability of the muscle; sometimes it stops after only a few millimeters and at other times travels many centimeters or even the entire length of the intestinal tract.

Contraction of Intestinal Muscle. The smooth muscle of the gastrointestinal tract exhibits *tonic contraction* and *rhythmic contraction*, both of which are characteristic of most types of smooth muscle, as discussed in Chapter 7.

Tonic contraction is continuous, lasting minute after minute or even hour after hour, sometimes increasing or decreasing in intensity but nevertheless continuing. This contraction may be caused by a series of action potentials or by non-electrogenic stimulation by hormones or ionic changes. The intensity of tonic contraction in each segment of the gut determines the amount of steady pressure in the segment, and tonic contraction of the sphincters determines the amount of resistance offered at the sphincters to the movement of intestinal contents. In this way the *pyloric*, the *ileocecal*, and the *anal sphincters* all help to regulate food movement in the gut.

In different parts of the gut, the rhythmic contractions of the gastrointestinal smooth muscle occur at rates as rapid as 12 times per minute or as slow as 3 times per minute. These frequencies are determined by slow waves in the electrical potentials of the muscle, waves that are distinct from the action potentials but that cause rhythmic entraining of the action potentials, as explained in Chapter 7. The rhythmic contractions are responsible for the phasic functions of the gastrointestinal tract, such as mixing the food with the secretions or the peristaltic propulsion of food, as discussed later in the chapter.

INNERVATION OF THE GUT—THE ENTERIC NERVOUS SYSTEM

The gastrointestinal tract has an intrinsic nervous system of its own, called the *enteric nervous system*, that begins in the esophagus and extends all the way to the anus. This system controls most gastrointestinal functions, especially gastrointestinal movements and secretions. On the other hand, both parasympathetic and sympathetic nervous signals to the gastrointestinal tract from the brain can strongly alter the degree of activity of this enteric nervous system.

The Myenteric and Submucosal Plexuses. The enteric nervous system is composed principally of two layers of neurons and appropriate connecting fibers: the outer layer, called the *myenteric plexus*, or *Auerbach's plexus*, lies between the longitudinal and circular muscle of the gut wall; the inner layer, called the *submucosal plexus*, or *Meissner's plexus*, lies in the submucosa. The myenteric plexus mainly controls the *gastrointestinal movements*, whereas the submucosal plexus is important in controlling *secretion* and *blood flow* and also subserves many *sensory functions*, receiving signals principally from the gut epithelium and from stretch receptors in the gut wall.

Most often, stimulation of the myenteric plexus increases the motor activity of the gut, causing four principal effects: (1) increased tonic contraction, or tone, of the gut wall, (2) increased intensity of the rhythmic contraction, (3) slightly increased rate of rhythmic contraction, and (4) increased velocity of conduction of excitatory waves along the gut wall. On the other hand, some myenteric plexus fibers are inhibitory rather than excitatory; these fibers secrete an inhibitory transmitter, possibly VIP (vasoactive intestinal polypeptide) or some other peptide. A large share of the excitatory fibers are *cholinergic*—that is, they secrete *acetylcholine*, though some secrete other excitatory transmitters. Transmitters that have been identified in the enteric plexuses, though their functions are mainly unknown, include *ATP, substance P, enkephalin, somatostatin, serotonin, bombesin*, and *neurotensin*.

Autonomic Control of the Gastrointestinal Tract. The gastrointestinal tract receives extensive parasympathetic and sympathetic nerves that are capable of altering the overall activity of the entire gut or of specific parts of it, particularly its upper end down to the stomach and its distal end from the mid-colon region to the anus.

Parasympathetic Innervation. The parasympathetic supply to the gut is divided into *cranial* and *sacral divisions*, which were discussed in Chapter 38. Except for a few parasympathetic fibers to the mouth and pharyngeal regions of the alimentary tract, the cranial parasympathetics are transmitted almost entirely in the *vagus nerves*. These fibers provide extensive innervation to the esophagus and stomach and, to a much lesser extent, to the small intestine, gallbladder, and first half of the large intestine. The sacral parasympathetics originate in the second and third sacral segments of the spinal cord and pass through the *pelvic nerves* to the distal half of the large intestine. The sigmoidal, rectal, and anal regions of the large intestine are considerably better supplied with parasympathetic fibers than are the other portions. These fibers function especially in the defecation reflexes, which are discussed later in the chapter.

The postganglionic neurons of the parasympathetic system are mainly located in the myenteric and submucosal plexuses, so that stimulation of the parasympathetic nerves causes a general increase in activity of the entire enteric nervous system. This is turn enhances the activity of most gastrointestinal functions, but not all, for some of the enteric neurons are inhibitory and therefore inhibit certain of the functions.

Sympathetic Innervation. The sympathetic fibers to the gastrointestinal tract originate in the spinal cord between the segments T-8 and L-2. The preganglionic fibers, after leaving the cord, enter the sympathetic chains and pass through the chains to outlying ganglia, such as the *celiac ganglion* and various *mesenteric ganglia*. Here the postganglionic neuron bodies are located, and postganglionic fibers spread from them along with the blood vessels to all parts of the gut, terminating principally on neurons in the enteric nervous system. The sympathetics innervate essentially all portions of the gastrointestinal tract rather than being more extensively supplied to the most orad and most analward portions as is true of the parasympathetics. The sympathetic nerve endings secrete *norepinephrine*.

In general, stimulation of the sympathetic nervous system inhibits activity in the gastrointestinal tract, causing effects essentially opposite to those of the parasympathetic system. Thus, strong stimulation of the sympathetic system can totally block movement of food through the gastrointestinal tract.

FUNCTIONAL TYPES OF MOVEMENTS IN THE GASTROINTESTINAL TRACT

Two basic types of movements occur in the gastrointestinal tract: (1) *mixing movements*, which keep the intestinal contents thoroughly mixed at all times, and (2) *propulsive movements*, which cause food to move forward along the tract at an appropriate rate for digestion and absorption.

THE MIXING MOVEMENTS

In most parts of the alimentary tract, the mixing movements are caused by *local contractions of small segments of the gut wall*. These movements are modified in different parts of the gastrointestinal tract, as discussed separately later in the chapter.

THE PROPULSIVE MOVEMENTS—PERISTALSIS

The basic propulsive movement of the gastrointestinal tract is *peristalsis*, which is illustrated in Figure 42–3. A contractile ring appears around the gut and then moves forward; this is analogous to putting one's fingers around a thin distended tube then constricting the fingers and moving them forward along the tube. Obviously, any material in front of the contractile ring is moved forward.

Peristalsis is an inherent property of many syncytial smooth muscle tubes; stimulation at any point can cause a contractile ring to spread along the tube. Thus, peristalsis occurs in (1) the gastrointestinal tract, (2) the bile ducts, (3) other glandular ducts

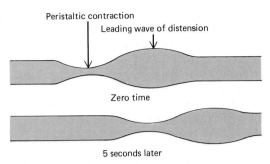

Peristaltic contraction

Leading wave of distension

Zero time

5 seconds later

Figure 42–3. Peristalsis.

throughout the body, (4) the ureters, and (5) most other smooth muscle tubes.

The usual stimulus for peristalsis is *distention*. That is, if a large amount of food collects at any point in the gut, the distention stimulates the gut wall 2 to 3 cm above this point, and a contractile ring appears that initiates a peristaltic movement.

Function of the Myenteric Plexus in Peristalsis. Even though peristalsis is a basic characteristic of all tubular smooth muscle structures, it occurs only weakly in portions of the gastrointestinal tract in which the myenteric plexus is absent, and it is greatly depressed or completely blocked in the entire gut when the person is treated with atropine to paralyze the cholinergic nerve endings of the myenteric plexus. Furthermore, since the myenteric plexus is principally under the control of the parasympathetic nerves, the intensity of peristalsis and its velocity of conduction can be altered by parasympathetic stimulation.

Therefore, *even though the basic phenomenon of peristalsis does not necessarily require the myenteric nerve plexus, effectual peristalsis does require an active myenteric plexus.*

INGESTION OF FOOD

The amount of food that a person ingests is determined principally by the intrinsic desire for food called *hunger*, and the type of food that he or she preferentially seeks is determined by his or her *appetite*. These mechanisms in themselves are extremely important automatic regulatory systems for maintaining an adequate nutritional supply for the body, and they are discussed in Chapter 48 in relation to nutrition of the body. The present discussion is confined to the actual mechanical aspects of food ingestion, including especially *mastication* and *swallowing*.

MASTICATION (CHEWING)

The teeth are admirably designed for chewing, the anterior teeth (incisors) providing a strong cutting action, and the posterior teeth (molars) a grinding action. All the jaw muscles working together can close the teeth with forces as great as 55 pounds on the incisors and 200 pounds on the molars. When this force is applied to a small object, such as a small

seed between the molars, the actual force *per square inch* may be several thousand pounds.

Most of the muscles of chewing are innervated by the motor branch of the 5th cranial nerve, and the chewing process is controlled by nuclei in the brain stem. Stimulation of an area in the reticular formation near the brain stem centers for taste can cause continual rhythmic chewing movements. Also, stimulation of areas in the hypothalamus, in the amygdaloid nuclei, and even in the cerebral cortex near the sensory areas for taste and smell can cause chewing.

Much of the chewing process is caused by the *chewing reflex*, which may be explained as follows: The presence of a bolus of food in the mouth causes reflex inhibition of the muscles of mastication, which allows the lower jaw to drop. The sudden drop in turn initiates a stretch reflex of the jaw muscles that leads to *rebound* contraction. This automatically raises the jaw to cause closure of the teeth, but it also again compresses the bolus against the linings of the mouth, which inhibits the jaw muscles once more, allowing the jaw to drop and rebound another time, and this process is repeated again and again.

Chewing of the food is important for digestion of all foods, but it is especially important for most fruits, raw vegetables, and grains because these have undigestible cellulose membranes around their nutrient portions that must be broken before the food can be utilized. Chewing aids in the digestion of food for the following simple reason: Since the *digestive enzymes act mainly on the surfaces of food particles*, the rate of digestion is highly dependent on the total surface area exposed to the intestinal secretions. Also, grinding the food to a very fine particulate consistency prevents excoriation of the gastrointestinal tract and increases the ease with which food is emptied from the stomach into the small intestine and thence into all succeeding segments of the gut.

SWALLOWING (DEGLUTITION)

Swallowing is a complicated mechanism, principally because most of the time the pharynx subserves other functions besides swallowing. It is converted for only a few seconds at a time into a tract for propulsion of food. Especially, it is important that respiration not be seriously compromised during swallowing.

In general, swallowing can be divided into (1) the *voluntary stage*, which initiates the swallowing process; (2) the *pharyngeal stage*, which is involuntary and constitutes the passage of food through the pharynx into the esophagus; and (3) the *esophageal stage*, another involuntary phase, which promotes passage of food from the pharynx to the stomach.

Voluntary Stage of Swallowing. When the food is ready for swallowing, it is voluntarily squeezed or rolled posteriorly in the mouth by pressure of the tongue upward and backward against the palate, as shown in Figure 42–4. Thus, the tongue forces the bolus of food into the pharynx. From here on, the process of swallowing becomes entirely, or almost entirely, automatic and ordinarily cannot be stopped.

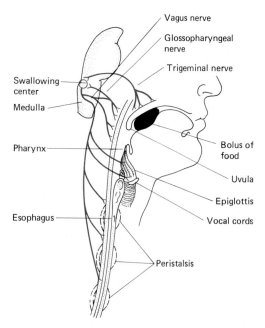

Figure 42–4. The swallowing mechanism.

Pharyngeal Stage of Swallowing. When the bolus of food is pushed backward in the mouth, it stimulates *swallowing receptor areas* all around the opening of the pharynx, especially on the tonsillar pillars, and impulses from these areas pass to the brain stem to initiate a series of automatic pharyngeal muscular contractions, as follows:

1. The soft palate is pulled upward to close the posterior nares, in this way preventing reflux of food into the nasal cavities.

2. The palatopharyngeal folds on either side of the pharynx are pulled medialward to approximate each other. In this way, these folds form a sagittal slit through which the food must pass into the posterior pharynx. This slit performs a selective action, allowing food that has been masticated properly to pass with ease while impeding the passage of large objects.

3. The vocal cords of the larynx are strongly approximated, and the epiglottis swings backward over the superior opening of the larynx. Both of these effects prevent passage of food into the trachea.

4. The entire larynx is pulled upward and forward by muscles attached to the hyoid bone: this movement of the larynx stretches the opening of the esophagus. At the same time, the upper 3 to 4 cm of the esophagus, an area called the *upper esophageal sphincter*, relaxes, thus allowing food to move easily and freely from the posterior pharynx into the upper esophagus. This sphincter, between swallows, remains tonically and strongly contracted, thereby preventing air from going into the esophagus during respiration.

5. At the same time that the larynx is raised and the upper esophageal sphincter is relaxed, the pharyngeal constrictor muscles contract, giving rise to a rapid peristaltic wave that passes downward over the pharyngeal muscles and into the esophagus and propels the food into the esophagus.

To summarize the mechanics of the pharyngeal stage of swallowing—the trachea is closed, the esophagus is opened, and a fast peristaltic wave originating in the pharynx then forces the bolus of food into the upper esophagus, the entire process occurring in one to two seconds.

Nervous Control of the Pharyngeal Stage of Swallowing. The most sensitive tactile areas of the pharynx for initiation of the pharyngeal stage of swallowing lie in a ring around the pharyngeal opening, with greatest sensitivity in the tonsillar pillars. Impulses are transmitted from these areas through the sensory portions of the trigeminal and glossopharyngeal nerves into a region of the medulla oblongata closely associated with the *tractus solitarius*, which receives essentially all sensory impulses from the mouth.

The successive stages of the swallowing process are then automatically controlled in orderly sequence by a neuronal area in the reticular substance of the medulla and lower portion of the pons. The sequence of the swallowing reflex remains the same from one swallow to the next, and the timing of the entire cycle also remains constant from one swallow to the next. The area in the medulla and the lower pons that controls swallowing is called the *deglutition* or *swallowing center*.

The motor impulses from the swallowing center to the pharynx and upper esophagus that cause swallowing are transmitted by the 5th, 9th, 10th, and 12th cranial nerves and even by a few of the superior cervical nerves.

In summary the pharyngeal stage of swallowing is principally a reflex act. It is rarely initiated by direct stimuli to the swallowing center from higher regions of the central nervous system. Instead, it is initiated by voluntary movement of food into the back of the mouth, which in turn elicits the swallowing reflex.

Esophageal Stage of Swallowing. The esophagus functions primarily to conduct food from the pharynx to the stomach, and its movements are organized specifically for this function.

Normally, the esophagus exhibits two types of peristaltic movements—*primary peristalsis* and *secondary peristalsis*. Primary peristalsis is simply a continuation of the peristaltic wave that begins in the pharynx and spreads into the esophagus during the pharyngeal stage of swallowing. This wave passes all the way from the pharynx to the stomach in approximately five to ten seconds. If the primary peristaltic wave fails to move all the food that has entered the esophagus on into the stomach, secondary peristaltic waves result from distention of the esophagus by the retained food. These waves are essentially the same as the primary peristaltic waves, except that they originate in the esophagus itself rather than in the pharynx. Secondary peristaltic waves continue to be initiated until all the food has emptied into the stomach.

The primary peristaltic waves of the esophagus are controlled almost entirely by vagal reflexes that are part of the overall swallowing mechanism. These reflexes are transmitted through *vagal afferent fibers* from the esophagus to the medulla and then back again to the esophagus through *vagal efferent fibers*.

FUNCTION OF THE LOWER ESOPHAGEAL SPHINCTER

At the lower end of the esophagus, 2 to 5 cm above its juncture with the stomach, the circular muscle of the esophagus functions as a *lower esophageal sphincter*. Anatomically, this sphincter is no different from the remainder of the esophageal muscle. However, physiologically, it remains tonically constricted, in contrast to the midportions of the esophagus, which normally remain completely relaxed. Yet when a peristaltic swallowing wave passes down the esophagus, "receptive relaxation," caused by myenteric nerve signals, relaxes the lower esophageal sphincter ahead of the peristaltic wave, and allows easy propulsion of swallowed food on into the stomach.

A principal function of the lower esophageal sphincter is to prevent reflux of stomach contents into the esophagus. The stomach contents are highly acidic and contain many proteolytic enzymes. The esophageal mucosa, except in the lower eighth of the esophagus, is not capable of resisting for long the digestive action of gastric secretions. Fortunately, the tonic constriction of the lower esophageal sphincter prevents significant reflux of stomach contents into the esophagus except under abnormal conditions.

MOTOR FUNCTIONS OF THE STOMACH

The motor functions of the stomach are three: (1) storage of large quantities of food until it can be accommodated in the lower portion of the gastrointestinal tract, (2) mixing of this food with gastric secretions until it forms a semifluid mixture called *chyme*, and (3) slow emptying of the food from the stomach into the small intestine at a rate suitable for proper digestion and absorption by the small intestine.

Figure 42–5 illustrates the basic anatomy of the stomach. Physiologically, the stomach can be divided into two major parts: (1) the *corpus*, or *body*, and (2) the *antrum*. The *fundus*, located at the upper end of the body of the stomach, is often considered by anatomists to be a separate entity from the body, but from a physiological point of view, the fundus is mainly a functional part of the body.

STORAGE FUNCTION OF THE STOMACH

As food enters the stomach, it forms concentric circles in the body and fundus of the stomach, the newest food lying closest to the esophageal opening and the oldest lying nearest the wall of the stomach. Normally, the body and fundus of the stomach have relatively little tone in their muscular wall, so that they can bulge progressively outward, thereby accom-

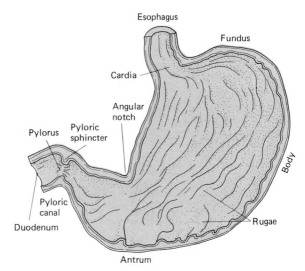

Figure 42–5. Physiologic anatomy of the stomach.

modating progressively greater quantities of food up to a limit of about 1 liter.

MIXING IN THE STOMACH

The digestive juices of the stomach are secreted by the *gastric glands,* which cover almost the entire outer wall of the body of the stomach. These secretions immediately come into contact with the stored food lying against the mucosal surface of the stomach. When the stomach is filled, weak *constrictor waves,* also called *mixing waves,* move along the stomach wall approximately once every 20 seconds. These waves move the gastric secretions and the outermost layer of food gradually toward the antral part of the stomach.

In addition to the mixing caused by the waves in the body of the stomach, mixing is also caused by peristaltic movements in the antral portion of the stomach. These movements cause mixing in the following way: Each time a peristaltic wave passes over the antrum toward the pylorus, it digs deeply into the contents of the antrum. Yet, the opening of the pylorus is small enough that only a few milliliters of antral contents are expelled into the duodenum with each peristaltic wave. Instead, most of the antral contents squirt backward through the peristaltic ring toward the body of the stomach. Thus, the moving peristaltic constrictive ring, combined with this reflux action, is an exceedingly important mixing mechanism of the stomach.

Chyme. After the food has become mixed with the stomach secretions, the resulting mixture that passes on down the gut is called *chyme.* The degree of fluidity of chyme depends on the relative amounts of food and stomach secretions and on the degree of digestion that has occurred. The appearance of chyme is that of a murky, milky semifluid or paste.

Propulsion of Food Through the Stomach. Strong peristaltic waves occur about 20 per cent of the time in the antrum of the stomach. These waves, when they occur, do so about once every 20 seconds, the same frequency as the mixing waves. As the stomach becomes progressively more empty, these intense waves begin farther and farther up the body of the stomach, gradually pinching off the lowermost portions of stored food, adding this food to the chyme in the antrum.

The peristaltic waves often exert as much as 50 to 70 cm of water pressure, which is about six times as powerful as the usual mixing waves.

EMPTYING OF THE STOMACH

Emptying of the stomach is normally opposed by resistance of the pylorus to the passage of food and is promoted by peristaltic waves in the antrum of the stomach. Usually, these two are reciprocally related—that is, those factors that increase antral peristalsis usually decrease the tone of the pyloric muscle.

Role of the Pylorus in Stomach Emptying. The pylorus normally remains almost, but not completely, closed because of tonic contraction of the pyloric muscle. The closing force is weak enough that water and other fluids empty from the stomach with ease. On the other hand, it is great enough to prevent movement of semisolid chyme into the duodenum except when a strong antral peristaltic wave forces the chyme through. On the other hand, the degree of constriction of the pyloric sphincter can increase or decrease under the influence of signals both from the stomach and from the duodenum, as we shall discuss subsequently.

Role of Antral Peristalsis in Stomach Emptying—The Pyloric Pump. The intensity of antral peristalsis, like the tone of the pyloric sphincter, also changes markedly in response to signals both from the stomach and from the duodenum. Therefore, the intensity of antral peristalsis is another principal factor determining the rate of stomach emptying.

When pyloric tone is normal, each *strong* antral peristaltic wave forces several milliliters of chyme into the duodenum. Thus, the peristaltic waves provide a pumping action that is frequently called the pyloric pump.

REGULATION OF STOMACH EMPTYING

The rate at which the stomach empties is regulated by signals both from the stomach and from the duodenum. The stomach signals are mainly twofold: (1) nervous signals caused by distention of the stomach by food and (2) the hormone *gastrin* released from the antral mucosa in response to the presence of certain types of food in the stomach. Both of these signals increase pyloric pumping force and at the same time inhibit the pylorus, thus promoting stomach emptying.

On the other hand, signals from the duodenum depress the pyloric pump and usually increase pyloric tone at the same time. In general, when an excess volume of chyme or excesses of certain types of chyme enter the duodenum, strong *negative* feedback signals, both *nervous* and *hormonal*, depress the pyloric pump and enhance pyloric sphincter tone. Obviously, these feedback signals prevent more chyme from entering the duodenum until that which has already been emptied from the stomach has been processed by the small intestine.

Effect of the Hormone Gastrin on Stomach Emptying. In the following chapter, we shall see that stretch as well as the presence of certain types of foods in the stomach—particularly meat—elicits release of the hormone called *gastrin* from the antral mucosa. Gastrin causes the secretion of highly acidic gastric juice by the gastric glands. Also, gastrin stimulates motor activity of the stomach. Most important, it enhances the activity of the pyloric pump while at the same time relaxing the pylorus. Thus, it is a strong influence for promoting stomach emptying.

The Inhibitory Effect of the Enterogastric Reflex from the Duodenum on Pyloric Activity. When chyme enters the duodenum, nervous reflex signals are transmitted back to the stomach to inhibit antral peristalsis and to increase the tone of the pylorus. This process is called the *enterogastric reflex*. It obviously acts to limit the emptying of the stomach until the small intestine can carry the chyme away. This reflex is both mediated by way of sympathetic nervous signals and by signals that pass all the way up the vagus nerve to the brain stem and then back again to the stomach, also by way of the vagus.

The types of factors that are continually monitored in the duodenum and that can elicit the enterogastric reflex include

1. The degree of distention of the duodenum
2. The presence of any degree of irritation of the duodenal mucosa
3. The degree of acidity of the duodenal chyme
4. The osmolality of the chyme
5. The presence of certain breakdown products in the chyme, especially breakdown products of proteins and, perhaps to a lesser extent, of fats

The enterogastric reflex is especially sensitive to the presence of irritants and acids in the duodenal chyme. For instance, whenever the pH of the chyme in the duodenum falls below approximately 3.5 to 4, this reflex is immediately elicited, which inhibits the pyloric pump and increases pyloric constriction, thus reducing or even further blocking the release of acidic stomach contents into the duodenum until the duodenal chyme can be neutralized by pancreatic and other secretions.

Inhibition of Gastric Emptying by Hormonal Feedback from the Duodenum—Role of Fats. Even when the enterogastric reflex has been blocked, excess amounts of chyme entering the duodenum will still inhibit stomach emptying. This effect is particularly powerful when the chyme contains large amounts of fat and is caused by several different hormones released from the mucosa of the upper small intestine. These hormones are absorbed into the blood and then carried to the stomach, where they inhibit antral peristalsis and increase pyloric tone.

One of the hormones is *cholecystokinin,* which is released from the mucosa of the jejunum in response to fatty substances in the chyme. This hormone acts as a competitive inhibitor to block the increased stomach motility caused by gastrin. Another hormone is *secretin,* which is released mainly from the duodenal mucosa in response to gastric acid released from the stomach through the pylorus. This hormone has a general but weak effect of decreasing gastrointestinal motility. Finally, a hormone called *gastric inhibitory peptide,* which is released from the upper small intestine in response mainly to fat in the chyme but to carbohydrates as well, is known also to inhibit gastric motility under some conditions.

Summary. Emptying of the stomach is controlled to a moderate degree by stomach factors such as the degree of filling in the stomach and the excitatory effect of gastrin on antral peristalsis. However, probably the most important control of stomach emptying resides in feedback signals from the duodenum, including both the enterogastric reflex and hormonal feedback. These two feedback signals work together to slow the rate of emptying when (a) too much chyme is already in the small intestine or (b) the chyme is excessively acid, contains too much protein or fat, is either hypotonic or hypertonic, or is irritating. In this way, the rate of stomach emptying is limited to that amount of chyme that the small intestine can process.

MOVEMENTS OF THE SMALL INTESTINE

The movements of the small intestine, as elsewhere in the gastrointestinal tract, can be divided into *mixing contractions* and *propulsive contractions.* However, to a great extent, this separation is artificial because essentially all movements of the small intestine cause at least some degree of both mixing and propulsion.

MIXING CONTRACTIONS (SEGMENTATION CONTRACTIONS)

When a portion of the small intestine becomes distended with chyme, this elicits localized concentric ringlike contractions spaced at intervals along the intestine. These rhythmic contractions occur at a rate of 11 to 12 per minute in the duodenum and at progressively slower rates down to 8 to 9 per minute in the terminal ileum. These contractions cause segmentation of the small intestine, as illustrated in Figure 42–6, dividing the intestines at times into regularly spaced segments that have the appearance of a chain of sausages. As one set of segmentation contractions relaxes, a new set begins, but the contractions this time occur at new points between the previous contractions. Therefore, the segmentation contractions "chop" the chyme many times a minute, in this way promoting the progressive mixing of the solid food particles with the secretions of the small intestine.

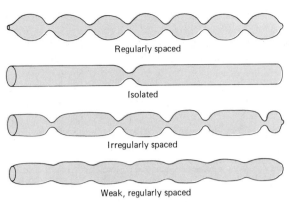

Regularly spaced

Isolated

Irregularly spaced

Weak, regularly spaced

Figure 42–6. Segmentation movements of the small intestine.

PROPULSIVE MOVEMENTS

Chyme is propelled through the small intestine by *peristaltic waves.* These can occur in any part of the small intestine, and they move analward at a velocity of 0.5 to 2 cm per second, much faster in the proximal intestine and much slower in the terminal intestine. However, the waves are normally very weak and usually die out after traveling only a few centimeters; therefore, movement of the chyme is slow. As a result, the net movement of the chyme along the small intestine averages only 1 cm per minute. This means that 3 to 5 hours are normally required for passage of chyme from the pylorus to the ileocecal valve.

Peristaltic activity of the small intestine is greatly increased after a meal. This is caused partly by the entry of chyme into the duodenum but also by a so-called *gastroenteric reflex* initiated by distention of the stomach and conducted principally through the myenteric plexus from the stomach down along the wall of the small intestine. This reflex increases the overall degree of excitability of the small intestine, including both increased motility and increased secretion.

The Peristaltic Reflex. The usual cause of peristalsis in the small intestine is distention. Circumferential stretch of the intestine excites receptors in the gut wall, and these elicit a local myenteric reflex that begins with contraction of the longitudinal muscle over a distance of several centimeters and is followed by contraction of the circular muscle. Simultaneously, the contractile process spreads in an anal direction by the process of peristalsis. Movement of the peristaltic contraction down the gut is controlled by the myenteric plexus; this forward movement does not occur when this plexus has been blocked by drugs or when the plexus has degenerated.

Very intense irritation of the intestinal mucosa, such as that occurring in some infectious processes, can elicit a so-called *peristaltic rush,* which is a series of powerful peristaltic waves that travel long distances in the small intestine in a few minutes. These waves can sweep the contents of the intestine into the colon and thereby relieve the small intestine of either irritants or excessive distention.

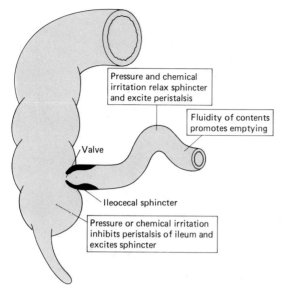

Figure 42–7. Emptying at the ileocecal valve.

The function of the peristaltic waves in the small intestine is not only to cause propulsion of the chyme toward the ileocecal valve but also to spread out the chyme along the intestinal mucosa.

FUNCTION OF THE ILEOCECAL VALVE

A principal function of the ileocecal valve is to prevent backflow of fecal contents from the colon into the small intestine. As illustrated in Figure 42–7, the lips of the ileocecal valve protrude into the lumen of the cecum and therefore are forcibly closed when the cecum fills. Usually, the valve can resist reverse pressure of as much as 50 to 60 cm water.

The wall of the ileum for several centimeters immediately preceding the ileocecal valve has a thickened muscular coat called the *ileocecal sphincter*. This sphincter normally remains mildly constricted and slows the emptying of ileal contents into the cecum except immediately following a meal, when a *gastroileal reflex* intensifies the peristalsis in the ileum. Also, the hormone *gastrin*, which is liberated from the stomach mucosa in response to food in the stomach, has a direct relaxant effect on the ileocecal sphincter, thus allowing rapid emptying. Even so, only about 1500 ml of chyme empties into the cecum each day. The resistance to emptying at the ileocecal valve prolongs the stay of chyme in the ileum and therefore facilitates absorption.

Control of the Ileocecal Sphincter. The degree of contraction of the ileocecal sphincter is controlled primarily by reflexes from the cecum. Whenever the cecum is distended, the degree of contraction of the ileocecal sphincter is intensified, which greatly delays emptying of additional chyme from the ileum. Also, any irritant in the cecum causes constriction of the ileocecal sphincter. For instance, when a person has an inflamed appendix, the irritation of this vestigial remnant of the cecum can cause such intense spasm of the ileocecal sphincter that it completely blocks

emptying of the ileum. These reflexes from the cecum to the ileocecal sphincter are mediated both by way of the myenteric plexus and through extrinsic nerves, especially reflexes by way of the prevertebral sympathetic ganglia.

MOVEMENTS OF THE COLON

The functions of the colon are (1) absorption of water and electrolytes from the chyme and (2) storage of fecal matter until it can be expelled. The proximal half of the colon, illustrated in Figure 42–8, is concerned principally with absorption, and the distal half with storage; since intense movements are not required for these functions, the movements of the colon are normally sluggish. Yet, even in a sluggish manner, the movements still have characteristics similar to those of the small intestine and can be divided once again into mixing movements and propulsive movements.

Mixing Movements—Haustrations. In the same manner that segmentation movements occur in the small intestine, large circular constrictions also occur in the large intestine. At each of these constriction points, about 2.5 cm of the circular muscle contracts, sometimes constricting the lumen of the colon to almost complete occlusion. At the same time, the longitudinal muscle of the colon, which is aggregated into three longitudinal strips called the *teniae coli*, contracts. These combined contractions of the circular and the longitudinal strips of smooth muscle cause the unstimulated portions of the large intestine to bulge outward into baglike sacs called *haustrations*. The haustral contractions, once initiated, usually reach peak intensity in about 30 seconds and then disappear during the next 60 seconds. They at times also move slowly analward during their period of contraction. After another few minutes, new haustral contractions occur nearby but not in the same areas. Therefore, the fecal material in the large intestine is slowly "dug" into and rolled over in much the same manner that one spades the earth. In this way, all the

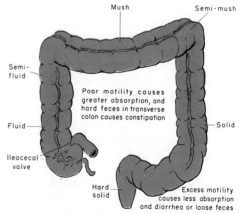

Figure 42–8. Absorptive and storage functions of the large intestine.

fecal material is gradually exposed to the surface of the large intestine, and fluid is progressively absorbed until only 80 to 150 ml of the 1500 ml daily load of chyme entering the colon is lost in the feces.

Propulsive Movements—Mass Movements. Peristaltic waves of the type seen in the small intestine do not occur in the colon. Instead, another type of movement, called *mass movement*, propels the fecal contents toward the anus. These movements usually occur only a few times each day, most abundantly for about 15 minutes during the first hour or so after eating breakfast.

A mass movement is characterized by the following sequence of events: First, a constrictive ring occurs at a distended or irritated point in the colon. Rapidly thereafter, the 20 or more cm of colon *distal* to the constriction contracts almost as a unit, forcing the fecal material in this segment *en masse* down the colon. The initiation of contraction is complete in about 30 seconds, and relaxation then occurs during the next two to three minutes. Mass movements can occur in any part of the colon, though they most often occur in the transverse or descending colon. When they have forced a mass of feces into the rectum, the desire for defecation is felt.

Initiation of Mass Movements by Gastrocolic and Duodenocolic Reflexes. The fact that mass movements occur after meals is caused at least partially by so-called *gastrocolic* and *duodenocolic reflexes*. These reflexes result from distention of the stomach and duodenum, and they are transmitted both through the myenteric plexus and probably even more strongly through the extrinsic autonomic nerves.

Irritation in the colon can also initiate intense mass movements. For instance, a person who has an ulcerated condition of the colon (*ulcerative colitis*) frequently has mass movements that persist almost all of the time.

DEFECATION

Most of the time the rectum is empty of feces. This circumstance results partly from the fact that a weak functional sphincter exists approximately 20 cm from the anus at the juncture between the sigmoid and the rectum. However, when a mass movement forces feces into the rectum, the process of defecation is normally initiated, including reflex contraction of the rectum, the sigmoid, and the descending colon, and also relaxation of the anal sphincters.

Continual dribble of fecal matter through the anus is prevented by tonic constriction of (1) the *internal anal sphincter*, a circular mass of smooth muscle that lies immediately inside the anus, and (2) the *external anal sphincter*, composed of striated voluntary muscle that surrounds and lies slightly distal to the internal sphincter and is controlled by the somatic nervous system and is therefore under voluntary, conscious, control.

Ordinarily, defecation results from the *defecation reflex*, the reflex pathway of which is illustrated in

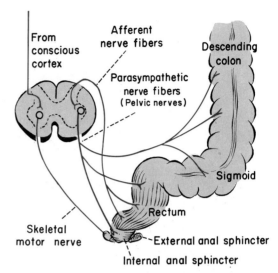

Figure 42–9. The afferent and efferent pathways of the parasympathetic mechanism for enhancing the defecation reflex.

Figure 42–9. When the sensory nerve fibers in the rectum are stimulated by stretch, signals are transmitted into the sacral portion of the spinal cord and thence, reflexly, back to the descending colon, sigmoid, rectum, and anus by way of parasympathetic nerve fibers in the pelvic nerves. These parasympathetic signals initiate strong peristaltic waves that are sometimes effective in emptying the large bowel all the way from the splenic flexure to the anus. Also, the afferent signals entering the spinal cord initiate other effects, such as taking a deep breath, closing the glottis, contracting the abdominal muscles to force downward the fecal contents of the colon, and at the same time, contracting the pelvic floor muscles, pulling outward and upward on the anus to evaginate the feces downward.

However, despite the defecation reflex, other effects are necessary before actual defecation occurs. Except in babies and mentally inept persons, the conscious mind voluntarily controls the external sphincter; the mind may inhibit its contraction and thereby allow defecation to occur, or the mind may contract the sphincter if the moment is not socially acceptable for defecation to occur. If the external sphincter is kept contracted, so that defecation does not occur, the defecation reflex dies out after a few minutes and usually will not return until an additional amount of feces enters the rectum, which may not be until several hours thereafter.

When it becomes convenient for the person to defecate, defecation reflexes can sometimes be initiated by taking a deep breath to move the diaphragm downward against the abdominal contents and then contracting the abdominal muscles to increase the pressure in the abdomen, thus forcing fecal contents into the rectum to elicit new reflexes. Unfortunately, reflexes initiated in this way are never as effective as those that arise naturally, for which reason people who inhibit their natural reflexes too often are likely to become severely constipated.

QUESTIONS

1. Describe the layers of the intestinal wall.
2. Give the characteristics of the smooth muscle in the intestinal wall, describing especially the *gap junctions* and their function.
3. Describe the *enteric nervous system,* and discuss its function in local control of gastrointestinal activity.
4. Explain the relationship of the *parasympathetic* and *sympathetic nervous systems* to the enteric nervous system of the gastrointestinal tract.
5. What are the two basic types of movement in the gastrointestinal tract, and what are their purposes?
6. Describe the mechanics of *mastication* and its control by the nervous system.
7. Describe the mechanics of *swallowing,* giving the sequential steps in the swallowing process.
8. Describe the nervous control of swallowing.
9. What is the role of the esophagus in swallowing, and how does the *lower esophageal sphincter* function?
10. What are the characteristics of the movements in the stomach, and how is *chyme* formed?
11. What are the roles of *pyloric tone* and *antral peristalsis* in stomach emptying?
12. Explain the control of stomach emptying by both *stomach factors* and *intestinal factors.*
13. What are the roles of *gastrin,* the *enterogastric reflex,* and the *intestinal hormones* in the control of stomach emptying?
14. Explain the differences between and the functions of the *segmentation contractions* and the *peristaltic movements* of the small intestine.
15. Describe the function of the *ileocecal valve* and its control.
16. Describe the mixing movements (the *haustrations*) and the propulsive movements (*mass movements*) of the colon.
17. Explain the mechanics of *defecation,* neural control of defecation, and function of the *defecation reflex.*

References

Bulbring, E., ed.: Smooth Muscle. An Assessment of Current Knowledge, Austin, University of Texas Press, 1981.
Chou, C. C.: Relationship between intestinal blood flow and motility. Ann Rev Physiol 44:29, 1982.
Donald, D. E.: Splanchnic circulation. In Shepherd, J. T., and Abboud, F. M., eds.: Handbook of Physiology. Sec. 2, Vol. 3. Bethesda, American Physiological Society, 1983, p. 219.
Gabella, G.: Structural apparatus for force transmission in smooth muscle. Physiol Rev 64:455, 1984.
Grossman, M. I.: Neural and hormonal regulation of gastrointestinal function: an overview. Annu Rev Physiol 41:27, 1979.
Hunt, J. N.: Mechanisms and disorders of gastric emptying. Annu Rev Med 34:219, 1983.
Kilmov, P. K.: Behavior of the organs of the digestive system. Neurosci Behav Physiol 14:333, 1984.
Loewenstein, W. R.: Junctional intercellular communication: the cell-to-cell membrane channel. Physiol Rev 61:829, 1981.
Miller, A. J.: Deglutition. Physiol Rev 62:129, 1982.
Szurszewski, J. H.: Physiology of mammalian prevertebral ganglia. Ann Rev Physiol 43:53, 1981.
Weems, W. A.: The intestine as a fluid propelling system. Annu Rev Physiol 43:9, 1981.
Weisbrodt, N. W.: Patterns of intestinal motility. Annu Rev Physiol 43:21, 1981.
Wood, J. D.: Intrinsic neural control of intestinal motility. Annu Rev Physiol 43:33, 1981.

43
Secretory Functions of the Alimentary Tract

GENERAL PRINCIPLES OF GASTROINTESTINAL SECRETION
ANATOMICAL TYPES OF GLANDS
BASIC MECHANISM OF SECRETION BY GLANDULAR CELLS
LUBRICATING AND PROTECTIVE PROPERTIES OF MUCUS AND ITS IMPORTANCE IN THE GASTROINTESTINAL TRACT
SECRETION OF SALIVA
ESOPHAGEAL SECRETION
GASTRIC SECRETION
CHARACTERISTICS OF THE GASTRIC SECRETIONS
REGULATION OF GASTRIC SECRETION BY NERVOUS AND HORMONAL MECHANISMS
PANCREATIC SECRETION
REGULATION OF PANCREATIC SECRETION

SECRETION OF BILE BY THE LIVER
PHYSIOLOGICAL ANATOMY OF THE LIVER
THE BILE SALTS AND THEIR FUNCTIONS
EXCRETION OF BILIRUBIN IN THE BILE
SECRETION OF CHOLESTEROL: GALLSTONE FORMATION
SECRETIONS OF THE SMALL INTESTINE
SECRETION OF MUCUS BY BRUNNER'S GLANDS AND BY MUCOUS CELLS OF THE INTESTINAL SURFACE
SECRETION OF THE INTESTINAL DIGESTIVE JUICES—THE CRYPTS OF LIEBERKÜHN
REGULATION OF SECRETION OF THE SMALL INTESTINE
SECRETIONS OF THE LARGE INTESTINE

Throughout the gastrointestinal tract, secretions serve two functions: First, digestive enzymes are secreted in most areas from the mouth to the distal end of the ileum. Second, mucous glands, from the mouth to the anus, provide mucus for lubrication and protection of all parts of the alimentary tract.

Most digestive secretions are formed only in response to the presence of food in the alimentary tract, and the quantity secreted in each segment of the tract is almost exactly the amount needed for proper digestion. Furthermore, in some portions of the gastrointestinal tract even the types of enzymes and other constituents of the secretions are varied in accordance with the types of food present. The purpose of the present chapter, therefore, is to describe the different alimentary secretions, their functions, and the regulation of their production.

GENERAL PRINCIPLES OF GASTROINTESTINAL SECRETION

ANATOMICAL TYPES OF GLANDS

Several types of glands provide the different types of secretions in the gastrointestinal tract. First, on the surface of the epithelium in most parts of the gastrointestinal tract are literally billions of *single cell mucous glands,* called *mucous cells,* or sometimes *goblet cells.* They simply extrude their mucus directly into the lumen of the gastrointestinal tract.

Second, most surface areas of the gastrointestinal tract are lined by pits that represent invaginations of the epithelium into the submucosa. In the small intestine, these pits, called *crypts of Lieberkühn,* are deep and contain specialized secretory cells. (One of

497

these is illustrated in Figure 43–11). They are lined with goblet cells that produce mucus and with other epithelial cells that produce mainly serous fluids.

Third, in the stomach and upper duodenum are found large numbers of deep *tubular glands*. A typical tubular gland is illustrated in Figure 43–4, which shows an acid- and pepsinogen-secreting gland of the stomach.

Fourth, also associated with the gastrointestinal tract are several complex glands—the *salivary glands*, the *pancreas*, and the *liver*—which provide secretions for digestion or emulsification of food. These glands lie completely outside the walls of the gastrointestinal tract and are described later.

BASIC MECHANISM OF SECRETION BY GLANDULAR CELLS

Secretion of Organic Substances. Though all the basic mechanisms by which glandular cells form different secretions and then extrude them to the exterior are not known, experimental evidence points to the following basic principles of secretion by glandular cells, as illustrated in Figure 43–1.

1. The nutrient material needed for formation of the secretion must diffuse or be actively transported from the capillary into the base of the glandular cell.

2. Many *mitochondria* located inside the cell, near its base, provide oxidative energy for formation of adenosine triphosphate.

3. Energy from the adenosine triphosphate, along with appropriate nutrients, is then used for synthesis of the organic substances, which occurs almost entirely on or near the *endoplasmic reticulum*. The *ribosomes* adherent to this reticulum are specifically responsible for formation of proteins.

4. The secretory materials are transported into and through the tubules of the endoplasmic reticulum, passing in about 20 minutes all the way to the vesicles of the Golgi complex, which lies near the secretory ends of the cells.

5. The materials then are modified, added to, concentrated, and discharged into the cytoplasm in the form of *secretory vesicles* that are stored in the apical ends of the secretory cells.

6. These vesicles remain stored until nervous or hormonal control signals cause them to extrude their contents through the cell's surface.

Water and Electrolyte Secretion in Response to Nervous Stimulation. A second necessity for glandular secretion is sufficient water and electrolytes to be secreted along with the organic substances. The following is a postulated method by which nervous stimulation causes water and salts to pass through the glandular cells in great profusion, washing the organic substances through the secretory border of the cells at the same time:

(1) Nerve stimulation has the specific effect on the *basal* portion of the cell membrane of causing active transport of chloride ions to the interior. (2) The resulting increase in electronegativity inside the cell then causes positive ions also to move to the interior of the cell. (3) The excess of both of these ions inside the cell creates osmotic force that pulls water to the interior, thereby increasing the hydrostatic pressure inside the cell and causing the cell itself to swell. (4) The pressure in the cell then results in minute ruptures of the secretory border of the cell and causes flushing of water, electrolytes, and organic materials out of the secretory end of the glandular cell and into the lumen of the gland.

LUBRICATING AND PROTECTIVE PROPERTIES OF MUCUS AND ITS IMPORTANCE IN THE GASTROINTESTINAL TRACT

Mucus is a thick secretion composed mainly of water, electrolytes, and a mixture of several glycoproteins. Mucus has several important characteristics that make it both an excellent lubricant and a protectant for the wall of the gut. *First*, mucus has adherent qualities that make it adhere tightly to the food or other particles and also to spread as a thin film over the food surfaces. *Second*, it has sufficient *body* to enable it to coat the wall of the gut and prevent actual contact of food particles with the mucosa. *Third*, mucus has a low resistance to slippage—that is, it is an excellent lubricant—so that the particles can slide along the epithelium with great ease. *Fourth*, mucus causes fecal particles to adhere to each other to form the fecal masses that are expelled during a bowel movement. *Fifth*, mucus is strongly resistant to digestion by the gastrointestinal enzymes. And, *sixth*, the glycoproteins of mucus have amphoteric properties and are therefore capable of buffering small amounts of either acids or alkalis; also, mucus usually contains moderate quantities of bicarbonate ions, which specifically neutralize acids.

In summary, mucus has the ability to allow easy slippage of food along the gastrointestinal tract and also to prevent excoriative or chemical damage to the epithelium. One becomes acutely aware of the lubri-

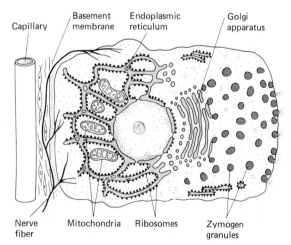

Figure 43–1. Typical function of a glandular cell in formation and secretion of enzymes or other secretory substances.

Labels: Capillary, Basement membrane, Endoplasmic reticulum, Golgi apparatus, Nerve fiber, Mitochondria, Ribosomes, Zymogen granules

cating qualities of mucus when his salivary glands fail to secrete saliva, for under these circumstances it is extremely difficult to swallow solid food even when it is taken with large amounts of water.

SECRETION OF SALIVA

The Salivary Glands; Characteristics of Saliva. The principal glands of salivation are the *parotid, submandibular,* and *sublingual* glands; in addition, there are many small *buccal* glands. The daily secretion of saliva normally ranges between 800 and 1500 ml, as shown in Table 43–1.

Saliva contains two major types of protein secretion: (1) a *serous secretion* containing *ptyalin* (an α-amylase), which is an enzyme for digesting starches, and (2) *mucous secretion* containing *mucus* for lubricating purposes. The parotid glands secrete entirely the serous type, and the submandibular glands secrete both the serous type and mucus. The sublingual and buccal glands secrete only mucus. Saliva has a pH between 6.0 and 7.4, a favorable range for the digestive action of ptyalin.

Secretion of Ions in the Saliva. Saliva contains especially large quantities of potassium and bicarbonate ions. On the other hand, the concentrations of both sodium and chloride ions are considerably less in saliva than in plasma. One can understand these special concentrations of ions in the saliva from the following description of the mechanism for its secretion.

Figure 43–2 illustrates secretion by the submandibular gland, a typical *compound gland* containing both *acini* and *salivary ducts.* Salivary secretion is a two-stage operation; the first stage involves the acini, and the second the salivary ducts. The acini release *primary secretion* that contains ptyalin or mucus or both in a solution of ions in concentrations not greatly different from those of typical extracellular fluid. However, as the primary secretion flows through the ducts, two major active transport processes take place that markedly modify the ionic composition of the saliva.

First, *sodium ions* are actively reabsorbed from all the salivary ducts, and *potassium ions* are actively secreted, but at a slower rate, in exchange for the

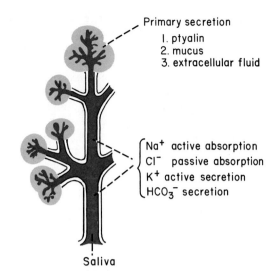

Figure 43–2. Formation and secretion of saliva by a salivary gland.

sodium. Therefore, the sodium concentration of the saliva is greatly reduced whereas the potassium ion concentration increases. The great excess of sodium reabsorption over potassium secretion creates negativity of about −70 mv in the salivary ducts, and this causes chloride ions to be reabsorbed passively; therefore, the chloride ion concentration falls to a very low level along with the decrease in sodium ion concentration.

Second, *bicarbonate ions* are secreted by the ductal epithelium into the lumen of the duct. This is probably an active secretory process, though little is known about its details.

The net result of these active transport processes is that, under resting conditions, the concentrations of sodium and chloride ions in the saliva are only about 15 mEq/liter each, approximately 1/7 to 1/10 their concentrations in plasma. On the other hand, the concentration of potassium ions is about 30 mEq/liter, seven times as great as its concentration in plasma, and the concentration of bicarbonate ions is 50 to 70 mEq/liter, about two to three times that of plasma.

During maximal salivation, the salivary ionic concentrations change considerably because the rate of formation of primary secretion by the acini can increase as much as 20-fold. As a result, this secretion then flows through the ducts so rapidly that the ductal reconditioning of the secretion is considerably reduced. Therefore, when copious quantities of saliva are secreted, the sodium chloride concentration rises to about one half to two thirds that of plasma, whereas the potassium concentration falls to only four times that of plasma.

In the presence of excess aldosterone secretion, the sodium and chloride reabsorption and the potassium secretion become greatly increased, so that the sodium chloride concentration in the saliva is sometimes reduced almost to zero while the potassium concentration increases still more.

Table 43–1. DAILY SECRETION OF GASTROINTESTINAL JUICES

	Daily Volume (ml)	pH
Saliva	1000	6.0–7.0
Gastric secretion	1500	1.0–3.5
Pancreatic secretion	1000	8.0–8.3
Bile	1000	7.8
Small intestinal secretion	1800	7.5–8.0
Brunner's gland secretion	200	8.0–8.9
Large intestinal secretion	200	7.5–8.0
Total	6700	

Function of Saliva for Oral Hygiene. Under basal conditions about 0.5 ml/min of saliva, almost entirely of the mucous type, is secreted all the time. This secretion plays an exceedingly important role in maintaining healthy oral tissues. The mouth is loaded with pathogenic bacteria that can easily destroy tissues and can also cause dental caries. However, saliva helps to prevent the deteriorative processes in several ways: First, the flow of saliva itself helps to wash away the pathogenic bacteria as well as the food particles that provide their metabolic support. Second, the saliva, also contains several factors that actually destroy bacteria, including *thiocyanate ions* and several *proteolytic enzymes* that (a) attack the bacteria, (b) aid the thiocyanate ions to enter the bacteria, where they in turn become bactericidal, and (c) digest food particles, thus helping further to remove the bacterial metabolic support. Third, saliva often contains significant amounts of protein antibodies that can destroy the oral bacteria, including those that cause dental caries.

Therefore, in the absence of salivation, the oral tissues become ulcerated and otherwise infected, and caries of the teeth become rampant.

Nervous Regulation of Salivary Secretion. Figure 43–3 illustrates the nervous pathways for regulation of salivation, showing that the salivary glands are controlled mainly by *parasympathetic nervous signals* from the *salivatory nuclei*. The salivatory nuclei are located approximately at the juncture of the medulla and the pons and are excited by both taste and tactile stimuli from the tongue and other areas of the mouth. Many taste stimuli, especially the sour taste, elicit copious secretion of saliva—often as much as 5 to 8 ml per minute or 8 to 20 times the basal rate of secretion. Also, certain tactile stimuli, such as the presence of smooth objects in the mouth (a pebble,

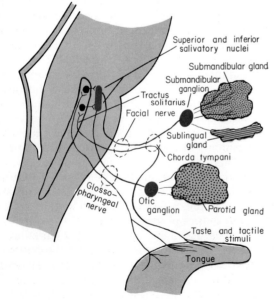

Figure 43–3. Nervous regulation of salivary secretion.

for instance), cause marked salivation, while rough objects cause less salivation and occasionally even inhibit salivation.

Salivation can also be stimulated or inhibited by impulses arriving in the salivatory nuclei from higher centers of the central nervous system. For instance, when a person smells or eats favorite foods, salivation is greater than when disliked food is smelled or eaten.

ESOPHAGEAL SECRETION

The esophageal secretions are entirely mucoid in character and principally provide lubrication for swallowing. The main body of the esophagus is lined with many *simple mucous glands,* but at the gastric end and to a lesser extent in the initial portion of the esophagus, there are many *compound mucous glands.* The mucus secreted by the compound glands in the upper esophagus prevents mucosal excoriation by the newly entering food, whereas the compound glands near the esophagogastric junction protect the esophageal wall from digestion by gastric juices that reflux into the lower esophagus. Despite this protection, a peptic ulcer at times may occur at the gastric end of the esophagus.

GASTRIC SECRETION

CHARACTERISTICS OF THE GASTRIC SECRETIONS

In addition to the mucus-secreting cells that line the surface of the stomach, the stomach mucosa has two different types of tubular glands: the *oxyntic* (or *gastric*) *glands* and the *pyloric glands.* The oxyntic, which means acid-forming, glands, secrete *hydrochloric acid, pepsinogen, intrinsic factor,* and *mucus;* and the pyloric glands secrete mainly *mucus* for protection of the pyloric mucosa but also some *pepsinogen* and the hormone *gastrin.* The oxyntic glands are located over the entire wall of the body and fundus of the stomach except along the lesser curvature, and the pyloric glands are located in the antral portion of the stomach.

The Secretions from the Oxyntic Glands. A typical oxyntic gland is shown in Figure 43–4. It is composed of three different types of cells: the *mucous neck cells,* which secrete mainly mucus but also some pepsinogen; the *peptic* (or *chief*) *cells,* which secrete large quantities of pepsinogen; and the *oxyntic* (or *parietal*) *cells*, which secrete hydrochloric acid and intrinsic factor.

Basic Mechanism of Hydrochloric Acid Secretion. The oxyntic cells secrete an electrolytic solution containing a maximum of about 160 millimoles of hydrochloric acid per liter. The pH of this acid solution is approximately 0.8, which illustrates its extreme acidity. At this pH the hydrogen ion concentration is about 3 million times that of the arterial blood.

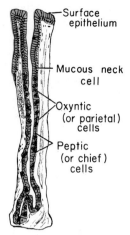

Figure 43–4. An oxyntic gland from the body or fundus of the stomach.

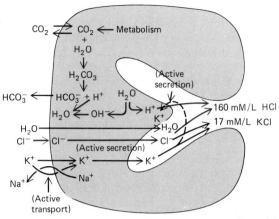

Figure 43–6. Postulated mechanism for the secretion of hydrochloric acid.

Figure 43–5 illustrates the basic structure of an oxyntic cell, showing that it contains a system of *intracellular canaliculi*. The hydrochloric acid is formed at the membranes of these canaliculi and then conducted through openings to the exterior.

Different suggestions for the precise mechanism of hydrochloric acid formation have been offered. One of these is illustrated in Figure 43–6 and consists of the following steps:

1. Chloride ion is actively transported from the cytoplasm of the oxyntic cell into the lumen of the canaliculus. This process creates a negative potential of -40 to -70 millivolts in the canaliculus, which in turn causes passive diffusion of positively charged potassium ions from the cell cytoplasm also into the canaliculus. Thus, in effect, *potassium chloride* enters the canaliculus.

2. Water is dissociated into hydrogen ions and hydroxyl ions in the cell cytoplasm. The hydrogen ion is then actively secreted into the canaliculus in exchange for potassium ions; this active exchange process is catalyzed by H^+-K^+ ATPase. Thus, most of the potassium ions that had been secreted are reabsorbed, and hydrogen ions take their place in the canaliculus.

3. Water passes through the cell and into the canaliculus by osmosis. Thus the final secretion entering the canaliculus is *a solution containing hydrochloric acid in a concentration of 160 millimoles per liter and potassium chloride in a concentration of 17 millimoles per liter.*

4. Finally, several steps involving carbon dioxide and carbonic acid cause removal of the excess hydroxyl ions from the cell.

Secretion of Pepsin. The principal enzyme secreted by the *peptic cells* is *pepsin*. This enzyme is formed inside the cells in the form of *pepsinogen,* which has no digestive activity. However, once pepsinogen is secreted and comes in contact with previously formed pepsin in the presence of hydrochloric acid, it is immediately activated to form active pepsin. In this process the pepsinogen molecule, having a molecular weight of about 42,500, yields the pepsin molecule, having a molecular weight of about 35,000.

Pepsin is an active proteolytic enzyme (for digesting proteins) in a highly acid medium (optimum pH = 2.0), but above a pH of about 5 it has little proteolytic activity and soon becomes completely inactivated. Therefore, hydrochloric acid secretion is just as necessary as pepsin secretion for protein digestion in the stomach.

Secretion of Mucus in the Stomach. The pyloric glands are structurally similar to the oxyntic glands, but contain very few peptic and oxyntic cells. Instead, they contain mainly mucous cells that are identical with the mucous neck cells of the gastric glands. These cells secrete a thin mucus that protects the stomach wall from digestion by the gastric enzymes.

In addition, the surface of the stomach mucosa has a continuous layer of mucous cells that secrete large quantities of a far more *viscid and alkaline mucus*

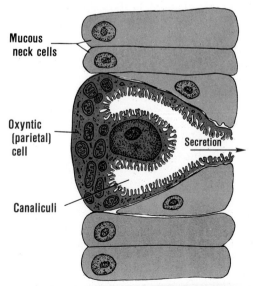

Figure 43–5. Anatomy of the canaliculi in an oxyntic (parietal) cell.

that coats the mucosa with a mucous gel layer over 1 mm thick, thus providing a major shell of protection for the stomach wall as well as contributing to lubrication of food transport. Even the slightest irritation of the mucosa directly stimulates the mucous cells to secrete copious quantities of this thick, viscid mucus.

REGULATION OF GASTRIC SECRETION BY NERVOUS AND HORMONAL MECHANISMS

Gastric secretion is regulated by both nervous and hormonal mechanisms; nervous regulation is effected through the parasympathetic fibers of the vagus nerves as well as through local enteric nervous system reflexes, and hormonal regulation takes place mainly in response to the hormone *gastrin*. Thus, regulation of gastric secretion is different from the regulation of salivary secretion, which is effected entirely by nervous mechanisms.

Vagal Stimulation of Gastric Secretion

Nervous signals to cause gastric secretion originate in the dorsal motor nuclei of the vagi and pass via the vagus nerves to the enteric nervous system of the stomach wall and thence to the oxyntic glands. In response these glands secrete vast quantities of both pepsin and acid, but with a higher proportion of pepsin than in gastric juice elicited in other ways.

Stimulation of Gastric Secretion by Gastrin

When food enters the stomach, it causes the antral portion of the stomach mucosa to secrete the hormone gastrin. This hormone is secreted by *gastrin cells,* also called *G cells,* in the pyloric glands. Gastrin is a large peptide secreted in two forms, a large form called *G-34,* containing 34 amino acids, and a smaller form, *G-17,* containing 17 amino acids. Though both of these forms are important, the smaller is more abundant.

The food causes release of this hormone in two ways: (1) The actual bulk of the food distends the stomach, and this causes the hormone gastrin to be released from the antral mucosa. (2) Certain substances called *secretagogues*—such as food extractives, partially digested proteins, alcohol (in low concentration), caffeine, and so forth—also cause gastrin to be liberated from the antral mucosa.

Both of these stimuli—the distension and the chemical action of the secretagogues—elicit gastrin release by means of a local nerve reflex. That is, they stimulate sensory nerve fibers in the stomach epithelim that in turn synapse with the enteric nervous system. The latter then transmits efferent signals to the gastrin cells, causing them to secrete the gastrin. Therefore, any factor that blocks this reflex will also block the formation of gastrin. For instance, anesthetization of the gastric mucosa to block the sensory stimuli will prevent gastrin release; administration of atropine, which blocks the action on the gastrin cells of the acetylcholine released by the enteric nerves, will also prevent gastrin release.

Gastrin is absorbed into the blood and carried to the oxyntic glands in the body of the stomach, where it stimulates mainly the oxyntic cells but, to a lesser extent, the peptic cells. The oxyntic cells increase their rate of hydrochloric acid secretion as much as eightfold, and the peptic cells increase their rate of enzyme secretion two- to fourfold.

The rate of secretion in response to gastrin is somewhat less than to vagal stimulation, 200 ml per hour in contrast to about 500 ml per hour, indicating

Glu- Gly- Pro- Trp- Leu- Glu- Glu- Glu- Glu- Glu- Ala- Tyr- Gly- Trp- Met- Asp- Phe- NH$_2$

$$HSO_3$$

Gastrin

Lys- (Ala, Gly, Pro, Ser)- Arg- Val- (Ile, Met, Ser)- Lys- Asn- (Asn, Gln, His, Leu$_2$, Pro, Ser$_2$)- Arg- Ile- (Asp, Ser)- Arg- Asp- Tyr- Met- Gly- Trp- Met- Asp- Phe- NH$_2$

$$HSO_3$$

Cholecystokinin

His- Ser- Asp- Gly- Thr- Phe- Thr- Ser- Glu- Leu- Ser- Arg- Leu- Arg- Asp- Ser- Ala- Arg- Leu- Gln- Arg- Leu- Leu- Gln- Gly- Leu- Val- NH$_2$

Secretin

that the gastrin mechanism is a less potent acute mechanism for stimulation of stomach secretion than is vagal stimulation. However, the gastrin mechanism usually continues for several hours in contrast with a much shorter period of time for vagal stimulation. Therefore, as a whole, it is likely that the gastrin mechanism is equally as important as, if not more so than, the vagal mechanism for control of gastric secretion.

Role of Histamine in Controlling Gastric Secretion. *Histamine,* an amino acid derivative, also stimulates gastric secretion. When the histamine receptors of the oxyntic glands are blocked with the histamine antagonist drug *cimetidine,* not only does this block the stimulatory effect of histamine on gastric secretion, it blocks the effect of gastrin as well. Therefore, it is believed that local gastric mucosal histamine is prerequisite for the sitmulatory function of gastrin—perhaps gastrin causes the release of histamine and it is the histamine that actually causes the secretion.

Chemical Composition of Gastrin and Other Gastrointestinal Hormones. Illustrated are the amino acid compositions of *gastrin-17,* as well as *cholecystokinin* and *secretin,* which are discussed later in the chapter. Note that all are polypeptides and that the last five amino acids in the gastrin and cholecystokinin molecular chains are exactly the same. The activity resides in the terminal four amino acids of gastrin and in the terminal eight amino acids for cholecystokinin; all the amino acids are essential in secretin. A synthetic gastrin, composed of the terminal four amino acids of natural gastrins plus the amino acid alanine, has all the same physiological properties as the natural gastrins. This synthetic product is called *pentagastrin.*

Feedback Inhibition of Gastric Acid Secretion When Stomach Acidity Is Too Great

When the acidity of the gastric juices increases to the highly acid pH of 2.0, the gastrin mechanism for stimulating gastric secretion becomes totally blocked. This effect probably results form two different factors. First, greatly enhanced acidity depresses or blocks the extraction of gastrin itself from the antral mucosa. Second, the acid seems to cause an inhibitory nervous reflex that inhibits gastric acid secretion.

Obviously, this feedback inhibition of the gastric glands plays an important role in protecting the stomach against excessively acid secretions, which would readily cause peptic ulceration. in addition to this protective effect, the feedback mechanism is also important in maintaining optimal pH for function of the peptic enzymes in the digestive process, because whenever the pH rises above 2.5 to 3.5, gastrin begins to be secreted again and more acid is secreted.

Inhibition by Intestinal Factors. The presence of food in the small intestine initiates an *enterogastric reflex,* transmitted through the enteric nerve plexus, the sympathetic nerves, and the vagus nerves, that inhibits stomach secretion. This reflex is part of the complex mechanism discussed in the preceding chapter for slowing stomach emptying when the intestines are already filled.

Also, the presence of acids, fats, protein breakdown products, hyper- or hypo-osmotic fluids, or any irritating factor in the upper small intestine causes the release of several intestinal hormones that inhibit gastric secretion. Three of these are *secretin, cholecystokinin,* and *gastric inhibitory peptide.* These, too, were discussed in the previous chapter.

The functional purpose of the inhibition of gastric secretion by intestinal factors is to slow the release of chyme from the stomach when the small intestine is already filled.

PANCREATIC SECRETION

Characteristics of Pancreatic Juice. The pancreas is a large compound gland similar to the salivary gland. It lies parallel to the stomach and secretes its juice into the duodenum a few centimeters beyond the pylorus.

Pancreatic juice contains enzymes for digesting all three major types of food: proteins, carbohydrates, and fats. It also contains large quantities of bicarbonate ions, which play an important role in neutralizing the acid chyme emptied by the stomach into the duodenum.

The proteolytic enzymes are *trypsin, chymotrypsin, carboxypolypeptidase, ribonuclease,* and *deoxyribonuclease.* By far the most abundant of these is trypsin. The first three split whole and partially digested proteins, while the nucleases split the two types of nucleic acids: ribonucleic and deoxyribonucleic acids.

The digestive enzyme for carbohydrates is *pancreatic amylase,* which hydrolyzes starches, glycogen, and most other carbohydrates except cellulose, mainly to form disaccharides.

The main enzymes for fat digestion are *pancreatic lipase,* which is capable of hydrolyzing neutral fat into fatty acids and monoglycerides; *cholesterol esterase* which causes hydrolysis of cholesterol esters; and *phospholipase,* which splits fatty acids from phospholipids.

When synthesized in the pancreatic cells, the proteolytic enzymes are in the inactive forms *trypsinogen, chymotrypsinogen,* and *procarboxypolypeptidase.* These become activated only after they are secreted into the intestinal tract. Trypsinogen is activated by an enzyme called *enterokinase,* which is secreted by the intestinal mucosa when chyme comes in contact with the mucosa. Also, trypsinogen can be autocatalytically activated by trypsin that has already been formed. Chymotrypsinogen is activated by trypsin to form chymotrypsin, and procarboxypolypeptidase is activated in a similar manner.

Secretion of Bicarbonate Ions. The enzymes of the pancreatic juice are secreted entirely by the acini of the pancreatic glands. On the other hand, two other important components of pancreatic juice, water and bicarbonate ions, are secreted *mainly by the epithelial cells of the small ductules* leading from the acini. The bicarbonate ion concentration can rise to as high as 145 mEq/liter, a value approximately five times that of bicarbonate ions in the plasma. Obviously, this provides a large quantity of alkaline ions in the pancreatic juice, which serves to neutralize the acid in the chyme emptied into the duodenum from the stomach.

REGULATION OF PANCREATIC SECRETION

Pancreatic secretion, like gastric secretion, is regulated by both nervous and hormonal mechanisms. However, in this case, hormonal regulation is the more important.

Nervous Regulation. At the same time that the vagus nerve stimulates stomach secretion, parasympathetic impulses are simultaneously transmitted along the vagus nerves to the pancreas, resulting in secretion of moderate amounts of enzymes into the pancreatic acini. However, little secretion actually flows through the pancreatic ducts to the intestine because little water and few electrolytes are secreted along with the enzymes. Therefore, most of the enzymes are temporarily stored in the acini.

Hormonal Regulation. After food enters the small intestine, pancreatic secretion becomes copious, mainly in response to the hormone *secretin*. In addition, a second hormone, *cholecystokinin*, causes still more secretion of the enzymes.

Stimulation of Secretion of Copious Quantities of Bicarbonate Solution by Secretin—Neutralization of the Acidic Chyme. Secretin is a polypeptide containing 27 amino acids that is present in the mucosa of the upper small intestine in an inactive form, *prosecretin*. When acid chyme enters the intestine, it causes the release and activation of secretin, which is subsequently absorbed into the blood. The one constituent of chyme that causes greatest secretin release is hydrochloric acid, though almost any type of food will cause at least some release.

Secretin causes the pancreas to secrete large quantities of fluid containing a high concentration of bicarbonate ion (up to 145 mEq per liter) but a low concentration of chloride ion.

The secretin mechanism is especially important for two reasons: *First*, secretin is released in especially large quantities from the mucosa of the small intestine any time the pH of the duodenal contents falls below 4.5. This immediately causes large quantities of pancreatic juice containing abundant amounts of sodium bicarbonate to be secreted, which results in the following reaction in the duodenum:

$$HCL + NaHCO_3 \rightarrow NaCl + H_2CO_3$$

Thus, the acid is neutralized by reacting with the bicarbonate. In turn, the carbonic acid immediately dissociates into carbon dioxide and water, and the carbon dioxide is absorbed into the body fluids, thus leaving a neutral solution of sodium chloride in the duodenum. And, because the pH now rises back toward neutrality, the peptic activity of the gastric juice is immediately blocked. Since the mucosa of the small intestine cannot withstand the intense digestive properties of gastric juice, this is a highly important protective mechanism against the development of duodenal ulcers, which will be discussed in further detail in the following chapter.

A *second* importance of bicarbonate secretion by the pancreas is to provide an appropriate pH for action of the pancreatic enzymes. All of these function optimally in a slightly alkaline or neutral medium. The pH of the pancreatic secretion averages 8.0.

Cholecystokinin—Control of Enzyme Secretion by the Pancreas. The presence of food in the upper small intestine also causes a second hormone, cholecystokinin, a polypeptide containing 33 amino acids, to be released from the mucosa. This release results especially from the presence of *fats* and also *proteoses* and *peptones*, which are products of partial protein digestion; however, acid will also cause its release in smaller quantities. Cholecystokinin, like secretin, passes by way of the blood to the pancreas but, instead of causing water and bicarbonate secretion, causes secretion of large quantities of digestive enzymes, an effect similar to that of vagal stimulation.

Figure 43–7 summarizes the overall regulation of pancreatic secretion. The total amount secreted each day is about 1200 ml.

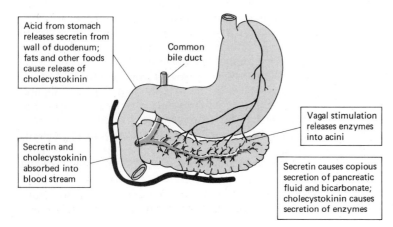

Acid from stomach releases secretin from wall of duodenum; fats and other foods cause release of cholecystokinin

Common bile duct

Vagal stimulation releases enzymes into acini

Secretin and cholecystokinin absorbed into blood stream

Secretin causes copious secretion of pancreatic fluid and bicarbonate; cholecystokinin causes secretion of enzymes

Figure 43–7. Regulation of pancreatic secretion.

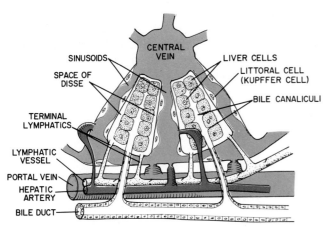

Figure 43-8. Basic structure of a liver lobule showing the hepatic cellular plates, the blood vessels, the bile-collecting system, and the lymph flow system comprised of the spaces of Disse and the interlobular lymphatics. (Reprinted from Guyton, Taylor, and Granger [as modified from Elias]: Dynamics of the Body Fluids. Philadelphia, W. B. Saunders Co., 1975.)

SECRETION OF BILE BY THE LIVER

PHYSIOLOGICAL ANATOMY OF THE LIVER

The basic functional unit of the liver is the liver lobule, which is a cylindrical structure several millimeters in length and 0.8 to 2 mm in diameter.

The liver lobule, illustrated in Figure 43-8, is constructed around a *central vein* and is composed principally of many *hepatic cellular plates* that radiate centrifugally from the central vein like spokes in a wheel. Between the adjacent cells of each hepatic plate lie small *bile canaliculi* into which the hepatic cells secrete *bile*; the canaliculi in turn empty into *terminal bile ducts* in the septa between the adjacent liver lobules.

Also in the septa are small *portal venules* that receive their blood from the portal veins. From these venules blood flows into flat, branching *hepatic sinusoids* between the hepatic plates, and thence into the central vein of the lobule. Thus, the hepatic cells are exposed continuously to portal venous blood.

In addition to the portal venules, there are also *hepatic arterioles* in the interlobular septa. They supply arterial blood to the septal tissues, and most of them also empty directly into the hepatic sinusoids.

Hepatic Secretion of Bile

All the hepatic cells continually form *bile*. This is secreted into the *bile canaliculi*, whence it flows into the *terminal bile ducts,* then into progressively larger ducts, finally reaching the *hepatic duct* and *common bile duct*. From here the bile either empties directly into the duodenum or is diverted into the gallbladder.

Storage of Bile in the Gallbladder. Though bile is secreted continuously by the liver cells, it is normally diverted into the gallbladder and temporarily stored there until needed in the duodenum. The total secretion each day is between 700 and 1200 ml, while the

maximum volume of the gallbladder is only 40 to 70 ml. Nevertheless, as much as 12 hours bile secretion can be stored, because water, sodium, chloride, and most other small electrolytes are continuously absorbed by the gallbladder mucosa. The absorption obviously concentrates those bile constituents that are not absorbed, including the bile salts, cholesterol, and bilirubin. Bile is normally concentrated about fivefold, but it can be concentrated up to a maximum of 10- to 12-fold.

Emptying of the Gallbladder. Two basic conditions are necessary for the gallbladder to empty: (1) The sphincter of Oddi—a smooth muscle constrictor that surrounds the opening of the common bile duct into the duodenum—must relax to allow bile to flow from this duct into the duodenum, and (2) the gallbladder itself must contract to provide the force required to move the bile along the common duct. After a meal, particularly one that contains a high concentration of fat, both these effects take place in the following manner:

First, the fat (also to a less extent partially digested protein) in the food entering the small intestine causes release of the hormone *cholecystokinin* from the intestinal mucosa. The cholecystokinin in turn, is absorbed into the blood, and in addition to its effect of causing enzyme secretion in the pancreas, it causes specific contraction of the gallbladder muscle. This contraction provides the pressure that forces bile toward the duodenum.

Second, when the gallbladder contracts, the sphincter of Oddi becomes inhibited as a result of either a neurogenic or a myogenic reflex from the gallbladder to the sphincter of Oddi. This inhibition may also be, to some extent, a direct effect of cholecystokinin, which directly causes the sphincter to relax.

Third, the presence of food in the duodenum causes the degree of peristalsis in the duodenal wall to increase. Each time a peristaltic wave travels toward the sphincter of Oddi, this sphincter, along with the adjacent intestinal wall, momentarily relaxes because of the phenomenon of "receptive relaxation" that travels ahead of the peristaltic contraction wave. If the bile in the common bile duct is under sufficient pressure, a small quantity of the bile squirts into the duodenum during each peristaltic wave.

In summary, the gallbladder empties its store of concentrated bile into the duodenum mainly in response to the cholecystokinin stimulus. When there is no fat in the meal, the gallbladder empties poorly, but when adequate quantities of fat are present, the gallbladder empties completely in about one hour.

Figure 43-9 summarizes the secretion of bile, its storage in the gallbladder, and its release from the bladder to the gut.

Composition of Bile. Table 43-2 gives the composition of bile when it is first secreted by the liver and then after it has been concentrated in the gallbladder. This table shows that the most abundant substance secreted in the bile is the *bile salts*, but also secreted or excreted in large concentrations are *bilirubin,*

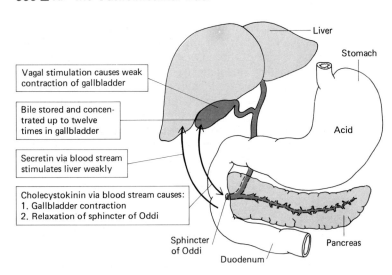

Vagal stimulation causes weak contraction of gallbladder

Bile stored and concentrated up to twelve times in gallbladder

Secretin via blood stream stimulates liver weakly

Cholecystokinin via blood stream causes:
1. Gallbladder contraction
2. Relaxation of sphincter of Oddi

Liver

Stomach

Acid

Sphincter of Oddi

Duodenum

Pancreas

Figure 43–9. Mechanisms of liver secretion and gallbladder emptying.

cholesterol, lecithin, and the usual *electrolytes* of plasma. Water and large portions of the electrolytes are reabsorbed by the gallbladder mucosa, but essentially all the other constituents, including especially the bile salts and lipid substances such as cholesterol, are not reabsorbed and therefore become highly concentrated in the gallbladder bile.

THE BILE SALTS AND THEIR FUNCTIONS

The liver cells form about 0.5 gram of *bile salts* daily. They have two important actions in the intestinal tract. First, they have a detergent action on the fat particles in the food, which decreases the surface tension of the particles and allows the mechanical agitation in the intestinal tract to break the fat globules into minute sizes. This action is called the *emulsifying function* of bile salts. Second, and even more important than the emulsifying function, bile salts help in the absorption of fatty acids, monoglycerides, cholesterol, and other lipids from the intestinal tract. This function will be discussed in detail in the following chapter.

EXCRETION OF BILIRUBIN IN THE BILE

In addition to secreting substances synthesized by the liver itself, the liver cells also *excrete* a number

of substances formed elsewhere in the body. Among the most important of these is *bilirubin*, which is one of the major end-products of hemoglobin decomposition when the red blood cells have outlived their usefulness, as was pointed out in Chapter 19.

Jaundice. The word *jaundice* means a yellowish tint to the body tissues, including yellowness of the skin and also of the deep tissues. The cause of jaundice is large quantities of bilirubin in the extracellular fluids. The normal plasma concentration of bilirubin averages 0.5 mg per 100 ml of plasma. However, in certain abnormal conditions it can rise to as high as 40 mg per 100 ml.

The common causes of jaundice are (1) increased destruction of red blood cells, with rapid release of bilirubin into the blood or (2) obstruction of the bile ducts or damage to the liver cells, so that the usual amounts of bilirubin cannot be excreted into the gastrointestinal tract. These two types are called, respectively, *hemolytic jaundice* and *obstructive jaundice*.

SECRETION OF CHOLESTEROL: GALLSTONE FORMATION

Bile salts are formed in the hepatic cells from cholesterol, which also is synthesized in these same cells. In the process of secreting the bile salts, about one tenth as much cholesterol as bile salts is secreted into the bile as well. No specific function is known for the cholesterol in the bile, and it is presumed that this is simply a by-product of bile salt formation and secretion.

Cholesterol is almost insoluble in pure water, but the bile salts and lecithin in bile combine physically with the cholesterol to form ultramicroscopic *micelles* that are soluble. When the bile becomes concentrated in the gallbladder, the bile salts and lecithin are concentrated along with the cholesterol, keeping the cholesterol in solution. Under abnormal conditions, however, the cholesterol may precipitate, resulting in the formation of *gallstones*, as shown in Figure 43–

Table 43–2. COMPOSITION OF BILE

	Liver Bile		Gallbladder Bile	
Water	97.5	gm/dl	92	gm/dl
Bile salts	1.1	gm/dl	6	gm/dl
Bilirubin	0.04	gm/dl	0.3	gm/dl
Cholesterol	0.1	gm/dl	0.3 to 0.9	gm/dl
Fatty acids	0.12	gm/dl	0.3 to 1.2	gm/dl
Lecithin	0.04	gm/dl	0.3	gm/dl
Na^+	145	mEq/L	130	mEq/L
K^+	5	mEq/L	12	mEq/L
Ca^+	5	mEq/L	23	mEq/L
Cl^-	100	mEq/L	25	mEq/L
HCO_3^-	28	mEq/L	10	mEq/L

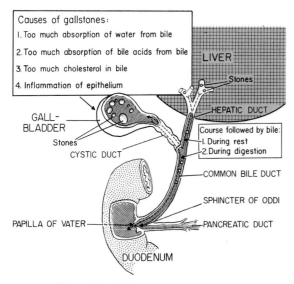

Causes of gallstones:
1. Too much absorption of water from bile
2. Too much absorption of bile acids from bile
3. Too much cholesterol in bile
4. Inflammation of epithelium

LIVER
Stones
HEPATIC DUCT

Course followed by bile:
1. During rest
2. During digestion

GALL-BLADDER
Stones
CYSTIC DUCT
COMMON BILE DUCT
SPHINCTER OF ODDI
PAPILLA OF VATER
PANCREATIC DUCT
DUODENUM

Figure 43–10. Formation of gallstones.

10. The different conditions that can cause cholesterol precipitation are these: (1) too much absorption of water from the bile, (2) too much absorption of bile salts and lecithin from the bile, (3) too much secretion of cholesterol in the bile, or (4) inflammation of the epithelium of the gallbladder. The latter two require special explanation, as follows:

The amount of cholesterol in the bile is determined partly by the quantity of fat that a person eats, for the hepatic cells synthesize cholesterol as one of the products of fat metabolism in the body. For this reason, persons on a high fat diet over a period of many years are prone to the development of gallstones.

Inflammation of the gallbladder epithelium often results from low grade chronic infection; this changes the absorptive characteristics of the gallbladder mucosa, sometimes allowing excessive absorption of water, bile salts, or other substances that are necessary to keep the cholesterol in solution. As a result, cholesterol begins to precipitate, usually forming many small crystals of cholesterol on the surface of the inflamed mucosa. These, in turn, act as nidi for further precipitation of cholesterol, and the crystals grow larger and larger. Occasionally tremendous numbers of sandlike stones develop, but much more frequently these coalesce to form a few large gallstones, or even a single stone that fills the entire gallbladder.

SECRETIONS OF THE SMALL INTESTINE

SECRETION OF MUCUS BY BRUNNER'S GLANDS AND BY MUCOUS CELLS OF THE INTESTINAL SURFACE

An extensive array of compound mucous glands, called *Brunner's glands*, is located in the mucosa of the first few centimeters of the duodenum, mainly between the pylorus and the papilla of Vater, where the pancreatic juice and bile empty into the duodenum from the common bile duct. These glands secrete mucus in response to (1) direct tactile stimuli or irritating stimuli of the overlying duodenal epithelium, (2) vagal stimulation, which causes secretion concurrently with increase in stomach secretion, and (3) intestinal hormones, especially secretin. The function of the mucus secreted by Brunner's glands is to protect the duodenal wall from digestion by the gastric juice, and the rapid and intense response of these glands to irritating stimuli is especially geared to this purpose.

Brunner's glands are inhibited by sympathetic stimulation; therefore, such stimulation is likely to leave the duodenal bulb unprotected and is perhaps one of the factors that cause this area of the gastrointestinal tract to be the site of peptic ulcers in about 50 per cent of cases.

Mucus is also secreted in large quantities by mucous cells spread extensively over the surface of the intestinal mucosa. This secretion results principally from direct tactile or chemical stimulation of the mucosa by the chyme. Additional mucus is also secreted by the mucous cells in the intestinal glands called the crypts of Lieberkühn. This secretion is probably controlled mainly by local reflexes of the enteric nervous system.

SECRETION OF THE INTESTINAL DIGESTIVE JUICES—THE CRYPTS OF LIEBERKÜHN

Located on the entire surface of the small intestine, with the exception of the Brunner's gland area of the duodenum, are small crypts that dip deeply into the mucosa, called *crypts of Lieberkühn*, one of which is illustrated in Figure 43–11. The intestinal secretions are formed by the epithelial cells in these crypts at a rate of about 1800 ml per day. The secretions are almost pure extracellular fluid, and they have a slightly alkaline pH, in the range of 7.5 to 8.0. They are rapidly reabsorbed by the intestinal villi. This

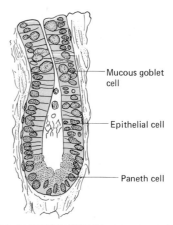

Mucous goblet cell

Epithelial cell

Paneth cell

Figure 43–11. A crypt of Lieberkühn, found in all parts of the small intestine between the villi, which secretes almost pure extracellular fluid.

circulation of fluid from the crypts to the villi supplies a watery vehicle for absorption of substances from the small intestine, which is one of the primary functions of the small intestine, as is discussed in the following chapter.

Enzymes in the Small Intestinal Secretion. When secretions of the small intestine are collected without cellular debris, they have almost no enzymes. However, the epithelial cells of the intestinal mucosa do contain large quantities of digestive enzymes that normally digest food substances *while* they are being absorbed through the epithelium. These enzymes are the following: (1) several different *peptidases* for splitting polypeptides into amino acids, (2) four enzymes for splitting disaccharides into monosaccharides—*sucrase, maltase, isomaltase* and *lactase*—and (3) small amounts of *intestinal lipase* for splitting neutral fats into monoglycerides and fatty acids. Most if not all of these enzymes are in the brush border of the epithelial cells. Therefore, they presumably catalyze hydrolysis of the foods on the outside surfaces of the microvilli prior to absorption of the end-products of digestion.

REGULATION OF SECRETION OF THE SMALL INTESTINE

By far the most important means for regulating secretion of the small intestine is various local nervous reflexes caused mainly by distention or tactile or irritative stimuli. Therefore, for the most part, secretion in the small intestine occurs simply in response to the presence of chyme in the intestine—the greater the amount of chyme, the greater the secretion.

SECRETIONS OF THE LARGE INTESTINE

Mucus Secretion. The mucosa of the large intestine, like that of the small intestine, is lined with crypts of Lieberkühn, but unlike the small intestine, there are no villi. Also, the epithelial cells contain essentially no enzymes. Instead, the crypts are lined almost entirely by mucous cells. On the surface epithelium of the large intestine are large numbers of mucous cells dispersed among the other epithelial cells.

Therefore, the preponderant secretion in the large intestine is mucus containing large amounts of bicarbonate ions. Its rate of secretion is regulated principally by direct, tactile stimulation of the mucous cells on the surface of the mucosa and by local nervous reflexes to the mucous cells in the crypts of Lieberkühn. However, stimulation of the *pelvic nerves*, which carry the parasympathetic innervation to the distal half of the large intestine, also causes marked increase in the secretion of mucus. This secretion occurs along with an increase in motility, discussed in the preceding chapter. Therefore, during extreme parasympathetic stimulation, often caused by severe emotional disturbance, so much mucus may be secreted into the large intestine that the person has a bowel movement of ropy mucus as often as every 30 minutes; the mucus contains little or no fecal material.

Mucus in the large intestine obviously protects the wall against excoriation, but in addition, it provides the adherent medium for holding fecal matter together. Furthermore, it protects the intestinal wall from the great amount of bacterial activity that takes place inside the feces, and the mucus, plus its alkalinity (pH of 8.0), also provides a barrier to keep acids formed deep in the feces from attacking the intestinal wall.

Secretion of Water and Electrolytes in Response to Irritation. Whenever a segment of the large intestine becomes intensely irritated, as occurs when bacterial infection becomes rampant during *bacterial enteritis*, the mucosa then secretes large quantities of water and electrolytes in addition to the normal viscid solution of mucus. These substances act to dilute the irritating factors and to cause rapid movement of the feces toward the anus. The usual result is *diarrhea*, with loss of large quantities of water and electrolytes but also earlier recovery from the disease than would otherwise occur.

QUESTIONS

1. Explain the basic mechanisms by which glandular cells secrete organic substances, and also explain the nervous control of water and electrolyte secretion.
2. What are the special characteristics of *mucus* that make it extremely important for lubrication and protection of the gastrointestinal tract?
3. Describe a salivary gland and explain the secretory processes of the *acini* and the *salivary ducts.*
4. Explain why the electrolytic composition of *saliva* is quite different from the electrolytic composition of plasma.
5. What roles does saliva play in maintaining *oral hygiene*?
6. Describe the nervous regulation of salivary secretion.
7. Explain the mechanism for secretion of hydrochloric acid by the *oxyntic cells* of the *oxyntic glands* in the stomach.
8. How is *pepsin* secreted, how is it activated, and what are its properties?
9. Explain both the *vagal* and the *gastrin mechanisms* for control of gastric secretion.
10. Give general descriptions of the chemical compositions of *gastrin, cholecystokinin,* and *secretin.*
11. What is the role of histamine in controlling gastric secretion, and how does the drug *cimetidine* block the gastrin mechanism for stimulating gastric secretion?
12. What are the roles of *gastric pH* and of different *intestinal factors* in the control of gastric secretion?
13. Describe the types of secretion and the mechanisms for

secretion of the different components of pancreatic juice.

14. Describe the regulation of secretion of *water* and *sodium bicarbonate* by the pancreas; also, explain the function of sodium bicarbonate in the duodenum.
15. Explain the control of secretion of *enzymes* by the pancreas.
16. Give the physiological anatomy of the liver, and explain the secretion of bile.
17. Explain the storage and concentration of bile in the *gallbladder,* and explain the control over emptying of the gallbladder.

18. Discuss the ultimate fates of the bile salts, the bilirubin, and the cholesterol that are secreted in the bile. Why and how are gallstones formed?
19. Explain the characteristics of the small intestinal secretions and the manner in which these secretions are regulated.
20. What are the specific characteristics of the large intestinal secretions, and how is large intestinal secretion regulated?

References

Berglindh, T.: The mammalian gastric parietal cell in vitro. Annu Rev Physiol 46:377, 1984.

Brooks, F.: Disease of the Exocrine Pancreas. Philadelphia, W. B. Saunders Co., 1980.

Burnham, D. B., and Williams, J. A.: Stimulus-secretion coupling in pancreatic acinar cells. J Pediatr Gastroenterol Nutr 3(Suppl. 1):S1, 1984.

Flemstrom, G., and Garner, A.: Some characteristics of duodenal epithelium. Ciba Found Symp 109:94, 1984.

Forte, J. G., et al.: Mechanisms of gastric H^+ and Cl^- transport. Annu Rev Physiol 42:111, 1980.

Ginsberg, B. L., and House, C. R.: Stimulus-response coupling in gland cells. Annu Rev Biophys Bioeng 9:55, 1980.

Guth, P. H.: Stomach blood flow and acid secretion. Annu Rev Physiol 44:3, 1982.

Hersey, S. J., et al.: Cellular control of pepsinogen secretion. Annu Rev Physiol 46:393, 1984.

Jerzy Glass, G. B.: Gastrointestinal Hormones. New York, Raven Press, 1980.

Lundgren, O.: Microcirculation of the gastrointestinal tract and pancreas.

In Renkin, E. M., and Michel, C. C., eds.: Handbook of Physiology. Sec. 2, Vol. 4. Bethesda, American Physiological Society, 1984, p. 799.

Malinowska, D. H., and Sachs, G.: Cellular mechanisms of acid secretion. Clin Gastroenterol 13:309, 1984.

Reichen, J., and Paumgartner, G.: Excretory function of the liver. In Javitt, N. B., ed.: Internal Review of Physiology: Liver and Biliary Tract Physiology I. Vol. 21. Baltimore, University Park Press, 1980, p. 103.

Salen, G., and Shefer, S.: Bile acid synthesis. Annu Rev Physiol 45:679, 1983.

Schulz, I., and Stolze, H. H.: The exocrine pancreas: the role of secretagogues, cyclic nucleotides and calcium in enzyme secretion. Annu Rev Physiol 42:127, 1980.

Shepherd, A. P.: Local control of intestinal oxygenation and blood flow. Annu Rev Physiol 44:13, 1982.

Strange, R. C.: Hepatic bile flow. Physiol Rev 64:1055, 1984.

Williams, J. A.: Regulatory mechanisms in pancreas and salivary acini. Annu Rev Physiol 46:361, 1984.

Willingham, M. C., and Pastan, I.: Endocytosis and exocytosis: current concepts of vesicle traffic in animal cells. Int Rev Cytol 92:51, 1984.

44

Digestion and Absorption in the Gastrointestinal Tract; Gastrointestinal Disorders

DIGESTION OF THE VARIOUS FOODS
  DIGESTION OF CARBOHYDRATES
  DIGESTION OF FATS
  DIGESTION OF PROTEINS
BASIC PRINCIPLES OF
  GASTROINTESTINAL ABSORPTION
  ANATOMICAL BASIS OF ABSORPTION
  BASIC MECHANISMS OF
    ABSORPTION
ABSORPTION IN THE SMALL INTESTINE
  ABSORPTION OF WATER
  ABSORPTION OF THE IONS
  ABSORPTION OF NUTRIENTS

ABSORPTION IN THE LARGE INTESTINE;
  FORMATION OF THE FECES
GASTROINTESTINAL DISORDERS
  GASTRITIS
  PEPTIC ULCER
  MALABSORPTION FROM THE SMALL
    INTESTINE—SPRUE
  CONSTIPATION
  DIARRHEA
  VOMITING
  GASES IN THE GASTROINTESTINAL
    TRACT (FLATUS)

The foods on which the body lives, with the exception of small quantities of substances such as vitamins and minerals, can be classified as carbohydrates, fats, and proteins. However, these generally cannot be absorbed in their natural forms through the gastrointestinal mucosa and, for this reason, are useless as nutrients without preliminary digestion. Therefore, this chapter discusses, first, the processes by which carbohydrates, fats, and proteins are digested into compounds small enough for absorption and, second, the mechanisms by which the digestive endproducts, as well as water, electrolytes, and other substances, are absorbed.

DIGESTION OF THE VARIOUS FOODS

Hydrolysis as the Basic Process of Digestion. Almost all the carbohydrates of the diet are either *large polysaccharides* or *disaccharides, both of which are combinations of monosaccharides*, bound to each other. The carbohydrates are digested into their constituent monosaccharides; to do this, specific enzymes combine hydrogen and hydroxyl ions, derived from water, with the poly- and disaccharides and thereby separate the monosaccharides from each other. This process, called *hydrolysis*, occurs as follows:

$$R'' - R' + H_2O \rightarrow R''OH + R'H$$

Almost the entire fat portion of the diet consists of triglycerides (neutral fats), which are combinations of three *fatty acid* molecules with a single *glycerol* molecule. Digestion of the triglycerides consists of fat-digesting enzymes that split fatty acid molecules away from the glycerol. Here again, the process is one of hydrolysis.

Finally, proteins are formed from *amino acids* that are bound together by means of *peptide linkages*. And digestion of proteins also involves the process of hydrolysis, the proteolytic enzymes combining hydroxyl and hydrogen ions derived from water with the protein molecules to split them into their constituent amino acids.

Therefore, the chemistry of digestion is really simple, for in the case of all three major types of food, the same basic process of *hydrolysis* is involved. The only difference is in the enzymes required to promote the reactions for each type of food.

All the digestive enzymes are proteins. Their secretion by the different gastrointestinal glands is discussed in the preceding chapter.

DIGESTION OF CARBOHYDRATES

Only three major sources of carbohydrates exist in the normal human diet. These are sucrose, which is the disaccharide known popularly as cane sugar; lactose, which is a disaccharide in milk; and starches, which are large polysaccharides present in almost all foods, particularly in the grains.

Figure 44–1 gives a schema for digestion of the principal carbohydrates. This shows that the starches are first hydrolyzed to maltose, a disaccharide, or other small glucose polymers. Then these, along with the other major disaccharides, lactose and sucrose, are hydrolyzed into the monosaccharides *glucose*, *galactose*, and *fructose*.

Hydrolysis of starches begins in the mouth under the influence of the enzyme *ptyalin*, which is secreted mainly in the saliva from the parotid gland. The hydrochloric acid of the stomach provides a slight amount of additional hydrolysis. Finally, the major share of hydrolysis occurs in the upper part of the small intestine under the influence of the enzyme *pancreatic amylase*.

The enzymes *lactase, sucrase, maltase,* and *α-dextrinase* for splitting disaccharides and small glucose polymers are located in the microvilli of the brush border of the epithelial cells. The disaccharides and small polymers are digested into monosaccharides as they come in contact with or diffuse into the microvilli. The digestive products, the monosaccharides *glucose, galactose,* and *fructose,* are then immediately absorbed into the portal blood.

DIGESTION OF FATS

By far the most common fats of the diet are the neutral fats, also known as *triglycerides,* each molecule of which is composed of a glycerol nucleus and three fatty acids. Neutral fat is found in food of both animal origin and plant origin.

In the usual diet are also small quantities of *phospholipids, cholesterol,* and *cholesterol esters.* The phospholipids and cholesterol esters contain fatty acid and therefore can be considered fats themselves. Cholesterol, on the other hand, is a sterol compound containing no fatty acid, but it does exhibit some of the physical and chemical characteristics of fats; also it is derived from fats, and it is metabolized similarly to fats. Therefore, cholesterol is considered from a dietary point of view to be a fat.

Though a minute amount of fat can be digested in the stomach under the influence of gastric lipase, 95 to 99 per cent of all fat digestion occurs in the small intestine, mainly under the influence of *pancreatic lipase.*

Emulsification of Fat by Bile Salts. The first step in fat digestion is to break the fat globules into small sizes so that the digestive enzymes, which are not fat soluble, can act on the globule surfaces. This process is called *emulsification* of the fat, and it is achieved under the influence of bile salts that are secreted in the bile by the liver. The bile salts act as a detergent, greatly decreasing the interfacial tension of the fat. With a low interfacial tension, the gastrointestinal mixing movements can break the globules of fat into finer and finer particles, with the total surface area of the fat increasing by a factor of two every time the diameters of the fat globules are decreased by one-half.

Digestion of Fat by Pancreatic Lipase and Enteric Lipase. Under the influence of *pancreatic lipase,* most of the fat is split into *monoglycerides* and *fatty acids,* as shown in Figure 44–2. A small portion does not proceed to the monoglyceride stage, but this portion usually is poorly absorbed or not absorbed at all.

The epithelial cells of the small intestine contain a small quantity of lipase, known as *enteric lipase.* This probably causes a very slight additional amount of fat digestion.

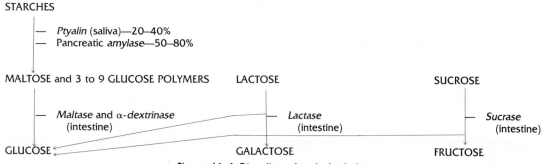

STARCHES

— *Ptyalin* (saliva)—20–40%
— Pancreatic *amylase*—50–80%

MALTOSE and 3 to 9 GLUCOSE POLYMERS   LACTOSE   SUCROSE

— *Maltase* and α-*dextrinase* (intestine)   *Lactase* (intestine)   *Sucrase* (intestine)

GLUCOSE   GALACTOSE   FRUCTOSE

Figure 44–1. Digestion of carbohydrates.

Fat —(Bile + Agitation)→ Emulsified fat

Emulsified fat —*Pancreatic lipase*→ Fatty acids and 2-Monoglycerides

Figure 44–2. Digestion of fats.

Role of Bile Salts in Accelerating Fat Digestion—Formation of Micelles. The hydrolysis of triglycerides is a highly reversible process; therefore, accumulation of monoglycerides and free fatty acids in the vicinity of digesting fats very quickly blocks further digestion. Fortunately, the bile salts play an important role in removing the monosaccharides and the free fatty acids from the vicinity of the digesting fat globules almost as rapidly as these end-products of digestion are formed. This removal occurs in the following way:

Bile salts have the propensity to form *micelles*, which are small spherical globules about 2.5 nanometers in diameter and are composed of 20 to 40 molecules of bile salt. The micelles develop because each bile salt molecule is composed of a sterol nucleus that is highly fat soluble and a polar group that is highly water soluble. The sterol nuclei of these 20 to 40 bile salt molecules of the micelle aggregate to form a small fat globule in the middle of the micelle. This formation causes the polar groups to project outward to cover the surface of the micelle. Since these polar groups are negatively charged, they allow the entire micelle globule to become dissolved in the water of the digestive fluids and to remain in solution despite the very large size of the micelle.

During triglyceride digestion, as rapidly as the monoglycerides and free fatty acids are formed, they become dissolved in the fatty portion of the micelles, which immediately removes these end-products of digestion from the vicinity of the digesting fat globules. Consequently, the digestive process can proceed unabated.

The bile salt micelles also act as a transport medium to carry the monoglycerides and the free fatty acids to the brush borders of the epithelial cells. There the monoglycerides and free fatty acids are absorbed, as will be discussed later. On delivery of these substances to the brush border, the bile salts are released back into the chyme to be used again and again for this "ferrying" process.

DIGESTION OF PROTEINS

The dietary proteins are derived almost entirely from meats and vegetables, and they are digested primarily in the stomach and upper part of the small intestine.

As illustrated in Figure 44–3, protein digestion begins in the stomach, the enzyme *pepsin* splitting the proteins into *proteoses, peptones,* and large *polypeptides.* This enzyme functions only in a highly acid medium, acting best at a pH of about 2.5. Therefore, the hydrochloric acid secreted in the stomach is essential for this digestive process.

Proteins —*pepsin*→ {Proteoses, Peptones, Polypeptides}

—*trypsin, chymotrypsin, carboxypolypeptidase*→ {Polypeptides + Amino acids} —*peptidases*→ Amino acids

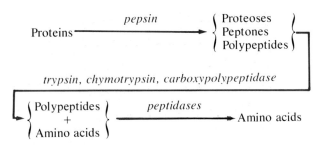

Figure 44–3. Digestion of proteins.

Pepsin is especially important for its ability to digest collagen, an albuminoid that is little affected by other digestive enzymes. Since collagen is a major constituent of the fibrous tissue in meat, it is essential that this substance be digested so that the remainder of the meat can be attacked by the other digestive enzymes.

The proteins are further digested in the upper part of the small intestine under the influence of the pancreatic enzymes *trypsin, chymotrypsin,* and *carboxypolypeptidases.* The final product of this digestion is mainly *small polypeptides* plus a few *amino acids.*

Finally, the small polypeptides are digested into amino acids when they come in contact with the epithelial cells of the small intestine. These cells contain several enzymes (*peptidases*) that convert the remaining protein products into *amino acids.*

When food has been properly masticated and is not eaten in too large a quantity at any one time, about 98 per cent of the protein finally becomes amino acids.

BASIC PRINCIPLES OF GASTROINTESTINAL ABSORPTION

ANATOMICAL BASIS OF ABSORPTION

The total quantity of fluid that must be absorbed each day is equal to the ingested fluid (about 1.5 liters) plus that secreted in the various gastrointestinal juices (about 7 liters). Together these come to a total of 8 to 9 liters. All but about 1.5 liters is absorbed in the small intestine, leaving only 1.5 liters to pass through the ileocecal valve into the colon each day.

The stomach is a poor absorptive area of the gastrointestinal tract. Only a few highly lipid-soluble substances, such as alcohol and some drugs, can be absorbed in small quantities.

The Absorptive Surface of the Intestinal Mucosa—The Villi. Figure 44–4 illustrates the absorptive surface of the intestinal mucosa, showing many folds called *valvulae conniventes*; these increase the surface area of the absorptive mucosa about threefold.

Also, located over the entire surface of the small intestine, from approximately the point at which the common bile duct empties into the duodenum down to the ileocecal valve, are literally millions of small *villi*, which project about 1 mm from the surface of

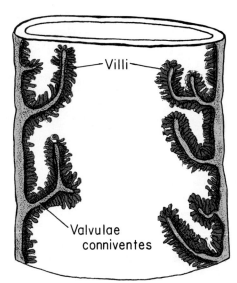

Figure 44–4. A longitudinal section of the small intestine, showing the valvulae conniventes covered by villi.

the mucosa, as shown on the surfaces of the valvulae conniventes in Figure 44–4 and in detail in Figure 44–5. These villi enhance the absorptive area another tenfold.

Finally, the epithelial cells on the surface of the villi are characterized by a brush border, consisting of about 600 *microvilli* 1 μ in length and 0.1 μ in diameter protruding from each cell; these are illustrated in the electron micrograph in Figure 44–6. These microvilli increase the surface area exposed to the intestinal materials another 20-fold. Thus, the combination of the valvulae conniventes, the villi, and the microvilli increases the absorptive area of the mucosa about 600-fold, making a very large total area of about 250 square meters for the entire small intestine.

Figure 44–5 illustrates the general organization of a villus, emphasizing especially the advantageous arrangement of the vascular system for absorption of fluid and dissolved material into the portal blood and the arrangement of the *central lacteal* for absorption into the lymphatics.

BASIC MECHANISMS OF ABSORPTION

Absorption through the gastrointestinal mucosa occurs by *active transport* and by *diffusion*, as is also true for other membranes. The physical principles of these processes were explained in Chapter 4.

Briefly, active transport provides energy to move a substance across a membrane. Therefore, the substance can be moved against a concentration gradient or against an electrical potential. On the other hand, the term *diffusion* means simply transport of substances through the membrane as a result of molecular movement *along*, rather than against, an electrochemical gradient.

ABSORPTION IN THE SMALL INTESTINE

Normally, the substances absorbed from the small intestine each day consist of several hundred grams of carbohydrates, 100 or more grams of fat, 50 to 100 grams of amino acids, 50 to 100 grams of ions, and 7 to 8 liters of water. However, the absorptive *capacity* of the *small intestine* is far greater than this: as much as several kilograms of carbohydrates per day, 500 to 1000 grams of fat per day, 500 to 700 grams of amino acids per day, and 20 or more liters of water per day. In addition, the *large intestine* can absorb still more water and ions, though almost no nutrients.

ABSORPTION OF WATER

Isosmotic Absorption. Water is transported through the intestinal membrane entirely by the process of *diffusion*. Furthermore, this diffusion obeys the usual laws of osmosis.

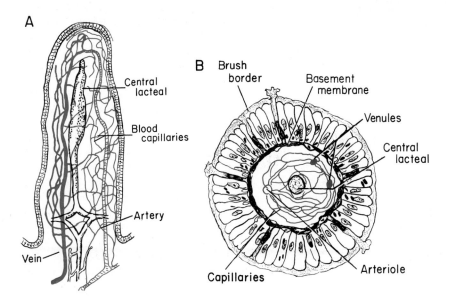

Figure 44–5. Functional organization of the villus. *A,* Longitudinal section. *B,* Cross-section showing the epithelial cells and basement membrane.

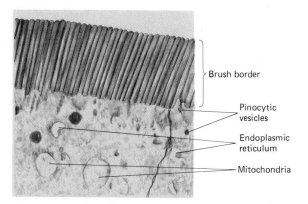

Figure 44–6. Brush border of the gastrointestinal epithelial cell, showing, also, pinocytic vesicles, mitochondria, and endoplasmic reticulum lying immediately beneath the brush border. (Courtesy of Dr. William Lockwood.)

As dissolved substances are actively transported from the lumen of the gut into the blood this decreases the osmotic pressure of the chyme while increasing the osmotic pressure on the other side of the membrane, thus creating an osmotic gradient that moves water through the membrane as well. Water diffuses so readily through the intestinal membrane that it almost instantaneously "follows" the transported substances into the circulation. Therefore, as ions and nutrients are absorbed, an isosmotic equivalent of water is also absorbed. In this way, not only are the ions and nutrients almost entirely absorbed before the chyme passes through the small intestine, but so is almost all the water too.

ABSORPTION OF THE IONS

Active Transport of Sodium. Twenty to thirty grams of sodium are secreted into the intestinal secretions each day. In addition, many people eat 5 to 8 grams of sodium normally daily. Combining these two, the small intestine absorbs 25 to 35 grams of sodium each day, which amounts to about one seventh of all the sodium that is present in the body.

The basic mechanism of sodium absorption from the intestine is illustrated in Figure 44–7. The prin-

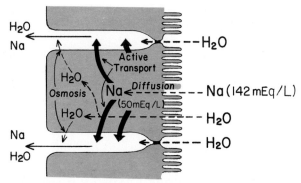

Figure 44–7. Absorption of sodium through the intestinal epithelium. Note also the osmotic absorption of water—that is, the water "follows" the sodium through the epithelial membrane.

ciples of this mechanism, which were discussed in Chapter 4, are essentially the same as those for absorption of sodium from the renal tubules, as discussed in Chapter 24. The motive power for the sodium absorption is provided by active transport of sodium from inside the epithelial cells, through the side walls of these cells, into the intercellular spaces. This is illustrated by the heavy black arrows in Figure 44–7. This active transport obeys the usual laws for such transport: It requires a carrier, it requires energy, and it is catalyzed by an appropriate ATPase carrier-enzyme in the cell membrane.

The next step in the transport process is osmosis of water into the intercellular spaces. This movement is caused by the osmotic gradient created by the elevated concentration of ions in the intercellular space. Most of this osmosis occurs through the "tight junctions," which actually are not so tight, between the apical borders of the epithelial cells, but a smaller proportion occurs through the cells themselves. The osmotic movement of water creates a flow of fluid into the intercellular space, then through the basement membrane of the epithelium, and finally into the circulating blood of the villi. New water diffuses along with sodium through the brush border of the epithelial cell to replenish the water that flows into the intercellular spaces.

Transport of Chloride. In most parts of the small intestine chloride transport is by passive diffusion. The transport of the positively charged sodium ions through the epithelium creates electronegativity in the chyme and electropositivity on the basal side of the epithelial cells. Then chloride ions move along this electrical gradient to "follow" the sodium ions.

However, the epithelial cells of the distal ileum and of the large intestine have the special capability of actively absorbing chloride ions. This occurs by means of a tightly coupled active transport mechanism in which an equivalent number of bicarbonate ions are secreted. The purpose of this mechanism is probably to provide bicarbonate ions for neutralization of acidic products formed by bacteria—especially in the large intestine.

Absorption of Other Ions. Calcium ions are actively absorbed, especially from the duodenum, and calcium ion absorption is exactly controlled in relation to the need of the body for calcium by parathyroid hormone secreted by the parathyroid glands and by vitamin D. These effects are discussed in Chapter 53.

Iron ions are also actively absorbed from the small intestine. The principles of iron absorption and its regulation in proportion to the body's need for iron were discussed in Chapter 19.

Potassium, magnesium, phosphate, and probably still other ions can also be actively absorbed through the muscosa.

ABSORPTION OF NUTRIENTS

Absorption of Carbohydrates. Essentially all the carbohydrates are absorbed in the form of monosaccharides, only a small fraction of a per cent being absorbed as disaccharides and almost none as larger carbohydrate compounds. Furthermore, little carbohydrate absorption results from diffusion, for the pores of the mucosa through which diffusion occurs are essentially impermeable to water-soluble solutes with molecular weights greater than 100.

Mechanism of Monosaccharide Absorption. We still do not know the precise mechanism of monosaccharide absorption, but we do know that most monosaccharide transport becomes blocked whenever sodium transport is blocked. Therefore, it is assumed that the energy required for most monosaccharide transport is actually provided by the sodium transport system. A theory that attempts to explain this process is the following: It is known that a carrier of glucose and some other monosaccharides, especially galactose, is present in the brush border of the epithelial cell. However, this carrier will not transport the glucose in the absence of sodium transport. Therefore, it is believed that the carrier has receptor sites for both a glucose molecule and a sodium ion and that the carrier will not transport the glucose to the inside of the cell if the receptor site for sodium is not simultaneously filled. The energy for movement of the carrier from the exterior of the membrane to the interior is derived from the difference in sodium concentration between the outside and inside of the cell. That is, as sodium diffuses to the inside of the cell it "drags" the carrier and the glucose along with it, thus providing the energy for transport of the glucose. For obvious reasons, this explanation is called the *sodium co-transport theory* for glucose transport.

Absorption of Proteins. Almost all proteins are absorbed in the form of amino acids. Four different carrier systems transport different amino acids—one transports *neutral amino acids*, a second transports *basic amino acids*, a third transports *acidic amino acids*, and a fourth has specificity for the two amino acids *proline* and *hydroxyproline*.

Amino acid transport, like glucose transport, occurs only in the presence of simultaneous sodium transport. Furthermore, the carrier systems for amino acid transport, like those for glucose, are in the brush border of the epithelial cell. It is believed that amino acids are transported by the same *sodium co-transport mechanism* as that explained above for glucose transport. That is, the theory postulates that the carrier has receptor sites for both an amino acid molecule and a sodium ion. Only when both of the sites are filled will the carrier move to the interior of the cell. Because of the sodium gradient across the brush border, the sodium diffusion to the cell interior pulls the carrier and its attached amino acid to the interior. Therefore, amino acid concentration increases within the cell, and it then diffuses through the sides or base of the cell into the portal blood.

Absorption of Fats. Earlier in this chapter it was pointed out that when fats are digested to form monoglycerides and free fatty acids, both of these digestive end-products become dissolved mainly in the lipid portion of the bile acid micelles. Because of the small dimensions of these micelles and also because of their highly charged exterior, they are soluble in the chyme. In this form the monoglycerides and the fatty acids are transported to the surfaces of the intestinal epithelial cells. On coming in contact with these surfaces, both the monoglycerides and the fatty acids immediately diffuse through the epithelial membrane, leaving the bile acid micelles still in the chyme. The micelles then diffuse back into the chyme and absorb still more monoglycerides and fatty acids, and similarly transport these also to the epithelial cells. Thus, the bile acids perform a ferrying function that is highly important for fat absorption. In the presence of an abundance of bile acids, approximately 97 per cent of the fat is absorbed; in the absence of bile acids, only 50 to 60 per cent is normally absorbed.

The mechanism for absorption of the monoglycerides and fatty acids through the brush border is based on the fact that both of these substances are highly lipid-soluble. Therefore, they become dissolved in the membrane and diffuse to the interior of the cell.

After entering the epithelial cell, the fatty acids and monoglycerides are taken up by the smooth endoplasmic reticulum, and here they are mainly recombined to form new triglycerides. However, a few of the monoglycerides are further digested into glycerol and fatty acids by an epithelial cell lipase, and the fatty acids are then combined with newly synthesized glycerol to form entirely new triglycerides rather than simply recombining with absorbed monoglycerides.

Once formed, the triglycerides aggregate within the endoplasmic reticulum into globules, along with absorbed cholesterol, absorbed phospholipids, and small amounts of newly synthesized cholesterol and phospholipids. The phospholipids arrange themselves in these globules with the fatty portion of the phospholipid toward the center and the polar portions located on the surface. This arrangement provides an electrically charged surface that makes the globules miscible with the fluids of the cell. In addition, small amounts of β-*lipoprotein*, also synthesized by the endoplasmic reticulum, coat part of the surface of each globule. In this form the globule diffuses to the side of the epithelial cell and is excreted by the process of cellular *exocytosis* into the space between the cells; from there it passes into the lymph in the central lacteal of the villus. These globules are then called *chylomicrons*.

Transport of the Chylomicrons in the Lymph. From the central lacteals of the villi, the chylomicrons are propelled along with the lymph by the lymphatic pump upward through the thoracic duct to be emptied into the great veins of the neck.

ABSORPTION IN THE LARGE INTESTINE; FORMATION OF THE FECES

Approximately 1500 ml of chyme passes through the ileocecal valve into the large intestine each day.

Most of the water and electrolytes in this are absorbed in the colon, leaving only 50 to 200 ml of fluid to be excreted in the feces.

Most of the absorption in the large intestine occurs in the proximal half of the colon, giving this portion the name *absorbing colon*, while the distal colon functions principally for storage and is therefore called the *storage colon*.

Absorption and Secretion of Electrolytes and Water. The mucosa of the large intestine, like that of the small intestine, has a very high capacity for active absorption of sodium, and the electrical potential gradient across the epithelium created by the absorption of the sodium causes chloride absorption as well. In addition, as in the distal portion of the small intestine, the mucosa of the large intestine actively secretes bicarbonate ions while it simultaneously actively absorbs a small amount of additional chloride ions. The bicarbonate helps to neutralize the acidic end-products of bacterial action in the colon.

The absorption of sodium and chloride ions creates an osmotic gradient across the large intestinal mucosa, which in turn causes absorption of water.

Bacterial Action in the Colon. Numerous bacteria, especially colon bacilli, are present in the absorbing colon. Substances formed as a result of bacterial activity are vitamin K, vitamin B_{12}, thiamin, riboflavin, and various gases that contribute to *flatus* in the colon. Vitamin K is especially important, for the amount of this vitamin in the ingested foods is normally insufficient to maintain adequate blood coagulation.

Composition of the Feces. The feces normally are about three-fourths water and one-fourth solid matter composed of about 30 per cent dead bacteria, 10 to 20 per cent fat, 10 to 20 per cent inorganic matter, 2 to 3 per cent protein, and 30 per cent undigested roughage of the food and dried constituents of digestive juices, such as bile pigment and sloughed epithelial cells.

The brown color of feces is caused by *stercobilin* and *urobilin*, which are derivatives of bilirubin. The odor is caused principally by the products of bacterial action; these vary from one person to another, depending on each person's colonic bacterial flora and on the type of food eaten. The actual odoriferous products include indole, skatole, mercaptans, and *hydrogen sulfide*.

GASTROINTESTINAL DISORDERS

GASTRITIS

Gastritis means inflammation of the gastric mucosa. This is exceedingly common in the population as a whole, especially in the later years of adult life.

The inflammation of gastritis may be merely superficial and therefore not very harmful, or it may penetrate deeply into the gastric mucosa, and in many longstanding cases it causes almost complete atrophy of the gastric mucosa. In a few cases, gastritis can be very acute and severe, with ulcerative excoriation of the stomach mucosa by the stomach's own peptic secretions.

The cause of gastritis in most instances is not known. In the past it was ascribed mainly to irritant foods, but the present clinical belief is that almost no food can be as irritant to the gastric mucosa as the normal acid-pepsin gastric juices themselves. Therefore, patients with gastritis are usually told to eat almost any food that will not cause nausea or burning epigastric pain. Yet, a few substances can be very damaging to the protective gastric mucosal barrier—that is, to the viscid mucous glands and tight epithelial junctions between the gastric lining cells—often leading to severe acute or chronic gastritis. The two most common of these substances are *alcohol* and *aspirin*.

Gastric Atrophy. In many persons who have chronic gastritis, the mucosa gradually becomes atrophic until little or no gastric gland activity remains. It is also believed that some persons develop autoimmunity against their own gastric mucosa, which leads eventually to gastric atrophy. Loss of the stomach secretions in gastric atrophy leads to *achlorhydria* and, occasionally, to *pernicious anemia*.

Achlorhydria means simply that the stomach fails to secrete hydrochloric acid. Usually, when acid is not secreted, pepsin also is not secreted, and, even if it is, the lack of acid prevents it from functioning because pepsin requires an acid medium for activity. Obviously, then, essentially all digestive function in the stomach is lost when achlorhydria is present.

Pernicious Anemia in Gastric Atrophy. Pernicious anemia, which was discussed in Chapter 19, is a common accompaniment of achlorhydria and gastric atrophy. The normal gastric secretions contain a glycoprotein called *intrinsic factor*, which is secreted by the oxyntic cells (the HCl-producing cells) and which must be present for adequate absorption of vitamin B_{12} from the ileum. The intrinsic factor combines with vitamin B_{12}, and the complex then binds with receptors on the surfaces of the ileal epithelial cells, a necessary step in the absorption of vitamin B_{12}. In the absence of intrinsic factor, an adequate amount of vitamin B_{12} is not made available from the foods. As a result *maturation failure* occurs in the formation of red blood cells in the bone marrow, resulting in pernicious anemia.

Pernicious anemia also occurs frequently when most of the stomach has been removed for treatment of either stomach ulcer or stomach cancer or when the ileum, where vitamin B_{12} is almost entirely absorbed, is removed.

PEPTIC ULCER

A peptic ulcer is an excoriated area of the mucosa caused by the digestive action of gastric juice. Figure 44–8 illustrates the points in the gastrointestinal tract at which peptic ulcers frequently occur, showing that by far the most frequent site of peptic ulcers is in the first few centimeters of the duodenum. In addition, peptic ulcers frequently occur along the lesser curva-

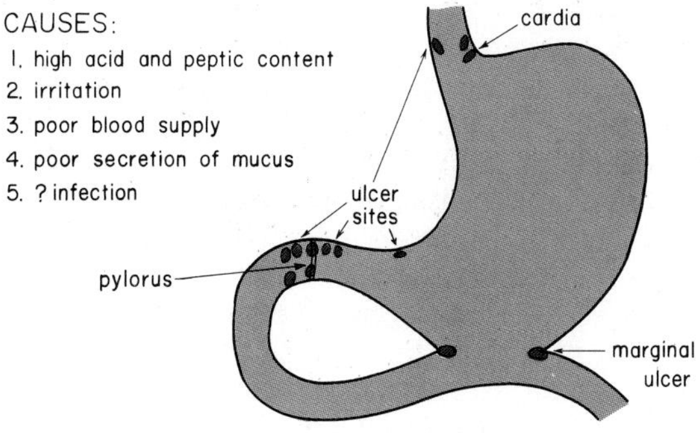

CAUSES:
1. high acid and peptic content
2. irritation
3. poor blood supply
4. poor secretion of mucus
5. ? infection

cardia

ulcer
sites

pylorus

marginal
ulcer

Figure 44-8. Peptic ulcer.

ture of the antral end of the stomach or, more rarely, in the lower end of the esophagus, where there is often reflux of stomach juices.

Basic Cause of Peptic Ulceration. The usual cause of peptic ulceration is too much secretion of gastric juice in relation to the degree of protection afforded by the mucous lining of the stomach and duodenum and by neutralization of the gastric acid by duodenal juices. It will be recalled that all areas normally exposed to gastric juices are well supplied with mucous glands, beginning with the compound mucous glands of the lower esophagus, including the mucous cell coating of the stomach mucosa, the mucous neck cells of the gastric glands, the deep pyloric glands that secrete mainly mucus, and, finally, the glands of Brunner in the upper duodenum, which secrete a highly alkaline mucus.

In addition to the mucus protection of the mucosa, the duodenum is also protected by the alkalinity of the pancreatic secretion, which contains large quantities of sodium bicarbonate that neutralize the hydrochloric acid of the gastric juice, thus inactivating the pepsin and thereby preventing digestion of the mucosa. Two additional mechanisms insure that this neutralization of gastric juices is complete:

1. When excess acid enters the duodenum, it reflexly inhibits gastric secretion and peristalsis in the stomach, thereby decreasing the rate of gastric emptying. This allows increased time for pancreatic secretion to enter the duodenum to neutralize the acid already present. After neutralization has taken place, the reflex subsides and more stomach contents are emptied.

2. The presence of acid in the small intestine liberates secretin from the intestinal mucosa. The secretin then passes by way of the blood to the pancreas to promote rapid secretion of pancreatic juice, which contains a high concentration of sodium bicarbonate, thus making more sodium bicarbonate available for neutralization of the acid. These mechanisms were discussed in detail in Chapters 42 and 43 in relation to gastrointestinal motility and secretion.

Causes of Peptic Ulcer in the Human Being. About 85 per cent of the patients with peptic ulcer *of the duodenum* secrete approximately two times as much

gastric acid following injection of a test dose of *pentagastrin* as do normal persons. Therefore, it is believed that the ulcers in these patients are caused by excessive secretion of acid and pepsin by the gastric glands. In the 15 per cent of the patients who secrete normal amounts of acid, it is presumed that one of four other abnormalities is the usual cause: (a) possible secretion of an abnormal mucus that has less than normal protective value, (b) diminished secretion of mucus, (c) failure of the normal duodenal-gastric feedback mechanisms to limit the rate of gastric emptying into the duodenum, or (d) failure of the secretin-pancreatic feedback mechanism to cause the secretion of enough alkaline pancreatic juice to neutralize the gastric juice as it enters the duodenum.

The development of peptic ulcers is strongly hereditary. For instance, the offspring of persons who secrete excessive amounts of gastric acid, like their parents, tend to secrete excessive amounts of acid. Also the offspring of patients who have diminished mucosal protection have a strong hereditary tendency to develop peptic ulceration as well.

Paradoxically, *gastric* ulcers, in contradistinction to duodenal ulcers, often occur in pateints who have normal or low secretion of hydrochloric acid. However, these patients almost invariably have an associated gastritis, indicating that ulceration in the stomach almost certainly results from reduced resistance of the stomach mucosa to digestion rather than to excess secretion of gastric juice. Stomach ulceration frequently results in patients who have ingested large quantities of substances such as aspirin or alcohol that reduce the mucosal resistance.

Physiology of Treatment. The usual medical treatment for peptic ulcer is a combination of (1) reduction of stressful situations that might lead to excessive acid secretion, (2) administration of antacid drugs to neutralize much of the acid in the stomach secretions, (3) adminstration of the drug *cimetidine*, which blocks the action of gastrin in stimulating gastric juice secretion, (4) interdiction against smoking because statistical studies have shown that smokers are several times as prone to have peptic ulcers as are nonsmokers, and (5) removal of such ulcer-causing factors as alcohol, aspirin, or other substances that might irritate the gastroduodenal mucosa.

Surgical treatment of peptic ulceration is usually by one or both of two procedures: (1) *vagotomy* or (2) *removal of a portion of the stomach*. Fortunately, however, since the advent of the drug cimetidine, the more drastic surgical procedures are employed far less frequently than in the past.

Vagotomy means section of the vagus nerves to the stomach; this temporarily blocks almost all secretion of acid and pepsin by the stomach and often cures the ulcer or ulcers within a week after the operation is performed. Unfortunately, though, a large amount of basal stomach secretion returns after a few months, and in many patients the ulcer also returns. Also, *gastric atony* usually follows section of both vagus trunks; this can be very distressing, since stomach motility is often reduced so much that gastric emptying becomes minimal, leading to partial or sometimes almost total pyloric obstruction. To prevent this occurrence, the surgeon often removes the stomach antrum and pylorus, and the body of the stomach is connected directly to the proximal end of the duodenum.

In the past, large numbers of patients were treated by removing the lower three fourths to four fifths of the stomach and then anastomosing the stomach to the jejunum. If less than this amount of the stomach is removed, far too much gastric juice continues to be secreted, and a *marginal ulcer* soon develops where the stomach is anastomosed to the intestine. Fortunately, since the advent of the drug cimetidine, this very severe procedure is rarely required in present-day therapy of peptic ulcer.

MALABSORPTION FROM THE SMALL INTESTINE—SPRUE

Occasionally, nutrients are not adequately absorbed from the small intestine even though the food is well digested. Several different diseases can cause decreased absorbability of the mucosa; these are often classified together under the general heading of *sprue*. Obviously, also, malabsorption can occur when large portions of the small intestine have been removed.

One type of sprue, called variously by the names *idiopathic sprue, celiac disease* (in children), or *gluten enteropathy*, results from the toxic effects of *gluten* present in certain types of grains, especially *wheat* and *rye*. The gluten causes destruction of the villi in some susceptible persons, perhaps as a result of an immunological or allergic reaction. The villi become blunted or disappear altogether, thus greatly reducing the absorptive area of the gut. Removal of wheat and rye flour from the diet, especially in children with this disease, frequently results in an apparently miraculous cure within weeks.

Malabsorption in Sprue. In the early stages of sprue, the absorption of fats is more impaired than the absorption of other digestive products. The fat appears in the stools almost entirely in the form of soaps rather than undigested neutral fat, illustrating that the problem is one of absorption, not of digestion. In this stage of sprue, the condition is frequently called *idiopathic steatorrhea*, which means simply excess fats in the stools as a result of unknown causes.

In more severe cases of sprue, the absorption of proteins, carbohydrates, calcium, vitamin K, folic acid, and vitamin B_{12} as well as many other important substances becomes greatly impaired. As a result, the person suffers (1) severe nutritional deficiency, often developing severe wasting of the tissues, (2) osteomalacia (demineralization of the bones because of calcium lack), (3) inadequate blood coagulation due to lack of vitamin K, and (4) macrocytic anemia of the pernicious anemia type, owing to diminished vitamin B_{12} and folic acid absorption.

CONSTIPATION

Constipation means slow movement of feces through the large intestine, and it is often associated with large quantities of dry, hard feces in the descending colon that accumulate because of the long time allowed for absorption of fluid.

A frequent cause of constipation is irregular bowel habits that have developed through a life-time of inhibition of the normal defecation reflexes. The newborn child is rarely constipated, but part of his training in the early years of life requires that he learn to control defecation, and this control is effected by inhibiting the natural defecation reflexes. Clinical experience shows that if one fails to allow defecation to occur when the defecation reflexes are excited or if one overuses laxatives to take the place of natural bowel function, the reflexes themselves become progressively less strong over a period of time and the colon often becomes *atonic*. For this reason, if a person establishes regular bowel habits early in life, usually defecating in the morning after breakfast when the gastrocolic and duodenocolic reflexes cause mass movements in the large intestine, he can generally prevent the development of constipation in later life.

DIARRHEA

Diarrhea, the opposite of constipation, results from rapid movement of fecal matter through the large intestine. The major cause of diarrhea is infection in the gastrointestinal tract, which is called *enteritis*.

In usual infectious diarrhea, the infection is most extensive in the large intestine and the distal end of the ileum. Everywhere that the infection is present, the mucosa becomes extensively irritated, and its rate of secretion becomes greatly enhanced. In addition, the motility of the intestinal wall usually increases many fold. As a result, large quantities of fluid are made available for washing the infectious agent toward the anus, and at the same time strong propulsive movements propel this fluid forward. Obviously, this is an important mechanism for ridding the intestinal tract of the debilitating infection.

Of special interest is the diarrhea caused by *cholera*. The cholera toxin directly stimulates excessive secretion of electrolytes and fluid from the crypts of Lieberkühn in the distal ileum and colon, and it specifically enhances the bicarbonate-chloride exchange mechanism, causing extreme quantities of sodium bicarbonate to be secreted into the intestinal tract. The loss of fluid and electrolytes can be so debilitating within a day or so that death ensues. Therefore, the most important basis of therapy is simply to replace the fluid and electrolytes as rapidly as they are lost. With proper and simple therapy of this type, almost no cholera patients die, but without treatment, 50 per cent or more do.

VOMITING

Vomiting is the means by which the upper gastrointestinal tract rids itself of its contents when the gut becomes excessively irritated, overdistended, or even overexcitable. The stimuli that cause vomiting can originate in any part of the gastrointestinal tract, though distention or irritation of the duodenum provides the strongest stimulus. Impulses are transmitted by both vagal and sympathetic afferents to the *vomiting center* of the medulla, which lies near the tractus solitarius at approximately the level of the dorsal motor nucleus of the vagus. Appropriate motor reactions are then instituted to cause the vomiting act, and the motor impulses that cause the actual vomiting are transmitted from the vomiting center through the fifth, seventh, ninth, tenth, and twelfth cranial nerves to the upper gastrointestinal tract and through the spinal nerves to the diaphragm and abdominal muscles.

The Vomiting Act. Once the vomiting center has been sufficiently stimulated and the vomiting act instituted, the first effects are (1) a deep inspiratory breath, (2) raising of the hyoid bone and the larynx to pull the upper esophageal sphincter open, (3) closing of the glottis, and (4) lifting of the soft palate to close the posterior nares. Next comes a strong downward contraction of the diaphragm along with simultaneous contraction of all the abdominal muscles. This obviously squeezes the stomach between the two sets of muscles, building the intragastric pressure to a high level. Finally, the lower esophageal sphincter relaxes, allowing expulsion of the gastric contents upward through the esophagus.

Thus, the vomiting act results from a squeezing action of the muscles of the abdomen associated with sudden opening of the esophageal sphincters so that the gastric contents can be expelled.

GASES IN THE GASTROINTESTINAL TRACT (FLATUS)

Gases can enter the gastrointestinal tract from three sources: (1) swallowed air, (2) the result of bacterial action, and (3) diffusion from the blood into the gastrointestinal tract.

Most gases in the stomach are nitrogen and oxygen derived from swallowed air, and a large proportion of these are expelled by belching.

Only small amounts of gas are usually present in the small intestine, and these are composed principally of air that passes from the stomach into the intestinal tract.

In the large intestine, the greater proportion of the gases is derived from bacterial action; these gases include especially *carbon dioxide, methane,* and *hydrogen.* When the methane and hydrogen become suitably mixed with oxygen from swallowed air, an actual explosive mixture is occasionally formed.

Certain foods are known to cause greater amounts of flatus from the large intestine than others—beans, cabbage, onions, cauliflower, corn, and certain highly irritant foods such as vinegar. Some of these foods—beans, for instance—serve as a suitable medium for gas-forming bacteria, especially because they contain fermentable types of carbohydrates that are poorly absorbed.

The amounts of gases entering or forming in the large intestine each day averages 7 to 10 liters, whereas the average amount expelled is usually only about 0.6 liter. The remainder is absorbed through the intestinal mucosa. Most often, a person expels large quantities of gases not because of excessive bacterial activity but because of excessive motility of the large intestine caused by intestinal irritation. This moves the gases on through the large intestine before they can be absorbed.

QUESTIONS

1. Explain why *hydrolysis* is the means by which essentially all digestion in the gastrointestinal tract takes place.
2. Give the schema for digestion of *carbohydrates.*
3. Give the schema for digestion of *fats.*
4. What is the role of *bile salts* in fat digestion?
5. Give the schema for digestion of *proteins.*
6. Describe the absorptive surface of the *intestinal mucosa,* including the detailed anatomy of a *villus.*
7. What is meant by *isosmotic absorption* of water?
8. Describe the active absorption of sodium ions by the intestinal epithelium. Why does this cause passive absorption of chloride ions?
9. Describe the *co-transport mechanism* for absorption of glucose and amino acids.
10. Explain the absorption of fats by the intestinal epithelium and the formation of *chylomicrons* that are then transported in the thoracic duct lymph.
11. What are the special characteristics of absorption in the large intestine, and how is this related to the formation of feces?
12. Describe the clinical conditions of *gastritis, gastric atrophy,* and the *pernicious* anemia that occurs in patients with gastric atrophy.
13. What is a *peptic ulcer,* what are its causes, and why do most peptic ulcers occur in the first few centimeters of the duodenum? Explain the medical and surgical treatment of peptic ulcers.
14. What is the cause of *idiopathic sprue,* and what are its effects?
15. What are the causes of *constipation* and *diarrhea?*
16. Give the mechanism of *vomiting,* including its nervous control.
17. Explain the occurrence of gases in the gastrointestinal tract, and how are these different at different levels of the tract?

References

Digestion and Absorption

Bickel, H., ed.: Digestion and Absorption of Nutrients. Ft. Lee, NJ, J. K. Burgess, 1983.

Christensen, H. N: The regulation of amino acid and sugar absorption by diet. Nutr Rev 42:237, 1984.

Cummings, J. H.: Chronic absorption: The importance of short chain fatty acids in man. Scand J Gastroenterol (Suppl) 93:89, 1984.

Donowitz, M. et al.: Cytosol free Ca^{++} in the regulation of active intestinal Na and Cl transport. KROC Found Ser 17:171, 1984.

Gardner, M. L.: Intestinal assimilation of intact peptides and proteins from the diet—a neglected field? Biol Rev 59:289, 1984.

Kenny, A. J., and Maroux, S.: Topology of microvillar membrane hydrolases of kidney and intestine. Physiol Rev 62:91, 1982.

Mailman, D.: Relationships between intestinal absorption and hemodynamics. Annu Rev Physiol 44:43, 1982.

Norum, K. R. et al.: Transport of cholesterol. Physiol Rev 63:1343, 1983.

Ockner, R. K., and Isselbacher, K. J.: Recent concepts of intestinal fat absorption. Rev Physiol Biochem Pharmacol 71:107, 1984.

Schultz, S. G.: A cellular model for active sodium absorption by mammalian colon. Annu Rev Physiol 46:435, 1984.

Smith, P. L. and McCabe, R. D.: Mechanisms and regulation of transcellular potassium transport by the colon. Am J Physiol 247:G445, 1984.

Stevens, B. R. et al.: Intestinal transport of amino acids and sugars: advances using membrane vesicles. Annu Rev Physiol 46:417, 1984.

Gastrointestinal Disorders

Awouters, F. et al.: Pharmacology of antidiarrheal drugs. Annu Rev Pharmacol Toxicol 23:279, 1983.

Berglinch, T.: The mammalian gastric parietal cell in vitro. Annu Rev Physiol 46:377, 1984.

Castell, D. O.: Calcium-channel blocking agents for gastrointestinal disorders. Am J Cardiol 55:210B, 1985.

Cook, G. C.: Topical Gastroenterology. New York, Oxford University Press, 1980.

Giannella, R. A.: Pathogenesis of acute bacterial diarrheal disorders. Annu Rev Med 32:341, 1981.

Guth, P. H.: Pathogenesis of gastric mucosal injury. Annu Rev Med 33:183, 1982.

Kestenbaum, D., and Behar, J.: Pathogenesis, diagnosis, and management of reflux esophagitis. Annu Rev Med 32:443, 1981.

McCarthy, D. M.: Zollinger-Ellison syndrome. Annu Rev Med 33:197, 1982.

Shearman, D. J., ed.: Diseases of the Gastrointestinal Tract and Liver. New York, Churchill Livingstone, 1982.

Strickland, R. G., and Jewell, D. P.: Immunoregulatory mechanisms in nonspecific inflammatory bowel disease. Annu Rev Med 34:195, 1983.

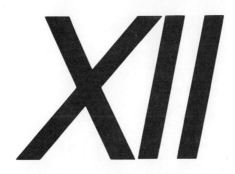

METABOLISM AND TEMPERATURE REGULATION

45 ■ Metabolism of Carbohydrates and Formation of Adenosine Triphosphate

46 ■ Lipid and Protein Metabolism

47 ■ Energetics, Metabolic Rate, and Regulation of Body Temperature

48 ■ Dietary Balances, Regulation of Feeding, Obesity, and Vitamins

45

Metabolism of Carbohydrates and Formation of Adenosine Triphosphate

ROLE OF ADENOSINE TRIPHOSPHATE
  (ATP) IN METABOLISM
TRANSPORT OF MONOSACCHARIDES
  THROUGH THE CELL MEMBRANE
  ENHANCEMENT OF GLUCOSE
    TRANSPORT BY INSULIN
  PHOSPHORYLATION OF GLUCOSE
STORAGE OF GLYCOGEN IN LIVER
  AND MUSCLE
  GLYCOGENESIS
  GLYCOGENOLYSIS
RELEASE OF ENERGY FROM THE
  GLUCOSE MOLECULE BY THE
  GLYCOLYTIC PATHWAY
  GLYCOLYSIS AND THE FORMATION
    OF PYRUVIC ACID
  CONVERSION OF PYRUVIC ACID TO
    ACETYL COENZYME A

THE CITRIC ACID CYCLE
FORMATION OF ATP BY OXIDATIVE
  PHOSPHORYLATION
SUMMARY OF ATP FORMATION
  DURING THE BREAKDOWN OF
  GLUCOSE
CONTROL OF GLYCOLYSIS AND
  OXIDATION BY ADENOSINE
  DIPHOSPHATE (ADP)
ANAEROBIC RELEASE OF ENERGY—
  ANAEROBIC GLYCOLYSIS
RELEASE OF ENERGY FROM GLUCOSE
  BY THE PHOSPHOGLUCONATE
  PATHWAY
FORMATION OF CARBOHYDRATES
  FROM PROTEINS AND FATS—
  GLUCONEOGENESIS
BLOOD GLUCOSE

The next few chapters deal with metabolism in the body, which means the chemical processes that make it possible for the cells to continue living. It is not the purpose of this textbook, however, to present the chemical details of all the various cellular reactions, for this lies in the discipline of biochemistry. Instead, these chapters are devoted to (1) a review of the principal chemical processes of the cell and (2) an analysis of their physiological implications, especially in relation to the manner in which they fit into the overall concept of homeostasis.

ROLE OF ADENOSINE TRIPHOSPHATE (ATP) IN METABOLISM

A great proportion of the chemical reactions in the cells is concerned with making the energy in foods

available to the various physiological systems of the cell. For instance, energy is required for (1) muscular activity, (2) secretion by the glands, (3) maintenance of membrane potentials in the nerve and muscle fibers, (4) synthesis of substances in the cells, and (5) absorption of foods from the gastrointestinal tract. The substance adenosine triphosphate (ATP) plays a key role in making the energy of the foods available for all of these purposes.

ATP, a labile chemical compound present in all cells, has the chemical structure shown on page 523.

From this formula it can be seen that ATP is a combination of adenine, ribose, and three phosphate radicals. The last two phosphate radicals are connected with the remainder of the molecule by so-called *high energy bonds*, which are indicated by the symbol $\sim$. The amount of free energy in each of

522

NH₂

ADENINE

RIBOSE

TRIPHOSPHATE

$$CH_2-O-\overset{O}{\underset{O^-}{P}}-O\sim\overset{O}{\underset{O^-}{P}}-O\sim\overset{O}{\underset{O^-}{P}}-O^-$$

OH   OH

these high energy bonds per mole of ATP is approximately 7300 calories per mole under standard conditions but 12,000 calories under the conditions of temperature and concentrations of the reactants in the body. Therefore, removal of each phosphate radical liberates 12,000 calories of energy. After loss of one phosphate radical from ATP, the compound becomes *adenosine diphosphate* (ADP), and after loss of the second phosphate radical the compound becomes *adenosine monophosphate* (AMP). The interconversions between ATP, ADP, and AMP are the following:

$$ATP \underset{+\ 12,000\ cal.}{\overset{-\ 12,000\ cal.}{\rightleftarrows}} \left\{ \begin{array}{c} ADP \\ + \\ PO_4 \end{array} \right\} \underset{+\ 12,000\ cal.}{\overset{-\ 12,000\ cal.}{\rightleftarrows}} \left\{ \begin{array}{c} AMP \\ + \\ 2PO_4 \end{array} \right\}$$

ATP is present everywhere in the cytoplasm and nucleoplasm of all cells, and essentially all the physiological mechanisms that require energy for operation obtain it directly from the ATP (or some other similar high energy compound—guanosine triphosphate, GTP, for example). In turn, the food in the cells is gradually oxidized, and the released energy is used to re-form the ATP, thus always maintaining a supply of this substance.

In summary, ATP is an intermediary compound that has the peculiar ability of entering into many coupled reactions—reactions with the food to extract energy and reactions in relation to many physiological mechanisms to provide energy for their operation. For this reason, ATP has frequently been called the energy *currency* of the body that can be gained and spent again and again.

The principal purpose of the present chapter is to explain how the energy from carbohydrates can be used to form ATP (or GTP) in the cells. At least 99 per cent of all the carbohydrates utilized by the body is used for this purpose.

TRANSPORT OF MONOSACCHARIDES THROUGH THE CELL MEMBRANE

From the previous chapter it will be recalled that the final products of carbohydrate digestion in the alimentary tract are almost entirely glucose, fructose, and galactose, with glucose representing by far the major share of these. These three monosaccharides are absorbed into the portal blood and, after passing through the blood sinuses of the liver, are carried everywhere in the body by the circulatory system. But before they can be used by the cells, they must be transported through the cell membrane into the cellular cytoplasm.

Monosaccharides cannot diffuse through the usual pores of the cell membrane, for the maximum molecular weight of substances that can do this is about 100, whereas glucose, fructose, and galactose all have molecular weights of 180. Yet glucose and some of the other monosaccharides combine with a *protein carrier* in the membrane that then allows them to diffuse freely to the inside of the cell. After passing through the membrane they become dissociated from the carrier. The transport mechanism is one of *facilitated diffusion* and not of active transport. These concepts are discussed in more detail in Chapter 4.

ENHANCEMENT OF GLUCOSE TRANSPORT BY INSULIN

The rate of glucose transport through the cell membrane is greatly increased by insulin. When large amounts of insulin are secreted by the pancreas, the rate of glucose transport into most cells increases to as much as ten times the rate of transport when no insulin at all is secreted. The amounts of glucose that can diffuse to the insides of most cells of the body in the absence of insulin, with the unique exceptions of the liver and the brain, are far too little to supply anywhere near the amount of glucose normally required for energy metabolism. Therefore, in effect, the rate of carbohydrate utilization by the body is controlled by the rate of insulin secretion in the pancreas. The functions of insulin and its control of carbohydrate metabolism will be discussed more fully in Chapter 52.

PHOSPHORYLATION OF GLUCOSE

Immediately upon entry into the cells, glucose combines with a phosphate radical in accordance with the following reaction:

$$\text{glucose} \xrightarrow[\text{+ ATP}]{\text{glucokinase or hexokinase}} \text{glucose 6-phosphate}$$

This phosphorylation is promoted by the enzyme *glucokinase* in the liver or *hexokinase* in most other cells.

The phosphorylation of glucose is almost completely irreversible except in the liver cells, the renal tubular epithelium, and the intestinal epithelial cells in which glucose phosphatase is available for reversing the reaction. Therefore, in most tissues of the body, phosphorylation serves to *capture* the glucose in the cell—once *in* the cell, the glucose will not diffuse back out except from those special cells that have the necessary phosphatase.

Conversion of Fructose and Galactose into Glucose. In liver cells appropriate enzymes are available to promote interconversions between the monosaccharides, and the dynamics of the reactions are such that when the liver releases the monosaccharides back into the blood, the final product of these interconversions is almost entirely glucose. Also, in the case of fructose, much of it is converted into glucose as it is absorbed through the intestinal epithelial cells into the portal blood. Therefore, essentially all of the monosaccharides that circulate in the blood are the final conversion product, glucose.

STORAGE OF GLYCOGEN IN LIVER AND MUSCLE

After absorption into the cells, glucose can be used immediately for release of energy to the cells, or it can be stored in the form of *glycogen*, which is a large polymer of glucose.

All cells of the body are capable of storing at least some glycogen, but certain cells can store large amounts, especially the liver cells, which can store up to 5 to 8 per cent of their weight as glycogen, and muscle cells, which can store up to 1 to 3 per cent as glycogen. The glycogen molecules can be polymerized to almost any molecular weight, the average molecular weight being five million or more; most of the glycogen precipitates in the form of solid granules.

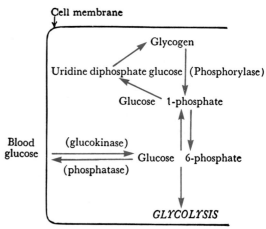

Figure 45–1. The chemical reactions of glycogenesis and glycogenolysis, showing also the interconversions between blood glucose and liver glycogen. (The phosphatase required for release of glucose from the cell is absent in muscle cells.)

GLYCOGENESIS

Glycogenesis is the process of glycogen formation, the chemical reactions of which are illustrated in Figure 45–1. From this figure it can be seen that *glucose 6-phosphate* first becomes *glucose 1-phosphate;* this is then converted to *uridine diphosphate glucose,* which is converted into glycogen. Several specific enzymes are required to cause these conversions. Any monosaccharide that can be converted into glucose obviously can enter into the reactions, and certain smaller compounds, including *lactic acid, glycerol, pyruvic acid,* and *some deaminated amino acids,* can also be converted into glucose or closely allied compounds and thence into glycogen.

GLYCOGENOLYSIS

Glycogenolysis means the breakdown of glycogen to re-form glucose in the cells. Glycogenolysis does not occur by reversal of the same chemical reactions that serve to form glycogen; instead, each succeeding glucose molecule on each branch of the glycogen polymer is split away by the process of *phosphorylation* catalyzed by the enzyme *phosphorylase.*

Under resting conditions, the phosphorylase is in an inactive form, so that glycogen can be stored but not reconverted into glucose. When it is necessary to re-form glucose from glycogen, therefore, the phosphorylase must first be activated. This activation is accomplished in the following ways:

Activation of Phosphorylase by Epinephrine and Glucagon. Two hormones, epinephrine and glucagon, can specifically activate phosphorylase and thereby cause rapid glycogenolysis. The initial effect of each of these hormones is to increase the formation of *cyclic adenosine monophosphate (cAMP)* in the cells. This substance then initiates a cascade of chemical reactions that activate the phosphorylase, a process discussed in more detail in Chapter 52.

Epinephrine is released by the adrenal medullae when the sympathetic nervous system is stimulated. The epinephrine than activates phosphorylase, thus making glucose available for rapid metabolism. This function of epinephrine occurs markedly both in liver cells and in muscle, thereby contributing, along with other effects of sympathetic stimulation, to preparation of the body for action, as discussed in Chapter 38.

Glucagon is a hormone secreted by the *alpha cells* of the pancreas when the blood glucose concentration falls low. It stimulates the formation of cAMP mainly in the liver and thereby activates phosphorylase. Its effect is primarily to dump glucose out of the liver into the blood, thereby elevating blood glucose concentration. The function of glucagon in blood glucose regulation is discussed in Chapter 52.

Transport of Glucose Out of Liver Cells. The cells of the liver contain *phosphatase*, an enzyme that can split phosphate away from glucose 6-phosphate and therefore make the glucose available for retransport out of the cells into the interstitial fluids. Therefore, when glucose is formed in the liver as a result of glycogenolysis, most of it immediately passes into the blood. Thus, liver glycogenolysis causes an immediate rise in blood glucose concentration. Glycogenolysis in most other cells of the body, especially in the muscle cells, simply makes increased amounts of glucose 6-phosphate available inside the cells and increases the local rate of glucose utilization, but it does not release the glucose into the extracellular fluids because the required phosphatase is not available to dephosphorylate the glucose 6-phosphate.

RELEASE OF ENERGY FROM THE GLUCOSE MOLECULE BY THE GLYCOLYTIC PATHWAY

Complete oxidation of 1 mole of glucose releases 686,000 calories of energy, but only 12,000 calories of energy are required to form 1 mole of adenosine triphosphate (ATP). Therefore, it would be extremely wasteful of energy if glucose should be decomposed all the way into water and carbon dioxide at once while forming only a single ATP molecule. Fortunately, cells contain an extensive series of different protein enzymes that cause the glucose molecule to split a little at a time in many successive steps, with its energy released in small packets to form one molecule of ATP at a time, forming a total of 38 moles of ATP for each mole of glucose utilized by the cells.

The purpose of the present section is to describe the basic principles by which the glucose molecule is progressively dissected and its energy released to form ATP.

GLYCOLYSIS AND THE FORMATION OF PYRUVIC ACID

By far the most important means by which energy is released from the glucose molecule is the process of *glycolysis*, followed by *oxidation of the end-products of glycolysis*. *Glycolysis* means splitting of the glucose molecule to form two molecules of pyruvic acid. This process occurs by ten successive steps of chemical reactions, illustrated in Figure 45–2. Each step is catalyzed by at least one specific protein enzyme. Note that glucose is first converted into fructose 1,6-phosphate and then split into two three–carbon atom molecules, each of which is then converted through five successive steps into pyruvic acid.

Formation of Adenosine Triphosphate (ATP) During Glycolysis. Despite the many chemical reactions in the glycolytic series, little energy is released. However, 2 moles of ATP are formed for each mole of glucose utilized. This amounts to 24,000 calories of energy stored in the form of ATP, but during glycolysis a total of 56,000 calories of energy is lost from the original glucose, giving an overall *efficiency* for ATP formation of 43 per cent. The remaining 57 per cent of the energy is lost in the form of heat.

CONVERSION OF PYRUVIC ACID TO ACETYL COENZYME A

The next stage in the degradation of glucose is conversion of its two derivative pyruvic acid molecules into two molecules of *acetyl coenzyme A* (acetyl Co-A) in accordance with the following reaction:

$$2 \; CH_3 \!-\! \overset{\displaystyle O}{\overset{\|}{C}} \!-\! COOH \; + \; 2 \; Co\text{-}A\!-\!SH$$
$$\text{(Pyruvic Acid)} \qquad \text{(Coenzyme A)}$$

$$\longrightarrow 2 \; CH_3 \!-\! \overset{\displaystyle O}{\overset{\|}{C}} \!-\! S\!-\!Co\text{-}A \; + \; 2CO_2 \; + \; 4H$$
$$\text{(Acetyl Co-A)}$$

From this reaction it can be seen that two carbon dioxide molecules and four hydrogen atoms are released, while the remainders of the two pyruvic acid molecules combine with coenzyme A, a derivative of the vitamin pantothenic acid, to form two molecules of acetyl Co-A. In this conversion, no ATP is formed, but six molecules of ATP are produced when the four hydrogen atoms are later oxidized, as is discussed in a later section.

THE CITRIC ACID CYCLE

The next stage in the degradation of the glucose molecule is called the *citric acid cycle* (also called the *tricarboxylic acid cycle,* or the *Krebs cycle*). This is a sequence of chemical reactions in which the acetyl

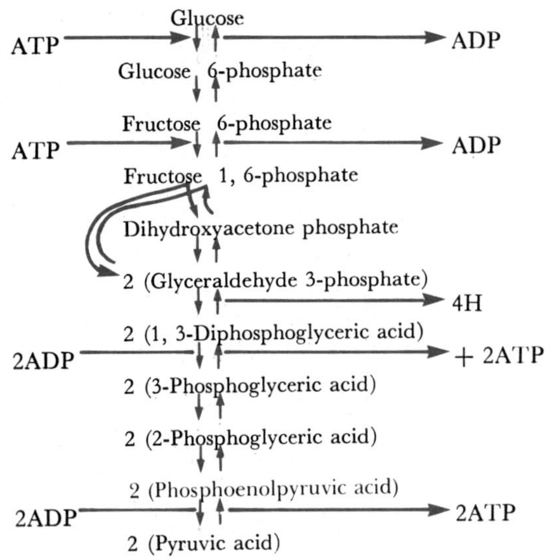

Glucose

ATP ——————→ ADP

Glucose 6-phosphate

Fructose 6-phosphate

ATP ——————→ ADP

Fructose 1, 6-phosphate

Dihydroxyacetone phosphate

2 (Glyceraldehyde 3-phosphate) ——————→ 4H

2 (1, 3-Diphosphoglyceric acid)

2ADP ——————→ + 2ATP

2 (3-Phosphoglyceric acid)

2 (2-Phosphoglyceric acid)

2 (Phosphoenolpyruvic acid)

2ADP ——————→ 2ATP

2 (Pyruvic acid)

Net reaction:

$$Glucose + 2ADP + 2PO_4^{---} \longrightarrow 2 \text{ Pyruvic acid} + 2ATP + 4H$$

Figure 45–2. The sequence of chemical reactions responsible for glycolysis.

portion of acetyl Co-A is degraded to carbon dioxide and hydrogen atoms. These reactions all occur *in the matrix of the mitochondrion.* The released hydrogen atoms are subsequently oxidized, as discussed later, releasing tremendous amounts of energy to form ATP.

Figure 45–3 shows the different stages of the chemical reactions in the citric acid cycle. The substances to the left are added during the chemical reactions, and the products of the chemical reactions are shown to the right. Note at the top of the column that the cycle begins with *oxaloacetic acid,* and then at the bottom of the chain of reactions *oxaloacetic acid* is formed once again. Thus, the cycle can continue indefinitely.

In the initial stage of the citric acid cycle, *acetyl Co-A* combines with *oxaloacetic acid* to form *citric acid.* The coenzyme A portion of the acetyl Co-A is released and can be used again and again for the formation of still more quantities of acetyl Co-A from pyruvic acid. The acetyl portion, however, becomes an integral part of the citric acid molecule. During the successive stages of the citric acid cycle, several molecules of water are added, and *carbon dioxide* and *hydrogen atoms* are released at various stages in the cycle, as shown on the right in the figure.

The net results of the entire citric acid cycle are shown at the bottom of Figure 45–3, illustrating that for each molecule of glucose originally metabolized, 2 acetyl Co-A molecules enter into the citric acid cycle along with 6 molecules of water. These molecules are then degraded into 4 carbon dioxide molecules, 16 hydrogen atoms, and 2 molecules of coenzyme A.

Formation of ATP in the Citric Acid Cycle. No large amount of energy is released during the citric acid cycle itself. However, for each molecule of glucose metabolized, 2 molecules of ATP are formed.

FORMATION OF ATP BY OXIDATIVE PHOSPHORYLATION

Despite all the complexities of glycolysis and the citric acid cycle, pitifully small amounts of ATP are formed during these processes—only 2 ATP molecules in the glycolysis scheme and another 2 in the citric acid cycle. Instead, almost 95 per cent of the final ATP is formed during subsequent oxidation of the hydrogen atoms that are released during these earlier stages of glucose degradation. Indeed, the principal function of all these earlier stages is to make the hydrogen of the glucose molecule available in a form that can be utilized for oxidation.

Oxidation of hydrogen is accomplished by a series of enzymatically catalyzed reactions that (a) change the hydrogen atoms into hydrogen ions and electrons and (b) use the electrons eventually to change the dissolved oxygen of the fluids into hydroxyl ions. Then the hydrogen and hydroxyl ions combine to form water. During this sequence of oxidative reactions, tremendous quantities of energy are released to form ATP. Formation of ATP in this manner is called *oxidative phosphorylation.* It occurs entirely in the mitochondria by a highly specialized process called the chemiosmotic mechanism.

The Chemiosmotic Mechanism for Forming ATP

Ionization of Hydrogen, the Electron Transport Chain, and Formation of Water. The first step in oxidative phosphorylation is to ionize the hydrogen atoms that are removed from the food substrates. These hydrogen atoms are removed in pairs during glycolysis and in the citric acid cycle; one immediately becomes a hydrogen ion, H^+, and the other combines with NAD^+ to form NADH. The upper portion of

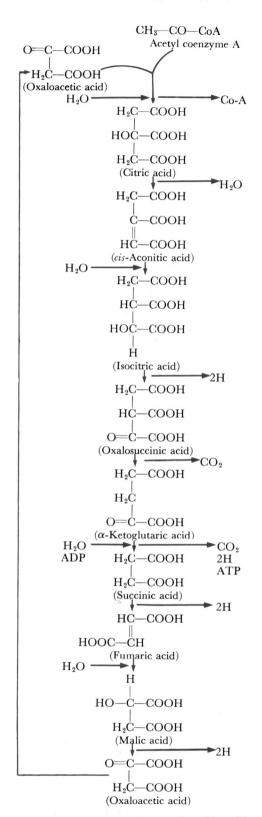

Figure 45–3. The chemical reactions of the citric acid cycle, showing the release of carbon dioxide and an especially large number of hydrogen atoms during the cycle.

Net reaction per molecule of glucose:

2 Acetyl-CoA + 6H_2O + 2ADP →

4CO_2 + 16H + 2CoA + 2ATP

Figure 45–4 shows in color the subsequent disposition of the NADH and H^+ in the mitochondrion. The initial effect is to release the other hydrogen atom bound with NAD to form another hydrogen ion, H^+; this process also reconstitutes NAD^+, which will be reused again and again.

During these changes, the electrons that are removed from the hydrogen atoms to cause their ionization immediately enter an *electron transport chain* that is an integral part of the inner membrane (the shelf membrane) of the mitochondrion. This transport chain consists of a series of electron acceptors that can be reversibly reduced or oxidized by accepting or giving up electrons. The important members of this electron transport chain include *flavoprotein, several iron sulfide proteins, ubiquinone,* and *cytochromes B, C_1, C, A, and A_3.* Each electron is shuttled from one of these acceptors to the next until it finally reaches cytochrome A_3, which is called *cytochrome oxidase* because it is capable, by giving up two electrons, of causing elemental oxygen to combine with hydrogen ions to form water.

Thus, Figure 45–4 illustrates transport of electrons through the electron chain and their ultimate use by cytochrome oxidase to cause the formation of water molecules. During the transport of these electrons through the electron transport chain, energy is released that is later used to cause synthesis of ATP, as follows:

Hydrogen Ion Pumping by the Electron Transport Chain. The energy released as the electrons pass

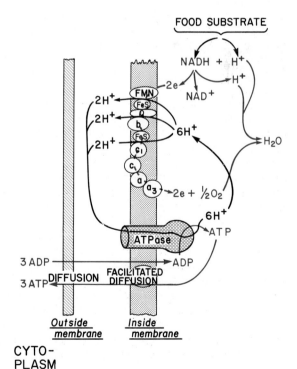

Figure 45–4. The chemiosmotic theory of oxidative phosphorylation for forming great quantities of ATP.

through the electron transport chain is used to pump hydrogen ions from the inner matrix of the mitochondrion into the space between the inner and outer mitochondrial membranes. The shift creates a high concentration of hydrogen ions in this space, and it also creates a strong negative electrical potential in the inner matrix.

Formation of ATP. The final step in oxidative phosphorylation is to convert ADP into ATP. This conversion occurs in conjunction with a large protein molecule with a knoblike head that protrudes all the way through the inner mitochondrial membrane and into the inner matrix. This molecule is an ATPase, the physical nature of which is illustrated in Figure 45–4. It is called *ATP synthetase*. It is postulated that the high concentration of hydrogen ions in the space between the two mitochondrial membranes and the large electrical potential difference across the inner membrane cause the hydrogen ions to flow into the mitochondrial matrix *through the substance of the ATPase molecule*. In doing so, energy derived from this hydrogen ion flow is utilized by the ATPase to convert ADP into ATP by combining an ADP with a phosphate radical, at the same time forming an additional high energy phosphate bond.

For each two electrons that pass through the entire electron transport chain (representing the ionization of two hydrogen atoms), up to three ATP molecules are synthesized.

SUMMARY OF ATP FORMATION DURING THE BREAKDOWN OF GLUCOSE

We can now determine the total number of ATP molecules formed by the energy from one molecule of glucose. The number is
1. Two during glycolysis
2. Two during the citric acid cycle and
3. During oxidative phosphorylation, 34, making a total of *38 ATP molecules* formed for each molecule of glucose degraded to carbon dioxide and water. Thus, 456,000 calories of energy are stored in the form of ATP, while 686,000 calories are released during the complete oxidation of each mole of glucose. This represents an overall *efficiency* of energy transfer of 66 per cent. The remaining 34 per cent of the energy becomes heat and therefore cannot be used by the cells to perform specific functions.

CONTROL OF GLYCOLYSIS AND OXIDATION BY ADENOSINE DIPHOSPHATE (ADP)

Continuous release of energy from glucose when the energy is not needed by the cells would be an extremely wasteful process. Fortunately, glycolysis and the subsequent oxidation of hydrogen atoms is continuously controlled in accordance with the needs of the cells for ATP. This control is accomplished only partially in the following manner:

Referring back to the various chemical reactions, we see that at different stages *ADP* is converted into *ATP. If ADP is not available at many of these stages, the reactions cannot occur, and the degradation of the glucose molecule is stopped.* Therefore, once all the ADP in the cells has been converted to ATP, the entire glycolytic and oxidative process stops. Then when more ATP is used to perform different physiological functions in the cell, new ADP is formed, which automatically turns on glycolysis and oxidation once more. In this way, essentially a full store of ATP is automatically maintained all the time, except when the activity of the cell becomes so great that ATP is used more rapidly than it can be formed.

ANAEROBIC RELEASE OF ENERGY— ANAEROBIC GLYCOLYSIS

Occasionally, oxygen becomes either unavailable or insufficient, so that cellular oxidation of glucose cannot take place. Yet, even under these conditions, a small amount of energy can still be released to the cells by glycolysis, for the chemical reactions in the glycolytic breakdown of glucose to pyruvic acid do not require oxygen. Unfortunately, this process is extremely wasteful of glucose because only 24,000 calories of energy are used to form ATP for each mole of glucose utilized, which represents only a little over 3 per cent of the total energy in the glucose molecule. Nevertheless, this release of glycolytic energy to the cells can be a lifesaving measure for a few minutes when oxygen becomes unavailable.

Formation of Lactic Acid During Anaerobic Glycolysis. The *law of mass action* states that as the end-products of a chemical reaction build up in a reacting medium the rate of the reaction approaches zero. The two end-products of the glycolytic reactions (see Figure 45–2) are (1) pyruvic acid and (2) hydrogen atoms in the forms NADH and H^+. The buildup of excessive amounts of these would stop the glycolytic process and prevent further formation of ATP. Fortunately, when their quantities begin to be excessive, these end-products react with each other to form lactic acid, in accordance with the following equation.

$$CH_3 - \overset{\displaystyle O}{\overset{\|}{C}} - COOH + NADH + H^+$$
(Pyruvic acid)

$$\xrightarrow[\text{dehydrogenase}]{\text{lactic}} CH_3 - \overset{\displaystyle OH}{\underset{\displaystyle H}{\overset{|}{\underset{|}{C}}}} - COOH + NAD^+$$
(Lactic acid)

Thus, under anaerobic conditions, by far the larger portion of the pyruvic acid is converted into lactic acid, which diffuses readily out of the cells into the extracellular fluids and even into the intracellular fluids of other less active cells. Therefore, lactic acid represents a type of "sinkhole" into which the glycolytic end-products can disappear, allowing glycolysis to proceed far longer than would be possible if the pyruvic acid and hydrogen were not removed from the reacting medium. Indeed, glycolysis could proceed for only a few seconds without this conversion. Instead, it can proceed for several minutes, supplying the body with considerable quantities of ATP even in the absence of respiratory oxygen.

When a person begins to breathe oxygen again after a period of anaerobic metabolism, the extra NADH and H^+ as well as the extra pyruvic acid that have built up in the body fluids are rapidly oxidized, mainly in the liver, thereby undergoing great reduction in their concentrations. As a result, the chemical reaction for formation of lactic acid immediately reverses itself, the lactic acid once again becoming pyruvic acid, which is eventually oxidized.

RELEASE OF ENERGY FROM GLUCOSE BY THE PHOSPHOGLUCONATE PATHWAY

Though essentially all the carbohydrates utilized by the muscles are degraded to pyruvic acid by glycolysis and then converted to carbon dioxide and hydrogen atoms by the citric acid cycle, this glycolytic and citric acid schema is not the only means by which glucose can be degraded to provide energy. A second important schema for glucose breakdown is called the *phosphogluconate pathway*. Though this process is not discussed here, it is responsible for as much as 30 per cent of the glucose breakdown in the liver and for even more than that in fat cells. It is especially important in providing energy and some of the substrates required for conversion of carbohydrates into fat, as will be discussed in the following chapter.

FORMATION OF CARBOHYDRATES FROM PROTEINS AND FATS— GLUCONEOGENESIS

When the body's stores of carbohydrates decrease below normal, moderate quantities of glucose can be formed from *amino acids* and from the *glycerol* portion of fat. This process is called *gluconeogenesis*. Approximately 60 per cent of the amino acids in the body proteins can easily be converted into carbohydrates, while the remaining 40 per cent have chemical configurations that make this difficult. Each amino acid is converted into glucose by a slightly different chemical process. For instance, alanine can be converted directly into pyruvic acid simply by deamination; the pyruvic acid then is converted into glucose by the liver.

Regulation of Gluconeogenesis. Diminished carbohydrates in the cells and decreased blood sugar are the basic stimuli that set off an increase in the rate of gluconeogenesis. The diminished carbohydrates can directly cause reversal of many of the glycolytic and phosphogluconate reactions, thus allowing conversion of deaminated amino acids and glycerol into carbohydrates. However, in addition, several of the hormones secreted by the endocrine glands are especially important in this regulation, as follows:

Effect of Corticotropin and Glucocorticoids on Gluconeogenesis. When normal quantities of carbohydrates are not available to the cells, the anterior pituitary gland, for reasons not yet completely understood, begins to secrete increased quantities of corticotropin, which stimulate the adrenal cortex to produce large quantities of *glucocorticoid hormones,* especially *cortisol*. In turn, cortisol mobilizes proteins from essentially all cells of the body, making them available in the form of amino acids in the body fluids. A high proportion of these immediately becomes deaminated in the liver and therefore provides ideal substrates for conversion into glucose. Thus, one of the most important means by which gluconeogenesis is promoted is through the release of glucocorticoids from the adrenal cortex.

Effect of Thyroxine on Gluconeogenesis. Thyroxine, secreted by the thyroid gland, also increases the rate of gluconeogenesis, though to a much smaller extent. This, too, is believed to result principally from mobilization of proteins from the cells. However, it may also result to some extent from the mobilization of fats from the fat depots, the glycerol portion of the fats being converted into glucose.

BLOOD GLUCOSE

The normal blood glucose concentration in a person who has not eaten a meal within the past three to four hours is approximately 90 mg per 100 ml of blood, and even after a meal containing large amounts of carbohydrates, this concentration rarely rises above 140 mg unless the person has diabetes mellitus.

The regulation of blood glucose concentration is intimately related to insulin and glucagon; this subject will be discussed fully in Chapter 52 in relation to the functions of these two hormones.

QUESTIONS

1. Describe the special features of the ATP molecule that allow it to function as an *energy currency*. At body temperature and at the concentrations of ATP found in the body cells, how much energy is present in each high energy phosphate bond per mole of ATP?

2. How is *glucose* transported through the cell membrane, and what is the effect of *insulin* on this transport?

3. How does *phosphorylation of glucose* cause the capture of glucose in the cell?

4. What is the composition of *glycogen,* and what is its role in cells, especially in the liver and in muscle?
5. Explain glycogenolysis and the release of glucose from liver when the glucose is needed elsewhere in the body.
6. Explain, in general, the *glycolytic pathway* for dissolution of the glucose molecule.
7. Describe the conversion of *pyruvic acid* to *acetyl coenzyme A* and the role of the *citric acid cycle* in converting the acetyl portion of the acetyl coenzyme A into carbon dioxide and hydrogen atoms.
8. Explain the *chemiosmotic mechanism* for formation of ATP in the *mitochondria.*

9. What percentage of the ATP normally used by the cell is formed by *oxidative phosphorylation?*
10. How does the concentration of *adenosine diphosphate* in the cells determine the rate of glycolysis?
11. Explain the mechanism and importance of *anaerobic glycolysis;* also explain the formation of *lactic acid* and tell why this is important to anaerobic glycolysis.
12. Explain what is meant by *gluconeogenesis,* how it is controlled, and its importance.
13. What is the normal resting blood glucose concentration, and how high does this rise after meals in the normal person?

References

Baer, H. P., and Drummond, G. I., eds.: Physiological and Regulatory Functions of Adenosine and Adenine Nucleotides. New York, Raven Press, 1979.

Butler, T. M., and Davies, R. E.: High-energy phosphates in smooth muscle. In Bohr, D. F., et al., eds.: Handbook of Physiology. Sec. 2, Vol. 2. Baltimore, Williams & Wilkins, 1980, p. 237.

Cornish-Bowden, A.: Fundamentals of Enzyme Kinetics. Boston, Butterworths, 1979.

Dickerson, R. E.: Cytochrome C and the evolution of energy metabolism. Sci Am 242(3):136, 1980.

Felig, P.: Disorders of carbohydrate metabolism. In Bondy, P. K., and Rosenberg, L. E., eds.: Metabolic Control and Disease, 8th ed. Philadelphia, W. B. Saunders Co., 1980, p. 276.

Friedmann, H. C., ed.: Enzymes. Stroudsburg, Pa., Dowden, Hutchinson & Ross, 1980.

Frohman, L. A.: CNS peptides and glucoregulation. Annu Rev Physiol 45:95, 1983.

Golinick, P. D.: Metabolism of substrates: Energy substrate metabolism during exercise and as modified by training. Fed Proc 44:353, 1985.

Hems, D. A., and Whitton, P. D.: Control of hepatic glycogenolysis. Physiol Rev 60:1, 1980.

Hetenyi, G., Jr., et al.: Turnover and precursor-product relationships of nonlipid metabolites. Physiol Rev 63:606, 1983.

Jacquez, J. A.: Red blood cell as glucose-carrier: significance for placental and cerebral glucose transfer. Am J Physiol 246:R289, 1984.

Kraus-Friedmann, N.: Hormonal regulation of hepatic gluconeogenesis. Physiol Rev 64:170, 1984.

Oomura, Y., and Yoshimatsu, H.: Neural network of glucose monitoring system. J Auton Nerv Syst 10:359, 1984.

Storlien, L. H.: The role of the ventromedial hypothalamic area in periprandial glucoregulation. Life-Sci 36:505, 1985.

Wang, J. H.: Coupling of proton flux to the hydrolysis and synthesis of ATP. Annu Rev Biophys Bioeng 12:21, 1983.

Wynn, C. H.: The Structure and Function of Enzymes, 2nd ed. Baltimore, University Park Press, 1979.

46

Lipid and Protein Metabolism

TRANSPORT OF LIPIDS IN THE BLOOD
  TRANSPORT FROM THE
    GASTROINTESTINAL TRACT—THE
    CHYLOMICRONS
TRANSPORT OF FATTY ACIDS IN
  COMBINATION WITH
  ALBUMIN—FREE FATTY ACID
  THE LIPOPROTEINS
THE FAT DEPOSITS
  ADIPOSE TISSUE
  THE LIVER LIPIDS
USE OF TRIGLYCERIDES FOR ENERGY
  AND FORMATION OF ADENOSINE
  TRIPHOSPHATE (ATP)
  FORMATION OF ACETOACETIC ACID
    IN THE LIVER AND ITS TRANSPORT
    IN THE BLOOD
  SYNTHESIS OF TRIGLYCERIDES FROM
    CARBOHYDRATES
  SYNTHESIS OF TRIGLYCERIDES FROM
    PROTEINS
  HORMONAL REGULATION OF FAT
    UTILIZATION

PHOSPHOLIPIDS AND CHOLESTEROL
  PHOSPHOLIPIDS
  CHOLESTEROL
  STRUCTURAL FUNCTIONS OF
    PHOSPHOLIPIDS AND
    CHOLESTEROL
ATHEROSCLEROSIS
THE BODY PROTEINS
  THE AMINO ACIDS
  FIBROUS PROTEINS
TRANSPORT AND STORAGE OF AMINO
  ACIDS
  THE BLOOD AMINO ACIDS
  STORAGE OF AMINO ACIDS AS
    PROTEINS IN THE CELLS
  THE PLASMA PROTEINS
CHEMISTRY OF PROTEIN SYNTHESIS
USE OF PROTEINS FOR ENERGY
  OBLIGATORY DEGRADATION OF
    PROTEINS

Several different chemical compounds in the food and in the body are classified as *lipids*. These include (1) *neutral fat*, known also as *triglycerides*, (2) *phospholipids*, (3) *cholesterol*, and (4) a few others of less importance. These substances have certain similar physical and chemical properties—especially, they are miscible with each other. Chemically, the basic lipid moiety of both the triglycerides and the phospholipids is *fatty acids*, which are simply long-chain hydrocarbon organic acids. Though cholesterol does not contain fatty acid, its sterol nucleus is synthesized from degradation products of fatty acid molecules, thus giving it many of the physical and chemical properties of other lipid substances.

The triglycerides are used in the body mainly to provide energy for the different metabolic processes; this function they share almost equally with the carbohydrates. However, some lipids, especially cholesterol, the phospholipids, and derivatives of these, are used throughout the body to provide other intracellular functions.

Basic Chemical Structure of Triglycerides (Neutral Fat). Since most of this chapter deals with utilization of triglycerides for energy, the following basic structure of the triglyceride molecule must be understood:

$$CH_3—(CH_2)_{16}—COO—CH_2$$
$$CH_3—(CH_2)_{16}—COO—CH$$
$$CH_3—(CH_2)_{16}—COO—CH_2$$
Tristearin

Note that three long-chain fatty acid molecules are bound with one molecule of glycerol.

TRANSPORT OF LIPIDS IN THE BLOOD

TRANSPORT FROM THE GASTROINTESTINAL TRACT—THE CHYLOMICRONS

It will be recalled from Chapter 44 that essentially all the fats of the diet are absorbed into the lymph in the form of *chylomicrons*, which have a size averaging 0.4 micron. The chylomicrons are then transported up the thoracic duct and emptied into the venous blood at the juncture of the jugular and subclavian veins.

Removal of the Chylomicrons from the Blood. The chylomicrons are removed from the plasma within an hour or so. Most are removed from the circulating blood as they pass through the capillaries of adipose tissue and the liver. The membranes of the fat cells contain large quantities of an enzyme called *lipoprotein lipase*. This enzyme hydrolyzes the triglycerides of the chylomicrons into fatty acids and glycerol. The fatty acids, being highly miscible with the membranes of the cells, immediately diffuse into the fat cells. Once within these cells, the fatty acids are resynthesized into triglycerides, new glycerol being supplied by the metabolic processes of the fat cells, as will be discussed later in the chapter.

TRANSPORT OF FATTY ACIDS IN COMBINATION WITH ALBUMIN—FREE FATTY ACID

When the fat that has been stored in the fat cells is to be used elsewhere in the body, usually for providing energy, it must first be transported to the other tissues. It is transported almost entirely in the form of *free fatty acid*, which is achieved by hydrolysis of the triglycerides stored in the fat cells, once again into fatty acids and glycerol. Although the stimulus for initiating this hydrolysis is not completely understood, it is known that a cellular lipase called *hormone-sensitive triglyceride lipase* becomes activated by one of several different means, and this activated lipase promotes rapid hydrolysis of the triglycerides.

On leaving the fat cells, the fatty acids ionize strongly in the plasma and immediately combine with albumin of the plasma proteins. The fatty acid bound with proteins in this manner is called *free fatty acid* or *nonesterified fatty acid* (or simply *FFA* or *NEFA*) to distinguish it from other fatty acids in the plasma that exist in the form of esters of glycerol, cholesterol, or other substances.

The concentration of free fatty acid in the plasma under resting conditions is about 15 mg per 100 ml of plasma, which is a total of only 0.45 gram of fatty acids in the entire circulatory system. Yet, strangely enough, even this small amount accounts for almost all of the transport of lipids from one part of the body to another, for the following reasons:

(1) Despite the minute amount of free fatty acid in the blood, its rate of turnover is extremely rapid, *half the plasma fatty acid being replaced by new fatty acid every two to three minutes*. One can calculate that at this rate over half of all the energy required by the body can be provided by the free fatty acid transported even without increasing the free fatty acid concentration. (2) All conditions that increase the rate of utilization of fat for cellular energy also increase the free fatty acid concentration in the blood; this concentration sometimes increases as much as five- to eightfold. Especially does this occur in starvation and in diabetes when a person is not using or cannot use carbohydrates for energy.

THE LIPOPROTEINS

In the postabsorptive state—that is, when no chylomicrons are in the blood—over 95 per cent of all the lipids in the plasma (in terms of mass, but *not* in terms of rate of transport) are in the form of lipoproteins, which are small particles much smaller than chylomicrons but similar in composition, containing mixtures of *triglycerides, phospholipids, cholesterol,* and *protein*. The protein in the mixture averages about one fourth to one third of the total constituents, and lipids form the remainder. The total concentration of lipoproteins in the plasma averages about 700 mg per 100 ml and can be broken down into the following average concentrations of the individual constituents:

	mg/100 ml of plasma
Cholesterol	180
Phospholipids	160
Triglycerides	160
Lipoprotein protein	200

Types of Lipoproteins. Chylomicrons sometimes are also classified as lipoproteins because they contain both lipids and protein. In addition to the chylomicrons, however, there are three other major classes of lipoprotein: (1) *very low density lipoproteins*, which contain high concentrations of triglycerides and moderate concentrations of both phospholipids and cholesterol; (2) *low density lipoproteins*, which contain relatively few triglycerides but a very high percentage of cholesterol; and (3) *high density lipoproteins*, which contain about 50 per cent protein with smaller concentrations of the lipids.

Formation of the Lipoproteins. The lipoproteins are formed almost entirely in the liver, which is in keeping with the fact that most plasma phospholipids, cholesterol, and triglycerides (except those in the chylomicrons) are synthesized in the liver.

Function of the Lipoproteins. The principal function of the lipoproteins in the plasma is to transport lipids throughout the body. For instance, the turnover of triglycerides in the lipoproteins is as much as several grams per hour and perhaps half this much turnover of cholesterol and phospholipids.

Triglycerides are synthesized mainly from carbohydrates in the liver and are transported to the adipose tissue and other peripheral tissues in the *very low density lipoproteins*. The *low density lipoproteins* are the residuals of the very low density lipoproteins after they have delivered most of their triglycerides to the adipose tissue, leaving large concentrations of cholesterol and phospholipids in the low density lipoproteins. On the other hand, the *high density lipoproteins* transport cholesterol away from the peripheral tissues and to the liver; therefore, this type of lipoprotein plays a very important role in preventing the development of atherosclerosis, which we shall discuss later in the chapter.

THE FAT DEPOSITS

ADIPOSE TISSUE

Large quantities of fat are frequently stored in two major tissues of the body, the adipose tissue and the liver. The adipose tissue is usually called the *fat deposits*, or simply the *fat depots*.

The major function of adipose tissue is storage of triglycerides until these are needed to provide energy elsewhere in the body. However, a subsidiary function is to provide heat insulation for the body, as is discussed in Chapter 47.

The Fat Cells. The fat cells of adipose tissue are modified fibroblasts that are capable of storing almost pure triglycerides in quantities equal to 80 to 95 per cent of their volume.

Fat cells can also synthesize small quantities of fatty acids and triglycerides from carbohydrates, this function supplementing the synthesis of fat in the liver, as discussed later in the chapter.

Exchange of Fat Between the Adipose Tissue and the Blood—Tissue Lipases. As discussed previously, large quantities of lipases are present in adipose tissue. Some of these enzymes catalyze the deposition of triglycerides derived from the chylomicrons and other lipoproteins. Others, when activated by hormones, cause splitting of the triglycerides of the fat cells to release free fatty acids. Because of rapid exchanges of the fatty acids, the triglycerides in the fat cells are renewed approximately once every two to three weeks, which means that the fat stored in the tissues today is not the same fat that was stored last month, thus emphasizing the dynamic state of the storage fat.

THE LIVER LIPIDS

The principal functions of the liver in lipid metabolism are (1) to degrade fatty acids into small compounds that can be used for energy, (2) to synthesize triglycerides mainly from carbohydrates and, to a lesser extent, from proteins, and (3) to synthesize other lipids from fatty acids, especially cholesterol and phospholipids.

The liver cells, in addition to containing triglycerides, contain large quantities of phospholipids and cholesterol, which are continually synthesized by the liver. Also, the liver cells are much more capable than other tissues of desaturating fatty acids, so that the liver triglycerides normally are much more unsaturated than the triglycerides of the adipose tissue. This capability of the liver to desaturate fatty acids seems to be functionally important to all the tissues of the body, because many of the structural members of all cells contain reasonable quantities of desaturated fats, and their principal source is the liver. This desaturation is accomplished by a *dehydrogenase* in the liver cells.

USE OF TRIGLYCERIDES FOR ENERGY AND FORMATION OF ADENOSINE TRIPHOSPHATE (ATP)

Approximately 40 to 45 per cent of the calories in the normal American diet are derived from fats, which amount is about equal to the calories derived from carbohydrates. Therefore, the use of fats by the body for energy is just as important as the use of carbohydrates. In addition, much of the carbohydrates ingested with each meal is converted into triglycerides, then stored, and later utilized as triglycerides for energy.

Entry of Fatty Acids into the Mitochondria. The degradation and oxidation of fatty acids occur only in the mitochondria. Therefore, the first step in the utilization of the fatty acids is their transport into the mitochondria. This is an enzyme-catalyzed process that employs *carnitine* as a carrier substance. Once inside the mitochondria, the fatty acid splits away from the carnitine and is then oxidized.

Degradation of Fatty Acid to Acetyl Coenzyme A by Beta Oxidation. The fatty acid molecule is degraded in the mitochondria by progressive release of 2-carbon segments to form acetyl coenzyme A (acetyl Co-A). This process is illustrated in Figure 46–1; it is called the *beta oxidation* mechanism for degradation of fatty acids. Each time the reactions of this schema go through a complete cycle, beginning at the top left-hand corner of the figure and proceeding to the bottom right-hand corner, a new acetyl Co-A molecule is formed, and the fatty acid chain becomes two carbon atoms shorter. The process is repeated again and again until the entire fatty acid molecule is split into acetyl Co-A. For instance, from each molecule of stearic acid, nine molecules of acetyl Co-A are formed.

Oxidation of Acetyl Co-A. The acetyl Co-A molecules formed by this beta oxidation of fatty acids enter the citric acid cycle, as explained in the preceding chapter and are degraded into carbon dioxide and hydrogen atoms. The hydrogen is subsequently oxidized by the oxidative enzymes of the mitochondria to form ATP.

Quantity of ATP Formed by Oxidation of Fatty Acid. In Figure 46–1 note that 4 hydrogen atoms are released each time a molecule of acetyl Co-A is formed from the fatty acid chain. Then additional hydrogen is released in the citric acid cycle. The oxidation of all these hydrogen atoms gives rise to the formation of 139 molecules of ATP *for each stearic acid molecule oxidized*. Also, another 7 mol-

(1) $RCH_2CH_2CH_2COOH + Co\text{-}A + ATP \xrightleftharpoons{\text{thiokinase}} RCH_2CH_2CH_2COCo\text{-}A + AMP + \text{Pyrophosphate}$
    (Fatty acid)   (Fatty acyl Co-A)

(2) $RCH_2CH_2CH_2COCo\text{-}A + FAD \xrightarrow{\text{acyl dehydrogenase}} RCH_2CH{=}CHCOCo\text{-}A + FADH_2$
    (Fatty acyl Co-A)

(3) $RCH_2CH{=}CHCOCo\text{-}A + H_2O \xrightleftharpoons{\text{enoyl hydrase}} RCH_2CHOHCH_2COCo\text{-}A$

(4) $RCH_2CHOHCH_2COCo\text{-}A + NAD^+ \xrightleftharpoons[\text{dehydrogenase}]{\beta\text{-hydroxyacyl}} RCH_2COCH_2COCo\text{-}A + NADH + H^+$

(5) $RCH_2COCH_2COCo\text{-}A + Co\text{-}A \xrightleftharpoons{\text{thiolase}} RCH_2COCo\text{-}A + CH_3COCo\text{-}A$
                                            (Fatty acyl Co-A)(Acetyl Co-A)

Figure 46–1. Beta oxidation of fatty acids to yield acetylcoenzyme A.

ecules of ATP are formed in other ways during this entire process, making a total of 146 molecules of ATP.

FORMATION OF ACETOACETIC ACID IN THE LIVER AND ITS TRANSPORT IN THE BLOOD

A large share of the degradation of fatty acids into acetyl Co-A occurs in the liver. However, the liver uses only a small proportion of the acetyl Co-A for its own intrinsic metabolic processes. Instead, pairs of acetyl Co-A condense to form molecules of *acetoacetic acid*, as follows:

$$2CH_3COCo\text{-}A + H_2O$$
Acetyl Co-A

$$\xrightleftharpoons[\text{other cells}]{\text{liver cells}}$$

$$CH_3COCH_2COOH + 2HCo\text{-}A$$
Acetoacetic acid

Then a large part of the acetoacetic acid is converted into β-*hydroxybutyric acid,* and minute quantities to *acetone,* in accordance with the following reactions:

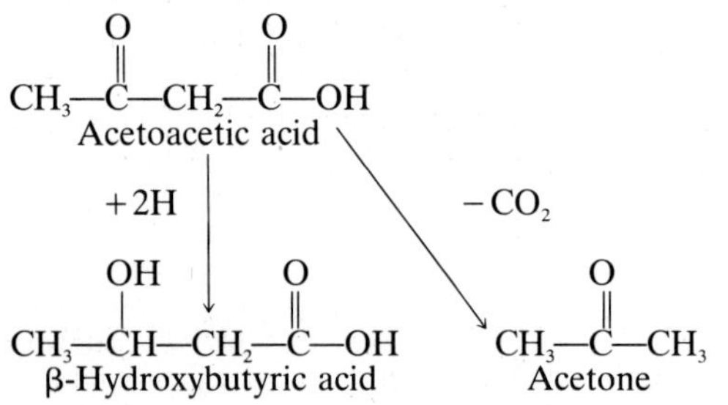

$$CH_3-\overset{\overset{\displaystyle O}{\|}}{C}-CH_2-\overset{\overset{\displaystyle O}{\|}}{C}-OH$$
Acetoacetic acid

$$+2H \qquad\qquad -CO_2$$

$$CH_3-\overset{\overset{\displaystyle OH}{|}}{C}H-CH_2-\overset{\overset{\displaystyle O}{\|}}{C}-OH \qquad CH_3-\overset{\overset{\displaystyle O}{\|}}{C}-CH_3$$
β-Hydroxybutyric acid   Acetone

The acetoacetic acid and β-hydroxybutyric acid then freely diffuse through the liver cell membranes and are transported by the blood to the peripheral tissues. Here they again diffuse into the cells, where reverse reactions occur and acetyl Co-A molecules are formed. These in turn enter the citric acid cycle and are oxidized for energy, as explained previously.

SYNTHESIS OF TRIGLYCERIDES FROM CARBOHYDRATES

Whenever a greater quantity of carbohydrates enters the body than can be used immediately for energy or stored in the form of glycogen, the excess is rapidly converted into triglycerides and is then stored in this form in the adipose tissue. Most triglyceride synthesis occurs in the liver, but smaller quantities are also synthesized in the adipose tissue. The triglycerides that are formed in the liver are then mainly transported by the lipoproteins to the adipose tissue to be stored until needed for energy.

Conversion of Acetyl Co-A into Fatty Acids. The first step in the synthesis of triglycerides is conversion of carbohydrates into acetyl Co-A. It will be recalled from the preceding chapter that this conversion occurs during the normal degradation of glucose by the glycolytic system. It will also be remembered from earlier in this chapter that fatty acids are actually large polymers of the acetyl portion of acetyl Co-A. Therefore, without going into the details of the chemical reactions, it is easy to understand how acetyl Co-A can be converted into fatty acids.

Combination of Fatty Acids with α-Glycerophosphate to Form Triglycerides. Once the synthesized fatty acid chains have grown to contain 14 to 18 carbon atoms, they then automatically bind with glycerol to form triglycerides.

The glycerol portion of the triglyceride is furnished by α-glycerophosphate, which is also a product derived from the glycolytic schema of glucose degradation, illustrated in Figure 45–2 (Chapter 45).

The real importance of this mechanism for formation of triglycerides is that the whole process is controlled to a great extent by the concentration of α-glycerophosphate, which in turn is determined by the availability of carbohydrates. When carbohydrates form large quantities of α-glycerophosphate, the equilibrium shifts to promote formation and storage of triglycerides.

Importance of Fat Synthesis and Storage. Fat synthesis from carbohydrates is especially important for two reasons: (1) The ability of the different cells of the body to store carbohydrates in the form of glycogen is generally slight; only a few hundred grams of glycogen are stored in the liver, the skeletal muscles, and all other tissues of the body put together. Therefore, fat synthesis provides a means by which the energy of excess ingested carbohydrates (and proteins, too) can be stored for later use. Indeed, the average person has about 200 times as much energy stored in the form of fat as in the form of carbohydrate. (2) Each gram of fat contains approximately two and one fourth times as many calories of useable energy as each gram of glycogen. Therefore, for a given weight gain, a person can store far more energy in the form of fat than in the form of carbohydrate, which is important when an animal must be highly motile to survive.

SYNTHESIS OF TRIGLYCERIDES FROM PROTEINS

Many amino acids can be converted into acetyl Co-A, as will be discussed later in the chapter. Obviously, this too can be converted into triglycerides. Therefore, when persons have more proteins in their diet than their tissues can use as proteins or directly for energy, a large share of the excess is stored as fat.

HORMONAL REGULATION OF FAT UTILIZATION

At least seven of the hormones secreted by the endocrine glands have marked effects on fat utilization.

Probably the most dramatic increase that occurs in fat utilization is that observed during heavy exercise. This results almost entirely from rapid release of *epinephrine* and *norepinephrine* by the adrenal medullae during exercise, as a result of sympathetic stimulation. These two hormones directly activate *hormone-sensitive triglyceride lipase*, which is present in abundance in the fat cells. This activated hormone then causes very rapid breakdown of triglycerides and mobilization of fatty acids. Sometimes the free fatty acid concentration in the blood rises as much as five- to eightfold. Other types of stress that activate the sympathetic nervous system will increase fatty acid mobilization and utilization in a similar manner.

Stress also causes large quantities of *corticotropin* to be released by the anterior pituitary gland, and this release in turn causes the adrenal cortex to secrete excessive quantities of *glucocorticoids*. Both the corticotropin and glucocorticoids activate either the same hormone-sensitive triglyceride lipase as that activated by epinephrine and norepinephrine or a similar lipase, which therefore is still another mechanism for increasing the release of fatty acids from fat tissue.

Growth hormone has an effect similar to but less effective than that of corticotropin and glucocorticoids in activating the hormone-sensitive lipase. Therefore, growth hormone can also have a mild fat-mobilizing effect.

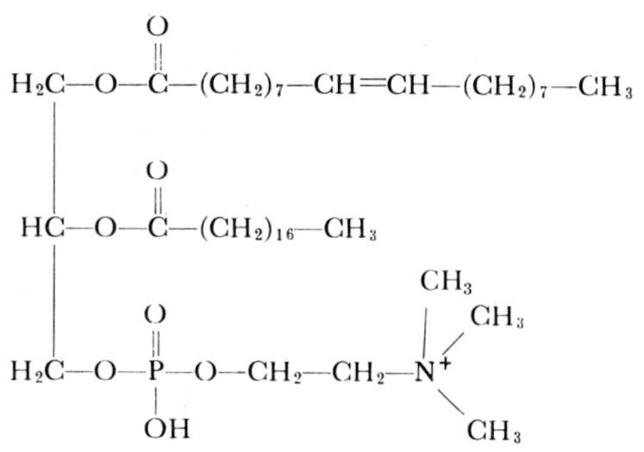

Figure 46–2. A lecithin.

Lack of insulin also activates hormone-sensitive lipase and therefore causes rapid mobilization of fatty acids. When carbohydrates are not available in the diet, insulin secretion diminishes, and this in turn promotes fatty acid metabolism.

Finally, *thyroid hormone* causes rapid mobilization of fat, a process that is believed to result indirectly from an increased rate of energy metabolism in all cells of the body under the influence of this hormone.

The effects of the different hormones on metabolism are discussed further in the chapters dealing with each of them.

PHOSPHOLIPIDS AND CHOLESTEROL

PHOSPHOLIPIDS

The three major types of body phospholipids are the *lecithins*, the *cephalins*, and the *sphingomyelins*. A lecithin is shown in Figure 46–2.

Phospholipids always contain one or more fatty acid molecules and one phosphoric acid radical, and they usually contain a nitrogenous base. Though the chemical structures of phospholipids vary somewhat, their physical properties are similar, for they are lipid soluble, are transported together in lipoproteins in the blood, and seem to be utilized similarly throughout the body for various structural purposes.

Phospholipids are formed in essentially all cells of the body, though certain cells have a special ability to form them. Probably 90 per cent or more of the phospholipids enter the blood in the lipoproteins that are formed in the liver cells.

CHOLESTEROL

Cholesterol, the formula of which is illustrated in Figure 46–3, is present in the diet of all persons, and it can be absorbed from the gastrointestinal tract into the intestinal lymph. It is highly fat soluble but only slightly soluble in water, and it is capable of forming esters with fatty acids. Indeed, approximately 70 per cent of the cholesterol of the plasma is in the form of cholesterol esters.

Besides the cholesterol absorbed each day from the gastrointestinal tract, which is called *exogenous cholesterol*, a large quanity, called *endogenous choles-*

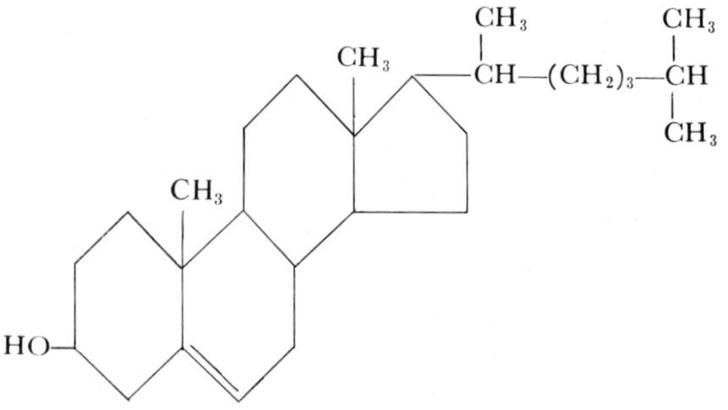

Figure 46–3. Cholesterol.

terol, is formed in the cells of the body. Essentially all the endogenous cholesterol that circulates in the lipoproteins of the plasma is formed by the liver, but all the other cells of the body form at least some cholesterol.

STRUCTURAL FUNCTIONS OF PHOSPHOLIPIDS AND CHOLESTEROL

In Chapter 2 it was pointed out that large quantities of phospholipids and cholesterol are present in the cell membrane as well as in the membranes of the internal organelles of all cells.

For membranes to be formed, substances that are not soluble in water must be available, and in general, the only substances in the body that are not soluble in water (besides the inorganic substances of bone) are mainly the lipids and some proteins. Thus, the physical integrity of cells throughout the body is based mainly on phospholipids, triglycerides, cholesterol, and certain insoluble proteins. Some phospholipids are somewhat water soluble as well as lipid soluble, which gives them the important property of helping to decrease the interfacial tension between the membranes and the surrounding fluids.

Another fact indicating that phospholipids and cholesterol are mainly concerned with the formation of structural elements of the cells is the slow turnover rate of these substances. For instance, phospholipids formed in the brain remain there for many months or perhaps even for years.

ATHEROSCLEROSIS

Atherosclerosis is principally a disease of the large arteries in which lipid deposits called *atheromatous plaques* appear in the intimal and subintimal layers of the arteries. These plaques contain an especially large amount of cholesterol and often are simply called *cholesterol deposits*. They are also associated with degenerative changes in the arterial wall. In a later stage of the disease, fibroblasts infiltrate the degenerative areas and cause progressive sclerosis of the arteries. In addition, calcium often precipitates with the lipids to develop *calcified plaques*. When these two processes occur, the arteries become extremely hard, and the disease is then called *arteriosclerosis*, or simply "hardening of the arteries."

Obviously, arteriosclerotic arteries lose most of their distensibility, and because of the degenerative areas, they are easily ruptured. Also, the atheromatous plaques often break through the intima and protrude into the flowing blood, and the roughness of their surfaces causes blood clots to develop, with resultant thrombus or embolus formation (see Chapter 21). Almost half of all human beings die of some complication of arteriosclerosis; approximately two thirds of these deaths are caused by thrombosis of one or more coronary arteries and the remaining one third by thrombosis or hemorrhage of vessels in other organs of the body—especially the brain, kidneys, liver, gastrointestinal tract, limbs, and so forth.

Effects of Age, Sex, and Heredity on Atherosclerosis. Atherosclerosis is mainly a disease of old age, but small atheromatous plaques can almost always be found in the arteries of young adults. Therefore, the full-blown disease is a culmination of a lifetime of lipid deposition rather than deposition over a few years.

Far more men die of atherosclerotic heart disease than do women. This is especially true of men younger than 50. For this reason, it is possible that the male sex hormone accelerates the development of atherosclerosis, or that the female sex hormone *protects* a person from atherosclerosis.

Atherosclerosis and atherosclerotic heart disease are highly hereditary in some families. In some instances, this is related to an inherited hypercholesterolemia, the excess cholesterol occurring almost entirely in the *low density lipoproteins*. The liver is unable to remove cholesterol from these lipoproteins. Therefore, much of the excess cholesterol is deposited in the arterial wall. Inheritance of the tendency to atherosclerosis is sometimes caused by dominant genes, which means that once this dominant trait enters a family a high incidence of the disease occurs among the offspring.

Relationship of Dietary Fat to Atherosclerosis in the Human Being. A high fat, high calorie diet, especially one containing cholesterol and saturated fats, greatly increases one's chances of developing atherosclerosis. Therefore, decreasing the fat and the calories in the diet can help greatly in protecting against atherosclerosis. Indeed, life insurance statistics show that the rate of mortality—mainly from coronary disease—of normal or low weight middle age and older persons is about half the mortality rate of overweight subjects of the same age.

THE BODY PROTEINS

About three quarters of the body solids are proteins. These include *structural proteins, enzymes, genes, proteins that transport oxygen, proteins of the muscle that cause contraction*, and many other types that perform specific functions both intracellularly and extracellularly throughout the body.

The basic chemical properties that explain the diverse functions of proteins are so extensive that they constitute a major portion of the entire discipline of biochemistry. For this reason, the present discussion is confined to the general aspects of protein metabolism.

THE AMINO ACIDS

The principal constituents of proteins are amino acids, 20 of which are present in the body in significant quantities. Figure 46–4 illustrates the chemical for-

mulas of these 20 amino acids, showing that they all have two features in common: Each amino acid has an acidic group (—COOH) and a nitrogen radical that lies in close association with the acidic radical, usually represented by the amino group (—NH$_2$).

Peptide Linkages and Peptide Chains. In proteins, the amino acids are aggregated into long chains by means of so-called *peptide linkages*, one of which is illustrated by the reaction on the following page:

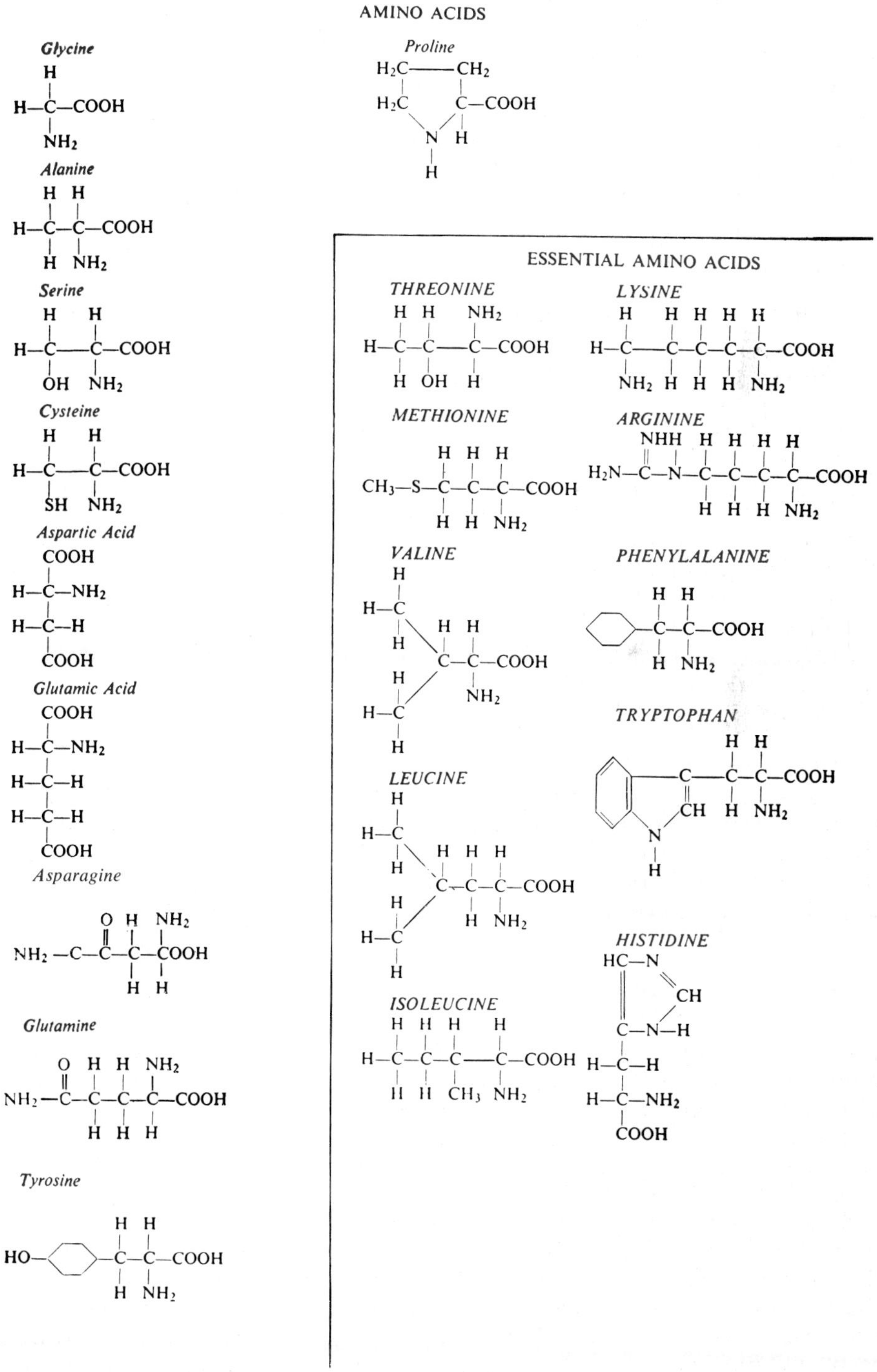

Figure 46–4. The amino acids, showing the 10 essential amino acids, which cannot be synthesized at all or in sufficient quantity in the body.

$$NH_2 \qquad\qquad NH_2$$
$$R{-}CH{-}COOH + R'{-}CH{-}COOH$$

$$NH_2$$
$$\longrightarrow R{-}CH{-}CO \qquad\qquad + H_2O$$
$$NH$$
$$R'{-}CH{-}COOH$$

Note that in this reaction the amino radical of one amino acid combines with the carboxyl radical of the other amino acid. A hydrogen atom is released from the amino radical, a hydroxyl radical is released from the carboxyl radical, and these two combine to form a molecule of water. Note that after the peptide linkage has been formed, an amino radical and a carboxyl radical are still in the new molecule, both of which are capable of combining with additional amino acids to form a *peptide chain.* Some complicated protein molecules have as many as a hundred thousand amino acids joined principally by peptide linkages, and even the smallest protein usually has more than 20 amino acids joined by peptide linkages.

FIBROUS PROTEINS

Many of the highly complex proteins are fibrillar and are called fibrous proteins. In these, many separate chains are held together in parallel bundles by cross-linkages. Major types of fibrous proteins are (1) *collagens,* which are the basic structural proteins of connective tissue, tendons, cartilage, and bone; (2) *elastins,* which are the elastic fibers of tendons, arteries, and connective tissue; (3) *keratins,* which are the structural proteins of hair and nails; and (4) *actin* and *myosin,* the contractile proteins of muscle.

TRANSPORT AND STORAGE OF AMINO ACIDS

THE BLOOD AMINO ACIDS

The normal concentration of amino acids in the blood is between 35 and 65 mg per 100 ml of plasma. This is an average of about 2 mg per 100 ml for each of the 20 amino acids, though some are present in far greater concentrations than others. Since the amino acids are relatively strong acids, they exist in the blood principally in the ionized state and account for 2 to 3 milliequivalents of the negative ions in the blood.

Fate of Amino Acids Absorbed from the Gastrointestinal Tract. It will be recalled from Chapter 44 that the end-products of protein digestion in the gastrointestinal tract are almost entirely amino acids and that polypeptide or protein molecules are only rarely absorbed into the blood. Immediately after a meal, the amino acid concentration in the blood rises, but the rise is usually only a few milligrams per 100 ml because, after entering the blood, the excess amino acids are absorbed within five to ten minutes by cells throughout the entire body. Therefore, almost never do large concentrations of amino acids accumulate in the blood. Nevertheless, the turnover rate of the amino acids is so rapid that many grams of proteins in the form of amino acids can be carried from one part of the body to another each hour.

Transport of Amino Acids into the Cells. The molecules of essentially all the amino acids are much too large to diffuse through the pores of the cell membranes. Instead, the amino acids are transported through the membrane only by active transport or facilitated diffusion, utilizing carrier mechanisms. The nature of the carrier mechanisms is still poorly understood, but some are discussed in Chapter 4.

STORAGE OF AMINO ACIDS AS PROTEINS IN THE CELLS

Almost immediately after entry into the cells, amino acids are conjugated under the influence of intracellular enzymes into cellular proteins, so that the concentration of amino acids inside the cells probably always remains low. Thus, so far as is known, storage of large quantities of amino acids as such probably does not occur in the cells; instead, they are mainly stored in the form of actual proteins. Yet many intracellular proteins can be rapidly decomposed again into amino acids under the influence of intracellular lysosomal digestive enzymes, and these amino acids in turn can be transported again from the cell into the blood. The proteins that can be thus decomposed include many cellular enzymes as well as some other functioning proteins. However, most of the structural proteins such as collagen and muscle contractile proteins do not participate significantly in this reversible storage of amino acids.

Some tissues of the body participate in the storage of amino acids to a greater extent than others. For instance, the liver, which is a large organ and also has special systems for processing amino acids, stores large quantities of labile proteins; this is also true of the kidney and the intestinal mucosa.

Release of Amino Acids from the Cells and Regulation of Plasma Amino Acid Concentration. Whenever the plasma amino acid concentration falls below its normal level, amino acids are transported out of the cells to replenish the supply in the plasma. Simultaneously, intracellular proteins are degraded back into amino acids.

The plasma concentration of each type of amino acid is maintained at a reasonably constant value. Later it will be noted that the various hormones secreted by the endocrine glands are able to alter the balance between tissue proteins and circulating amino acids; growth hormone and insulin increase the formation of tissue proteins, while the adrenocortical glucocorticoid hormones increase the concentration of circulating amino acids.

THE PLASMA PROTEINS

The three major types of protein in the plasma are *albumin, globulin,* and *fibrinogen.* The principal function of albumin is to provide *colloid osmotic pressure,* which in turn prevents plasma loss from the capillaries, as discussed in Chapter 22. The globulins perform a number of enzymatic functions in the plasma itself, but more important than this, they are mainly responsible for both natural and acquired *immunity* against invading organisms, a subject discussed in Chapter 20. The fibrinogen polymerizes into long, branching fibrin threads during *blood coagulation,* thereby forming blood clots that help to repair leaks in the circulatory system, discussed in Chapter 21.

Formation of the Plasma Proteins. Essentially all the albumin and fibrinogen in the plasma proteins, as well as about one half of the globulins, are formed in the liver. The remainder of the globulins are formed principally in the lymphoid tissues and bone marrow. These are mainly the *gamma globulins* that constitute the antibodies.

The rate of plasma protein formation by the liver can be extremely high, as much as 50 grams per day. Certain disease conditions often cause rapid loss of plasma proteins; severe burns that denude large surface areas cause loss of many liters of plasma through the denuded areas each day. The rapid production of plasma proteins by the liver is obviously valuable in preventing death in such states. Furthermore, occasionally, a person with severe renal disease loses as much as 20 grams of plasma protein in the urine each day for months, and these are continually replaced.

Use of Plasma Proteins by the Tissue. When the tissues become depleted of proteins, the plasma proteins can act as a source for rapid replacement of these proteins. Indeed, whole plasma proteins can be imbibed *in toto* by the liver cells and macrophages; then they are split into amino acids that are transported back into the blood and utilized throughout the body to build cellular proteins. In this way, therefore, the plasma proteins function as a labile protein storage medium and represent a rapidly available source of amino acids whenever a particular tissue requires them.

CHEMISTRY OF PROTEIN SYNTHESIS

Proteins are synthesized in all cells of the body, and the functional characteristics of each cell are dependent upon the types of protein that it can form. Basically, the genes of the cells control the protein types and thereby control the functions of the cell. This regulation of cellular function by the genes was discussed in detail in Chapter 3. Chemically, two basic processes must be accomplished for the synthesis of proteins; these are (1) synthesis of the amino acids and (2) appropriate conjugation of the amino acids to form the respective types of whole proteins in each individual cell.

Essential and Nonessential Amino Acids. Ten of the twenty amino acids normally present in animal proteins can be synthesized in the cells, while the other ten either cannot be synthesized at all or are synthesized in quantities too small to supply the body's needs. The first group of amino acids is called *nonessential,* while the second group is called *essential amino acids* because these must be present in the diet if protein formation is to take place in the body. Use of the word *essential* does not mean that the other 10 amino acids are not equally essential in the formation of the proteins, but only that these others are not essential in the diet.

Synthesis of the nonessential amino acids depends on the formation, first, of appropriate α-keto acids, which are the precursors of the respective amino acids. For instance, *pyruvic acid,* which is formed in large quantities during the glycolytic breakdown of glucose, is the keto acid precursor of the amino acid *alanine.* Then, by the simple process of *transamination,* an amino radical is transferred to the α-keto acid to form the alanine molecule while the keto oxygen is transferred to the donor of the amino radical.

Formation of Proteins from Amino Acids. Once the appropriate amino acids are present in a cell, whole proteins are synthesized rapidly. However, each peptide linkage requires from 500 to 4000 calories of energy, and this must be supplied from ATP and GTP (guanosine triphosphate) in the cell. Protein formation proceeds through two steps: (1) "activation" of each amino acid, during which the amino acid is "energized" by energy derived from ATP and GTP, and (2) alignment of the amino acids into the peptide chains, a function that is under control of the DNA-RNA system of each individual cell. Both of these processes were discussed in Chapter 3. Indeed, the formation of cellular proteins is the basis of life itself and is so important that the reader would do well to review Chapter 3.

USE OF PROTEINS FOR ENERGY

There is an upper limit to the amount of protein that can accumulate in each particular type of cell. Once the cells are filled to their limits, the feedback controls of the DNA-RNA system block further protein synthesis, as explained in Chapter 3, and any additional amino acids in the body fluids are degraded and used for energy or are stored, as fat. This degradation occurs almost entirely in the liver, and it begins with the process known as deamination.

Deamination. Deamination means removal of the amino groups from the amino acids. This can occur by several different means, two of which are especially important: (1) transamination, which means transfer of the amino group to some acceptor substance (as explained earlier in relation to the synthesis of amino acids) and (2) oxidative deamination.

The greatest amount of deamination occurs by the following transamination schema:

$$\alpha\text{-ketoglutaric acid } + \text{ amino acid}$$
$$\text{glutamic acid } + \alpha\text{-keto acid}$$
$$+ NAD^+ + H_2O$$
$$\longrightarrow NADH + H^+ + NH_3$$

Note from this schema that the amino group from the amino acid is transferred to α-ketoglutaric acid, which then becomes glutamic acid. The glutamic acid can then transfer the amino group to still other substances or can release it in the form of ammonia. In the process of losing the amino group, the glutamic acid once again becomes α-ketoglutaric acid, so that the cycle can be repeated again and again.

Urea Formation by the Liver. The ammonia released during deamination is removed from the blood almost entirely by conversion into urea, two molecules of ammonia and one molecule of carbon dioxide combining in accordance with the following net reaction:

$$2NH_3 + CO_2 \rightarrow H_2N\!-\!\underset{\underset{O}{\|}}{C}\!-\!NH_2 + H_2O$$

Essentially all urea formed in the human body is synthesized in the liver. In the absence of the liver or in serious liver disease, ammonia accumulates in the blood. This in turn is extremely toxic, especially to the brain, often leading to a state called *hepatic coma.*

The stages in the formation of urea are essentially the following:

Ornithine $+ CO_2 + NH_3$
$\xrightarrow{\;\;\;\;\;\;\;\;\;\;\;}$ Citrulline
$- H_2O$
$+ NH_3$
$- H_2O$
Arginine
$+ H_2O$
(Arginase)
Urea

The reaction begins with the amino acid derivative *ornithine*, which combines with one molecule of carbon dioxide and one molecule of ammonia to form a second substance, *citrulline*. This in turn combines with still another molecule of ammonia to form *arginine*, which then splits into *ornithine* and *urea*. The urea diffuses from the liver cells into the body fluids and is excreted by the kidneys, while the ornithine is reused in the cycle again and again.

Oxidation of Deaminated Amino Acids. Once the amino acids have been deaminated, the resulting keto acid products can in most instances be oxidized to release energy for metabolic purposes. This usually involves two processes: (1) The keto acid is changed into an appropriate chemical substance that can enter the citric acid cycle, and (2) this substance is then degraded by this cycle in the same manner that acetyl Co-A derived from carbohydrate and fat metabolism is degraded.

In general, the amount of adenosine triphosphate formed for each gram of protein that is oxidized is slightly less than that formed for each gram of glucose oxidized.

Gluconeogenesis and Ketogenesis. Certain deaminated amino acids are similar to the breakdown products that result from glucose and fatty acid metabolism. For instance, deaminated alanine is pyruvic acid. Obviously, it can be converted into glucose or glycogen; or it can be converted into acetyl Co-A, which can then be polymerized into fatty acids. Also, two molecules of acetyl Co-A can condense to form acetoacetic acid, which is one of the so-called keto acids, as explained earlier in the chapter.

The conversion of amino acids into glucose or glycogen is called *gluconeogenesis,* and the conversion of amino acids into keto acids or fatty acids is called *ketogenesis.* Eighteen of twenty of the deaminated amino acids have chemical structures that allow them to be converted into glucose, and nineteen can be converted into fats—five directly and the other fourteen by becoming carbohydrate first and then becoming fat.

OBLIGATORY DEGRADATION OF PROTEINS

When a person eats no proteins, a certain proportion of his own body proteins continues to be degraded into amino acids, deaminated, and oxidized. This process involves 20 to 30 grams of protein each day, which is called the *obligatory loss* of proteins. Therefore, to prevent a net loss of protein from the body, one must ingest at least 20 to 30 grams of protein each day, and to be on the safe side 60 to 75 grams is usually recommended.

Effect of Starvation on Protein Degradation. Except for the excess protein in the diet or the 20 to 30 grams of obligatory protein degradation each day, the body normally uses almost entirely carbohydrates or fats for energy as long as they are available. However, after several weeks of starvation, when the quantity of stored fats begins to run out, the amino acids of the blood begin to be rapidly deaminated and oxidized for energy. From this point on, the proteins of the tissues degrade rapidly—as much as 125 grams daily—and the cellular functions deteriorate precipitously.

Because carbohydrate and fat utilization for energy occurs in preference to protein utilization, carbohydrates and fats are called *protein sparers.*

QUESTIONS

1. Explain how *fatty acid molecules* combine with *glycerol* to form *triglycerides*.
2. Describe the transport of fats from the digestive tract to the blood and their ultimate deposition in the fat stores of the body.
3. Explain how tremendous quantities of fatty acids can be transported in the free fatty acid form by the plasma protein *albumin* even though the concentration of these fatty acids is very slight.
4. Explain what is meant by a *lipoprotein,* and also explain in general the function of lipoproteins in the blood.
5. Describe the storage and release of fats from *adipose tissue,* including the function of *hormone-sensitive lipase.*
6. Explain the general schema for beta oxidation of the fatty acid molecule.
7. What is the role of *acetoacetic acid* in the transport of fat degradation products to peripheral cells?
8. How are carbohydrates converted into triglycerides, and what controls this process?
9. Explain how the different hormones affect fat utilization.
10. What are the functions of *phospholipids* and *chlolesterol* in the body?
11. Describe the development of *atherosclerosis* and *arteriosclerosis* in the arteries of older persons, and explain the effects of age, sex, heredity, and diet on these processes.
12. Explain the *peptide linkage* mechanism for the formation of *peptide chains.*
13. How are amino acids transported in the blood, and how are they stored in cells?
14. Explain how amino acids stored in cells can be released for use elsewhere in the body, and also explain how the plasma proteins can be used to provide amino acids for the body's cells.
15. What is meant by an *essential amino acid*?
16. Explain the processes of *deamination* and *urea formation* as one of the initial steps in the utilization of proteins for energy.
17. What is meant by *gluconeogenesis* and *ketogenesis* in relation to the utilization of amino acids?
18. What is meant by the *obligatory loss of proteins*? How great is this loss normally, and how great can it become in starvation?

References

Lipid Metabolism

Benditt, E. P.: The origin of atherosclerosis. Sci Am 236(2):74, 1977.

Bisgaier, C., and Glickman, R. M.: Intestinal synthesis, secretion, and transport of lipoproteins. Annu Rev Physiol 45:625, 1983.

Bremer, J.: Carnitine—metabolism and functions. Physiol Rev 63:1420, 1983.

Carey, M. C., et al.: Lipid digestion and absorption. Annu Rev Physiol 45:651, 1983.

Chan, L.: Hormonal control of apolipoprotein synthesis. Annu Rev Physiol 45:615, 1983.

Fitzgerald, F. T.: The problem of obesity. Annu Rev Physiol 32:21, 1981.

Golinick, P. D.: Metabolism of substrates: energy substrate metabolism during exercise and as modified by training. Fed Proc 44:353, 1985.

Grundy, S. M.: Absorption and metabolism of dietary cholesterol. Annu Rev Nutr 3:71, 1983.

Havel, R. J., and Kane, J. P.: Therapy of hyperlipidemic states. Annu Rev Med 33:417, 1982.

Kane J. P.: Apolipoprotein B: structural and metabolic heterogeneity. Annu Rev Physiol 45:637, 1983.

Parmley, W. W., et al.: Modification of experimental atherosclerosis by calcium-channel blockers. Am J Cardiol 55:165B, 1985.

Rosenberg, R. D.: Role of heparin and heparinlike molecules in thrombosis and atherosclerosis. Fed Proc 44:404, 1985.

Royce, S. M., et al.: The influence of dietary isomeric and saturated fatty acids on atherosclerosis and eicosanoid synthesis in swine. Am J Clin Nutr 39:215, 1984.

Samuel, P., et al.: The role of diet in the etiology and treatment of atherosclerosis. Annu Rev Med 34:179, 1983.

Stallones, R. A.: Ischemic heart disease and lipids in blood and diet. Annu Rev Nutr 3:155, 1983.

Wight, T. N.: Proteoglycans in pathological conditions: atherosclerosis. Fed Proc 44:381, 1985.

Protein Metabolism

Benevenga, N. J., and Steele, R. D.: Adverse effects of excessive consumption of amino acids. Annu Rev Nutr 4:157, 1984.

Christensen, H. N.: Interorgan amino acid nutrition. Physiol Rev 62:1193, 1982.

Dohm, G. L., et al.: Protein metabolism during endurance exercise. Fed Proc 44:348, 1985.

Friedmann, H. C., ed.: Enzymes. Stroudsburg, Pa., Dowden, Hutchinson & Ross, 1980.

Gevers, W.: Protein metabolism of the heart. J Mol Cell Cardiol 16:3, 1984.

Kinney, J. M., and Elwyn, D. H.: Protein metabolism and injury. Annu Rev Nutr 3:433, 1983.

Rosenberg, L. E., and Scriver, C. R.: Disorders of amino acid metabolism. In Bondy, P. K., and Rosenberg, L. E., eds.: Metabolic Control and Disease, 8th Ed. Philadelphia, W. B. Saunders Co., 1980, p. 583.

Rothschild, M. A.: Albumin synthesis. In Javitt, N. B., ed.: International Review of Physiology: Liver and Biliary Tract Physiology I. Vol. 21. Baltimore, University Park Press, 1980, p. 249.

Sugden, P. H.: The effects of hormonal factors on cardiac protein turnover. Adv Myocardiol 5:105, 1985.

Visek, W. J.: An update of concepts of essential amino acids. Annu Rev Neurosci 5:137, 1982.

Waterlow, J. C., ed.: Nitrogen Metabolism in Man. New York, Elsevier Science Publishing Co., 1982.

47

Energetics, Metabolic Rate, and Regulation of Body Temperature

IMPORTANCE OF ADENOSINE
   TRIPHOSPHATE (ATP) IN METABOLISM
   PHOSPHOCREATINE AS A STORAGE
      DEPOT FOR ENERGY
   SUMMARY OF ENERGY UTILIZATION
      BY THE CELLS
   MEASUREMENT OF THE METABOLIC
      RATE-INDIRECT CALORIMETRY
   FACTORS THAT AFFECT THE
      METABOLIC RATE
   THE BASAL METABOLIC RATE
THE BODY TEMPERATURE
BALANCE BETWEEN HEAT PRODUCTION
   AND HEAT LOSS
   HEAT LOSS
   SWEATING AND ITS REGULATION BY
      THE AUTONOMIC NERVOUS
      SYSTEM
   THE INSULATOR SYSTEM OF THE
      BODY
   FLOW OF BLOOD TO THE SKIN AND
      HEAT TRANSFER FROM THE BODY
      CORE

REGULATION OF BODY TEMPERATURE
   INTEGRATION OF HEAT AND COLD
      THERMOSTATIC SIGNALS IN THE
      HYPOTHALAMUS—THE
      HYPOTHALAMIC THERMOSTAT
   MECHANISMS OF INCREASED HEAT
      LOSS WHEN THE BODY BECOMES
      OVERHEATED
   MECHANISMS OF HEAT
      CONSERVATION AND INCREASED
      HEAT PRODUCTION WHEN THE
      BODY BECOMES COOLED
   BEHAVIORAL CONTROL OF BODY
      TEMPERATURE
ABNORMALITIES OF BODY
   TEMPERATURE REGULATION
   FEVER
   EXPOSURE OF THE BODY TO
      EXTREME COLD

IMPORTANCE OF ADENOSINE TRIPHOSPHATE (ATP) IN METABOLISM

In the last few chapters it has been pointed out that carbohydrates, fats, and proteins can all be used by the cells to synthesize large quantities of ATP and that the ATP can in turn be used as an energy source for many other cellular functions. The attribute of ATP that makes it highly valuable as a means of energy currency is the large quantity of free energy (about 12,000 calories per mole under physiological conditions) vested in each of its two high energy phosphate bonds. The amount of energy in each bond, when liberated by decomposition of one molecule of ATP, is enough to cause almost any step of any chemical reaction in the body to take place if

appropriate transfer of the energy is achieved. Some chemical reactions that require ATP energy use only a few hundred of the available 12,000 calories, and the remainder of this energy is then lost in the form of heat. Yet even this inefficiency in the utilization of energy is better than lack of the ability to energize the necessary chemical reactions at all.

Throughout this book we have listed many functions of ATP. So we will list here only its principal functions, which are

1. To energize the synthesis of important cellular components

2. To energize muscle contraction

3. To energize active transport across membranes for (a) absorption from the intestinal tract, (b) absorption from the renal tubules, (c) formation of

glandular secretions, and (d) establish ionic concentration gradients in nerves which in turn provide the energy required for nerve impulse transmission.

PHOSPHOCREATINE AS A STORAGE DEPOT FOR ENERGY

Despite the paramount importance of ATP as a coupling agent for energy transfer, this substance is not the most abundant store of high energy phosphate bonds in the cells. On the contrary, phosphocreatine, which also contains high energy phosphate bonds, is several times as abundant, at least in muscle. The high energy bond of phosphocreatine contains about 13,000 calories per mole under conditions in the body (38° C and low concentrations of the reactants). This is not greatly different from the 12,000 calories per mole in each of the two high energy phosphate bonds of ATP. The formula for phosphocreatine is the following:

$$HOOC\!-\!CH_2\!-\!\overset{\displaystyle CH_3}{\underset{\displaystyle N}{|}}\!-\!\overset{\displaystyle NH}{\underset{\displaystyle C}{\|}}\!-\!\overset{\displaystyle H}{\underset{\displaystyle N}{|}}\!\sim\!\overset{\displaystyle O}{\underset{\displaystyle \underset{\displaystyle H}{|}}{\overset{\displaystyle \|}{P}}}\!-\!OH$$

Phosphocreatine, unlike ATP, cannot act as a coupling agent for transfer of energy between the foods and the functional cellular systems. But it can transfer energy interchangeably with ATP. When extra amounts of ATP are available in the cell, much of its energy is utilized to synthesize phosphocreatine, thus building up this storehouse of energy. Then when the ATP begins to be used up, the energy in the phosphocreatine is transferred rapidly back to ATP and then from the ATP to the functional systems of the cells.

The higher energy level of the high energy phosphate bond in phosphocreatine, 13,000 in comparison with 12,000 calories per mole, causes the reaction between phosphocreatine and ATP to proceed to an equilibrium state very much in favor of ATP. Therefore, the slightest utilization of ATP by the cells calls forth the energy from the phosphocreatine to synthesize new ATP. This effect keeps the concentration of ATP at almost peak level as long as any phosphocreatine remains in the cell. Therefore, one can call phosphocreatine an ATP "buffer" compound.

SUMMARY OF ENERGY UTILIZATION BY THE CELLS

With the background of the past few chapters and the preceding discussion, we can now synthesize a composite picture of overall energy utilization by the cells as illustrated in Figure 47–1. This figure shows the utilization of glycogen and glucose to form ATP, which is called anaerobic metabolism because it does not require oxygen; the figure also shows the aerobic utilization of compounds derived from carbohydrates,

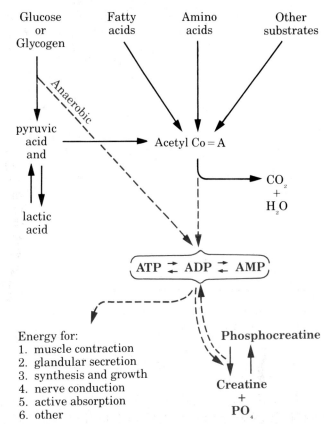

Figure 47–1. Overall scheme of energy transfer from foods to the adenylic acid system and then to the functional elements of the cells.

fats, proteins, and other substances for the formation of still additional ATP. In turn, ATP is in reversible equilibrium with phosphocreatine in the cells, and since large quantities of phosphocreatine are present in the cell, much of the energy of the cell is stockpiled in this energy storehouse.

Energy from ATP can be utilized by the differently functioning systems of the cells to promote the formation of chemical linkages, and these linkages represent stored energy. But we also noted in our discussions of proteins in Chapter 46 that there is continuous turnover of proteins, some being degraded while others are being formed. When the proteins are degraded, the energy stored in the peptide linkage is released in the form of heat into the body.

Now let us consider the energy used for muscle activity. Much of this energy simply overcomes the viscosity of the muscles themselves or of the surrounding tissues so that the limbs can move. The viscous movement in turn causes friction within the tissues, which generates heat.

We might also consider the energy expended by the heart in pumping blood. The blood distends the arterial system, the distention in itself representing a reservoir of potential energy. However, as the blood flows through the peripheral vessels, the friction of the different layers of blood flowing over each other and the friction of the blood against the walls of the vessels turns this energy into heat.

Therefore, we can say that essentially all the energy expended by the body is converted into heat. The only real exception to this occurs when the muscles are used to perform some form of work outside the body. For instance, when the muscles elevate an object to a height or carry the person's body up steps, a type of potential energy outside the body is thus created by raising a mass against gravity. But, on the whole, this normally averages no more than one per cent of the energy metabolism of the body. Therefore, measuring the body's heat production is an excellent means for studying the body's overall metabolism.

The Calorie. To discuss the metabolic rate and related subjects intelligently, it is necessary to use some unit for expressing the quantity of energy released from the different foods or expended by the different functional processes of the body. Most often, the *Calorie* is the unit used for this purpose. It will be recalled that 1 *calorie,* spelled with a lower case *c,* is the quantity of heat required to raise the temperature of 1 gram of water 1° C. The calorie is much too small a unit for ease of expression in speaking of energy in the body. Consequently the kilocalorie, or in common parlance the large Calorie, (with a capital C), which is equivalent to 1000 calories, is the unit ordinarily used.

MEASUREMENT OF THE METABOLIC RATE—INDIRECT CALORIMETRY

Indirect Calorimetry. Since more than 95 per cent of the energy expended in the body is derived from reaction of oxygen with the different foods, the metabolic rate can be calculated with a high degree of accuracy from the rate of oxygen utilization. For the average diet, the *quantity of energy liberated per liter of oxygen utilized in the body averages approximately 4.825 Calories*, and this rarely varies from the average more than plus or minus 3 per cent. Therefore, using this *energy equivalent* of oxygen, one can calculate approximately the rate of heat liberation in the body from the quantity of oxygen utilized in a given period of time. This procedure is called *indirect calorimetry.*

The Metabolator. Figure 47-2 illustrates the metabolator usually used for indirect calorimetry. This apparatus contains a floating drum, under which there is an oxygen chamber connected to a mouthpiece through two flexible tubes. Valves in these tubes allow air to pass from the oxygen chamber into the mouth through one tube, while the expired air is directed through the second tube. Before this expired air re-enters the oxygen chamber, it flows through a container filled with pellets of soda lime, which combines chemically with the carbon dioxide in the expired air. Therefore, as oxygen is used by the person's body and the carbon dioxide is absorbed by the soda lime, the floating oxygen chamber, which is precisely balanced by a weight, gradually sinks in the water, owing to the oxygen loss. This chamber is coupled to a pen that records on a moving paper drum the rate at which the chamber sinks in the water and thereby records the rate at which the body utilizes oxygen.

FACTORS THAT AFFECT THE METABOLIC RATE

Factors that increase the chemical activity in the cells also increase the metabolic rate. Some of these are the following.

Exercise. The factor that causes by far the most dramatic effect on metabolic rate is strenuous exercise. Short bursts of maximal muscle contraction in any single muscle liberate as much as a hundred times its normal resting amount of heat for a few seconds at a time. In the entire body, however, maximal muscle exercise can increase the overall heat production of the body for a few seconds to about 50 times normal or can sustain it for several minutes to about 20 times normal in the well-trained athlete, which is an increase in metabolic rate to 2000 per cent of normal.

Energy Requirements for Daily Activities. When an average man weighing 70 kilograms lies in bed all day, he utilizes approximately 1650 Calories of energy. The process of eating increases the amount of energy utilized by an additional 200 or more Calories,

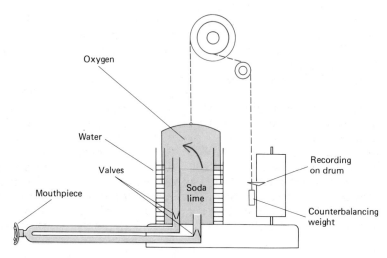

Figure 47-2. The metabolator.

Table 47–1. ENERGY EXPENDITURE PER HOUR DURING DIFFERENT TYPES OF ACTIVITY FOR A 70-KILOGRAM MAN

Form of Activity	Calories per Hour
Sleeping	65
Awake lying still	77
Sitting at rest	100
Standing relaxed	105
Dressing and undressing	118
Tailoring	135
Typewriting rapidly	140
Light exercise	170
Walking slowly (2.6 miles per hour)	200
Carpentry, metal working, industrial painting	240
Active exercise	290
Strenuous exercise	450
Sawing wood	480
Swimming	500
Running (5.3 miles per hour)	570
Very strenuous exercise	600
Walking very fast (5.3 miles per hour)	650
Walking up stairs	1100

Extracted from data compiled by Professor M. S. Rose.

so that the same man lying in bed and also eating a reasonable diet requires a dietary intake of approximately 1850 Calories per day.

Table 47–1 illustrates the rates of energy utilization while one performs different types of activities. Note that walking up stairs requires approximately 17 times as much energy as lying in bed asleep. In general, over a 24-hour period a laborer can achieve a maximum rate of energy utilization as great as 6000 to 7000 Calories—in other words as much as three and a half times the basal rate of metabolism.

Thyroid Hormone. When the thyroid gland secretes maximal quantities of thyroxine, the metabolic rate sometimes rises to as much as 60 to 100 per cent above normal. On the other hand, total loss of thyroid secretion decreases the metabolic rate to as low as 50 to 60 per cent of normal. These effects can readily be explained by the basic function of thyroxine, which is to increase the rates of activity of almost all the chemical reactions in all cells of the body. This relationship between thyroxine and metabolic rate will be discussed in much greater detail in Chapter 50 in relation to thyroid function, because one of the useful methods for diagnosing abnormal rates of thyroid secretion is to determine the basal metabolic rate of the patient.

Sympathetic Stimulation. Stimulation of the sympathetic nervous system with liberation of norepinephrine and epinephrine increases the metabolic rates of most tissues of the body. These hormones directly affect cells to cause glycogenolysis, and this, with other intracellular effects of these hormones, increases cellular activity.

Maximal stimulation of the sympathetic nervous system can increase the metabolic rate in some lower animals as much as several hundred per cent, but the magnitude of this effect in human beings is in question. It is probably 15 per cent or less in the adult but as much as 100 per cent in the newborn child.

THE BASAL METABOLIC RATE

The Basal Metabolic Rate as a Method for Comparing Metabolic Rates Between Individuals. It is often important to measure the inherent activity of the tissues independently of exercise and other extraneous factors that would make it impossible to compare one person's metabolic rate with another's. To do so the metabolic rate is measured under so-called *basal conditions*; this rate is called the *basal metabolic rate*. For the normal adult the average basal metabolic rate is about 70 Calories per hour.

The following basal conditions are necessary for measuring the basal metabolic rate:

1. No food for at least 12 hours
2. A night of restful sleep before determination
3. No strenuous exercise after the night of restful sleep, and complete rest in a reclining position for at least 30 minutes prior to actual determination
4. Elimination of all psychic and physical factors that cause excitement
5. Air temperature comfortable and somewhere between the limits of 68° and 80° F.

Constancy of the Basal Metabolic Rate From Person to Person. When the basal metabolic rate is measured in a wide variety of different persons and comparisons are made within single age, weight, and sex groups, 85 per cent of normal persons have been found to have basal metabolic rates within 10 per cent of the mean. Thus, it is obvious that measurements of metabolic rates performed under basal conditions offer an excellent means for comparing the rates of metabolism from one person to another.

THE BODY TEMPERATURE

The temperature of the inside of the body—that is, in the "core" of the body—remains almost exactly constant, within ± 1° F, day in and day out except when a person develops a febrile illness. Indeed, a person can be exposed while nude to temperatures as low as 55° F or as high as 140° F in dry air and still maintain an almost constant internal body temperature. Therefore, it is obvious that the mechanisms for control of body temperature represent a beautifully designed control system.

The Normal Body Temperature. No single temperature level can be considered normal, for measurements in many normal persons have shown a *range* of normal temperatures, as illustrated in Figure 47–3, from approximately 97° F to over 99° F. When measured by rectum, the values are approximately 1° F greater than the oral temperatures. The average normal temperature is generally considered to be 98.6° F (37° C). However, when excessive heat is produced in the body by strenuous exercise, the rectal

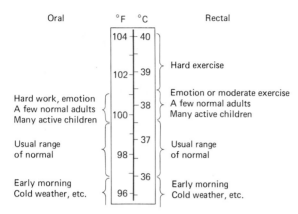

Figure 47–3. Estimated range of body temperature in normal persons. (From DuBois: Fever. Charles C Thomas, Springfield, Illinois.)

temperature can rise to as high as 101° to 104° F for short periods of time.

BALANCE BETWEEN HEAT PRODUCTION AND HEAT LOSS

Heat is continuously being produced in the body as a by-product of metabolism, and body heat is also continuously being lost to the surroundings. When the rate of heat production is exactly equal to the rate of loss, the person is said to be in *heat balance*. But when the two rates are out of equilibrium, body heat, and body temperature as well, will obviously either increase or decrease.

HEAT LOSS

The various methods by which heat is lost from the body are shown pictorially in Figure 47–4. These include *radiation, conduction,* and *evaporation*. Also, *convection* of the air plays a major role in heat loss by both conduction and evaporation. The amount of heat lost by each of these different mechanisms obviously varies with atmospheric conditions.

Radiation. As illustrated in Figure 47–4, a nude person in a room maintained at normal temperature loses about 60 per cent of his total heat loss by radiation.

Loss of heat by radiation means loss in the form of infrared heat rays, electromagnetic waves that radiate from the body to any surroundings that are colder than the body itself. This loss increases as the temperature of the surroundings decreases.

Conduction. Usually, only minute quantities of heat—perhaps about 3 per cent of the total—are lost from the body by direct conduction from the body to other objects, such as a chair or a bed. However, loss of heat by *conduction to air* does represent a sizeable proportion of the body's heat loss even under normal conditions. It will be recalled that heat is actually the kinetic energy of molecular motion, and the molecules that compose the skin of the body are continu-

ously undergoing vibratory motion. Thus, the vibratory motion of the skin molecules can cause increased velocity of motion of the air molecules that come into direct contact with the skin. But once the temperature of the air immediately adjacent to the skin approaches the temperature of the skin, little additional exchange of heat from the body to the air can occur. Therefore, conduction of heat from the body to the air is self-limited unless the heated air moves away from the skin so that new, unheated air is continuously brought in contact with the skin, a phenomenon called *convection*.

Convection. Movement of air is known as convection, and the removal of heat from the body by convection air currents is commonly called heat loss by convection. Actually, the heat must first be *conducted* to the air and then carried away by the convection currents.

A small amount of convection almost always occurs around the body because of the tendency for the air adjacent to the skin to rise as it becomes heated. Therefore, a nude person seated in a comfortable room loses about 12 per cent of his heat by conduction to the air and then by convection away from the body.

Evaporation. When water evaporates from the body surface, 0.58 Calorie of heat is lost for each gram of water that evaporates. Water evaporates *insensibly* from the skin and lungs at a rate of about 600 ml per day. This causes continuous heat loss at a rate of 12 to 16 Calories per hour. Unfortunately, this insensible evaporation of water directly through the skin and lungs cannot be controlled for purposes of temperature regulation because it results from continuous diffusion of water molecules regardless of body temperature. However, additional evaporative loss of heat can be controlled by regulating the rate of sweating, which is discussed below.

Evaporation as a Necessary Refrigeration Mechanism at High Air Temperatures. In the preceding discussions of radiation and conduction, it was noted that as long as the body temperature is greater than that of the surroundings, heat is lost by radiation and conduction; but when the temperature of the surroundings is greater than that of the skin, instead of losing heat, the body gains heat by radiation and conduction from the surroundings. Under these conditions, *the only means by which the body can rid itself of heat is evaporation*. Therefore, any factor that prevents adequate evaporation when the sur-

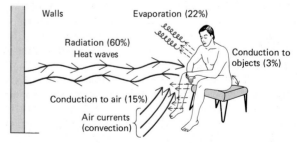

Figure 47–4. Mechanisms of heat loss from the body.

rounding temperatures are higher than body temperature permits the body temperature to rise to abnormally high levels. This circumstance occurs occasionally in human beings who are born with congenital absence of sweat glands. These persons can withstand cold temperatures as well as a normal person can, but they are likely to die of heat stroke in tropical zones, for without the evaporative refrigeration system, the body temperatures will remain at levels greater than those of the surroundings.

SWEATING AND ITS REGULATION BY THE AUTONOMIC NERVOUS SYSTEM

When the body becomes overheated, large quantities of sweat are secreted onto the surface of the skin by the sweat glands to provide rapid *evaporative cooling* of the body. Stimulation of the preoptic area in the anterior part of the hypothalamus excites sweating. The impulses from this area that cause sweating are transmitted in the autonomic pathways to the cord and thence through the sympathetic outflow to the sweat glands in the skin everywhere in the body.

Rate of Sweating. In cold weather the rate of sweat production is essentially zero, but in very hot weather the maximum rate of sweat production is from 0.7 liter per hour in an unacclimatized person to 1.5 to 2 liters per hour in a person maximally acclimatized to heat. Thus, during maximal sweating, a person can lose more than 3 pounds of body weight per hour.

Mechanism of Sweat Secretion. The sweat gland, illustrated in Figure 47–5, is a tubular structure consisting of two parts: (1) a deep *coiled portion* that secretes the sweat and (2) a *duct portion* passing outward to the surface of the skin. As is true of the salivary glands, the secretory portion of the sweat gland emits a fluid called the *precursor secretion*; then certain constituents of this fluid are altered as it flows through the duct.

The precursor secretion is an active secretory product of the epithelial cells lining the coiled portion of the sweat gland. Cholinergic sympathetic nerve fibers ending on or near the glandular cells elicit the secretion.

Since large amounts of sodium chloride are lost in the sweat, it is especially important to know how the sweat glands handle sodium and chloride during the secretory process. When the rate of sweat secretion is very low, the sodium and chloride concentrations of the sweat are also very low, because most of these ions are reabsorbed from the precursor secretion before it reaches the surface of the body; their concentrations are sometimes as low as 5 mEq per liter each. On the other hand, when the rate of secretion becomes progressively greater, the rate of sodium chloride reabsorption does not increase commensurately, so that the concentrations in the sweat of the normal unacclimatized person then usually rise to maximum levels of about 60 mEq per liter, or nearly half the levels in plasma.

Effect of Aldosterone on Sodium Loss in the

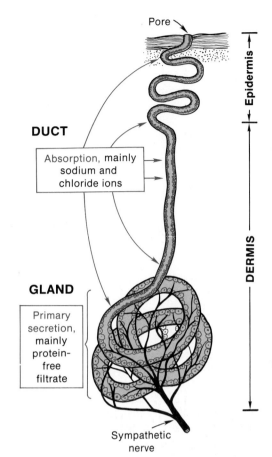

Figure 47–5. A sweat gland innervated by a sympathetic nerve. A *primary secretion* is formed by the glandular portion, but much if not most of the electrolytes are reabsorbed in the duct, leaving a dilute, watery secretion.

Sweat—Acclimatization to Heat. Aldosterone functions in much the same way in the sweat glands as in the renal tubules; that is, it increases the rate of active reabsorption of sodium by the ducts. The reabsorption of sodium also carries chloride ions along as well because of the electrical gradient that develops across the epithelium when sodium is reabsorbed. The importance of this aldosterone effect is to minimize loss of sodium chloride in the sweat when the blood sodium chloride concentration is already low.

Extreme sweating, which often occurs in continuously hot surroundings, can deplete the extracellular fluids of electrolytes, particularly of sodium and chloride. A person who sweats profusely may lose as much as 15 to 20 grams of sodium chloride each day until he becomes acclimatized to the heat. On the other hand, after four to six weeks of acclimatization the loss of sodium chloride may be as little as 3 to 5 grams per day. This change occurs because of increased aldosterone secretion resulting from depletion of the salt reserves of the body.

THE INSULATOR SYSTEM OF THE BODY

The skin, the subcutaneous tissues, and especially the fat of the subcutaneous tissues are a heat insulator for the body. The fat is especially important because it conducts heat only *one third* as readily as other tissues. When no blood is flowing from the heated internal organs to the skin, the insulating properties of the male body are approximately equal to three quarters of the insulating properties of a usual suit of clothes. In women this insulation is still better.

Because most body heat is produced in the deeper portions of the body—the body "core"—the insulation beneath the skin is an effective means for maintaining normal core temperatures, even though it allows the temperature of the skin to approach the temperature of the surroundings.

FLOW OF BLOOD TO THE SKIN AND HEAT TRANSFER FROM THE BODY CORE

A high rate of blood flow to the skin causes heat to be conducted from the internal core of the body to the skin with great efficiency. Blood vessels penetrate the subcutaneous insulator tissues and are distributed profusely in the subpapillary portions of the skin. Indeed, immediately beneath the skin over the entire body is an extensive venous plexus that functions continually in body heat control. In the most exposed areas of the body—hands, feet, and ears—blood is supplied through direct *arteriovenous anastomoses* from the arterioles to this venous plexus. The rate of blood flow is controlled by the sympathetic nervous system as a means to control heat loss from the body. This flow can vary tremendously—from barely above zero in cold weather to as much as 30 per cent of the total cardiac output in hot weather.

Obviously, therefore, the skin is an effective "radiator" system, and the flow of blood to the skin is the principal mechanism of heat transfer from the body core to the skin.

REGULATION OF BODY TEMPERATURE

Figure 47–6 illustrates approximately what happens to the temperature of the nude body after a few hours' exposure to dry, still air ranging from 30° to 170° F. Obviously, the precise dimensions of this curve vary, depending on the movement of air, the amount of moisture in the air, and even the nature of the surroundings. However, in general, between approximately 55° and 140° F in dry air, the nude body is capable of maintaining for long periods of time a normal body core temperature somewhere between 97° and 100° F.

The temperature of the body is regulated almost entirely by nervous feedback control mechanisms, and almost all of them operate through a *temperature regulating center* located in the *hypothalamus*. However, for these feedback mechanisms to operate temperature detectors must also exist to determine when the body temperature becomes either too hot or too cold. Some of these receptors are the following.

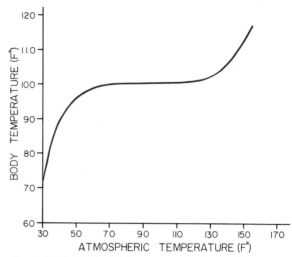

Figure 47–6. Effect of high and low atmospheric temperature for several hours' duration on the internal body temperature, showing that the internal body temperature remains stable despite wide changes in atmospheric temperature.

Temperature Receptors. Probably the most important temperature receptors for control of body temperature are many special *heat-sensitive neurons* located *in the preoptic area of the hypothalamus.* These neurons increase their impulse output as the temperature rises and decrease their output when the temperature decreases. The firing rate sometimes increases as much as tenfold with an increase in body temperature of 10° C.

In addition to these heat-sensitive neurons of the preoptic area, other important receptors sensitive to temperature include the following: (1) *skin temperature receptors*, both *warmth* and *cold receptors*, (but four to ten times as many cold as warmth receptors) that transmit nerve impulses into the spinal cord and thence to the hypothalamic region of the brain to help control body temperature; and (2) *receptors in the spinal cord, in the abdomen, and possibly in other internal structures* of the body that also transmit signals—mainly cold signals—to the central nervous system to help control body temperature.

Experiments in recent years have shown that the preoptic receptors play the greatest role in temperature control when the body temperature rises above normal. But at low temperatures, the peripheral cold receptors are perhaps of equal importance.

INTEGRATION OF HEAT AND COLD THERMOSTATIC SIGNALS IN THE HYPOTHALAMUS—THE HYPOTHALAMIC THERMOSTAT

The signals that arise in peripheral receptors are transmitted to the *posterior hypothalamus,* where they are integrated with the receptor signals from the preoptic area to give the final efferent signals for controlling heat loss and heat production. Therefore, we generally speak of the overall hypothalamic tem-

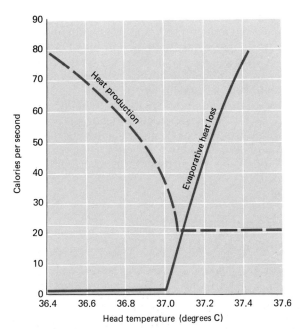

Figure 47–7. Effect of hypothalamic temperature on (1) evaporative heat loss from the body and (2) heat production caused primarily by muscular activity and shivering. This figure demonstrates the extremely critical temperature level at which increased heat loss begins and increased heat production stops. (Drawn from data in Benzinger, Kitzinger, and Pratt, in Hardy [ed.]: Temperature, Part 3, p. 637. Reinhold Publishing Corp.)

perature control mechanism as the *hypothalamic thermostat.*

Figure 47–7 illustrates the effectiveness of the hypothalamic thermostat in initiating temperature regulatory changes when the body temperature rises too high or falls too low. The solid curve shows that as the head temperature increases—almost precisely at 37° C (98.4° F)—sweating begins and then increases rapidly as the temperature rises still higher. On the other hand, sweating ceases at any temperature below this same critical level of 37° C.

Likewise, the hypothalamic thermostat controls the rate of heat production, which is illustrated by the dashed curve. At any temperature above 37.1° C, the heat production remains almost exactly constant, but whenever the temperature falls below this level, the various mechanisms for increasing heat production become markedly activated, especially an increase in muscular activity which culminates in shivering.

MECHANISMS OF INCREASED HEAT LOSS WHEN THE BODY BECOMES OVERHEATED

Overheating the preoptic thermostatic area increases the rate of heat loss from the body in two principal ways: (1) by stimulating the sweat glands to cause evaporative heat loss from the body and (2) by inhibiting sympathetic centers in the posterior hypothalamus that normally constrict the skin vessels; this inhibition allows vasodilatation and, consequently, greatly increased loss of heat from the skin.

MECHANISMS OF HEAT CONSERVATION AND INCREASED HEAT PRODUCTION WHEN THE BODY BECOMES COOLED

When the body core is cooled below approximately 37° C, special mechanisms are set into play to conserve the heat that is already in the body, and still other mechanisms are set into play to increase the rate of heat production, as follows:

Heat Conservation

Vasoconstriction in the Skin. One of the first effects to cause heat conservation is intense vasoconstriction of the skin vessels over the entire body. The posterior hypothalamus strongly activates the sympathetic nervous signals to the skin vessels, and intense skin vasoconstriction occurs throughout the body. This vasoconstriction obviously prevents the conduction of heat from the internal core of the body to the skin. Consequently, with maximal vasoconstriction the only heat that can leave the body is that which can be conducted directly through the fat insulator layers of the skin. This mechanism can reduce the heat loss from the skin as much as eightfold and therefore conserves the quantity of heat in the body.

Piloerection. A second means by which heat is conserved when the hypothalamus is cooled is piloerection—that is, the hairs "stand on end." Obviously, this effect is not important in the human being because of the paucity of hair, but in lower animals the upright projection of the hairs in cold weather entraps a thick layer of *insulator air* next to the skin so that the transfer of heat to the surroundings is greatly depressed.

Abolition of Sweating. Sweating is completely abolished by cooling the preoptic thermostat below about 37° C (98.6° F). This obviously causes evaporative cooling of the body to cease except for that resulting from insensible evaporation.

Increased Production of Heat. Heat production is increased in three separate ways when the temperature of the body thermostat falls below 37° C.

Hypothalamic Stimulation of Shivering. Located in the dorsomedial portion of the posterior hypothalamus near the wall of the third ventricle is an area called the *primary motor center for shivering.* This area is normally inhibited by heat signals from the preoptic thermostatic area but is driven by cold signals from the skin and spinal cord. Therefore, in response to cold, this center becomes activated and transmits impulses through bilateral tracts, down the brain stem, into the lateral columns of the spinal cord, and finally to the anterior motoneurons. These impulses are nonrhythmic and do not cause the actual muscle shaking. Instead, they increase the tone of the skeletal muscles throughout the body and also increase the sensitivity of the muscle spindle stretch reflex. When the tone has risen above a certain critical level, shivering begins. This is believed to result from feedback oscillation of the stretch reflex mechanism. During maximum shivering, body heat production can rise to as high as four to five times normal.

Sympathetic Chemical Excitation of Heat Production. Either sympathetic stimulation or circulating epinephrine (and norepinephrine to a slight extent) in the blood can cause an immediate increase in the rate of cellular metabolism; this effect is called *chemical thermogenesis.* However, as discussed earlier in the chapter, in the adult it is rare for chemical thermogenesis to increase the rate of heat production more than 10 to 15 per cent. However, in infants chemical thermogenesis can increase the rate of heat production as much as 100 per cent, which is probably a very important factor in maintaining normal body temperature in the newborn.

Increased Thyroxine Output as a Cause of Increased Heat Production. Cooling the preoptic area of the hypothalamus also increases the production of the neurosecretory *thyrotropin-releasing hormone* by the hypothalamus. This hormone is carried by way of the hypothalamic portal veins to the adenohypophysis, where it stimulates the secretion of *thyrotropin.* Thyrotropin, in turn, stimulates increased output of thyroxine by the thyroid gland, as will be explained in Chapter 50. The increased thyroxine increases the rate of cellular metabolism throughout the body. However, this increase in metabolism through the thyroid mechanism does not occur immediately but requires several weeks for the thyroid gland to hypertrophy before it reaches its new level of thyroxine secretion.

Exposure of animals to extreme cold for several weeks can cause their thyroid glands to increase in size as much as 20 to 40 per cent. Unfortunately, however, human beings rarely allow themselves to be exposed to the same degree of cold as that to which animals have been subjected. Therefore, we still do not know, quantitatively, how important the thyroid method of adaptation to cold is in the human being.

BEHAVIORAL CONTROL OF BODY TEMPERATURE

Aside from the hypothalamic thermostatic mechanism for body temperature control, the body has still another neural mechanism that is usually even more potent. This mechanism is behavioral control of temperature, which can be explained as follows: Whenever the internal body temperature becomes too high, signals from the preoptic area of the brain give one a psychic sensation of being overheated. Whenever the body becomes too cold, signals from the skin and perhaps from other peripheral receptors elicit the feeling of cold discomfort. Therefore, one makes appropriate environmental adjustments to reestablish comfort. This is a much more powerful system of body temperature control than most physiologists have recognized in the past; indeed, for human beings it is the only really effective mechanism for body heat control in severely cold environs.

Regulation of Internal Body Temperature After Cutting the Spinal Cord. After cutting of the spinal cord in the neck above the level at which sympathetic nerves leave the cord, regulation of body temperature becomes extremely poor, for the hypothalamus can then no longer control either skin blood flow or the degree of sweating anywhere in the body. Therefore, in persons with this condition, body temperature must be regulated principally by the patient's psychic response to cold and hot sensations in the head region. That is, if the person feels too hot or develops a headache from the heat, he or she knows that cooler surroundings should be selected; and, conversely, cold sensations mean that warmer surroundings are needed.

ABNORMALITIES OF BODY TEMPERATURE REGULATION

FEVER

Fever, which means a body temperature above the usual range of normal, may be caused by abnormalities in the brain itself, by toxic substances that affect the temperature regulating centers, by bacterial diseases, by brain tumors, or by dehydration.

Resetting the Hypothalamic Thermostat in Febrile Diseases—Effect of Pyrogens

Many proteins, breakdown products of proteins, and certain other substances, such as lipopolysaccharide toxins secreted by bacteria, can cause the "set point" of the hypothalamic thermostat to rise. Substances that cause this effect are called *pyrogens.* It is pyrogens secreted by toxic bacteria or released from degenerating tissues of the body that cause fever during disease conditions. When the set point of the hypothalamic thermostat becomes increased to a higher level than normal, all the mechanisms for raising the body temperature are brought into play, including heat conservation and increased heat production. Within a few hours after the thermostat has been set to a higher level, the body temperature also approaches this new level.

To give one an idea of the extremely powerful effect of pyrogens in resetting the hypothalamic thermostat, as little as a few nanograms of some purified bacterial pyrogens injected into a person can cause severe fever.

Characteristics of Febrile Conditions

Chills. When the thermostat setting is suddenly changed from the normal level to a higher-than-normal level as a result of tissue destruction, pyrogenic substances, or dehydration, the body temperature usually takes several hours to reach the new temperature setting. For instance, the temperature setting of the hypothalamic thermostat, as illustrated in Figure 47–8, might suddenly rise to 103° F. Because the blood temperature is less than the temperature setting of the hypothalamic thermostat, the usual

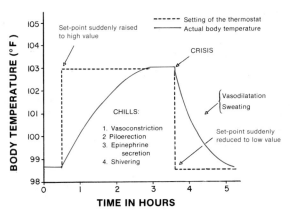

Figure 47–8. Effects of changing the setting of the "hypothalamic thermostat."

autonomic responses that cause elevation of body temperature occur. During this period chills cause the person to feel extremely cold even though body temperature may already be above normal. Also, the skin is cold because of vasoconstriction, and the body shakes from shivering. The chills continue until body temperature rises to the hypothalamic setting of 103° F. Then, when the temperature of the body reaches this level, the person no longer experiences chills but feels neither cold nor hot. As long as the factor that is causing the hypothalamic thermostat to be set at this high level continues its effect, the body temperature is regulated more or less in the usual manner but at the higher temperature level.

The Crisis or "Flush." If the factor that is causing the high temperature is suddenly removed, the set-point of the hypothalamic thermostat suddenly returns to the normal lower level, as illustrated in Figure 47–8. In this instance, the blood temperature is still 103° F, but the hypothalamus is now attempting to regulate the body temperature at 98.6° F. This situation is analogous to excessive heating of the normal preoptic area, which causes *intense sweating* and sudden development of a *hot skin* because of vasodilatation everywhere. This sudden change of events in a febrile disease is known as the crisis or, more appropriately, the flush. Before the advent of antibiotics, the doctor always awaited the crisis, for once this occurred he or she knew immediately that the patient's temperature would soon be falling.

Heat Stroke

The limits of extreme heat that one can stand depend almost entirely on whether the heat is dry or wet. If the air is completely dry and sufficient convection air currents are flowing to promote rapid evaporation from the body, a person can withstand several hours of air temperature at 150° F with no apparent ill effects. On the other hand, if the air is 100 per cent humidified or if the body is in water, the body temperature begins to rise whenever the environmental temperature rises above approximately 94° F. If the person is performing very heavy work, the critical temperature level may fall to 85° to 90° F in these humid surroundings.

Unfortunately, there is a limit to the rate at which the body can lose heat even with maximal sweating. Furthermore, when the hypothalamus becomes heated beyond a critical temperature, its heat-regulatory ability then becomes depressed and sweating diminishes. As a result, a high body temperature tends to perpetuate itself unless measures are taken specifically to decrease body heat.

When the body temperature rises into the range of 106° to 108° F, the person is likely to develop *heat stroke*. The symptoms include dizziness, abdominal distress, sometimes delirium, and, eventually, loss of consciousness if the body temperature is not soon decreased. Many of these symptoms probably result from a mild degree of *circulatory shock* brought on by the excessive loss of fluid and electrolytes in the sweat before the onset of symptoms. However, the hyperpyrexia itself is also exceedingly damaging to the body tissues, especially the brain, and therefore is undoubtedly responsible for many of the effects. In fact, even a few minutes of very high body temperature can sometimes be fatal. For this reason, many authorities recommend immediate treatment of heat stroke by placing the person in an ice-water bath. However, because this often induces uncontrollable shivering with considerable increase in rate of heat production, others have suggested that sponge-cooling of the skin is likely to be more effective for rapidly decreasing the body core temperature.

Harmful Effects of the High Temperature. When the body temperature rises above 106° to 108° F, the parenchyma of many cells begins to be damaged. The pathological findings in a person who dies of hyperpyrexia are local hemorrhages and parenchymatous degeneration of cells throughout the entire body but especially in the brain. Unfortunately, once neuronal cells are destroyed, they can never be replaced. Damage to the liver, kidneys, and other body organs can often be so great that failure of one or more of these organs eventually causes death, sometimes not till several days after the heat stroke.

Antipyretics. Aspirin, antipyrine, aminopyrine, and a number of other substances known as antipyretics have an effect on the hypothalamic thermostat opposite to that of the pyrogens. In other words, they cause the setting of the thermostat to be lowered, causing the body temperature to fall, though usually not more than a degree or so. Aspirin is especially effective in lowering the hypothalamic setting when pyrogens have raised the setting, but aspirin will not lower the normal temperature. On the other hand, amninopyrine will decrease even the normal body temperature. Obviously, these drugs can be used to prevent damage to the body from excessively high body temperature in feverish conditions.

EXPOSURE OF THE BODY TO EXTREME COLD

A person exposed to ice water for approximately 20 to 30 minutes ordinarily dies because of heart standstill or heart fibrillation unless treated immediately. By that time, the internal body temperature has fallen to about 77° F. Yet if the victim is warmed rapidly by application of external heat, his or her life can often be saved.

Once the body temperature has fallen below 85° F, the ability of the hypothalamus to regulate temperature is completely lost, and it is greatly impaired even when the body temperature falls below approximately 94° F. Part of the reason for this loss of temperature regulation is that the rate of heat production in each cell is greatly depressed by the low temperature. Also, sleepiness and even coma, which depress the activity of the central nervous system heat-control mechanisms and prevent shivering, are likely to develop. This loss of temperature regulation obviously further accelerates the decrease in body temperature and rapidly leads to death.

QUESTIONS

1. Why does the concentration of *ATP* remain almost at the maximal level until all the *phosphocreatine* in a cell has been depleted?
2. What is meant by the function of phosphocreatine to "buffer" the concentration of ATP?
3. Explain the function of the *metabolator* and the physiological principles of *indirect calorimetry*.
4. How do the following factors affect the *metabolic rate:* exercise, thyroid hormone, and sympathetic stimulation?
5. In measuring the *basal metabolic rate*, what are the *basal conditions* that are prerequisite?
6. Explain how each of the following factors contributes to heat loss from the body: *radiation, conduction, convection,* and *evaporation*.
7. Why is evaporation necessary for the maintenance of body temperature when the temperature of the body's surroundings is greater than body temperature? Describe the sweat gland and its formation of sweat.
8. Why is the normal concentration of sodium chloride in the sweat very low and why does this become even lower in heat acclimatization? What is the role of aldosterone in heat acclimatization of the sweating process?
9. Explain the *heat insulator system* of the body and how heat is transferred from the body core to the skin. What regulates the rate at which heat is transferred to the skin?
10. What are the different *temperature receptors* of the body?
11. Describe the organization of the *hypothalamus* for the control of body temperature. What is meant by the *hypothalamic thermostat*?
12. List the mechanisms by which the body conserves heat and increases heat production when the body becomes cooled.
13. Describe the mechanism of *shivering*.
14. What is meant by *chemical excitation of heat production*?
15. How does *behavior* enter into the control of temperature?
16. What is meant by *fever*, and what are pyrogens?
17. Why do chills occur when the set point of the *hypothalamic thermostat* is suddenly increased to a level greater than the present body temperature?
18. Explain the cause of the *crisis* or flush.
19. What is meant by *heat stroke*, and how does it affect the body?
20. Explain the deleterious effects on the body caused by extreme cold.

References

Energetics and Metabolic Rate

Atkins, G. L.: An Outline of Energy Metabolism in Man. Philadelphia, International Ideas, 1981.
Baldwin, R. L., and Bywater, A. C.: Nutritional energetics of animals. Annu Rev Nutr 4:101, 1984.
Becker, D. J.: The endocrine responses to protein-calorie malnutrition. Annu Rev Nutr 3:187, 1983.
Durnin, J. V.: Energy balance in childhood and adolescence. Proc Nutr Soc 43:271, 1984.
Golinick, P. D.: Metabolism of substrates: energy substrate metabolism during exercise and as modified by training. Fed Proc 44:353, 1985.
Guyton, A. C., and Farrish, C. A.: A rapidly responding continuous oxygen consumption recorder. J Appl Physiol 14:143, 1959.
Magnen, J. L.: Body energy balance and food intake: a neuroendocrine regulatory mechanism. Physiol Rev 63:314, 1983.
Nicholls, D. G., and Locke, R. M.: Thermogenic mechanisms in brown fat. Physiol Rev 64:1, 1984.

Regulation of Body Temperature

Brengelmann, G. L.: Circulatory adjustments to exercise and heat stress. Annu Rev Physiol 45:191, 1983.
Calder, W. A., III: Scaling of physiological processes in homeothermic animals. Annu Rev Physiol 43:301, 1981.
Crawshaw, L. I.: Temperature regulation in vertebrates. Annu Rev Physiol 42:473, 1980.
Galanter, E.: Detection and discrimination of environmental change. In Darian-Smith, I., ed.: Handbook of Physiology. Sec. 1, Vol. 3. Bethesda, American Physiological Society, 1984, p. 103.
Hales, J. E., ed.: Thermal Physiology. New York, Raven Press, 1984.
Hellon, R.: Thermoreceptors. In Shepherd, J. T., and Abboud, F. M., eds.: Handbook of Physiology. Sec. 1, Vol. 3. Bethesda, American Physiological Society, 1983, p. 659.
Prosser, C. L., and Nelson, D. O.: The role of nervous systems in temperature adaptation of poikilotherms. Annu Rev Physiol 43:281, 1981.
Quinton, P. M.: Sweating and its disorders. Annu Rev Med 34:453, 1983.
Rowell, L. B.: Cardiovascular adjustments to thermal stress. In Shepherd, J. T., and Abboud, F. M., eds.: Handbook of Physiology. Sec. 2, Vol. 3. Bethesda, American Physiological Society, 1983, p. 967.

48

Dietary Balances, Regulation of Feeding, Obesity, and Vitamins

DIETARY BALANCES
REGULATION OF FOOD INTAKE
   NEURAL CENTERS FOR REGULATION
     OF FOOD INTAKE
   FACTORS THAT REGULATE FOOD
     INTAKE
OBESITY
   ABNORMAL FEEDING REGULATION
     AS A PATHOLOGICAL CAUSE OF
     OBESITY
STARVATION
VITAMINS
   VITAMIN A

THIAMINE (VITAMIN B_1)
NIACIN
RIBOFLAVIN (VITAMIN B_2)
VITAMIN B_{12}
FOLIC ACID (PTEROYLGLUTAMIC
   ACID)
PYRIDOXINE (VITAMIN B_6)
PANTOTHENIC ACID
ASCORBIC ACID (VITAMIN C)
VITAMIN D
VITAMIN E
VITAMIN K

The intake of food must always be sufficient to supply the metabolic needs of the body and yet not enough to cause obesity. Also, since foods contain different proportions of proteins, carbohydrates, and fats, appropriate balance must be maintained between these different types of food so that all segments of the body's metabolic systems can be supplied with the requisite materials. This chapter therefore discusses especially the problems of balance between the major types of food and the intrinsic homeostatic mechanisms of the body that cause the intake of food to be regulated in accordance with the body's metabolic need.

DIETARY BALANCES

Energy Available in Foods. The energy liberated from each gram of carbohydrate as it is oxidized to carbon dioxide and water is 4.1 Calories (kilocalories), and that liberated from fat is 9.3 Calories. The energy liberated from metabolism of the average protein in the diet as each gram is oxidized to carbon dioxide, water, and urea is 4.35 Calories. Also, these different substances vary in the average percentage absorbed from the gastrointestinal tract: approximately 98 per cent of the carbohydrate, 95 per cent of the fat, and 92 per cent of the protein. Therefore, in round figures the average *physiologically available energy* in each gram of the three different foodstuffs in the diet is:

	Calories
Carbohydrates	4.0
Fat	9.0
Protein	4.0

Average Composition of the Diet. The average American receives approximately 15 per cent of his energy from protein, about 40 per cent from fat, and 45 per cent from carbohydrates. In most other parts of the world, the quantity of energy derived from carbohydrates far exceeds that derived from both proteins and fats. Indeed, in some parts of Mongolia, the energy received from fats and proteins combined is said to be no greater than 15 to 20 per cent.

Daily Requirement for Protein. Twenty to 30 grams of body proteins are degraded and used for energy daily. Therefore, all cells must continue to synthesize

553

new proteins to take the place of those that are being destroyed, and a supply of protein is needed in the diet for this purpose. An average man can maintain his normal stores of protein provided that his *daily intake is above 30 to 55 grams.*

Partial Proteins. Another factor that must be considered in analyzing the proteins of the diet is whether the dietary proteins are *complete* or *partial* proteins. Complete proteins have compositions of amino acids in appropriate proportion to each other so that all the amino acids can be properly used by the human body. In general, proteins derived from animal foodstuffs are more nearly complete than are proteins derived from vegetable and grain sources. When partial proteins are in the diet, an increased minimal quantity of protein is necessary in the daily rations to maintain protein balance. A particular example of this occurs in the diet of many African natives who subsist primarily on a corn meal diet. The protein of corn is almost totally lacking in the amino acid tryptophan, which means that this diet in effect is almost completely protein deficient because, if any single amino acid that is needed to make animal proteins is missing, protein synthesis stops entirely, and the remaining amino acids are used for energy instead. As a result, many Africans, especially the children, develop the protein deficiency syndrome called *kwashiorkor,* which consists of failure to grow, lethargy, depressed mentality, and hypoprotein edema.

Study of the Balance Between Fat and Carbohydrate Utilization— The Respiratory Quotient

When glucose is oxidized, the number of molecules of carbon dioxide liberated is exactly equal to the number of oxygen molecules necessary for the oxidative process. This *ratio of carbon dioxide output to oxygen usage* is called the *respiratory quotient.* Thus, for glucose the respiratory quotient is 1.00. On the other hand, oxidation of triolein (the most abundant fat in the body) liberates 57 carbon dioxide molecules while 80 oxygen molecules are being utilized. Consequently, the respiratory quotient in this instance is 0.71. Finally, oxidation of alanine liberates five carbon dioxide molecules for every six oxygen molecules, giving a respiratory quotient of 0.83.

Because only a small part of one's metabolic energy is derived from protein and because the respiratory quotient of protein is approximately midway between the respiratory quotients of fat and carbohydrate (see preceding paragraph), one can estimate reasonably well the relative quantities of fat and carbohydrate being metabolized by the body by simply measuring the respiratory quotient—that is, by measuring the respiratory intake of oxygen and the output of carbon dioxide. For instance, if the respiratory quotient is approximately 0.71, the body is burning almost entirely fat to the exclusion of carbohydrates. If, on the other hand, the respiratory quotient is 1.00, the body is probably metabolizing almost entirely carbohydrate

to the exclusion of fat. Finally, a respiratory quotient of 0.85 indicates approximately equal utilization of carbohydrate and fat.

REGULATION OF FOOD INTAKE

Hunger. The term *hunger* means a craving for food, and it is associated with a number of objective sensations. For instance, in a person who has not had food for many hours, the stomach undergoes intense rhythmic contractions called *hunger contractions.* These cause a tight or a gnawing feeling in the pit of the stomach and sometimes actually cause pain called *hunger pangs.* In addition to the hunger pangs, the hungry person also becomes more tense and restless than usual.

Some physiologists actually define hunger as the tonic contractions of the stomach. However, even after the stomach is completely removed, the psychic sensations of hunger still occur, and craving for food still makes the person search for an adequate food supply.

Appetite. The term *appetite* is often used in the same sense as hunger except that it usually implies desire for specific types of food instead of food in general. Therefore, appetite helps determine the quality of food a person eats.

Satiety. Satiety is the opposite of hunger. It means a feeling of fulfillment of the quest for food. Satiety usually results from a filling meal, particularly when the person's nutritional storage depots, the adipose tissue and the glycogen stores, are already filled.

NEURAL CENTERS FOR REGULATION OF FOOD INTAKE

Hunger and Satiety Centers. Stimulation of the *lateral hypothalamus* causes an animal to eat voraciously, while stimulation of the *ventromedial nuclei of the hypothalamus* causes complete satiety, and even in the presence of highly appetizing food an animal will nevertheless refuse to eat if this area is stimulated. Conversely, a destructive lesion of the ventromedial nuclei causes exactly the same effect as stimulation of the lateral hypothalamic nuclei—that is, voracious and continued eating until the animal becomes extremely obese, sometimes as large as four times normal in size. Lesions of the lateral hypothalamic nuclei cause exactly the opposite effects—complete lack of desire for food and progressive inanition of the animal. Therefore, we can label the lateral nuclei of the hypothalamus the *hunger,* or the *feeding, center* and the ventromedial nuclei of the hypothalamus the *satiety center.*

The feeding center operates by directly exciting the emotional drive to search for food. On the other hand, it is believed that the satiety center operates primarily by inhibiting the feeding center.

Other Neural Centers That Enter Into Feeding. If the brain is removed above the mesencephalon, the animal can still perform the basic mechanical features of the feeding process. It can salivate, lick its lips, chew food, and swallow. Therefore, the actual mechanics of feeding are all controlled by centers in the lower brain stem. The function of the hunger center in the hypothalamus, then, is to control the quantity of food intake and to excite the lower centers to activity.

Higher centers than the hypothalamus also play important roles in the control of feeding, particularly in the control of appetite. These centers include especially the *amygdala* and some cortical areas of the limbic system, all of which are closely coupled with the hypothalamus. It will be recalled from the discussion of the sense of smell that the amygdala is one of the major parts of the olfactory nervous system. Destructive lesions in the amygdala have demonstrated that some of its areas greatly increase feeding, while others inhibit feeding. In addition, stimulation of some areas of the amygdala elicits the mechanical act of feeding. However, the most important effect of destruction of the amygdala on both sides of the brain is a "psychic blindness" in the choice of foods. In other words, the animal (and presumably the human being as well) loses or at least partially loses the mechanism of appetite control over the type and quality of food that is eaten.

The cortical regions of the limbic system, including the infraorbital regions, the hippocampal gyrus, and the cingulate gyrus, all have areas that when stimulated can either increase or decrease feeding activities. These areas seem especially to play a role in an animal's drive to search for food when hungry. It is presumed that these centers are also responsible, probably operating in association with the amygdala and hypothalamus, for determining the quality of food that is eaten. For instance, a previous unpleasant experience with almost any type of food often destroys a person's appetite for that food thereafter.

FACTORS THAT REGULATE FOOD INTAKE

We can divide the regulation of food into (1) *nutritional regulation*, which is concerned with maintenance of normal quantities of nutrient stores in the body, and (2) *alimentary regulation*, which is concerned with the immediate effects of feeding on the alimentary tract and is sometimes called *peripheral, alimentary,* or *short-term regulation.*

Nutritional Regulation. An animal that has been starved for a long time and is then presented with unlimited food eats a far greater quantity than does an animal that has been on a regular diet. Conversely, an animal that has been force-fed for several weeks eats little when allowed to eat according to its own desires. Thus, the feeding center in the hypothalamus is geared to the nutritional status of the body. Some of the nutritional factors that control the degree of activity of the feeding center are the following:

Availability of Glucose to the Body Cells—The Glucostatic Theory of Hunger and of Feeding Regulation. It has long been known that a decrease in blood glucose concentration is associated with devel-

opment of hunger, which has led to the so-called *glucostatic theory of hunger and of feeding regulation,* as follows: When the blood glucose level falls too low, this automatically causes the animal to increase its feeding, which eventually returns the glucose concentration back toward normal. There are two particular observations that also support the glucostatic theory: (1) An increase in blood glucose level increases the measured electrical activity in the satiety center in the ventromedial nuclei of the hypothalamus and simultaneously decreases the electrical activity in the feeding center of the lateral nuclei. (2) Chemical studies show that the ventromedial nuclei (the satiety center) concentrate glucose while other areas of the hypothalamus fail to concentrate glucose; therefore, it is assumed that increased glucose stores in the body limit feeding by increasing the degree of satiety.

Effect of Blood Amino Acid Concentration on Feeding. An increase in amino acid concentration in the blood also reduces feeding, and a decrease enhances feeding. In general, though, this effect is not as powerful as the glucostatic mechanism.

Effect of Fat Metabolites on Feeding—Long-term Regulation. The overall degree of feeding varies almost inversely with the amount of adipose tissue in the body. That is, as the quantity of adipose tissue increases, the rate of feeding decreases. Therefore, many physiologists believe that *long-term regulation* of feeding is controlled mainly by fat metabolites of an undiscovered nature. This is called the lipostatic theory of feeding regulation. In support of this is the fact that the long-term average concentration of free fatty acids in the blood is directly proportional to the quantity of adipose tissue in the body. Therefore, it is likely that the free fatty acids or some other similar fat metabolites act in the same manner as glucose and amino acids to cause a negative feedback regulatory effect on feeding. It is also possible, if not probable, that this mechanism is by far the most important long-term regulator of feeding.

Summary of Long-term Regulation. Even though our information on the different feedback factors in long-term feeding regulation is imprecise, we can make the following general statement: When the nutrient stores of the body fall below normal, the feeding center of the hypothalamus becomes highly active and the person exhibits increased hunger; on the other hand, when the nutrient stores are abundant, the person loses hunger and develops a state of satiety.

Alimentary Regulation (Short-term, Nonmetabolic Regulation). The degree of hunger or satiety can be temporarily increased or decreased by habit. For instance, the normal person has the habit of eating three meals a day, and when one is missed he or she is likely to develop a state of hunger at mealtime despite completely adequate nutritional stores in the tissues. But, in addition to habit, several other short-term physiological stimuli mainly related to the alimentary tract can alter one's desire for food for several hours at a time, as follows.

Gastrointestinal Filling. When the gastrointestinal

tract becomes distended, especially the stomach or the duodenum, inhibitory signals temporarily suppress the feeding center, thereby reducing the desire for food. This effect probably depends mainly on sensory signals transmitted through the vagi, but part of the effect still persists after the vagi and the sympathetic nerves from the upper gastrointestinal tract have been severed. Therefore, somatic sensory signals from the stretched abdomen may also play a role. And recently it has been found that short-term hormonal feedback also suppresses feeding, for the hormone *cholecystokinin,* which is released mainly in response to fat entering the duodenum, has a strong effect on inhibition of further eating.

Obviously, these mechanisms are of particular importance in bringing one's feeding to a halt during a heavy meal.

Metering of Food by Head Receptors. When a person with an esophageal fistula is fed large quantities of food, even though this food is immediately lost again to the exterior, the degree of hunger is decreased after a reasonable quantity of food has passed through the mouth. This effect occurs despite the fact that the gastrointestinal tract does not in the least become filled. Therefore, it is postulated that various "head factors" related to feeding, such as chewing, salivation, swallowing, and tasting, "meter" the food as it passes through the mouth, and after a certain amount has passed through, the hypothalamic feeding center becomes inhibited.

Importance of Having Both Long- and Short-term Regulatory Systems for Feeding. The long-term regulatory system, especially the lipostatic feedback mechanism, obviously helps an animal to maintain constant stores of nutrients in its tissues, preventing them from becoming too little or too great. On the other hand, the short-term regulatory stimuli make the animal feed only when the gastrointestinal tract is receptive to food. Thus, food passes through the gastrointestinal tract fairly continuously, so that its digestive, absorptive, and storage mechanisms can all work at a steady pace rather than only when the animal needs food for energy. Indeed, the digestive, absorptive, and storage mechanisms can increase their rates of activity above normal only four- to fivefold, whereas the rate of usage of stored nutrients for energy sometimes increases to 20 times normal.

It is important, then, that feeding should occur rather continuously (but at a rate that the gastrointestinal tract can accommodate), regulated principally by the short-term mechanisms. However, it is also important that the intensity of the daily rhythmic feeding habits be modulated up or down by the long-term regulatory system, based on the level of nutrient stores in the body.

OBESITY

Energy Input Versus Energy Output. When greater quantities of energy in the form of food enter the body than are expended, the body weight increases. Therefore, obesity is obviously caused by excess en-

ergy input over energy output. For each 9.3 Calories excess energy entering the body, 1 gram of fat is stored.

Excess energy input occurs *only during the developing phase of obesity;* once a person has already become obese, all that is required of him to remain obese is that his energy input equal his energy output. For the person to reduce, the output must be *greater* than the input. Indeed, studies of obese persons, once they have become obese, show that their intake of food is almost exactly the same as that of normal weight persons.

Effect of Muscular Activity on Energy Output. About one third of the energy used each day by a normal person goes into muscular activity, though in the laborer doing heavy work as much as two thirds and occasionally three fourths is used in this way. Since muscular activity is by far the most important means by which energy is expended in the body, it is frequently said that obesity results from *too high a ratio of food intake to daily exercise.*

ABNORMAL FEEDING REGULATION AS A PATHOLOGICAL CAUSE OF OBESITY

The preceding discussion of the mechanisms that regulate feeding have emphasized that the rate of feeding is normally regulated in proportion to the nutrient stores in the body. When these stores begin to approach an optimal level in a normal person, feeding is automatically reduced to prevent overstorage. However, in most obese persons this is not true, for feeding does not automatically slacken until body weight is far above normal. Therefore, in effect, obesity is often caused by an abnormality of the feeding regulatory mechanism. This can result from either psychogenic factors that affect the regulation or actual abnormalities of the hypothalamus itself.

Psychogenic Obesity. Studies of obese patients show that a large proportion of obesity results from psychogenic factors. Perhaps the most common psychogenic factor contributing to obesity is the prevalent idea that healthy eating habits require three meals a day and that each meal must be filling. Many children are forced into this habit by overly solicitous parents, and these children continue to practice it throughout their lives.

Genetic Factors in Obesity. Obesity definitely runs in families. Furthermore, identical twins usually maintain weight levels within 2 pounds of each other throughout life if they live under similar conditions, or within 5 pounds if their conditions of life differ markedly. This might result partly from eating habits engendered during childhood, but it is generally believed that this close similarity between twins is genetically controlled.

The genes can cause abnormal feeding in several different ways, including (1) a genetic abnormality of the feeding center that sets the level of nutrient storage high or low or (2) abnormal hereditary psychic factors that either whet the appetite or cause a person to eat as a "release" mechanism.

A genetic abnormality in the *chemistry of fat storage* is also known to cause obesity in a certain strain of rats. In these rats, fat is easily stored in the adipose tissue, but the quantity of hormone-sensitive lipase in the adipose tissue is greatly reduced, so that little of the fat can be removed. In addition, the rats develop hyperinsulinism, which promotes fat storage. This combination obviously results in a one-way path, the fat continuously being deposited but never released. This, too, is another possible mechanism of obesity in some human beings.

Childhood Overnutrition as a Possible Cause of Obesity. The rate of formation of new fat cells is especially rapid in the first few years of life, and the greater the rate of fat storage the greater becomes the number of fat cells. In obese children the number of fat cells is often as much as three times that in normal children. After adolescence, the number of fat cells remains almost identically the same throughout the remainder of life. Therefore, it has been suggested that overfeeding children, especially in infancy, can lead to a lifetime of obesity. The person who has excess fat cells is thought to have a higher setting of the hypothalamic feedback autoregulatory mechanism for control of adipose tissues.

In persons who become obese in middle or old age, most of the obesity results from hypertrophy of already existing fat cells. This type of obesity is far more susceptible to treatment than is the life-long type.

STARVATION

Depletion of Food Stores in the Body Tissues During Starvation. Even though the tissues preferentially use carbohydrate for energy instead of fat and protein, the quantity of carbohydrate stores of the body is only a few hundred grams (mainly glycogen in the liver and muscles), and it can supply the energy required for body function for only about half a day. Therefore, except for the first few hours of starvation, the major effects are progressive depletion of tissue fat and protein. Since fat is the prime source of energy, its rate of depletion continues unabated, as illustrated in Figure 48–1, until most of the fat stores in the body are gone.

Protein undergoes three different phases of depletion: rapid depletion at first, then greatly slowed depletion, and finally rapid depletion again, shortly before death. The initial rapid depletion is caused by conversion of protein to glucose in the liver by the process of gluconeogenesis. The glucose thus formed (about two thirds of it) is used to supply energy to the brain, which under normal circumstances utilizes almost no metabolic substrate for energy other than glucose. However, after the readily mobilizable protein stores have been depleted during the early phase of starvation, the remaining protein is not so easily removed from the tissues. At this time, the rate of gluconeogenesis decreases to one third to one fifth its previous rate, and the rate of depletion of protein

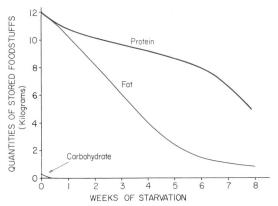

Figure 48–1. Effect of starvation on the food stores of the body.

becomes greatly decreased, as illustrated in Figure 48–1. The diminished availability of glucose then initiates a series of events leading to *ketosis*, which means greatly increased formation of ketone bodies, as described in Chapter 46. Fortunately, the ketone bodies (mainly acetoacetic acid and hydroxybutyric acid), like glucose, can cross the blood-brain barrier and can be utilized by the brain cells for energy. Therefore, approximately two thirds of the brain's energy now is derived from these ketone bodies. This sequence of events thus leads to at least partial preservation of the protein stores of the body.

However, there finally comes a time when the fat stores also are almost totally depleted, and the only remaining source of energy is proteins. At that time, protein stores once again enter a stage of rapid depletion. Since the proteins are essential for maintenance of cellular function, death ordinarily ensues when the proteins of the body have been depleted to approximately one half their normal level.

VITAMINS

Daily Requirements of Vitamins. A vitamin is an organic compound needed in small quantities for operation of normal bodily metabolism and that cannot be manufactured in the cells of the body. When lacking in the diet, vitamins can cause specific metabolic deficits.

Table 48–1 lists the amounts of important vitamins

Table 48–1. REQUIRED DAILY AMOUNTS OF THE VITAMINS

A	5000 IU*
Thiamine	1.5 mg
Riboflavin	1.8 mg
Niacin	20 mg
Ascorbic acid	45 mg
D	400 IU*
E	15 IU*
K	none
Folic acid	0.4 mg
B_{12}	3 μg
Pyridoxine	2 mg
Pantothenic acid	unknown

*IU = international units.

required daily by the average adult. These requirements vary considerably, depending on such factors as (a) body size, (b) rate of growth, (c) amount of exercise, (d) disease and fever, and (e) special need for vitamin D in pregnant or lactating women. Also, a number of metabolic deficits occur pathologically in which the vitamins themselves cannot be utilized properly in the body; in such conditions the requirement for one or more specific vitamins may be extreme.

VITAMIN A

Vitamin A precursors occur in abundance in many different vegetable foods. These are the yellow and red *carotenoid pigments*, which, since they have chemical structures similar to that of vitamin A, can be changed into vitamin A in the human body. Vitamin A exists in the body mainly as *retinol*.

The basic function of vitamin A in the metabolism of the body is not known except in relation to its use in formation of the retinal photochemicals (discussed in Chapter 39). Nevertheless, vitamin A is also necessary for normal growth of most cells of the body and especially for normal growth and proliferation of the different types of epithelial cells. When vitamin A is lacking, the epithelial structures of the body tend to become stratified and keratinized. Therefore, vitamin A deficiency manifests itself by (1) scaliness of the skin and sometimes acne, (2) failure of growth of young animals, (3) failure of reproduction in many animals, associated especially with atrophy of the germinal epithelium of the testes and sometimes with interruption of the female sexual cycle, and (4) keratinization of the cornea with resultant corneal opacity and blindness.

THIAMINE (VITAMIN B₁)

Thiamine operates in the metabolic systems of the body principally as *thiamine pyrophosphate*; this compound functions as a *cocarboxylase*, operating mainly for decarboxylation of pyruvic acid, which was discussed in Chapter 45.

Thiamine deficiency causes decreased utilization of pyruvic acid and some amino acids by the tissues but increased utilization of fats. Thus, thiamine is specifically needed for final metabolism of carbohydrates and many amino acids. Probably the decreased utilization of these nutrients is responsible for the debilities associated with thiamine deficiency.

Thiamine Deficiency and the Nervous System. The central nervous system depends almost entirely on the metabolism of carbohydrates for its energy. In thiamine deficiency the utilization of glucose by nervous tissue may be decreased as much as 50 to 60 per cent. Therefore, it is readily understandable that thiamine deficiency can greatly impair function of the central nervous system. The neuronal cells of the central nervous system frequently show chromatolysis and swelling during thiamine deficiency, changes that

are characteristic of neuronal cells with poor nutrition.

Also, thiamine deficiency can cause *degeneration of myelin sheaths* of nerve fibers both in the peripheral nerves and in the central nervous system. The lesions in the peripheral nerves frequently cause these nerves to become extremely irritable, resulting in polyneuritis characterized by pain radiating along the course of one or more peripheral nerves. Also, in severe thiamine deficiency, the peripheral nerve fibers and fiber tracts in the cord can degenerate to such an extent that *paralysis* occasionally results.

Thiamine Deficiency and the Cardiovascular System. Thiamine deficiency also weakens the heart muscle, so that a person with severe thiamine deficiency sometimes develops *cardiac failure*. *Peripheral edema* and *ascites* also occur to a major extent in some persons with thiamine deficiency, partly because of the cardiac failure but also because thiamine deficiency causes arteriolar dilatation.

Thiamine Deficiency and the Gastrointestinal Tract. Among the gastrointestinal symptoms caused by thiamine deficiency are indigestion, severe constipation, anorexia, gastric atony, and hypochlorhydria. All these effects possibly result from failure of the smooth muscle and glands of the gastrointestinal tract to derive sufficient energy from carbohydrate metabolism.

The overall picture of thiamine deficiency, including polyneuritis, cardiovascular symptoms, and gastrointestinal disorders, is frequently referred to as *beriberi*—especially when the cardiovascular symptoms predominate.

NIACIN

Niacin, also called *nicotinic acid*, functions in the body as coenzymes in the forms of nicotinamide adenine dinucleotide (NAD) and nicotinamide adenine dinucleotide phosphate (NADP). These coenzymes are hydrogen acceptors, which combine with hydrogen atoms as they are removed from food substrates by many different types of dehydrogenases. When a deficiency of niacin exists, the normal rate of dehydrogenation cannot be maintained; therefore, oxidation of the hydrogen and consequent delivery of energy from the foodstuffs to the functioning elements of the cells likewise cannot occur at normal rates.

Because NAD and NADP operate in all cells of the body, it is understandable that lack of niacin can cause multiple symptoms. Clinically, niacin deficiency causes mainly gastrointestinal symptoms, neurological symptoms, and a characteristic dermatitis. Pathological lesions appear in many parts of the central nervous system, and permanent dementia or any of many different types of psychoses may result. Also, the skin develops a cracked, pigmented scaliness in areas that are exposed to mechanical irritation or to sun irradiation; thus, the skin is unable to repair the different types of irritative damage. Finally, niacin deficiency causes intense irritation and inflammation of the mucous membranes of the mouth and other portions of the gastrointestinal tract, thus instituting many digestive abnormalities.

The clinical entity called pellagra is caused mainly by niacin dificiency. Pellagra is greatly exacerbated in persons on a corn diet (such as many of the natives of Africa) because corn in deficient in the amino acid tryptophan, which can be converted in limited quantities to niacin in the body.

RIBOFLAVIN (VITAMIN B₂)

Riboflavin normally combines in the tissues with phosphoric acid to form two coenzymes, *flavin mononucleotide* (FMN), and *flavin adenine dinucleotide* (FAD). These in turn operate as hydrogen carriers in several of the important oxidative systems of the body.

Deficiency of riboflavin in lower animals causes severe *dermatitis*; *vomiting*; *diarrhea*; *muscular spasticity*, which finally becomes muscular weakness; and then *death* preceded by coma and declining body temperature. Thus, severe riboflavin deficiency can cause many of the same effects as lack of niacin in the diet; presumably the debilities that result in each instance are due to generally depressed oxidative processes within the cells.

In the human being, riboflavin deficiency has never been known to be severe enough to cause the marked debilities noted in animal experiments, but mild riboflavin deficiency is probably common. Perhaps the most common characteristic lesion of riboflavin deficiency is *cheilosis*, which is inflammation and cracking at the angles of the mouth. In addition, a fine, scaly dermatitis often occurs at the angles of the nares, and keratitis of the cornea may occur, with invasion of the cornea by small blood vessels.

Though its manifestations are usually relatively mild, riboflavin deficiency frequently occurs in association with lack of thiamine or niacin. Therefore, many deficiency syndromes, including pellagra, beriberi, sprue, and kwashiorkor, are probably due to a combined insufficiency of several of the vitamins and also of protein.

VITAMIN B₁₂

Several different *cobalamin* compounds exhibit so-called vitamin B₁₂ activity.

Vitamin B₁₂ performs many metabolic functions, acting as a hydrogen acceptor coenzyme. For instance, it performs this function in the conversion of amino acids and similar compounds into other substances. Its most important function is to act as a coenzyme for reducing ribonucleotides to deoxyribonucleotides, a step that is important in the formation of genes and that could explain the two major functions of vitamin B₁₂: (1) promotion of growth and (2) red blood cell maturation. This latter function was described in Chapter 19.

A particular effect of vitamin B₁₂ deficiency, pernicious anemia, is often demyelination of the large nerve fibers of the spinal cord, especially of the posterior columns and occasionally of the lateral columns. As a result, persons with pernicious anemia (caused by failure of red cell maturation) frequently have much simultaneous loss of peripheral sensation and, in severe cases, even become paralyzed.

FOLIC ACID (PTEROYLGLUTAMIC ACID)

Several different pteroylglutamic acids exhibit the "folic acid effect." Folic acid functions as a carrier of hydroxymethyl and formyl groups. Perhaps its most important use in the body is in the synthesis of purines and thymine, which are required for formation of deoxyribonucleic acid. Therefore, folic acid is required for reproduction of the cellular genes. This perhaps explains one of the most important functions of folic acid—that is, to promote growth.

Folic acid is an even more potent growth promoter than vitamin B₁₂, and, like vitamin B₁₂, is also important for the maturation of red blood cells, as discussed in Chapter 19. However, vitamin B₁₂ and folic acid each perform specific and different functions in promoting growth and maturation of red blood cells.

PYRIDOXINE (VITAMIN B₆)

Pyridoxine exists in the form of *pyridoxal phosphate* in the cells and functions as a coenzyme for many different chemical reactions relating to amino acid and protein metabolism. Its most important role is that of coenzyme in transamination for the synthesis of amino acids. Also, it is believed to act in the transport of some amino acids across cell membranes.

In the human being, pyridoxine deficiency has been known to cause convulsions, dermatitis, and gastrointestinal disturbances such as nausea and vomiting in children. However, this deficiency is rare.

PANTOTHENIC ACID

Pantothenic acid mainly is incorporated in the body into coenzyme A, which has many metabolic roles in the cells. Two of these discussed in Chapters 45 and 46 are (1) acetylation of decarboxylated pyruvic acid to form acetyl Co-A prior to its entry into the citric acid cycle and (2) degradation of fatty acid molecules into multiple molecules of acetyl Co-A by the process of "beta" oxidation. Thus, lack of pantothenic acid can lead to depressed metabolism of both carbohydrates and fats.

However, in the human being, no definite deficiency syndrome has been proved, presumably because of wide occurrence of this vitamin in almost all foods and because small amounts of the vitamin can probably be synthesized in the body. Nevertheless, this does not mean that pantothenic acid is not of value in the metabolic systems of the body; indeed, it is perhaps as necessary as any other vitamin.

ASCORBIC ACID (VITAMIN C)

Asorbic acid is essential for activating the enzyme *prolyl hydroxylase* that promotes the hydroxylation step in the formation of hydroxyproline, an integral constituent of collagen. Without ascorbic acid the collagen that is formed is defective and weak. Therefore, this vitamin is essential for growth of subcutaneous tissue, cartilage, bone, and teeth.

Deficiency of ascorbic acid for 20 to 30 weeks, as occurred frequently during long sailing voyages in olden days, causes *scurvy*, some effects of which are the following:

One of the most important effects of scurvy is *failure of wounds to heal*. This is caused by failure of the cells to deposit collagen fibrils and intercellular cement substances. As a result, healing of a wound may require several months instead of the several days ordinarily necessary.

Lack of ascorbic acid causes *cessation of bone growth*. The cells of the growing epiphyses continue to proliferate, but no new matrix is laid down between the cells, and the bones fracture easily at the point of growth because of failure to ossify. Also, when an already ossified bone fractures in a person with ascorbic acid deficiency, the osteoblasts cannot secrete a new matrix for the deposition of new bone. Consequently, the fractured bone does not heal.

The *blood vessel walls become extremely fragile* in scurvy because of failure of the endothelial cells to cement together properly and to form the collagen fibrils normally present in vessel walls. The capillaries especially are likely to rupture, and as a result, many small petechial hemorrhages occur throughout the body. The hemorrhages beneath the skin cause purpuric blotches, sometimes over the entire body.

In extreme scurvy the muscle cells sometimes fragment; lesions of the gums with loosening of the teeth occur; infections of the mouth develop; vomiting of blood, bloody stools, and cerebral hemorrhage all may result; and, finally, high fever often develops before death.

VITAMIN D

Vitamin D increases calcium absorption from the gastrointestinal tract and also helps to control calcium deposition in the bone. The mechanism by which vitamin D increases calcium absorption is to promote active transport of calcium through the epithelium of the ileum. It increases the formation of a calcium-binding protein in the epithelial cells that aids in calcium absorption. The specific functions of vitamin D in relation to overall body calcium metabolism and to bone formation are presented in Chapter 53.

VITAMIN E

Several related compounds exhibit so-called vitamin E activity. Only rare instances of vitamin E deficiency occur in human beings. In lower animals, lack of vitamin E can cause degeneration of the germinal epithelium in the testis and therefore can cause male sterility. Lack of vitamin E can also cause resorption of a fetus after conception in the female. Because of these deficiency effects, vitamin E is sometimes called the antisterility vitamin.

Vitamin E deficiency in animals can also cause paralysis of the hindquarters, and pathological changes occur in the muscles similar to those found in muscular dystrophy patients. However, administration of vitamin E to these patients has not proved to be of any benefit.

Finally, as is true of almost all the vitamins, deficiency of vitamin E prevents normal growth.

Vitamin E is believed to function mainly in relation to unsaturated fatty acids, preventing oxidation of the unsaturated fats. In the absence of vitamin E, the quantity of unsaturated fats in the cells becomes diminished, causing abnormal structure and function of such cellular organelles as the mitochondria, the lysosomes, and even the cell membrane.

VITAMIN K

Vitamin K is necessary for the formation by the liver of prothrombin, factor VII (proconvertin), factor IX, and factor X, all of which are important in blood coagulation. Therefore, when vitamin K deficiency occurs, blood clotting is retarded. The function of this vitamin has been presented in greater detail in Chapter 21.

Several different compounds, both natural and synthetic, exhibit vitamin K activity. Because vitamin K is synthesized by bacteria in the colon, a dietary source of this vitamin is not usually necessary; but when the bacteria of the colon are destroyed by administration of large quantities of antibiotic drugs, vitamin K deficiency occurs rapidly because of the paucity of this compound in the normal diet.

QUESTIONS

1. Approximately how much *physiologically available energy* can be derived from each one of the three foodstuffs in the diet: carbohydrates, fat, and protein?
2. What is meant by a *partial protein*, and why are far greater quantities of protein required to maintain protein balance when partial proteins are eaten?
3. How can one use the *respiratory quotient* to determine the relative utilization of carbohyrates and fat by the metabolic systems of the body?
4. Describe the location of the *hunger* and *satiety centers* in the hypothalamus.

5. How does the *amygdala* contribute to the control of feeding?
6. Explain the *glucostatic* and *lipostatic theories* of feeding regulation.
7. Why is it important to have both a *long-term mechanism* for feeding regulation and a *short-term mechanism*? What are the different mechanisms of short-term regulation?
8. In a person who is very obese but has reached a stable weight level, what is the status of this person's energy input-output balance?
9. Explain the role of each of the following factors in *obesity*: psychological status of the person, genetic factors, and childhood overnutrition.
10. In *starvation*, how long do the carbohydrate stores last, and what is the sequence of protein depletion during the starvation period?
11. Describe the functions and the clinical effects of deficits of each of the following vitamins: (a) Vitamin A, (b) Thiamine, (c) Niacin, (d) Riboflavin, (e) Vitamin B$_{12}$, (f) Folic acid, (g) Pyridoxine, (h) Pantothenic acid, (i) Ascorbic acid, (j) Vitamin D, (k) Vitamin E, (l) Vitamin K.

References

Anderson, K. E., et al.: Nutrient regulation of chemical metabolism in humans. Fed Proc 44:130, 1985.

Brennan, M. R.: Total parenteral nutrition in the management of the cancer patient. Annu Rev Med 32:233, 1981.

Brownell, K. D.: The psychology and physiology of obesity: implications for screening and treatment. J Am Diet Assoc 84:406, 1984.

Christensen, H. N.: The regulation of amino acid and sugar absorption by diet. Nutr Rev 42:237, 1984.

Cunningham, J. J.: Introduction to Nutritional Physiology. Philadelphia, G. F. Stickley, 1983.

Forbes, R. M., and Erdman, J. W., Jr.: Biovailability of trace mineral elements. Annu Rev Nutr 3:213, 1983.

Gershwin, M. E.: Nutrition and Immunity. New York, Academic Press, 1985.

Henderson, L. M.: Niacin. Annu Rev Nutr 3:289, 1983.

Hunt, S. M., et al.: Nutrition: Principles and Clinical Practice. New York, John Wiley & Sons, 1980.

LeBow, M. D.: Weight Control: The Behavioural Strategies. New York, John Wiley & Sons, 1980.

MacLean: Pediatric Nutrition in Clinical Practice. Menlo Park, Addison-Wesley Publishing Co., 1984.

Magnen, J. L.: Body energy balance and food intake: a neuroendocrine regulatory mechanism. Physiol Rev 63:314, 1983.

Morr, M. L.: Introductory Foods. New York, Macmillan Publishing Co., 1985.

Nielsen, F. H.: Ultratrace elements in nutrition. Annu Rev Nutr 4:21, 1984.

Olson, R. E.: The function and metabolism of vitamin K. Annu Rev Nutr 4:281, 1984.

Oomura, Y., and Yoshimatsu, H.: Neural network of glucose monitoring system. J Auton Nerv Syst 10:359, 1984.

Ryan, U. S.: Structural bases for metabolic activity. Annu Rev Physiol 44:223, 1982.

Shoden, R. J., and Griffin, W. S.: Fundamentals of Clinical Nutrition. New York, McGraw-Hill, 1980.

Storlien, L. H.: The role of the ventromedial hypothalamic area in periprandial glucoregulation. Life Sci 360:505, 1985.

Sullivan, A. C., and Gruen, R. K.: Mechanisms of appetite modulation by drugs. Fed Proc 44:139, 1985.

Swan, P. B.: Food consumption by individuals in the United States: two major surveys. Annu Rev Nutr 3:413, 1983.

Wolf, G.: Multiple functions of vitamin A. Physiol Rev 64:873, 1984.

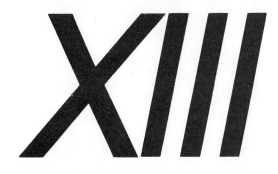

ENDOCRINOLOGY AND REPRODUCTION

49 ■ Introduction to Endocrinology; the Pituitary Hormones

50 ■ The Thyroid Metabolic Hormones

51 ■ The Adrenal Cortical Hormones

52 ■ Insulin, Glucagon, and Diabetes Mellitus

53 ■ Parathyroid Hormone, Calcitonin, Calcium and Phosphate Metabolism, Vitamin D, Bone, and Teeth

54 ■ Reproductive Functions of the Male, the Male Sex Hormones, and the Pineal Gland

55 ■ Prepregnancy Reproductive Functions in the Female and the Female Hormones

56 ■ Pregnancy, Lactation, and Fetal and Neonatal Physiology

49

Introduction to Endocrinology; the Pituitary Hormones

NATURE OF A HORMONE
MECHANISMS OF HORMONAL ACTION
  HORMONE RECEPTORS AND THEIR
    ACTIVATION
  THE CYCLIC AMP MECHANISM FOR
    CONTROLLING CELL FUNCTION—
    A "SECOND MESSENGER" FOR
    HORMONE MEDIATION
  ACTION OF STEROID HORMONES
    ON THE GENES TO CAUSE
    PROTEIN SYNTHESIS
MEASUREMENT OF HORMONE
  CONCENTRATIONS IN THE BLOOD—
  RADIOIMMUNOASSAY
THE PITUITARY GLAND, ITS MULTIPLE
  CONTROL FUNCTIONS, AND ITS
  RELATIONSHIP TO THE
  HYPOTHALAMUS
  CONTROL OF PITUITARY SECRETION
    BY THE HYPOTHALAMUS
THE ANTERIOR PITUITARY GLAND AND
  ITS REGULATION BY HYPOTHALAMIC-
  RELEASING HORMONES

THE HYPOTHALAMIC-HYPOPHYSIAL
  PORTAL SYSTEM
PHYSIOLOGICAL FUNCTIONS OF THE
  ANTERIOR PITUITARY HORMONES
PHYSIOLOGICAL FUNCTIONS OF
  GROWTH HORMONE
  METABOLIC EFFECTS OF GROWTH
    HORMONE
  STIMULATION OF CARTILAGE AND
    BONE GROWTH—ROLE OF THE
    SOMATOMEDINS
  REGULATION OF GROWTH
    HORMONE SECRETION
  ABNORMALITIES OF GROWTH
    HORMONE SECRETION
THE POSTERIOR PITUITARY GLAND AND
  ITS RELATION TO THE
  HYPOTHALAMUS
  PHYSIOLOGICAL FUNCTIONS OF
    ANTIDIURETIC HORMONE
    (VASOPRESSIN)
  OXYTOCIC HORMONE

The functions of the body are regulated by two major control systems: (1) the nervous system, which has been discussed, and (2) the hormonal, or endocrine, system. In general, the hormonal system is concerned principally with control of the metabolic functions of the body, controlling the rates of chemical reactions in the cells, the transport of substances through cell membranes, or other aspects of cellular metabolism such as growth and secretion. Some hormonal effects occur in seconds, while others require several days simply to start, and then they continue for weeks, months, or even years.

Many interrelationships exist between the hormonal and nervous systems. For instance, at least two glands, the *adrenal medullae* and the *posterior pituitary gland*, secrete their hormones only in re-sponse to nerve stimuli, and a few of the anterior pituitary hormones are secreted to a significant extent only in response to nervous activity in the hypothalamus (detailed later in this chapter).

NATURE OF A HORMONE

A hormone is a chemical substance that is secreted into the body fluids by one cell or a group of cells and that exerts a physiological *control* effect on other cells of the body.

At many points in this text we have already discussed different hormones, some of which are called *local hormones,* and others, *general hormones.* Examples of local hormones are *acetylcholine*, released at the parasympathetic and skeletal nerve endings;

secretin, released by the duodenal wall and transported in the blood to the pancreas to cause an alkaline, watery pancreatic secretion; and *cholecystokinin*, released in the small intestine to cause contraction of the gallbladder and to promote enzyme secretion by the pancreas. These hormones obviously have specific local effects, hence the name local hormones.

On the other hand, the general hormones are secreted by specific *endocrine glands* located at different places in the body as illustrated in Figure 49–1. These hormones are secreted into the blood, and they cause physiological actions in distant tissues. A few of the general hormones affect all, or almost all, cells of the body; examples are *growth hormone* from the adenohypophysis and *thyroid hormone* from the thyroid gland. Other general hormones, however, primarily affect specific tissues; for instance, *corticotropin* from the anterior pituitary gland specifically stimulates the adrenal cortex, and the *ovarian hormones* have specific effects on the uterine endometrium. The tissues affected specifically in this way are called *target tissues*. Many examples of target organs will become apparent in the following chapters on endocrinology.

The following general hormones have proved to be of major significance and are discussed in detail in this and the following chapters:

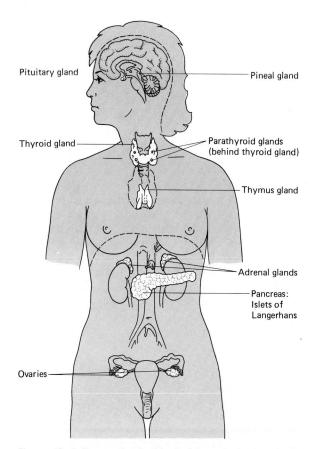

Pituitary gland

Pineal gland

Thyroid gland

Parathyroid glands (behind thyroid gland)

Thymus gland

Adrenal glands

Pancreas: Islets of Langerhans

Ovaries

Figure 49–1. The anatomical loci of the principal endocrine glands of the body.

Anterior Pituitary Hormones

1. *Growth hormone* causes growth of almost all cells and tissues of the body.

2. *Adrenocorticotropin* causes the adrenal cortex to secrete adrenocortical hormones.

3. *Thyroid-stimulating hormone* causes the thyroid gland to secrete thyroxine and triiodothyronine.

4. *Follicle-stimulating hormone* causes growth of follicles in the ovaries prior to ovulation; also promotes the formation of sperm in the testes.

5. *Luteinizing hormone* plays an important role in causing ovulation; also causes secretion of female sex hormones by the ovaries and testosterone by the testes.

6. *Prolactin* promotes development of the breasts and secretion of milk.

Posterior Pituitary Hormones

1. *Antidiuretic hormone* (also called *vasopressin*) causes the kidneys to retain water, thus increasing the water content of the body; also, in high concentrations, causes constriction of the blood vessels throughout the body and elevates the blood pressure.

2. *Oxytocin* contracts the uterus during the birthing process, thus helping expel the baby; it also contracts myoepithelial cells in the breasts, thereby expressing milk from the breasts when the baby suckles.

Adrenal Cortex Hormones

1. *Cortisol* has multiple metabolic functions for control of the metabolism of proteins, carbohydrates, and fats.

2. *Aldosterone* reduces sodium excretion by the kidneys and increases potassium excretion, thus increasing sodium in the body while decreasing the amount of potassium.

Thyroid Gland Hormones

(1, 2). *Thyroxine* and *triiodothyronine* increase the rates of chemical reactions in almost all cells of the body, thus increasing the general level of body metabolism.

3. *Calcitonin* promotes the deposition of calcium in the bones and thereby decreases calcium concentration in the extracellular fluid.

Hormones of the Islets of Langerhans in the Pancreas

1. *Insulin* promotes glucose entry into most cells of the body, in this way controlling the rate of metabolism of most carbohydrates.

2. *Glucagon* increases the release of glucose from the liver into the circulating body fluids.

Hormones of the Ovaries

1. *Estrogens* stimulate the development of the female sex organs, the breasts, and various secondary sexual characteristics.

2. *Progesterone* stimulates secretion of "uterine milk" by the uterine endometrial glands; also helps

promote development of the secretory apparatus of the breasts.

Hormones of the Testes

1. *Testosterone* stimulates growth of the male sex organs; also promotes the development of male secondary sex characteristics.

Parathyroid Gland Hormones

1. *Parathormone* controls the calcium ion concentration of the body by controlling (a) absorption of calcium from the gut, (b) excretion of calcium by the kidneys, and (c) release of calcium from the bones.

Placental Hormones

1. *Human chorionic gonadotropin* promotes growth of the corpus luteum and secretion of estrogens and progesterone by the corpus luteum.

2. *Estrogens* promote growth of the mother's sex organs and of some of the tissues of the fetus.

3. *Progesterone* probably promotes development of some of the fetal tissues and organs; helps promote development of the secretory apparatus of the mother's breasts.

4. *Human somatomammotropin* probably promotes growth of some fetal tissues as well as aiding in the development of the mother's breasts.

MECHANISMS OF HORMONAL ACTION

HORMONE RECEPTORS AND THEIR ACTIVATION

The endocrine hormones almost never act directly on the intracellular machinery to control the different cellular chemical reactions; instead, they almost invariably first combine with *hormone receptors* on the membrane surfaces of the cells or inside the cells. The combination of hormone and receptor then usually initiates a cascade of reactions in the cell.

Either all or almost all hormonal receptors are very large proteins, and each receptor is almost always highly specific for a single hormone.

Activation of the Receptors. The receptors in their unbound state usually are inactive, and the intracellular mechanisms that are associated with them are also inactive. However, in a few instances the unbound receptor, are in the active form, and when bound with the hormone they become inhibited.

Activation of a receptor occurs in different ways for different types of receptors. For instance, in Chapter 31 we discussed the many types of receptors located in the postsynaptic membranes of neurons and activated by the synaptic hormones called transmitter substances. The transmitter substance combines with the receptor and causes a conformational change of the receptor molecule; this in turn alters the membrane permeability to one or more ions, especially sodium, chloride, potassium, and calcium ions. A few of the general endocrine hormones also function in this same way—for instance, epinephrine and norepinephrine change the membrane permeability in certain of their target tissues.

In addition to this occasional direct effect of hormone receptors to change cell membrane permeability, there are also two very important general mechanisms by which a large share of the hormones function: (1) by *activating the cyclic AMP system of the cells,* which in turn activates multiple other intracellular functions, or (2) by *activating the genes of the cell,* which causes the formation of intracellular proteins that in turn initiate specific cellular functions. These two general mechanisms are described as follows:

THE CYCLIC AMP MECHANISM FOR CONTROLLING CELL FUNCTION— A "SECOND MESSENGER" FOR HORMONE MEDIATION

Many hormones exert their effects on cells by first causing the substance *cyclic 3′, 5′-adenosine monophosphate* (cyclic AMP) to be formed in the cell. Once formed, the cyclic AMP causes the hormonal effects inside the cell. Thus, *cyclic AMP is an intracellular hormonal mediator.* It is also frequently called a "second messenger" for hormone mediation—the "first messenger" being the original stimulating hormone.

The cyclic AMP mechanism has been shown to be a way in which all the following hormones (and many more) can stimulate their target tissues:

1. Adrenocorticotropin
2. Thyroid-stimulating hormone
3. Luteinizing hormone
4. Follicle-stimulating hormone
5. Vasopressin
6. Parathyroid hormone
7. Glucagon
8. Catecholamines
9. Secretin
10. The hypothalamic-releasing hormones

Figure 49–2 illustrates the function of the cyclic AMP mechanism in more detail. The stimulating hormone first binds with a specific receptor for that hormone on the membrane surface of the target cell. Then this combination of hormone and receptor activates the protein enzyme *adenyl cyclase,* which is also located in the membrane and is either bound directly with the receptor protein or closely associated with it. A large portion of the adenyl cyclase enzyme protrudes through the inner surface of the membrane into the cytoplasm and, when activated, causes immediate *conversion of much of the cytoplasmic ATP into cyclic AMP.*

Once cyclic AMP is formed inside the cell, it activates still other enzymes. In fact, it usually activates a *cascade of enzymes.* That is, a first enzyme is activated, and this activates another enzyme, which activates still a third, and so forth. The importance of this mechanism is that only a few molecules of activated adenyl cyclase in the cell membrane can

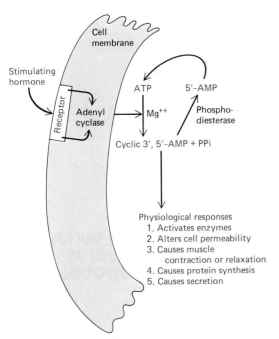

Figure 49–2. The cyclic AMP mechanism by which many hormones exert their control of cell function.

cause many more molecules of the second enzyme to be activated, and these can cause still many times that number of molecules of the third enzyme to be activated, and so forth. In this way, even the slightest amount of hormone acting on the cell surface can initiate a very powerful cascading activating force for the entire cell.

The specific action that occurs in response to cyclic AMP in each type of target cell depends upon the nature of the intracellular machinery, some cells having one set of enzymes and other cells having other enzymes. Therefore, different functions are elicited in different target cells—such functions as

1. initiating synthesis of specific intracellular chemicals

2. causing muscle contraction or relaxation

3. initiating secretion by the cells

4. altering the cell permeability

5. and many other possible effects.

Thus, a thyroid cell stimulated by cyclic AMP forms the metabolic hormones thyroxine and triiodothyronine, whereas the same cyclic AMP in an adrenocortical cell causes secretion of the adrenocortical steroid hormones. On the other hand, cyclic AMP affects epithelial cells of the renal tubules by increasing their permeability to water.

Role of Calcium Ions and Calmodulin as Another Second Messenger System. Another second messenger system operates in response to the entry of calcium ions into cells caused by a hormone that acts on membrane receptors that open calcium channels. On entering the cell, the calcium ions bind with a protein called *calmodulin*. A conformational change occurs that activates the calmodulin, causing multiple effects inside the cell in the same way that cyclic

AMP functions. For instance, calmodulin activates many other enzymes in addition to those activated by cyclic AMP, thus causing an additional set of intracellular metabolic reactions. One of the specific functions of calmodulin is to activate myosin kinase that then acts directly on the myosin of smooth muscle to cause smooth muscle contraction.

ACTION OF STEROID HORMONES ON THE GENES TO CAUSE PROTEIN SYNTHESIS

A second major means by which some hormones act—specifically, the steroid hormones secreted by the adrenal cortex, the ovaries, and the testes—is to cause synthesis of proteins in target cells; some of these proteins are enzymes that in turn activate other functions of the cells.

The sequence of events in steroid function is the following:

1. The steroid hormone enters the cytoplasm of the cell, where it binds with a specific *receptor protein*.

2. The combined receptor protein–hormone then diffuses, or is transported, into the nucleus.

3. The combination then activates specific genes to form messenger RNA.

4. The messenger RNA diffuses into the cytoplasm, where it promotes the translation process at the ribosomes to form new proteins.

To give an example, aldosterone, one of the hormones secreted by the adrenal cortex, enters the cytoplasm of renal tubular cells, which contain its specific receptor protein. Then the outlined sequence of events ensues. After about 45 minutes, proteins that promote sodium reabsorption from the tubules and potassium secretion into the tubules begin to appear in the renal tubular cells. Thus, there is a characteristic delay in the final action of the steroid hormone of 45 minutes to several hours, which is in marked contrast to the almost instantaneous action of some of the peptide and peptide-derived hormones that stimulate cells by the cyclic AMP mechanism.

Action of the Thyroid Hormones in the Cell Nucleus. The thyroid hormones thyroxine and triiodothyronine also activate the genetic mechanisms for formation of many different types of intracellular proteins—probably a hundred or more. Many of these are enzymes that promote enhanced intracellular metabolic activity, as we shall discuss more fully in Chapter 50.

MEASUREMENT OF HORMONE CONCENTRATIONS IN THE BLOOD— RADIOIMMUNOASSAY

Most hormones are present in the blood in extremely minute quantities, some in concentrations as low as one millionth of a milligram (1 picogram) per milliliter. Therefore, except in a few instances, it has been almost impossible to measure these concentra-

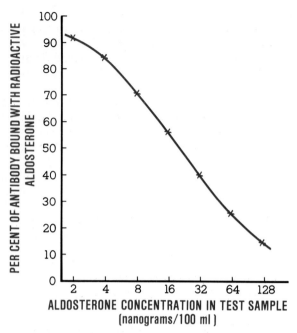

Figure 49–3. A "standard curve" for radioimmunoassay of aldosterone. (Courtesy of Dr. Manis Smith.)

tions by usual chemical means. Fortunately, though, an extremely sensitive method was developed about two decades ago that revolutionized the measurement of hormones, their precursors, and their metabolic end-products. This is the method of *radioimmunoassay*.

The principle of radioimmunoassay is as follows:

First, an antibody is developed that is highly specific for the hormone to be measured.

Second, a small quantity of this antibody is simultaneously mixed with (a) a quantity of fluid (from the person) containing the hormone to be measured and (b) an appropriate amount of purified standard hormone of the same type that has been tagged with a radioactive isotope. However, one specific condition must be met: there must be too little antibody to bind completely both the tagged hormone and the hormone in the fluid to be assayed. Therefore, the natural hormone in the assay fluid and the radioactive standard hormone *compete for the binding sites* on the antibody. In the process of competing, the quantity of each of the two hormones that binds is proportional to its concentration.

Third, after binding has reached equilibrium, the antibody-hormone complex is separated from the remainder of the solution, and the quantity of radioactive hormone bound with antibody is measured by radioactive counting techniques. If a *large amount of radioactive hormone* has bound with the antibody, then it is clear that there was only a *small amount of natural hormone* to compete with the radioactive hormone, and therefore the concentration of the natural hormone in the assayed fluid was small. Conversely, if only a small amount of radioactive hormone was bound, it is clear that there was a very

large amount of natural hormone to compete for the binding sites.

Fourth, to make the assay highly quantitative, the radioimmunoassay procedure is performed also for standard solutions of untagged hormone at several different concentration levels. Then, a standard curve is plotted as illustrated in Figure 49–3. By comparing the radioactive counts recorded from the original assay procedure with the standard curve, one can determine within an error of ± 10 to 15 per cent the concentration of the hormone in the assayed fluid. As little as one trillionth of a gram of hormone is often assayed in this way.

THE PITUITARY GLAND, ITS MULTIPLE CONTROL FUNCTIONS, AND ITS RELATIONSHIP TO THE HYPOTHALAMUS

The *pituitary gland* (Fig. 49–4), also called the *hypophysis,* is a small gland—less than 1 cm in diameter and about 0.5 to 1 gram in weight—that lies in the *sella turcica* at the base of the brain and is connected with the hypothalamus by the *pituitary* (or *hypophysial*) *stalk.* Physiologically, the pituitary gland is divisible into two distinct portions: the *anterior pituitary,* also known as the *adenohypophysis,* and the posterior pituitary, also known as the *neurohypophysis.*

Six very important hormones plus several less important ones are secreted by the *anterior* pituitary, and two important hormones are secreted by the *posterior* pituitary. The hormones of the anterior pituitary play major roles in the control of metabolic functions throughout the body, as shown in Figure 49–5; thus: (1) *Growth hormone* promotes growth by affecting many metabolic functions throughout the body, especially protein formation. (2) *Adrenocorticotropin* controls the secretion of some of the adre-

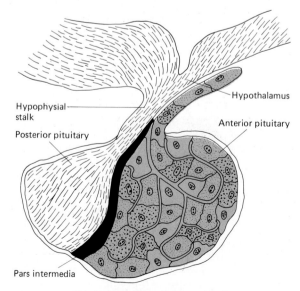

Figure 49–4. The pituitary gland.

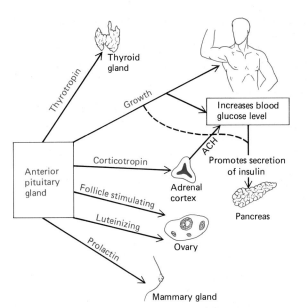

Figure 49–5. Metabolic functions of the anterior pituitary hormones.

nocortical hormones, which in turn affect the metabolism of glucose, proteins, and fats. (3) *Thyroid-stimulating hormone* controls the rate of secretion of thyroxine by the thyroid gland, and thyroxine in turn controls the rates of most chemical reactions of the entire body. (4) *Prolactin* promotes mammary gland development and milk production. And two separate gonadotropic hormones, (5) *follicle-stimulating hormone* and (6) *luteinizing hormone*, control growth of the gonads as well as their reproductive activities.

The two hormones secreted by the posterior pituitary play other roles: (1) *Antidiuretic hormone* controls the rate of water excretion into the urine and in this way helps to control the concentration of water in the body fluids. (2) *Oxytocin* (a) contracts the alveoli of the breasts, thereby helping to deliver milk from the glands of the breast to the nipples during suckling, and (b) contracts the uterus, thus helping in delivery of the baby at the end of gestation.

CONTROL OF PITUITARY SECRETION BY THE HYPOTHALAMUS

Secretion from the posterior pituitary is controlled by nerve fibers originating in the hypothalamus and terminating in the posterior pituitary. In contrast, secretion by the anterior pituitary is controlled by hormones called *hypothalamic-releasing* and *inhibitory hormones* (or *factors*) secreted within the hypothalamus itself and then conducted to the anterior pituitary through minute blood vessels called *hypothalamic-hypophysial portal vessels*. In the anterior pituitary, these releasing and inhibitory hormones act on the glandular cells to control their secretion. This system of control will be discussed in detail later in the chapter.

The hypothalamus receives signals from almost all

possible sources in the nervous system. Thus, when a person is exposed to pain, a portion of the pain signal is transmitted into the hypothalamus. Likewise, when a person experiences some powerful depressing or exciting thought, a portion of the signal is transmitted into the hypothalamus. Olfactory stimuli denoting pleasant or unpleasant smells transmit strong signal components through the amygdaloid nuclei into the hypothalamus. *Even the concentrations of nutrients, electrolytes, water, and various hormones* in the blood excite or inhibit various portions of the hypothalamus. Thus, the hypothalamus is a collecting center for information concerned with the well-being of the body, and in turn much of this information is used to control secretion by the pituitary gland.

THE ANTERIOR PITUITARY GLAND AND ITS REGULATION BY HYPOTHALAMIC–RELEASING HORMONES

The anterior pituitary gland contains at least five different types of secretory cells. Usually, there is one cell type for each major hormone formed in this gland. Using special stains attached to high affinity antibodies that bind with the distinctive hormones, these various cell types can be differentiated one from another. The only major exception to this general rule is that the same cell type seems to secrete both luteinizing hormone and follicle-stimulating hormone.

THE HYPOTHALAMIC-HYPOPHYSIAL PORTAL SYSTEM

The anterior pituitary is a highly vascular gland with extensive capillary sinuses among the glandular cells. Almost all of the blood that enters these sinuses passes first through a capillary bed in the tissue of the lower hypothalamus and then through small *hypothalamic-hypophysial portal vessels* into the anterior pituitary sinuses. Thus, Figure 49–6 illustrates a small artery supplying the lowermost portion of the

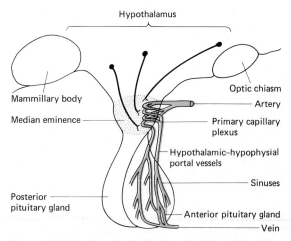

Figure 49–6. The hypothalamic-hypophysial portal system.

hypothalamus, called the *median eminence*. Small vascular tufts project into the substance of the median eminence and then return to its surface, coalescing to form the hypothalamic-hypophysial portal vessels. These in turn pass downward along the pituitary stalk to supply the anterior pituitary sinuses.

Secretion of Hypothalamic-Releasing and Inhibitory Hormones in the Median Eminence. Special neurons in the hypothalamus synthesize and secrete hormones called *hypothalamic-releasing* and *inhibitory hormones* (or *releasing* and *inhibitory factors*) that control the secretion of the anterior pituitary hormones. These neurons originate in various parts of the hypothalamus and send their nerve fibers into the median eminence. The endings of these fibers are different from most endings in the central nervous system in that their function is not to transmit signals from one neuron to another but merely to secrete the hypothalamic-releasing and inhibitory hormones into the tissue fluids. These hormones are immediately absorbed into the hypothalamic-hypophysial portal capillaries and carried directly to the sinuses of the anterior pituitary gland.

Function of the Releasing and Inhibitory Hormones. The function of the releasing and inhibitory hormones is to control the secretion of the anterior pituitary hormones. For each type of anterior pituitary hormone there is usually a corresponding hypothalamic-releasing hormone; for some of the anterior pituitary hormones there is also a corresponding hypothalamic inhibitory hormone. For most of the anterior pituitary hormones, it is the releasing hormones that are important; but for prolactin, the inhibitory hormone probably exerts most control. The hypothalamic-releasing and inhibitory hormones that are of major importance are

1. *Thyroid-stimulating hormone–releasing hormone* (TRH), which causes release by the anterior pituitary gland of thyroid-stimulating hormone

2. *Corticotropin-releasing factor* (CRF), which causes release of adrenocorticotropin

3. *Growth hormone–releasing hormone* (GHRH), which causes release of growth hormone

4. *Luteinizing hormone–releasing hormone* (LRH), which causes release of both luteinizing hormone and follicle-stimulating hormone

5. *Prolactin inhibitory factor* (PIF), which causes inhibition of prolactin secretion.

PHYSIOLOGICAL FUNCTIONS OF THE ANTERIOR PITUITARY HORMONES

All of the major anterior pituitary hormones besides growth hormone exert their effects by stimulating "target glands"—the thyroid gland, the adrenal cortex, the ovaries, the testicles, and the mammary glands. The functions of each of the anterior pituitary hormones, except for growth hormone, are so intimately concerned with the functions of the respective target glands that their functions will be discussed in

subsequent chapters along with the functions of these target glands. Growth hormone, in contrast to other hormones, does not function through a target gland but instead exerts effects on all or almost all tissues of the body.

PHYSIOLOGICAL FUNCTIONS OF GROWTH HORMONE

Growth hormone (GH), also called *somatotropic hormone* (SH) or *somatotropin*, is a small protein molecule containing 191 amino acids in a single chain and having a molecular weight of 22,005. It causes growth of all tissues of the body that are capable of growing. It promotes both increased sizes of the cells and increased mitosis with development of increased numbers of cells. As an example, Figure 49–7 illustrates weight charts of two growing rats, one of which received daily injections of growth hormone, compared with a litter-mate that did not receive growth hormone.

METABOLIC EFFECTS OF GROWTH HORMONE

Aside from its general effect of causing growth, growth hormone has many specific metabolic effects as well, including especially:

1. Increased rate of protein synthesis in all cells of the body

2. Increased mobilization of fatty acids from adipose tissue, and increased use of the fatty acids for energy

3. Decreased rate of glucose utilization throughout the body

Thus, in effect, growth hormone enhances the body protein, uses up the fat stores, and conserves carbohydrate. It is probable that the increased rate of growth results mainly from the increased rate of protein synthesis.

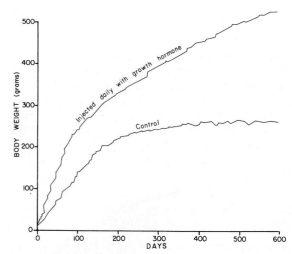

Figure 49–7. Comparison of weight gain of a rat injected daily with growth hormone with that of a normal rat.

Role of Growth Hormone in Promoting Protein Deposition

Although the most important basis for the increased protein deposition caused by growth hormone is not known, a series of different effects are known, all of which can lead to enhanced protein. These effects are

1. Enhancement of Amino Acid Transport Through the Cell Membranes. Growth hormone directly enhances transport of at least some and perhaps most amino acids through the cell membranes to the interior of the cells. This increases the concentrations of the amino acids in the cells and is presumed to be at least partly responsible for the increased protein synthesis.

2. Enhancement of Protein Synthesis by the Ribosomes. Even when the amino acids are not increased, growth hormone still causes protein to be synthesized in increased amounts in the cells. This is believed to be partly due to a direct effect on the ribosomal machinery, making it produce greater numbers of protein molecules.

3. Increased Formation of RNA. Over more prolonged periods of time, growth hormone also stimulates the transcription process in the nucleus, causing formation of increased quantities of RNA. This in turn promotes protein synthesis.

4. Decreased Catabolism of Protein and Amino Acids. In addition to the increase in protein synthesis, there is a decrease in the breakdown of protein and in the utilization of protein and amino acids for energy. A possible, if not probable, reason for this effect is that growth hormone also mobilizes large quantities of free fatty acids from the adipose tissue, and these in turn are used to supply most of the energy for the body cells; thus growth hormone acts as a potent "protein sparer."

Summary. Growth hormone enhances almost all facets of amino acid uptake and protein synthesis by cells while at the same time reducing the breakdown of proteins.

Effect of Growth Hormone in Enhancing Fat Utilization for Energy

Growth hormone has a specific effect in causing release of fatty acids from adipose tissue and therefore increasing the fatty acid concentration in the body fluids. In addition, in the tissues it enhances the conversion of fatty acids to acetyl-CoA, with subsequent utilization of this product for energy. Therefore, under the influence of growth hormone, fat is utilized for energy in preference to both carbohydrates and proteins.

Effect of Growth Hormone on Carbohydrate Metabolism

Growth hormone has three major effects on cellular metabolism of glucose. These effects are (1) decreased utilization of glucose for energy, (2) marked enhancement of glycogen deposition in the cells, and (3) diminished uptake of glucose by the cells.

Decreased Glucose Utilization for Energy. Unfortunately, we do not know the precise mechanism by which growth hormone decreases glucose utilization by the cells. However, the decrease probably results partially from the increased mobilization and utilization of fatty acids for energy caused by growth hormone. That is, the fatty acids form large quantities of acetyl-CoA, which in turn initiate feedback effects that block the glycolytic breakdown of glucose and glycogen.

Enhancement of Glycogen Deposition. Since glucose and glycogen cannot be utilized for energy, the glucose that does enter the cells is rapidly polymerized into glycogen and deposited. Therefore, the cells rapidly become saturated with glycogen and can store no more.

Diminished Uptake of Glucose by the Cells and Increased Blood Glucose Concentration. When growth hormone is first administered to an animal, the cellular uptake of glucose is enhanced and the blood glucose concentration falls slightly. However, as the cells become saturated with glycogen and their utilization of glucose for energy decreases, further uptake of glucose then becomes greatly diminished. Without normal cellular uptake, the blood concentration of glucose increases, sometimes to as high as 50 to 100 per cent above normal.

STIMULATION OF CARTILAGE AND BONE GROWTH—ROLE OF THE SOMATOMEDINS

Though we have discussed at length the role of growth hormone in causing growth, growth hormone does not have a *direct* effect on the growth of the skeletal elements cartilage and bone. For instance, when growth hormone is applied directly to cartilage chondrocytes cultured outside the body, no discernible proliferation or enlargement of the chondrocytes occurs, even though growth hormone injected into the intact animal does cause such proliferation and growth. To make a long story short, it has been found that growth hormone acts indirectly on cartilage and bone by causing the liver to form several small proteins called *somatomedins*, with molecular weights varying between 4500 and 7500. These somatomedins then act on the cartilage and bone to promote their growth. Their basic function is that one or more of them is required for deposition of chondroitin sulfate and collagen, both of which are necessary for cartilage and bone growth.

Other Metabolic and Growth Functions of the Somatomedins. Though growth hormone can cause all the metabolic effects that we have discussed thus far, except cartilage and bone growth, when added directly to tissues removed from the body, the concentrations of growth hormone that are required to cause these actions are often many times as great as those known to exist in the body. On the other hand, the different somatomedins in very small concentrations can cause essentially all the same effects as the direct actions of growth hormone. Therefore, it is probable that most of the metabolic functions of growth hormone are caused not by its direct effects on the tissues, but indirectly through the somatomedins.

REGULATION OF GROWTH HORMONE SECRETION

For many years it was believed that growth hormone was secreted primarily during the period of growth but then disappeared from the blood at adolescence. However, this belief has proved to be very far from the truth, because after adolescence secretion continues at a rate almost as great as that in childhood. Furthermore, the rate of growth hormone secretion can increase within minutes in relation to the person's state of nutrition or stress—during starvation, hypoglycemia, exercise, excitement, and trauma.

The normal concentration of growth hormone in the plasma of an adult is about 3 nanograms per milliliter and in the child about 5 nanograms per milliliter. However, these values often increase to as high as 50 nanograms per milliliter after depletion of the body stores of proteins or carbohydrates. Under acute conditions, hypoglycemia is a far more potent stimulator of growth hormone secretion than is a decrease in the amino acid concentration in the blood. On the other hand, in chronic conditions the degree of cellular protein depletion seems to be more correlated with the level of growth hormone secretion than is the availability of glucose. For instance, the extremely high levels of growth hormone that occur during starvation are very closely related to the amount of protein depletion.

Thus, it is almost certain that growth hormone secretion is controlled moment by moment by the nutritional and stress status of the body, and it seems that the most important factor in the control of growth hormone secretion is the level of cell protein, though changes in blood glucose concentration can also cause extremely rapid and dramatic alterations in growth hormone secretion. Consequently, it can be postulated that growth hormone operates in a feedback control system as follows: When the tissues begin to suffer from malnutrition, especially from poor protein nutrition, large quantities of growth hormone are secreted. Growth hormone, in turn, promotes the synthesis of new proteins, while at the same time conserving the protein already present in the cells.

Role of the Hypothalamus and Growth Hormone–Releasing Hormone (GHRH). All of these feedback effects that control growth hormone secretion are believed to be mediated through the hypothalamus. The hypothalamus secretes *growth hormone–releasing hormone* (GHRH), which in turn causes the anterior pituitary to secrete the growth hormone. The hypothalamic center that causes growth hormone secretion is the *ventromedial nucleus,* the same nucleus that helps to control other aspects of metabolism, such as the level of hunger and feeding.

ABNORMALITIES OF GROWTH HORMONE SECRETION

Dwarfism. Some instances of dwarfism result from deficiency of anterior pituitary secretion of growth hormone during childhood. In general, the features of the body develop in appropriate proportion to each other, but the rate of development is greatly decreased. A child who has reached the age of 10 may have the bodily development of a child of 4 to 5, whereas the same person on reaching the age of 20 may have the bodily development of a child of 7 to 10.

Two thirds of the pituitary dwarfs do not pass through puberty and do not secrete a sufficient quantity of gonadotropic hormones to develop adult sexual functions. In one third, however, the deficiency is of growth hormone alone; these individuals do mature sexually and occasionally reproduce.

Giantism. Occasionally, the growth hormone-producing cells of the anterior pituitary become excessively active, and sometimes even growth hormone cell (acidophilic cell) tumors occur in the gland. As a result, large quantities of growth hormone are produced. All body tissues grow rapidly, including the bones, and if the epiphyses of the long bones have not already become fused with the shafts—that is, if this occurs before adolescence—height increases, so that the person becomes a giant with a height up to 8 to 9 feet.

Most giants, unfortunately, eventually develop hypopituitarism if they remain untreated, because the tumor of the pituitary gland grows until the gland itself is destroyed. This general deficiency of pituitary hormones, if untreated, usually causes death in early adulthood. However, once giantism is diagnosed, further development of the disease can usually be blocked by microsurgical removal of the tumor from the pituitary gland or by irradiation of the gland.

Acromegaly. If a growth hormone cell tumor occurs after adolescence—that is, after the epiphyses of the long bones have fused with the shafts—the person cannot grow taller; but his soft tissues can continue to grow, and the bones can grow in thickness. This condition is known as *acromegaly.* Enlargement is especially marked in the small bones of the hands and feet and in the *membranous bones,* including the cranium, the nose, the bosses on the forehead, the supraorbital ridges, the lower jawbone, and portions of the vertebrae, for their growth does not cease at adolescence anyway. Consequently, as illustrated in Figure 49–8 (a typical acromegalic), the jaw protrudes forward, sometimes as much as a half inch; the forehead slants forward because of excess development of the supraorbital ridges; and the nose increases to as much as twice normal size. Also, the foot requires a size 14 or larger shoe, and the fingers become extremely thickened, so that the hand devel-

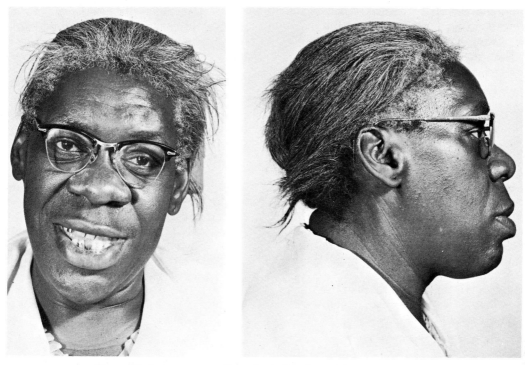

Figure 49–8. An acromegalic patient. (Courtesy of Dr. Herbert Langford.)

ops a size almost twice normal. In addition to these effects, changes in the vertebrae ordinarily cause a hunched back. Finally, many soft tissue organs, such as the tongue, the liver, and especially the kidneys, become greatly enlarged.

THE POSTERIOR PITUITARY GLAND AND ITS RELATION TO THE HYPOTHALAMUS

The *posterior pituitary gland,* also called the *neurohypophysis,* is composed mainly of glia-like cells called *pituicytes.* However, the pituicytes do not secrete hormones; they act simply as a supporting structure for large numbers of *terminal nerve fibers* and *terminal nerve endings* from nerve tracts that originate in the *supraoptic* and *paraventricular nuclei* of the hypothalamus, as shown in Figure 49–9. These tracts pass to the neurohypophysis through the *pituitary stalk* (hypophysial stalk). The nerve endings are bulbous knobs that lie on the surfaces of capillaries onto which they secrete the two posterior pituitary hormones: (1) *antidiuretic hormone* (ADH), also called *vasopressin,* and (2) *oxytocin.* Both of these hormones are small polypeptides, each containing nine amino acids. They are identical with each other except for two of the amino acids.

If the pituitary stalk is cut near the pituitary gland, leaving the entire hypothalamus intact, the posterior pituitary hormones continue, after a transient decrease for a few days, to be secreted almost normally, but they are then secreted by the cut ends of the fibers within the hypothalamus and not by the nerve endings in the posterior pituitary. The reason for this is that the hormones are initially synthesized in the cell bodies of the neurons in the supraoptic and paraventricular nuclei and are then transported to the nerve endings in the posterior pituitary gland, requiring several days to reach the gland.

ADH is formed primarily in the supraoptic nuclei, while *oxytocin is formed primarily in the paraventricular nuclei.* However, each of these two nuclei can synthesize approximately one sixth as much of the second hormone as the primary hormone.

Under resting conditions, large quantities of both ADH and oxytocin accumulate in the nerve endings of the posterior pituitary gland. Then, when nerve impulses are transmitted downward along the fibers

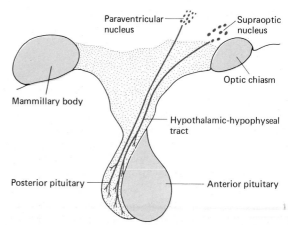

Figure 49–9. Hypothalamic control of the posterior pituitary.

from the supraoptic and paraventricular nuclei, the hormones are immediately released from the nerve endings and are absorbed into the adjacent capillaries.

PHYSIOLOGICAL FUNCTIONS OF ANTIDIURETIC HORMONE (VASOPRESSIN)

Extremely minute quantities of antidiuretic hormone (ADH)—as little as 2 nanograms—when injected into a person can cause antidiuresis, that is, decreased excretion of water by the kidneys. This antidiuretic effect was discussed in detail in Chapter 25. Briefly, in the absence of ADH, the collecting ducts and collecting tubules are almost totally impermeable to water, which prevents significant reabsorption of water and therefore allows extreme loss of water into the urine. On the other hand, in the presence of ADH, the permeability of these ducts to water increases greatly and allows most of the water in the tubular fluid to be reabsorbed, thereby conserving water in the body.

Regulation of ADH Production

Osmotic Regulation. When the body fluids become highly concentrated, the supraoptic nuclei become excited, impulses are transmitted to the posterior pituitary, and ADH is secreted. This hormone then passes by way of the blood to the kidneys, where it increases the permeability of the collecting tubules and ducts to water. As a result, most of the water is reabsorbed from the tubular fluid, while electrolytes continue to be lost into the urine. This effect dilutes the extracellular fluids, returning them to a normal osmotic composition. The details of this mechanism were also discussed in Chapter 25 in relation to body fluid electrolyte control.

Stimulation of ADH Secretion When the Blood

Volume Decreases—Pressor Effect of ADH. ADH in moderate concentrations has a very potent effect of constricting the arterioles and therefore of increasing the arterial pressure. Also, one of the most powerful stimuli of all for increasing the secretion of ADH is severe loss of blood volume. As little as 10 per cent loss of blood will promote a moderate increase in ADH secretion, and 25 per cent or more blood loss can cause as much as 20 to 50 times normal rates of secretion.

The increased secretion is believed to result mainly from the low pressure caused in the atria of the heart by the low blood volume. The relaxation of the atrial stretch receptors supposedly elicits the increase in ADH secretion. However, the baroreceptors of the carotid, aortic, and pulmonary regions also participate in this control of ADH secretion.

The marked secretion of ADH following hemorrhage perhaps plays a very important role in the homeostasis of arterial pressure. Because ADH has this potent pressor effect, it is also called *vasopressin*.

OXYTOCIC HORMONE

Effect on the Uterus. An oxytocic substance is one that causes contraction of the pregnant uterus. The hormone *oxytocin*, in accordance with its name, powerfully stimulates the pregnant uterus, especially toward the end of gestation. Therefore many obstetricians believe that this hormone is at least partially responsible for effecting the birth of the baby. This will be discussed in Chapter 56 in relation to reproduction and pregnancy.

Effect of Oxytocin on Milk Ejection. Oxytocin also has an especially important function in the process of lactation, for this hormone causes milk to be expressed from the alveoli into the ducts so that the baby can obtain it by suckling. This, too, will be discussed in Chapter 56.

QUESTIONS

1. Explain the role of *membrane receptors* in the activation of tissue cells by hormones.
2. Describe the *cyclic AMP mechanism* as a second messenger system for controlling cell function.
3. Explain the role of *calmodulin* as a second messenger system.
4. Explain how steroid hormones and thyroid hormone act on the *cell genes* to cause their hormonal effects.
5. Describe the relationship of the pituitary gland to the hypothalamus, especially the *hypothalamic-hypophysial portal system*.
6. What are the important *releasing* and *inhibitory hormones* secreted by the hypothalamus, and what are their functions?
7. How does growth hormone promote *protein deposition*?
8. What is the effect of growth hormone on *fat mobilization* and utilization for energy?
9. What are the effects of growth hormone on *carbohydrate metabolism*?
10. Explain the role of the *somatomedins* in promoting bone and cartilage growth as well as other possible functions of growth hormone.
11. What are the principal metabolic and nervous factors that can cause increased growth hormone secretion? How do the hypothalamus and *growth hormone–releasing hormone* function in the control of growth hormone secretion?
12. Explain the causes of pituitary *dwarfism*, *giantism*, and *acromegaly*.
13. Describe the secretion and the release of the posterior pituitary hormones.
14. What are the principal functions of *antidiuretic hormone*?
15. What are the principal functions of *oxytocic* hormone?

References

General Endocrinology

Aurbach, G. D.: Polypeptide and amine hormone regulation of adenylate cyclase. Annu Rev Physiol 44:653, 1982.

Blackshear, P. J.: Key References in Endocrinology. An Annotated Guide. New York, Churchill Livingstone, 1982.

Cheung, W. Y.: Calmodulin: its potential role in cell proliferation and heavy metal toxicity. Fed Proc 43:2995, 1984.

Dawson, K. G.: Endocrine physiology of electrolyte metabolism. Drugs 28(Suppl. 1):98, 1984.

Douglass, J., et al.: Polyprotein gene expression: generation of diversity of neuroendocrine peptides. Annu Rev Biochem 53:665, 1984.

Gustafsson, J.-A., et al.: Central control of prolactin and estrogen receptors in rat liver—expression of a novel endocrine system, the hypothalamo-pituitary-liver axis. Annu Rev Pharmacol Toxicol 23:259, 1983.

Hall, P. F.: The role of the cytoskeleton in hormone action. Can J Biochem Cell Biol 62:653, 1984.

Kupfermann, I.: Role of cyclic nucleotides in excitable cells. Annu Rev Physiol 42:629, 1980.

Means, A. R., and Chafouleas, J. G.: Calmodulin in endocrine cells. Annu Rev Physiol 44:667, 1982.

Means, A. R., et al.: Physiological implications of the presence, distribution, and regulation of calmodulin in eukaryotic cells. Physiol Rev 62:1, 1982.

Poste, G.: New insights into receptor regulation. J Appl Physiol 57:1297, 1984.

Rasmussen, H., and Barrett, P. Q.: Calcium messenger system: an integrated view. Physiol Rev 64:938, 1984.

Roth, J., and Taylor, S. I.: Receptors for peptide hormones: alterations in diseases of humans. Annu Rev Physiol 44:639, 1982.

Sherman, M. R., and Stevens, J.: Structure of mammalian steroid receptors: evolving concepts and methodological developments. Annu Rev Physiol 46:83, 1984.

Stiles, G. L., et al.: β-Adrenergic receptors: biochemical mechanisms of physiological regulation. Physiol Rev 64:661, 1984.

Tixier-Vidal, A., and Gourdji, D.: Mechanism of action of synthetic hypothalamic peptides on anterior pituitary cells. Physiol Rev *61*:974, 1981.

Yalow, R. W.: Radioimmunoassay. Annu Rev Biophys Bioeng 9:327, 1980.

Pituitary Hormones

Brownstein, M. J.: Biosynthesis of vasopressin and oxytocin. Annu Rev Physiol 45:129, 1983.

Chawla, R. K., et al.: Structural variants for human growth hormone: biochemical, genetic, and clinical aspects. Annu Rev Med 34:519, 1983.

Chrousos, G. P., et al.: NIH Conference: Clinical applications of corticotropin-releasing factor. Ann Intern Med 102:344, 1985.

Conn, P. M., et al.: Gonadotropin-releasing hormone: molecular and cell biology, physiology, and clinical applications. Fed Proc 43:2351, 1984.

Gann, D. S., et al.: Neural interaction in control of adrenocorticotropin. Fed Proc 44:161, 1985.

Handler, J. S., and Orloff, J.: Antidiuretic hormone. Annu Rev Physiol 43:611, 1981.

Johnston, F. E., et al., eds.: Human Physical Growth and Maturation: Methodologies and Factors. New York, Plenum Press, 1980.

Lewis, U. J.: Variants of growth hormone and prolactin and their posttranslational modifications. Annu Rev Physiol 46:33, 1984.

Menninger, R. P.: Current concepts of volume receptor regulation of vasopressin release. Fed Proc 4:55, 1985.

Nissley, S. P., and Rechler, M. M.: Somatomedin/insulin-like growth factor tissue receptors. Clin Endocrinol Metab 13:43, 1984.

Oriordan, J. L.: Recent Advances in Endocrinology and Metabolism. New York, Churchill Livingstone, 1982.

Rennels, E. G., and Herbert, D. C.: Functional correlates of anterior pituitary cytology. In Greep, R. O., ed.: International Review of Physiology: Reproductive Physiology III. Vol. 22. Baltimore, University Park Press, 1980, p. 1.

Sawyer, W. H., and Manning, M.: The use of antagonists of vasopressin in studies of its physiological functions. Fed Proc 44:78, 1985.

Sklar, A. H., and Schrier, R. W.: Central nervous system mediators of vasopressin release. Physiol Rev 63:1243, 1983.

Swanson, L. W., and Sawchenko, P. E.: Hypothalamic integration: organization of the paraventricular and supraoptic nuclei. Ann Rev Neurosci 6:269, 1983.

Wass, J. A. H., and Besser, G. M.: The medical management of hormone-secreting tumors of the pituitary. Annu Rev Med 34:283, 1983.

50

The Thyroid
Metabolic Hormones

FORMATION AND SECRETION OF THE THYROID HORMONES
REQUIREMENTS OF IODINE FOR FORMATION OF THYROXINE
THE IODIDE PUMP (IODIDE TRAPPING)
THYROGLOBULIN AND THE CHEMISTRY OF THYROXINE AND TRIIODOTHYRONINE FORMATION
RELEASE OF THYROXINE AND TRIIODOTHYRONINE FROM THYROGLOBULIN
TRANSPORT OF THYROXINE AND TRIIODOTHYRONINE TO THE TISSUES

FUNCTIONS OF THE THYROID HORMONES IN THE TISSUES
GENERAL INCREASE IN METABOLIC RATE
EFFECTS OF THYROID HORMONE ON GROWTH
EFFECTS OF THYROID HORMONE ON SPECIFIC PHYSIOLOGICAL MECHANISMS
REGULATION OF THYROID HORMONE SECRETION
DISEASES OF THE THYROID
HYPERTHYROIDISM
HYPOTHYROIDISM

The thyroid gland, which is located immediately below the larynx on either side of and anterior to the trachea, secretes large amounts of two hormones, *thyroxine* and *triiodothyronine*, that have a profound effect on the metabolic rate of the body. It also secretes *calcitonin*, a hormone that is important for calcium metabolism and which will be considered in Chapter 53. Complete lack of thyroid secretion usually causes the basal metabolic rate to fall to about 40 per cent below normal, and extreme excesses of thyroid secretion can cause the basal metabolic rate to rise as high as 60 to 100 per cent above normal. Thyroid secretion is controlled primarily by thyroid-stimulating hormone secreted by the anterior pituitary gland.

The purpose of this chapter is to discuss the formation and secretion of the thyroid hormones, their functions in the metabolic schema of the body, and the regulation of their secretion.

FORMATION AND SECRETION OF THE THYROID HORMONES

The most abundant of the hormones secreted by the thyroid gland is *thyroxine*. However, moderate amounts of *triiodothyronine* are also secreted. The functions of these two hormones are qualitatively the same, but they differ in rapidity and intensity of action. Triiodothyronine is about four times as potent as thyroxine, but it is present in the blood in smaller quantities and persists for a much shorter time than does thyroxine.

Physiological Anatomy of the Thyroid Gland. The thyroid gland is composed, as shown in Figure 50–1, of large numbers of closed *follicles* filled with a secretory substance called *colloid* and lined with *cuboidal epithelioid cells* that secrete into the interior of the follicles. The major constituent of colloid is a large glycoprotein, *thyroglobulin*, which contains the thyroid hormones as part of its molecule. Once the secretion has entered the follicles, the thyroid hormones must be absorbed back through the follicular epithelium into the blood before they can function in the body, which is a very slow process.

REQUIREMENTS OF IODINE FOR FORMATION OF THYROXINE

To form normal quantities of thyroxine, approximately 50 mg of ingested iodine are required *each year*, or approximately *1 mg per week*. To prevent

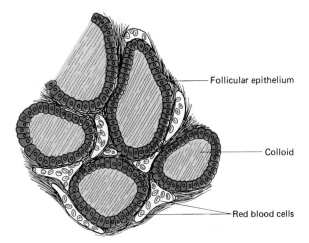

Figure 50–1. Microscopic appearance of the thyroid gland, showing the secretion of thyroglobulin into the follicles.

iodine deficiency, common table salt is iodized with one part sodium iodide to every 100,000 parts sodium chloride.

THE IODIDE PUMP (IODIDE TRAPPING)

The first stage in the formation of thyroid hormones, as shown in Figure 50–2, is the transfer of iodides from the extracellular fluid into the thyroid glandular cells and thence into the follicle. The basal membrane of the thyroid cell has a specific ability to transport iodides actively to the interior of the cell; this is called the *iodide pump*, or *iodide trapping*. In a normal gland, the iodide pump can concentrate the iodide ion to about 30 times its concentration in the blood. However, when the thyroid gland becomes maximally active, the concentration ratio can rise to several times this value.

THYROGLOBULIN AND THE CHEMISTRY OF THYROXINE AND TRIIODOTHYRONINE FORMATION

Formation and Secretion of Thyroglobulin by the Thyroid Cells. The thyroid cells are typical protein-secreting glandular cells, as illustrated in Figure 50–2. The endoplasmic reticulum and the Golgi complex synthesize and secrete into the follicles a large glycoprotein molecule with a molecular weight of 660,000 called *thyroglobulin*.

Each molecule of thyroglobulin contains 140 tyrosine amino acids, and these are the major substrates that combine with iodine to form the thyroid hormones. These hormones form *within* the thyroglobulin molecule. That is, the tyrosine amino acid residues, as well as the thyroxine and triiodothyronine hormones formed from them, remain a part of the thyroglobulin molecule during the entire synthesis of the thyroid hormones.

In addition to secreting the thyroglobulin, the glandular cells also provide the iodine, the enzymes, and the other substances necessary for thyroid hormone synthesis.

Oxidation of the Iodide Ion. An essential step in the formation of the thyroid hormones is conversion of the iodide ions to an *oxidized form of iodine* that is then capable of combining directly with the amino acid tyrosine. This oxidation of iodine is promoted by the enzyme *peroxidase* and the accompanying *hydrogen peroxide*, which together provide a potent system capable of oxidizing iodides. The peroxidase is located either in the apical membrane of the cell or in the cytoplasm immediately adjacent to this membrane, thus providing the oxidized iodine at exactly the point in the cell where the thyroglobulin molecule first issues from the Golgi apparatus.

Iodination of Tyrosine and Formation of the Thyroid Hormones—Organification of Thyroglobulin. The binding of iodine with the thyroglobulin molecule is called *organification* of the thyroglobulin. Oxidized iodine even in the molecular form will bind directly but slowly with the amino acid tyrosine, but in the thyroid cell, the oxidized iodine is associated with an *iodinase* enzyme that causes the process to occur in seconds or minutes. Therefore, almost as rapidly as the thyroglobulin molecule is released from the Golgi apparatus or as it is secreted through the apical cell membrane into the follicle, iodine binds with about one sixth of the tyrosine residues within the thyroglobulin molecule.

Figure 50–3 illustrates the successive stages of iodination of tyrosine and the final formation of the two important thyroid hormones, thyroxine and triiodothyronine. Tyrosine is first iodized to form *monoiodotyrosine* and then to form *diiodotyrosine*. Then during the next few minutes, hours, and days, more and more of the diiodotyrosine residues become *coupled* with each other. The product of the coupling reaction is the molecule *thyroxine*, which also remains part of the thyroglobulin molecule. Or, one molecule of monoiodotyrosine couples with one molecule of diiodotyrosine to form *triiodothyronine*.

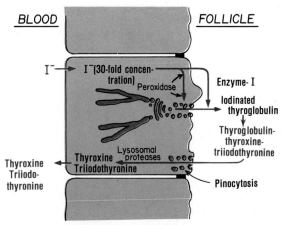

Figure 50–2. Thyroid cellular mechanisms for iodine transport, thyroxine (and triiodothyronine) formation, and thyroxine (and triiodothyronine) release into the blood.

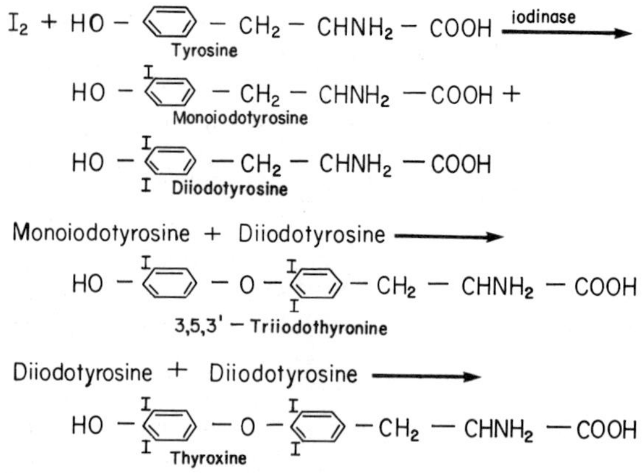

$$I_2 + HO - \langle hexagon \rangle - CH_2 - CHNH_2 - COOH \xrightarrow{iodinase}$$
Tyrosine

$$HO - \overset{I}{\underset{}{\langle hexagon \rangle}} - CH_2 - CHNH_2 - COOH +$$
Monoiodotyrosine

$$HO - \overset{I}{\underset{I}{\langle hexagon \rangle}} - CH_2 - CHNH_2 - COOH$$
Diiodotyrosine

$$\text{Monoiodotyrosine} + \text{Diiodotyrosine} \longrightarrow$$

$$HO - \overset{I}{\langle hexagon \rangle} - O - \overset{I}{\underset{I}{\langle hexagon \rangle}} - CH_2 - CHNH_2 - COOH$$
3,5,3' − Triiodothyronine

$$\text{Diiodotyrosine} + \text{Diiodotyrosine} \longrightarrow$$

$$HO - \overset{I}{\underset{I}{\langle hexagon \rangle}} - O - \overset{I}{\underset{I}{\langle hexagon \rangle}} - CH_2 - CHNH_2 - COOH$$
Thyroxine

Figure 50–3. Chemistry of thyroxine and triiodothyronine formation.

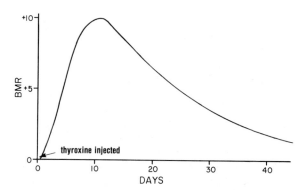

Figure 50–4. Prolonged effect on the basal metabolic rate caused by administering a single large dose of thyroxine.

Storage of Thyroglobulin. After synthesis of the thyroid hormones has run its course, each thyroglobulin molecule contains from 5 to 6 thyroxine molecules, and there is an average of one triiodothyronine molecule for every ten molecules of thyroxine. In this form the thyroid hormones are often stored in the follicles for several months. In fact, the total amount stored is sufficient to supply the body with its normal requirements of thyroid hormones for one to three months. Therefore, even when synthesis of thyroid hormone ceases entirely, the effects of deficiency might not be observed for several months.

RELEASE OF THYROXINE AND TRIIODOTHYRONINE FROM THYROGLOBULIN

Thyroglobulin itself is not released into the circulating blood; instead, the thyroxine and triiodothyronine are first cleaved from the thyroglobulin molecule, and then these free hormones are released. This process occurs as follows: The apical surface of the thyroid cells continually sends out pseudopod extensions that close around small portions of the colloid to form pinocytic vesicles. Then lysosomes immediately fuse with these vesicles to form digestive vesicles containing the digestive enzymes from the lysosomes mixed with the colloid. The *proteinases* among these enzymes digest the thyroglobulin molecules and release the thyroxine and triiodothyronine, which then diffuse through the base of the thyroid cell into the surrounding capillaries. In this way, the thyroid hormones are released into the blood.

TRANSPORT OF THYROXINE AND TRIIODOTHYRONINE TO THE TISSUES

Binding of Thyroxine and Triiodothyronine with the Plasma Proteins. On entering the blood, all but minute portions of the thyroxine and triiodothyronine combine immediately with several of the plasma proteins, especially with *thyroxine-binding globulin*, which is a glycoprotein. Then, half of the thyroxine bound with the proteins is released to the tissue cells approximately every 6 days, whereas half of the

triiodothyronine—because of its lower affinity for the proteins—is released to the cells in approximately 1.3 days.

On entering the cells, both of these hormones again bind with intracellular proteins, the thyroxine once again binding more strongly than the triiodothyronine. They therefore are again stored, but this time in the functional cells themselves, and they are used slowly over a period of days or weeks.

Latency and Duration of Action of the Thyroid Hormones. After injection of a large quantity of thyroxine into a human being, essentially no effect on the metabolic rate can be discerned for two to three days, thereby illustrating that there is a *long latent period* before thyroxine activity begins. Once activity does begin, it increases progressively and reaches a maximum in 10 to 12 days, as shown in Figure 50–4. Thereafter, activity decreases, with a half-time of about 15 days. Some of the activity still persists as long as 6 weeks to 2 months later.

The actions of triiodothyronine occur about 4 times as rapidly as those of thyroxine, with a latent period as short as 6 to 12 hours and maximum cellular activity occurring within 2 to 3 days.

A large part of the latency and prolonged period of action of these hormones is caused by their binding with proteins both in the plasma and in the tissue cells, followed by their slow release. However, we shall see in subsequent discussions that part of the latent period also results from the manner in which these hormones perform their functions in the cells themselves.

FUNCTIONS OF THE THYROID HORMONES IN THE TISSUES

The thyroid hormones have two major effects on the body: (1) an increase in the overall metabolic rate and (2) in children, stimulation of growth.

GENERAL INCREASE IN METABOLIC RATE

The thyroid hormones increase the metabolic activities of almost all tissues of the body. The basal metabolic rate can increase to as much as 60 to 100 per cent above normal when large quantities of the hormones are secreted. The rate of utilization of foods for energy is greatly accelerated. The rate of protein synthesis is at times increased while at the same time the rate of protein catabolism is also increased. The growth rate of young persons is greatly accelerated. The mental processes are excited, and the activity of many endocrine glands is often increased. Yet despite the fact that we know all these many changes in metabolism are under the influence of the thyroid hormones, the basic mechanism (or mechanisms) by which they act is much less well known. However, some of the possible mechanisms of action of the thyroid hormones are described in the following sections.

Effect of Thyroid Hormones in Causing Increased Protein Synthesis. When either thyroxine or triiodothyronine is given to an animal, protein synthesis increases in almost all tissues of the body. The first stage of the increased protein synthesis results from stimulation of the *translation* process—that is, increase in the rate of formation of proteins by the ribosomes. The second stage occurs hours to days later and is caused by increased RNA synthesis by the genes, the process of *transcription*, which leads to a generalized increase in synthesis of many types of proteins within the cells. This stimulation of the genes occurs in the following way: (1) The thyroid hormone, probably mainly triiodothyronine derived from deiodinated thyroxine within the cell, combines with a receptor protein in the cell nucleus. (2) This combination, or a product of it, then activates a large portion of the cellular genes to cause RNA formation and subsequent protein formation.

Effect of Thyroid Hormones on the Cellular Enzyme Systems. Within a week or so following administration of the thyroid hormones, at least 100 and probably many more intracellular enzymes are increased in quantity. As an example, one enzyme, α-glycerophosphate dehydrogenase, can be increased to an activity six times its normal level. Since this enzyme is particularly important in the degradation of carbohydrates, its increase could help to explain the rapid utilization of carbohydrates under the influence of thyroxine. Also, the oxidative enzymes and the elements of the electron transport system, both of which are normally found in mitochondria, are greatly increased.

Effect of Thyroid Hormones on Mitochondria. When thyroxine or triiodothyronine is given to an animal, the mitochondria in most cells of the body increase in size and also in number. Furthermore, the total membrane surface of the mitochondria increases almost directly in proportion to the increase in metabolic rate of the whole animal. Therefore, it seems almost to be an obvious deduction that the principal function of thyroxine might be simply to increase the number and activity of mitochondria and that these in turn increase the rate of formation of ATP to energize cellular function. Unfortunately, though, the increase in number and activity of mitochondria could as well be the *result* of increased activity of the cells as the cause of the increase.

Effect of Thyroid Hormone in Increasing Active Transport of Ions Through Cell Membranes. One of the enzymes that becomes increased in response to thyroid hormone is *Na-K ATPase*, which is the cell membrane transport protein for moving sodium and potassium ions through the membrane. Therefore, increase of this enzyme increases the rate of transport of both sodium and potassium through the cell membranes of some tissues. Since this process utilizes energy and also increases the amount of heat produced in the body, it has been suggested that this might be one of the mechanisms by which thyroid hormone increases the body's metabolic rate.

Summary. It is clear that we know many effects that occur in the cells throughout the body under the influence of thyroid hormone. Yet, a specific metabolic mechanism that leads to all of these effects has been elusive. At present, the most likely basic function of the thyroid hormones is their capability to activate the DNA transcription process in the cell nucleus with the resulting formation of many new cellular proteins, many of which are metabolic enzymes.

EFFECTS OF THYROID HORMONE ON GROWTH

Thyroid hormone has both general and specific effects on growth. For instance, it has long been known that thyroid hormone is essential for the metamorphic change of the tadpole into the frog. In the human being, the effect of thyroid hormone on growth is manifest mainly in growing children. In those with hypothyroidism, the rate of growth is greatly retarded. In those with hyperthyroidism, excessive skeletal growth often occurs, causing the child to become considerably taller than otherwise. However, the epiphyses close at an early age, so that the duration of growth, and the eventual height of the adult, may be shortened.

The growth-promoting effect of thyroid hormone is presumably based on its ability to promote protein synthesis. (On the other hand, a great excess of thyroid hormone can cause more rapid catabolism than synthesis of protein, so that the protein stores are then actually mobilized and amino acids released into the extracellular fluids.)

EFFECTS OF THYROID HORMONE ON SPECIFIC PHYSIOLOGICAL MECHANISMS

Effect on Carbohydrate Metabolism. Thyroid hormone stimulates almost all aspects of carbohydrate metabolism, including rapid uptake of glucose by the cells, enhanced glycolysis, enhanced gluconeogenesis, increased rate of absorption from the gastrointestinal tract, and even increased insulin secretion with its resultant secondary effects on carbohydrate metabolism. All of these effects probably result from the overall increase in enzymes caused by thyroid hormone.

Effect on Fat Metabolism. Essentially all aspects of fat metabolism are also enhanced under the influence of thyroid hormone. Since fats are the major source of long-term energy supplies, the fat stores of the body are depleted to a greater extent than are most of the other tissue elements when there is excess secretion of thyroid hormone; in particular, lipids are mobilized from the fat tissue, which increases the free fatty acid concentration in the plasma, and thyroid hormone also greatly accelerates the oxidation of free fatty acids by the cells.

Effect on Body Weight. Greatly increased thyroid hormone production in the fully grown person almost always decreases the body weight, and greatly decreased production almost always increases the body weight; but these effects do not always occur, because thyroid hormone increases the appetite, and this may overbalance the change in the metabolic rate.

Effect on the Cardiovascular System. Increased metabolism in the tissues causes more rapid utilization of oxygen than normal and causes greater than normal quantities of metabolic end-products to be released from the tissues. These effects cause vasodilatation in most of the body tissues, thus increasing blood flow in almost all areas of the body, Especially does the rate of blood flow in the skin increase because of the increased necessity for heat elimination.

As a consequence of the increased blood flow to the constituent parts of the body, the cardiac output and heart rate also increase, sometimes to 50 per cent or more above normal when excessive thyroid hormone is present.

The increased cardiac output resulting from thyroid hormone tends to increase the arterial pressure. On the other hand, dilatation of the peripheral blood vessels due to the local effects of thyroid hormone and to excessive body heat tends to decrease the pressure. Therefore, the mean arterial pressure usually is unchanged, though there often is increased pulse pressure.

Effect on Respiration. The increased rate of metabolism caused by thyroid hormone increases the utilization of oxygen and the formation of carbon dioxide; these effects activate all the mechanisms that increase the rate and depth of respiration.

Effect on the Gastrointestinal Tract. In addition to increased rate of absorption of foodstuffs, thyroid hormone also increases both the rate of secretion of the digestive juices and the motility of the gastrointestinal tract. Often, diarrhea results. Also, associated with this increased secretion and motility is an increased appetite, so that the food intake usually increases. Lack of thyroid hormone causes constipation.

Effect on the Central Nervous System. In general, thyroid hormone increases the rapidity of cerebration, while, on the other hand, lack of thyroid hormone decreases this function. The hyperthyroid individual is likely to develop extreme nervousness and is likely to have many psychoneurotic tendencies, such as anxiety complexes, extreme worry, or paranoias.

Muscle Tremor. One of the most characteristic signs of hyperthyroidism is a fine muscle tremor. This is not the coarse tremor that occurs in Parkinson's disease or in shivering, for it occurs at the rapid frequency of 10 to 15 times per second. The tremor can be observed easily by placing a sheet of paper on the extended fingers and noting the degree of vibration of the paper. The cause of this tremor is probably increased activity in the areas of the cord that control muscle tone. The tremor is an excellent means for assessing the degree of thyroid hormone effect on the central nervous system.

Effect on Sleep. Because of the exhausting effect of thyroid hormone on the musculature and on the central nervous system, the hyperthyroid person often has a feeling of constant tiredness; but because of the excitable effects of thyroid hormone on the nervous system, it is difficult to sleep. On the other hand, extreme somnolence is characteristic of hypothyroidism.

REGULATION OF THYROID HORMONE SECRETION

To maintain normal metabolic activity in the body, precisely the right amount of thyroid hormone must be secreted all the time, and to provide this, specific feedback mechanisms operate through the hypothalamus and anterior pituitary gland to control the rate of thyroid secretion. This system is illustrated in Figure 50–5 and can be explained as follows:

Effects of Thyroid-Stimulating Hormone on Thyroid Secretion. Thyroid-stimulating hormone (TSH), also known as *thyrotropin*, is an anterior pituitary hormone, a glycoprotein with a molecular weight of about 28,000; it increases the secretion of thyroxine and triiodothyronine by the thyroid gland. Its specific effects on the thyroid gland are (1) increased proteo-

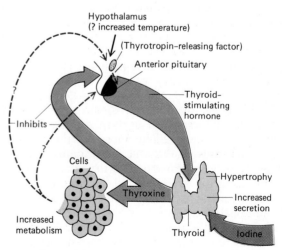

Figure 50–5. Regulation of thyroid secretion.

lysis of the thyroglobulin in the follicles, with resultant release of thyroid hormone into the circulating blood and diminishment of the follicular substance itself; (2) increased activity of the iodide pump, which increases the rate of iodide trapping in the glandular cells, increasing the ratio of intracellular to extracellular iodide concentration severalfold; (3) increased iodination of tyrosine and increased coupling to form the thyroid hormones; (4) both increased size and secretory activity of the thyroid cells; and (5) increased number of thyroid cells, plus a change from cuboidal to columnar cells with much infolding of the thyroid epithelium into the follicles. In summary, thyroid-stimulating hormone *increases all the known activities of the thyroid glandular cells.*

Role of Cyclic AMP in the Stimulatory Effects of TSH. In an attempt to explain the many and varied effects of thyroid-stimulating hormone on the thyroid cell, a single primary action of this hormone has been sought for years. Recent experiments have shown that the hormone almost certainly does have such a single primary effect, which is to activate *adenyl cyclase* in the membrane of the thyroid cell. This in turn causes formation in the cell of *cyclic AMP,* which then acts as a *second messenger* to activate almost all systems of the thyroid cell. The result is both an immediate increase in release of the thyroid hormones followed by prolonged growth of the thyroid glandular tissue itself. This method of controlling thyroid cell activity is similar to the function of cyclic AMP in many other target tissues of the body.

Hypothalamic Regulation of TSH Secretion by the Anterior Pituitary—Thyrotropin-Releasing Hormone (TRH)

Electrical stimulation of several areas of the hypothalamus, but most particularly of the paraventricular nuclei, increases the anterior pituitary secretion of TSH and correspondingly increases the activity of the thyroid gland. This control of anterior pituitary secretion is exerted by a hypothalamic hormone, *thyrotropin-releasing hormone* (TRH), which is secreted by nerve endings in the median eminence of the hypothalamus and then is transported from there to the anterior pituitary in the hypothalamic-hypophysial portal blood, as explained in Chapter 49. TRH has been obtained in pure form, and it has proved to be a very simple substance, a tripeptide amide—*pyroglutamyl-histidyl-proline-amide.*

TRH has the direct effect on the anterior pituitary gland cells of increasing their output of thyroid-stimulating hormone. When the portal system from the hypothalamus to the anterior pituitary gland is completely blocked, so that TRH cannot reach the anterior pituitary gland, the rate of secretion of TSH by the anterior pituitary is greatly decreased but not reduced to zero.

Effects of Cold and Other Neurogenic Stimuli on TSH Secretion. One of the best-known stimuli for increasing the rate of TSH secretion by the anterior pituitary is exposure of an animal to cold. Exposure of rats for several weeks sometimes increases the output of thyroid hormones more than 100 per cent, and can increase the basal metabolic rate as much as 50 per cent. Indeed, even human beings moving to arctic regions have been known to develop basal metabolic rates 15 to 20 per cent above normal.

Various emotional reactions can also affect the output of TRH and TSH and can therefore indirectly affect the secretion of thyroid hormone.

Neither the emotional effects nor the effect of cold is observed when the hypophysial stalk is cut, illustrating that both of these effects are mediated by way of the hypothalamus.

Inverse Feedback Effect of Thyroid Hormone on Anterior Pituitary Secretion of TSH—Feedback Regulation of Thyroid Secretion. Increased thyroid hormone in the body fluids decreases the secretion of TSH by the anterior pituitary. When the rate of thyroid hormone secretion rises to about 1.75 times normal, the rate of TSH secretion falls essentially to zero. Most of this depressant effect occurs even when the anterior pituitary has been completely separated from the hypothalamus, but the effect is somewhat greater if the hypothalamus and hypothalamic-hypophysial portal system are intact. Therefore, it is probable that increased thyroid hormone inhibits anterior pituitary secretion of TSH in two different ways: (1) a direct effect on the anterior pituitary itself and (2) a weaker effect acting through the hypothalamus.

Regardless of the mechanism of the feedback, its effect is to maintain an almost constant concentration of free thyroid hormone in the circulating body fluids. For instance, during periods of heavy exercise, thyroid hormone is consumed much more rapidly than under resting conditions; yet, because of appropriate feedback control, the rate of secretion of thyroid hormone rises to equal the rate of consumption, and the blood thyroid hormone concentration remains almost exactly constant.

DISEASES OF THE THYROID

HYPERTHYROIDISM

Most effects of hyperthyroidism are obvious from the preceding discussion of the various physiologic effects of thyroid hormone. However, some specific effects should be mentioned especially in connection with the development and treatment of hyperthyroidism.

Causes of Hyperthyroidism (Toxic Goiter, Thyrotoxicosis, Graves's Disease). In the patient with hyperthyroidism, the entire thyroid gland is usually markedly hyperplastic. It is increased to two to three times normal size, with tremendous folding of the follicular cell lining into the follicles, so that the number of cells is increased several times as much as the size of the gland. Also, each cell increases its rate of secretion severalfold; radioactive iodine uptake studies indicate that these hyperplastic glands secrete thyroid hormone at a rate as great as 5 to 15 times normal.

These changes in the thyroid gland are similar to those caused by excessive thyroid-stimulating hormone. However, radioimmunoassay studies have shown the plasma TSH concentrations usually to be less than normal rather than enhanced, and often to be essentially zero. On the other hand, one or more globulin antibodies having actions similar to that of TSH are found in the blood of almost all these patients. These antibodies bind with the thyroid cell membranes, and it is believed that they bind with the same membrane receptors that bind TSH and that this induces continual activation of the cells, with resultant development of the hyperthyroidism. One of these antibodies, found in 50 to 80 per cent of thyrotoxic patients, is called *long-acting thyroid stimulator* (LATS).

The antibodies that cause hyperthyroidism almost certainly develop as the result of autoimmunity that has developed against thyroid tissue. Presumably, at some time in the history of the person an excess of thyroid cell antigens has been released from the thyroid cells, and this has resulted in the formation of antibodies against the thyroid gland itself.

Symptoms of Hyperthyroidism. The symptoms of hyperthyroidism are obvious from the preceding discussion of the physiology of the thyroid hormones: intolerance to heat, increased sweating, mild to extreme weight loss, varying degrees of diarrhea, muscular weakness, nervousness and other psychic disorders, extreme fatigue yet with inability to sleep, and tremor of the hands.

Exophthalmos. Most, but not all, persons with hyperthyroidism develop some degree of protrusion of the eyeballs, as illustrated in Figure 50–6. This condition is called *exophthalmos.*

The cause of the protrusion is edematous swelling of the retro-orbital tissues and degeneration of the extraocular muscles. The factor or factors that initiate

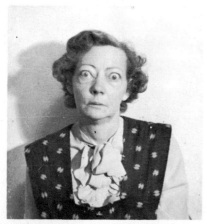

Figure 50–6. Patient with exophthalmic hyperthyroidism. Note protrusion of the eyes and retraction of the superior eyelids. The basal metabolic rate was +40. (Courtesy of Dr. Leonard Posey.)

these changes is still in serious dispute. In most patients, antibodies can be found in the blood that react with the retro-orbital tissues. Therefore, there is much reason to believe that exophthalmos, like hyperthyroidism itself, is an autoimmune process. Usually, the exophthalmos disappears or at least greatly ameliorates with treatment of the hyperthyroidism.

Diagnostic Tests for Hyperthyroidism. In the usual patient with hyperthyroidism, the most accurate diagnostic test is direct measurement of the concentration of "free" thyroxine in the plasma using appropriate radioimmunoassay procedures.

Other tests that are frequently used are these:

1. The basal metabolic rate is usually increased to + 30 to + 60 in severe hyperthyroidism.

2. The rate of uptake of a standard injected dose of radioactive iodine by the normal thyroid gland, when measured by a calibrated radioactive detector placed over the neck, is about 4 per cent per hour. In the hyperthyroid person, this can rise to as high as 20 to 25 per cent per hour.

Physiology of Treatment in Hyperthyroidism. The most direct treatment of hyperthyroidism is surgical removal of the thyroid gland. However, treatment of less severe cases can be achieved with antithyroid drugs such as propylthiouracil, a drug that blocks the formation of thyroid hormones in the thyroid cells.

HYPOTHYROIDISM

The effects of hypothyroidism, in general, are opposite to those of hyperthyroidism, but here again, a few physiological mechanisms peculiar to hypothyroidism are involved.

Endemic Colloid Goiter. The term *goiter* means a greatly enlarged thyroid gland. As was pointed out in the discussion of iodine metabolism, about 50 mg of iodine is needed each year for the formation of adequate quantities of thyroid hormone. In certain areas of the world, notably in the Swiss Alps and in the Great Lakes region of the United States, insufficient iodine is present in the soil for the foodstuffs to contain even this minute quantity of iodine. Therefore, prior to the introduction of iodized table salt, many persons living in these areas developed extremely large thyroid glands called *endemic goiters.*

The mechanism for development of the large endemic goiters is the following: Lack of iodine prevents production of thyroid hormone by the thyroid gland; as a result, no hormone is available to inhibit production of TSH by the anterior pituitary and this allows the pituitary to secrete excessively large quantities of TSH. The TSH then causes the thyroid cells to secrete tremendous amounts of thyroglobulin (colloid) into the follicles, and the gland grows larger and larger. But unfortunately, owing to lack of iodine, increased thyroxine and triiodothyronine production does not occur. The follicles become tremendous in size, and the thyroid gland may increase to as large as 300 to 500 grams or more, which is more than ten times the normal size.

Idiopathic Nontoxic Colloid Goiter. Enlarged thyroid glands almost identical with those of endemic colloid goiter frequently develop even when the affected persons receive sufficient quantities of iodine in their diets. These goitrous glands may secrete normal quantities of thyroid hormones, but more frequently the secretion of hormone is depressed, as in endemic colloid goiter.

The exact cause of the enlarged thyroid gland in patients with idiopathic colloid goiter is not known, but most of these patients show signs of mild thyroiditis; therefore, it has been suggested that thyroiditis causes slight hypothyroidism, which then leads to increased TSH secretion and progressive growth of the noninflamed portions of the gland. This could explain why these glands usually are very nodular, with some portions of the gland growing while other portions are being destroyed by thyroiditis.

In some persons with colloid goiter, the thyroid glands have abnormal enzyme systems, which leads to diminished thyroid hormone formation and resultant excess stimulation of the thyroid gland by TSH. And, finally, some foods contain *goitrogenic substances* that have a propylthiouracil-type of antithyroid activity, thus also leading to TSH-stimulated enlargement of the thyroid gland. Such goitrogenic substances are found in some varieties of turnips and cabbages.

Characteristics of Hypothyroidism. Whether hypothyroidism is due to endemic colloid goiter, idiopathic colloid goiter, destruction of the thyroid gland by irritation, surgical removal of the thyroid gland, or destruction of the thyroid gland by various other diseases, the physiological effects are the same. These include extreme somnolence with 14 to 16 hours of sleep a day; extreme muscular sluggishness, slowed heart rate, decreased cardiac output; decreased blood volume; increased weight; constipation; mental sluggishness; failure of many trophic functions in the body as evidenced by depressed growth of hair and scaliness of the skin; development of a frog-like husky voice; and, in severe cases, development of an edematous appearance throughout the body called myxedema.

Myxedema. The patient with almost total lack of thyroid function develops *myxedema.* Figure 50–7 shows such a patient with bagginess under the eyes and swelling of the face. In this condition, for reasons not yet explained, greatly increased quantities of proteoglycans, containing mainly hyaluronic acid, collect in the interstitial spaces and form an edema characterized by a myxomatous gel in the interstitial spaces.

Arteriosclerosis in Hypothyroidism. Lack of thyroid hormone increases the quantity of blood lipids, with especially large amounts of cholesterol, and the increase in blood cholesterol is usually associated with atherosclerosis and arteriosclerosis. Therefore, many hypothyroid patients, particularly those with myxedema, develop severe arteriosclerosis, which results in peripheral vascular disease, deafness, and

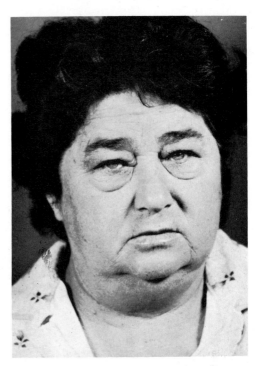

Figure 50–7. Patient with myxedema. (Courtesy of Dr. Herbert Langford.)

often extreme coronary sclerosis with consequent early demise.

Diagnostic Tests in Hypothyroidism. The tests already described for diagnosis of hyperthyroidism give the opposite results in hypothyroidism. The free thyroxine in the blood is low. The basal metabolic rate in myxedema ranges between -30 and -40. And the rate of radioactive iodine uptake by the thyroid gland (except in iodine deficiency hypothyroidism) measures less than 1 per cent per hour rather than the normal of approximately 4 per cent per hour. However, just as important for diagnosis as the various diagnostic tests are the characteristic symptoms of hypothyroidism just discussed.

Treatment of Hypothyroidism. Figure 50–4 shows the effect of thyroid hormone on the basal metabolic rate, illustrating that the hormone normally has a duration of action of more than one month. Consequently, it is easy to maintain a steady level of thyroid hormone activity in the body by daily oral ingestion of a tablet or so of desiccated thyroid gland or thyroid extract. Furthermore, proper treatment of the hypothyroid patient results in such complete normality that formerly myxedematous patients properly treated have lived into their 90's after treatment for over 50 years.

Cretinism. Cretinism is the condition caused by extreme hypothyroidism during infancy and childhood, and it is characterized especially by failure of growth. Cretinism results fron congenital lack of a thyroid gland (*congenital cretinism*), from failure of the thyroid gland to produce thyroid hormone because of a genetic deficiency of the gland, or from iodine lack in the diet (*endemic cretinism*). The severity of endemic cretinism varies greatly, depending on the amount of iodine in the diet, and whole populations of an endemic area have been shown to have cretinoid tendencies.

A newborn baby without a thyroid gland may have absolutely normal appearance and function because it had been supplied with thyroid hormone by the mother while *in utero*, but a few weeks after birth its movements become sluggish, and both its physical and mental growth are greatly retarded. Treatment of the cretin at any time usually causes normal return to physical growth, but unless the cretin is treated within a few months after birth, its mental growth will be permanently retarded.

QUESTIONS

1. Explain the anatomy of both secretion and absorption into the blood of the thyroid metabolic hormones.
2. What is the importance of *iodide trapping* for the formation of thyroid hormones?
3. Give the chemical steps required for the formation of thyroid hormone within the structure of *thyroglobulin*.
4. Explain the storage of thyroglobulin and the release of the thyroid metabolic hormones from the thyroglobulin into the circulating blood.
5. How are *thyroxine* and *triiodothyronine* transported to the tissues?
6. Explain the mechanism by which thyroid hormones cause increased protein synthesis in cells and tell how this affects the metabolic rate of the body.
7. What is the effect of the thyroid hormones on the cellular *enzyme systems*, especially on the enzyme systems of the *mitochondria*?
8. What is the effect of thyroid hormone on growth, especially in children?
9. Explain briefly the effects of thyroid hormone on carbohydrate metabolism, fat metabolism, body weight, function of the cardiovascular system, function of the gastrointestinal tract, function of the central nervous system, muscle tremor, and sleep.
10. What are the chemical compositions of *TRH* and *TSH*, and what are their respective functions in the control of thyroid hormone secretion?
11. What are the feedback mechanisms from the body that play important roles in the regulation of thyroid hormone secretion?
12. Explain the causes and effects of *hypothyroidism*.
13. What is *exophthalmos*, and what is its cause?
14. What is meant by *endemic colloid goiter*, and what is its cause?
15. What are the causes of *hypothyroidism*, and what are its effects on the body?
16. What is *myxedema*, and why does it develop in severe hypothyroidism?
17. What are the characteristics of *cretinism*, and how does the lack of thyroid hormones cause this abnormality?

References

Bayliss, R. I.: Thyroid Disease. New York, Oxford University Press, 1982.

Chopra, I. J., and Solomon, D. H.: Pathogenesis of hyperthyroidism. Annu Rev Med 34:267, 1983.

DeGroot, L. J.: Thyroid hormone action. In DeGroot, L. J., et al., eds.: Endocrinology. Vol. 1. New York, Grune & Stratton, 1979, p. 357.

Ho, K. L.: Basophilic degeneration of skeletal muscle in hypothyroid myopathy. Histochemical and ultrastructural studies. Arch Pathol Lab Med 108:239, 1984.

King, D. B., and May, J. D.: Thyroidal influence on body growth. J Exp Zool 232:453, 1984.

Kourides, I. A., et al.: The regulation and organization of thyroid stimulating hormone genes. Recent Prog Horm Res 40:79, 1984.

Krieger, D. T., ed.: Current Therapy in Endocrinology, 1983–1984. St. Louis, C. V. Mosby, 1983.

Lenzen, S., and Bailey, C. J.: Thyroid hormones, gonadal and adrenocortical steroids and the function of the islets of Langerhans. Endocr Rev 5:411, 1984.

Matovinovic, J.: Endemic goiter and cretinism at the dawn of the third millennium. Annu Rev Nutr 3:341, 1983.

McClung, M. R., and Greer, M. A.: Treatment of hyperthyroidism. Annu Rev Med 31:385, 1980.

McKenzie, J. M., and Zakarija, M.: Hyperthyroidism. In DeGroot, L. J., et al., eds.: Endocrinology. Vol. 1. New York, Grune & Stratton, 1979, p. 429.

Oppenheimer, J. H.: Thyroid hormone action at the nuclear level. Ann Intern Med 102:374, 1985.

Robbins, J., et al.: The thyroid and iodine metabolism. In Bondy, P. K., and Rosenberg, L. E., eds.: Metabolic Control and Disease, 8th ed. Philadelphia, W. B. Saunders Co., 1980, p. 1325.

Stanbury, J. B., ed.: Endemic Goiter and Endemic Cretinism. New York, John Wiley & Sons, 1980.

Utiger, R. D.: Hypothyroidism. In DeGroot, L. J., et al., eds.: Endocrinology. Vol. 1. New York, Grune & Stratton, 1979, p. 471.

51

The Adrenocortical Hormones

CHEMISTRY OF THE
  ADRENOCORTICAL HORMONES
FUNCTIONS OF THE
  MINERALOCORTICOIDS—
  ALDOSTERONE
RENAL EFFECTS OF ALDOSTERONE
CELLULAR MECHANISM OF
  ALDOSTERONE ACTION
REGULATION OF ALDOSTERONE
  SECRETION
FUNCTIONS OF THE
  GLUCOCORTICOIDS
EFFECTS OF CORTISOL ON
  CARBOHYDRATE METABOLISM
EFFECTS OF CORTISOL ON PROTEIN
  METABOLISM
EFFECTS OF CORTISOL ON FAT
  METABOLISM

OTHER EFFECTS OF CORTISOL
REGULATION OF CORTISOL
  SECRETION—
  ADRENOCORTICOTROPIC
  HORMONE (ACTH)
SECRETION OF MELANOCYTE-
  STIMULATING HORMONE (MSH)
  ALONG WITH ACTH
ABNORMALITIES OF ADRENOCORTICAL
  SECRETION
HYPOADRENALISM—ADDISON'S
  DISEASE
HYPERADRENALISM—CUSHING'S
  SYNDROME
PRIMARY ALDOSTERONISM

The two *adrenal glands,* each of which weighs about 4 grams, lie at the superior poles of the two kidneys. Each gland is composed of two distinct parts, the *adrenal medulla* and the *adrenal cortex.* The adrenal medulla, the central 20 per cent of the gland, is functionally related to the sympathetic nervous system; it secretes the hormones *epinephrine* and *norepinephrine* in response to sympathetic stimulation. In turn, these hormones cause almost the same effects as direct stimulation of the sympathetic nerves in all parts of the body. These hormones and their effects were discussed in detail in Chapter 38 in relation to the sympathetic nervous system.

The adrenal cortex secretes an entirely different group of hormones, called *corticosteroids.* These hormones are all synthesized from the steroid cholesterol, and they all have similar chemical formulas. However, very slight differences in their molecular structures give them several very different but very important functions.

Mineralocorticoids and Glucocorticoids. Two major types of adrenocortical hormones, the *mineralocorticoids* and the *glucocorticoids,* are secreted by the adrenal cortex. In addition to these, small amounts of sex hormones are secreted, especially *androgenic hormones,* which exhibit approximately the same effects in the body as the male sex hormone testoster-

one. These are normally of only slight importance, though in certain abnormalities of the adrenal cortices, extreme quantities can be secreted, and can then result in masculinizing effects.

The *mineralocorticoids* have gained this name because they especially affect the electrolytes of the extracellular fluids—sodium and potassium, in particular. The *glucocorticoids* have gained their name because they exhibit an important effect in increasing blood glucose concentration. However, the glucocorticoids have additional effects on both protein and fat metabolism that likely are equally important if not more so to body function than are their effects on carbohydrate metabolism.

Over 30 different steroids have been isolated from the adrenal cortex, but only two of these are of exceptional importance to the endocrine function of the human body—*aldosterone*, which is the principal mineralocorticoid, and *cortisol*, which is the principal glucocorticoid.

CHEMISTRY OF THE ADRENOCORTICAL HORMONES

Figure 51–1 illustrates the chemical formulas of aldosterone and cortisol. *Aldosterone* has an oxygen atom bound at the number 18 carbon of the choles-

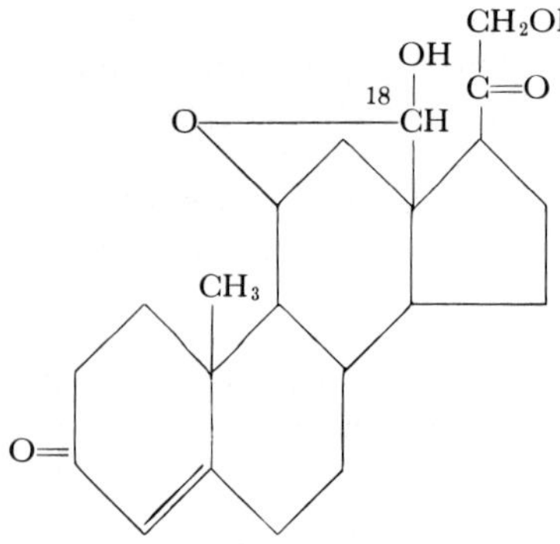

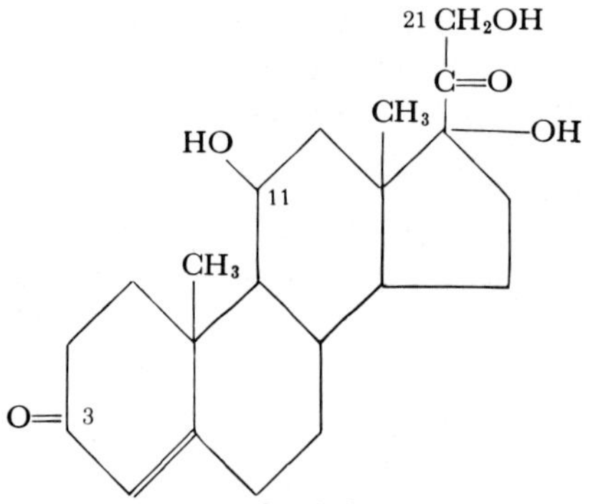

Figure 51-1. The two important corticosteroids.

terol nucleus that is most important in providing the mineralocorticoid activity of aldosterone. The glucocorticoid activity of *cortisol* is provided principally by the presence of a keto-oxygen on carbon number 3 and the hydroxylation of carbon numbers 11 and 21.

In addition to aldosterone and cortisol, which respectively are the principal mineralocorticoid and glucocorticoid hormones, still other steroids having one or both of these activities are normally secreted in small amounts by the adrenal cortex. And several additional potent steroid hormones not normally formed in the adrenal glands have been synthesized and are used in various forms of therapy. The more important of these adrenocortical hormones are the following:

Mineralocorticoids

Aldosterone (very potent, accounts for 95 per cent or more of mineralocorticoid activity)

Desoxycorticosterone (one fifteenth as potent as aldosterone, very small quantities secreted)

Corticosterone (slight activity)

9α-Fludrocortisone (synthetic, slightly more potent than aldosterone)

Glucocorticoids

Cortisol (very potent, accounts for about 95 per cent of all glucocorticoid activity)

Corticosterone (about 4 per cent of total glucocorticoid activity, but much less potent than cortisol)

Cortisone (synthetic, almost as potent as cortisol)

Prednisone (synthetic, four times as potent as cortisol)

Dexamethasone (synthetic, 30 times as potent as cortisol)

FUNCTIONS OF THE MINERALOCORTICOIDS— ALDOSTERONE

Loss of adrenocortical secretion usually causes death within three days to two weeks unless the person receives extensive salt therapy or mineralocorticoid therapy. Without mineralocorticoids, the potassium ion concentration of the extracellular fluid rises markedly, the sodium and chloride concentrations decrease, and the total extracellular fluid volume and blood volume also become reduced. The person

soon develops diminished cardiac output, which proceeds to a shocklike state followed by death. This entire sequence can be prevented by the administration of aldosterone or some other mineralocorticoid. Therefore, the mineralocorticoids are said to be the "life-saving" portion of the adrenocortical hormones, while the glucocorticoids are of particular importance in helping a person resist different types of stresses, as discussed later in the chapter.

Aldosterone exerts at least 95 per cent of the mineralocorticoid activity of the adrenocortical secretion, but cortisol, the major glucocorticoid secreted by the adrenal cortex, also provides a small amount of mineralocorticoid activity.

RENAL EFFECTS OF ALDOSTERONE

By far the most important function of aldosterone is to cause transport of sodium and potassium through the renal tubular walls and, to a smaller extent, transport of hydrogen ions. The mechanisms of these effects were discussed in detail in Chapter 24. However, let us summarize briefly the renal and body fluid effects of aldosterone.

Effect on Tubular Reabsorption of Sodium and Tubular Secretion of Potassium. It will be recalled from Chapter 24 that aldosterone causes an exchange transport of sodium and potassium—that is, absorption of sodium and simultaneous excretion of potassium by the tubular epithelial cells—in both the distal tubule and the collecting duct. Therefore, aldosterone causes sodium to be conserved in the extracellular fluid while potassium is excreted into the urine.

A high concentration of aldosterone in the plasma can decrease the sodium loss into the urine to as little as a few milligrams a day. At the same time, potassium loss into the urine increases manyfold.

Conversely, total lack of aldosterone secretion can cause loss of as much as 20 grams of sodium in the urine a day, an amount equal to one fifth of all the sodium in the body. But, at the same time, potassium is conserved tenaciously.

Therefore, the net effect of excess aldosterone in the plasma is to increase the total quantity of sodium in the extracellular fluid while decreasing the potassium. In turn, the increase in tubular reabsorption causes water reabsorption as well, mainly because the absorbed sodium causes osmosis of water through the tubular epithelium. Thus, an excess of aldosterone can increase the extracellular fluid volume to as much as 10 to 20 per cent above normal, or the volume may decrease to as low as 20 to 25 per cent below normal in the absence of aldosterone.

Hypokalemia and Muscle Paralysis; Hyperkalemia and Cardiac Toxicity. The excessive loss of potassium ions from the extracellular fluid into the urine under the influence of aldosterone causes a serious decrease in the plasma potassium concentration, often from the normal value of 4.5 mEq/liter to as low as 1 to 2 mEq/liter. This condition is called *hypokalemia*. When the potassium ion concentration falls below approximately one half normal, muscle paralysis or at least severe muscle weakness often develops. This is caused by effects on the nerve and muscle fiber membranes (see Chapter 5), which prevent transmission of action potentials.

On the other hand, when aldosterone is deficient, the extracellular fluid potassium ion concentration can rise above normal. When it rises to approximately double normal, serious cardiac toxicity, including weakness of contraction and arrhythmia, becomes evident: a still slightly higher concentration of potassium leads inevitably to cardiac death.

Effect of Aldosterone on Increasing Tubular Hydrogen Ion Secretion, with Resultant Mild Alkalosis. Though aldosterone mainly causes potassium to be secreted into the tubules in exchange for sodium reabsorption, to a much smaller extent it also causes tubular secretion of hydrogen ions in exchange for sodium. The obvious effect is to decrease the hydrogen ion concentration in the extracellular fluid. However, this effect is not a strong one, usually causing only a mild degree of alkalosis.

Effect of Aldosterone on Circulatory Function. In the absence of aldosterone secretion, a decrease in extracellular fluid volume to 20 to 25 per cent below normal and a comparable decrease in plasma volume cause circulatory shock to develop rapidly. Indeed, in complete lack of aldosterone, a person not treated with extra intake of salt, administration of a mineralocorticoid drug, or both is likely to die of circulatory shock within as few as four to eight days.

In the case of hypersecretion of aldosterone, not only is the extracellular fluid volume increased but blood volume and cardiac output are increased as well. Each of these can increase to as much as 20 to 30 per cent above normal in the first few days of excess aldosterone secretion, but after compensations occur, the volumes and the cardiac output usually return to no more than 5 to 10 per cent above normal. Nevertheless, over a prolonged period of time even these small increases are sufficient to cause moderate to severe hypertension, as we discuss later in the chapter in relation to primary aldosteronism.

CELLULAR MECHANISM OF ALDOSTERONE ACTION

Although for many years we have known the overall effects of mineralocorticoids on the body, the basic action of aldosterone on the tubular cells to increase transport of sodium is still only partly understood. The sequence of events that leads to increased sodium reabsorption seems to be the following:

First, because of its lipid solubility in the cellular membranes, aldosterone diffuses to the interior of the tubular epithelial cells.

Second, in the cytoplasm of the tubular cells, aldosterone combines with a highly specific cytoplasmic *receptor protein*, a protein with a stereomolecular configuration that allows only aldosterone or extremely similar compounds to combine.

Third, the aldosterone-receptor complex diffuses into the nucleus, where it may undergo further alterations, and then it induces specific portions of the DNA to form one or more types of messenger RNA related to the process of sodium and potassium transport.

Fourth, the messenger RNA diffuses back into the cytoplasm, where in conjunction with the ribosomes, it causes protein formation. The protein formed is one or more enzymes, or carrier substances, required for sodium and potassium transport, probably a specific ATPase that catalyzes energy transfer from cytoplasmic ATP to the sodium-potassium transport mechanism of the cell membrane.

Thus, aldosterone does not have an immediate effect on sodium and potassium transport, but must await the sequence of events that leads to the formation of the specific intracellular substance or substances required for transport. Approximately 20 to 30 minutes are required before new RNA appears in the cells, and approximately 45 minutes are required before the rates of sodium and potassium transport begin to increase; the effect reaches maximum in several hours.

REGULATION OF ALDOSTERONE SECRETION

The regulation of aldosterone secretion is so deeply intertwined with the regulation of extracellular fluid electrolyte concentrations, extracellular fluid volume, blood volume, arterial pressure, and many special aspects of renal function that it is not possible to discuss the regulation of aldosterone secretion independently of all of these other factors. This subject has already been presented in Chapter 25, to which the reader is referred. However, it is important to list here, also, the most important factors that are presently known to play essential roles in the regulation of aldosterone. In the probable order of their importance they are:

1. Potassium ion concentration of the extracellular fluid
2. Renin-angiotensin system
3. Quantity of body sodium
4. Adrenocorticotropic hormone (ACTH)

This very potent effect of potassium ions is exceedingly important because it establishes a powerful feedback mechanism for control of extracellular fluid potassium ion concentration as follows: (1) An increase in potassium ion concentration causes increased secretion of aldosterone. (2) The aldosterone in turn potently affects the kidneys, causing enhanced excretion of potassium. (3) Therefore, the potassium ion concentration returns to normal. This effect of potassium ions on aldosterone secretion results from a direct influence of the potassium ions on the adrenocortical cells themselves, though the intracellular mechanism is unknown.

When an animal or human being is placed on a sodium deficient diet, after several days the rate of aldosterone secretion increases markedly even though the sodium ion concentration of the body fluids does not fall significantly. Suggestions as to the cause of this phenomenon have included the following:

1. The diminished sodium leads to diminished extracellular fluid volume, with resultant diminished cardiac output and renal blood flow. This causes enhanced formation of angiotensin, and the angiotensin stimulates aldosterone secretion.

2. Lack of sodium causes retention of potassium by the kidneys. The elevated potassium could then cause the increased aldosterone secretion.

3. A few experiments have suggested that diminished sodium concentration possibly causes the anterior pituitary gland to secrete some substance (not ACTH) that affects the adrenal glands to increase aldosterone secretion. For the present, this substance is called the *unidentified pituitary factor*.

Effect of the Renin-Angiotensin System on Aldosterone Secretion. Infusion of moderate amounts of angiotensin into an animal can cause acute increases in aldosterone secretion of as much as 8-fold. However, if the angiotensin infusion is continued, the rate of aldosterone secretion falls in about 12 hours to only 50 to 100 per cent above normal. Yet, even so, in many clinical conditions the renin-angiotensin system is the cause of excessive aldosterone secretion because tremendous quantities of angiotensin are often formed.

FUNCTIONS OF THE GLUCOCORTICOIDS

Even though mineralocorticoids can save the life of an acutely adrenalectomized animal, the animal still is far from normal. Instead, its metabolic systems for utilization of carbohydrates, proteins, and fats are considerably deranged. Furthermore, without glucocorticoids the animal cannot resist different types of physical or even mental stress, and minor illnesses such as respiratory tract infections can lead to death. Therefore, the glucocorticoids have functions just as important to long-continued life of the animal as do the mineralocorticoids. These functions are explained in the following sections.

At least 95 per cent of the glucocorticoid activity of the adrenocortical secretions results from the secretion of *cortisol,* also known as *hydrocortisone.* In addition, a small amount of glucocorticoid activity is provided by *corticosterone* that is secreted in very small amounts.

EFFECTS OF CORTISOL ON CARBOHYDRATE METABOLISM

Stimulation of Gluconeogenesis. By far the best-known metabolic effect of cortisol and other glucocorticoids on metabolism is their ability to stimulate gluconeogenesis by the liver, often increasing the rate of gluconeogenesis as much as six- to tenfold. This results mainly from two different effects of cortisol:

First, all the enzymes required to convert amino acids into glucose are increased in the liver cells. This results from the effect of the glucocorticoids to activate DNA transcription in the liver cell nuclei in the same way that aldosterone functions in the renal tubular cells, with formation of messenger RNAs that in turn lead to the array of enzymes required for gluconeogenesis.

Second, cortisol causes mobilization of amino acids from the extrahepatic tissues, mainly from muscle. As a result, more amino acids become available in the plasma to enter into the gluconeogenesis process of the liver and thereby to promote the formation of glucose.

Decreased Glucose Utilization by the Cells. Cortisol also causes a moderate decrease in the rate of glucose utilization by the cells. Though the cause of this decrease is unknown, most physiologists believe that somewhere between the point of entry of glucose into the cells and its final degradation cortisol directly delays the rate of glucose utilization.

Also, it is known that glucocorticoids slightly depress glucose transport into the cells, which could be an additional factor that depresses cellular glucose utilization.

Elevated Blood Glucose Concentration, and Adrenal Diabetes. Both the increased rate of gluconeogenesis and the moderate reduction in rate of glucose utilization by the cells cause the blood glucose concentration to rise. The increased blood glucose concentration is occasionally so great—50 per cent or more above normal—that the condition is called *adrenal diabetes* (meaning elevated blood glucose concentration); it has many similarities to pituitary diabetes, which was discussed in Chapter 49 but is quite different from the diabetes caused by insulin deficiency.

EFFECTS OF CORTISOL ON PROTEIN METABOLISM

Reduction in Cellular Protein. One of the principal effects of cortisol on the metabolic systems of the body is reduction of the protein stores in essentially all body cells except those of the liver. This reduction is caused both by decreased protein synthesis and increased catabolism of protein already in the cells. Both of these effects may possibly result from decreased amino acid transport into extrahepatic tissues, discussed below, but this probably is not the only cause, since cortisol also depresses the formation of RNA in many extrahepatic tissues, including especially muscle and lymphoid tissue.

Increased Liver and Plasma Proteins Caused by Cortisol. Coincidently with the reduced proteins elsewhere in the body, the liver proteins become enhanced. Furthermore, the plasma proteins (which are produced by the liver and then released into the blood) are also increased. These are exceptions to the protein depletion that occurs elsewhere in the body. This difference is probably caused by enhancement of the liver enzymes required for protein synthesis.

Increased Blood Amino Acids, Diminished Transport of Amino Acids into Extrahepatic Cells, and Enhanced Transport into Hepatic Cells. Recent studies in isolated tissues have demonstrated that cortisol depresses amino acid transport into muscle cells and perhaps into other extrahepatic cells. But, in contrast, it enhances transport into liver cells.

The increased plasma concentration of amino acids, plus the fact that cortisol enhances transport of amino acids into the hepatic cells, could also account for expanded utilization of amino acids by the liver in the presence of cortisol—such effects as (1) increased rate of deamination of amino acids by the liver, (2) increased protein synthesis in the liver, (3) increased formation of plasma proteins by the liver, and (4) increased conversion of amino acids to glucose—that is, enhanced gluconeogenesis.

Thus, it is possible that many of the effects of cortisol on the metabolic systems of the body can be explained very simply from this ability of cortisol to mobilize amino acids.

EFFECTS OF CORTISOL ON FAT METABOLISM

Mobilization of Fatty Acids. In much the same manner that cortisol promotes amino acid mobilization from muscle, it also promotes mobilization of fatty acids from adipose tissue. This in turn increases the concentration of free fatty acids in the plasma, which also increases their utilization for energy. Cortisol moderately enhances the oxidation of fatty acids in the cells as well, perhaps as a secondary result of the reduced availability of glycolytic products for metabolism.

The increased mobilization of fats, combined with their increased oxidation in the cells, is one of the factors that help to shift the metabolic systems of the cells from utilization of glucose for energy to utilization of fatty acids instead in times of starvation or other stresses. This cortisol mechanism, however, requires several hours to become fully developed—not nearly so rapid or powerful an effect as the similar shift elicited by a decrease in insulin, as discussed in the following chapter. Nevertheless, it is probably an important factor for long-term conservation of body glucose and glycogen.

OTHER EFFECTS OF CORTISOL

Function of Cortisol in Different Types of Stress. It is amazing that almost any type of stress, whether physical or neurogenic, causes an immediate and marked increase in ACTH (adrenocorticotropic hormone) secretion by the anterior pituitary gland, followed within minutes by greatly increased secretion of cortisol by the adrenal gland. Some of the types of stress that increase cortisol release are the following:

1. Trauma of almost any type
2. Infection
3. Intense heat or cold
4. Injection of norepinephrine and other sympathomimetic drugs
5. Surgery
6. Injection of a necrotizing substance beneath the skin
7. Restraint of an animal that prevents movement
8. Almost any debilitating disease

Thus, a wide variety of nonspecific stimuli can cause marked increase in the rate of cortisol secretion by the adrenal cortex.

Yet even though we know that cortisol secretion often increases greatly in stressful situations, we still are not sure why this is of significant benefit to the animal. One guess, which is probably as good as any other, is that the glucocorticoids cause rapid mobilization of amino acids and fats from their cellular stores, making these available both for energy and for synthesis of other compounds needed by the different tissues of the body. Indeed, it is well known that when proteins are released from most of the tissue cells, the liver cells can use the mobilized amino acids to form both glucose and new proteins. It has also been shown that damaged tissues momentarily depleted of proteins can also utilize the newly available amino acids to form new proteins that are essential to the lives of the cells. Or perhaps the amino acids are used to synthesize such essential intracellular substances as purines, pyrimidines, and creatine phosphate, which are necessary for maintenance of cellular life.

Anti-Inflammatory Effects of Cortisol. When tissues are damaged by trauma, by infection with bacteria, or in almost any other way, they almost always become inflamed. In some conditions the inflammation is more damaging than the trauma or disease itself. Administration of large amounts of cortisol can usually block this inflammation or even reverse many of its effects once it has begun.

Basically, there are five main stages of inflammation: (1) release from the damaged tissue cells of chemical substances that activate the inflammation process—chemicals such as histamine, bradykinin, and proteolytic enzymes; (2) an increase in blood flow in the inflamed area caused by some of the released products from the tissues, a condition called *erythema*; (3) leakage of large quantities of almost pure plasma out of the capillaries into the damaged areas, followed by clotting of the tissue fluid, which causes a *nonpitting type of edema*; (4) infiltration of the area by leukocytes; and, finally, (5) tissue healing, which is often accomplished at least partially by ingrowth of fibrous tissue.

One of the most important anti-inflammatory effects of cortisol is its ability to cause *stabilization of the lysosomal membranes*. That is, cortisol makes it much more difficult than normal for the membranes of the lysosomes to rupture. Therefore, most of the proteolytic enzymes released by damaged cells that cause inflammation and that are mainly formed in the lysosomes are released in greatly decreased quantity.

Even after inflammation has become well established, administration of cortisol can often reduce inflammation within hours to several days. The immediate effect is to block most of the factors that are promoting the inflammation. Then the rate of healing is also increased. This probably results from those same factors that allow the body to resist many other types of physical stress when large quantities of cortisol are secreted; perhaps the enhancement of healing results from the mobilization of amino acids and their use to repair the damaged tissues; perhaps it results from increased amounts of glucose and fatty acids available for cellular energy; or perhaps it depends on some catalytic effect of cortisol to inactivate or remove inflammatory products.

Regardless of the precise mechanisms by which the anti-inflammatory effect occurs, this effect of cortisol can play a major role in combating certain types of diseases, such as rheumatoid arthritis, rheumatic fever, and acute glomerulonephritis. All of these are characterized by severe local inflammation, and the harmful effects to the body are caused mainly by the inflammation itself, not by other aspects of the disease. When cortisol or other glucocorticoids are administered to patients with these diseases, the inflammation almost invariably subsides within 24 to 48 hours. And even though the cortisol does not correct the basic disease condition but merely prevents the damaging effects of the inflammatory response, this alone can be a life-saving measure.

REGULATION OF CORTISOL SECRETION—ADRENOCORTICOTROPIC HORMONE (ACTH)

Control of Cortisol Secretion by ACTH. Unlike aldosterone secretion by the adrenal cortex, which is controlled mainly by potassium and angiotensin acting directly on the adrenocortical cells themselves, almost no stimuli have *direct* effects on the adrenal cells to control cortisol secretion. Instead, secretion of cortisol is controlled almost entirely by *adrenocorticotropic hormone* (ACTH) secreted by the anterior pituitary gland, as illustrated in Figure 51–2. This hormone, also called *corticotropin* or *adrenocorticotropin*, is *a large polypeptide chain* composed of 39 amino acids. It also enhances the production of adrenal androgens by the adrenal cortex. Small amounts of ACTH are required for aldosterone secretion, providing a permissive role that allows the other more important factors to exert their more powerful controls.

Control of ACTH Secretion by the Hypothalamus—Corticotropin-Releasing Factor (CRF). In the same way that other pituitary hormones are controlled by releasing hormones, or factors, from the hypothalamus, so also does an important releasing

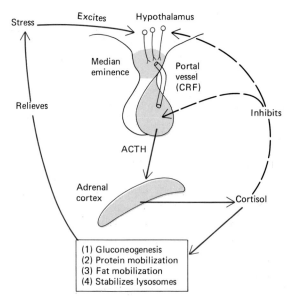

Figure 51–2. Mechanism for regulation of glucocorticoid secretion.

factor control ACTH secretion. This is called *corticotropin-releasing factor* (CRF). It is *a small peptide* that is secreted into the primary capillary plexus of the hypophysial portal system in the median eminence of the hypothalamus and then carried to the anterior pituitary gland, where it induces ACTH secretion.

The anterior pituitary gland can secrete only small quantities of ACTH in the absence of CRF. Instead, most conditions that cause high ACTH secretory rates initiate this secretion by signals that begin in the hypothalamus and then are transmitted by CRF to the anterior pituitary gland.

Effect of Physiological Stress on ACTH Secretion. It was pointed out earlier in the chapter that almost any type of physical or mental stress can lead within minutes to greatly enhanced secretion of ACTH and consequently of cortisol as well, often increasing cortisol secretion as much as 20-fold. This effect is illustrated forcefully by the curves in Figure 51–3, which shows a manyfold increase in plasma corticosterone concentration in a rat within minutes after tibia and fibula had been broken (corticosterone is the principal glucocorticoid secreted by the rat adrenal in place of cortisol). It is believed that pain stimuli caused by the stress are first transmitted upward through the brain stem to the perifornical area of the hypothalamus and from here into the medial basal hypothalamus and eventually to the median eminence, as shown in Figure 51–2, in which CRF is secreted into the hypophysial portal system. Within minutes the entire control sequence leads to large quantities of the glucocorticoids in the blood.

Inhibitory Effect of Cortisol on the Hypothalamus and the Anterior Pituitary—Decreased ACTH Secretion. Cortisol has direct negative feedback *effects* on (1) the hypothalamus, decreasing the formation of CRF, and (2) the anterior pituitary gland, decreasing the formation of ACTH. These feedbacks help to regulate the plasma concentration of cortisol. That

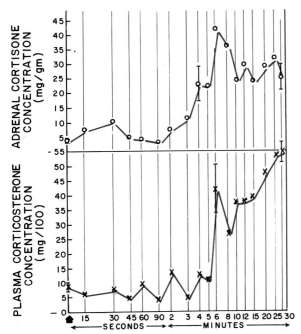

Figure 51–3. Rapid reaction of the adrenal cortex of a rat to stress caused by fracture of the tibia and fibula. (Courtesy of Drs. Guillemin, Dear, and Lipscomb.)

is, whenever the concentration becomes too great, these feedbacks automatically reduce this concentration back toward a normal control level.

Summary of the Control System. Figure 51–2 illustrates the overall system for control of cortisol secretion. The central key to this control is the excitation of the hypothalamus by different types of stress. These stresses activate the entire system to cause rapid release of cortisol, and the cortisol in turn initiates a series of metabolic effects directed toward relieving the damaging nature of the stressful state. In addition, there is also direct feedback of the cortisol to the hypothalamus and anterior pituitary gland to stabilize the concentration of cortisol in the plasma at times when the body is not experiencing stress. However, the stress stimuli are the prepotent ones; they can always break through this direct inhibitory feedback control of cortisol.

SECRETION OF MELANOCYTE-STIMULATING HORMONE (MSH) ALONG WITH ACTH

When ACTH is secreted by the anterior pituitary gland, several other hormones with similar chemical structures are secreted simultaneously, including especially *melanocyte-stimulating hormone* (MSH). Under normal conditions this hormone is not known to be secreted in enough quantity to have a significant effect on the body, but this may not be true when the rate of secretion of ACTH is very high, as occurs in Addison's disease, which will be discussed later. Melanocyte-stimulating hormone occurs in two forms, an *alpha* and a *beta* form. This alpha form has exactly the same chemical structure as the first 13 amino acids of the 39 amino acid ACTH polypeptide chain.

MSH causes the *melanocytes*, which are located in abundance at the border between the dermis and the epidermis of the skin, to form the pigment *melanin* and to disperse in the cells of the epidermis. Injection of melanocyte-stimulating hormone into a person over a period of eight to ten days can cause intense darkening of the skin. The effect is much greater in persons with genetically dark skins than in light-skinned persons.

In some lower animals, an intermediate "lobe" of the pituitary gland, called the *pars intermedia*, is highly developed, lying between the anterior and the posterior pituitary lobes. This lobe secretes an especially large amount of melanocyte-stimulating hormone. Furthermore, this secretion is independently controlled by the hypothalamus in response to the amount of light to which an animal is exposed or to other environmental factors. For instance, some arctic animals develop darkened fur in the summer yet have entirely white fur in the winter.

ACTH, because of its similarity to MSH, has about one thirtieth as much melanocyte-stimulating effect as MSH. Furthermore, because the quantities of MSH secreted in the human being are extremely small, while those of ACTH are large, it is likely that ACTH is considerably more important normally than MSH in determining the amount of melanin in the skin.

ABNORMALITIES OF ADRENOCORTICAL SECRETION

HYPOADRENALISM—ADDISON'S DISEASE

Addison's disease results from failure of the adrenal cortices to produce adrenocortical hormones, and this failure in turn is most frequently caused by *primary atrophy* of the adrenal cortices, probably resulting from autoimmunity against the cortices, but also frequently caused by tuberculous destruction of the adrenal glands or invasion of the adrenal cortices by cancer. Basically, the disturbances in Addison's disease are these:

Mineralocorticoid Deficiency. Lack of aldosterone secretion greatly decreases sodium reabsorption and consequently allows sodium ions, chloride ions, and water to be lost into the urine in profusion. The net result is a greatly decreased extracellular fluid volume. Furthermore, the person develops hyperkalemia and acidosis because of failure of potassium and hydrogen ions to be secreted in exchange for sodium reabsorption.

As the extracellular fluid becomes depleted, the plasma volume falls, the red blood cell concentration rises markedly, the cardiac output decreases, and the patient dies in shock. Death usually occurs in the untreated patient four days to two weeks after complete cessation of mineralocorticoid secretion.

Glucocorticoid Deficiency. Loss of cortisol secretion makes it impossible for the person with Addison's disease to maintain normal blood glucose concentration between meals because of an inability to synthesize significant quantities of glucose by gluconeogenesis. Furthermore, lack of cortisol reduces the mobilization of both proteins and fats from the tissues, thereby depressing many other metabolic functions of the body. This sluggishness of energy mobilization when cortisol is not available is one of the major detrimental effects of glucocorticoid lack. However, even when excess quantities of glucose and other nutrients are available, the person's muscles are still weak, indicating that glucocorticoids are also needed to maintain other metabolic functions of the tissues besides simply energy metabolism.

Lack of adequate glucocorticoid secretion also makes the person with Addison's disease highly susceptible to the deteriorating effects of different types of stress, and even a mild respiratory infection can sometimes cause death.

Treatment of Persons with Addison's Disease. The untreated person with full-blown Addison's disease dies within a few days because of consuming weakness and eventual circulatory shock. Yet such a person can usually live for years if small quantities of mineralocorticoids and glucocorticoids are administered daily—about 0.1 milligram of fludrocortisone (a very potent synthetic mineralocorticoid) and 30 milligrams of cortisol. A high salt intake is also necessary.

The Addisonian Crisis. As noted earlier in the chapter, great quantities of glucocorticoids are occasionally secreted in response to different types of physical or mental stress. In the person with Addison's disease, the output of glucocorticoids does not increase during stress. Yet whenever such a person is specifically subjected to different types of trauma, disease, or other stresses such as surgical operations, he or she is likely to develop an acute need for excessive amounts of glucocorticoids and must be given as much as 10 or more times the normal quantities in order to prevent death.

This critical need for extra glucocorticoids and the associated severe debility in times of stress is called *Addisonian crisis.*

HYPERADRENALISM— CUSHING'S SYNDROME

Hypersecretion of cortisol by the adrenal cortex causes a complex of hormonal effects called Cushing's syndrome, resulting from either a cortisol-secreting tumor of one adrenal cortex or general hyperplasia of both adrenal cortices. The hyperplasia in turn is usually caused by increased secretion of ACTH by the anterior pituitary. Most abnormalities of Cushing's syndrome are ascribable to abnormal amounts of cortisol, but increased secretion of androgens is often of significance as well.

A special characteristic of Cushing's syndrome is mobilization of fat from the lower part of the body, with concomitant extra deposition of fat in the thoracic region, giving rise to a so-called "buffalo" torso. The excess secretion of steroids also leads to an edematous appearance of the face, and the androgenic potency of some of the hormones causes acne and hirsutism (excess growth of facial hair). The total appearance of the face is freqently described as a "moon face," as illustrated to the left in Figure 51–4 in a patient with Cushing's syndrome prior to treatment.

Effects on Carbohydrate and Protein Metabolism. The abundance of glucocorticoids secreted in Cushing's syndrome causes increased blood glucose concentration, sometimes to values as high as 200 mg per 100 ml of blood after meals, which is called

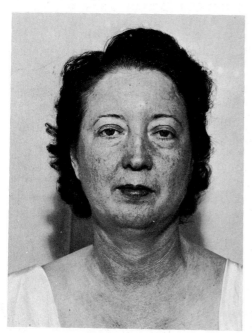
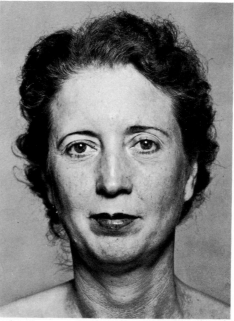

Figure 51–4. A person with Cushing's disease before subtotal adrenalectomy (left) and after subtotal adrenalectomy (right). (Courtesy of Dr. Leonard Posey.)

adrenal diabetes. This effect results mainly from enhanced gluconeogenesis.

The effects of glucocorticoids on protein catabolism in Cushing's syndrome are often profound, causing greatly decreased proteins almost everywhere in the body except for the liver and the plasma. The loss of protein from the muscles in particular causes severe weakness. The loss of protein synthesis in the lymphoid tissues leads to a diminished immunity system, so that many of these patients die of infections. Even the collagen fibers in the subcutaneous tissue are diminished, so that the subcutaneous tissues tear easily, resulting in development of large *purplish striae*; these are actually scars where the subcutaneous tissues have torn apart. In addition, lack of protein deposition in the bones causes *osteoporosis* with consequent weakness of the bones.

Treatment of Cushing's Syndrome. Treatment in Cushing's syndrome consists of removing an adrenal tumor if this is the cause or of decreasing the secretion of ACTH if possible. Hypertrophied pituitary glands or even small tumors in the pituitary gland that oversecrete ACTH can be surgically or microsurgically removed or can be destroyed by radiation. If ACTH secretion cannot easily be decreased, the only satisfactory treatment usually is bilateral total or partial adrenalectomy followed by the administration of adrenal steroids to make up for any insufficiency that develops.

PRIMARY ALDOSTERONISM

Occasionally, a small tumor of the zona glomerulosa cells (cells located on the outer surface of the adrenal cortex) occurs and secretes large amounts of aldosterone. The effects of the excess aldosterone are those discussed earlier in the chapter. The most important effects are hypokalemia, slight increase in extracellular fluid volume and blood volume, very slight increase in plasma sodium concentration (usually not over a 2 to 3 per cent increase), and moderate to severe hypertension. Especially interesting in primary aldosteronism are occasional periods of muscular paralysis caused by the hypokalemia. The paralysis is caused by a depressant effect of the hypokalemia on action potential transmission, as explained in Chapter 5.

Treatment of primary aldosteronism is usually surgical removal of the adrenal tumor.

QUESTIONS

1. What is the difference between the *adrenal medulla* and the *adrenal cortex*?
2. Describe, in general, the chemistry of the *adrenocortical hormones*.
3. Why are the adrenocortical hormones divided into *mineralocorticoids* and *glucocorticoids*?
4. What are the effects of *aldosterone* on sodium absorption and potassium secretion by the renal tubules?
5. How does *hypokalemia* cause muscle paralysis? On the other hand, how does *hypokalemia* cause cardiac toxicity?
6. Explain the cellular mechanism for aldosterone action.
7. Review briefly the regulation of aldosterone secretion. What are the specific effects of potassium ions and angiotensin on aldosterone secretion?
8. What are the most important glucocorticoids secreted by the body?
9. What are the effects of *cortisol* on carbohydrate metabolism? How does cortisol increase *gluconeogenesis*?
10. What is the effect of cortisol on protein metabolism, especially on the *mobilization of amino acids* from the peripheral tissues, and what are its effects on liver proteins and plasma proteins?
11. What are the effects of cortisol on fat metabolism?
12. Explain what we know about the role of cortisol in protecting the body against different types of stress.
13. What is the role of cortisol in neutralizing the effects of inflammation, and why is this important?
14. What are the chemical characteristics of *CRF* and *ACTH*, and how do these function in the control of glucocorticoid secretion by the adrenal cortex?
15. What are the feedback effects from the body that help to control secretion of ACTH by the anterior pituitary gland and therefore control the secretion of glucocorticoids?
16. What is the relationship of ACTH to *melanocyte-stimulating hormone*, and what are the effects of both of these on body pigmentation?
17. What are the causes of *Addison's disease*, and what are the functional abnormalities of the body that it causes?
18. What are the causes of and the functional abnormalities caused by *Cushing's syndrome*?
19. What are the clinical characteristics of *primary aldosteronism*, and what are the physiological mechanisms of these effects?

References

Bondy, P. K.: The adrenal cortex. In Bondy, P. K., and Rosenberg, L. E., eds.: Metabolic Control and Disease, 8th ed. Philadelphia, W. B. Saunders Co., 1980, p. 1427.

Chrousos, G. P., et al.: NIH Conference: Clinical applications of corticotropin-releasing factor. Ann Intern Med 102:344, 1985.

Fanestil, D. D., and Park, C. S.: Steroid hormones and the kidney. Annu Rev Physiol 43:637, 1981.

Gann, D. S., et al.: Neural interaction in control of adrenocorticotropin. Fed Proc 44:161, 1985.

Hall, J. E., et al.: Control of arterial pressure and renal function during glucocorticoid excess in dogs. Hypertension 2:139, 1980.

James, V. H., ed.: The Adrenal Gland. New York, Raven Press, 1979.

Keller-Wood, M. E., and Dallman, M. F.: Corticosteroid inhibition of ACTH secretion. Endocr Rev 5:1, 1984.

Kraus-Friedmann, N.: Hormonal regulation of hepatic gluconeogenesis. Physiol Rev 64:170, 1984.

Lan, N. C., et al.: Mechanisms of glucocorticoid hormone action. J Steroid Biochem 20:77, 1984.

Miller, M.: Assessment of hormonal disorders of water metabolism. Clin Lab Med 4:729, 1984.

Rousseau, G. G.: Control of gene expression by glucocorticoid hormones. Biochem J 224:1, 1984.

Schmidt, T. J., and Litwack, G.: Activation of the glucocorticoid-receptor complex. Physiol Rev 62:1131, 1982.

Seron-Ferre, M., and Jaffe, R. B.: The fetal adrenal gland. Annu Rev Physiol 43:141, 1981.

Smith, P. L., and McCabe, R. D.: Mechanism and regulation of transcellular potassium transport by the colon. Am J Physiol 247:G445, 1984.

Young, D. B., and Guyton, A. C.: Steady state aldosterone dose-response relationships. Circ Res 40(2):138, 1977.

52

Insulin, Glucagon, and Diabetes Mellitus

INSULIN
    EFFECT OF INSULIN ON
        CARBOHYDRATE METABOLISM
    EFFECT OF INSULIN ON FAT
        METABOLISM
    EFFECT OF INSULIN ON PROTEIN
        METABOLISM AND GROWTH
    CONTROL OF INSULIN SECRETION
    ROLE OF INSULIN IN SWITCHING
        BETWEEN CARBOHYDRATE AND
        LIPID METABOLISM

GLUCAGON AND ITS FUNCTIONS
    REGULATION OF GLUCAGON
        SECRETION
SUMMARY OF BLOOD GLUCOSE
    REGULATION
DIABETES MELLITUS
    PATHOLOGICAL PHYSIOLOGY OF
        DIABETES
    TREATMENT OF DIABETES
    DIABETIC COMA

The pancreas, in addition to its digestive functions, secretes two important hormones, *insulin* and *glucagon*. The purpose of this chapter is to discuss the functions of these hormones in regulating glucose, lipid, and protein metabolism, also to discuss briefly the disease *diabetes mellitus,* which is caused by hyposecretion of insulin.

Physiologic Anatomy of the Pancreas. The pancreas is composed of two major types of tissues, as shown in Figure 52–1: (1) the *acini,* which secrete digestive juices into the duodenum, and (2) the *islets of Langerhans,* which secrete insulin and glucagon directly into the blood. The digestive secretions of the pancreas were discussed in Chapter 43.

The islets of Langerhans of the human being contain three major types of cells, the *alpha, beta,* and *delta* cells, which are distinguished from one another by their structure and staining characteristics. The beta cells secrete insulin, the alpha cells secrete glucagon, and the delta cells secrete somatostatin, the important functions of which are still not entirely clear.

INSULIN

Insulin is a very large polypeptide (small protein) with a molecular weight of 5808 in the case of human insulin. It is composed of two amino acid chains connected to each other by disulfide linkages.

Before insulin can exert its function it must first bind with a large *receptor protein* in the cell membrane, as explained later in the chapter.

EFFECT OF INSULIN ON CARBOHYDRATE METABOLISM

Immediately after a high-carbohydrate meal, the glucose that is absorbed into the blood causes rapid secretion of insulin. The insulin in turn causes rapid uptake, storage, and use of glucose by almost all tissues of the body, but especially by the liver, muscles, and fat tissues. Therefore, let us discuss each of these.

Effect of Insulin in Promoting Liver Uptake, Storage, and Use of Glucose

One of the most important effects of insulin is to cause most of the glucose absorbed after a meal to be stored almost immediately in the liver in the form of glycogen. Then, between meals, when insulin is not available and the blood glucose concentration begins to fall, the liver glycogen is split back into glucose, which is released into the blood again to keep the blood glucose concentration from falling too low.

Insulin

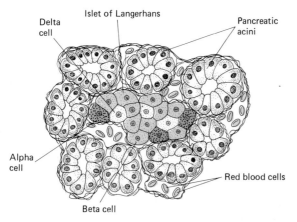

Figure 52–1. Physiologic anatomy of the pancreas.

The mechanism by which insulin causes glucose uptake and storage in the liver includes several almost simultaneous steps:

1. Insulin *inhibits phosphorylase*, the enzyme that causes liver glycogen to split into glucose.

2. Insulin causes *enhanced uptake of glucose* from the blood by the liver cells. It does so by *increasing the activity of the enzyme glucokinase*, which is the enzyme that causes the initial phosphorylation of glucose after it diffuses into the liver cells. Once phosphorylated, the glucose is trapped inside the liver cells, because phosphorylated glucose cannot diffuse back through the cell membrane.

3. Insulin also increases the activities of the enzymes that promote glycogen synthesis.

The net effect of the above actions is to increase the amount of glycogen in the liver. The glycogen can increase to a total of about 5 to 6 per cent of the liver mass, which is equivalent to almost 100 grams of stored glycogen.

Release of Glycogen from the Liver Between Meals. After the meal is over and the blood glucose begins to fall to a low level, several events now transpire that cause the liver to release glucose back into the circulating blood.

1. The decreasing blood glucose causes the pancreas to decrease its insulin secretion.

2. The lack of insulin then reverses all the effects listed above for glycogen storage.

3. The lack of insulin also activates the enzyme *phosphorylase*, which causes the splitting of glycogen into *glucose phosphate*.

4. The enzyme *glucose phosphatase* causes the phosphate radical to split away from the glucose, and this allows the free glucose to diffuse back into the blood.

Thus, the liver removes glucose from the blood when it is present in excess after a meal and returns it to the blood when it is needed between meals. Ordinarily, about 60 per cent of the glucose in the meal is stored in this way in the liver.

Other Effects of Liver on Carbohydrate Metabolism in the Liver. Insulin also *promotes the conversion of liver glucose into fatty acids,* and these fatty acids are subsequently transported to the adipose tissue and deposited as fat. This process will be discussed in relation to insulin effects on fat metabolism. Insulin also *inhibits gluconeogenesis.* It does so mainly by decreasing the activities of the liver enzymes required for gluconeogenesis.

Effect of Insulin in Promoting Glucose Metabolism in Muscle

During most of the day, muscle tissue depends not on glucose for its energy but instead on fatty acids. The principal reason for this is that the normal *resting muscle* membrane is almost impermeable to glucose except when the muscle fiber is stimulated by insulin. And, between meals, the amount of insulin that is secreted is too small to promote the entry of significant amounts of glucose into the muscle cells.

However, under two conditions the muscles do utilize large amounts of glucose for energy. One is during periods of heavy exercise. This usage of glucose does not require large amounts of insulin because the exercising muscle fibers, for reasons not understood, become highly permeable to glucose even in the absence of insulin because of the contraction process itself.

The second condition for muscle usage of large amounts of glucose occurs during the few hours after a meal. At this time the blood glucose concentration is high; also, the pancreas is secreting large quantities of insulin, and the extra insulin causes rapid transport of glucose into the muscle cells.

Storage of Glycogen in Muscle. If the muscles are not exercising during the period following a meal and yet glucose is transported into the muscle cells in great abundance, much of the glucose is stored in the form of muscle glycogen instead of being used for energy. However, the concentration of muscle glycogen rarely rises much above 1 to 2 per cent rather than the possible 5 to 6 per cent in liver cells. The glycogen can later be used for energy by the muscle.

Muscle glycogen is different from liver glycogen in that it cannot be reconverted into glucose and released into the body fluids. The reason for this is that there is no glucose phosphatase in muscle cells, in contrast to liver cells.

Mechanism by Which Insulin Promotes Glucose Transport Through the Muscle Cell Membrane. Insulin promotes glucose transport into muscle cells quite differently from transport into liver cells. Transport into the liver results mainly from a trapping mechanism caused by phosphorylation of the glucose under the influence of glucokinase. However, this is only a minor factor in the insulin effect on glucose transport into muscle cells. Of more importance, insulin directly affects the muscle cell membrane to facilitate glucose transport. This is illustrated by the experimental results depicted in Figure 52–2. This

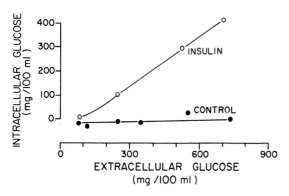

Figure 52–2. Effect of insulin in enhancing the concentration of glucose inside muscle cells. Note that in the absence of insulin (control) the intracellular glucose concentration remained near zero despite very high extracellular glucose concentrations. (From Park, Morgan, Kaji, et al., *In* Eisenstein, ed.: The Biochemical Aspects of Hormone Action. Boston, Little, Brown & Co.)

experiment was performed in muscle cells at a temperature of 4° C, a temperature at which glucose, upon entering the cell, cannot be phosphorylated. The lower curve, labeled *control*, shows the concentration of free glucose measured inside the cell, illustrating that the glucose concentration remained almost exactly zero despite increases in extracellular glucose concentration up to as high as 750 mg/100 ml. In contrast, the curve labeled *insulin* illustrates that the intracellular glucose concentration rose to as high as 400 mg/100 ml when insulin was added. Thus it is clear that insulin can increase the rate of transport of glucose into the resting muscle cell by at least 15- to 20-fold.

As pointed out in the discussion of glucose transport through the cell membrane in Chapter 4, glucose cannot pass through the usual membrane pores but instead must be transported by a specific carrier protein. Figure 52–3 depicts the generally accepted

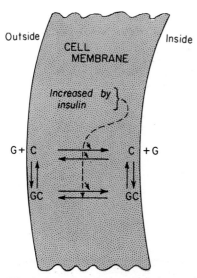

Figure 52–3. Effect of insulin in increasing glucose transport in either direction through the cell membrane.

method by which this is achieved, showing that glucose combines with a carrier substance in the cell membrane and then diffuses in association with the carrier to the inside of the membrane. Then the glucose is released to the interior of the cell. The carrier is then used again and again to transport additional quantities of glucose.

Glucose transport through the cell membrane does not occur against a concentration gradient. That is, once the glucose concentration inside the cell rises as high as the glucose concentration on the outside, additional glucose will not be transported to the interior. Therefore, the transport process is one of *facilitated diffusion*, which means simply that the carrier facilitates the diffusion of glucose through the membrane but cannot impart energy to the transport process to cause glucose movement against an energy gradient.

The manner in which insulin enhances facilitated diffusion of glucose is still largely unknown. All that is known is that the insulin combines with a receptor protein in the cell membrane—a protein having a molecular weight of about 300,000. This may be the glucose carrier itself, or it may be merely the first step in a chain of events that leads to activation of the carrier system. The insulin increases the glucose transport within seconds, suggesting either a rapid direct action on the cell membrane itself or some other equally rapid mechanism.

Lack of Effect of Insulin on Glucose Uptake and Usage by the Brain

The brain is quite different from most other tissues of the body in that insulin has little or no effect on uptake or use of glucose. Instead, the brain cells are permeable to glucose without the intermediation of insulin.

The brain cells normally use only glucose for energy. Therefore, it is essential that the blood glucose level be always maintained above a critical level, which is one of the important functions of the blood glucose control system. When the blood glucose does fall too low—into the range of 20 to 50 mg/100 ml—symptoms of *hypoglycemic shock* develop, characterized by progressive irritability that leads to fainting, convulsions, and even coma.

EFFECT OF INSULIN ON FAT METABOLISM

Though not quite as dramatic as the acute effects of insulin on carbohydrate metabolism, insulin also affects fat metabolism in ways that, in the long run, are perhaps even more important. Especially dramatic is the long-term effect of insulin lack in causing extreme atherosclerosis, often leading to heart attacks, cerebral strokes, and other vascular accidents. But, first, let us discuss the acute effects of insulin on fat metabolism.

Effect of Insulin Excess on Fat Synthesis and Storage

Insulin has several different effects that lead to fat storage in adipose tissue. One is the simple fact that insulin increases the rate of utilization of glucose by many of the body's tissues, thus functioning as a fat sparer. However, insulin also promotes fatty acid synthesis. Most of this synthesis occurs in the liver cells, and the fatty acids are then transported to the adipose cells to be stored. However, a small part of the synthesis occurs in the fat cells themselves. The different factors that lead to increased fatty acid synthesis in the liver include these:

1. Insulin increases the transport of glucose into the liver cells. Then the glucose is split to pyruvate in the glycolytic pathway, and the pyruvate is subsequently converted to acetyl-CoA, the substrate from which fatty acids are synthesized.

2. An excess of *citrate* and *isocitrate ions* is formed by the citric acid cycle when excess amounts of glucose are being used for energy. These ions then have a direct effect in activating *acetyl-CoA carboxylase,* the enzyme required to initiate the first stage of fatty acid synthesis.

3. The fatty acids are then transported from the liver to the adipose cells, where they are stored.

Effect of Insulin on Storage of Fat in the Adipose Cells. Insulin has very much the same effect in adipose cells as in the liver in causing synthesis of fatty acids. However, only about one tenth as much glucose is transported into human fat cells as into the liver, so that the amount of fatty acids synthesized in adipose cells is rather small compared with the amount formed in the liver.

Yet insulin has two other essential effects that are required for fat storage in adipose cells:

1. Insulin *inhibits the action of hormone-sensitive lipase.* Since this is the enzyme that causes hydrolysis of the triglycerides in fat cells, the release of fatty acids into the circulating blood is therefore inhibited.

2. Insulin *promotes glucose transport into the fat cells* in exactly the same way that it promotes glucose transport into muscle cells. The glucose is then utilized to synthesize fatty acids, as noted above, but, more important, it also forms another substance that is essential to the storage of fat. During the glycolytic breakdown of glucose, large quantities of the substance α-*glycerophosphate* are formed. This substance supplies the *glycerol* that binds with fatty acids to form triglycerides, the storage form of fat in adipose cells. Therefore, when insulin is not available to promote glucose entry into the fat cells, fat storage is greatly inhibited or blocked, even when large amounts of fatty acid are available.

Increased Metabolic Use of Fat Caused by Insulin Lack

All aspects of fat metabolism are greatly enhanced in the absence of insulin. This occurs even normally between meals when secretion of insulin is minimal, but it becomes extreme in diabetes when secretion of insulin is almost zero. The resulting effects are these:

Lipolysis of Storage Fat and Release of Free Fatty Acids During Insulin Lack. In the absence of insulin, all the effects of insulin just noted that cause storage of fat are reversed. The most important effect is that the enzyme *hormone-sensitive lipase* in the fat cells becomes strongly activated. This causes hydrolysis of the stored triglycerides, releasing large quantities of fatty acids and glycerol into the circulating blood. Consequently, the plasma concentration of free fatty acids rises within minutes to hours. This free fatty acid then becomes the main energy substrate used by essentially all tissues of the body except the brain. Figure 52–4 illustrates the effect of insulin lack on the plasma concentrations of free fatty acids, glucose, and acetoacetic acid. Note that immediately after removal of the pancreas the free fatty acid concentration in the plasma begins to rise, increasing considerably more rapidly even than the concentration of glucose.

Effect of Insulin Lack on Plasma Lipid Concentrations. The excess of fatty acids available to the liver also promotes conversion of some of the fatty acids into phospholipids and cholesterol, two of the major products of fat metabolism. These two substances, along with some of the triglycerides formed in the liver, are then discharged into the blood in the lipoproteins. Occasionally, the plasma lipoproteins increase as much as threefold, giving a total concentration of plasma lipids of as much as 2 per cent rather than the normal 0.6 per cent. This high lipid concentration—especially the high concentration of cholesterol—leads to rapid development of atherosclerosis in persons with serious diabetes.

Ketogenic and Acidotic Effects of Insulin Lack. Insulin lack also causes excessive amounts of *acetoacetic acid* to be formed in the liver cells. This results

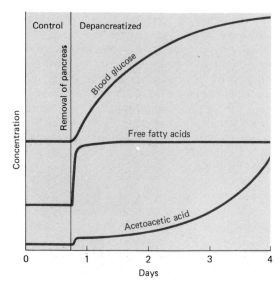

Figure 52–4. Effect of removing the pancreas on the concentrations of blood glucose, plasma free fatty acids, and acetoacetic acid.

from the rapid breakdown of fatty acids in the liver to form extreme amounts of acetyl-CoA. A part of this acetyl-CoA can be utilized for energy in the liver, but the excess is condensed to form acetoacetic acid, which in turn is released into the circulating blood. As explained in Chapter 46, some of the acetoacetic acid is also converted into β-hydroxybutyric acid and *acetone*. These two substances, along with the acetoacetic acid are called *ketone bodies*, and their presence in large quantities in the body fluids is called *ketosis*. We shall see later that the acetoacetic acid and the β-hydroxybutyric acid can cause extreme *acidosis* and *coma* in patients with severe diabetes. In the absence of heroic treatment, this almost always leads to death.

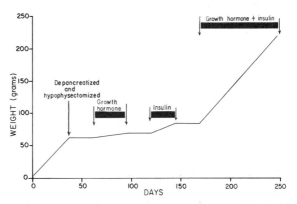

Figure 52–5. Effect of (a) growth hormone, (b) insulin, and (c) growth hormone plus insulin on growth in a depancreatized and hypophysectomized rat.

EFFECT OF INSULIN ON PROTEIN METABOLISM AND GROWTH

Effect of Insulin on Protein Synthesis and Storage. During the few hours following a meal when excess quantities of nutrients are available in the circulating blood, not only carbohydrates and fats but proteins as well are stored in the tissues; insulin is required for this to occur. The manner in which insulin causes protein storage is not as well understood as the mechanism for both glucose and fat storage. Some of the known facts are these:

1. Insulin causes active transport of many of the amino acids into the cells. Thus insulin shares with growth hormone the capability of increasing the uptake of amino acids into cells.

2. Insulin directly affects the ribosomes to *increase the translation of messenger RNA*, thus forming new proteins. In some unexplained way, insulin turns on the ribosomal machinery. In the absence of insulin, the ribosomes simply stop working, almost as if insulin operates an "on-off" mechanism.

3. Over a longer period of time, insulin also *increases the rate of transcription of DNA* in the cell nuclei, thus forming increased quantities of RNA. Eventually, it also increases the rate of formation of new DNA and even reproduction of cells. All these effects promote still more protein synthesis.

4. Insulin also *inhibits the catabolism of proteins*, thus decreasing the rate of amino acid release from the cells, especially from the muscle cells. Presumably, this results from some ability of the insulin to diminish the normal degradation of proteins by the cellular lysosomes.

5. In the liver, insulin *depresses the rate of gluconeogenesis* by decreasing the activity of the enzymes that promote gluconeogenesis. Since the substrates most used for synthesis of glucose by the process of gluconeogenesis are the plasma amino acids, this suppression of gluconeogenesis conserves the amino acids in the protein stores of the body.

In summary, insulin greatly enhances the rate of protein formation and also prevents the degradation of proteins.

Protein Depletion and Increased Plasma Amino Acids Caused by Insulin Lack. All protein storage comes to a complete halt when insulin is not available. The catabolism of proteins increases, protein synthesis stops, and large quantities of amino acids are dumped into the plasma. The plasma amino acid concentration rises considerably, and most of the excess amino acids are used either directly for energy or as substrates for gluconeogenesis. This degradation of the amino acids also leads to enhanced urea excretion in the urine. The resulting protein wasting is one of the most serious of all the effects of severe diabetes mellitus. It can lead to extreme muscle weakness as well as to many deranged functions of the organs.

Effect of Insulin on Growth—Its Synergistic Effect with Growth Hormone. Because insulin is required for the synthesis of proteins, it is just as essential for growth of an animal as is growth hormone. This is illustrated in Figure 52–5, which shows that a depancreatized and hypophysectomized rat without therapy hardly grew at all. Furthermore, neither growth hormone nor insulin administered singly caused significant growth. Yet a combination of both of these hormones did cause dramatic growth. It thus appears that the two hormones function synergistically to promote growth, each performing a separate, specific function. Perhaps part of the necessity for both hormones results from the fact that each promotes cellular uptake of a different selection of amino acids, all of which are required if growth is to be achieved.

CONTROL OF INSULIN SECRETION

Insulin secretion is controlled mainly by the blood glucose concentration. However, blood amino acids and other factors also play important roles, as we shall see.

Stimulation of Insulin Secretion by Blood Glucose. At the normal fasting level of blood glucose of 80 to 90 mg/100 ml, the rate of insulin secretion is minimal. However, as the concentration of blood glucose rises above 100 mg/100 ml of blood, the rate of insulin secretion rises within minutes, reaching a peak some 10 to 30 times the basal level at blood glucose concentrations between 400 and 600 mg/100 ml. Thus, the increase in insulin secretion under a glucose stimulus is dramatic both in its rapidity and in the tremendous level of secretion achieved. Furthermore, the turn-off of insulin secretion is almost equally rapid, occurring within minutes after reduction in blood glucose concentration back to the fasting level.

This response of insulin secretion to an elevated blood glucose concentration provides an extremely important feedback mechanism for regulating the blood glucose concentration. That is, the rise in blood glucose increases insulin secretion, and the insulin in turn causes transport of glucose into the liver, muscle, and other cells, thereby reducing the blood glucose concentration back toward the normal value.

Effect of Amino Acids on Insulin Secretion. In addition to glucose stimulation of insulin secretion, some of the amino acids have a similar effect. However, this effect differs from glucose stimulation of insulin secretion in the following way: Amino acids administered in the absence of a rise in blood glucose cause only a small increase in insulin secretion. However, when administered at the same time that the blood glucose concentration is elevated, the glucose-induced secretion of insulin may be as much as doubled. Thus, the amino acids very strongly *potentiate* the glucose stimulus for insulin secretion.

The stimulation of insulin secretion by amino acids seems to be a purposeful response, because the insulin in turn promotes transport of the amino acids into the tissue cells and also promotes intracellular formation of protein. That is, the insulin is important for proper utilization of the excess amino acids as well as excess glucose.

Gastrointestinal Hormones. A mixture of several important gastrointestinal hormones—*gastrin, secretin, cholecystokinin,* and *gastric inhibitory peptide*—will cause a moderate increase in insulin secretion. These hormones are released in the gastrointestinal tract after a person eats a meal. They seem to cause an anticipatory increase in blood insulin in preparation for the glucose and amino acids to be absorbed from the meal. These gastrointestinal hormones almost double the rate of insulin secretion following an average meal.

ROLE OF INSULIN IN SWITCHING BETWEEN CARBOHYDRATE AND LIPID METABOLISM

From the above discussions it should be clear that insulin promotes the utilization of carbohydrates for energy and depresses the utilization of fats. Conversely, lack of insulin causes fat utilization mainly to the exclusion of glucose utilization, except by brain tissue. Furthermore, the signal that controls this rapid switching mechanism is principally the blood glucose concentration. When the glucose concentration is low, insulin secretion is suppressed, and fat is utilized almost exclusively for energy everywhere except in the brain; when the glucose concentration is high, insulin secretion is stimulated, and carbohydrate is utilized instead of fat until the excess blood glucose is stored. Therefore, one of the most important functional roles of insulin in the body is to control which of these two foods, from moment to moment, will be utilized by the cells for energy.

GLUCAGON AND ITS FUNCTIONS

Glucagon, a hormone secreted by the alpha cells of the islets of Langerhans, has several functions that are opposite to those of insulin. Most important of these is its effect to *increase* the blood glucose concentration.

Like insulin, glucagon is a large polypeptide. It has a molecular weight of 3485 and is composed of a chain of 29 amino acids. On injection of purified glucagon into an animal, a profound *hyper*glycemic effect occurs. One microgram of glucagon per kilogram body weight can elevate the blood glucose concentration approximately 20 mg/100 ml of blood in about 20 minutes. For this reason, glucagon is frequently called *hyperglycemic factor*.

The two major effects of glucagon on glucose metabolism are (1) breakdown of liver glycogen (*glycogenolysis*) and (2) increased *gluconeogenesis*.

Glycogenolysis and Increased Blood Glucose Concentration Caused by Glucagon. The most dramatic effect of glucagon is its ability to cause glycogenolysis in the liver, which in turn increases the blood glucose concentration within minutes.

Glucagon does this by the following complex cascade of events:

1. It activates *adenyl cyclase* in the liver cell membrane
2. Which causes the formation of *cyclic AMP*
3. Which activates *protein kinase regulator protein*
4. Which activates *protein kinase*
5. Which activates *phosphorylase b kinase*
6. Which converts *phosphorylase b* into *phosphorylase a*
7. Which promotes the degradation of glycogen into glucose-1-phosphate
8. Which then is dephosphorylated and the glucose released from the liver cells.

This sequence of events is exceedingly important for several reasons. First, it is one of the most thoroughly studied of all the *second messenger* functions of cyclic AMP. Second, it illustrates a cascading system in which each succeeding product is produced in greater quantity than the preceding product; therefore the sequence represents a potent *amplifying* mechanism, which explains how only a few micrograms of glucagon can have the extreme effect of causing hyperglycemia.

Infusion of glucagon for about four hours can cause such intensive liver glycogenolysis that all of the liver stores of glycogen become totally depleted.

Gluconeogenesis Caused by Glucagon. Even after all the glycogen in the liver has been exhausted under the influence of glucagon, continued infusion of this hormone causes continued hyperglycemia. This results from an effect of glucagon that increases the rate of gluconeogenesis in the liver cells. Unfortunately, the precise mechanism of this effect is unknown, but it is believed to result mainly from activation of the enzymes that are required in gluconeogenesis.

Glucagon-Like Effect of Epinephrine. Epinephrine (and to a slight extent norepinephrine as well) is also a potent promoter of liver glycogenolysis, having an effect almost exactly the same as that of glucagon, though not quite as strong.

REGULATION OF GLUCAGON SECRETION

Effect of Blood Glucose Concentration. Changes in blood glucose concentration have exactly the opposite effect on glucagon secretion as on insulin secretion. That is, a *decrease* in blood glucose increases glucagon secretion. When the blood glucose falls to as low as 70 mg/100 ml of blood, the pancreas secretes large quantities of glucagon. The glucagon rapidly mobilizes glucose from the liver; thus glucagon helps to protect against hypoglycemia.

Effect of Amino Acids. Amino acids enhance the secretion of glucagon, an effect exactly opposite to that of glucose. The physiological importance of this consequence is that it helps to prevent the hypoglycemia that would otherwise result when a meal of pure protein is ingested, because the amino acids from the protein enhance insulin secretion and thereby tend to decrease blood glucose. The increased glucagon secretion seems to nullify this effect.

SUMMARY OF BLOOD GLUCOSE REGULATION

In the normal person the blood glucose concentration is very narrowly controlled, usually in a range between 80 and 90 mg/100 ml of blood in the fasting person each morning before breakfast. This concentration increases to 120 to 140 mg/100 ml during the first hour or so following a meal, but the feedback systems for control of blood glucose return the glucose concentration very rapidly back to the control level, usually within two hours after the last absorption of carbohydrates. Conversely, in starvation the gluconeogenesis function of the liver provides the glucose that is required to maintain the fasting blood glucose level.

The mechanisms for achieving this high degree of control have been presented in this chapter. However, let us summarize these briefly:

1. The liver functions as a very important *blood glucose–buffer system*. That is, when the blood glucose rises to a very high concentration following a meal and the rate of insulin secretion also increases, as much as two thirds of the glucose absorbed from the gut is almost immediately stored in the liver in the form of glycogen. Then during the succeeding hours, when both the blood glucose concentration and the rate of insulin secretion fall, the liver releases the glucose back into the blood.

2. It is very clear that both insulin and glucagon function as important and separate feedback control systems for maintaining a normal blood glucose concentration. When the concentration level rises too high, insulin is secreted; the insulin in turn causes the blood glucose concentration to decrease toward normal. Conversely, a decrease in blood glucose stimulates glucagon secretion; the glucagon then functions in the opposite direction to increase the glucose toward normal. Under most normal conditions, the insulin feedback mechanism is much more important than the glucagon mechanism.

3. Also, in hypoglycemia a direct effect of low blood glucose on the hypothalamus stimulates the sympathetic nervous system. In turn, the epinephrine secreted by the adrenal glands causes still further release of glucose from the liver. This, too, helps to protect against severe hypoglycemia.

4. And, finally, over a period of hours and days, both growth hormone and cortisol are secreted in response to prolonged hypoglycemia, and they both decrease the rate of glucose utilization by most cells of the body. This, too, helps to return the blood glucose concentration toward normal.

Importance of Blood Glucose Regulation. One might ask, Why is it important to maintain a constant blood glucose concentration, particularly since most tissues can shift to utilization of fats and proteins for energy in the absence of glucose? The answer is that glucose is the *only* nutrient that normally can be utilized by the *brain, retina,* and *germinal epithelium of the gonads* in sufficient quantities to supply them with their required energy. Therefore, it is important to maintain a blood glucose concentration at a sufficiently high level to provide this necessary nutrition.

Most of the glucose formed by gluconeogenesis during the interdigestive period is used for metabolism in the brain. Indeed, it is important that the pancreas not secrete any insulin during this time, for otherwise the scant supplies of glucose that are available would all go into the muscles and other peripheral tissues, leaving the brain without its normal nutritive source.

DIABETES MELLITUS

Diabetes mellitus is caused by diminished rate of insulin secretion by the beta cells of the islets of Langerhans. It is usually divided into two different types: *juvenile diabetes,* which usually but not always begins in early life, and *maturity-onset diabetes,* which begins in later life, mainly in obese persons.

Heredity plays an important role in the development of both types of diabetes. The juvenile type results in some instances from hereditary predisposition to development of antibodies against the beta cells or to simple degeneration of these cells. Maturity-onset diabetes is apparently caused by degeneration or suppression of the beta cells, as a result of more rapid aging, in susceptible persons. Obesity predisposes a person to this type of diabetes for two reasons: (1) There are fewer insulin receptors on many of the body's cells in obesity, so that the metabolic effect of the insulin that is present is insufficient to perform the usual insulin functions. (2) The beta cells of the islets of Langerhans are less responsive in obesity to high glucose concentrations, so that less insulin is secreted.

PATHOLOGICAL PHYSIOLOGY OF DIABETES

Blood Glucose Concentration. Most of the pathological conditions in diabetes mellitus can be attributed to one of the following three major effects of insulin lack: (1) decreased utilization of glucose by the body cells, with a resultant increase in blood glucose concentration to as high as 300 to 1200 mg per 100 ml; (2) markedly increased mobilization of fats from the fat storage areas, causing abnormal fat metabolism as well as deposition of lipids in the vascular walls, resulting in atherosclerosis; and (3) depletion of protein in the tissues of the body.

However, in addition, some special pathophysiological problems occur in diabetes mellitus that are not so readily apparent. These are the following:

Loss of Glucose and Water in the Urine of the Diabetic Person. When the quantity of glucose entering the kidney tubules in the glomerular filtrate rises above approximately 225 mg per minute, a significant proportion of the glucose begins to spill into the urine. If normal quantities of glomerular filtrate are formed per minute, glucose spillage will occur when the blood glucose level rises over 180 mg/100 ml. Consequently, it is frequently stated that the blood threshold for the appearance of glucose in the urine is approximately 180 mg/100 ml.

The loss of glucose in the urine causes *diuresis*, which means loss of an excessive amount of water in the urine, because of the osmotic effect of glucose in the tubules to prevent tubular reabsorption of water. The overall effect is dehydration of the extracellular space, which then causes dehydration of the intracellular spaces as well. Thus, one of the important features of diabetes is a tendency for extracellular and intracellular dehydration to develop, and these states are often associated with collapse of the circulation.

Acidosis in Diabetes. The shift from carbohydrate to fat metabolism in diabetes has already been discussed. When the body depends almost entirely on fat for energy, the level of acetoacetic acid and β-hydroxybutyric acid in the body fluids may rise from 1 mEq/liter to as high as 10 mEq/liter. This is obviously likely to result in acidosis.

A second consequence, which is usually even more important in causing acidosis than is the direct in-crease in keto acids, is a decrease in sodium concentration caused in the following way: Keto acids have a low threshold for excretion by the kidneys; therefore, when the keto acid level rises in diabetes, as much as 100 to 200 grams of keto acids can be excreted in the urine each day. Because these are strong acids, only a very small amount can be excreted in the acidic form; instead, they are excreted in combination with sodium derived from the extracellular fluid. As a result, the sodium concentration in the extracellular fluid usually decreases, and much of the sodium is replaced by increased quantities of hydrogen ions, thus adding greatly to the acidosis.

Obviously, all the usual reactions that occur in metabolic acidosis take place in diabetic acidosis, including *rapid and deep breathing*. But, most important of all, the acidosis can lead to *coma* and death, as discussed later.

TREATMENT OF DIABETES

The theory of treatment of diabetes mellitus is based on the administration of enough insulin to enable the patient's metabolism of carbohydrate, fat, and protein to be as nearly normal as possible. Optimal therapy can prevent most acute effects of diabetes and can greatly delay the chronic effects as well.

Ordinarily, the severely diabetic patient is given a single dose of a long-acting insulin (a preparation that releases insulin slowly) each day; this increases overall carbohydrate metabolism throughout the day. Then additional quantities of regular insulin (a short-acting preparation lasting only a few hours) are given at those times of the day when the blood glucose level tends to rise too high—meal times, for example. Thus each patient is established on an individualized routine of treatment.

Diet of the Diabetic. The insulin requirements of a diabetic are established with the patient on a standard diet containing normal, well-controlled amounts of carbohydrates, for any change in the quantity of carbohydrate intake changes the requirements for insulin. In a normal person, the pancreas has the ability to adjust the quantity of insulin produced to the intake of carbohydrate; but in the completely diabetic person, this control function has been totally lost.

In the obesity maturity-onset type of diabetes, the disease can often be controlled by weight reduction alone. The decreased fat reduces the insulin requirements, and the pancreas can supply the need.

Relationship of Treatment to Arteriosclerosis. Diabetic patients have an extremely strong tendency to develop atherosclerosis, arteriosclerosis, severe coronary heart disease, and multiple microcirculatory lesions. Indeed, those who have relatively poorly controlled diabetes throughout childhood are likely to die of heart disease in their twenties.

In the early days of treating diabetes, the tendency was to reduce drastically the carbohydrates in the diet so that the insulin requirements would be minimized. This procedure kept the blood sugar level down to normal values and prevented loss of glucose in the urine, but it did not prevent the abnormalities of fat metabolism. Consequently, the tendency at present is to allow the patient an almost normal carbohydrate diet and then to give simultaneously large quantities of insulin to metabolize the carbohydrates. This depresses the rate of fat metabolism and also depresses the high level of blood cholesterol that occurs in diabetes as a result of abnormal fat metabolism.

Because the complications of diabetes—such as atherosclerosis, greatly increased susceptibility to infection, diabetic retinopathy, cataracts, hypertension, and chronic renal disease—are more closely associated with the level of the blood lipids than with the level of blood glucose, it is the object of many clinics treating diabetes to administer sufficient glucose and insulin to bring the concentrations of the blood lipids near to normal.

DIABETIC COMA

If diabetes is not controlled satisfactorily, severe dehydration and acidosis may result; sometimes, even when the person is receiving treatment, sporadic changes in metabolic rates of the cells, such as might occur during bouts of fever, can also precipitate dehydration and acidosis.

If the pH of the body fluids falls below approximately 7.0, the diabetic person develops coma. Also, in addition to the acidosis, dehydration is believed to exacerbate the coma. Once the diabetic person reaches this stage, the outcome is usually fatal unless immediate treatment is provided.

Physiological Basis of Treating Diabetic Coma. The patient with diabetic coma is extremely refractory to insulin because acidic plasma has an *insulin antagonist*, an alpha globulin, that opposes the action of the insulin. Also, the very high free fatty acid and acetoacetic acid levels in the blood inhibit cellular usage of glucose, as discussed earlier. Therefore, instead of the 60 to 80 units of insulin per day usually necessary for control of severe diabetes, several times this much insulin must often be given the first day of treatment of coma.

Administration of insulin often will not by itself reverse the abnormal physiology in diabetic coma. In addition, it is usually necessary to correct both the dehydration and acidosis immediately. The dehydration is ordinarily corrected by rapidly administering large quantities of sodium chloride solution, and the acidosis is often corrected by administering sodium bicarbonate or sodium lactate solution.

QUESTIONS

1. Give the physiologic anatomy of the pancreas for secreting the pancreatic hormones.
2. What is the chemical nature of *insulin*?
3. Explain the effect of insulin on glucose uptake by the liver and later release from the liver back into the blood.
4. Explain the role of insulin in increasing the utilization of glucose by muscle. How does insulin increase *membrane transport* of glucose?
5. What is the effect of insulin on glucose uptake by the brain?
6. Explain the effect of insulin on *storage of fat* in the adipose tissues.
7. Explain the effects of *lack of insulin* on the *release of fatty acids* from the fat tissues as well as on the *increase in plasma lipid concentrations*.
8. How does insulin promote *growth*, and why does *insulin lack* cause *protein depletion* in the cells and weakness of muscles?
9. Explain the control of insulin secretion by the blood glucose concentration.
10. What other factors help to control insulin secretion?
11. Explain the important role of insulin for switching between carbohydrate and lipid metabolism.
12. Explain the *cascade method* by which extremely minute quantities of *glucagon* can cause marked release of glucose from the liver.
13. Explain the factors that control glucagon secretion.
14. Discuss the overall integration of the different hormonal and metabolic systems in the control of blood glucose concentration.
15. In *diabetes* what happens to the following factors: blood glucose concentration, rate of urine excretion, concentration of glucose in the urine, acid-base balance of the body fluids, blood concentration of cholesterol and other lipids, and state of body hydration?
16. What is the basic goal of current treatment of diabetes, and how is this achieved by the use of diet, *short-acting insulin*, and *long-acting insulin*?
17. What are the characteristics of *diabetic coma*, and what is the physiology of its treatment?

References

Bennett, P. H.: The diagnosis of diabetes: new international classification and diagnostic criteria. Annu Rev Med 34:295, 1983.

Cudworth, A. G., et al.: Etiology of type I diabetes mellitus: heterogeneity and immunological events leading to clinical onset. Annu Rev Med 34:13, 1983.

Czech, M. P.: New perspectives on the mechanism of insulin action. Recent Prog Horm Res 40:347, 1984.

Fain, J. N.: Insulin secretion and action. Metabolism 33:672, 1984.

Flier, J. S.: Insulin receptors and insulin resistance. Annu Rev Med 34:145, 1983.

Gammeltoft, S.: Insulin receptors: Binding kinetics and structure-function relationship of insulin. Physiol Rev 64:1321, 1984.

Guyton, J. R., et al.: A model of glucose-insulin homeostasis in man that incorporates the heterogeneous fast pool theory of pancreatic insulin release. Diabetes 27:1027, 1978.

Hedeskov, C. J.: Mechanism of glucose-induced insulin secretion. Physiol Rev 60:442, 1980.

Howell, S. L., and Tyhurst, M.: Insulin secretion: the effector system. Experientia 40:1098, 1984.

Jacobs, S., and Cuatrecasas, P.: Insulin receptors. Annu Rev Pharmacol Toxicol 23:461, 1983.

Kraus-Friedmann, N.: Hormonal regulation of hepatic gluconeogenesis. Physiol Rev 64:170, 1984.

Malaisse, W. J., et al.: Coupling factors in nutrient-induced insulin release. Experientia 40:1035, 1984.

Ward, W. K., et al.: Pathophysiology of insulin secretion in noninsulin dependent diabetes mellitus. Diabetes Care 7:491, 1984.

Wolheim, C. B., and Sharp, G. W. G.: Regulation of insulin release by calcium. Physiol Rev 61:914, 1981.

53

Parathyroid Hormone, Calcitonin, Calcium and Phosphate Metabolism, Vitamin D, Bone, and Teeth

CALCIUM AND PHOSPHATE IN
  EXTRACELLULAR FLUID AND
  PLASMA—FUNCTION OF VITAMIN D
  *ABSORPTION OF CALCIUM AND
    PHOSPHATE*
  *VITAMIN D AND ITS ROLE IN
    CALCIUM ABSORPTION*
  *CALCIUM IN PLASMA AND
    INTERSTITIAL FLUID*
  *INORGANIC PHOSPHATE IN
    EXTRACELLULAR FLUIDS*
  *EFFECTS OF ABNORMAL CALCIUM
    CONCENTRATION IN THE BODY
    FLUIDS*
BONE AND ITS RELATIONSHIPS WITH
  EXTRACELLULAR CALCIUM AND
  PHOSPHATES
  *PRECIPITATION AND ABSORPTION OF
    CALCIUM AND PHOSPHATE IN
    BONE—EQUILIBRIUM WITH THE
    EXTRACELLULAR FLUIDS*
  EXCHANGEABLE CALCIUM
  *DEPOSITION AND ABSORPTION OF
    BONE—REMODELING OF BONE*

PARATHYROID HORMONE
  *EFFECT OF PARATHYROID HORMONE
    ON CALCIUM AND PHOSPHATE
    CONCENTRATIONS IN
    EXTRACELLULAR FLUID*
  *CONTROL OF PARATHYROID
    SECRETION BY CALCIUM ION
    CONCENTRATION*
  *INTESTINAL AND RENAL CONTROL
    OF PLASMA CALCIUM
    CONCENTRATION—ROLE OF
    PARATHYROID HORMONE*
CALCITONIN
PHYSIOLOGY OF PARATHYROID AND
  BONE DISEASES
  HYPOPARATHYROIDISM
  HYPERPARATHYROIDISM
  RICKETS
PHYSIOLOGY OF THE TEETH
  *FUNCTIONS OF THE DIFFERENT PARTS
    OF THE TEETH*
  DENTITION
  MINERAL EXCHANGE IN TEETH
  DENTAL ABNORMALITIES

The physiology of both parathyroid hormone and the hormone calcitonin is closely related to calcium and phosphate metabolism, the function of vitamin D, and the formation of bone and teeth. Therefore these are discussed together in the present chapter.

CALCIUM AND PHOSPHATE IN EXTRACELLULAR FLUID AND PLASMA—FUNCTION OF VITAMIN D

ABSORPTION OF CALCIUM AND PHOSPHATE

By far the major sources of calcium in the diet are milk and milk products, which are also major sources of phosphate, but phosphate is also present in many other dietary foods, including especially the meats.

Calcium is poorly absorbed from the intestinal tract because of the relative insolubility of many of its compounds and also because bivalent cations are poorly absorbed through the intestinal mucosa. On the other hand, phosphate is absorbed exceedingly well most of the time except when excess calcium is in the diet; the calcium tends to form almost insoluble calcium phosphate compounds in the intestines that fail to be absorbed but instead pass on through the bowels to be excreted in the feces. In other words, the major problem in the absorption of calcium and phosphate is actually a problem of calcium absorption alone, for if this is absorbed, phosphate will also be absorbed.

About seven eighths of the daily intake of calcium is not absorbed and therefore is excreted in the feces; the remaining one eighth is eventually excreted in the urine.

VITAMIN D AND ITS ROLE IN CALCIUM ABSORPTION

Vitamin D has a potent effect to increase calcium absorption from the intestinal tract; it also has important effects on both bone deposition and bone reabsorption, as will be discussed later in the chapter. However, vitamin D itself is not the active substance that actually causes these effects. Instead, the vitamin D must first be converted through a succession of reactions in the liver and the kidney to the final active product, *1,25-dihydroxycholecalciferol.* Figure 53–1 illustrates the succession of steps that leads to the formation of this substance from vitamin D. Some of the important features of this schema are the following stages.

The Vitamin D Compounds. Several different compounds derived from sterols belong to the vitamin D family, and they all perform more or less the same functions. The most important of them is *cholecalciferol,* called vitamin D_3. Most of this substance is formed in the skin as a result of irradiation of *7-dehydrocholesterol* by ultraviolet light from the sun. Consequently, appropriate exposure to the sun prevents vitamin D deficiency.

Conversion of Cholecalciferol to 25-Hydroxycholecalciferol in the Liver and Its Feedback Control.

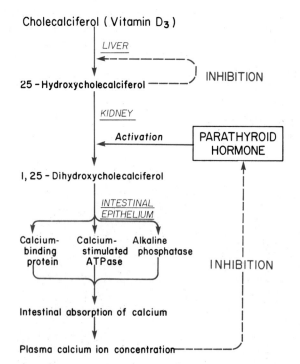

Figure 53–1. Activation of vitamin D_3 to form *1,25-dihydroxycholecalciferol;* and the role of vitamin D in controlling the plasma calcium concentration.

The first step in the activation of cholecalciferol is to convert it to 25-hydroxycholecalciferol; this conversion occurs in the liver. The process, however, is a limited one, because the 25-hydroxycholecalciferol itself has a feedback inhibitory effect on the conversion reactions. This feedback effect is extremely important for two reasons.

First, the feedback mechanism regulates very precisely the concentration of 25-hydroxycholecalciferol in the plasma. The intake of vitamin D_3 can change many fold, and yet the concentration of 25-hydroxycholecalciferol still remains within a few percentage points of its normal mean value. Obviously, this high degree of feedback control prevents excessive action of vitamin D_3 when it is present in too high a concentration.

Second, this controlled conversion of vitamin D_3 to 25-hydroxycholecalciferol conserves the vitamin D_3 for future use, because once converted, it persists in the body for only a short time, whereas in the vitamin D_3 form it can be stored in the liver for as long as several months.

Formation of 1,25-Dihydroxycholecalciferol in the Kidneys and Its Control by Parathyroid Hormone. Figure 53–1 illustrates that 25-hydroxycholecalciferol is converted in the kidneys to 1,25-dihydroxycholecalciferol. This latter substance is the active form of vitamin D; none of the previous products in the schema of Figure 53–1 have very much vitamin D effect. Therefore in the absence of the kidneys, vitamin D is almost totally ineffective.

Note also in Figure 53–1 that the conversion of 25-hydroxycholecalciferol to 1,25-dihydroxycholecalciferol requires parathyroid hormone. In the absence of this hormone, either none or almost none of the 1,25-dihydroxycholecalciferol is formed. Therefore, parathyroid hormone exerts a potent effect in determining the functional effects of vitamin D in the body, specifically its effects on calcium absorption in the intestines and its effect on bone.

Hormonal Effect of 1,25-Dihydroxycholecalciferol on the Intestinal Epithelium in Promoting Calcium Absorption. 1,25-Dihydroxycholecalciferol has several effects on the intestinal epithelium to promote intestinal absorption of calcium. Probably the most important of these effects is that it causes formation of a *calcium-binding protein* in the intestinal epithelial cells. The rate of calcium absorption seems to be directly proportional to the quantity of this calcium-binding protein. Furthermore, this protein remains in the cells for several weeks after the 1,25-dihydroxycholecalciferol has been removed from the body, thus causing a prolonged effect on calcium absorption.

Other effects of 1,25-dihydroxycholecalciferol that might play a role in promoting calcium absorption are (1) the formation of a calcium-stimulated ATPase in the brush border of the epithelial cells and (2) the formation of an alkaline phosphatase in the epithelial cells. Unfortunately, the precise details of calcium absorption are still unknown.

Feedback Effect of Calcium Ion Concentration on the Formation of 1,25-Dihydroxycholecalciferol.

Later in the chapter we shall see that the rate of secretion of parathyroid hormone is controlled almost entirely and very potently by the plasma calcium ion concentration. When the calcium ion concentration rises, this immediately inhibits parathyroid hormone secretion; in the absence of this hormone, 1,25-dihydroxycholecalciferol cannot be formed in the kidney. Thus, this is a *negative* feedback mechanism for control of the plasma concentration of 1,25-dihydroxycholecalciferol and also of the plasma calcium ion concentration. That is, an increase in the calcium ion concentration decreases the vitamin D effect, decreases the absorption of calcium from the intestinal tract, and thus returns the calcium ion concentration to its normal value.

CALCIUM IN PLASMA AND INTERSTITIAL FLUID

The concentration of calcium in plasma is approximately 9.4 mg/100 ml, normally varying between 9.0 and 10.0 mg/100 ml. This is equivalent to approximately 2.4 millimoles per liter. It is apparent from these limits that the calcium level in the plasma is regulated within narrow limits, and mainly by parathyroid hormone, as discussed later in the chapter.

The calcium in the plasma is present in three different forms, as shown in Figure 53–2. (1) Approximately 40 per cent of the calcium is combined with the plasma proteins and consequently is not diffusible through the capillary membrane. (2) Approximately 10 per cent of the calcium (0.2 mM per liter) is diffusible through the capillary membrane but is combined with other substances of the plasma and interstitial fluids (citrate and phosphate, for instance) in such a manner that it is not ionized. (3) The remaining 50 per cent of the calcium in the plasma is both diffusible through the capillary membrane and ionized. Thus, the plasma and interstitial fluids have a normal *calcium ion concentration of approximately*

1.2 mM per liter. This ionic calcium is important for most functions of calcium in the body, including its effect on the heart, on the nervous system, and on bone formation.

INORGANIC PHOSPHATE IN EXTRACELLULAR FLUIDS

Inorganic phosphate in the plasma is mainly in two forms: HPO_4^{--} and $H_2PO_4^-$. The concentration of both of these together is approximately 1.3 mM per liter. Because it is difficult to determine chemically the exact ratio of HPO_4^{--} to $H_2PO_4^-$ in the blood, ordinarily the total quantity of phosphate is expressed in terms of milligrams of *phosphorus* per 100 ml of blood. The average total quantity of inorganic phosphorus represented by both phosphate ions is about 4 mg per 100 ml.

EFFECTS OF ABNORMAL CALCIUM CONCENTRATION IN THE BODY FLUIDS

Tetany Resulting from Hypocalcemia. When the extracellular fluid concentration of calcium ions falls below normal, the nervous system becomes progressively more excitable because of increased neuronal membrane permeability. Especially, the peripheral nerve fibers become so excitable that they begin to discharge spontaneously, initiating nerve impulses that pass to the peripheral skeletal muscles, where they elicit tetanic contraction. Consequently, hypocalcemia causes tetany.

Figure 53–3 illustrates tetany in the hand, which usually occurs before generalized tetany develops. This is called *carpopedal spasm.*

Acute hypocalcemia in the human being ordinarily causes essentially no other significant effects besides tetany, because tetany kills the patient before other effects can develop. Tetany ordinarily occurs when the blood concentration of calcium falls from its normal level of 9.4 mg to approximately 6 mg per 100 ml, which is only 35 per cent below the normal calcium concentration, and it is usually lethal at about 4 mg per 100 ml.

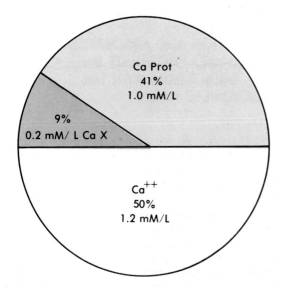

Figure 53–2. Distribution of ionic calcium (*Ca⁺⁺*), diffusible but un-ionized calcium (*Ca X*), and calcium proteinate (*Ca Prot*) in blood plasma.

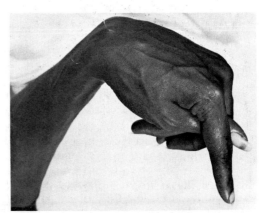

Figure 53–3. Hypocalcemic tetany in the hand, called "carpopedal spasm." (Courtesy of Dr. Herbert Langford.)

In experimental animals, in which the level of calcium can be reduced beyond the normal lethal stage, extreme hypocalcemia can cause marked dilatation of the heart, changes in cellular enzyme activities, increased cell membrane permeability in other cells besides nerve cells, and impaired blood clotting.

Hypercalcemia. When the level of calcium in the body fluids rises above normal, the nervous system is depressed, and reflex activities of the central nervous system become sluggish. Also, increased calcium ion concentration causes constipation and lack of appetite, probably because of depressed contractility of the muscular walls of the gastrointestinal tract.

The depressive effects of an increased calcium level begin to appear when the blood level of calcium rises above approximately 12 mg per 100 ml, and they can become marked as the calcium level rises above 15 mg per 100 ml. When the level of calcium rises above approximately 17 mg per 100 ml in the body fluids, calcium phosphate is likely to precipitate throughout the blood and soft tissues, an effect that can be rapidly lethal.

BONE AND ITS RELATIONSHIPS WITH EXTRACELLULAR CALCIUM AND PHOSPHATES

Bone is composed of a tough *organic matrix* that is greatly strengthened by deposits of *calcium salts.* Average *compact bone* contains by weight approximately 30 per cent matrix and 70 per cent salts. However, *newly formed bone* may have a considerably higher percentage of matrix in relation to salts.

The Organic Matrix of Bone. The organic matrix of bone is 90 to 95 per cent *collagen fibers,* and the remainder is a homogeneous medium called *ground substance.* The collagen fibers extend primarily along the lines of tensional force. These fibers give bone its great tensile strength.

The ground substance is composed of extracellular fluid plus *proteoglycans,* especially *chondroitin sulfate* and *hyaluronic acid.* The precise function of these is not known, though perhaps they help to control the deposition of calcium salts.

The Bone Salts. The crystalline salts deposited in the organic matrix of bone are composed principally of *calcium* and *phosphate,* and the formula for the major crystalline salts, known as *hydroxyapatites,* is the following:

$$Ca^{++}_{10-x}(H_3O^+)_{2x} \cdot (PO_4)_6(OH^-)_2$$

Each crystal—about 400 Å long, 10 to 30 Å thick, and 100 Å wide—is shaped like a long, flat plate. The relative ratio of calcium to phosphorus can vary markedly under different nutritional conditions, the Ca/P ratio on a weight basis varying between 1.3 and 2.0.

Magnesium, sodium, potassium, and *carbonate* ions are also present among the bone salts, though x-ray diffraction studies fail to show definite crystals formed by them. Therefore, they are believed to be adsorbed to the surfaces of the hydroxyapatite crystals rather than organized into distinct crystals of their own. This ability of many different types of ions to adsorb to bone crystals extends to many ions normally foreign to bone, such as *strontium, uranium, plutonium* and the *other transuranic elements, lead, gold, other heavy metals,* and *at least 9 out of 14 of the major radioactive products released by explosion of the hydrogen bomb.* Deposition of radioactive substances in the bone can cause prolonged irradiation of the bone tissues, and if a sufficient amount is deposited, an osteogenic sarcoma almost invariably eventually develops.

Tensile and Compressive Strength of Bone. Each collagen fiber of bone is composed of repeating periodic segments every 640 Å along its length; hydroxyapatite crystals lie adjacent to each segment of the fiber bound tightly to it. This intimate bonding prevents "shear" in the bone; that is, it prevents the crystals and collagen fibers from slipping out of place, which is essential in providing strength to the bone. In addition, the segments of adjacent collagen fibers overlap each other, also causing the hydroxyapatite crystals to be overlapped like bricks keyed to each other in a brick wall.

The collagen fibers of bone, like those of tendons, have great tensile strength, while the calcium salts, which are similar in physical properties to marble, have great compressional strength. These combined properties, plus the degree of bondage between the collagen fibers and the crystals, provide a bony structure that has both extreme tensile and compressional strength. Thus, bones are constructed in exactly the same way that reinforced concrete is constructed. The steel of reinforced concrete provides the tensile strength, while the cement, sand, and rock provide the compressional strength. Indeed, the compressional strength of bone is greater than, and the tensile strength approaches, that of reinforced concrete.

PRECIPITATION AND ABSORPTION OF CALCIUM AND PHOSPHATE IN BONE—EQUILIBRIUM WITH THE EXTRACELLULAR FLUIDS

Supersaturated State of Calcium and Phosphate Ions in Extracellular Fluids with Respect to Hydroxyapatite. The concentrations of calcium and phosphate ions in extracellular fluid are considerably greater than those required to cause precipitation of hydroxyapatite. However, because of the large number of ions required to form a single molecule of hydroxyapatite, it is very difficult for all of these ions to come together simultaneously. Therefore, hydroxyapatite crystals fail to precipitate in tissues other than bone, despite the state of supersaturation of the ions.

Mechanism of Bone Calcification. The initial stage of bone production is the secretion of collagen and ground substance by the *osteoblasts*. The collagen polymerizes rapidly to form collagen fibers, and the resultant tissue becomes *osteoid*, a cartilage-like material but differing from cartilage in that calcium salts precipitate in it. As the osteoid is formed, some osteoblasts become entrapped in it, and these are called *osteocytes*.

Within a few days after the osteoid is formed, calcium salts begin to precipitate on the surfaces of the collagen fibers. The precipitates appear at periodic intervals along each collagen fiber, forming minute nidi that gradually over a period of days and weeks grow into the finished product, *hydroxyapatite crystals*.

The initial calcium salts to be deposited are not hydroxyapatite crystals but amorphous compounds (noncrystalline), probably a mixture of such salts as $CaHPO_4 \cdot 2H_2O$, $Ca_3(PO_4)_2 \cdot 3H_2O$, and others. Then by a process of substitution and addition of atoms, these salts are reshaped into the hydroxyapatite crystals.

It is still not known what causes calcium salts to be deposited in osteoid. One theory holds that at the time of formation the collagen fibers are specially constituted in advance for causing precipitation of calcium salts. It is also believed that the osteoblasts secrete a substance into the osteoid to neutralize an inhibitor that normally prevents hydroxyapatite crystallization. Once the inhibitor has been neutralized, the natural affinity of the collagen fibers for calcium salts supposedly causes the precipitation. In support of this theory is the fact that properly prepared collagen fibers from tissues of the body other than bone will also cause precipitation of hydroxyapatite crystals from plasma.

EXCHANGEABLE CALCIUM

If soluble calcium salts are injected intravenously, the calcium ion concentration can be made to increase immediately to very high levels. However, within 20 minutes to an hour or so, the calcium ion concentration returns to normal. Likewise, if large quantities of calcium ions are removed from the circulating body fluids, the calcium ion concentration again returns to normal within 20 minutes to an hour or so. These effects result from the fact that the bone and other body tissues contain a type of *exchangeable* calcium that is always in equilibrium with the calcium ions in the extracellular fluids. Most of this exchangeable calcium is in the bone, and it normally amounts to about 0.4 to 1.0 per cent of the total bone calcium. Most of this calcium is probably deposited in the bones by the process of adsorption or in the form of readily mobilizable salts such as $CaHPO_4$ and the other amorphous salts.

The importance of exchangeable calcium to the body is that it provides a rapid buffering mechanism to keep the calcium ion concentration in the extracellular fluids from rising to excessive levels or falling to very low levels under transient conditions of excess or diminished availability of calcium.

DEPOSITION AND ABSORPTION OF BONE— REMODELING OF BONE

Deposition of Bone by the Osteoblasts. Bone is continually being deposited by *osteoblasts*, and it is continually being absorbed where *osteoclasts* are active. Osteoblasts are found on the outer surfaces of the bones and in the bone cavities. A small amount of osteoblastic activity occurs continually in all living bones (on about 4 per cent of all surfaces in adult bone), so that at least some new bone is being formed constantly.

Absorption of Bone—Function of the Osteoclasts. Bone is also being continually absorbed in the presence of osteoclasts, which are normally active at any one time on about 1 per cent of the bone surfaces. Later in this chapter we will see that parathyroid hormone controls the bone absorptive activity of osteoclasts.

Histologically, bone absorption occurs immediately adjacent to the osteoclasts, as illustrated in Figure 53–4. The mechanism of this absorption is believed to be the following: The osteoclasts send out villous-like projections toward the bone and from these "villi" secrete two types of substances: (1) proteolytic enzymes, released from the lysosomes of the osteoclasts, and (2) several acids, including citric acid and lactic acid. The enzymes presumably digest or dissolute the organic matrix of the bone, while the acids cause solution of the bone salts. Also, whole fragments of bone salts and collagen are literally gobbled up (phagocytosed) by the "villi" and then digested within the osteoclasts.

Equilibrium Between Bone Deposition and Absorption. Normally, except in growing bones, the rates of bone deposition and absorption are equal to

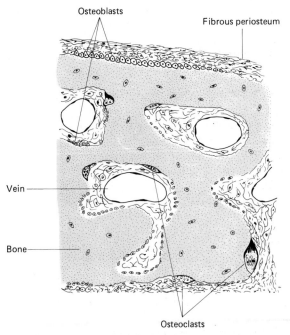

Figure 53–4. Osteoblastic and osteoclastic activity in the same bone.

each other, so that the total mass of bone remains constant. Usually, osteoclasts exist in large masses, and once a mass of osteoclasts begins to develop, it usually eats away at the bone for about three weeks, eating out a tunnel that may be as great as 1 mm in diameter and several mm in length. At the end of this time, the osteoclasts disappear, and the tunnel is invaded by osteoblasts instead. Bone deposition then occurs for several months, the new bone being laid down in successive layers on the inner surfaces of the cavity until the tunnel is filled. Deposition of new bone ceases when the bone begins to encroach on the blood vessels supplying the area. The canal through which these vessels run, called the *haversian canal,* therefore, is all that remains of the original cavity. Each new area of bone deposited in this way is called an *osteon,* shown in Figure 53–5.

Value of Continual Remodeling of Bone. The continual deposition and absorption of bone have a number of physiologically important functions. First, bone ordinarily adjusts its strength in proportion to the degree of bone stress. Consequently, bones thicken when subjected to heavy loads. Second, even the shape of the bone can be rearranged for proper support of mechanical forces by deposition and absorption of bone in accordance with stress patterns. Third, new organic matrix is needed as the old organic matrix degenerates. In this manner the normal toughness of bone is maintained. Indeed, the bones of children, in whom the rate of deposition and absorption is rapid, show little brittleness in comparison with the bones of old age, at which time the rates of deposition and absorption are slow.

Control of the Rate of Bone Deposition by Bone Stress. Bone is deposited in proportion to the com-

pressional load that the bone must carry. For instance, the bones of athletes become considerably heavier than those of nonathletes. Also, if a person has one leg in a cast but continues to walk on the opposite leg, the bone of the leg in the cast becomes thin and decalcified, while the opposite bone remains thick and normally calcified. Therefore, continual physical stress stimulates osteoblastic deposition of bone.

The deposition of bone at points of compressional stress has been suggested to be caused by a *piezo-electric* effect, as follows: Compression of bone causes a negative potential at the compressed site and a positive potential elsewhere in the bone. It has been shown that minute quantities of current flowing in bone cause osteoblastic activity at the negative end of the current flow, which could explain the increased bone deposition at compression sites.

Repair of a Fracture. A fracture of a bone in some way maximally activates all the periosteal and intraosseous osteoblasts involved in the break. Immense numbers of new obsteoblasts are formed almost immediately from *osteoprogenitor cells,* which are bone stem cells. Therefore, within a short time a large bulge of osteoblastic tissue and new organic bone matrix, followed shortly by the deposition of calcium salts, develops between the two broken ends of the bone. This is called a *callus.* It is reshaped into an appropriate structural bone during the ensuing months.

PARATHYROID HORMONE

For many years it has been known that increased activity of the parathyroid gland causes rapid absorption of calcium salts from the bones with resultant hypercalcemia in the extracellular fluid; conversely, hypofunction of the parathyroid glands causes hypocalcemia, often with resultant tetany, as described earlier in the chapter. Also, parathyroid hormone is important in phosphate metabolism as well as in calcium metabolism.

Physiological Anatomy of the Parathyroid Glands. Normally there are four parathyroid glands in the human being; these are located immediately behind the thyroid gland—one behind each of the upper and each of the lower poles of the thyroid. Each parathyroid gland is approximately 6 mm long, 3 mm wide, and 2 mm thick and has a macroscopic appearance of dark brown fat; for this reason the parathyroid glands are difficult to locate.

Removal of half the parathyroid glands usually causes little physiological abnormality. However, removal of three out of four normal glands usually causes transient hypoparathyroidism. But even a small quantity of remaining parathyroid tissue is usually capable of enough hypertrophy to perform the function of all the glands.

The parathyroid gland of the adult human being, illustrated in Figure 53–6, contains mainly *chief cells* and *oxyphil cells,* but oxyphil cells are absent in many

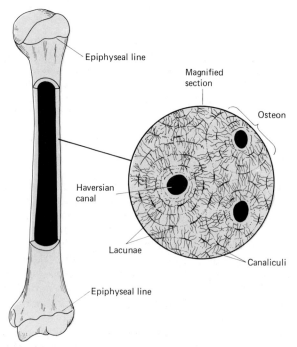

Figure 53–5. The structure of bone.

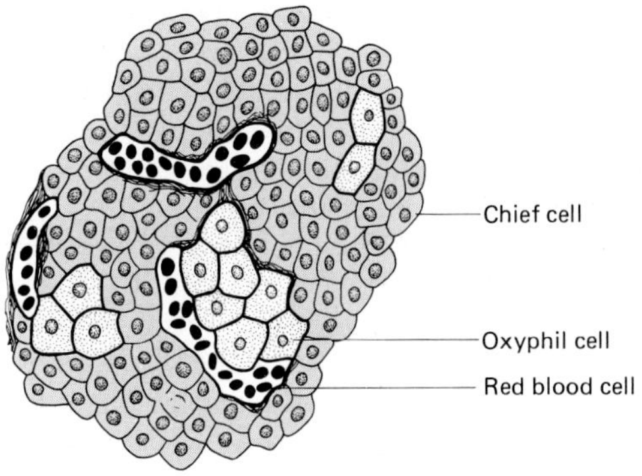

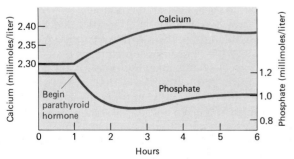

Figure 53–6. Histological structure of a parathyroid gland.

animals and in young humans. The chief cells secrete most of the parathyroid hormone. The function of the oxyphil cells is not certain; they are probably aged chief cells that still secrete some hormone.

Chemistry of Parathyroid Hormone. Parathyroid hormone has been isolated in a pure form. It is a small protein with a molecular weight of approximately 9500 and is composed of a polypeptide chain of 84 amino acids.

EFFECT OF PARATHYROID HORMONE ON CALCIUM AND PHOSPHATE CONCENTRATIONS IN EXTRACELLULAR FLUID

Figure 53–7 illustrates the effects on blood calcium and phosphate concentrations caused by suddenly beginning to infuse parathyroid hormone into an animal and continuing the infusion for an indefinite period of time. Note that at the onset of infusion the calcium ion concentration begins to rise and reaches a plateau level in about 4 hours. On the other hand, the phosphate concentration falls and reaches a depressed plateau level within an hour or two. The rise in calcium concentration is caused principally by (1) a direct effect of parathyroid hormone in causing calcium and phosphate absorption from the bone and (2) an effect on the kidneys to decrease the excretion of calcium in the urine. The decline in phosphate concentration, on the other hand, is caused by a very strong effect of parathyroid hormone on the kidney

Figure 53–7. Approximate changes in calcium and phosphate concentrations during the first five hours of parathyroid hormone infusion at a moderate rate.

resulting in excessive renal phosphate excretion that is usually great enough to override the increased phosphate absorption from the bone.

Calcium and Phosphate Absorption from Bone Caused by Parathyroid Hormone

Parathyroid hormone seems to have two separate effects on bone in causing absorption of calcium and phosphate. One effect, very rapid, takes place in minutes and probably results from activation of the already existing bone cells to promote the calcium and phosphate absorption. The second phase is a much slower one, requiring several days or even weeks to become fully developed, and it results from the proliferation of osteoclasts, followed by greatly increased osteoclastic reabsorption of the bone itself, not merely absorption of calcium phosphate salts from the bone.

The Rapid Phase of Calcium and Phosphate Absorption—Osteolysis. When large quantities of parathyroid hormone are injected, the calcium ion concentration in the blood begins to rise within minutes, long before any new bone cells can be developed. Histological studies have shown that the parathyroid hormone causes removal of bone salts from the bone matrix in the vicinity of the osteocytes lying within the bone itself and also in the vicinity of the osteoblasts along the bone surface. Yet, strangely enough, one does not usually think of either osteoblasts or osteocytes functioning to cause bone salt absorption, because both these types of cells are osteoblastic in nature and are normally associated with bone deposition and its calcification. However, recent studies have shown that the osteoblasts and osteocytes form a system of interconnected cells that spreads over all the bone surfaces except the small surface areas that are adjacent to the osteoclasts. Also, long filmy processes extend from osteocyte to osteocyte throughout the bone structure, and these processes also connect with the surface osteocytes and osteoblasts. This extensive system is called the *osteocytic membrane system*, and it is believed to provide a membrane that separates the bone itself from the extracellular fluid. Between the osteocytic membrane and the bone is a small amount of fluid called simply *bone fluid*. Indirect experiments suggest that the osteocytic membrane pumps calcium ions from the bone fluid into the extracellular fluid, creating a calcium ion concentration in the bone fluid only one third of that in the extracellular fluid. When the osteocytic pump becomes excessively activated, the bone fluid calcium concentration falls even lower, and calcium phosphate salts are then absorbed from the bone. This effect is called *osteolysis*, and it occurs without absorption of the bone matrix. When the pump is inactivated, the bone fluid calcium concentration rises to a higher level, and calcium phosphate salts are then redeposited in the matrix.

But where does parathyroid hormone fit into this picture? It seems that parathyroid hormone can strongly activate the calcium pump, thereby causing rapid removal of calcium phosphate salts from the amorphous bone crystals that lie near the osteocytic membrane. The parathyroid hormone is believed to stimulate calcium absorption by increasing the calcium permeability of the bone fluid side of the osteocytic membrane, thus allowing calcium ions to diffuse into the membrane cells from the bone fluid. Then the calcium pump on the other side of the cell membrane transfers the calcium ions the rest of the way into the extracellular fluid.

The Slow Phase of Bone Absorption and Calcium Phosphate Release—Activation of the Osteoclasts. A much better-known effect of parathyroid hormone is activation of the osteoclasts. These in turn set about their usual task of gobbling up the bone.

Activation of the osteoclastic system occurs in two stages: (1) immediate activation of the osteoclasts that are already formed and (2) formation of new osteoclasts from *osteoprogenitor cells.* Usually, several days of excess parathyroid hormone cause the osteoclastic system to become well developed, but it can continue to grow for literally months under the influence of very strong parathyroid hormone stimulation.

Bone contains such great amounts of calcium in comparison with the total amount in all the extracellular fluids (about 1000 times as much) that even when parathyroid hormone causes a great rise in calcium concentration in the fluids, it is impossible to discern any immediate effect at all on the bones. Yet prolonged administration or secretion of parathyroid hormone finally results in evident absorption in all the bones with development of large cavities filled with very large, multinucleated osteoclasts.

Effect of Parathyroid Hormone on Phosphate and Calcium Excretion by the Kidneys

Administration of parathyroid hormone causes immediate and rapid loss of phosphate in the urine. This effect is caused by diminished renal tubular reabsorption of phosphate ions.

Parathyroid hormone also causes renal tubular *reabsorption* of calcium at the same time that it diminishes phosphate reabsorption. Were it not for this effect of parathyroid hormone on the kidneys to increase calcium reabsorption, the continual loss of calcium into the urine would eventually deplete the bones of this mineral.

Effect of Vitamin D on Bone and Its Relation to Parathyroid Activity

Vitamin D plays important roles in both bone absorption and bone deposition. Administration of extreme quantities of vitamin D causes absorption of bone in much the same way that administration of parathyroid hormone does. Also, in the absence of vitamin D, the effect of parathyroid hormone in causing bone absorption is greatly reduced or even prevented. Therefore, it is possible, if not likely, that parathyroid hormone functions in bone the same way that it functions in the kidneys and intestines—that is, by causing the conversion of vitamin D to 1,25-dihydroxycholecalciferol, which in turn acts to cause the bone absorption.

Vitamin D in much smaller amounts promotes bone calcification. Obviously, one of the ways in which it does so is to increase calcium and phosphate absorption from the intestines. However, even in the absence of such increase, it still enhances the mineralization of bone. Here again, the mechanism of the effect is unknown, but it probably results from the ability of 1,25-dihydroxycholecalciferol to cause transport of calcium ions through cell membranes—perhaps through the osteoblastic or osteocytic cell membranes.

CONTROL OF PARATHYROID SECRETION BY CALCIUM ION CONCENTRATION

Even the slightest decrease in calcium ion concentration in the extracellular fluid causes the parathyroid glands to increase their rate of secretion and eventually to hypertrophy. For instance, the parathyroid glands become greatly enlarged in *rickets,* in which the level of calcium is usually depressed only a few per cent; they also become greatly enlarged in pregnancy, even though the decrease in calcium ion concentration in the mother's extracellular fluid is hardly measurable; and they are greatly enlarged during lactation because calcium is used for milk formation.

On the other hand, any condition that increases the calcium ion concentration causes decreased activity and reduced size of the parathyroid glands. Such conditions include (1) excess quantities of calcium in the diet, (2) increased vitamin D in the diet, and (3) bone absorption caused by factors other than parathyroid hormone (for example, bone absorption caused by disuse of the bones).

Figure 53–8 illustrates quantitatively the relationship between plasma calcium concentration and plasma parathyroid hormone concentration. The solid curve shows the acute relationship when the calcium concentration is changed over a period of a few hours. This shows that a decrease in calcium concentration from 9.4 to 8.4 mg/100 ml doubles or triples the plasma parathyroid hormone. On the other hand, the approximate chronic relationship that one finds when the calcium ion concentration changes over a period of many weeks, thus allowing time for the glands to hypertrophy, is illustrated by the dashed line; this illustrates that chronically, approximately a 1 per cent decrease in calcium can give as much as a 100 per cent increase in parathyroid hormone. Obviously, this is the basis of the body's extremely potent feedback system for control of plasma calcium ion concentration.

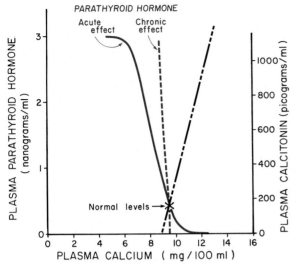

Figure 53–8. Approximate effect of plasma calcium concentration on the plasma concentrations of parathyroid hormone and calcitonin. Note especially that long-term, chronic changes of only a small percentage in calcium concentration can cause as much as 100 per cent change in parathyroid hormone concentration.

INTESTINAL AND RENAL CONTROL OF PLASMA CALCIUM CONCENTRATION—ROLE OF PARATHYROID HORMONE

Though it is frequently stated that the absorption and deposition of calcium in bone is *the* long-term controller of blood calcium ion concentration, this is true only as long as the bone does not become saturated with calcium or totally depleted. However, since the bone does have these limits, it is actually a large reservoir for long-term *buffering* of calcium ion concentration over a period of months or years. It is not, however, the eventual long-term controller of plasma calcium concentration. Instead, this control is achieved by the control of absorption and excretion by the intestines and kidneys.

It has already been pointed out that an increase in parathyroid hormone causes an increase in net absorption of calcium from the intestines and also causes increased reabsorption of calcium from the renal tubules. When the bone has become saturated with calcium salts and can no longer function as a depository of additional calcium ions, the slight excess of extracellular calcium ions reduces parathyroid secretion, which then decreases calcium absorption in both the intestines and kidney tubules. Conversely, when the bone has even a slight deficit of calcium salts, parathyroid secretion increases; this increase can allow for maintenance of almost normal plasma calcium concentration by increasing calcium absorption from both the intestines and kidney tubules.

CALCITONIN

About 25 years ago, a new hormone that has effects on blood calcium opposite to those of parathyroid hormone was discovered. This hormone was named *calcitonin*, because it reduces the blood calcium ion concentration. It is secreted in the human being not by the parathyroid glands but instead by the thyroid gland, by *parafollicular cells,* or C cells, in the interstitium between the thyroid follicles.

Calcitonin is a large polypeptide with a molecular weight of approximately 3400; it has a chain of 32 amino acids.

Effect of Calcitonin in Decreasing Plasma Calcium Concentration. In young animals, calcitonin decreases blood calcium ion concentration very rapidly, beginning within minutes after injection of the calcitonin. Thus the effect of calcitonin on blood calcium ion concentration is exactly opposite that of parathyroid hormone, and it occurs several times as rapidly.

Calcitonin reduces plasma calcium concentration in three separate ways:

1. The immediate effect is to decrease the osteolytic effect of the osteocytic membrane throughout the bone, thus shifting the balance in favor of deposition of calcium in the rapidly exchangeable pool of bone calcium salts.

2. The second effect, which can be seen within about an hour, is an increase in osteoblastic activity. However, this is a transient effect, lasting not more than a few days.

3. The third and most prolonged effect of calcitonin is to prevent formation of new osteoclasts from the osteoprogenitor cells.

Calcitonin has only a weak effect on plasma calcium concentration in the adult human being. The reason for this is simply that the daily rates of bone absorption and deposition of calcium are small, and the stimulatory effect of calcitonin cannot alter the rates enough to make much difference.

Effect of Plasma Calcium Concentration on the Secretion of Calcitonin

An increase in plasma calcium concentration of about 10 per cent causes an immediate three- to sixfold increase in the rate of secretion of calcitonin, which is illustrated by the dot-dash line of Figure 53–8. This provides a second hormonal feedback mechanism for controlling the plasma calcium ion concentration, but one that works exactly opposite to the parathyroid hormone system. That is, an increase in calcium concentration causes increased calcitonin secretion, and the increased calcitonin in turn reduces the plasma calcium concentration back toward normal.

However, there are two major differences between the calcitonin and the parathyroid feedback systems. First, the calcitonin mechanism operates more rapidly, reaching peak activity in less than an hour, in contrast with the 3 to 4 hours required for peak activity to be attained following the onset of parathyroid secretion.

The second difference is that the calcitonin mechanism acts mainly as a short-term regulator and has little long-term effect, month in and month out, on calcium ion concentration—contrary to the powerful long-term effect of the parathyroid hormone system. As was pointed out above, the calcitonin mechanism is a very weak one in the normal human adult, anyway. Therefore, over a prolonged period of time it is almost entirely the parathyroid system that sets the long-term level of calcium ions in the extracellular fluid.

PHYSIOLOGY OF PARATHYROID AND BONE DISEASES

HYPOPARATHYROIDISM

When the parathyroid glands do not secrete sufficient parathyroid hormone, the osteoclasts of the bone become almost totally inactive. As a result, bone reabsorption is so depressed that the level of calcium in the body fluids decreases.

If the parathyroid glands are suddenly removed, the calcium level in the blood falls from the normal of 9.4 mg/100 ml to 6 to 7 mg/100 ml within two to three days. When this level is reached, the usual signs of tetany develop. Among the muscles of the body that are especially sensitive to tetanic spasm are the laryngeal muscles. Laryngeal spasm obstructs respiration, which is a usual cause of death in tetany unless appropriate treatment is applied.

Treatment of Hypoparathyroidism

Parathyroid Hormone (Parathormone). Parathyroid hormone is occasionally used for treating hypoparathyroidism. However, because of the expense of this hormone, because its effect lasts only a few hours, and because the tendency of the body to develop immune bodies against it makes it progressively less active in the body, treatment of hypoparathyroidism with parathyroid hormone is rare in present-day therapy.

Vitamin D and Calcium Therapy. In most patients administration of extremely large quantities of vitamin D, as high as 100,000 units per day, along with 1 to 2 grams of calcium, will suffice to keep the calcium ion concentration in a normal range. At times it may be necessary to administer 1,25-dihydroxycholecalciferol instead of the nonactivated form of vitamin D because of its much more potent and rapid action, but this can also cause unwanted effects, because it is sometimes difficult to prevent overactivity by this activated form of vitamin D.

HYPERPARATHYROIDISM

One cause of hyperparathyroidism is a tumor in one of the parathyroid glands.

In hyperparathyroidism extreme osteoclastic activity occurs in the bones, and this elevates the calcium ion concentration in the extracellular fluid while usually (but not always) depressing the concentration of phosphate ions because of increased renal excretion of phosphate.

In severe hyperparathyroidism, the osteoclastic absorption of bone soon far outstrips osteoblastic deposition, and the bone may be eaten away almost entirely. Indeed, often the reason a hyperparathyroid person comes to the doctor is a broken bone. X-rays of the bones show extensive decalcification, and occasionally, large punched-out cystic areas of the bones, that are filled with osteoclasts in the form of so-called giant cell tumors. Obviously, multiple fractures of the weakened bones result from only slight trauma.

The obvious treatment of hyperparathyroidism is surgical removal of the parathyroid tumor, but this is a difficult procedure because these tumors are often only a few millimeters in size and are difficult to find at operation.

RICKETS

Rickets occurs mainly in children as a result of calcium or phosphate deficiency *in the extracellular fluid.* Yet, ordinarily, rickets is not due to lack of calcium or phosphate in the diet but instead to a deficiency of vitamin D. However, if the child is properly exposed to sunlight, the ultraviolet rays will form enough vitamin D_3 (cholecalciferol) in the skin to prevent rickets by promoting calcium and phosphate absorption from the intestines as discussed earlier in the chapter.

Children who remain indoors through the winter generally do not receive adequate quantities of vitamin D without some supplementary therapy in the diet. Rickets tends to occur especially in the spring months because vitamin D formed during the preceding summer can be stored for several months in the liver, and also, calcium and phosphorus absorption from the bones must take place for several months before clinical signs of rickets become apparent.

Effect of Rickets on Bone. During prolonged deficiency of calcium and phosphate in the body fluids, increased parathyroid hormone secretion protects the body against hypocalcemia by causing osteoclastic absorption of the bone; this in turn causes the bone to become progressively weaker and imposes marked physical stress on the bone, resulting in rapid osteoblastic activity. The osteoblasts lay down large quantities of organic bone matrix, osteoid, which does not become calcified because the calcium and phosphate concentrations are insufficient to cause calcification. Consequently, the newly formed, uncalcified osteoid gradually takes the place of other bone that is being reabsorbed.

Obviously, hyperplasia of the parathyroid glands is marked in rickets because of the decreased blood calcium level.

Tetany in Rickets. In the early stages of rickets, tetany almost never occurs, because the parathyroid glands continually stimulate osteoclastic absorption of bone and therefore maintain an almost normal level of calcium in the body fluids. However, when the bones become exhausted of calcium, the level of calcium may fall rapidly. As the blood level of calcium falls below 7 mg/100 ml, the usual signs of tetany develop, and the child may die of tetanic laryngeal spasm unless intravenous calcium is administered, which relieves the tetany immediately.

Treatment of Rickets. The treatment of rickets depends on supplying adequate calcium and phosphate in the diet and also on administering vitamin D.

Osteomalacia. Osteomalacia is considered the adult form of rickets and indeed is frequently called adult rickets.

Normal adults rarely have dietary lack of vitamin D or calcium, because large quantities of calcium are not needed for bone growth as in children. However, lack of vitamin D and calcium occasionally occurs as a result of steatorrhea (failure to absorb fat), for vitamin D is fat soluble, and calcium tends to form insoluble soaps with fat; consequently, in steatorrhea vitamin D and calcium tend to pass into the feces. Under these conditions an adult occasionally has such poor calcium and phosphate absorption that adult rickets can occur. Though this almost never causes tetany, it does often cause severe bone debility.

PHYSIOLOGY OF THE TEETH

The teeth cut, grind, and mix the food. To perform these functions, the jaws have powerful muscles capable of providing an occlusive force of as much as 50 to 100 pounds between the front teeth and as much as 150 to 200 pounds for the jaw teeth. Also, the upper and lower teeth are provided with projections and facets that interdigitate, so that each set of teeth fits with the other. This fitting is called *occlusion*, and it allows even small particles of food to be caught and ground between the tooth surfaces.

FUNCTIONS OF THE DIFFERENT PARTS OF THE TEETH

Figure 53–9 illustrates a sagittal section of a tooth, showing its major functional parts: the *enamel, dentine, cementum,* and *pulp*. The tooth can also be divided into the *crown*, which is the portion that protrudes out of the gum into the mouth, and the *root*, which is the portion that protrudes into the bony socket of the jaw. The collar between the crown and the root where the tooth is surrounded by gum is called the *neck*.

Dentine. The main body of the tooth is composed of dentine, which has a strong, bony structure. Dentine is made up principally of hydroxyapatite crystals similar to those in the bone but much more dense. These are embedded in a strong meshwork of collagen fibers. In other words, the principal constituents of dentine are very much the same as those of bone.

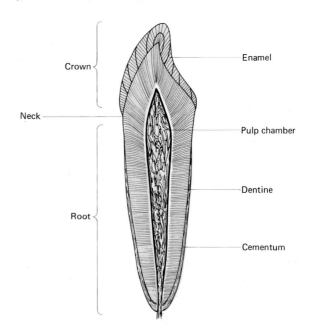

Figure 53–9. Functional parts of a tooth.

The major difference is its histological organization, for dentine does not contain any osteoblasts, osteoclasts, or spaces for blood vessels or nerves. Instead, it is deposited and nourished by a layer of cells called *odontoblasts*, which line its inner surface along the wall of the pulp cavity.

The calcium salts in dentine make it extremely resistant to compressional forces, while the collagen fibers make it tough and resistant to tensional forces that might result when the teeth are struck by solid objects.

Enamel. The outer surface of the tooth is covered by a layer of enamel that is formed prior to eruption of the tooth by special epithelial cells called *ameloblasts*. Once the tooth has erupted, no more enamel is formed. Enamel is composed of very large and extremely dense crystals of hydroxyapatite with adsorbed carbonate, magnesium, sodium, potassium, and other ions embedded in a meshwork of very strong and almost completely insoluble protein fibers that are similar to (but not identical with) the keratin of hair. The dense crystalline structure of the salts makes the enamel extremely hard, much harder than the dentine. Also, the special protein fiber meshwork makes enamel very resistant to acids, enzymes, and other corrosive agents, because this protein is one of the most insoluble and resistant proteins known.

Cementum. Cementum is a bony substance secreted by cells of the *periodontal membrane*, which lines the tooth socket. Many collagen fibers pass directly from the bone of the jaw, through the periodontal membrane, and then into the cementum. These collagen fibers and the cementum hold the tooth in place. When the teeth are exposed to excessive strain, the layer of cementum becomes thicker and stronger. Also, it increases in thickness and strength with age, causing the teeth to become progressively more firmly seated in the jaws as one reaches adulthood and grows older.

Pulp. The inside of each tooth is filled with pulp, which in turn is composed of connective tissue with an abundant supply of nerves, blood vessels, and lymphatics. The cells lining the surface of the pulp cavity are the odontoblasts, which, during the formative years of the tooth, lay down the dentine but at the same time encroach more and more on the pulp cavity, making it smaller. In later life the dentine stops growing, and the pulp cavity thereafter remains essentially constant in size. However, the odontoblasts are still viable and send projections into small *dentinal tubules* that penetrate all the way through the dentine; they are of importance for providing nutrition and probably for exchange of calcium, phosphate, and other minerals.

DENTITION

All human beings and most other mammals develop two sets of teeth during a lifetime. The first teeth are called the *deciduous teeth*, or *milk teeth*, and they number 20 in the human being. These erupt between the seventh month and second year of life, and they last until the sixth to the thirteenth year. After each deciduous tooth is lost, a permanent tooth replaces it, and an additional 8 to 12 molars appear posteriorly in the jaw, making the total number of permanent teeth 28 to 32, depending on whether the four *wisdom teeth* finally appear, which does not occur in everyone.

Formation of the Teeth. Figure 53–10 illustrates the formation and eruption of teeth. Figure 53–10A shows invagination of the oral epithelium into the *dental lamina*; this is followed by the development of a tooth-producing organ. The outer epithelial cells form ameloblasts, which form the enamel on the outside of the tooth. The inner epithelial cells invaginate upward to form a pulp cavity and also to form the odontoblasts that secrete dentine. Thus, enamel is formed on the outside of the tooth, and dentine is formed on the inside, giving rise to an early tooth as illustrated in Figure 53–10B.

Eruption of Teeth. During early childhood, the teeth begin to protrude from the jaw bone through the oral epithelium into the mouth. The cause of eruption is unknown, though several theories have been offered in an attempt to explain this phenomenon. The most likely theory is that growth of the tooth root as well as the bone underneath the tooth progressively shoves the tooth forward.

Development of the Permanent Teeth. During embryonic life, a tooth-forming organ also develops in the dental lamina for each permanent tooth that will be needed after the deciduous teeth are gone. These tooth-producing organs slowly form the permanent teeth throughout the first 6 to 20 years of life. When each permanent tooth becomes fully formed, it, like the deciduous tooth, pushes upward through the bone of the jaw. In so doing it erodes the root of the deciduous tooth and eventually causes it to loosen and fall out. Soon thereafter, the permanent tooth erupts to take the place of the original one.

Metabolic Factors in Development of the Teeth. The rate of development and the speed of eruption of teeth can be accelerated by both thyroid and growth hormones. Also, the deposition of salts in the early forming teeth is affected considerably by various factors of metabolism, such as the availability of calcium and phosphate in the diet, the amount of vitamin D present, and the rate of parathyroid hormone secretion. When all these factors are normal, the dentine and enamel will be correspondingly healthy, but when they are deficient, the calcification of the teeth also may be defective so that the teeth will be abnormal throughout life.

MINERAL EXCHANGE IN TEETH

The salts of teeth, like those of bone, are composed basically of hydroxyapatite with adsorbed carbonates and various cations bound together in a hard crystalline substance. Also, new salts are constantly being deposited while old salts are being reabsorbed from the teeth, as also occurs in bone. However, experiments indicate that deposition and reabsorption occur

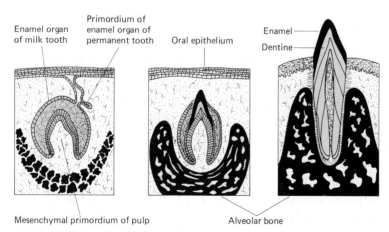

Enamel organ of milk tooth
Primordium of enamel organ of permanent tooth
Oral epithelium
Enamel
Dentine
Mesenchymal primordium of pulp
Alveolar bone

A **B** **C**

Figure 53–10. *A,* Primordial tooth organ. *B,* The developing tooth. *C,* The erupting tooth.

mainly in the dentine and cementum, while very little occurs in the enamel. Much of what does occur in the enamel is by exchange of minerals with the saliva rather than the fluids of the pulp cavity. The rate of absorption and deposition of minerals in the cementum is approximately equal to that in the surrounding bone of the jaw, while the rate of deposition and absorption of minerals in the dentine is only one third that of bone. The cementum has characteristics almost identical with those of usual bone, including the presence of osteoblasts and osteoclasts, while dentine does not have these characteristics, as explained above; this difference undoubtedly accounts for the varying rates of mineral exchange.

The mechanism by which minerals are deposited and reabsorbed from the dentine is not clear. It is probable that the small processes of the odontoblasts that protrude into the tubules of the dentine are capable of absorbing salts and then of providing new salts to take the place of the old.

In summary, rapid mineral exchange occurs in the dentine and cementum of teeth, though the mechanism of this exchange in dentine is unknown. On the other hand, enamel exhibits extremely slow mineral exchange so that it maintains most of its original mineral complement throughout life.

DENTAL ABNORMALITIES

The two most common dental abnormalities are *caries* and *malocclusion*. Caries means erosions of the teeth, whereas malocclusion means failure of the projections of the upper and lower teeth to interdigitate properly.

Caries and the Role of Fluorine. It is generally agreed by research investigators that dental caries results from the action of bacteria on the teeth, the most common of which is *Streptococcus mutans*. The first event in the development of caries is the deposit of *plaque*, a film of precipitated products of saliva and food, on the teeth. Large numbers of bacteria inhabit this plaque and are readily available to cause caries. However, these bacteria depend to a great extent on carbohydrates for their food. When carbohydrates are available, their metabolic systems are strongly activated and they also multiply. In addition, they form acids, particularly lactic acid, and proteolytic enzymes. The acids are the major culprit in the causation of caries, because the calcium salts of teeth are slowly dissolved in a highly acid medium. And once the salts have been absorbed, the remaining organic matrix is rapidly digested by the proteolytic enzymes.

Enamel is far more resistant to demineralization by acids than is dentine, primarily because the crystals of enamel are very dense and also are about 200 times as large as the dentine crystals. Therefore, the enamel of the tooth is the primary barrier to the development of caries. Once the carious process has penetrated through the enamel to the dentine, it then proceeds many times as rapidly because of the high degree of solubility of the dentine salts.

Because of the dependence of the caries causing bacteria on carbohydrates, it is frequently taught that a diet high in carbohydrate content will lead to excessive development of caries. However, it is not the quantity of carbohydrate ingested but instead the frequency with which it is eaten that is important. If eaten in many small portions throughout the day, as in the form of candy, the bacteria are supplied with their preferential metabolic substrate for many hours of the day, and the development of caries is extreme. If the carbohydrates, even though in large amounts, are eaten only at mealtimes, the extensiveness of the caries is greatly reduced.

The teeth of some people are more resistant to caries than those of others. Studies show that teeth of children who drink water containing small amounts of fluorine develop enamel that is more resistant to caries than the enamel in children who drink water not containing fluorine. Fluorine does not make the enamel harder than usual, but instead it displaces hydroxyl ions in the hydroxyapatite crystals, which in turn makes the enamel several times less soluble. It is also believed that the fluorine might be toxic to some of the bacteria as well. Finally, when small pits do develop in the enamel, fluorine is believed to promote deposition of calcium phosphate to "heal" the enamel surface. Regardless of the precise means by which fluorine protects the teeth, it is known that small amounts of fluorine deposited in enamel make teeth about three times as resistant to caries as are teeth without fluorine.

Malocclusion. Malocclusion is usually caused by a hereditary abnormality that causes the teeth of one jaw to grow to an abnormal position. In malocclusion, the teeth cannot perform their normal grinding or cutting action adequately. Occasionally malocclusion also results in abnormal displacement of the lower jaw in relation to the upper jaw, causing such undesirable effects as pain in the mandibular joint or deterioration of the teeth.

The orthodontist can often correct malocclusion by applying prolonged gentle pressure against the teeth with appropriate braces. The gentle pressure causes absorption of alveolar jaw bone on the compressed side of the tooth socket and deposition of new bone on the tensional side of the socket. In this way the tooth gradually moves to a new position as directed by the applied pressure.

QUESTIONS

1. Explain the steps by which *vitamin D* is converted into *1,25-dihydroxycholecalciferol*. What is the role of parathyroid hormone in this conversion?
2. What is the feedback mechanism in the conversion process of the above question that keeps the concentration of 1,25-dihydroxycholecalciferol at a reasonably constant level?
3. How does 1,25-dihydroxycholecalciferol function to

control the absorption of calcium from the intestinal tract?

4. What proportion of the calcium in the plasma is in ionic form?

5. What are the effects on the body of *hypocalcemia* and *hypercalcemia*?

6. Describe the way in which the organic matrix of bone and the bone salts are structured to provide both compressional strength and tensional strength of the bone.

7. What is the composition of *hydroxyapatite*?

8. During bone calcification, what salts are first laid down in the bone, and how are these converted to hydroxyapatite?

9. What is meant by *exchangeable calcium*, and how does it function to buffer the calcium concentration of the extracellular fluid?

10. Explain the histological mechanisms by which bone is continually being remodeled. What is the value of continual remodeling of bone?

11. What is the chemical composition of *parathyroid hormone*?

12. What is the effect of parathyroid hormone on plasma calcium and plasma phosphate concentrations? How does parathyroid hormone act on the bone to cause calcium removal? What is the difference between the rapid phase and the slow phase of calcium and phosphate absorption?

13. What is the effect of parathyroid hormone on calcium and phosphate excretion by the kidneys?

14. Describe the effect of plasma calcium ion concentration on the rate of parathyroid hormone secretion. How does this function as a means for negative feedback control of the calcium ion concentration?

15. What is the chemical composition of *calcitonin*, and where is it formed in the body?

16. How do the functions of calcitonin differ from those of parathyroid hormone?

17. In *hypoparathyroidism*, what causes tetany?

18. In *hyperparathyroidism*, why is it that the first symptom of the disease is often a broken bone?

19. In *rickets*, why is it that *tetany* and symptoms of *bone weakness* and *lack of bone growth* occur in the spring months of the year? Describe the effects of rickets on the bones.

20. Describe the functional parts of the *teeth*.

21. What are the special characteristics of enamel that make it highly resistant to the development of caries?

22. How does *mineral exchange* occur in the different parts of teeth?

23. Describe the cause and development of *caries*. What is the role of *fluorine* in preventing caries?

References

Angus, Z. S., et al.: PTH, calcitonin, cyclic nucleotides, and the kidney. Annu Rev Physiol 43:583, 1981.

Avioli, L. V.: Calcium and osteoporosis. Annu Rev Nutr 4:471, 1984.

DeLuca, H. F.: Recent advances in the metabolism of vitamin D. Annu Rev Physiol 43:199, 1981.

Fraser, D. R.: Regulation of the metabolism of vitamin D. Physiol Rev 60:551, 1980.

Habener, J. F.: Regulation of parathyroid hormone secretion and biosynthesis. Annu Rev Physiol 43:211, 1981.

Habener, J. F., et al.: Parathyroid hormone: biochemical aspects of biosynthesis, secretion, action, and metabolism. Physiol Rev 64:985, 1984.

Henry, H. L., and Norman, A. W.: Vitamin D: metabolism and biological actions. Annu Rev Nutr 4:493, 1984.

Kumar, R.: Metabolism of 1,25-dihydroxyvitamin D_3. Physiol Rev 64:478, 1984.

Newman, H. N.: Dental Plaque: the Ecology of the Flora on Human Teeth. Springfield, Ill., Charles C Thomas, 1980.

Pitkin, R. M.: Calcium metabolism in pregnancy and the perinatal period: a review. Am J Obstet Gynecol 151:99, 1985.

Raisz, L. G., and Kream, B. E.: Hormonal control of skeletal growth. Annu Rev Physiol 43:2225, 1981.

Rao, G. S.: Dietary intake and bioavailability of fluoride. Annu Rev Nutr 4:115, 1984.

Richmond, V. L.: Thirty years of fluoridation: a review. Am J Clin Nutr 41:129, 1985.

Ryan, K. J.: Postmenopausal estrogen use. Annu Rev Med 33:171, 1982.

Stewart, A. F., and Broadus, A. E.: The regulation of renal calcium excretion: an approach to hypercalciuria. Annu Rev Med 32:457, 1981.

Talmage, R. V., and Cooper, C. W.: Physiology and mode of action of calcitonin. In DeGroot, L. J., et al., eds.: Endocrinology. Vol. 2. New York, Grune & Stratton, 1979, p. 647.

Wasserman, R. H., and Fullmer, C. S.: Calcium transport proteins, calcium absorption, and vitamin D. Annu Rev Physiol 45:375, 1983.

54

Reproductive Functions of the Male, the Male Sex Hormones, and the Pineal Gland

SPERMATOGENESIS
  THE STEPS OF SPERMATOGENESIS
  FUNCTION OF THE SEMINAL
    VESICLES
  FUNCTION OF THE PROSTATE GLAND
  SEMEN
THE MALE SEXUAL ACT
  NEURONAL STIMULUS FOR
    PERFORMANCE OF THE MALE
    SEXUAL ACT
  STAGES OF THE MALE SEXUAL ACT
TESTOSTERONE AND OTHER MALE SEX
  HORMONES
  FUNCTIONS OF TESTOSTERONE

BASIC INTRACELLULAR MECHANISM
  OF ACTION OF TESTOSTERONE
CONTROL OF MALE SEXUAL
  FUNCTIONS BY THE
  GONADOTROPIC
  HORMONES—FSH AND LH
ABNORMALITIES OF MALE SEXUAL
  FUNCTION
  THE PROSTATE GLAND AND ITS
    ABNORMALITIES
  TESTICULAR TUMORS AND
    HYPERGONADISM IN THE MALE
THE PINEAL GLAND—ITS FUNCTION IN
  CONTROLLING SEASONAL FERTILITY

The reproductive functions of the male can be divided into three major subdivisions: first, spermatogenesis, which means simply the formation of sperm; second, performance of the male sexual act; and third, regulation of male sexual functions by the various hormones. Associated with these reproductive functions are the effects of the male sex hormones on the accessory sexual organs, on cellular metabolism, on growth, and on other functions of the body.

Physiologic Anatomy of the Male Sexual Organs. Figure 54–1 illustrates the various portions of the male reproductive system. The testis is composed of about 100 coiled *seminiferous tubules*, each about three quarters of a meter long, in which the sperm are formed. The sperm then empty into the *epididymis*, another coiled tube approximately 6 meters long. The epididymis leads into the *vas deferens*, which enlarges into the *ampulla of the vas deferens* immediately before the vas enters the body of the *prostate gland*. A *seminal vesicle*, one located on each side of the prostate, empties into the prostatic end of the ampulla, and the contents from both the ampulla and the seminal vesicle pass into an *ejaculatory duct* leading through the body of the prostate gland to empty into the *internal urethra. Prostate ducts* in turn empty from the prostate gland into the ejaculatory duct. Finally, the *urethra* is the last connecting link from the testis to the exterior. The urethra is supplied with mucus derived from a large number of minute *urethral glands* located along its entire extent and even more so from bilateral *bulbourethral glands* located near the origin of the urethra.

SPERMATOGENESIS

Spermatogenesis occurs in all the seminiferous tubules during active sexual life, beginning at an average age of 13 as the result of stimulation by anterior pituitary gonadotropic hormones and continuing throughout the remainder of life.

619

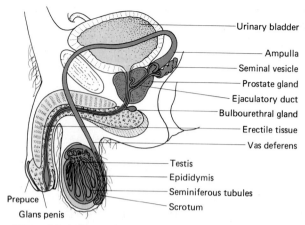

Figure 54–1. The male reproductive system. (Modified from Bloom and Fawcett: A Textbook of Histology. 10th ed. Philadelphia, W. B. Saunders Company, 1985.)

THE STEPS OF SPERMATOGENESIS

The seminiferous tubules, one of which is illustrated in Figure 54–2A, contain a large number of small to medium-sized germinal epithelial cells called *spermatogonia*, which are located in two to three layers along the outer border of the tubular epithelium. These continually proliferate to replenish themselves, and a portion of them differentiate through definite stages of development to form sperm, as shown in Figure 54–2B.

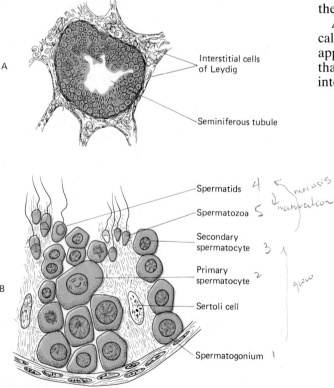

Figure 54–2. *A,* Cross-section of a seminiferous tubule. *B,* Spermatogenesis. (Modified from Arey: Developmental Anatomy. 7th ed. Philadelphia, W. B. Saunders Company, 1974.)

The first stage in spermatogenesis is growth of some spermatogonia to form considerably enlarged cells called *spermatocytes*. Then the spermatocyte divides by the process of *meiosis* (in which there is no formation of new chromosomes, only separation of the chromosomal pairs) to form two *spermatids*, each containing 23 chromosomes. The spermatids do not divide again but instead mature for several weeks to become spermatozoa.

The Sex Chromosomes. In each spermatogonium one of the 23 pairs of chromosomes carries the genetic information that determines the sex of the eventual offspring. This pair is composed of one X chromosome, which is called the *female chromosome*, and one Y chromosome, the *male chromosome*. During meiotic division the sex-determining chromosomes are distributed between the spermatids, so that half of the sperm become *male sperm* containing the Y chromosome and the other half *female sperm* containing the X chromosome. The sex of the offspring is determined by which of these two types of sperm fertilizes the ovum. This will be discussed further in Chapter 56.

Formation of Sperm. When the spermatids are first formed, they still have the usual characteristics of epithelioid cells, but soon most of the cytoplasm disappears, and each spermatid begins to elongate into a spermatozoon, illustrated in Figure 54–3, composed of a *head, neck, body,* and *tail*. To form the head, the nuclear material is condensed into a compact mass, and the cell membrane contracts around the nucleus. It is this nuclear material that fertilizes the ovum.

At the front of the sperm head is a small structure called the *acrosome*, which is formed from the Golgi apparatus and contains hyaluronidase and proteases that play important roles in the entry of the sperm into the ovum.

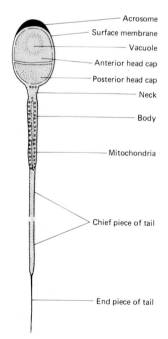

Figure 54–3. Structure of the human spermatozoon.

The *centrioles* are aggregated in the neck of the sperm, and the *mitochondria* are arranged in a spiral in the body.

Extending beyond the body is a long tail, which is mainly an outgrowth of one of the centrioles. This has almost the same structure as a cilium, which was described in detail in Chapter 2. The tail contains two paired microtubules down the center and nine double microtubules arranged around the border. This whole structure is called the *axoneme.*

To and fro movement of the tail (flagellar movement) provides motility for the sperm. This movement is believed to result from a rhythmic longitudinal sliding motion between the anterior and posterior tubules that make up the axoneme. Normal sperm move in a straight line at a velocity of 1 to 4 mm per minute.

Function of the Sertoli Cells. The Sertoli cells of the germinal epithelium, known also as the *sustentacular cells*, are illustrated in Figure 54–2B. These cells are large, extending from the base of the seminiferous epithelium all the way to the lumen of the tubule. The spermatids attach themselves to the Sertoli cells, and a specific relationship exists between the two cells that causes the spermatids to change into spermatozoa. The Sertoli cells provide nutrient material, hormones, and possibly also enzymes that are necessary for causing appropriate changes in the spermatids. The Sertoli cells also remove the excess cytoplasm as the spermatids are converted to spermatozoa, a process called *spermiation.*

Maturation of Sperm in the Epididymis. Following formation in the seminiferous tubules, the sperm pass into the *epididymis.* Sperm removed from the seminiferous tubules are completely nonmotile, and they cannot fertilize an ovum. However, after the sperm have been in the epididymis for some 18 hours to 10 days, they develop the capability of motility, even though some inhibitory factor still prevents motility until after ejaculation. The sperm also become capable of fertilizing the ovum, a process called *maturation.* The epididymis secretes a copious quantity of fluid containing hormones, enzymes, and special nutrients that may be important or even essential for sperm maturation.

Storage of Sperm. A small quantity of sperm can be stored in the epididymis, but most sperm are stored in the vas deferens and ampulla of the vas deferens. They can remain stored, maintaining their fertility, in these areas for several months, though it is doubtful that during normal sexual activity such prolonged storage ordinarily occurs. Indeed, with excessive sexual activity storage may be no longer than a few days at most.

Physiology of the Mature Sperm. The usual motile and fertile sperm are capable of flagellated movement through the fluid media at a rate of approximately 1 to 4 mm per minute. Furthermore, *normal* sperm tend to travel in a straight, rotating line rather than in circles. The activity of sperm is greatly enhanced in neutral and slightly alkaline media such as exist in the ejaculated semen, but it is greatly depressed in mildly acid media, and strong acid media can cause rapid death of sperm. Though sperm can live for many weeks in the genital ducts of the testes, the life of sperm in the female genital tract is only one to two days.

FUNCTION OF THE SEMINAL VESICLES

The seminal vesicles are secretory glands lined with an epithelium that secretes a mucoid material containing an abundance of *fructose* and other nutrient substances, as well as large quantities of *prostaglandins* and *fibrinogen.* During the process of ejaculation, each seminal vesicle empties its contents into the ejaculatory duct shortly after the vas deferens empties the sperm. This adds greatly to the bulk of the ejaculated semen, and the fructose and other substances in the seminal fluid are of considerable nutrient value for the ejaculated sperm until one of them fertilizes the ovum. The prostaglandins are believed to aid fertilization in two ways: (1) by reacting with the cervical mucus to make it more receptive to sperm and (2) possibly causing reverse peristaltic contractions in the uterus and fallopian tubes to move the sperm toward the ovaries (a few sperm reach the upper end of the fallopian tubes within five minutes).

FUNCTION OF THE PROSTATE GLAND

The prostate gland secretes a thin, milky, alkaline fluid containing citric acid, calcium, and several other substances. During emission, the capsule of the prostate gland contracts simultaneously with the contractions of the vas deferens and seminal vesicles, so that the thin, milky fluid adds to the bulk of the semen. The alkaline characteristic of the prostatic fluid may be quite important for successful fertilization of the ovum, because the fluid of the vas deferens is relatively acidic owing to the presence of metabolic end-products of the sperm and, consequently, inhibits sperm motility and fertility. Also, the vaginal secretions of the female are acidic (pH of 3.5 to 4.0). Sperm do not become optimally motile until the pH of the surrounding fluids rises to approximately 6 to 6.5. Consequently, it is probable that prostatic fluid neutralizes the acidity of these other fluids after ejaculation and greatly enhances the motility and fertility of the sperm.

SEMEN

Semen, which is ejaculated during the male sexual act, is composed of the fluids from the vas deferens, the seminal vesicles, the prostate gland, and the mucous glands, especially the bulbourethral glands. The major bulk of the semen is seminal vesicle fluid (about 60 per cent), which is the last to be ejaculated and serves to wash the sperm out of the ejaculatory duct and urethra. The average pH of the combined semen is approximately 7.5, the alkaline prostatic fluid having neutralized the mild acidity of the other portions of the semen. The prostatic fluid gives the semen a milky appearance, while fluid from the seminal vesicle and from the mucous glands gives the semen a mucoid consistency. Indeed, a clotting enzyme of the prostatic fluid causes the fibrinogen of the seminal vesicle fluid to form a weak coagulum, which then dissolves during the next 15 to 20 minutes because of lysis by a fibrinolysin formed from a prostatic profibrinolysin. In the early minutes after ejaculation, the sperm remain relatively immobile, possibly because of the viscosity of the coagulum. However, after the coagulum dissolutes, the sperm simultaneously become highly motile.

Though sperm can live for many weeks in the male genital ducts, once they are ejaculated in the semen, their maximal life span is only 24 to 48 hours at body temperature. At lowered temperatures, however, semen may be stored for several weeks, and when frozen at temperatures below $-100°$ C, sperm have been preserved for years.

Effect of Sperm Count on Fertility. The usual quantity of semen ejaculated at each coitus averages approximately 3.5 ml, and in each milliliter of semen is an average of approximately 120 million sperm, though even in normal persons this number can vary from 35 million to 200 million. Therefore, an average of 400 million sperm are usually present in each ejaculate. When the number of sperm in each milliliter falls below approximately 20,000,000, the person is likely to be infertile. Thus, even though only a single sperm is necessary to fertilize the ovum, the ejaculate must contain a tremendous number of sperm for at least one to fertilize the ovum. A possible reason for this requirement is the following:

Function of Hyaluronidase and Proteinases Secreted by the Sperm for the Process of Fertilization. Stored in the acrosomes of the sperm are large quantities of hyaluronidase and proteinases. Hyaluronidase is an enzyme that depolymerizes the hyaluronic acid polymers that are present in large quantities in the intercellular cement substance; proteinases can dissolute the proteins of tissues.

When the ovum is expelled from the follicle of the ovary into the abdominal cavity, it carries with it several layers of cells. Before a sperm can reach the ovum to fertilize it, these cells must be removed; it is believed that the hyaluronidase and proteinases released by the acrosomes play at least some role (in addition to that played by sodium bicarbonate in the fallopian tube secretions) in causing these cells to break away from the ovum, thus allowing the sperm to reach the surface of the ovum. When sperm are insufficient in number, the man is often sterile. It has been postulated that this sterility results from insufficient enzymes to help remove the cell layers from the ovum.

Another possible function of the proteinases is to allow the sperm to penetrate the mucus that frequently forms in the cervix of the uterus. The proteinases act as mucolytic enzymes that presumably proceed in advance of the sperm and create channels through the mucous plug. It is believed that this deficiency of the appropriate enzymes to perform this function is occasionally responsible for male sterility.

THE MALE SEXUAL ACT

NEURONAL STIMULUS FOR PERFORMANCE OF THE MALE SEXUAL ACT

The most important nerve signals for initiating the male sexual act originate in the glans penis, for the glans contains a highly organized sensory end-organ system that transmits into the central nervous system a special modality of sensation called *sexual sensation*. The massaging action of intercourse on the glans stimulates the sensory end-organs, and the sexual sensations in turn pass through the pudendal nerve, thence through the sacral plexus into the sacral portion of the spinal cord, and finally up the cord to undefined areas of the cerebrum. Impulses may also enter the spinal cord from areas adjacent to the penis to aid in stimulating the sexual act. For instance, stimulation of the anal epithelium, the scrotum, and perineal structures in general can all send impulses into the cord which add to the sexual sensation. Sexual sensations can even originate in internal structures, such as irritated areas of the urethra, the bladder, the prostate, the seminal vesicles, the testes, and the vas deferens. Indeed, one of the causes of "sexual drive" is probably overfilling of the sexual organs with secretions. Infection and inflammation of these sexual organs sometimes cause almost continual sexual desire, and aphrodisiac drugs, such as cantharides, increase the sexual desire by irritating the bladder and urethral mucosa.

The Psychic Element of Male Sexual Stimulation. Appropriate psychic stimuli can greatly enhance the ability of a person to perform the sexual act. Simply thinking sexual thoughts or even dreaming that the act of intercourse is being performed can cause the male sexual act to occur and to culminate in ejaculation. Indeed, *nocturnal emissions* during dreams occur in many males during some stages of sexual life, especially during the teens.

Integration of the Male Sexual Act in the Spinal Cord. Though psychic factors usually play an important part in the male sexual act and can actually initiate it, the cerebrum is probably not absolutely necessary for its performance, for appropriate genital stimulation can cause ejaculation in some animals and in an occasional human being after their spinal cords have been cut above the lumbar region. Therefore, the male sexual act results from inherent reflex mechanisms integrated in the sacral and lumbar spinal cord, and these mechanisms can be activated by either psychic or direct sexual stimulation or both.

STAGES OF THE MALE SEXUAL ACT

Erection; Role of the Parasympathetic Nerves. Erection is the first effect of male sexual stimulation, and the degree of erection is proportional to the degree of stimulation, whether this be psychic or physical.

Erection is caused by parasympathetic impulses that pass from the sacral portion of the spinal cord to the penis. These parasympathetic impulses dilate the arteries of the penis, thus allowing arterial blood to flow under high pressure into the *erectile tissue* of the penis, illustrated in Figure 54–4. This erectile tissue is composed of large, cavernous venous sinusoids, which are normally relatively empty but become dilated tremendously when arterial blood flows into them under pressure. Also, these erectile bodies are surrounded by strong fibrous coats; therefore, high pressure within the sinusoids causes ballooning of the erectile tissue to such an extent that the penis becomes hard and elongated.

Lubrication, a Parasympathetic Function. During sexual stimulation, parasympathetic impulses, in addition to promoting erection, cause the urethral glands and the bulbourethral glands to secrete mucus. This mucus flows through the urethra during intercourse to aid in the lubrication of coitus. However, most of the lubrication of coitus is provided by the female sexual organs rather than by the male. Without satisfactory lubrication, the male sexual act is rarely successful because unlubricated intercourse causes pain impulses that inhibit rather than excite sexual sensations.

Emission and Ejaculation; Role of the Sympathetic Nerves. Emission and ejaculation are the culmination of the male sexual act. When the sexual stimulus becomes extremely intense, the reflex centers of the spinal cord begin to emit *sympathetic impulses* that leave the cord at L-1 and L-2 and pass to the genital organs to initiate *emission*, the forerunner of ejaculation.

Emission is believed to begin with contraction of the vas deferens and the ampulla to cause expulsion of sperm into the internal urethra. Then, contractions in the seminal vesicles and the muscular coat of the prostate gland expel seminal fluid and prostatic fluid, forcing the sperm forward. All these fluids mix with the mucus already secreted by the bulbourethral glands to form the semen. The process to this point is *emission*.

The filling of the internal urethra then elicits signals that are transmitted through the pudendal nerves to the sacral regions of the cord. In turn, signals from the sacral cord further excite the rhythmic contraction of the internal genital organs and also cause contraction of the ischiocavernosus and bulbocavernosus skeletal muscles that compress the bases of the penile erectile tissue. These effects together cause rhythmic, wavelike increases in pressure in the genital ducts and urethra, which project the semen from the urethra to the exterior. This process is called *ejaculation*. At the same time, rhythmic contractions of the pelvic muscles and even of some of the muscles of the body trunk cause thrusting movements of the pelvis and penis, which also help propel the semen into the deepest recesses of the vagina and perhaps even through the cervix into the uterus.

This entire period of emission and ejaculation is called the *male orgasm.* At its termination, the male sexual excitement disappears almost entirely within one to two minutes and erection ceases, a process called *resolution.*

TESTOSTERONE AND OTHER MALE SEX HORMONES

Secretion of Testosterone by the Interstitial Cells of the Testes. The testes secrete several male sex hormones, which are collectively called *androgens.* However, one of these, *testosterone*, is so much more abundant and potent than the others that it can be considered to be the significant hormone responsible for the male hormonal effects.

Testosterone is formed by the *interstitial cells of Leydig,* which lie in the interstices between the seminiferous tubules, as illustrated in Figure 54–5, and constitute about 20 per cent of the mass of the adult testes. Interstitial cells in the testes are not numerous in a child, but they *are* numerous in a newborn male infant and also in the adult male any time after

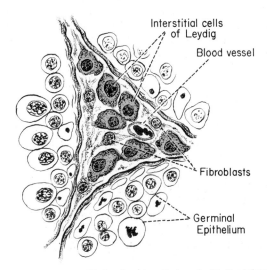

Figure 54–5. Interstitial cells of Leydig located in the interstices between the seminiferous tubules. (Modified from Bloom and Fawcett: Textbook of Histology. 10th ed. Philadelphia, W. B. Saunders Company, 1985.)

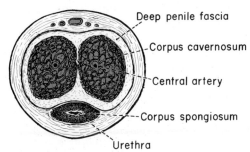

Figure 54–4. Erectile tissue of the penis.

puberty; at both these times the testes secrete large quantities of testosterone.

Secretion of Androgens Elsewhere in the Body. The term *androgen* is used synonymously with the term male sex hormone, but it also includes male sex hormones produced elsewhere in the body besides the testes. For instance, the adrenal gland secretes at least five different androgens, though the total masculinizing activity of all these is normally so slight that they do not cause significant masculine characteristics even in women. But when an adrenal tumor of the androgen-producing cells occurs, the quantity of androgenic hormones may become great enough to cause all the usual male secondary sexual characteristics.

Chemistry of Testosterone. All androgens are steroid compounds, as illustrated by the formula in Figure 54–6 for *testosterone* and its closely related hormone, *dihydrotestosterone*. Both in the testes and in the adrenals, the androgens can be synthesized either from cholesterol or directly from acetyl coenzyme A.

Metabolism of Testosterone. After secretion by the testes, testosterone, most of it loosely bound with plasma protein, circulates in the blood for not over 15 to 30 minutes before it either becomes fixed to the tissues or is degraded into inactive products that are subsequently excreted.

Much of the testosterone that becomes fixed to the tissues is converted within the cells to dihydrotestosterone, which is also shown in Figure 54–6; it is in this form that testosterone performs many of its intracellular functions.

Degradation and Excretion of Testosterone. The testosterone that does not become fixed to the tissues is rapidly converted, mainly by the liver, into *androsterone* and *dehydroepiandrosterone* and is simultaneously conjugated either as glucuronides or sulfates (glucuronides, particularly). These are excreted either in the bile into the intestinal tract or into the urine.

FUNCTIONS OF TESTOSTERONE

In general, testosterone is responsible for the distinguishing characteristics of the masculine body. Even during fetal life, the testes are stimulated by chorionic gonadotropin from the placenta to produce

a small quantity of testosterone, but essentially no testosterone is produced during childhood until approximately the age of 10 to 13. Then testosterone production increases rapidly at the onset of puberty and lasts throughout most of the remainder of life, dwindling rapidly beyond the age of 40 to perhaps one third to one fifth the peak value by the age of 80.

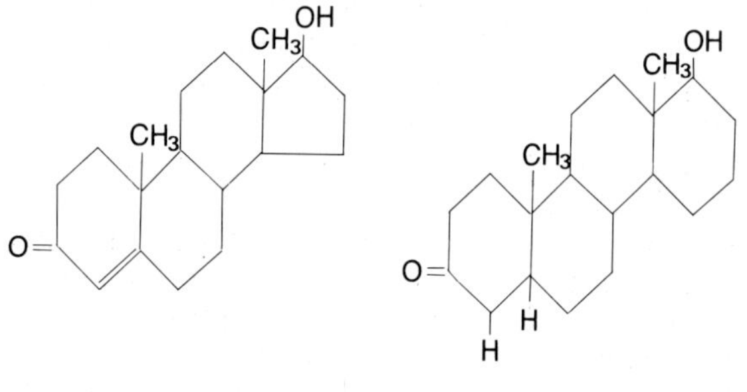

Functions of Testosterone During Fetal Development. Testosterone begins to be elaborated by the male at about the second month of embryonic life. Injection of large quantities of male sex hormone into gravid animals causes development of male sexual organs in the fetus even when the fetus is female. Also, removal of the fetal testes in a male fetus causes development of female sexual organs. Therefore, the presence or absence of testosterone in the fetus is the determining factor in the development of male or female genital organs and characteristics. That is, testosterone secreted by the genital ridges and the subsequently developing testes is responsible for the development of the male sex characteristics, including the growth of a penis and a scrotum rather than the formation of a clitoris and a vagina. Also, it causes development of the prostate gland, the seminal vesicles, and the male genital ducts, while at the same time suppressing the formation of female genital organs.

Effect on the Descent of the Testes. The testes usually descend into the scrotum during the last two months of pregnancy, when the testes are secreting adequate quantities of testosterone. If a male child is born with undescended testes, administration of testosterone will often cause the testes to descend in the usual manner if the inguinal canals are large enough to allow the testes to pass. Or administration of gonadotropic hormones, which stimulate the interstitial cells of the testes to produce testosterone, can also cause the testes to descend. Thus, the stimulus for descent of the testes is testosterone, indicating again that testosterone is an important hormone for male sexual development during fetal life.

Effect of Testosterone on Development of Adult Primary and Secondary Sexual Characteristics. Testosterone secretion after puberty causes the penis, the scrotum, and the testes all to enlarge about eightfold until about the age of 20. In addition, testosterone causes the secondary sexual characteristics of the male to develop at the same time, beginning at puberty and ending at maturity. These secondary sexual characteristics, in addition to the sexual organs themselves, distinguish the male from the female as follows:

Distribution of Body Hair. Testosterone causes growth of hair (1) over the pubis, (2) on the face, (3) usually on the chest, and (4) less often on other regions of the body, such as the back. It also causes the hair on most other portions of the body to become more prolific.

Baldness. Testosterone in some men decreases the growth of hair on the top of the head; a man who does not have functional testes does not become bald.

Figure 54–6. Testosterone and dihydrotestosterone.

Testosterone   Dihydrotestosterone

However, many virile men never become bald, for baldness is a result of two factors: first, a *genetic background* for the development of baldness and, second, superimposed on this genetic background, *large quantities of androgenic hormones.* A woman who has the appropriate genetic background and who develops a long-sustained androgenic tumor becomes bald in the same manner as a man.

Effect on the Voice. Testosterone secreted by the testes or injected into the body causes hypertrophy of the laryngeal mucosa and enlargement of the larynx. These effects cause at first a relatively discordant, "cracking" voice, but this gradually changes into the typical masculine lower-pitched voice.

Effect on the Skin. Testosterone increases the thickness of the skin over the entire body and increases the ruggedness of the subcutaneous tissues.

Effect on Protein Formation and Muscular Development. One of the most important male characteristics is the development of increasing musculature following puberty. This is associated with increased protein in other parts of the body as well. Many of the changes in the skin are due to deposition of proteins in the skin, and the changes in the voice even result, at least partly, from the protein anabolic function of testosterone.

Because of the very great effect that testosterone has on the body musculature, it (or more usually a synthetic androgen instead) is widely used by athletes to improve their muscular performance. This practice is to be severely deprecated because of prolonged harmful effects of excess testosterone, as we shall discuss in Chapter 57 in relation to sports physiology. Testosterone is also frequently used in old age as a "youth hormone" to improve muscle strength and vigor.

Effect on Bone Growth and Calcium Retention. Following puberty or following prolonged injection of testosterone, the bones grow considerably in thickness and also deposit substantial amounts of calcium salts. Thus, testosterone increases the total quantity of bone matrix, and this also causes calcium retention. The increase in bone matrix is believed to result from the general protein anabolic function of testosterone.

When great quantities of testosterone (or any other androgen) are secreted in the still-growing child, the rate of bone growth increases markedly, causing a spurt in total body growth as well. However, the testosterone also causes the epiphyses of the long bones to unite with the shafts of the bones at an early age in life. Therefore, despite the rapidity of growth, the early uniting of the epiphyses prevents the person from growing as tall as he would grow were testosterone not secreted at all. Even in normal men the final adult height is slightly less than that which would have been attained had the person been castrated prior to puberty.

Effect on the Red Blood Cells. The average man has about 700,000 more red blood cells per cubic millimeter than the average woman. However, this difference may be due partly to increased metabolic rate following testosterone administration rather than to a direct effect of testosterone on red blood cell production.

BASIC INTRACELLULAR MECHANISM OF ACTION OF TESTOSTERONE

Probably all or almost all the effects just listed result from increased rate of protein formation in the target cells. This has been studied extensively in the prostate gland, one of the organs that is most affected by testosterone. In this gland, testosterone enters the cells within a few minutes after secretion, is there converted to *dihydrotestosterone*, and binds with a cytoplasmic receptor protein. This combination then migrates to the nucleus, where it binds with a nuclear protein and induces the DNA-RNA transcription process. Within 30 minutes RNA polymerase has become activated, and the concentration of RNA begins to increase in the cells; this is followed by progressive increase in cellular protein. After several days the quantity of DNA in the gland has also increased, and there has been a simultaneous increase in the number of prostatic cells.

Therefore, it is assumed that testosterone greatly stimulates production of proteins in general, though increasing more specifically those proteins in target organs or tissues responsible for the development of male sexual characteristics.

CONTROL OF MALE SEXUAL FUNCTIONS BY THE GONADOTROPIC HORMONES— FSH AND LH

The anterior pituitary gland secretes two major gonadotropic hormones: (1) *follicle-stimulating hormone* (FSH) and (2) *luteinizing hormone* (LH). Both of these play major roles in the control of male sexual function.

Regulation of Testosterone Production by LH. Testosterone is produced by the interstitial cells of Leydig when the testes are stimulated by LH from the pituitary gland, and the quantity of testosterone secreted varies approximately in proportion to the amount of LH available.

Injection of purified LH into a child causes fibroblasts in the interstitial areas of the testes to develop into interstitial cells of Leydig, though mature Leydig cells are not normally found in the child's testes until after the age of approximately 10.

Effect of Human Chorionic Gonadotropin on the Fetal Testes. During gestation the placenta secretes large quantities of *human chorionic gonadotropin*, a hormone that has almost the same properties as LH. This hormone stimulates the formation of interstitial cells in the testes of the fetus and causes testosterone secretion. As pointed out earlier in the chapter, the secretion of testosterone during fetal life is necessary for promoting formation of male sexual organs.

Regulation of Spermatogenesis by FSH and Testosterone. The conversion of spermatogonia into spermatocytes in the seminiferous tubules is stimulated by FSH from the anterior pituitary gland. This probably results from the effect of FSH to stimulate the Sertoli cells, which are responsible for converting the spermatids into sperm, a process called *spermiation*. In addition, FSH causes the Sertoli cells to secrete estrogens, which may also help to promote spermatogenesis.

However, FSH cannot by itself cause complete formation of spermatozoa. For spermatogenesis to proceed to completion, testosterone must be secreted simultaneously by the interstitial cells. Thus testosterone diffusing from the interstitial cells into the seminiferous tubules apparently is necessary for final maturation of the spermatozoa. Because testosterone is secreted by the interstitial cells under the influence of LH, both FSH and LH must be secreted by the anterior pituitary gland if spermatogenesis is to occur.

Regulation of Pituitary Secretion of LH and FSH by the Hypothalamus. The gonadotropins, like corticotropin and thyrotropin, are secreted by the anterior pituitary gland mainly in response to nervous activity in the hypothalamus. For instance, psychic stimuli can affect fertility of the male animal, as exemplified by the fact that transporting a bull under uncomfortable conditions can often cause almost complete temporary sterility. In the human being, too, it is known that various psychic stimuli feeding into the hypothalamus can cause marked excitatory or inhibitory effects on gonadotropin secretion, in this way sometimes greatly altering the degree of fertility.

Luteinizing Hormone–Releasing Hormone (LHRH), the Hypothalamic Hormone That Stimulates Gonadotropin Secretion. In both the male and the female, the hypothalamus controls gonadotropin secretion by way of the hypothalamic-hypophysial portal system, as discussed in Chapter 49. Though there are two different gonadotropic hormones, luteinizing hormone and follicle-stimulating hormone, only one hypothalamic-releasing hormone has been discovered; this is called *luteinizing hormone–releasing hormone* (LHRH). Though this hormone has an especially strong effect on inducing luteinizing hormone secretion by the anterior pituitary gland, it also has a potent effect in causing follicle-stimulating hormone secretion as well. For this reason it is often also called *gonadotropin-releasing hormone.*

Reciprocal Inhibition of Hypothalamic–Anterior Pituitary Secretion of Gonadotropic Hormones by Testicular Hormones

Feedback Control of Testosterone Secretion. The following negative feedback control system operates continuously to control very precisely the rate of testosterone secretion:

1. The hypothalamus secretes *luteinizing hormone–releasing hormone*, which stimulates the anterior pituitary gland to secrete *luteinizing hormone.*

2. Luteinizing hormone in turn stimulates *hyperplasia of the Leydig cells* of the testes and also stimulates production of *testosterone* by these cells.

3. The testosterone in turn feeds back *negatively* to the hypothalamus, inhibiting production of luteinizing hormone–releasing hormone. This obviously limits the rate at which testosterone will be produced. On the other hand, when testosterone production is too low, lack of inhibition of the hypothalamus leads to return of testosterone secretion to the normal level.

Feedback Control of Spermatogenesis—Role of Inhibin. It is known, too, that spermatogenesis by the testes inhibits the secretion of FSH. It is believed that the Sertoli cells secrete a hormone that has a direct inhibitory effect mainly on the anterior pituitary gland (but perhaps slightly on the hypothalamus as well) to inhibit the secretion of FSH. A glycoprotein hormone having a molecular weight between 10,000 and 30,000 and called *inhibin* has been isolated from cultured Sertoli cells and is probably responsible for most of the feedback control of FSH secretion and of spermatogenesis. This feedback cycle is the following:

1. Follicle-stimulating hormone stimulates the Sertoli cells that provide nutrition for the developing spermatozoa.

2. The Sertoli cells release inhibin that in turn feeds back negatively to the anterior pituitary gland to inhibit the production of FSH. Thus, this feedback cycle maintains a constant rate of spermatogenesis, without underproduction or overproduction, that is required for male reproductive function.

Puberty and Regulation of Its Onset. During the first ten years of life, the male child secretes almost no gonadotropins and consequently almost no testosterone. Then, at the age of about 10, the anterior pituitary gland begins to secrete progressively increasing quantities of gonadotropins, and this is followed by a corresponding increase in testicular function. By approximately the age of 13, the male child reaches full adult sexual capability. This period of change is called *puberty*.

The cause of the onset of puberty is the following: *During childhood, the hypothalamus simply does not secrete significant amounts of luteinizing hormone–releasing hormone.* Then, for reasons not understood, some maturation process in the brain causes the hypothalamus to begin secreting LHRH at the time of puberty. This secretion will not occur if the neuronal connections between the hypothalamus and other parts of the brain are not intact. Therefore, the present belief is that the maturation process probably occurs elsewhere in the brain instead of in the hypothalamus. One suggested locus is the amygdala.

ABNORMALITIES OF MALE SEXUAL FUNCTION

THE PROSTATE GLAND AND ITS ABNORMALITIES

The prostate gland remains relatively small throughout childhood but begins to grow at puberty under the stimulus of testosterone. This gland reaches an almost stationary size by the age of 20 and remains this size up to the age of approximately 50 years. At that time in some men, it begins to degenerate along with the decreased production of testosterone by the testes. A benign fibroadenoma frequently develops in the prostate in older men and causes urinary obstruction. This hypertrophy is not caused by testosterone.

Cancer of the prostate gland is an extremely common cause of death, resulting in approximately 2 to 3 per cent of all male deaths.

Once cancer of the prostate gland does occur, the cancerous cells are usually stimulated to more rapid growth by testosterone and are inhibited by removal of the testes so that testosterone cannot be formed. Also, prostatic cancer can usually be inhibited by administration of estrogens. Some patients who have prostatic cancer that has already metastasized to almost all the bones of the body can be successfully treated for a few months to years by removal of the testes, by estrogen therapy, or by both; following this therapy the metastases degenerate and the bones heal. This treatment does not completely stop the cancer but does slow it down and greatly diminishes the severe bone pain.

TESTICULAR TUMORS AND HYPERGONADISM IN THE MALE

An *interstitial cell tumor* on rare occasions develops in a testis, but when one does develop it sometimes produces as much as 100 times the normal quantity of testosterone. When such tumors develop in young children, they cause rapid growth of the musculature and bones but also early uniting of the epiphyses, so that the eventual adult height actually is less than that which would have been achieved otherwise. Obviously, such interstitial cell tumors cause excessive development of the sexual organs and of the secondary sexual characteristics. In the adult male, small interstitial cell tumors are difficult to diagnose because masculine features are already present.

Much more common than the interstitial cell tumors are tumors of the germinal epithelium. Because germinal cells are capable of differentiating into almost any type of cell, many of these tumors contain multiple types of tissue, such as placental tissue, hair, teeth, bone, and skin, all found together in the same tumorous mass called a *teratoma*. Often these tumors secrete no hormones, but if a significant quantity of placental tissue develops in the tumor, it may secrete large quantities of human chorionic gonadotropin that

has functions very similar to those of LH. Also, estrogenic hormones are frequently secreted by these tumors and cause the condition called *gynecomastia*, which means overgrowth of the breasts.

THE PINEAL GLAND—ITS FUNCTION IN CONTROLLING SEASONAL FERTILITY

The pineal gland is a small nervous tissue-glandular body protruding from the midbrain above and behind the superior colliculi. Some physiologists have claimed for many years that the pineal gland plays important roles in the control of sexual activities and reproduction, functions that still others have said were nothing more than the zealous imaginings of physiologists preoccupied with sexual delusions.

But now, after years of turmoil and dispute, it looks as though the sex advocates have at last won. For, in some lower animals in which the pineal gland has been removed or in which the nervous circuits to the pineal gland have been sectioned, the normal annual periods of seasonal fertility are lost. To these animals such seasonal fertility is very important because it allows birth of the offspring in the spring and summer months when survival is most likely. The mechanism of this effect is still not entirely clear, but it seems to be the following:

First, the pineal gland is controlled by nerve signals elicited by the amount of light seen by the eyes each day. For instance, in the hamster, more than 13 hours of darkness each day activates the pineal gland, while less than that amount of darkness fails to activate it.

Second, the pineal gland secretes *melatonin* and several other similar substances. Either melatonin or one of the other substances then passes either by way of the blood or through the fluid of the third ventricle to the anterior pituitary gland to *inhibit* gonadotropic hormone secretion, and the gonads become inhibited and even involuted. This is what occurs during the early winter months. But after about four months of dysfunction, the gonadotropic hormone secretion breaks through the inhibitory effect of the pineal gland, and the gonads become functional once more, ready for a full springtime of activity.

But does the pineal gland have a similar function in controlling reproduction in man? The answer to this is still far from known. However, tumors in the region of the pineal gland are often associated with serious hypo- or hypergonadal dysfunction. So perhaps the pineal gland does play at least some role in controlling sexual drive and reproduction in man.

QUESTIONS

1. Describe the physiological anatomy of the *testes* and the other male sex organs.
2. Give the steps of *spermatogenesis*.
3. What determines the sex of a *sperm*?
4. Give the characteristics of the mature sperm.

5. What is the function of the *Sertoli cells* during the formation of sperm?
6. What is the role of the *epididymis* during the maturation of the sperm?

7. What are the respective roles of the *seminal vesicles* and the *prostate gland* in the formation of *semen*?

8. What is the composition of semen?

9. What is the relationship of *sperm count* to *fertility*, and what role does the secretion by sperm of *hyaluronidase* and *proteinases* play in this effect?

10. What are the types of stimuli that can lead to sexual sensations and culmination of the sexual act?

11. What are the roles of the parasympathetic and the sympathetic nerves in *erection, lubrication,* and *emission* and *ejaculation*?

12. What is the chemistry of *testosterone*, and by what cells is it formed?

13. What are the functions of testosterone during fetal development?

14. What are the effects of testosterone on the male sexual organs during adolescence?

15. What are the effects of testosterone on body hair, baldness, the voice, the skin, muscle development, bone growth, and the red blood cells?

16. What is the basic intracellular mechanism by which testosterone performs most or all of its functions?

17. Explain the control of *testosterone secretion* by *LHRH* and *LH*. Give the feedback control mechanism that maintains a relatively constant rate of testosterone secretion.

18. Explain the effects of LHRH, FSH, LH, and testosterone in the control of *spermatogenesis.*

19. What is the feedback mechanism for control of spermatogenesis? How does the hormone *inhibin* enter into this?

20. What causes the onset of *puberty*?

21. Why are tumors of the germinal epithelium frequently of the *teratoma* type in which multiple types of body tissues are found, such as hair, teeth, skin, and so forth?

22. Explain how the *pineal gland* might control seasonal fertility in animals.

References

Arnold, A. P., and Gorski, R. A.: Gonadal steroid induction of structural sex differences in the central nervous system. Annu Rev Neurosci 7:413, 1984.

Brooks, D. E.: Metabolic activity in the epididymis and its regulation by androgens. Physiol Rev 61:515, 1981.

Conn, P. M., et al.: Gonadotropin-releasing hormone: molecular and cell biology, physiology, and clinical applications. Fed Proc 43:2351, 1984.

Griffin, J. E., and Wilson, J. D.: The testis. In Bondy, P. K., and Rosenberg, L. E., eds.: Metabolic Control and Disease, 8th ed. Philadelphia, W. B. Saunders Co., 1980, p. 1535.

Habenicht, U. F.: Hormonal Regulation of Testicular Descent. New York, Springer-Verlag, 1983.

Hawkins, D. F., and Elder, M. G.: Human Fertility Control: the Theory and Practice. Boston, Butterworths, 1979.

Janne, O. A., and Bardin, C. W.: Androgen and antiandrogen receptor binding. Annu Rev Physiol 46:107, 1984.

Krieger, D. T., ed.: Current Therapy in Endocrinology, 1983–1984. St. Louis, C. V. Mosby, 1983.

McCann, S. M.: Physiology and pharmacology of LHRH and somatostatin. Annu Rev Pharmacol Toxicol 22:491, 1982.

McEwen, B. S.: Binding and metabolism of sex steroids by the hypothalamic-pituitary unit: physiological implications. Annu Rev Physiol 42:97, 1980.

Means, A. R., et al.: Regulation of the testis Sertoli cell by follicle stimulating hormone. Annu Rev Physiol 42:59, 1980.

Negro, V. A., ed.: Male Reproduction and Fertility. New York, Raven Press, 1983.

Ochiai, K, ed.: Endocrine Correlates of Reproduction. New York, Springer-Verlag, 1984.

Odell, W. D.: The physiology of puberty: Disorders of the pubertal process. In DeGroot, L. J., et al., eds.: Endocrinology. Vol. 3. New York, Grune & Stratton, 1979, p. 1363.

Reiter, R. J., ed.: The Pineal and Reproduction. New York, S. Karger, 1978.

Ross, G. F., and Lipsett, M. B., eds.: Reproductive Endocrinology. Clinics in Endocrinology and Metabolism. London, W. B. Saunders Co., Nov., 1978.

Schiavi, R. C.: Male erectile disorders. Annu Rev Med 32:509, 1981.

Setchell, B. P.: The Mammalian Testis. N.Y., Cornell University Press, 1978.

Steinberger, A., and Steinberger, E., eds.: Testicular Development, Structure and Function. New York, Raven Press, 1980.

Thomas, J. A., and Singahl, R. L., eds.: Sex Hormone Receptors in Endocrine Organs. Baltimore, Urban & Schwarzenberg, 1980.

Waites, G. M. H., and Gladwell, R. T.: Physiological significance of fluid secretion in the testis and blood-testis barrier. Physiol Rev 62:624, 1982.

55

Prepregnancy Reproductive Functions in the Female and the Female Hormones

PHYSIOLOGICAL ANATOMY OF THE
FEMALE SEXUAL ORGANS
THE FEMALE HORMONAL SYSTEM
FUNCTION OF THE GONADOTROPIC
HORMONES TO CONTROL THE
MONTHLY OVARIAN CYCLE
FOLLICULAR GROWTH—FUNCTION
OF FSH
THE CORPUS LUTEUM—THE LUTEAL
PHASE OF THE OVARIAN CYCLE
SUMMARY
FUNCTIONS OF THE OVARIAN
HORMONES—ESTRADIOL AND
PROGESTERONE
CHEMISTRY OF THE SEX HORMONES
FUNCTIONS OF THE ESTROGENS—
EFFECTS ON THE PRIMARY AND
SECONDARY SEXUAL
CHARACTERISTICS

FUNCTIONS OF PROGESTERONE
THE ENDOMETRIAL CYCLE AND
MENSTRUATION
REGULATION OF THE FEMALE MONTHLY
RHYTHM; INTERPLAY BETWEEN THE
OVARIAN AND HYPOTHALAMIC-
PITUITARY HORMONES
FEEDBACK OSCILLATION OF THE
HYPOTHALAMIC-PITUITARY-
OVARIAN SYSTEM
PUBERTY
THE MENOPAUSE
ABNORMALITIES OF SECRETION BY THE
OVARIES
THE FEMALE SEXUAL ACT
FEMALE FERTILITY

The sexual and reproductive functions in the female can be divided into two major phases: first, preparation of the body for conception, and second, the period of gestation. The present chaper is concerned with the preparation of the body for gestation, and the following chapter presents the physiology of pregnancy.

PHYSIOLOGICAL ANATOMY OF THE FEMALE SEXUAL ORGANS

Figure 55–1 illustrates the principal organs of the human female reproductive tract, including the *ovaries*, the *fallopian tubes*, the *uterus*, and the *vagina*.

Reproduction begins with the development of ova in the ovaries. A single ovum is expelled from an ovarian follicle into the abdominal cavity in the middle of each monthly sexual cycle. This ovum then passes through one of the fallopian tubes into the uterus, and if it has been fertilized by a sperm, it implants in the uterus, where it develops into a fetus, a placenta, and fetal membranes.

At puberty, the two ovaries contain 300,000 to 400,000 ova. Each ovum surrounded by a single layer of *granulosa cells* is called a *primordial follicle*. During all the reproductive years of the female, only about 450 of these follicles develop enough to expel their ova; the remainder degenerate. At the end of reproductive capability, the *menopause*, only a few pri-

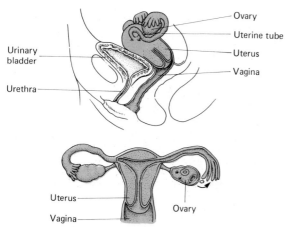

Figure 55–1. The female reproductive organs.

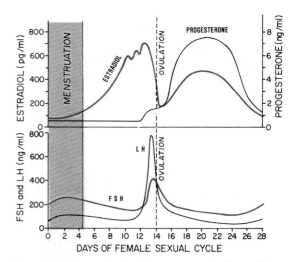

Figure 55–2. Approximate plasma concentrations of the gonadotropins and ovarian hormones during the normal female sexual cycle.

mordial follicles remain in the ovaries, and even these degenerate soon thereafter.

THE FEMALE HORMONAL SYSTEM

The female hormonal system, like that of the male, consists of three different hierarchies of hormones:

1. A hypothalamic releasing hormone: *luteinizing hormone–releasing hormone* (LHRH)

2. The anterior pituitary hormones: *follicle-stimulating hormone* (FSH) and *luteinizing hormone* (LH), both of which are secreted in response to the same releasing hormone from the hypothalamus

3. The ovarian hormones: *estrogen* and *progesterone*, which are secreted by the ovaries in response to the two hormones from the anterior pituitary gland

The various hormones are not secreted in constant, steady amounts but at drastically differing rates during different parts of the female sexual month, as will be explained later in the chapter.

Before it is possible to discuss the interplay between these different hormones, it is first necessary to describe some of their specific functions and their relationships to the function of the ovaries.

FUNCTION OF THE GONADOTROPIC HORMONES TO CONTROL THE MONTHLY OVARIAN CYCLE

The normal reproductive years of the female are characterized by monthly rhythmic changes in the rates of secretion of the female hormones and corresponding changes in the sexual organs themselves. This rhythmic pattern is called the *female sexual cycle* (or less accurately, the *menstrual cycle*). The duration of the cycle averages 28 days. It may be as short as 20 days or as long as 45 days even in completely normal women, though abnormal cycle length is occasionally associated with decreased fertility.

The two significant results of the female sexual cycle are: First, only a *single* mature ovum is normally

released from the ovaries each month, so that only a single fetus can begin to grow at a time. Second, the uterine endometrium is prepared for implantation of the fertilized ovum at the required time of the month.

The Gonadotropic Hormones. The ovarian changes during the sexual cycle are completely dependent on gonadotropic hormones secreted by the anterior pituitary gland. Ovaries that are not stimulated by gonadotropic hormones remain completely inactive, which is essentially the case throughout childhood, when almost no gonadotropic hormones are secreted. However, at the age of about 8, the pituitary begins secreting progressively more and more gonadotropic hormones, which culminates in the initiation of monthly sexual cycles between the ages of 11 and 15; this culmination is called *menarche*, and this period of life in the female is called *puberty*.

The anterior pituitary secretes two different hormones that are known to be essential for function of the ovaries: (1) *follicle-stimulating hormone* (FSH), and (2) *luteinizing hormone* (LH). Both of these are small glycoproteins having molecular weights of about 30,000.

During each month of the female sexual cycle, there is a cyclic increase and decrease of FSH and LH as illustrated in Figure 55–2. These cyclic variations in turn cause cyclic ovarian changes, which are explained in the following sections.

FOLLICULAR GROWTH—FUNCTION OF FSH

Figure 55–3 depicts the various stages of follicular growth in the ovaries, illustrating, first, the primordial follicle. Throughout childhood the primordial follicles do not grow, but at puberty, when FSH and LH from the anterior pituitary gland begin to be secreted in large quantities, the entire ovaries and especially the follicles within them begin to grow. The first stage of follicular growth is enlargement of the ovum itself and growth of additional layers of granulosa cells; the

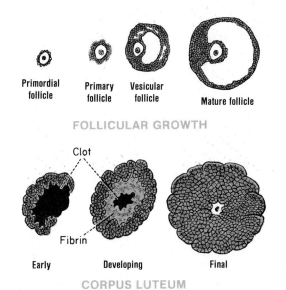

FOLLICULAR GROWTH

CORPUS LUTEUM

Figure 55–3. Stages of follicular growth in the ovary, showing also formation of the corpus luteum. (Modified from Arey: Developmental Anatomy. 7th ed. Philadelphia, W. B. Saunders Company, 1974.)

follicle is then known as the *primary follicle.* Then, a few weeks before ovulation still many more layers of granulosa cells develop, as well as several layers of *theca cells* around the granulosa cells. The theca cells originate from the stroma of the ovary and soon take on epithelioid characteristics. It is probably these cells that are destined to secrete most of the estrogens, while the granulosa cells will secrete progesterone.

The Vesicular Follicles. At the beginning of each month of the female sexual cycle, at the time of menstruation, the concentrations of FSH and LH increase. These hormones then cause accelerated growth of the theca and granulosa cells in about 20 of the ovarian follicles each month. These cells also secrete a *follicular fluid* that contains a high concentration of estrogen, one of the important female sex hormones discussed later. The accumulation of this fluid in the follicle causes an *antrum* to appear within the theca and granulosa cells, as illustrated in Figure 55–3.

After the antrum is formed, the theca and granulosa cells continue to proliferate, the rate of secretion accelerates, and each of the growing follicles is now called a *vesicular follicle.*

As the vesicular follicle enlarges, the theca and granulosa cells now develop mainly at one pole of the follicle. It is in this mass that the ovum is located.

Maturation of Only One Follicle, Atresia of the Remainder. After a week or more of growth—but before ovulation occurs—one of the follicles begins to outgrow all the others; the remainder begin to involute (a process called *atresia*), and these follicles are said to become *atretic.* The cause of the atresia is unknown, but it has been postulated to be the following: The one follicle that becomes more highly developed than the others also secretes more estrogen than the others. This causes feedback inhibition of secretion of the gonadotropic hormones FSH and LH

by the anterior pituitary gland. Lack of these hormones does not prevent further growth of the largest follicle because the large amount of locally secreted estrogen in this follicle has a self-stimulatory effect of causing it to continue growing. However, the lack of the FSH and LH stimulus to the less well-developed follicles causes these to stop growing and, indeed, to involute.

This process of atresia obviously is important in that it allows only one of the follicles to grow large enough to ovulate. This single follicle reaches a size of approximately 1 to 1.5 cm at the time of ovulation.

Ovulation

Ovulation in a woman with a normal 28-day female sexual cycle occurs 14 days after the onset of menstruation.

Shortly before ovulation the protruding outer wall of the follicle swells rapidly, and a small area in the center of the capsule, called the *stigma,* protrudes like a nipple. In another half hour or so, fluid begins to ooze from the follicle through the stigma. About two minutes later, the stigma ruptures widely, and a more viscous fluid that has occupied the central portion of the follicle is evaginated outward into the abdomen. This viscous fluid carries with it the ovum surrounded by several thousand granulosa cells called the *corona radiata.*

Need for LH in Ovulation—Preovulatory Surge of LH. Luteinizing hormone is necessary for final follicular growth and ovulation. Without this hormone, even though large quantities of FSH are available, the follicle will not progress to the stage of ovulation.

Approximately two days before ovulation, for reasons that are not completely known at present but that are discussed in more detail later in the chapter, the rate of secretion of LH by the anterior pituitary gland increases markedly, rising 6- to 10-fold and peaking about 18 hours before ovulation. FSH also increases about 2-fold at the same time, and these two hormones act synergistically to cause the extremely rapid swelling of the follicle that culminates in ovulation.

THE CORPUS LUTEUM—THE LUTEAL PHASE OF THE OVARIAN CYCLE

During the last day before ovulation and continuing for a day or so after ovulation, the granulosa cells, under the stimulation of luteinizing hormone, undergo rapid physical and chemical change, a process called *luteinization.* Thus, the mass of cells still remaining at the site of the ruptured follicle becomes the *corpus luteum,* which is illustrated at the bottom of Figure 55–3; this then secretes large quantities of the hormones progesterone and estrogen. These cells become greatly enlarged and develop lipid inclusions that give the cells a distinctive yellowish color, from which is derived the term *luteum,* which means *yellow.*

In the normal female, the corpus luteum grows to

approximately 1.5 cm, reaching this stage of development approximately 7 or 8 days following ovulation. After this, it begins to involute and loses its secretory function as well as its lipid characteristics approximately 12 days following ovulation, becoming then the so-called *corpus albicans,* which during the ensuing few weeks is replaced by connective tissue.

The Role of LH. The conversion of the granulosa cells into the *lutein cells* in the corpus luteum requires the presence of luteinizing hormone (LH). Indeed, this is the reason for its name. Also, in the presence of LH the degree of growth of the corpus luteum is enhanced, its secretion is greater, and its life is extended.

Termination of the Ovarian Cycle and Onset of the Next Cycle. After several days of the luteal phase of the ovarian cycle, the large amounts of estrogen and progesterone secreted by the corpus luteum cause a feedback effect to the hypothalamus to decrease the secretion of both FSH and LH. Therefore, during this period no new follicles begin to grow in the ovary. However, when the corpus luteum degenerates completely at the end of 12 days of its life (approximately on the 26th day of the female sexual cycle), the loss of feedback suppression now allows the anterior pituitary gland to secrete greatly increased quantities of FSH after another few days and moderately increased quantities of LH. The FSH and LH initiate growth of new follicles to begin a new ovarian cycle. At the same time, the paucity of secretion of progesterone and estrogen leads to menstruation by the uterus, as explained later.

SUMMARY

Approximately each 28 days, gonadotropic hormones from the anterior pituitary gland cause new follicles to begin to grow in the ovaries, one of which finally ovulates at the 14th day of the cycle. During growth of the follicles, estrogen is secreted.

Following ovulation, the secretory cells of the follicle develop into a corpus luteum, which secretes large quantities of both of the female hormones progesterone and estrogen. In another two weeks the corpus luteum degenerates, whereupon the ovarian hormones estrogen and progesterone decrease greatly and menstruation begins. A new ovarian cycle then follows.

FUNCTIONS OF THE OVARIAN HORMONES—ESTRADIOL AND PROGESTERONE

The two types of ovarian sex hormones are the *estrogens* and the *progestins.* By far the most important of the estrogens is the hormone *estradiol,* and by far the most important progestin is *progesterone.* The estrogens mainly promote proliferation and growth of specific sex-related cells in the body and are

responsible for development of most secondary sexual characteristics of the female. On the other hand, the progestins are concerned almost entirely with final preparation of the uterus for pregnancy and the breasts for lactation.

CHEMISTRY OF THE SEX HORMONES

The Estrogens. In the normal nonpregnant female, estrogens are secreted in major quantities only by the ovaries, though minute amounts are also secreted by the adrenal cortices. In pregnancy, tremendous quantities are also secreted by the placenta, as we shall discuss in the following chapter.

Only three estrogens are present in significant quantities in the plasma of the human female: β-*estradiol, estrone,* and *estriol,* the formulas for which are illustrated in Figure 55–4. The principal estrogen secreted by the ovaries is β-estradiol. Small amounts of estrone are also secreted, and estriol is an oxidative product derived from both estradiol and estrone, the conversion occurring mainly in the liver.

The estrogenic potency of β-estradiol is 12 times that of estrone and 80 times that of estriol. Considering these relative potencies, the total estrogenic effect of β-estradiol is usually many times that of the other two together. For this reason β-estradiol is considered to be the major estrogen, though the estrogenic effects of estrone are far from negligible.

The Progestins. By far the most important of the progestins is progesterone. However, small amounts of another progestin, *17-α-hydroxyprogesterone* also are secreted along with progesterone, and it has essentially the same effects. Yet for practical purposes, it is usually proper to consider progesterone to be the single important progestin.

In the normal nonpregnant female, progesterone is secreted in significant amounts only during the latter half of each ovarian cycle when it is secreted by the corpus luteum.

Synthesis of the Estrogens and Progestins. Note from the chemical formulas of the estrogens and progesterone in Figure 55–4 that all these are steroids. They are synthesized in the ovaries mainly from cholesterol derived from the blood but to a slight extent also from acetylcoenzyme A, multiple molecules of which can combine to form the appropriate steroid nucleus.

FUNCTIONS OF THE ESTROGENS—EFFECTS ON THE PRIMARY AND SECONDARY SEXUAL CHARACTERISTICS

The principal function of the estrogens is to cause cellular proliferation and growth of the tissues of the sexual organs and of other tissues related to reproduction.

Effect on the Sexual Organs. During childhood, estrogens are secreted only in small quantities, but following puberty the quantity of estrogens secreted under the influence of the pituitary gonadotropic

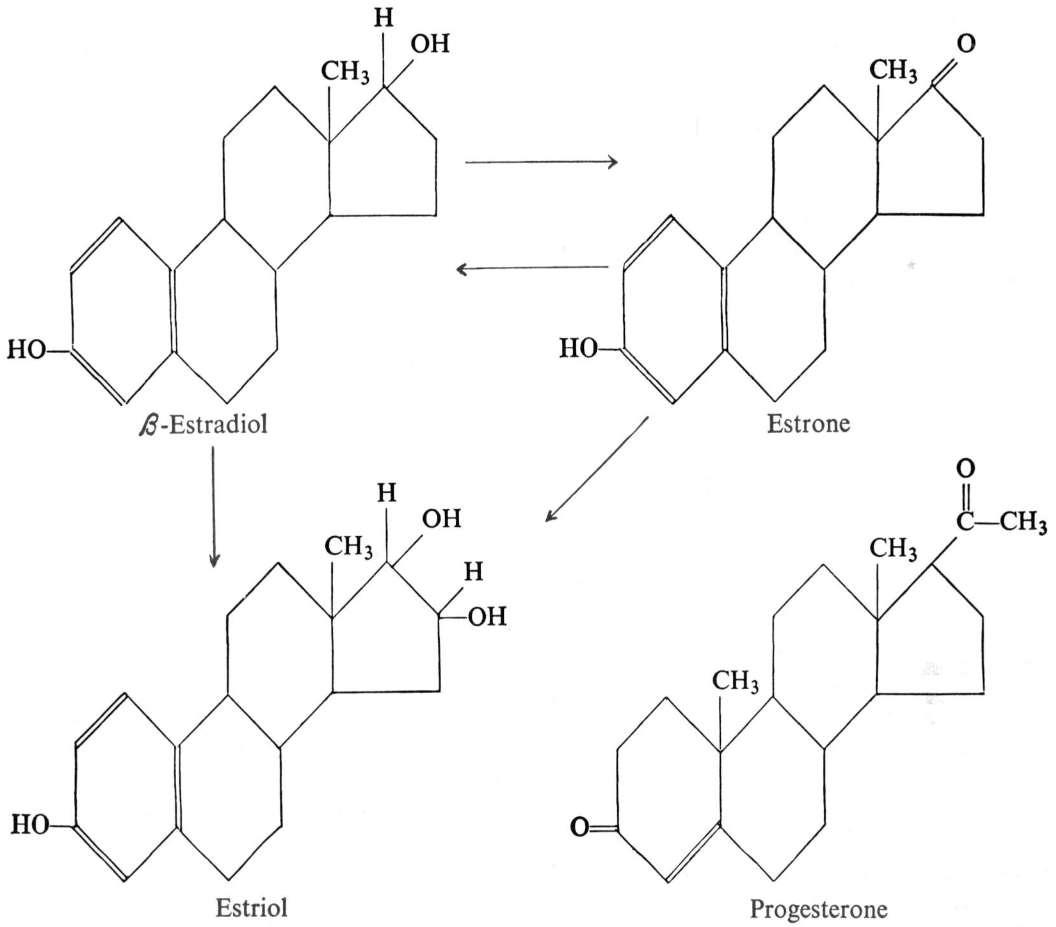

Figure 55–4. Chemical formulas of the principal female hormones.

hormones increases some 20-fold or more. At this time the female sexual organs change from those of a child to those of an adult. The fallopian tubes, uterus, and vagina all increase in size. Also, the external genitalia enlarge, with deposition of fat in the mons pubis and labia majora and with enlargement of the labia minora.

In addition, estrogens change the vaginal epithelium from a cuboidal into a stratified type, which is considerably more resistant to trauma and infection than is the prepubertal epithelium. More important, however, are the changes that take place in the endometrium under the influence of estrogens, for estrogens cause marked proliferation of the endometrium and development of the endometrial glands that will later be used to aid in nutrition of the implanting ovum. These effects are discussed later in the chapter in connection with the endometrial cycle.

Effect on the Breasts. Estrogens cause fat deposition in the breasts, development of the stromal tissues of the breasts, and growth of an extensive ductile system. The lobules and alveoli of the breast develop to a slight extent, but it is progesterone and prolactin that cause the determinative growth and function of these structures. In summary, the estrogens initiate growth of the breasts and the breasts' milk-producing apparatus, and they are also responsible for the characteristic external appearance of the mature female breast, but they do not complete the conversion of the breasts into milk-producing organs, a subject discussed in the following chapter.

Effect on the Skeleton. Estrogens cause increased osteoblastic activity. Therefore, at puberty, when the female enters her reproductive years, her height increases rapidly for several years. However, estrogens have another potent effect on skeletal growth: they cause early uniting of the epiphyses with the shafts of the long bones. This effect is much stronger in the female than is a similar effect of testosterone in the male. As a result, growth of the female usually ceases several years earlier than growth of the male. The female eunuch who is completely devoid of estrogen production usually grows several inches taller than the normal mature female because her epiphyses do not unite early.

Effect on Fat Deposition. Estrogens cause deposition of increased quantities of fat in the subcutaneous tissues. As a result, the overall specific gravity of the female body, as judged by flotation in water, is considerably less than that of the male body, which contains more protein and less fat. In addition to deposition of fat in the breasts and subcutaneous tissues, estrogens cause especially marked deposition of fat in the buttocks and thighs, causing the broadening of the hips that is characteristic of the feminine figure.

Effect on the Skin. Estrogens cause the skin to become more vascular than normal; this effect often results in greater bleeding of cut surfaces than is observed in men.

The Basic Intracellular Functions of Estrogens

After secretion by the ovaries, estrogens circulate in the blood for only a few minutes before they are delivered to the target cells. On entry into these cells, the estrogens combine within 10 to 15 seconds with a receptor protein in the cytoplasm and then, in combination with this protein, migrate to the nucleus. This immediately initiates the process of DNA-RNA transcription in specific chromosomal areas, and RNA begins to be produced within a few minutes. In addition, over a period of many hours, DNA also is produced, resulting eventually in division of the cell. The RNA diffuses into the cytoplasm, where it causes greatly increased protein formation and subsequently altered cellular function.

One of the principal differences between the estrogens and testosterone is that the effects of estrogens occur almost exclusively in certain target organs such as the uterus, the breasts, the skeleton, and certain fatty areas of the body, whereas testosterone has a more generalized effect throughout the body.

FUNCTIONS OF PROGESTERONE

Effect on the Uterus. By far the most important function of progesterone is *to promote secretory changes in the endometrium,* thus preparing the uterus for implantation of the fertilized ovum. This function is discussed later in connection with the endometrial cycle of the uterus.

Effect on the Fallopian Tubes. Progesterone also promotes secretory changes in the mucosal lining of the fallopian tubes. These secretions are important for nutrition of the fertilized, dividing ovum as it traverses the fallopian tube prior to implantation.

Effect on the Breasts. Progesterone promotes development of the lobules and alveoli of the breasts, causing the alveolar cells to proliferate, to enlarge, and to become secretory in nature. However, progesterone does not cause the alveoli actually to secrete milk, for, as discussed in the following chapter, milk is secreted only after the prepared breast is further stimulated by prolactin from the anterior pituitary.

Progesterone also causes the breasts to swell. Part of this swelling is due to the secretory development in the lobules and alveoli, but part also seems to result somewhat from increased fluid in the subcutaneous tissue itself.

THE ENDOMETRIAL CYCLE AND MENSTRUATION

Associated with the cyclic production of estrogens and progesterone by the ovaries is an endometrial

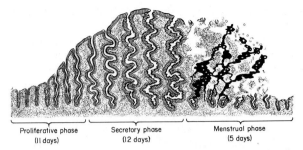

Proliferative phase (II days)   Secretory phase (12 days)   Menstrual phase (5 days)

Figure 55–5. Phases of endometrial growth and menstruation during each monthly female sexual cycle.

cycle operating through the following stages: first, proliferation of the uterine endometrium; second, secretory changes in the endometrium; and third, desquamation of the endometrium, which is known as *menstruation*. The various phases of the endometrial cycle are illustrated in Figure 55–5.

Proliferative Phase (Estrogen Phase) of the Endometrial Cycle. At the beginning of each menstrual cycle, most of the endometrium is desquamated by the process of menstruation. After menstruation, only a thin layer of endometrial stroma remains at the base of the original endometrium, and the only epithelial cells left are those located in the remaining deep portions of the glands and crypts of the endometrium. *Under the influence of estrogens,* secreted in increasing quantities by the vesicular follicles of the ovary during the first part of the ovarian cycle, the stromal cells and the epithelial cells proliferate rapidly. The endometrial surface is re-epithelialized within three to seven days after the beginning of menstruation. For the first two weeks of the sexual cycle—that is, until ovulation—the endometrium increases greatly in thickness, owing to increasing numbers of stromal cells and to progressive growth of the endometrial glands as well as ingrowth of blood vessels into the endometrium, all of which effects are promoted by the estrogens. At the time of ovulation the endometrium is approximately 2 to 3 mm thick.

Secretory Phase (Progestational Phase) of the Endometrial Cycle. During the latter half of the sexual cycle, progesterone as well as estrogens is secreted in large quantity by the corpus luteum. The estrogens cause slight additional cellular proliferation, and progesterone causes considerable swelling and secretory development of the endometrium. The glands increase in tortuosity, secretory substances accumulate in the glandular epithelial cells, and the glands secrete small quantities of endometrial fluid. Also, the cytoplasm of the stromal cells increases, lipid and glycogen deposits increase greatly in these cells, and the blood supply to the endometrium further increases in proportion to the developing secretory activity. The thickness of the endometrium approximately doubles during the secretory phase, so that toward the end of the monthly cycle the endometrium has a thickness of 4 to 6 mm.

The whole purpose of all these endometrial changes is to produce a highly secretory endometrium containing large amounts of stored nutrients that can provide appropriate conditions for implantation of a fertilized ovum during the latter half of the monthly cycle.

Menstruation. Approximately two days before the end of the monthly cycle, the ovarian hormones estrogens and progesterone decrease sharply to low levels of secretion, as was illustrated in Figure 55–2, and menstruation follows. Menstruation is caused by this sudden reduction in both progesterone and estrogens at the end of the monthly ovarian cycle. The first effect is decreased stimulation of the endometrial cells by these two hormones, followed rapidly by involution of the endometrium itself to about 65 per cent of its previous thickness. During the 24 hours preceding the onset of menstruation, the blood vessels leading to the mucosal layers of the endometrium become vasospastic, presumably because of some effect of the involution, such as release of a vasoconstrictor material. The vasospasm and loss of hormonal stimulation cause beginning necrosis in the endometrium. As a result, blood seeps into the vascular layer of the endometrium, the hemorrhagic areas growing over a period of 24 to 36 hours. Gradually, the necrotic outer layers of the endometrium separate from the uterus at the site of the hemorrhages, until, at approximately 48 hours following the onset of menstruation, all the superficial layers of the endometrium have desquamated. The desquamated tissue and blood in the uterine vault initiate uterine contractions that expel the uterine contents.

During normal menstruation, approximately 35 ml of blood and an additional 35 ml of serous fluid are lost. This menstrual fluid is normally nonclotting, because a *fibrinolysin* is released along with the necrotic endometrial material.

Within three to seven days after menstruation starts, the loss of blood ceases, for by this time the endometrium has become completely re-epithelialized.

REGULATION OF THE FEMALE MONTHLY RHYTHM: INTERPLAY BETWEEN THE OVARIAN AND THE HYPOTHALAMIC-PITUITARY HORMONES

Now that we have presented the major changes that occur during the female sexual cycle, we can attempt to explain the basic rhythmic mechanism that causes these variations.

Function of the Hypothalamus in the Regulation of Gonadotropin Secretion—the Hypothalamic Releasing Hormone. As was pointed out in Chapter 49, secretion of most of the anterior pituitary hormones is controlled by releasing hormones formed in the hypothalamus and transmitted to the anterior pituitary gland by way of the hypothalamic-hypophysial portal system. In the case of the gonadotropins, one releasing hormone, *luteotropic hormone–releasing hormone (LHRH)*, is especially important. This hormone has been purified and is a decapeptide having the following formula:

$$GLU\text{-}HIS\text{-}TRP\text{-}SER\text{-}TYR\text{-}GLY\text{-}\\LEU\text{-}ARG\text{-}PRO\text{-}GLY\text{-}NH_2$$

It has been found that the above purified LHRH causes release not only of luteinizing hormone but also of follicle-stimulating hormone. Therefore, LHRH is sometimes called simply *gonadotropin-releasing hormone (GnRH)*.

Effect of Psychic Factors on the Female Sexual Cycle. It is well known that the young woman on first leaving home to go to college experiences disruption or irregularity of the female sexual cycle almost as often as not. Likewise, serious stresses of almost any type can interfere with the cycle. Finally, in many lower animals no ovulation occurs at all until after copulation; the sexual excitation attendant to the sexual act initiates a sequence of events that leads first to secretion in the hypothalamus of LHRH, then to secretion of the anterior pituitary gonadotropins FSH and LH, and finally to secretion of the ovarian hormones and ovulation.

Negative Feedback Effect of Estrogen, Progesterone, and Inhibin on Secretion of Follicle-Stimulating Hormone and Luteinizing Hormone. Estrogen in small amounts and progesterone in large amounts inhibit the production of FSH and LH. Both these feedback effects seem to operate on the hypothalamus and the anterior pituitary gland as well.

In addition to the feedback effects of estrogen and progesterone, still another hormone also seems to be involved. This is *inhibin,* which is secreted along with the steroid sex hormones by the corpus luteum cells. Inhibin has the same effect in the female as in the male—inhibiting the secretion of FSH by the anterior pituitary gland, and also of LH to a lesser extent. Therefore, it is believed that inhibin might be especially important in causing the decrease in secretion of FSH and LH toward the end of the female sexual month.

Positive Feedback Effect of Estrogen Before Ovulation—the Preovulatory Luteinizing Hormone Surge. For reasons not completely understood, the anterior pituitary gland secretes greatly increased amounts of LH about 36 hours before ovulation. This effect, illustrated in Figure 55–2, apparently results from a *positive* feedback effect of estrogen in place of the normal negative feedback that occurs during the remainder of the female sexual cycle. Its precise cause is not known, but nevertheless it is an absolute necessary and integral part of the control mechanism. Without this preovulatory surge of luteinizing hormone, ovulation will not occur.

FEEDBACK OSCILLATION OF THE HYPOTHALAMIC-PITUITARY-OVARIAN SYSTEM

Now, after discussing much of the known information about the interrelationships of the different components of the female hormonal system, we can digress from the area of proven fact into the realm of speculation and attempt to explain the feedback oscillation that controls the rhythm of the female sexual cycle. It seems to operate in approximately the following sequence of three successive events:

1. The Postovulatory Secretion of the Ovarian Hormones and Depression of Gonadotropins. The easiest part of the cycle to explain is the events that occur during the postovulatory phase—between ovulation and the beginning of menstruation. During this time the corpus luteum secretes very large quantities of both progesterone and estrogen. Their combined effect on the hypothalamus is to inhibit the secretion of LHRH and therefore to cause strong negative feedback depression of secretion of the gonadotropins, both FSH and LH, during this period of time. These effects are illustrated in Figure 55–2. In addition, inhibin, also secreted by the corpus luteum, mainly inhibits the secretion of FSH by the anterior pituitary gland.

2. The Follicular Growth Phase. A few days before menstruation, the corpus luteum involutes, and the secretion of both estrogen and progesterone as well as inhibin decreases to a low ebb. This releases the hypothalamus from the feedback effect of the estrogen and progesterone, so that LHRH secretion increases again, followed in succession by a several hundred per cent increase in FSH and LH, also. These hormones initiate new follicular growth and progressively increased secretion of estrogen, reaching a peak of estrogen secretion at about 12.5 to 13 days after the onset of menstruation. During the first 11 to 12 days of this follicular growth, the rates of secretion of the gonadotropins FSH and LH decrease slightly and gradually; then comes a sudden increase—the preovulatory surge—in secretion of both of these hormones, leading to the ovulatory stage of the cycle.

3. Preovulatory Surge of LH and FSH, Ovulation. At approximately 11.5 to 12 days after the onset of menstruation, the decline in secretion of FSH and LH comes to an abrupt halt. It is believed that the high level of estrogens at this time causes a positive feedback effect, as explained earlier, which leads to a tremendous surge of secretion—especially of LH but to a lesser extent of FSH. Whatever the cause of this preovulatory LH and FSH stage, the LH leads to both ovulation and formation of the corpus luteum. Thus, the hormonal system begins a new round of the female sexual cycle.

PUBERTY

Puberty means the onset of adult sexual life, and as pointed out earlier in the chapter, it is caused by a gradual increase in gonadotropic hormone secretion by the pituitary, beginning approximately in the eighth year of life.

In the female, as in the male, the infantile pituitary gland and ovaries are capable of full function if appropriately stimulated. However, as is also true in the male and for reasons not yet understood, the hypothalamus does not secrete luteinizing hormone–releasing hormone during childhood. Experiments have shown that the hypothalamus itself is perfectly capable of secreting this hormone, but there is lack of the appropriate signal from some other brain area to cause the secretion. Therefore, it is now believed that the onset of puberty is initiated by some maturation process occurring elsewhere in the brain than the hypothalamus, perhaps somewhere in the limbic system.

THE MENOPAUSE

At an average age of approximately 45 to 50 years, the sexual cycles usually become irregular, and ovulation fails to occur during many of these cycles. After a few months to a few years, the cycles cease altogether. This cessation of the cycles is called the *menopause.*

The cause of the menopause is "burning out" of the ovaries. In other words, throughout a woman's sexual life many of the primordial follicles grow into vesicular follicles with each sexual cycle, and eventually almost all the ova either are ovulated (about 0.15 per cent of the total) or degenerate. Therefore at the age of about 45, only a few primordial follicles still remain to be stimulated by FSH and LH; the production of estrogens by the ovaries also decreases as the number of primordial follicles approaches zero. When estrogen production falls below a critical value, the estrogens can no longer inhibit the production of FSH and LH sufficiently to cause oscillatory cycles. Consequently, FSH and LH (mainly FSH) are produced thereafter in large and continuous quantities. Estrogens continue to be produced in subcritical quantities for a short time after the menopause, but over a few years, as the final remaining primordial follicles become atretic, the production of estrogens by the ovaries falls almost to zero.

ABNORMALITIES OF SECRETION BY THE OVARIES

Hypogonadism. Less than normal secretion by the ovaries can result from poorly formed ovaries or lack of ovaries. When ovaries are absent from birth or when they never become functional, *female eunuchism* occurs. In this condition the usual secondary sexual characteristics do not appear, and the sexual organs remain infantile. Especially characteristic of this condition is excessive growth of the long bones because the epiphyses do not unite with the shafts of these bones as early as in the normal adolescent woman. Consequently, the female eunuch is as tall as her male counterpart of similar genetic background, or perhaps even slightly taller.

When the ovaries of a fully developed woman are removed, the sexual organs regress to some extent, so that the uterus becomes almost infantile in size, the vagina becomes smaller, and the vaginal epithelium becomes thin and easily damaged. The breasts atrophy and become pendulous, and the pubic hair becomes considerably thinner. These same changes occur in the woman after the menopause.

Irregularity of Menses and Amenorrhea Due to Hypogonadism. The quantity of estrogens produced by the ovaries must rise above a critical value if they are to be capable of inhibiting the production of follicle-stimulating hormone sufficiently to cause an oscillatory sexual cycle. Consequently, in hypogonadism or when the gonads are secreting small quantities of estrogens as a result of other factors, the ovarian cycle likely will not occur normally. Instead, several months may elapse between menstrual periods, or menstruation may cease altogether (amenorrhea). Characteristically, ovulation often fails to occur in these prolonged ovarian cycles, presumably due to insufficient secretion of luteinizing hormone, which is necessary for ovulation.

Hypersecretion by the Ovaries. Extreme hypersecretion of hormones by the ovaries is a rare clinical entity, for excessive secretion of estrogens automatically decreases the production of gonadotropins by the pituitary, and this in turn limits the production of the ovarian hormones. Consequently, hypersecretion of feminizing hormones is recognized clinically only when a feminizing tumor develops.

Rarely, a granulosa cell tumor develops in an ovary, more often after menopause than before. Such a tumor secretes large quantities of estrogens, which exert the usual estrogenic effects, including hypertrophy of the uterine endometrium and irregular bleeding from it. In fact, bleeding is often the first indication that such a tumor exists.

THE FEMALE SEXUAL ACT

Stimulation of the Female Sexual Act. As is true in the male sexual act, successful performance of the female sexual act depends on both psychic stimulation and local sexual stimulation.

As is also true in the male, the thinking of erotic thoughts can lead to female sexual desire, and this aids greatly in the performance of the female sexual act. Such desire is probably based as much on one's background training as on physiological drive, though sexual drive does increase in proportion to the level of secretion of the sex hormones. Desire also changes during the sexual month, reaching a peak near the time of ovulation, probably because of the high levels of estrogen secretion during the preovulatory period.

Local sexual stimulation in women occurs in more or less the same manner as in men, for massage, irritation, or other types of stimulation of the perineal region, sexual organs, and urinary tract create sexual sensations. The *clitoris* is especially sensitive for initiating sexual sensations. As in the male, the sexual sensory signals are mediated to the sacral segments of the spinal cord through the pudendal nerve and

sacral plexus. Once these signals have entered the spinal cord, they are transmitted thence to the cerebrum. Also, local reflexes integrated in the sacral and lumbar spinal cord are at least partially responsible for female sexual reactions.

Female Erection and Lubrication. Located around the introitus and extending into the clitoris is erectile tissue almost identical with the erectile tissue of the penis. This erectile tissue, like that of the penis, is controlled by the parasympathetic nerves that pass through the pelvic nerves to the external genitalia. In the early phases of sexual stimulation, the parasympathetics dilate the arteries allowing rapid accumulation of blood in the erectile tissue, so that the introitus tightens around the penis; this aids the male greatly in his attainment of sufficient sexual stimulation for ejaculation to occur.

Parasympathetic signals also pass to the bilateral Bartholin's glands located beneath the labia minora to cause secretion of mucus immediately inside the introitus. This mucus is responsible for much of the lubrication during sexual intercourse, though much is also provided by mucus secreted by the vaginal epithelium and a small amount secreted from the male urethral glands. The lubrication in turn is necessary for establishing during intercourse a satisfactory massaging rather than an irritative sensation, which may be provoked by a dry vagina. Massaging constitutes the optimal type of sensation for evoking the appropriate reflexes that culminate in both the male and female climaxes.

The Female Orgasm. When local sexual stimulation reaches maximum intensity, and especially when the local sensations are supported by appropriate psychic conditioning signals from the cerebrum, reflexes are initiated that cause the female orgasm, also called the *female climax*. The female orgasm is analogous to emission and ejaculation in the male, and it perhaps helps promote fertilization of the ovum. Indeed, the human female is known to be somewhat more fertile when inseminated by normal sexual intercourse rather than by artificial methods, thus indicating an important function of the female orgasm. Possible effects that could result in greater fertility are:

First, during the orgasm the perineal muscles of the female contract rhythmically, which results from spinal cord reflexes similar to those that cause ejaculation in the male. It is possible, also, that reflexes involving the sympathetic nervous system increase uterine and fallopian tube motility during the orgasm, thus helping transport the sperm toward the ovum, but the information on this subject is scanty.

Second, in many lower animals, copulation causes the posterior pituitary gland to secrete oxytocin; this effect is probably mediated through the amygdaloid nuclei and then through the hypothalamus to the pituitary. The oxytocin in turn causes increased rhythmic contractility of the uterus, which has been postulated to cause rapid transport of the sperm. Sperm have been shown to traverse the entire length of the fallopian tube in the cow in approximately five minutes, a rate at least ten times as fast as that which the swimming motions of the sperm themselves could achieve. Whether or not this occurs in the human female is unknown.

In addition to the possible effects of the orgasm on fertilization, the intense sexual sensations that develop during the orgasm also pass to the cerebrum and cause intense muscle tension throughout the body. But after culmination of the sexual act, this gives way during the succeeding minutes to a sense of satisfaction characterized by relaxed peacefulness, an effect called *resolution*.

FEMALE FERTILITY

The Fertile Period of Each Sexual Cycle. The ovum remains viable and capable of being fertilized for probably no longer than 24 hours after it is expelled from the ovary. Therefore, sperm must be available soon after ovulation if fertilization is to take place. On the other hand, a few sperm can remain viable in the female reproductive tract for up to 72 hours, though most of them for not more than 24 hours. Therefore, for fertilization to take place, intercourse usually must occur some time between one day prior to ovulation and one day after ovulation.

The Rhythm Method of Contraception. A method of contraception often practiced is to avoid intercourse near the time of ovulation. The difficulty with this method is the impossibility of predicting the exact time of ovulation. Yet the interval between ovulation and the next succeeding onset of menstruation is almost always between 13 and 15 days. In other words, if the periodicity of the menstrual cycle is 28 days, ovulation usually occurs within one day of the 14th day of the cycle. If, on the other hand, the periodicity of the cycle is 40 days, ovulation usually occurs within one day of the 26th day of the cycle. Finally, if the periodicity of the cycle is 21 days, ovulation usually occurs within one day of the 7th day of the cycle. Therefore, it is usually stated that avoidance of intercourse for 4 days prior to the calculated day of ovulation and 3 days afterward prevents conception. But such a method of contraception can be used only when the periodicity of the menstrual cycle is regular.

Hormonal Suppression of Fertility—"The Pill." It has long been known that administration of either estrogen or progesterone, if given in appropriate quantity during the first half of the monthly female cycle, can inhibit ovulation. The reason for this is that administration of either of these can prevent the preovulatory surge of LH secretion by the pituitary gland, which, it will be recalled, is essential in causing ovulation.

The reason the administration of estrogen or progesterone prevents the preovulatory surge of LH secretion is not fully understood. However, experimental work has suggested that immediately before the surge occurs there is probably a sudden depression of estrogen secretion by the ovarian follicles, and that

this might be the necessary signal for causing the feedback effect that leads to the surge. Obviously, administration of the sex hormones could prevent the initial hormonal depression that might be the initiating signal for ovulation.

The problem in devising methods for hormonal suppression of ovulation has been to develop appropriate combinations of estrogens and progestins that will suppress ovulation but that will not cause unwanted effects of these two hormones. For instance, too much of either of the hormones can cause abnormal menstrual bleeding patterns. However, use of certain synthetic progestins in place of progesterone, especially the 19-norsteroids, along with small amounts of estrogens will usually prevent ovulation and yet also allow almost a normal pattern of menstruation. Therefore, almost all "pills" used for control of fertility consist of some combination of synthetic estrogens and synthetic progestins. The main reason for using synthetic estrogens and synthetic progestins is that the *natural* hormones are almost entirely destroyed by the liver within a short time after they are absorbed from the gastrointestinal tract into the portal circulation. However, many of the *synthetic* hormones can resist this destructive propensity of the liver, thus allowing oral administration.

The medication is usually begun in the early stages of the monthly cycle and continued beyond the time that ovulation normally would have occurred. Then the medication is stopped, allowing menstruation to occur and a new cycle to begin.

Anovulation and Female Sterility. Approximately one out of every six to ten marriages is infertile; in about 60 per cent of these, the infertility is due to female sterility.

Occasionally, no abnormality whatsoever can be discovered in the female genital organs, in which case it must be assumed that the infertility is due either to abnormal physiological function of the genital system or to abnormal genetic development of the ova themselves.

However, one of the most common causes of female sterility is failure to ovulate. This can result from either hyposecretion of gonadotropic hormones, in which case the intensity of the hormonal stimuli simply is not sufficient to cause ovulation, or from abnormal ovaries that will not allow ovulation. For instance, thick capsules occasionally exist on the outside of the ovaries and prevent ovulation.

Lack of ovulation caused by hyposecretion of the pituitary gonadotropic hormones can usually be treated by administration of *human chorionic gonadotropin,* a hormone that will be discussed in the following chapter and that is extracted from the human placenta. This hormone, though secreted by the placenta, has almost exactly the same effects as luteinizing hormone and therefore is a powerful stimulator of ovulation. However, excess use of this hormone can cause ovulation from many follicles simultaneously; and multiple births result. As many as eight children have been born to mothers treated for infertility with this hormone.

QUESTIONS

1. Describe the physiological anatomy of the female sexual organs.
2. Describe the monthly changes in the ovaries and control of the ovarian cycle by the *gonadotropic hormones.*
3. What are the characteristics of the *vesicular follicles,* what do they secrete, and what is their fate?
4. Describe *ovulation.* What are the roles of *FSH* and *LH* leading up to ovulation, and what is the role of the *preovulatory surge of LH*?
5. Describe the formation of the *corpus luteum,* its secretion of *progesterone* and *estrogen* and its control by LH.
6. Describe, in general, the chemistry of the estrogens and progesterone.
7. What are the effects of the estrogens on the female sex organs, the breasts, and the skin?
8. How do the estrogens function intracellularly to cause their hormonal effects?
9. What are the functional effects of progesterone on the uterus, the fallopian tubes, and the breasts?
10. Describe the monthly changes in the *uterine endometrium.* What are the roles of estrogen and progesterone in controlling the endometrial cycle?
11. Describe the sequential changes in the endometrium that cause menstruation and the hormonal effects that lead to menstruation.
12. Explain the role of the *hypothalamus* in secreting *LHRH* and the effect of this secretion to control the secretion of FSH and LH by the anterior pituitary gland. What is the cause of the preovulatory surge of luteinizing hormone?
13. Explain the sequential changes in LHRH, the anterior pituitary hormones, and the ovarian hormones that are responsible for the monthly *female sexual cycle.*
14. What leads to *puberty*?
15. What is the cause of the *menopause*?
16. What are the clinical characteristics of *hypogonadism*?
17. What are the clinical characteristics of *hypersecretion by the ovaries*?
18. Describe the sexual sensory signals that lead to female excitement during the sexual act.
19. What is the role of the parasympathetic nervous system in female *erection* and *lubrication*, and what is the possible role of the sympathetic nervous system in the female *orgasm*?
20. How can one spot with reasonable accuracy the few days of the female sexual cycle when the female will be fertile?
21. What is the physiological basis of hormonal *suppression of fertility*?
22. How can female sterility caused by *anovulation* frequently be treated with hormones?

References

Arnold, A. P., and Gorski, R. A.: Gonadal steroid induction of structural sex differences in the central nervous system. Annu Rev Neurosci 7:413, 1984.

Chambon, P., et al.: Promoter elements of genes coding for proteins and modulation of transcription by estrogens and progesterone. Recent Prog Horm Res 40:11, 1984.

Channing, C. P., et al.: Ovarian follicular and luteal physiology. In Greep, R. O., ed.: International Review of Physiology: Reproductive Physiology III. Vol. 22, Baltimore, University Park Press, 1980, p. 117.

Conn, P. M., et al.: Gonadotropin-releasing hormone: molecular and cell biology, physiology, and clinical applications. Fed Proc 43:2351, 1984.

Coutts, S. R., ed.: Functional Morphology of the Human Ovary. Baltimore, University Park Press, 1981.

Cummings, A. M., and Yochim, J. M.: Differentiation of the uterus in preparation for gestation: a model for the action of progesterone. J Theor Biol 106:353, 1984.

Kase, N. G., and Speroff, L.: The ovary. In Bondy, P. K., and Rosenberg, L. E., eds.: Metabolic Control and Disease, 8th ed. Philadelphia, W. B. Saunders Co., 1980, p. 1579.

McCann, S. M.: Physiology and pharmacology of LHRH and somatostatin. Annu Rev Pharmacol Toxicol 22:491, 1982.

McEwen, B. S., and Parsons, B.: Gonadal steroid action on the brain: neurochemistry and neuropharmacology. Annu Rev Pharmacol Toxicol 22:555, 1982.

Mishell, D. R., Jr., ed.: Long-Acting Steroid Contraception. New York, Raven Press, 1983.

Ochiai, K., ed.: Endocrine Correlates of Reproduction. New York, Springer-Verlag, 1984.

Pohl, C. R., and Knobil, E.: The role of the central nervous system in the control of ovarian function in higher primates. Annu Rev Physiol 44:583, 1982.

Reiter, E. O., and Grumbach, M. M.: Neuroendocrine control mechanisms and the onset of puberty. Annu Rev Physiol 44:595, 1982.

Richards, J. S.: Maturation of ovarian follicles: actions and interactions of pituitary andd ovarian hormones on follicular cell differentiation. Physiol Rev 60:51, 1980.

Schwartz, N. B., ed.: Dynamics of Ovarian Function. New York, Raven Press, 1981.

Serra, G. B., ed.: The Ovary. New York, Raven Press, 1983.

Weiss, G.: Relaxin. Annu Rev Physiol 46:43, 1984.

56

Pregnancy, Lactation, and Fetal and Neonatal Physiology

MATURATION OF THE OVUM
FERTILIZATION OF THE OVUM
TRANSPORT AND IMPLANTATION OF
    THE DEVELOPING OVUM
FUNCTION OF THE PLACENTA
DIFFUSION THROUGH THE
    PLACENTAL MEMBRANE
HORMONAL FACTORS IN PREGNANCY
HUMAN CHORIONIC
    GONADOTROPIN AND ITS
    EFFECTS—PERSISTENCE OF THE
    CORPUS LUTEUM AND
    PREVENTION OF MENSTRUATION
SECRETION OF ESTROGENS BY THE
    PLACENTA
SECRETION OF PROGESTERONE BY
    THE PLACENTA
HUMAN CHORIONIC
    SOMATOMAMMOTROPIN
RESPONSE OF THE MOTHER TO
PREGNANCY
PRE-ECLAMPSIA AND ECLAMPSIA
PARTURITION
INCREASED UTERINE CONTRACTILITY
    NEAR TERM
ONSET OF LABOR—A POSITIVE
    FEEDBACK THEORY FOR ITS
    INITIATION
ABDOMINAL MUSCLE
    CONTRACTIONS DURING LABOR

MECHANICS OF PARTURITION
SEPARATION AND DELIVERY OF THE
    PLACENTA
LABOR PAINS
INVOLUTION OF THE UTERUS
LACTATION
DEVELOPMENT OF THE BREASTS
INITIATION OF LACTATION—
    FUNCTION OF PROLACTIN
THE EJECTION (OR "LET-DOWN")
    PROCESS IN MILK
    SECRETION—FUNCTION OF
    OXYTOCIN
THE COMPOSITION OF MILK AND
    THE METABOLIC DRAIN ON THE
    MOTHER CAUSED BY LACTATION
GROWTH AND FUNCTIONAL
DEVELOPMENT OF THE FETUS
DEVELOPMENT OF THE FETAL
    ORGAN SYSTEMS
ADJUSTMENTS OF THE INFANT TO
EXTRAUTERINE LIFE
ONSET OF BREATHING
CIRCULATORY READJUSTMENTS AT
    BIRTH
SPECIAL FUNCTIONAL PROBLEMS IN
THE NEONATAL INFANT
SPECIAL PROBLEMS OF PREMATURITY

In the preceding two chapters, the sexual functions of the male and the female were described to the point of fertilization of the ovum. If the ovum becomes fertilized, a completely new sequence of events called *gestation*, or *pregnancy*, takes place, and the fertilized ovum eventually develops into a full-term fetus. The purpose of the present chapter is to discuss these events.

MATURATION OF THE OVUM

Shortly before the ovum is released from the follicle, each of the 23 pairs of chromosomes loses one of its partners, so that 23 *unpaired* chromosomes remain in the mature ovum. It is at this point that ovulation occurs, and soon thereafter, usually after the ovum enters the tip of the fallopian tube, fertilization occurs.

FERTILIZATION OF THE OVUM

After coitus, the first sperm are transported through the uterus to the ovarian end of the fallopian tubes within five to ten minutes. This is many times more rapid than the motility of the sperm themselves can account for, which indicates that propulsive movements of the uterus and fallopian tubes might be responsible for much of the sperm movement. Yet, even with this aid, of the nearly one-half billion sperm deposited in the vagina, only 1000 to 3000 succeed in traversing the fallopian tubes to reach the proximity of the ovum.

Only one sperm is required for fertilization of the ovum, the process of which is illustrated in Figure 56–1. Furthermore, almost never does more than one sperm enter the ovum for the following reason: The zona pellucida of the ovum has a lattice-type structure, and once this is punctured, some substance (perhaps one of the proteolytic enzymes of the sperm acrosome) diffuses throughout the lattice to prevent penetration by additional sperm. Indeed, many sperm do attempt to penetrate the zona pellucida but become inactivated after traveling only part way through.

Once a sperm enters the ovum, its head swells rapidly to form a *male pronucleus*, which is also illustrated in Figure 56–1. Later, the 23 chromosomes of the male pronucleus and the 23 of the *female pronucleus* align themselves to re-form a complete complement of 46 chromosomes (23 pairs) in the fertilized ovum.

Sex Determination. The sex of a child is determined by the type of sperm that fertilizes the ovum—that is, whether it is a male or a female sperm. It will be recalled from Chapter 54 that a male sperm carries a *Y sex chromosome* and *22 autosomal chromosomes*, while a female sperm carries the same 22 autosomal chromosomes but an *X sex chromosome*. On the other hand, the ovum always has an X sex chromosome, never a Y chromosome. After recombination

of the male and female pronuclei during fertilization, the fertilized ovum then contains 44 autosomal chromosomes and either 2 X chromosomes, which causes a female child to develop, or an X and a Y chromosome, which causes a male child to develop.

TRANSPORT AND IMPLANTATION OF THE DEVELOPING OVUM

Entry of the Ovum into the Fallopian Tube. When ovulation occurs, the ovum along with its attached granulosa cells, the *corona radiata*, is expelled directly into the peritoneal cavity and must then enter one of the fallopian tubes. The fimbriated end of each fallopian tube falls naturally around the ovaries, and the inner surfaces of the fimbriated tentacles are lined with ciliated epithelium, the *cilia* of which continuously beat toward the *ostium* of the fallopian tube. One can actually see a slow fluid current flowing toward the ostium. By this means the ovum enters one or the other fallopian tube.

Transport of the Ovum Through the Fallopian Tube. Fertilization of the ovum normally takes place soon after the ovum enters the fallopian tube. After fertilization has occurred, three to five days are normally required for transport of the ovum through the tube into the cavity of the uterus. This transport is effected mainly by a feeble fluid current in the fallopian tube resulting from action of the ciliated epithelium that lines the tube, the cilia always beating toward the uterus. It is possible also that weak contractions of the fallopian tube aid in the passage of the ovum.

This delayed transport of the ovum through the fallopian tube allows several stages of division to occur before the ovum enters the uterus. During this time, large quantities of secretions are formed by secretory cells that line the fallopian tube. These secretions are for nutrition of the developing ovum.

Implantation of the Ovum in the Uterus. After reaching the uterus, the developing ovum usually remains in the uterine cavity an additional two to five days before it implants in the endometrium, which means that implantation ordinarily occurs on the seventh or eighth day following ovulation. During this time the ovum obtains its nutrition from the endometrial secretions, called uterine milk. Figure 56–2 shows a very early stage of implantation, illustrating that the developing ovum is in the *blastocyst stage*. It has developed a cavity with the embryo, shown in color, developing along one wall of the cavity.

Implantation results from the action of *trophoblastic cells* that develop over the surface of the blastocyst. These cells secrete proteolytic enzymes that digest and liquefy the cells of the endometrium. Simultaneously, much of the fluid and nutrients thus released is actively absorbed into the blastocyst as a result of phagocytosis by the trophoblastic cells; these absorbed substances provide the sustenance for further growth of the blastocyst. Also, at the same time,

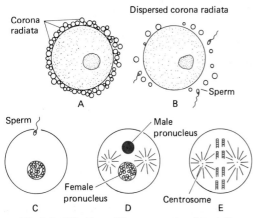

Figure 56–1. Fertillization of the ovum, showing *A,* the mature ovum surrounded by the corona radiata; *B,* dispersal of the corona radiata; *C,* entry of the sperm; *D,* formation of the male and female pronuclei; and *E,* reorganization of a full complement of chromosomes and beginning division of the ovum. (Modified from Arey: Developmental Anatomy, 7th ed. Philadelphia, W. B. Saunders Company, 1974.)

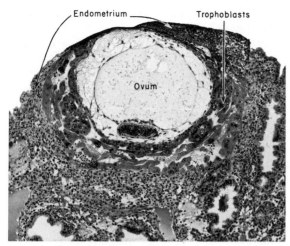

Figure 56–2. Implantation of the early human embryo, showing trophoblastic digestion and invasion of the endometrium. (Courtesy of Dr. Arthur Hertig.)

additional trophoblastic cells form cords of cells that extend into the deeper layers of the endometrium and attach to them. Thus, the blastocyst eats a hole in the endometrium and attaches to it at the same time.

Once implantation has taken place, the trophoblastic and underlying blastocyst cells proliferate rapidly; and they, along with cells from the mother's endometrium, form the placenta and the various membranes of pregnancy.

Early Intrauterine Nutrition of the Embryo. As the trophoblastic cells invade the endometrium, digesting and imbibing it, the stored nutrients in the large endometrial cells, called *decidual cells*, are used by the embryo for appropriate growth and development. During the first week after implantation, this is the only means by which the embryo can obtain any nutrients, and the embryo continues to obtain a large measure of its total nutrition in this way for 8 to 12 weeks, though the placenta also begins to provide slight amounts of nutrients after approximately the sixteenth day beyond fertilization (a little over a week after implantation).

FUNCTION OF THE PLACENTA

The structure of the placenta is illustrated in Figure 56–3. Note that the fetus's blood flows through two *umbilical arteries* to the capillaries of the villi, and thence back through the *umbilical vein* into the fetus. On the other hand, the mother's blood flows from the *uterine arteries* into large *blood sinuses* surrounding the villi and then back into the *uterine veins* of the mother.

The lower part of Figure 56–3 illustrates the relationship between the fetal blood of the villus and the blood of the mother in the fully developed placenta. The capillaries of the villus are lined with an extremely thin endothelium and are surrounded by a layer of *mesenchymal tissue* that is covered on the outside of the villus by a layer of *trophoblast cells*.

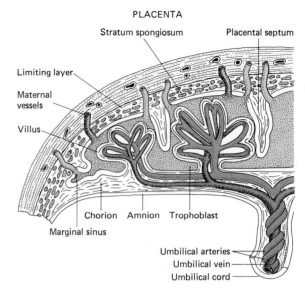

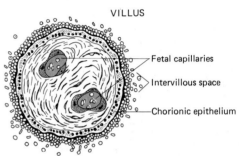

Figure 56–3. *Above:* Organization of the mature placenta. *Below:* Relationship of the fetal blood in the villus capillaries to the mother's blood in the intervillous spaces. (Modified from Clemente, C. O. (Ed.): Gray's Anatomy. Philadelphia, Lea & Febiger, 1985; and from Arey: Developmental Anatomy, 7th ed. Philadelphia, W. B. Saunders Company, 1974.)

DIFFUSION THROUGH THE PLACENTAL MEMBRANE

The major function of the placenta is to allow *diffusion* of foodstuffs from the mother's blood into the fetus's blood and diffusion of excretory products from the fetus back into the mother.

In the early months of development, placental permeability is relatively slight because the villar membranes have not yet been reduced to their minimum thickness. However, as the placenta becomes older, the permeability increases progressively until the last month or so of pregnancy.

Diffusion of Oxygen Through the Placental Membrane. Almost exactly the same principles are applicable for the diffusion of oxygen through the placental membrane as through the pulmonary membrane; these principles were discussed in Chapter 28. The dissolved oxygen in the blood of the large placental sinuses simply passes through the villar membrane into the fetal blood because of a pressure gradient of oxygen from the mother's blood to the fetus's blood. The mean P_{O_2} in the mother's blood in the placental sinuses is approximately 50 mm Hg toward the end of pregnancy, and the mean P_{O_2} in the blood leaving the villi and returning to the fetus after it has been oxygenated is about 30 mm Hg. Therefore, the mean pressure gradient for diffusion of oxygen through the placental membrane is about 20 mm Hg.

One might wonder how it is possible for a fetus to obtain sufficient oxygen when the fetal blood leaving the placenta has a Po₂ of only 30 mm Hg. However, most of the hemoglobin of the fetus is *fetal hemoglobin*, a type of hemoglobin synthesized in the fetus prior to birth. At low Po₂s fetal hemoglobin can carry as much as 20 to 30 per cent more oxygen than can maternal hemoglobin.

Also, the *hemoglobin concentration of the fetus is about 50 per cent greater than that of the mother*, which is also an important factor in enhancing the amount of oxygen transported to the fetal tissues.

Diffusion of Carbon Dioxide Through the Placental Membrane. Carbon dioxide is continuously formed in the tissues of the fetus in the same way that it is formed in maternal tissues. The only means for excreting the carbon dioxide is through the placenta. The Pco₂ builds up in the fetal blood until it is about 48 mm Hg, in contrast with 40 to 45 mm Hg in maternal blood. Thus, a small pressure gradient for carbon dioxide develops across the placental membrane, but this is sufficient to allow adequate diffusion of carbon dioxide from the fetal blood into the maternal blood, because the extreme solubility of carbon dioxide in the water of the placental membrane allows carbon dioxide to diffuse through this membrane about 20 times as rapidly as oxygen.

Diffusion of Foodstuffs Through the Placental Membrane. Other metabolic substrates needed by the fetus diffuse into the fetal blood in the same manner as oxygen. For instance, the glucose level in the fetal blood ordinarily is approximately 20 to 30 per cent lower than the glucose level in the maternal blood, for glucose is metabolized rapidly by the fetus. This in turn causes rapid diffusion of additional glucose from the maternal blood into the fetal blood.

Because of the high solubility of fatty acids in cell membranes, these too diffuse from the maternal blood into the fetal blood. Also, such substances as potassium, sodium, and chloride ions diffuse from the maternal blood into the fetal blood.

Active Absorption by the Placental Membrane. The cells that line the outer surfaces of the villi can also actively absorb certain nutrients from the maternal blood in the placenta during the first half of pregnancy at least and perhaps even throughout the entire pregnancy. For instance, the measured *amino acid* concentration of fetal blood is greater than that of maternal blood, and *calcium* and *inorganic phosphate* occur in greater concentration in fetal blood than in maternal blood. These effects indicate that the placental membrane has the ability to absorb actively at least small amounts of certain substances even during the latter part of pregnancy.

Excretion Through the Placental Membrane. In the same manner that carbon dioxide diffuses from the fetal blood into the maternal blood, other excretory products formed in the fetus diffuse into the maternal blood and then are excreted by the mother's kidneys along with her own excretory products. These include especially the waste products such as *urea, uric acid,* and *creatinine.* For instance, the level of urea in the fetal blood is only slightly greater than in maternal blood, because urea diffuses through the placental membrane with considerable ease.

HORMONAL FACTORS IN PREGNANCY

In pregnancy, the placenta forms large quantities of *human chorionic gonadotropin, estrogens, progesterone,* and *human chorionic somatomammotropin,* the first three of which, and perhaps the fourth as well, are essential to the continuance of pregnancy.

HUMAN CHORIONIC GONADOTROPIN AND ITS EFFECTS—PERSISTENCE OF THE CORPUS LUTEUM AND PREVENTION OF MENSTRUATION

Menstruation normally occurs approximately 14 days after ovulation, at which time most of the secretory endometrium of the uterus sloughs away from the uterine wall and is expelled to the exterior. If this were to happen after implantation of an ovum, the pregnancy would terminate. However, this is prevented by the secretion of human chorionic gonadotropin in the following manner:

Coincidently with the development of the trophoblast cells from the early dividing ovum, the hormone *human chorionic gonadotropin* is secreted into the fluids of the mother. As illustrated in Figure 56–4, the secretion of this hormone can first be measured 8 days after ovulation, just as the ovum is first implanting in the endometrium. Then the rate of secretion rises rapidly to reach a maximum approximately 8 weeks after ovulation, and decreases to a relatively low value by 16 to 20 weeks after ovulation.

Function of Human Chorionic Gonadotropin. Human chorionic gonadotropin is a glycoprotein having a molecular weight of 39,000 and very much the same molecular structure and function as the luteinizing hormone secreted by the pituitary. By far its most

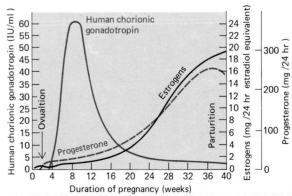

Figure 56–4. Rates of secretion of estrogens, progesterone, and chorionic gonadotropin at different stages of pregnancy.

important function is to prevent the normal involution of the corpus luteum at the end of the female sexual cycle. Instead, it causes the corpus luteum to secrete even larger quantities of its usual hormones, progesterone and estrogens. These excess hormones cause the endometrium to continue growing and to store large amounts of additional nutrients rather than to be passed in the menstruum.

If the corpus luteum is removed before approximately the seventh to eleventh week of pregnancy, spontaneous abortion usually occurs, but after this time the placenta itself secretes sufficient quantities of progesterone and estrogens to maintain pregnancy.

Effect of Human Chorionic Gonadotropin on the Fetal Testes. Human chorionic gonadotropin also exerts an *interstitial cell–stimulating effect* on the testes, thus resulting in the production of testosterone in male fetuses. This small secretion of testosterone during gestation is the factor that causes the fetus to grow male sex organs. Near the end of pregnancy, the testosterone secreted by the fetal testes also causes the testicles to descend into the scrotum.

SECRETION OF ESTROGENS BY THE PLACENTA

The placenta, like the corpus luteum, secretes both estrogens and progesterone. Figure 56–4 shows that the daily production of placental estrogens increases markedly to about 30 times normal toward the end of pregnancy.

Function of Estrogens in Pregnancy. In the discussions of estrogens in the preceding chapter it was pointed out that these hormones exert mainly a proliferative function on certain reproductive and associated organs. During pregnancy, the extreme quantities of estrogens cause (1) enlargement of the uterus, (2) enlargement of the breasts and growth of the breast glandular tissue, and (3) enlargement of the female external genitalia.

The estrogens also relax the various pelvic ligaments, so that the sacroiliac joints become relatively limber and the symphysis pubis becomes elastic. These changes facilitate easy passage of the fetus through the birth canal.

There is much reason to believe that estrogens also affect the development of the fetus during pregnancy, for example, by affecting the rate of cell reproduction in the early embryo.

SECRETION OF PROGESTERONE BY THE PLACENTA

Progesterone is also a hormone essential for pregnancy. In addition to being secreted in moderate quantities by the corpus luteum at the beginning of pregnancy, it is secreted in tremendous quantities by the placenta, averaging about one-quarter gram per day toward the end of pregnancy. Indeed, the rate of progesterone secretion increases by as much as 10-fold during the course of pregnancy, as illustrated in Figure 56–4.

The special effects of progesterone that are essential for normal progression of pregnancy are the following:

1. As pointed out earlier, progesterone causes decidual cells to develop in the uterine endometrium, and these cells then play an important role in the nutrition of the early embryo.

2. Progesterone has a special effect in decreasing the contractility of the gravid uterus, thus preventing uterine contractions from causing spontaneous abortion.

3. Progesterone also contributes to the development of the ovum even prior to implantation, for it specifically increases the secretions of the fallopian tubes and uterus to provide appropriate nutritive matter for the developing *morula* and *blastocyst*. There are some reasons to believe, too, that progesterone even affects cell cleavage in the early developing embryo.

4. The progesterone secreted during pregnancy also helps to prepare the breasts for lactation, as discussed later in the chapter.

HUMAN CHORIONIC SOMATOMAMMOTROPIN

Recently, a new hormone called *human chorionic somatomammotropin* has been discovered. This is a protein having a molecular weight of about 38,000 that begins to be secreted about the fifth week of pregnancy and increases progressively throughout the remainder of pregnancy. Human chorionic somatomammotropin has several important effects:

First, when administered to several different types of lower animals, human chorionic somatomammotropin causes at least partial development of the breasts.

Second, this hormone has weak actions similar to those of growth hormone, causing deposition of protein tissues in the same way that growth hormone does.

Third, human chorionic somatomammotropin has recently been found to have important actions on both glucose metabolism and fat metabolism in the mother, effects that perhaps are very important for nutrition of the fetus. The hormone causes decreased utilization of glucose by the mother, thereby making larger quantities of glucose available to the fetus. Furthermore, the hormone promotes release of free fatty acids from the fat stores of the mother, thus providing an alternative source of energy for her metabolism.

Therefore, it is beginning to appear that human chorionic somatomammotropin is a general metabolic hormone that has specific nutritional implications for both the mother and fetus.

RESPONSE OF THE MOTHER TO PREGNANCY

The presence of a growing fetus in the uterus adds an extra physiological load on the mother, and much of the response of the mother to pregnancy is due to this increased load. However, special effects include the following:

Blood Flow Through the Placenta; Cardiac Output. About 625 ml of blood flows through the maternal circulation of the placenta each minute during the latter stages of gestation. This flow increases the cardiac output in the same manner that arteriovenous shunts increase the output. This factor, plus a general increase in the mother's metabolism, increases her cardiac output to 30 to 40 per cent above normal.

Blood Volume of the Mother. The maternal blood volume shortly before term is approximately 30 per cent above normal. This increase occurs mainly because of increased secretion during pregnancy of aldosterone and estrogens, both of which cause increased fluid retention by the kidneys.

At the time of birth of the baby, the mother has approximately 1 to 2 liters of extra blood in her circulatory system. Only about one fourth of this amount is normally lost during delivery of the baby, thereby allowing a considerable safety factor for the mother.

Nutrition During Pregnancy. The growing fetus assumes priority for many of the nutritional elements in the mother's body, and many portions of the fetus continue to grow even if the mother does not eat a sufficiently nourishing diet.

By far the greatest growth of the fetus occurs during the last trimester of pregnancy; the weight of the child almost doubles during the last two months of pregnancy. Ordinarily, the mother does not absorb sufficient protein, calcium, phosphorus, and iron from the gastrointestinal tract during the last month of pregnancy to supply the fetus. However, from the beginning of pregnancy the mother's body has been storing these substances to be used during the latter months of pregnancy. Some of this storage is in the placenta, but most of it is in the normal storage depots of the mother.

If appropriate nutritional elements are not present in the mother's diet, a number of maternal deficiencies can occur during pregnancy. Such deficiencies often occur for calcium, phosphates, iron, and the vitamins. For example, approximately 375 mg of iron is needed by the fetus to form its blood, and an additional 600 mg is needed by the mother to form her own extra blood. The normal store of nonhemoglobin iron in the mother at the outset of pregnancy is often only 100 mg or so. Therefore, in general, the obstetrician supplements the diet of the mother with the needed substances. It is especially important that the mother receive large quantities of vitamin D, for although the total quantity of calcium utilized by the fetus is small, calcium even normally is poorly absorbed by the gastrointestinal tract. Finally, shortly before birth of the baby vitamin K is often added to the mother's diet so that the baby will have sufficient prothrombin to prevent postnatal hemorrhage.

The Amniotic Fluid and Its Formation. Normally, the volume of amniotic fluid (the fluid that surrounds the fetus in the uterus) is between 500 ml and 1 liter.

Studies with isotopes of the rate of formation of amniotic fluid show that on the average the water in amniotic fluid is completely replaced once every 3 hours, and the electrolytes sodium and potassium are replaced once every 15 hours. Yet, strangely enough, the sources of the fluid and the points of reabsorption are mainly unknown. A small portion of the fluid is derived from renal excretion by the fetus, and a small amount of absorption occurs by way of the fetal gastrointestinal tract. But about one half of the fluid turnover is believed to occur through the amniotic membranes.

PRE-ECLAMPSIA AND ECLAMPSIA

Approximately 4 per cent of all pregnant women develop a rapid rise in arterial blood pressure associated with loss of large amounts of protein in the urine at some time during the latter four months of pregnancy. This condition, called *preeclampsia*, is often also characterized by salt and water retention by the kidneys, weight gain, and development of edema. In addition, arterial spasm occurs in many parts of the body, most significantly in the kidneys, brain, and liver. Both the renal blood flow and the glomerular filtration rate are decreased, which is exactly opposite to the changes that occur in the normal pregnant woman. The renal effects are caused at least partly by thickened glomerular tufts that contain a fibrinoid deposit in the basement membranes.

Various attempts have been made to prove that preeclampsia is caused by excessive secretion of placental or adrenal hormones, but proof of a hormonal basis is still lacking. Indeed, a more plausible theory is that preeclampsia results from some type of autoimmunity or allergy resulting from the presence of the fetus. Indeed, the acute symptoms disappear within a few days after birth of the baby.

Eclampsia is a severe degree of preeclampsia characterized by extreme vascular spasticity throughout the body, clonic convulsions followed by coma, greatly decreased kidney output, malfunction of the liver, often extreme hypertension, and a generalized toxic condition of the body. Usually, it occurs shortly before parturition. Without treatment, a very high percentage of eclamptic patients die. However, with optimal and immediate use of rapidly acting vasodilating drugs to reduce the arterial pressure to normal, followed by immediate termination of pregnancy—by cesarean operation if necessary—the mortality has been reduced to 1 per cent or less.

PARTURITION

INCREASED UTERINE CONTRACTILITY NEAR TERM

Parturition simply means the process by which the baby is born. At the termination of pregnancy, the uterus becomes progressively more excitable until finally it begins strong rhythmic contractions with such force that the baby is expelled. The exact cause of the increased activity of the uterus is not known, but at least two major categories of effects lead up to the culminating contractions responsible for parturition; these are, first, progressive hormonal changes that cause increased excitability of the uterine musculature and, second, progressive mechanical changes.

Hormonal Factors That Cause Increased Uterine Contractility

Ratio of Estrogens to Progesterone. Progesterone inhibits uterine contractility during pregnancy, thereby helping to prevent expulsion of the fetus. On the other hand, estrogens have a definite tendency to increase the degree of uterine contractility. Both these hormones are secreted in progressively greater quantities throughout pregnancy, but from the seventh month onward, estrogen secretion increases more than progesterone secretion. Therefore, it has been postulated that the *estrogen to progesterone ratio* increases sufficiently toward the end of pregnancy to be at least partly responsible for the increased contractility of the uterus.

Effect of Oxytocin on the Uterus. Oxytocin is a hormone secreted by the posterior pituitary gland that specifically causes uterine contraction (see Chapter 49). Experiments in animals have shown that irritation or stretching of the uterine cervix, such as that occurring at the end of pregnancy, causes a neurogenic reflex to the neurohypophysis that increases the rate of oxytocin secretion. Therefore this hormone probably helps considerably to increase uterine contractions.

Mechanical Factors That Increase the Contractility of the Uterus

Stretch of the Uterine Musculature. Simply stretching smooth muscle organs usually increases their contractility. Furthermore, intermittent stretch, like that occurring repetitively in the uterus because of movements of the fetus, can also elicit smooth muscle contraction.

Note especially that twins are born on the average *19 days* earlier than a single child, which emphasizes the importance of mechanical stretch in promoting parturition.

Stretch or Irritation of the Cervix. There is much reason to believe that stretch or irritation of the uterine cervix is particularly important in directly eliciting uterine contractions. The mechanism of this effect is probably transmission of action potentials through the muscle of the uterus itself from the cervix to the body of the uterus.

ONSET OF LABOR—A POSITIVE FEEDBACK THEORY FOR ITS INITIATION

During most of the months of pregnancy, the uterus undergoes periodic episodes of weak and slow rhythmic contractions called *Braxton Hicks's contrac-*

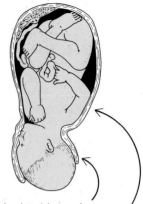

1. Baby's head stretches cervix...
2. Cervical stretch excites fundic contraction
3. Fundic contraction pushes baby down and stretches cervix some more...
4. Cycle repeats over and over again...

Figure 56–5. Theory for the onset of intensely strong contractions during labor.

tions. These become progressively stronger toward the end of pregnancy; and they eventually change rather suddenly, within hours, to exceptionally strong contractions that start stretching the cervix and, later, forcing the baby through the birth canal. This process is called *labor*, and the strong contractions that result in final parturition are called *labor contractions.*

On the basis of our new understanding of control systems in the past few years, a theory has been proposed for explaining the onset of labor based on positive feedback. This theory suggests that stretch of the cervix by the fetus's head finally becomes great enough to elicit a reflex increase in contractility of the uterine body. This pushes the baby forward, which stretches the cervix some more and initiates a new cycle. Thus, the process continues again and again until the baby is expelled. This theory is illustrated in Figure 56–5. We know at least two positive feedbacks that could lead to birth of the baby, as follows:

(1) Stretch of the cervix causes the entire body of the uterus to contract, and this stretches the cervix still more because of the downward thrust of the baby's head. (a) Cervical stretch also causes the pituitary gland to secrete oxytocin, which is still another cause of increased uterine contractility.

To summarize the theory, we can assume that multiple factors increase the contractility of the uterus toward the end of pregnancy. Eventually, a uterine contraction becomes strong enough to irritate the uterus enough to increase its contractility still more because of positive feedback, and to result in a second contraction stronger than the first, a third stronger than the second, and so forth. Once these contractions become strong enough to cause this type of increasing feedback, with each contraction greater than the one preceding, the process proceeds to completion.

ABDOMINAL MUSCLE CONTRACTIONS DURING LABOR

Once labor contractions become strong and painful, neurogenic reflexes, mainly from the birth canal to the spinal cord and thence back to the abdominal muscles, cause intense abdominal muscle contractions along with the uterine contractions. These abdominal contractions add greatly to the forces that cause expulsion of the baby.

MECHANICS OF PARTURITION

At the beginning of labor, strong contractions might occur only once every 30 minutes. As labor progresses, the contractions finally appear as often as once every one to three minutes, and the intensity of contraction increases greatly with only a short period of relaxation between contractions.

The combined contractions of the uterine and abdominal musculature during delivery of the baby cause a downward force on the fetus of approximately 25 pounds during each strong contraction. It is fortunate that the contractions of labor occur intermittently, because strong contractions impede or sometimes even stop blood flow through the placenta and would cause death of the fetus were the contractions continuous.

In 19 out of 20 births the head is the first part of the baby to be expelled; in most of the remaining instances the buttocks are presented first. The head acts as a wedge to open the structures of the birth canal as the fetus is forced downward from above.

The first major obstruction to expulsion of the fetus is the uterine cervix. Toward the end of pregnancy the cervix becomes soft, which allows it to stretch when labor pains cause the body of the uterus to contract. The so-called *first stage of labor* is the period of progressive cervical dilatation, which continues until the cervical opening is as large as the head of the fetus. This stage usually lasts 8 to 24 hours in the first pregnancy but often only a few minutes if the mother has had many pregnancies.

Once the cervix has dilated fully, the fetal membranes usually rupture, and the amniotic fluid is lost through the vagina. Then the fetus's head moves rapidly into the birth canal and, with additional force from above, continues to wedge its way through the canal until delivery is effected. This is called the *second stage of labor*; it may last from as little as a minute after many pregnancies up to half an hour or more in the first pregnancy.

SEPARATION AND DELIVERY OF THE PLACENTA

During the succeeding 10 to 45 minutes after birth of the baby, the uterus contracts to a very small size, which causes a *shearing* effect between the walls of the uterus and the placenta and consequent separation of the placenta from its implantation site. Separation of the placenta opens the placental sinuses and causes bleeding. However, the amount of bleeding is limited to an average of 350 ml by the following mechanism: The smooth muscle fibers of the uterine musculature are arranged in figure of eights around the blood vessels as they pass through the uterine wall. Therefore, contraction of the uterus following delivery of the baby constricts the vessels that had previously supplied blood to the placenta.

LABOR PAINS

With each uterine contraction, the mother experiences considerable pain. The pain in early labor is probably caused mainly by hypoxia of the uterine muscle resulting from compression of the blood vessels to the uterus. This pain is not felt when the sympathetic *hypogastric nerves*, which carry the sensory fibers leading from the uterus, have been sectioned. However, during the second stage of labor, when the fetus is being expelled through the birth canal, much more severe pain is caused by cervical stretch, perineal stretch, and stretch or tearing of structures in the vaginal canal itself. This pain is conducted by somatic nerves instead of by the hypogastric nerves.

INVOLUTION OF THE UTERUS

During the first four to five weeks following parturition, the uterus involutes. Its weight becomes less than one half its immediate postpartum weight within a week, and in four weeks the uterus may be as small as it had been prior to pregnancy. During early involution of the uterus the placental site on the endometrial surface autolyzes, causing a vaginal discharge known as lochia, which is first bloody and then serous, and continues for approximately a week and a half in all. After this time, the endometrial surface will have become re-epithelialized and ready for normal, nongravid sex life again.

LACTATION

DEVELOPMENT OF THE BREASTS

The breasts begin to develop at puberty; this development is stimulated by the estrogens of the monthly sexual cycles that stimulate growth of the stroma and ductile system plus deposition of fat to give mass to the breasts. However, much additional growth occurs during pregnancy, and the glandular tissue only then becomes completely developed for actual production of milk.

All through pregnancy, the tremendous quantities of estrogens secreted by the placenta—plus additional quantities of growth hormone, prolactin, and several other hormones—cause the ductile system of the breasts to grow and to branch. Simultaneously, the stroma of the breasts also increases, and large quantities of fat are laid down in the stroma.

Then the action of progesterone causes growth of the lobules, budding of alveoli, and development of secretory characteristics in the cells of the alveoli, most of which occurs in response to the very large amount of progesterone secreted by the placenta during pregnancy.

INITIATION OF LACTATION— FUNCTION OF PROLACTIN

Though estrogen and progestrone are essential for the physical development of the breasts during pregnancy, both of these hormones also have a specific effect to inhibit the actual secretion of milk. On the other hand, the hormone *prolactin* has exactly the opposite effect, promotion of the secretion of milk. This hormone is secreted by the mother's anterior pituitary gland, and its concentration in her blood rises steadily from the fifth week of pregnancy until birth of the baby, at which time it has risen to very high levels, usually about ten times the normal non-pregnant level. This is illustrated in Figure 56–6. In addition, the placenta secretes large quantities of *human chorionic somatomammotropin*, which also has mild lactogenic properties, thus supporting the prolactin from the mother's pituitary. Even so, only a few milliliters of fluid are secreted each day until after the baby is born. This fluid is called *colostrum*; it contains essentially the same concentrations of proteins and lactose as milk but almost no fat, and its maximum rate of production is about 1/100 the subsequent rate of milk production.

Immediately after the baby is born, the sudden loss of both estrogen and progesterone secretion by the placenta allows the lactogenic effect of the prolactin from the mother's pituitary gland to assume its natural milk-promoting role, and within two or three days, the breasts begin to secrete copious quantities of milk instead of colostrum.

Following birth of the baby, the *basal level* of prolactin secretion returns during the next few weeks to the nonpregnant level, as shown in Figure 56–6. However, each time the mother nurses her baby, nervous signals from the nipples to the hypothalamus cause approximately a tenfold surge in prolactin secretion lasting about one hour, which is also shown in the figure. The prolactin in turn acts on the breasts to provide the milk for the next nursing period. If this prolactin surge is absent, if it is blocked as a result of hypothalamic or pituitary damage, or if nursing does not continue, the breasts lose their ability to produce milk within a few days. However, milk production can continue for several years if the child continues to suckle, but the rate of milk formation normally decreases considerably within seven to nine months.

Hypothalamic Control of Prolactin Secretion. Though secretion of most of the anterior pituitary hormones is enhanced by neurosecretory releasing factors transmitted from the hypothalamus to the anterior pituitary gland through the hypothalamic-hypophysial portal system, the secretion of prolactin is normally controlled by an exactly opposite effect. That is, the hypothalamus synthesizes a *prolactin inhibitory factor* (PIF). Under normal conditions, large amounts of PIF are continuously transmitted to the anterior pituitary gland so that the normal rate of prolactin secretion is slight. However, it is believed that during lactation the formation of a *prolactin releasing factor* (PRF) may be formed intermittently at the time of nursing, causing the surges in prolactin secretion that occur at that time.

THE EJECTION (OR "LET-DOWN") PROCESS IN MILK SECRETION—FUNCTION OF OXYTOCIN

Milk is secreted continuously into the alveoli of the breasts, but milk does not flow easily from the alveoli into the ductile system and therefore does not continually leak from the breast nipples. Instead, the milk must be ejected, or "let-down" from the alveoli to the ducts before the baby can obtain it. This process is caused by a combined neurogenic and hormonal reflex involving the hormone *oxytocin* as follows:

When the baby suckles the breast, sensory signals are transmitted through somatic nerves to the spinal cord and then to the hypothalamus, there causing *oxytocin* secretion. This hormone flows in the blood to the breasts, where it causes the *myoepithelial cells* that surround the outer walls of the alveoli to contract, thereby expressing the milk from the alveoli into the ducts. Thus, within 30 seconds to a minute after a baby begins to suckle the breast, milk begins to flow. This process is called milk ejection, or milk let-down.

Suckling on one breast causes milk flow not only in that breast but also in the opposite breast. Also, it is especially interesting that the sound of the baby crying is often enough of a signal to cause milk ejection.

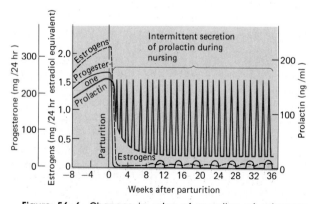

Figure 56–6. Changes in rates of secretion of estrogens, progesterone, and prolactin for 8 weeks prior to parturition and for 36 weeks thereafter. Note especially that prolactin secretion decreases back to basal levels within a few weeks, but that there are also intermittent periods of marked prolactin secretion (for about one hour at a time) during and after periods of nursing.

THE COMPOSITION OF MILK AND THE METABOLIC DRAIN ON THE MOTHER CAUSED BY LACTATION

Table 56–1 gives the contents of human milk and cow's milk.

At the height of lactation, 1.5 liters of milk may be formed each day. With this amount of lactation, great quantities of metabolic substrates are drained from the mother. For instance, approximately 50 grams of fat enter the milk each day, and approximately 100 grams of lactose, which must be derived from the mother's glucose. Also, some 2 to 3 grams of calcium phosphate may be lost each day, and unless the mother is drinking large quantities of milk and has an adequate intake of vitamin D, the output of calcium and phosphate by the lactating mammae will be much greater than the intake of these substances. To supply the excess calcium and phosphate, the parathyroid glands enlarge greatly, and the bones become progressively decalcified. The problem of decalcification is usually not very great during pregnancy, but it can be a distinct problem during lactation.

GROWTH AND FUNCTIONAL DEVELOPMENT OF THE FETUS

During the first two to three weeks, the fetus remains almost microscopic in size, but thereafter the dimensions of the fetus increase almost in proportion to age. At 12 weeks the length of the fetus is approximately 10 cm; at 20 weeks, approximately 25 cm, and at term (40 weeks), approximately 53 cm (about 21 inches). Because the weight of the fetus is proportional to the cube of the length, the weight increases approximately in proportion to the cube of the age of the fetus. Therefore, the weight of the fetus remains almost nothing during the first months and reaches only 1 pound at five and a half months of gestation. Then during the last trimester of pregnancy, the fetus gains tremendously, so that two months prior to birth the weight averages 3 pounds, at one month prior to birth 4.5 pounds, and at birth 7 pounds.

DEVELOPMENT OF THE FETAL ORGAN SYSTEMS

Within one month after fertilization of the ovum, all the different organs of the fetus are already at least partly formed, and during the next two to three months, the minute details of the different organs are established. Beyond the fourth month, the organs of the fetus are grossly the same as those of the newborn child, even including most of the smaller structures of the organs. However, cellular development of these structures is usually far from complete and requires the entire remaining five months of pregnancy for full maturation. Even at birth the cells of certain structures, particularly those of the nervous system, the kidneys, and the liver, still lack full development, as is discussed in more detail later in the chapter.

The Circulatory System. The human heart begins beating during the fourth week following fertilization, contracting at the rate of about 65 beats per minute. The rate increases steadily as the fetus grows and reaches approximately 140 per minute immediately before birth.

Formation of Blood Cells. Nucleated red blood cells begin to be formed in the yolk sac and mesothelial layers of the placenta at about the third week of fetal development. This is followed a week later by the formation of non-nucleated red blood cells by the fetal mesenchyme and by the endothelium of the fetal blood vessels. Then at approximately six weeks, the liver begins to form blood cells, and in the third month the spleen and other lymphoid tissues of the body also begin forming blood cells. Finally, from approximately the third month on, the bone marrow forms more and more red and white blood cells while the other structures completely lose their ability to form blood cells.

The Respiratory System. Obviously, respiration cannot occur during fetal life. However, respiratory movements do take place beginning at the end of the first trimester of pregnancy. Tactile stimuli or fetal asphyxia especially cause respiratory movements.

The Nervous System. Most of the peripheral reflexes of the fetus are well developed by the third to fourth month of pregnancy. However, some of the more imporant higher functions of the central nervous system are still undeveloped even at birth. Indeed, myelinization of some major tracts of the central nervous system becomes complete only after approximately a year of postnatal life.

The Gastrointestinal Tract. Even in midpregnancy the fetus ingests and absorbs large quantities of amniotic fluid, and during the latter two to three months, gastrointestinal function approaches that of the normal newborn infant. Small quantities of *meconium* are continually formed in the gastrointestinal tract and excreted from the bowels into the amniotic fluid. Meconium is composed partly of unabsorbed residue of amniotic fluid and partly of excretory products from the gastrointestinal mucosa and glands.

The Kidneys. The fetal kidneys are capable of excreting urine during at least the latter half of pregnancy, and urination occurs normally *in utero*. However, the renal control systems for regulation of extracellular fluid electrolyte balances and acid-base

Table 56–1. PERCENTAGE COMPOSITION OF MILK

	Human Milk	Cow's Milk
Water	88.5	87.0
Fat	3.3	3.5
Lactose	6.8	4.8
Casein	0.9	2.7
Lactalbumin and other protein	0.4	0.7
Ash	0.2	0.7

balance are almost nonexistent until after midfetal life and do not reach full development until about a month after birth.

ADJUSTMENTS OF THE INFANT TO EXTRAUTERINE LIFE

ONSET OF BREATHING

The most obvious effect of birth on the baby is loss of the placental connection with the mother and therefore loss of this means for metabolic support. And by far the most important immediate adjustment required of the infant is to begin breathing.

Cause of Breathing at Birth. Following completely normal delivery from a mother who has not been depressed by anesthetics, the child ordinarily begins to breathe immediately and has a completely normal respiratory rhythm from the outset. The promptness with which the fetus begins to breathe indicates that breathing is initiated by sudden exposure to the exterior world, probably resulting from a slightly asphyxiated state incident to the birth process but also from sensory impulses originating in the suddenly cooled skin. However, if the infant does not breathe immediately, its body becomes progressively more hypoxic and hypercapnic, which provides additional stimulus to the respiratory center and usually causes breathing within a few seconds to a few minutes after birth.

Delayed and Abnormal Breathing at Birth—Danger of Hypoxia. If the mother has been depressed by an anesthetic during delivery, which at least partially anesthetizes the child as well, respiration is likely to be delayed for several minutes, which illustrates the importance of using as little obstetrical anesthesia as feasible. Also, many infants who have had head trauma during delivery are slow to breathe or sometimes will not breathe at all. This can result from two possible effects: First, in a few infants, intracranial hemorrhage or brain contusion causes a concussion syndrome with a greatly depressed respiratory center. Second, and probably much more important, prolonged fetal hypoxia during delivery causes serious depression of the respiratory center. Hypoxia frequently occurs during delivery because of (1) compression of the umbilical cord, (2) premature separation of the placenta, (3) excessive contraction of the uterus, which cuts off blood flow to the placenta, or (4) excessive anesthesia of the mother.

Degree of Hypoxia that an Infant Can Tolerate. In the adult, failure to breathe for only four minutes often causes death, but a newborn infant often survives as long as 10 to 15 minutes of failure to breathe after birth. Unfortunately, though, permanent brain impairment often ensues if breathing is delayed more than 8 to 10 minutes. Indeed, actual lesions develop, mainly in brain stem areas, thus affecting many motor functions of the body. This is believed to be one of the causes of *cerebral palsy.*

Expansion of the Lungs at Birth. At birth, the walls of the alveoli are held together by the surface tension of the viscid fluid that fills them. More than 25 mm Hg of negative pressure is required to oppose the effects of this surface tension and therefore to open the alveoli for the first time. But once the alveoli are open, further respiration can be effected with relatively weak respiratory movements. Fortunately, the first inspirations of the newborn infant are extremely powerful, usually capable of creating as much as 50 mm Hg negative pressure in the intrapleural space.

Figure 56–7 illustrates the tremendous forces required to open the lungs at the onset of breathing. To the left is shown the pressure-volume curve (compliance curve) for the first breath after birth. Observe first the lowermost curve, which shows that the lungs do not expand at all until the negative pressure has reached −40 cm water (−30 mm Hg). Then as the negative pressure increases to −60 cm water, only about 40 ml of air enters the lungs. Then, to deflate the lungs, considerable positive pressure is required, probably because of the viscous resistance offered by the fluid in the bronchioles.

Note that the second breath is much easier. However, breathing does not become completely normal until about 40 minutes after birth, as shown by the third compliance curve, the shape of which compares favorably with that of the normal adult.

Respiratory Distress Syndrome. A few infants, especially premature infants, develop severe respiratory distress during the few hours to several days following birth and frequently succumb within the next day or so. The alveoli of these infants at death contain large quantities of proteinaceous fluid, almost as if pure plasma had leaked out of the capillaries into the alveoli.

One of the most characteristic findings in these infants is failure to secrete adequate quantities of *surfactant,* a substance normally secreted into the alveoli that decreases the surface tension of the alveolar fluid, therefore allowing the alveoli to open easily. The surfactant secreting cells (the type II alveolar epithelial cells) do not begin to secrete surfactant until the last one to three months of gestation. Therefore, many premature babies and some full-term babies are born without the capability of secreting surfactant, which therefore causes both a tendency

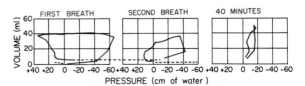

Figure 56–7. Pressure-volume curves of the lungs (compliance curves) of a newborn baby immediately after birth, showing (*a*) the extreme forces required for breathing during the first two breaths of life and (*b*) development of a nearly normal compliance within 40 minutes after birth. (From Smith: SCIENTIFIC AMERICAN, 209:32, 1963. ©1963 by Scientific American Inc. All rights reserved.)

of the lungs to collapse and to develop pulmonary edema. The role of surfactant in preventing these effects was discussed in Chapter 27.

CIRCULATORY READJUSTMENTS AT BIRTH

Almost as important as the onset of breathing at birth are the immediate circulatory adjustments that allow adequate blood flow through the lungs. Because the lungs are mainly nonfunctional during fetal life, it is not necessary for the fetal heart to pump much blood through the lungs. On the other hand, the fetal heart must pump large quantities of blood through the placenta. As illustrated in Figure 56–8, most of the blood entering the right atrium from the inferior vena cava is directed in a straight pathway across the posterior aspect of the right atrium and thence through the *foramen ovale* directly into the left atrium. Thus, the well-oxygenated blood from the placenta enters the left side of the heart without going through the right ventricle and lungs. Instead, it is pumped by the left ventricle mainly into the vessels of the head and forelimbs.

The blood entering the right atrium from the superior vena cava is directed downward through the tricuspid valve into the right ventricle. This blood is mainly deoxygenated blood from the head region of the fetus, and it is pumped by the right ventricle into the pulmonary artery. Then almost all of the blood passes through the *ductus arteriosus* into the descending aorta and through the two umbilical arteries into the placenta, where this deoxygenated blood becomes oxygenated.

Changes in the Fetal Circulation at Birth. The basic changes in the fetal circulation at birth were discussed in Chapter 17 in relation to congenital anomalies of the ductus arteriosus and foramen ovale that persist throughout life. Briefly, these are as follows:

First, the tremendous blood flow through the placenta ceases, which *approximately doubles the systemic vascular resistance at birth.* This obviously *increases the aortic pressure* as well as the pressures in the left ventricle and left atrium.

Second, the *pulmonary vascular resistance decreases greatly* as a result of expansion of the lungs. In the unexpanded fetal lungs, the blood vessels are compressed because of the small volume of the lungs. Immediately upon expansion these vessels are no longer compressed, and the resistance to blood flow decreases several fold. Also, in fetal life the hypoxia of the lungs causes considerable tonic vasoconstriction of the lung blood vessels, but vasodilation takes place when aeration of the lungs eliminates the hypoxia. These changes reduce the resistance of blood flow through the lungs as much as five fold, which obviously *reduces the pulmonary arterial pressure, the right ventricular pressure, and the right atrial pressure.*

Closure of the Foramen Ovale. The *low right atrial pressure* and the *high left atrial pressure* that occur secondary to the changes in pulmonary and systemic resistance at birth cause a tendency for blood to flow backward from the left atrium into the right atrium rather than the other direction, as occurred during fetal life. Consequently, the small valve that lies over the foramen ovale on the left side of the atrial septum closes over this opening, thereby preventing further flow.

Closure of the Ductus Arteriosus. Similar effects occur in relation to the ductus arteriosus, for the increased systemic resistance *elevates the aortic pressure* while the decreased pulmonary resistance *reduces the pulmonary arterial pressure.* As a consequence, immediately after birth, blood begins to flow backward from the aorta into the pulmonary artery rather than in the other direction as in fetal life. However, after only a few hours the muscular wall of the ductus arteriosus constricts markedly, and within one to eight days the constriction is sufficient to stop all blood flow. This is called *functional closure* of the ductus arteriosus. Then sometime during the next one to four months, the ductus arteriosus ordinarily becomes anatomically *occluded* by growth of fibrous tissue into its lumen.

Ductus closure almost certainly results from the increased oxygenation of the blood flowing through the ductus. In fetal life the P_{O_2} of the ductus blood is only 15 to 20 mm Hg, but it increases to about 100 mm Hg within a few hours after birth. Furthermore, many experiments have shown that the degree of contraction of the smooth muscle in the ductus wall is closely related to the availability of oxygen.

In one out of several thousand infants, the ductus

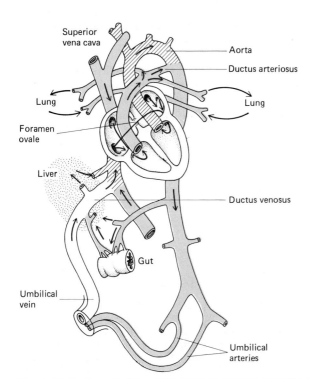

Figure 56–8. Organization of the fetal circulation. (Modified from Arey: Developmental Anatomy. 7th ed. Philadelphia, W. B. Saunders Company, 1974.)

fails to close, resulting in a *patent ductus arteriosus,* the consequences of which were discussed in Chapter 17.

SPECIAL FUNCTIONAL PROBLEMS IN THE NEONATAL INFANT

The most important characteristic of the newborn infant is instability of the various hormonal and neurogenic control systems. This results partly from the immature development of the different organs of the body and partly from the fact that the control systems simply have not become adjusted to the completely new way of life.

Cardiac Output. The cardiac output of the newborn infant averages 550 ml per minute, which is about two times as much in relation to body weight as in the adult. Occasionally, a child is born with an especially low cardiac output caused by hemorrhage through the placental membrane into the mother's blood prior to birth.

Arterial Pressure. The arterial pressure during the first day after birth averages about 70/50; it increases slowly during the next several months to approximately 90/60. Then there is a much slower rise during the subsequent years until the adult pressure of 120/80 is attained at adolescence.

Fluid Balance, Acid-Base Balance, and Renal Function. The rate of fluid intake and fluid excretion in the infant is seven times as great in relation to weight as in the adult, which means that even a slight alteration of fluid balance can cause rapidly developing abnormalities. Also, the rate of metabolism in the infant is two times as great in relation to body mass as in the adult, which means that two times as much acid is normally formed, leading to a tendency toward acidosis in the infant. Finally, functional development of the kidneys is not complete until approximately the end of the first month of life. For instance, the kidneys of the newborn can concentrate urine to only one and a half times the osmolality of the plasma instead of the normal three- to fourfold in the adult.

Therefore, considering the immaturity of the kidneys together with the marked fluid turnover and rapid formation of acid in the infant, one can readily understand that among the most important problems of infancy are acidosis and dehydration.

Liver Function. During the first few days of life, liver function may be quite deficient, as evidenced by the following effects:

1. The liver of the newborn conjugates bilirubin with glucuronic acid poorly and therefore excretes bilirubin only slightly during the first few days of life.

2. The liver of the newborn is deficient in forming plasma proteins, so that the plasma protein concentration falls in the first few weeks of life to 1 g/100 ml less than that for older children. Occasionally, the protein concentration falls so low that the infant actually develops hypoproteinemic edema.

3. The gluconeogenesis function of the liver is particularly deficient. As a result, the blood glucose level of the unfed newborn infant falls to about 30 to 40 mg/100 ml, and the infant must depend on its stored fats for energy until feeding can occur.

4. The liver of the newborn often also forms too little of the factors needed for normal blood coagulation.

Digestion, Absorption, and Metabolism of Energy Foods. In general, the ability of the newborn infant to digest, absorb, and metabolize foods is not different from that of the older child, with the following three exceptions:

First, secretion of pancreatic amylase in the newborn infant is deficient, so that the infant utilizes starches less adequately than do older children. However, the infant readily assimilates disaccharides and monosaccharides.

Second, absorption of fats from the gastrointestinal tract is somewhat less than in the older child. Consequently, milk with a high fat content, such as some varieties of cow's milk, is frequently inadequately utilized.

Third, because the liver functions are imperfect during at least the first week of life, the glucose concentration in the blood is unstable and often low.

Metabolic Rate and Body Temperature. The normal metabolic rate of the newborn in relation to body weight is about two times that of the adult, which accounts also for the two times as great cardiac output and two times as great minute respiratory volume in the infant.

However, since the body surface area is very large in relation to the body mass, heat is readily lost from the body. As a result, the body temperature of the newborn infant, particularly of the premature infant, falls. Figure 56–9 shows that the body temperature of even the normal infant falls several degrees during the first few hours after birth but returns to normal in seven to eight hours. Still, the body temperature regulatory mechanisms remain poor during the early days of life, at first allowing marked deviations in temperature, which are also illustrated in Figure 56–9.

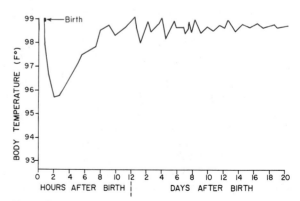

Figure 56–9. Fall in body temperature of the infant immediately after birth, and instability of body temperature during the first few days of life.

Nutritional Needs During the Early Weeks of Life. Three specific problems occur in the early nutrition of the infant, as follows:

Need for Calcium. In the newborn infant rapid ossification of the bones has only begun at birth, so that a ready supply of calcium is needed throughout infancy.

Need for Iron. If the mother has had adequate amounts of iron in her diet, the liver of the infant usually has stored enough iron to keep forming blood cells for four to six months after birth. But if the mother has had insufficient iron in her diet, anemia is likely to supervene in the infant after about three months of life. Therefore, administration of iron in some form is desirable by the second or third month of life.

Vitamin C Deficiency. Ascorbic acid (vitamin C) is not stored in significant quantities in the fetal tissues; yet it is required for proper formation of cartilage, bone, and other intercellular structures of the infant. Furthermore, milk, especially cow's milk, has poor supplies of ascorbic acid. For this reason, orange juice or other sources of ascorbic acid are usually prescribed by the third week of life.

Immunity. Fortunately, the newborn inherits much immunity from its mother because many antibodies diffuse from the mother's blood through the placenta into the fetus. However, the newborn itself does not form antibodies to a significant extent. By the end of the first month, the baby's gamma globulins, which contain the antibodies, have decreased to less than one half the original level, with a corresponding decrease in immunity. Therefore, the baby's own immunization processes begin to form antibodies, and the gamma globulin concentration returns essentially to normal by the age of 6 to 20 months.

Endocrine Problems. Ordinarily, the endocrine system of the infant is highly developed at birth, and the infant rarely exhibits any immediate endocrine abnormalities. However, there are special instances in which endocrinology of infancy is important.

1. If a pregnant mother bearing a *female child* is treated with an androgenic hormone or if she develops an androgenic tumor during pregnancy, the child will be born with a high degree of masculinization of its sexual organs, thus resulting in a type of *hermaphroditism.*

2. An infant born of a diabetic mother will have considerable hypertrophy and hyperfunction of its islets of Langerhans. As a consequence, the infant's blood glucose concentration may fall to as low as 20 mg per 100 ml or even lower shortly after birth. Fortunately, the newborn infant, unlike the adult, only rarely develops insulin shock or coma from this low level of blood glucose concentration.

Because of metabolic deficits in the diabetic mother, the fetus is often stunted in growth, and growth of the newborn infant and tissue maturation are often impaired. Also, there is a high rate of intrauterine mortality, and of those fetuses that do come to live birth, there is still a high mortality rate. Two-thirds of the infants who die succumb to the respiratory distress syndrome, which was described earlier in the chapter.

3. Occasionally, a child is born with hypofunctional adrenal cortices, perhaps resulting from *agenesis* of the glands or *exhaustion atrophy*, which can occur when the adrenal glands have been overstimulated.

SPECIAL PROBLEMS OF PREMATURITY

All the problems just noted for neonatal life are especially exacerbated in prematurity. These can be categorized under the following two headings: (1) immaturity of certain organ systems and (2) instability of the different homeostatic control systems. Because of these effects, a premature baby rarely lives if it is born more than two and a half to three months prior to term.

The respiratory system is especially likely to be underdeveloped in the premature infant. The vital capacity and the functional residual capacity of the lungs are unusually small in relation to the size of the infant. Also, surfactant secretion is seriously depressed. As a consequence, respiratory distress is a common cause of death. Also, the low functional residual capacity in the premature infant is often associated with periodic breathing of the Cheyne-Stokes type.

Another major problem of the premature infant is its inability to ingest and absorb adequate food. If the infant is more than two months premature, the digestive and absorptive systems are almost always inadequate. The absorption of fat is so poor that the premature infant must have a low fat diet. Furthermore, the premature infant has unusual difficulty in absorbing calcium and therefore can develop severe rickets before the difficulty is recognized. For this reason, special attention must be paid to adequate calcium and vitamin D intake.

Immaturity of the different organ systems in the premature infant creates a high degree of instability in the homeostatic systems of the body. For instance, the acid-base balance can vary tremendously, particularly when the food intake varies from time to time. And one of the particular problems of the premature infant is inability to maintain normal body temperature. Its temperature tends to approach that of its surroundings. At normal room temperature the baby's temperature may stabilize in the low 90's or even in the 80's. Statistical studies show that a body temperature maintained below 96° F is associated with a particularly high incidence of death, which explains the common use of the incubator in the treatment of prematurity.

QUESTIONS

1. Describe the *fertilization* of the ovum.
2. Describe the *transport* and *implantation* of the developing ovum.
3. How does the early-developing ovum derive its *nutrition* from the uterus?
4. In what ways is *diffusion* through the placental membrane similar to diffusion through the respiratory membrane?
5. Describe the diffusion of oxygen, carbon dioxide, and the various food substances through the placental membrane.
6. Explain the role of *human chorionic gonadotropin* in the maintenance of pregnancy during the first few weeks after fertilization.
7. What are the functions of the *estrogens* and the *progesterone* secreted by the placenta?
8. How does the mother respond to pregnancy in relation to each of the following factors: placental blood flow and cardiac output, mother's blood volume, mother's nutrition during pregnancy, and formation of amniotic fluid?
9. What are the characteristics of *pre-eclampsia* and *eclampsia*?
10. Discuss the factors that increase *uterine contractility* toward the end of pregnancy. How does increased contractility lead to a possible positive feedback cycle that culminates in labor and birth of the baby?
11. Describe the mechanics of *parturition*. What specific feedback mechanisms at the time of labor probably play major roles in enhancing the *labor contractions* and causing parturition to go to completion?
12. Discuss the factors that cause growth and development of the breasts and their glandular apparatus.
13. Explain the hormonal mechanisms that prevent *lactation* before birth but cause it to begin immediately after birth. What is the role of *prolactin* in maintaining the capability of the breasts to secrete milk for many months if the baby continues to suckle?
14. Explain the function of *oxytocin* in *milk ejection*.
15. What are some of the metabolic drains on the mother during lactation?
16. Which organs of the fetus are not fully developed at the time of birth?
17. Describe the onset of breathing. Why is *surfactant* important in this?
18. Explain the changes in pressure in different parts of the circulatory system immediately after birth that cause the immediate closure of the *foramen ovale* and the closure over a period of hours of the *ductus arteriosus*.
19. What are some of the special nutritional needs of the newborn child?
20. Explain what happens to the fetus when the mother is given an androgenic hormone or when she has diabetes.
21. What are some of the special problems of prematurity, especially problems related to the respiratory system and to the maintenance of body temperature?

References

Pregnancy and Lactation

Aynsley-Green, A.: Metabolic and endocrine interrelations in the human fetus and neonate. Am J Clin Nutr 41:399, 1985.
Challis, J. R. G.: Endocrinology of late pregnancy and parturition. In Greep, R. O., ed.: International Review of Physiology: Reproductive Physiology III. Vol. 22. Baltimore, University Park Press, 1980, p. 277.
Clark, D. A., et al.: Local active suppression by suppressor cells in the decidua: a review. Am J Reprod Immunol 5:78, 1984.
Conn, P. M., et al.: Gonadotropin-releasing hormone: molecular and cell biology, physiology, and clinical applications. Fed Proc 43:2351, 1984.
Cowie, A. T., et al.: Hormonal Control of Lactation. New York, Springer-Verlag, 1980.
Grant, N. F., and Worley, R.: Hypertension in Pregnancy: Concepts and Management. New York, Appleton-Century-Crofts, 1980.
Leong, D. A., et al.: Neuroendocrine control of prolactin secretion. Annu Rev Physiol 45:109, 1983.
Munro, H. N., et al.: The placenta in nutrition. Annu Rev Nutr 3:97, 1983.
Ochiai, K., ed.: Endocrine Correlates of Reproduction. New York, Springer-Verlag, 1984.
Pitkin, R. M.: Calcium metabolism in pregnancy and the perinatal period: a review. Am J Obstet Gynecol 151:99, 1985.
Sampson, D. A., and Jansen, G. R.: Protein and energy nutrition during lactation. Annu Rev Nutr 4:43, 1984.
Simpson, E. R., and MacDonald, P. C.: Endocrine physiology of the placenta. Annu Rev Physiol 43:163, 1981.
Tienhoven, A. V.: Reproductive Physiology of Vertebrates. Ithaca, Cornell University Press, 1982.

Fetal Neonatal Physiology

Aynsley-Green, A.: Metabolic and endocrine interrelations in the human fetus and neonate. Am J Clin Nutr 41:399, 1985.

Bissonnette, J. M., et al.: Regulation of cerebral blood flow in the fetus. J Dev Physiol 6:275, 1984.
Dallman, P. R.: Anemia of prematurity. Annu Rev Med 32:143, 1981.
Durnin, J. V.: Energy balance in childhood and adolescence. Proc Nutr Soc 43:271, 1984.
Fanaroff, A. A.: Behrman's Neonatal-Perinatal Medicine. Diseases of the Fetus and Infant. St. Louis, C. V. Mosby, 1983.
Gaull, G. E., et al.: Significance of growth modulators in human milk. Pediatrics 75:142, 1985.
Harding, R.: Function of the larynx in the fetus and newborn. Annu Rev Physiol 46:645, 1984.
Heymann, M. A., et al.: Factors affecting changes in the neonatal systemic circulation. Annu Rev Physiol 43:371, 1981.
King, D. B., and May, J. D.: Thyroidal influence on body growth. J Exp Zool 232:453, 1984.
Lotgering, F. K., et al.: Maternal and fetal responses to exercise during pregnancy. Physiol Rev 65:1, 1985.
Mendez, H.: Introduction to the study of pre- and postnatal growth in humans: a review. Am J Med Genet 20:63, 1985.
Mott, J. C., and Walker, D. W.: Neural and endocrine regulation of circulation in the fetus and newborn. In Shepherd, J. T., and Abboud, F. M., eds.: Handbook of Physiology. Sec. 2, Vol. 3. Bethesda, American Physiological Society, 1983, p. 837.
Read, D. J., and Henderson-Smart, D. J.: Regulation of breathing in the newborn during different behavioral states. Annu Rev Physiol 46:675, 1984.
Rigatto, H.: Control of ventilation in the newborn. Annu Rev Physiol 46:661, 1984.
Rosett, H. L.: Alcohol and the Fetus. A Clinical Perspective. New York, Oxford University Press, 1984.
Walker, D. W.: Peripheral and central chemoreceptors in the fetus and newborn. Annu Rev Physiol 46:687, 1984.

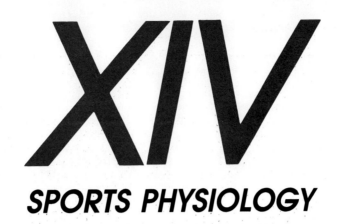

XIV

SPORTS PHYSIOLOGY

57 ■ Sports Physiology

57

Sports Physiology

THE MUSCLES IN EXERCISE
  STRENGTH, POWER, AND
    ENDURANCE OF MUSCLES
  THE MUSCLE METABOLISM SYSTEMS IN
    EXERCISE
RESPIRATION IN EXERCISE

THE CARDIOVASCULAR SYSTEM IN
  EXERCISE
BODY HEAT IN EXERCISE
BODY FLUIDS AND SALT IN EXERCISE
DRUGS AND ATHLETES

It is fitting to end this text with a chapter on sports physiology, because there are no normal stresses to which the body is exposed that even nearly approach the extreme stresses of heavy exercise. In fact, if some of the extremes of exercise were continued for even slightly prolonged periods of time, they might easily be lethal. Therefore, in the main, sports physiology is a discussion of the ultimate limits to which most of the bodily mechanisms can be stressed. To emphasize this, let us give one simple example: In a person who has extremely high fever that is approaching the level of lethality the body metabolism increases to about 100 per cent above normal. By comparison, the metabolism of the body during a marathon race increases to 2000 per cent above normal.

The Female and the Male Athlete

Most of the quantitative data given in this chapter is for the young male adult, not because it is desirable to know only these values but because it is only in this class of athletes that relatively complete measurements have been made. However, for those measurements which have been made in the female, almost identically the same basic physiological principles apply equally to women as to men except for quantitative differences. In general, most quantitative values—such as muscle strength, pulmonary ventilation, and cardiac output, all of which are related mainly to the muscle mass—will vary between two thirds and three quarters of the values recorded in men. However, these lower values do not translate into the same differential in athletic performance because the female body size is correspondingly smaller. A good indication of the relative performance capabilities of the female versus the male athlete comes from the relative times required for running the marathon race.

In a recent comparison, the top female performer had a running time about 12 per cent less than that of the top male performer. On the other hand, for some endurance events, women have proved to have capabilities superior to those of men. As an example, the record for the two-way swim across the English channel is presently held by a woman, not a man. Part of the reason for this has been reputed to be that the female has extra fat in her subcutaneous tissues to insulate her from the cold of the channel waters, but this certainly is not all of the reason, and it may be more wishful thinking of the male ego than fact.

The hormonal differences between woman and man certainly account for a large part if not most of the differences in athletic performance. *Testosterone* secreted by the male testicles has a powerful anabolic effect, which means that it causes greatly increased deposition of protein everywhere in the body, especially in the muscles. In fact, even the male who participates in very little sports activity but who nevertheless is well-endowed with testosterone will have muscles that grow to sizes 40 per cent or more greater than those of his female counterpart and with a corresponding increase in strength. Thus, the male who begins to train for sports activity already has a running start on the female.

The female sex hormone *estrogen* probably also accounts for some of the difference between female and male performance, though its effect is not nearly as great as that of testosterone. Estrogen is known to increase the deposition of fat in the female, especially in certain tissues such as the breasts, the hips, and the subcutaneous tissue. At least partly for this reason, the average nonathletic female has about 26 per cent body fat composition in contrast with the nonathletic male, who has about 15 per cent. In marathon runners who have trained themselves to the least amount of excess fat, the male has about 4 per cent body fat composition, and the female 6 per cent. Thus, either in the untrained or the trained state, the female usually averages about 50 per cent more body fat than the male. This obviously is a detriment to the highest levels of athletic performance in those events in which performance is dependent upon speed or bodily strength, but on the other hand it could be an aid in grueling endurance athletic events that require the fat for energy.

Estrogen plays another more insidious role in athletics, for it is the estrogen secreted by the female ovaries after puberty that makes the female stature smaller than that of the male. Immediately after puberty, the surge in estrogen secretion causes a rapid spurt of growth that usually makes the postpubertal female grow more rapidly than her male counterpart. On the other hand, this growth is short-lived because the epiphyseal cartilages of the long bones, which is where the growth occurs, rapidly run their course and actually disappear, allowing the epiphyses to unite with the shafts of the long bones—therefore, no further growth. As a result, the female frequently reaches her full height at an age of perhaps 15 to 17 years, whereas the male may continue to grow until the age of 19 to 21. This difference obviously looms large in most athletic events because the very design of athletic competition often gives the edge to those of greater body size.

Finally, one cannot neglect the effect of the sex hormones on temperament. There is no doubt that testosterone promotes aggressiveness and that estrogen is associated with a more mild temperament. Certainly a large part of competitive sports is the aggressive spirit that drives a person to his maximum effort, often at the expense of judicious restraint.

THE MUSCLES IN EXERCISE

STRENGTH, POWER, AND ENDURANCE OF MUSCLES

The final common denominator in athletic events is what the muscles can do for you—what strength they can give when it is needed, what power they can achieve in the performance of work, and how long they can continue in their activity.

The strength of a muscle is determined mainly by its size, with a *maximum contractile force between 2.5 kg and 3.5 kg per cm²* of muscle cross-sectional area. Thus, the male who is well laced with testosterone and therefore has correspondingly enlarged muscles will be much stronger than those persons without the testosterone advantage. Also, the athlete whose muscles have hypertrophied through an exercise training program likewise will have increased muscle strength because of increased muscle size.

To give an example of muscle strength, a world-class weight lifter might have a quadriceps muscle with a cross-sectional area as great as 150 cm². This would translate into a maximum contractile strength of 525 kg (or 1155 lb), with all this force applied to the patellar tendon. Therefore, one can readily understand how it is possible for this tendon to be ruptured or actually to be avulsed from its insertion into the tibia below the knee. Also, when such forces occur in tendons that span a joint, similar forces are also applied to the surfaces of the joints, or sometimes to ligaments spanning the joints, thus accounting for such happenings as displaced cartilages, compression fractures about the joint, or torn ligaments.

Yet, to make matters still worse, the *holding strength* of muscles is about 40 per cent greater than the contractile strength. That is, if a muscle is already contracted and a force then attempts to stretch out the muscle, about 40 per cent more force is required than can be achieved by a shortening contraction. Therefore, the force of 525 kg calculated previously for the patellar tendon becomes 735 kg (1617 lb). This obviously further compounds the problems of tendons, joints, and ligaments. It can also lead to internal tearing in the muscle itself. In fact, stretching of a maximally contracted muscle is one of the best ways to insure the highest degree of muscle soreness.

The *power* of muscle contraction is different from muscle strength, for power is a measure of the amount of work that the muscle can perform in a given period of time. This is determined not only by the strength of muscle contraction but also by its *velocity of contraction* and the number of times that it contracts each minute.

Muscle power is generally measured in *kilogram-meters (kg-m)/minute*. That is, a muscle that can lift a kilogram weight to a height of 1 m or that can move some object laterally against a force of 1 kg for a distance of a meter in 1 minute is said to have a power of 1 kg-m/minute. The maximum power that all of the muscles in the body of a highly trained athlete with all of the muscles working together can achieve is approximately the following:

First 10 to 15 seconds	7000 kg-m/minute
Next 1 minute	4000 kg-m/minute
Next half hour	1700 kg-m/minute

Thus, it is clear that a person has the capability of an extreme power surge for a short period of time, such as during a 100-m dash that can be completed entirely within the first 10 seconds, whereas for long-term endurance events, the power output of the muscles is only one fourth as great as during the initial power surge. Yet, this does not mean that one's athletic performance is four times as great during the initial power surge as it is for the next half hour, because the efficiency for translation of muscle power output into athletic performance is often much less during rapid activity than during less rapid but sustained activity. Thus, the velocity of the hundred meter dash is only 1¾ times as great as the velocity of the 30-minute race despite the 4-fold difference in short-term versus long-term muscle power capability.

The final characteristic of muscle performance is *endurance*. This, to a great extent, depends on the nutritive support for the muscle—more than anything else on the amount of glycogen that has been stored in the muscle prior to the period of exercise. A person on a high carbohydrate diet stores far more glycogen in his muscles than a person on either a mixed or a high fat diet. Therefore, endurance is greatly enhanced by a high carbohydrate diet. When athletes run at speeds typical for the marathon race, their endurance, as measured by the time that they can sustain the race until complete exhaustion, is approximately the following:

High carbohydrate diet	240 minutes
Mixed diet	120 minutes
High fat diet	85 minutes

The corresponding amounts of glycogen stored in the muscle are approximately the following:

High carbohydrate diet	33 g per kg of muscle
Mixed diet	17.5 g per kg of muscle
High fat diet	6 g per kg of muscle

THE MUSCLE METABOLIC SYSTEMS IN EXERCISE

The same basic metabolic systems are present in muscles as in all other parts of the body; these were discussed in detail in Chapters 45 through 48. However, special quantitative measures of the activities of three metabolic systems are exceedingly important in understanding the limits of physical activity.

The Phosphagen System

Adenosine Triphosphate. The basic source of energy for muscle contraction is adenosine triphosphate (ATP), which has the following basic formula.

$$Adenosine—PO_4 \sim PO_3 \sim PO_3$$

The bonds attaching the last two phosphate radicals to the molecule, designated by the symbol ~, are so-called *high energy phosphate bonds*. Each of these bonds stores about 12,000 calories of energy per mole of ATP (under the physical conditions of the body). Therefore, when one phosphate radical is removed from the molecule, 12,000 calories of energy that can

be used to energize the muscle contractile process are released. Then, when the second phosphate radical is removed, still another 12,000 calories become available. Removal of the first phosphate converts the ATP into *adenosine diphosphate* (ADP), and removal of the second converts this ADP into *adenosine monophosphate* (AMP).

Unfortunately, the amount of ATP present in the muscles, even in the well-trained athlete, is sufficient to sustain maximal muscle power for only 5 or 6 seconds, maybe enough for a 50-m dash. Therefore, except for a few seconds at a time, it is essential that new adenosine triphosphate be formed continuously, even during the performance of athletic events. Figure 57–1 illustrates the overall metabolic system, showing the breakdown of ATP first to ADP and then to AMP, with the release of energy to the muscles for contraction. To the left-hand side of the figure are illustrated the three different metabolic mechanisms that are responsible for reconstituting a continuous supply of adenosine triphosphate in the muscle fibers. These are the following:

Release of Energy from Phosphocreatine. Phosphocreatine is another chemical compound that has a high energy phosphate bond, with the following formula:

$$Creatine \sim PO_3$$

This can decompose to *creatine* and *phosphate ion*, as illustrated to the left in Figure 57–1, and in doing so releases large amounts of energy. In fact, the high-energy phosphate bond of phosphocreatine has slightly more energy than the bond of ATP. Therefore, the phosphocreatine can easily provide enough energy to reconstitute the high-energy bonds of the ATP. Furthermore, most muscle cells have two to three times as much phosphocreatine as ATP.

A special characteristic of energy transfer from phosphocreatine to ATP is that it occurs within a small fraction of a second. Therefore, in effect, all the energy stored in the muscle phosphocreatine is instantaneously available for muscle contraction, just as is the energy stored in the ATP.

The cell phosphocreatine plus its ATP are called the *phosphagen energy system*. These together can provide maximal muscle power for a period of 10 to 15 seconds, barely enough for the 100-m run. Thus

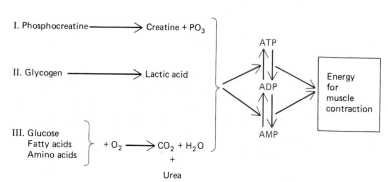

Figure 57–1. The three important metabolic systems that supply energy for muscle contraction.

the energy from the phosphagen system is used for maximal short bursts of muscle power.

The Glycogen–Lactic Acid System

The stored glycogen in muscle can be split into glucose, and the glucose then can be utilized for energy. The initial stage of this process, called *glycolysis,* occurs entirely without use of oxygen and therefore is said to be *anaerobic metabolism* (see Chapter 45). During glycolysis, each glucose molecule is split into two *pyruvic acid molecules,* and energy is released to form several ATP molecules. Ordinarily, the pyruvic acid then enters the mitochondria of the muscle cells and reacts with oxygen to form still many more ATP molecules. However, when there is insufficient oxygen for this second stage (the oxidative stage) of glucose metabolism to occur, most of the pyruvic acid is converted into *lactic acid,* which then diffuses out of the muscle cells into the interstitial fluid and blood. Therefore, in effect, much of the muscle glycogen becomes lactic acid, but in doing so considerable amounts of adenosine triphosphate are formed entirely without the consumption of oxygen.

Another characteristic of the glycogen–lactic acid system is that it can form ATP molecules about two and one-half times as rapidly as can the oxidative mechanism of the mitochondria. Therefore, when large amounts of adenosine triphosphate are required for moderate periods of muscle contraction, this anaerobic glycolysis mechanism can be used as a rapid source of energy. It is not as rapid as the phosphagen system but is about half as rapid.

Under optimal conditions the glycogen–lactic acid system can provide 30 to 40 seconds of excess muscle activity in addition to the 10 to 15 seconds provided by the phosphagen system.

The Aerobic System

The aerobic system means the oxidation of foodstuffs in the mitochondria to provide energy. That is, as illustrated to the left in Figure 57–1, glucose, fatty acids, and amino acids from the foods—after some intermediate processing—combine with oxygen to release tremendous amounts of energy that are used to convert AMP and ADP into ATP, as was discussed in Chapter 45.

In comparing this aerobic mechanism of energy supply with the glycogen–lactic acid system and the phosphagen system, the relative maximum rates of power generation in terms of ATP utilization are the following:

Aerobic system	1 M of ATP per minute
Glycogen–lactic acid system	2.5 M of ATP per minute
Phosphagen system	4 M of ATP per minute

On the other hand, when comparing the systems for endurance, the relative values are the following:

Phosphagen system	10 to 15 seconds
Glycogen–lactic acid system	30 to 40 seconds
Aerobic system	unlimited time (as long as nutrients last)

Thus, one can readily see that the phosphagen system is the one utilized by the muscle for power surges, and the aerobic system is required for prolonged athletic activity. In between is the glycogen–lactic acid system, which is especially important for giving extra power during such intermediate races as the 200- to 800-m runs.

What Types of Sports Utilize Which Energy Systems?

By considering the vigor of a sports activity and its duration, one can estimate very closely which of the energy systems are used for each activity. The following are various approximations.

Almost Entirely Phosphagen System
100-m dash
Jumping
Weight lifting
Diving
Football dashes
    Phosphagen and Glycogen–Lactic Acid Systems
200-m dash
Basketball
Baseball home run
Ice hockey
    Mainly Glycogen–Lactic Acid System
400-m dash
100-m swim
Tennis
Soccer
    Glycogen–Lactic Acid and Aerobic Systems
800-m dash
200-m swim
1500-m skating
Boxing
2000-m rowing
1500-m run
1-mi run
400-m swim
    Aerobic System
10,000-m skating
Cross-country running
Marathon run (26.2 mi, 42.2 km)
Jogging

Recovery of the Muscle Metabolic Systems After Exercise

Performance in athletic events is often determined by how rapidly the athlete can recover strength between surges of activity, and in general this means how rapidly the energy systems can recover. Each of these systems has its own characteristic rate of recovery, as follows:

The Phosphagen System. The total amount of energy in the phosphagen system in all the musculature of the well-trained male athlete's body is equivalent to about 0.6 M of ATP (about 0.3 M for the female), and this can be almost completely depleted in an average of 10 to 15 seconds of maximal muscle activity. However, the glycogen–lactic acid system can replenish this phosphagen system as rapidly as 2.5 M of ATP per minute, and the aerobic system can replenish it as rapidly as 1 M per minute. Therefore, in theory, it would be possible for these other energy systems to replenish fully the phosphagen system within 15 to 30 seconds after its full depletion, which would mean that a person could run a second 100-m dash in less than 1 minute after the first. However, in practice, this does not work quite that way because the other systems function at full force to replenish the phosphagen only when the phosphagen system is almost totally depleted. Instead, the phosphagen normally is replenished with a *half-time* of about 20 to 30 seconds. This means that for those events using the phosphagen system alone, such as high jumping, one could reasonably expect to have full replenishment of this system within about 3 to 5 minutes.

The Glycogen–Lactic Acid System. The limitation in the use of this system for energy is mainly the amount of lactic acid that the person can tolerate in his muscles and body fluids. Lactic acid causes extreme *fatigue,* which serves as a self limitation to further use of this system for energy. The amount of time required for replenishing this system, therefore, is determined by how rapidly the person can eliminate lactic acid from his body. Under most conditions, this is achieved with a half-time of about 20 to 30 minutes; therefore, as long as an hour after an athletic event has utilized the glycogen–lactic acid system to its fullest extent, this metabolic system still will not have achieved full recovery.

The Aerobic System—Short-Term Recovery and the Oxygen Debt. Recovery of the aerobic system has a short-term phase and a long-term phase, one lasting about an hour and the other several days. The short-term phase of recovery is a function of the so-called *oxygen debt,* illustrated in Figure 57–2. The oxygen debt is defined as the extra amount of oxygen that must be taken into the body after an athletic event to restore all the metabolic systems back to their full normal state. Oxygen debt can be accumulated in two different ways: First, part of this debt results from usage of oxygen that is already stored in different parts of the body. For instance, even normally about 0.3 liter of oxygen is stored in the muscles themselves combined with myoglobin, an oxygen-binding chemical substance similar to hemoglobin that is present in muscle fibers. In addition, almost 1 liter of oxygen is normally combined with all the hemoglobin in the blood, and another 0.5 liter is in the air of the lungs as well about 0.25 liter dissolved in all the body fluids. Most of this oxygen can be used by the muscles during exercise and therefore must be replenished after the exercise is over.

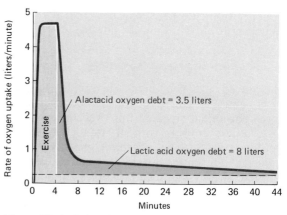

Figure 57–2. Rate of oxygen uptake by the lungs during maximal exercise for 4 minutes and then for almost 1 hour after the exercise is over. This figure demonstrates the principle of *oxygen debt.*

Second, oxygen debt can be accumulated by depletion of both the phosphagen and the glycogen–lactic acid systems. As much as 2 liters of oxygen are required to replenish a fully depleted phosphagen system, and as much as 8 liters to replenish a depleted glycogen–lactic acid system.

In toto, a person can develop an oxygen debt up to 10 to 12 liters, and this oxygen is repaid to the body for as long as an hour or more after periods of exhaustive exercise. Figure 57–2 illustrates that the repayment occurs in two different stages. First, that portion of the debt not related to the accumulation of lactic acid, called *alact-acid oxygen debt,* which means the oxygen needed to replenish the oxygen stores of the body as well as to replenish the phosphagen system, is usually fully repaid within 2 to 3 minutes. On the other hand, removal of the lactic acid from all the body fluids requires an hour or more, so that the *lactic acid oxygen debt,* which is usually by far the greater proportion of the total debt, continues to be repaid very slowly for at least an hour. Therefore, for those sports that deplete the glycogen–lactic acid metabolic system, one should allow for full recovery at least an hour and preferably 2 hours between events.

The mechanism of recovery of the glycogen–lactic acid system is simply to remove the lactic acid from the blood and other body fluids. This is achieved in two ways: First, some of the lactic acid is converted back into pyruvic acid and then metabolized directly by all the body tissues. Second, much of the lactic acid is converted into glucose by the liver, and the glucose in turn is used mainly to replenish the glycogen stores of the muscles.

The Aerobic System—Long-Term Recovery; Importance of Muscle Glycogen. Earlier in the chapter we discussed the importance of stored muscle glycogen for muscle endurance. This is true because glycogen is the food substrate of choice not only for the glycogen–lactic acid system but also for the aerobic oxidative energy system as well. The muscle endurance that can be achieved may be as long as 4 hours of exhaustive exercise in the athlete who has a high

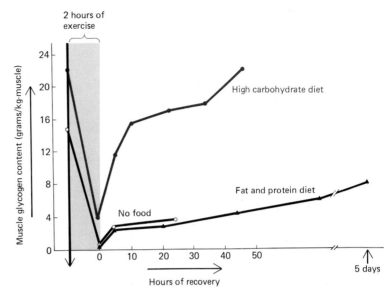

Figure 57–3. Effect of diet on the rate of muscle glycogen replenishment following prolonged exercise. (Reprinted from Fox: Sports Physiology. Philadelphia, Saunders College Publishing, 1979.)

concentration of muscle glycogen, or as little as 1.5 hours in the athlete with minimal muscle glycogen.

Recovery from exhaustive muscle glycogen depletion is not a simple matter, requiring hours to days rather than the seconds or minutes required for the phosphagen and glycogen–lactic acid metabolic systems. Figure 57–3 illustrates this recovery process under three different conditions: first, in persons on a high carbohydrate diet; second, in persons on a high fat/high protein diet; and, third, in persons with no food. Note that on the high carbohydrate diet, full-recovery occurred in approximately 2 days, whereas persons on the high fat/high protein diet or on no food at all showed extremely little recovery even after periods as long as 5 days. The message of this study is that it is important for an athlete not to participate in exhaustive exercise during the last 24 to 48 hours prior to a grueling athletic event.

Nutrients Used During Muscle Activity

Though we have emphasized the importance of a high carbohydrate diet and large stores of muscle glycogen for maximal athletic performance, this does not mean that only carbohydrates are used for muscle energy—it means simply that carbohydrates are used by preference. Actually, the muscles often use large amounts of fat in the form of *fatty acids* and *aceto-acetic acid* for energy (see Chapter 46) and also use to a much less extent proteins in the form of *amino acids*. In fact, even under the best conditions, in those endurance athletic events that last longer than 4 to 5 hours, the glycogen stores of the muscle become depleted and are then of little further use for energizing muscle contraction. Instead, the muscle now depends upon glucose that can be absorbed from the blood, which is limited, or upon energy from other sources, mainly from fats.

Figure 57–4 illustrates the approximate relative usage of carbohydrates and fat for energy during

prolonged exhaustive exercise under three different dietary conditions: high carbohydrate diet, mixed diet, and high fat diet. Note that most of the energy is derived from carbohydrate during the first few seconds or minutes of the exercise, but at the time of exhaustion, as much as 50 to 80 per cent of the energy is being derived from fats rather than carbohydrates.

Not all of the energy from carbohydrates comes from the stored muscle glycogen. In many persons almost as much glycogen is stored in the liver as in the muscles, and this can be released into the blood in the form of glucose, then taken up by the muscles as an energy source. In addition, glucose solutions given to an athlete to drink during the course of an athletic event (in optimal concentrations of 2 to 2.5 per cent) can provide as much as 30 to 40 per cent of the energy required during the event.

In essence, then, if muscle glycogen and blood glucose are available, these are the energy nutrients

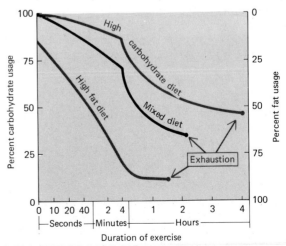

Figure 57–4. Effect of duration of exercise as well as type of diet on relative percentages of carbohydrate or fat used for energy by muscles. (Based partly on data in Fox: Sports Physiology. Philadelphia, Saunders College Publishing, 1979.)

of choice for intense muscle activity. Yet, even so, for a real endurance event one can expect fat to supply more than 50 per cent of the required energy after about the first 3 to 4 hours.

Effect of Athletic Training on Muscles and Muscle Performance

Importance of Resistance Training. One of the cardinal principles of muscle development during athletic training is the following: Muscles that function under no load, even if they are exercised for hours upon end, increase little in strength. At the other extreme, muscles that contract at or near their maximal force of contraction will develop strength very rapidly even if the contractions are performed only a few times each day. Utilizing this principle, experiments on muscle building have shown that 6 maximal or nearly maximal muscle contractions performed in three separate sets 3 days out of each week gives approximately optimal increase in muscle strength and without producing chronic muscle fatigue. The upper curve in Figure 57–5 illustrates the approximate percentage increase in strength that can be achieved in the previously untrained person by this optimal resistive training program, showing that the muscle strength increases about 30 per cent during the first 6 to 8 weeks but reaches a plateau after that time. Along with this increase in strength is approximately an equal percentage increase in muscle mass, which is called *muscle hypertrophy*.

Muscle Hypertrophy. The basic size of a person's muscles is determined mainly by heredity plus the level of testosterone secretion, which, in the male, causes considerably larger muscles than in the female. However, with training, the muscles can be hypertrophied perhaps an additional 30 to 60 per cent. Most of this hypertrophy results from increased diameter of the muscle fibers, but this is not entirely true, because greatly enlarged muscle fibers can split down the middle along their entire length to form entirely new fibers, thus increasing the numbers of fibers as well.

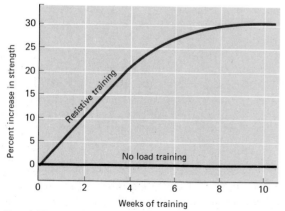

Figure 57–5. Approximate effect of optimal resistive exercise training on increase in muscle strength over a training period of 10 weeks.

The changes that occur inside the hypertrophied muscle fibers themselves include (1) increased numbers of myofibrils, proportionate to the degree of hypertrophy; (2) increased numbers and sizes of mitochondria; (3) as much as 25 to 40 per cent increase in the components of the phosphagen metabolic system, including both ATP and phosphocreatine, (4) as much as 100 per cent increase in stored glycogen, and (5) as much as 75 to 100 per cent increase in stored triglyceride (fat). In addition, the enzymes required for the oxidative metabolic system are increased, increasing the maximum oxidation rate and efficiency of the oxidative metabolic system as much as 45 per cent.

Fast Twitch and Slow Twitch Muscle Fibers

In the human being, all muscles have varying percentages of *fast twitch* and *slow twitch muscle fibers*. For instance, the gastrocnemius muscle has a higher preponderance of fast twitch fibers, which gives it the capability of very forceful and rapid contraction of the type used in jumping. On the other hand, the soleus muscle has a higher preponderance of slow twitch muscle fibers and therefore is said to be the muscle that is used to a greater extent for prolonged lower leg muscle activity.

The basic differences between the fast twitch and the slow twitch fibers are the following:

1. Fast twitch fibers are about two times as large in diameter.

2. The enzymes that promote rapid release of energy from the phosphagen and glycogen-lactic acid energy systems are two to three times as active in fast twitch fibers as in slow twitch fibers, thus making the maximal power that can be achieved by fast twitch fibers as great as two times that of slow twitch fibers.

3. Slow twitch fibers are mainly organized for endurance, especially for generation of aerobic energy. They have far more mitochondria than the fast twitch fibers. In addition, they contain considerably more myoglobin, a hemoglobin-like protein that combines with oxygen within the muscle fiber; and even more important, myoglobin increases the rate of diffusion of oxygen throughout the fiber by shuttling oxygen from one molecule of myoglobin to the next. In addition, the enzymes of the aerobic metabolic system are considerably more active in slow twitch fibers than in fast twitch fibers.

4. The number of capillaries per mass of fibers is greater in the vicinity of slow twitch fibers than in the vicinity of fast twitch fibers.

In summary, fast twitch fibers can deliver extreme amounts of power for short periods of time. On the other hand, slow twitch fibers provide endurance, delivering prolonged strength of contraction over much longer periods of time.

Hereditary Differences Among Athletes for Fast Twitch Versus Slow Twitch Muscle Fibers. Some persons have considerably more fast twitch than slow twitch fibers, and others have more slow twitch fibers; this obviously could determine to some extent the athletic capabilities of different individuals. Unfortunately, athletic training has not been shown to change the relative proportions of fast twitch and slow twitch fibers, however much an athlete might wish to develop one type of athletic prowess over another. Instead, this is an aspect of genetic inheritance that helps to determine which of athletics is most suited to each person; some people are born to be marathoners; others are born to be sprinters and jumpers. For example, the following are recorded percentages of fast twitch versus slow twitch fibers in the quadriceps muscles of different types of athletes:

	Fast Twitch	*Slow Twitch*
Marathoners	18	82
Swimmers	26	74
Average Male	55	45
Weight Lifters	55	45
Sprinters	63	37
Jumpers	63	37

RESPIRATION IN EXERCISE

Though one's respiratory ability is of relatively little concern for the performance of sprint types of athletics, it is critical for maximal performance in endurance athletics. Let us see how important it is:

Oxygen Consumption and Pulmonary Ventilation in Exercise. Normal oxygen consumption for a young adult male at rest is about 250 ml per minute. However, under maximal conditions this can be increased to approximately the following average levels:

Untrained average male	3600 ml per minute
Athletically trained average male	4000 ml per minute
Male marathon runners	5100 ml per minute

Figure 57–6 illustrates the relationship between oxygen consumption at different degrees of exercise and *total pulmonary ventilation*. It is clear from this figure, as would be expected, that there is a linear

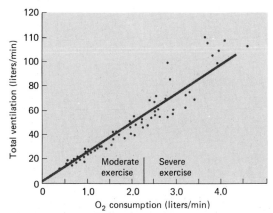

Figure 57–6. Effect of exercise on oxygen consumption and ventilatory rate. (From Gray: Pulmonary Ventilation and Its Physiological Regulation. Charles C Thomas, Publisher, Springfield, Ill.)

relationship. In round numbers, both oxygen consumption and total pulmonary ventilation increase about 20-fold between the resting state and maximum intensity of exercise.

The Limits of Pulmonary Ventilation. How severely do we stress our respiratory system during exercise? This can be answered by the following comparison for the normal male:

Pulmonary ventilation at maximal exercise	100 to 110 L per minute
Maximal breathing capacity	150 to 170 L per minute

Thus, the maximal breathing capacity is about 50 percent greater than the actual pulmonary ventilation during maximal exercise. This obviously provides an element of safety for the athlete, giving extra ventilation that can be called on in such conditions as (1) exercise at high altitudes, (2) exercise under very hot conditions, and (3) abnormalities in the respiratory system.

The important point is that the respiratory system is not normally the most limiting factor in the delivery of oxygen to the muscles during maximal muscle aerobic metabolism. We shall see shortly that the ability of the heart to pump blood to the muscles is a much greater limiting factor.

Effect of Training on $\dot{V}_{O_2}$ Max. The abbreviation for the rate of oxygen usage under maximal aerobic metabolism is $\dot{V}_{O_2}$ Max. Figure 57–7 illustrates the progressive effect of athletic training on $\dot{V}_{O_2}$ Max recorded in a group of subjects beginning at the level of no training and then pursuing the training program for 7 to 13 weeks. In this study, it is surprising that the $\dot{V}_{O_2}$ Max increased only about 10 per cent. Furthermore, the frequency of training, whether two times or five times per week, made little difference on the increase in $\dot{V}_{O_2}$ Max. Yet, as was pointed out earlier, the $\dot{V}_{O_2}$ Max of marathoners is about 45 per cent greater than that of the untrained person. Part of this greater $\dot{V}_{O_2}$ Max of the marathoner is genetically determined; that is, it is those persons who have greater chest sizes and stronger respiratory muscles who select themselves to become marathoners. However, it is also very likely that the very prolonged training of the marathoner does increase the $\dot{V}_{O_2}$ Max by values considerably greater than the 10 per cent that has been recorded in short-term experiments such as that in Figure 57–7.

The O_2 Diffusing Capacity of Athletes. The O_2 *diffusing capacity* is a measure of the rate at which oxygen can diffuse from the alveoli into the blood. This is expressed in terms of *milliliters of oxygen that will diffuse for each millimeter of mercury difference between alveolar partial pressure of oxygen and pulmonary blood oxygen pressure.* That is, if the partial pressure of oxygen in the alveoli is 91 mm Hg while the pressure in the blood is 90 mm Hg, the amount of oxygen that diffuses through the respiratory membrane each minute is the diffusing capacity. The following are measured values for different diffusing capacities:

Nonathlete at rest	23 ml per minute
Nonathlete during maximum exercise	48 ml per minute
Speed skaters during maximum exercise	64 ml per minute
Swimmers during maximum exercise	71 ml per minute
Oarsmen during maximum exercise	80 ml per minute

The most startling fact about these results is the almost threefold increase in diffusing capacity between the resting state and the state of maximum exercise. This results from the fact that blood flow through many of the pulmonary capillaries is very sluggish or even dormant in the resting state, whereas in exercise increased blood flow through the lungs causes all of the pulmonary capillaries to be perfused at their maximum level, thus providing far greater surface area through which oxygen can diffuse into the pulmonary capillary blood.

It is also clear from the above values that those athletes who require greater amounts of oxygen per minute have higher diffusing capacities. Is this because persons with naturally greater diffusing capacities choose these types of sports, or is it because something about the training procedures increases the diffusing capacity? The answer to this is not known, but one must believe that training does play some role in this, particularly the endurance types of training.

The Blood Gases During Exercise. Because of the great usage of oxygen by the muscles in exercise, one would expect the oxygen pressure of the arterial blood to decrease markedly during exercise and the carbon dioxide pressure of the venous blood to increase far above normal. However, this is not the case. Both of these remain nearly normal, illustrating the extreme ability of the respiratory system to provide very adequate aeration of the blood even in heavy exercise. This illustrates another very important point. The blood gases do not have to become abnormal for respiration to be stimulated in exercise. Instead, respiration is stimulated mainly by neurogenic mechanisms. Part of this stimulation results from direct stimulation of the respiratory center by the same nervous signals that are transmitted from the brain to the muscles to cause the exercise. And another part is believed to result from sensory signals transmitted into the respiratory center from the contracting muscles and moving joints. All this nervous stimulation of respiration is normally sufficient to provide almost exactly the proper increase in pulmonary ventilation to keep the blood respiratory gases—the oxygen and the carbon dioxide—almost normal.

Effect of Smoking on Pulmonary Ventilation in Exercise. It is widely stated that smoking can decrease an athlete's "wind." This is a very true statement for many reasons. First, one effect of nicotine is to cause constriction of the terminal bronchioles of the lungs, which increases the resistance to air flow into and out of the lungs. Second, the irritating effects of smoke cause increased fluid secretion in the bronchial tree as well as some swelling of the epithelial linings. Third, nicotine paralyzes the cilia on the surfaces of the respiratory epithelial cells that normally beat continuously to remove excess fluids and foreign particles. As a result, much debris accumulates in the respiratory passageways and adds further to the difficulty of breathing. Putting all these factors together, even the light smoker will feel respiratory strain during maximal exercise, and the level of performance obviously may be reduced.

Much more severe are the effects of chronic smoking, because there is hardly any chronic smoker who does not eventually develop some degree of emphysema. In this disease, the following occur: (1) chronic bronchitis, (2) obstruction of many of the terminal bronchioles, and (3) destruction of many alveolar walls. In severe emphysema, as much as four fifths of the respiratory membrane can be destroyed; then even the slightest exercise can cause respiratory distress. In fact, many such patients cannot even perform the athletic feat of walking across the floor of a single room without gasping for breath. Such is the indictment of smoking.

THE CARDIOVASCULAR SYSTEM IN EXERCISE

Muscle Blood Flow. The final common denominator of cardiovascular function in exercise is to deliver oxygen and other nutrients to the muscles. For this purpose, the muscle blood flow increases drastically during exercise. Figure 57–8 illustrates a recording of muscle blood flow in the leg calf of a person for a period of 6 minutes during strong intermittent contraction. Note the great increase in flow—about 13-fold—but note also that the flow decreased during each muscle contraction. There are two points that can be made from this study: (1) The actual contractile process itself temporarily decreases muscle blood flow because the contracting muscle compresses the intramuscular blood vessels; therefore, strong tonic contractions can cause rapid muscle fatigue because of lack of delivery of enough oxygen and nutrients during the continuous contraction. (2) The blood flow to muscles during exercise can increase markedly.

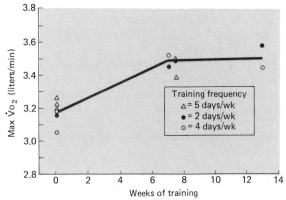

Figure 57–7. Increase in $\dot{V}_{O_2}$ Max over a period of 7 to 13 weeks of athletic training. (Reprinted from Fox: Sports Physiology. Philadelphia, Saunders College Publishing, 1979.)

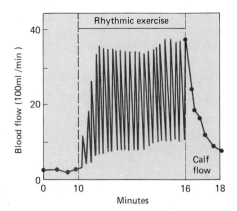

Figure 57–8. Effects of muscle exercise on blood flow in the calf of a leg during strong rhythmic contraction. The blood flow was much less during contraction than between contractions. (From Barcroft and Dornhorst: J Physiol 109:402, 1949.)

The following comparison illustrates the maximum increase in blood flow that can occur in the well-trained athlete:

Resting blood flow	3.6 ml per 100 g of muscle per minute
Blood flow during maximal exercise	90 ml per 100 g of muscle per minute

Thus, muscle blood flow can increase a maximum of about 25-fold during the most strenuous exercise. About half of this increase in flow results from intramuscular vasodilation caused by the direct effects of increased muscle metabolism, as was explained in Chapter 13. The other half results from multiple factors, the most important of which is probably the moderate increase in arterial blood pressure that occurs in exercise, usually about a 30 per cent increase. The increase in pressure not only forces more blood through the blood vessels, but it also stretches the walls of the arterioles and further reduces the vascular resistance. Therefore, a 30 per cent increase in blood pressure can often more than double the blood flow—in addition to the great increase in flow already caused by the metabolic vasodilation.

Work Output, Oxygen Consumption, and Cardiac Output During Exercise. Figure 57–9 illustrates the interrelationships between work output, oxygen consumption, and cardiac output during exercise. It is not surprising that all of these are directly related to each other, as shown by the linear functions, because the muscle work output increases oxygen consumption, and oxygen consumption in turn dilates the muscle blood vessels, thus increasing venous return and cardiac output. Typical cardiac outputs at several levels of exercise are the following:

Average young adult male at rest	5.5 L per minute
Maximum output during exercise in young untrained male	23 L per minute
Maximum output during exercise in male marathoner	30 L per minute

Thus the normal untrained person can increase his or her cardiac output a little over fourfold, and the

well-trained athlete about sixfold. Individual marathoners have been clocked at cardiac outputs as great as 35 to 40 liters per minute.

Effect of Training on Heart Hypertrophy and on Cardiac Output. From the above data, it is clear that marathoners can achieve maximum cardiac outputs about 40 per cent greater than those achieved by the untrained person. This results mainly from the fact that the heart chambers of marathoners enlarge about 40 per cent, and, along with enlargement of the chambers, the heart mass enlarges 40 per cent or more as well. Therefore, it is not only the skeletal muscles but also the heart that hypertrophy during athletic training. However, heart enlargement and increased pumping capacity occur only in the endurance types, not in the sprint types, of athletic training.

Even though the heart of the marathoner is considerably larger than that of the normal person, his resting cardiac output is almost exactly the same as in the normal person. However, this normal cardiac output is achieved by a large stroke volume at a reduced heart rate. Comparisons between the untrained person and the marathoner are the following:

		Stroke Volume	Heart Rate
Resting:	untrained	75 ml	75 beats per minute
	trained	105 ml	50 beats per minute
Maximum:	untrained	110 ml	195 beats per minute
	trained	162 ml	185 beats per minute

Thus, the heart pumping effectiveness of each heart beat is 40 to 50 per cent greater in the highly trained athlete than in the untrained person, but there is a corresponding decrease in heart rate at rest.

Role of Stroke Volume and Heart Rate in Increasing the Cardiac Output. Figure 57–10 illustrates the approximate changes in stroke volume and heart rate as the cardiac output increases from its resting level of about 5.5 liters per minute to 30 liters per minute in the marathon runner. The *stroke volume* increases from 105 ml to 162 ml, an increase of about 50 per

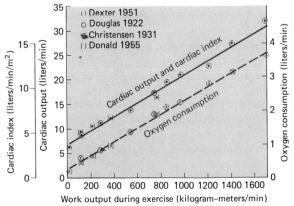

Figure 57–9. Relationship between cardiac output and work output (solid line) and between oxygen consumption and work output (dashed line) during different levels of exercise. (From Guyton, Jones, and Coleman: Circulatory Physiology: Cardiac Output and Its Regulation. Philadelphia, W. B. Saunders Company, 1973.)

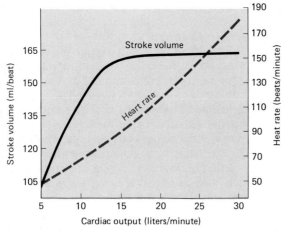

Figure 57–10. Approximate stroke volume output and heart rate at different levels of cardiac output in a marathon athlete.

cent, while the heart rate increases from 50 to 185 beats per minute, an increase of 270 per cent. Therefore, the heart rate increase accounts for by far the greater proportion of the increase in cardiac output than does the increase in stroke volume during strenuous exercise. The stroke volume reaches its maximum by the time the cardiac output has increased only halfway to its maximum. Any further increase in cardiac output must occur by increasing the heart rate.

Relationship of Cardiovascular Performance to V_{O_2} Max. During maximal exercise, both the heart rate and the stroke volume are increased to about 95 per cent of their maximal levels. Since the cardiac output is equal to stroke volume *times* heart rate, one finds that the cardiac output is about 90 per cent of the maximum that the person can achieve. This is in contrast to about 65 per cent of maximum for pulmonary ventilation. Therefore, one can readily see that the cardiovascular system is normally much more limiting on $\dot{V}_{O_2}$ Max than is the respiratory system. For this reason, it is frequently stated that the performance that can be achieved by the marathoner is mainly dependent on his heart, for this is the most limiting link in the delivery of adequate oxygen to the exercising muscles. Therefore, the 40 per cent advantage in maximum cardiac output that the marathoner has over the average untrained male is probably the most important physiological benefit of the marathoner's training program.

Effect of Heart Disease and Old Age on Athletic Performance. Because of the critical limitation that the cardiovascular system places on maximal performance in endurance athletics, one can readily understand that any type of heart disease that reduces the maximum cardiac output will cause an almost corresponding decrease in achievable muscle power. Therefore, a person with congestive heart failure frequently has difficulty achieving even the muscle power required to climb out of bed, much less to walk across the floor.

The maximum cardiac outputs of older persons also decrease considerably—as much as 50 per cent decrease between the teens and the age of eighty. Again, one finds that the maximum achievable muscle power is greatly reduced.

BODY HEAT IN EXERCISE

Almost all the energy released by the cellular metabolism of nutrients is eventually converted into body heat. This even applies to the energy that causes muscle contraction, for the following reasons: First, the maximum efficiency for conversion of nutrient energy into muscle work, even under the best of conditions, is only 20 to 25 per cent; the remainder of the nutrient energy is converted into heat during the course of the intracellular chemical reactions. Second, almost all of the energy that does go into creating muscle work still becomes body heat because all but a small portion of this energy is used for (1) overcoming viscous resistance to the movement of the muscles and joints, (2) overcoming the friction of the blood flowing through the blood vessels, and (3) other similar effects—all of which convert the muscle contractile energy into heat.

Now, recognizing that the oxygen consumption by the body can increase as much as 20- to 25-fold in the well-trained athlete and that the amount of heat liberated in the body is directly proportional to the oxygen consumption (as discussed in Chapter 47), one quickly realizes that tremendous amounts of heat are injected into the internal body during endurance athletic events.

Next, if this vast rate of heat flow into the body occurs on a very hot and humid day, so that the sweating mechanism cannot eliminate the heat, the athlete can easily develop an intolerable and even lethal situation called *heat stroke*.

Heat Stroke. During endurance athletics even under normal environmental conditions, the body temperature often rises from its normal level of 98.6°F to 102 to 103°F (37°C to 40°C). But, with very hot and humid conditions or great excesses of athletic clothing, the body temperature can then easily rise as high as 106 to 108°F. At this level the elevated temperature itself becomes destructive to tissue cells, especially to brain cells. When this happens, multiple symptoms begin to appear, including

1. Extreme weakness
2. Exhaustion
3. Headache
4. Dizziness
5. Nausea
6. Profuse sweating
7. Confusion
8. Staggering gait
9. Collapse
10. Unconsciousness

This whole complex is called heat stroke, and failure to treat it immediately can lead to death. In fact, even though the person has stopped the exercise, the temperature does not easily decrease by itself. One of the reasons is that at these high temperatures the temperature-regulating mechanism itself often fails. A second reason is that the high temperature approximately doubles the rates of all intracellular chemical reactions, thus liberating still more heat.

The treatment of heat stroke is to reduce the body temperature as rapidly as possible. The most practical way to do this is to remove all clothing, to maintain a spray of water on all surfaces of the body or continually to sponge the body, and to blow air over the body with a strong fan. Experiments have shown that these measures can reduce the temperature either as rapidly or almost as rapidly as any other procedure, though some physicians prefer total immersion of the body in ice water containing a mush of crushed ice if this could possibly be available.

BODY FLUIDS AND SALT IN EXERCISE

As much as 5- to 10-lb weight loss has been recorded in athletes in a period of 1 hour during endurance athletic events under hot and humid conditions. Essentially all of this weight loss results from loss of sweat. Loss of enough sweat to decrease body weight only 3 per cent can significantly diminish a person's performance, and 5 to 10 per cent rapid decrease in weight in this way can often be very serious, leading to muscle cramps, nausea, and other effects. Therefore, it is essential to replace fluid as it is lost.

Replacement of Salt and Potassium. Sweat contains a large amount of salt, for which reason it has long been stated that all athletes should take salt tablets when performing exercise on hot and humid days. Unfortunately, overuse of salt tablets has often led to more harm than good. Furthermore, if an athlete becomes acclimatized to the heat by progressive increase in athletic exposure over a period of 1 to 2 weeks rather than by performing maximal athletic feats on the first day, the sweat glands will also become acclimatized, so that the amount of salt lost in the sweat is only a small fraction of that prior to acclimatization. This sweat gland acclimatization results mainly from increased aldosterone secretion by the adrenal cortex. The aldosterone in turn has a direct effect on the sweat glands to increase the reabsorption of sodium chloride from the sweat before it issues onto the surface of the skin. Once the athlete is acclimatized to heat, only rarely do salt supplements need to be considered during athletic events.

On the other hand, recent experience by armed forces suddenly exposed to heavy exercise in the hot desert has demonstrated still another electrolyte problem—the problem of potassium loss. This results partly from the fact that the increased secretion of aldosterone during heat acclimatization increases the loss of potassium in the urine as well as some increase in potassium in the sweat. As a consequence of these new findings, some of the newer supplemental fluids for athletics, usually in the form of fruit juices, are beginning to contain properly proportioned amounts of potassium.

DRUGS AND ATHLETES

Without belaboring this issue, let us list some of the effects of drugs in athletics:

First, *caffeine* can increase athletic performance. In one experiment on a marathon runner, his running time for the marathon was reduced by 7 per cent by judicious use of caffeine in amounts similar to those found in a cup or so of coffee.

Second, use of *male sex hormones (androgens)* to increase muscle strength probably can increase athletic performance under some conditions, especially in women and in those men who are poorly endowed with normal testosterone secretion. Unfortunately, some of the synthetic testosterone analog preparations can cause liver damage, and, in men, any type of male sex hormone preparation can lead to decreased testicular function, including both decreased formation of sperm and decreased secretion of the person's own natural testosterone. In a woman, even more dire effects can occur because she is not normally adapted to the male sex hormone.

Other drugs, such as *amphetamines* and *cocaine*, have been reputed to increase one's athletic performance. However, it is equally true that overuse of these drugs can lead to deterioration of performance. Furthermore, actual experiments have failed to prove the value of such drugs. Some athletes have been known to die during athletic performance because of interaction between such drugs and the norepinephrine and epinephrine released by the sympathetic nervous system during exercise. One of the causes of death under these conditions is overexcitability of the heart, leading to ventricular fibrillation, which is lethal within seconds.

QUESTIONS

1. Discuss the differences between the female and the male athlete.
2. What is the relationship between muscle cross-sectional area and muscle strength?
3. How does muscle power differ from muscle strength?
4. Characterize the three important metabolic systems that supply energy in exercise.
5. Explain the mechanisms for recovery of each of the above three metabolic systems after they are depleted.

6. How do the different nutrients contribute to muscle energy during endurance athletics?
7. Explain the principles of muscle building and the changes in the muscle fibers during muscle hypertrophy.
8. What are the differences between fast twitch and slow twitch fibers?
9. Approximately how much can the untrained person and the trained person increase their rates of oxygen consumption above the resting level during maximum exercise?
10. What are the effects of maximum exercise on blood oxygen and carbon dioxide concentrations? Why do these effects occur?

11. How much can muscle blood flow increase during maximum exercise? What are the causes of this increase?
12. Explain the relationship between work output, oxygen consumption, and cardiac output during exercise.
13. What are the relationships of both respiratory and cardiovascular performance to $\dot{V}_{O_2}$ Max?
14. Discuss the perils of excess body heat during exercise.
15. Discuss the problems of fluid and electrolyte loss during exercise. Discuss their replacement.

References

Adams, G. M.: Exercise Physiology Primer. Costa Mesa, Calif., Custom Publishing Co., 1983.

Alexander, R. M.: Mechanics of skeleton and tendons. In Brooks, V. B., ed.: Handbook of Physiology. Sec. 1, Vol. 2. Bethesda, American Physiological Society, 1981, p. 17.

American Physiological Society: Skeletal Muscle. Baltimore, Waverly Press, 1983.

Blomqvist, C. G., and Saltin, B.: Cardiovascular adaptations to physical training. Annu Rev Physiol 45:169, 1983.

Brengelmann, G. L.: Circulatory adjustments to exercise and heat stress. Annu Rev Physiol 45:191, 1983.

Bye, P. T. P., et al.: Respiratory factors limiting exercise. Annu Rev Physiol 45:439, 1983.

Dohm, G. L., et al.: Protein metabolism during endurance exercise. Fed Proc 44:348, 1985.

Golinick, P. D.: Metabolism of substrates: energy substrate metabolism during exercise and as modified by training. Fed Proc 44:353, 1985.

Guyton, A. C., et al.: Circulatory Physiology: Cardiac Output and Its Regulation. 2nd ed. Philadelphia, W. B. Saunders Company, 1973.

Hockey, R.: Stress and Fatigue in Human Performance. New York, John Wiley & Sons, 1983.

Killian, K. J., and Campbell, E. J. M.: Dyspnea and exercise. Annu Rev Physiol 45:465, 1983.

Lamb, D. R.: Physiology of Exercises. Responses and Adaptations. New York, Macmillan Publishing Co., 1984.

McManus: Cardiovascular Complications of Exercise. Chicago, Year Book Medical Publishers, 1985.

Mitchell, J. H., et al.: The exercise pressor reflex: Its cardiovascular effects, afferent mechanisms, and control pathways. Annu Rev Physiol 45:229, 1983.

Partridge, L. D., and Benton, L. A.: Muscle, the motor. In Brooks, V. B., ed.: Handbook of Physiology. Sec. 1, Vol. 2. Bethesda, American Physiological Society, 1981, p. 43.

Rash, J.: Neuromuscular Atlas. New York, Praeger Publishers, 1984.

Rigotti, N. A., et al.: Exercise and coronary heart disease. Annu Rev Med 34:391, 1983.

Stone, H. L.: Control of the coronary circulation during exercise. Annu Rev Physiol 45:213, 1983.

Index

Note: Numbers in *italics* refer to figures; numbers followed by t refer to tables.

A (anisotropic) bands, 57, *58, 64*
A blood group, 213–214, 213t–214t
AB blood group, 213–214, 213t–214t
Abdomen, muscles of, in labor, 647
Abdominal recti muscles, in breathing, 295
Abdominal spasm, 393
Absorption, by placental membrane, 463
    gastrointestinal. See *Gastrointestinal absorption.*
    in kidney tubules, 249, 252–254, *252,* 255t
    of bone, 609–612, *610,* 614–615
    of calcium, 605–606, 611–612
    of iron, 198
    of minerals, in teeth, 616–617
    of phosphate, 605–606, 611–612
    tubular, aldosterone and, 586–587
Acceleratory forces, 335–336, *336*
    detection of, in vestibular apparatus, 397
Acclimatization, sweating and, 547
    to heat, 547, 667
    to high altitude, 334–335
Accommodation, visual, 449–450, *449–450*
    autonomic nervous system control by, 469–470, *469*
Acetoacetate, reabsorption of, 253
Acetoacetic acid, formation of, 534
    in diabetes mellitus, 285
    in insulin lack, 598–599, *598*
    in muscular activity, 661
Acetone, formation of, 534
    in insulin lack, 598–599
Acetyl CoA carboxylase, 597
Acetyl coenzyme A (acetyl CoA), condensation of, 534
    formation of, 525
        from fatty acid, 533, *534*
        in citric acid cycle, 526, *526*
    in fatty acid formation, 534
    oxidation of, 533
Acetylcholine, as cause of pain, 378
    as neurotransmitter, 349
    cardiac effects of, 93
    coronary blood flow control by, 170
    destruction of, 70, 441
    formation of, in reticular activating system, 427, *427*
    in action potential, 54
    in bronchioles, 300
    in enteric plexus, 488
    in neuromuscular transmission, 69–71, 349
    in sweating, 190
    in transmitter vesicle, 348
    inactivation of, 71. See also *Acetylcholinesterase; Cholinesterase.*

Acetylcholine (*Continued*)
    secretion of, 69–70, 441
        in smooth muscle, 75–76
    synthesis of, 348–349
Acetylcholine channels, 35, 70
Acetylcholine receptors, 442, 442t
Acetylcholinesterase, 69–70, 441
Achlorhydria, 516
Acid, definition of, 280
    fixed, 285
    gastric, 503
        in peptic ulcer, 517
Acid hydrolases, 11
Acid-base balance, 279–280
    abnormalities in, 285–286
    buffers in, 280–281
    in newborn, 652
    renal regulation of, 282–285, *282, 284*
    respiratory regulation of, 281–282, *281*
Acidosis, 279
    buffer systems and, 280
    in diabetes mellitus, 602–603
    in uremia, 287–288
    metabolic, 285–286
    renal correction of, 283
    respiratory, 285
        in deep sea diver, 338
    synaptic transmission effect of, 355
    treatment of, 286
Acini, in salivary gland, 499, *499*
    pancreatic, 503–504, 595, *596*
Acromegaly, 572–573, *573*
Acrosome, 620–621, *620*
ACTH. See *Adrenocorticotropic hormone.*
Actin, in mitosis, 29
    in platelets, 219
Actin filaments, anatomy of, 57–58, *58–59*
    in cardiac muscle, 80, *81*
    in skeletal muscle, 60–63, *60, 62*
    in smooth muscle, 72–73, *73*
    molecular characteristics of, 61, *61*
Action potential(s), 48–52
    at axon hillock, 352
    at node of Ranvier, 365, *365*
    depolarization stage of, 48
    excitation of, 54
    in cardiac muscle, 81–82, *81,* 99, *99*
    in sinoatrial node, 91, *91*
    in skeletal muscle contraction, 60
    in smooth muscle, 73–74, *74*
    initiation of, 50
    monophasic, 73–74, *74,* 99, *99*
    muscle, 63
    neurotransmitter release by, 348
    plateau in, 51–52, *52,* 73–74, *74*
    propagation of, 50–51, *50,* 82

Action potential(s) (*Continued*)
    recording of, *46, 48–50, 52, 54,* 55
    repetitive discharge and, 52, *52*
    repolarization stage of, 48
    resting stage of, 48
    spontaneous generation of, 74, *74*
Action tremor, 410
Activation gate, 48–49, *49*
Activator operator, 26, *26*
Activator protein, 26, *26*
Activator substance, genetic regulation by, 26
Active theory, of sleep, 430
Active transport, 13, 38–40. See also *Pump.*
    energetics of, 40
    in gastrointestinal absorption, 513
    in kidney tubule, 252, *252*
    mechanism of, 39–40, *39*
    membrane potential caused by, *45–46,* 46
    of sodium, 39, *39,* 579
        in kidney, 257–258, *258*
        in small intestine, 514, *514*
    saturation of, 40
    secondary, 40
        carrier proteins in, 40
    through cell membrane, 33, *33,* 38–40, *39–40*
    thyroid hormones and, 579
    vs. diffusion, 33
Acupuncture, 381
Adaptation, of sensory receptors, 365–367, *366*
    of thermal receptors, 384
    to light intensity, 457–458
Addison's disease, 591–592
    potassium concentration and, 277
    salt craving in, 275
Addisonian crisis, 592
Adenine, in ATP, 16
    in DNA, 21, *21–22*
    in RNA, *22,* 23
Adenohypophysis, 570
Adenosine, as vasodilator, 131, 170
    in muscle, 184
Adenosine diphosphate (ADP), ATP formation from, *527,* 528
    formation of, 16
    in actin filaments, 61
    in energy release, 523
    in glycolysis, 528
    in platelets, 219
    oxygen use and, 315, *315*
Adenosine monophosphate (AMP), in energy release, 523

Adenosine triphosphate (ATP), 12
  formation of, by oxidative phosphorylation, 526–528, *527*
    in aerobic system, *658*, 659
    in citric acid cycle, 526
    in glycogen–lactic acid system, *658*, 659
    in glycolysis, 525, *526*
    in lipid metabolism, 533–535, *534–535*
    in phosphagen system, *658*, 658, 660
  formula of, 16, *16*
  function of, 16–17, *17*
  in active transport, 39–40, *39*
  in body fluids, 270t
  in enteric plexus, 488
  in hormone mediation, 566, *567*
  in metabolism, 522–523
  in protein formation, 539
  in red blood cells, 198
  in skeletal muscle contraction, 62
  oxygen use and, 315
Adenyl cyclase, 76, 442, 580
  in hormone mediation, 566–567, *567*
  in water reabsorption, 259
ADH. See *Antidiuretic hormone*.
Adipose cells, insulin and, 597
Adipose tissue, 533
ADP. See *Adenosine diphosphate*.
Adrenal cortex, 585
  atrophy of, 591–592
  hormones of. See *Adrenocortical hormones*.
Adrenal diabetes, 588
Adrenal gland, abnormalities of, in newborn, 653
  androgen secretion by, 624
  blood flow in, 129, 130t
  tumor of, 593
Adrenal medulla, 585
  function of, 444
  sympathetic nerve endings in, 440
Adrenalectomy, in Cushing's syndrome, 593
Adrenergic fibers, 441–442
Adrenergic mediators, 441
Adrenergic receptors, 442, 442t
Adrenocortical hormones, 565, 585–593. See also specific hormone, e.g., *Aldosterone; Epinephrine; Norepinephrine*.
  abnormalities in, 591–592, *592*
  chemistry of, 585–586, *586*
  functions of, glucocorticoids, 588–591, *590–591*
  mineralocorticoids, 586–588
Adrenocorticotropic hormone (ACTH), 565, 587
  in cortisol regulation, 590–591, *590–591*
  in fat utilization, 535
  in gluconeogenesis, 529
Adrenocorticotropin. See *Adrenocorticotropic hormone*.
Aerobic system, *658*, 659–660, *660*, 662
Afferent arterioles, blood flow through, 248–250
  in glomerular filtration rate, 251, 263–264, *264*
Afferent lymphatics, 202, *202*
After-discharge, in crossed extensor reflex, 392
  in flexor reflex, 392
  in neuronal pool, 359–360, *359–360*
Age, arterial pressure and, 139–140, *140*
  athletic performance and, 666
  cardiac output and, 156–157, *157*
  in atherosclerosis, 536

Agglutination, in blood transfusion, 214
  of antigens, 209–210
Agglutinins, 213–214, 213t–214t
Agglutinogens, 213–214, 213t–214t
Agranulocytosis, 204
Air, alveolar, composition of, 306–307, 306t
  oxygen transport from, 311, *311*
  vapor pressure in, 306, 306t
  atmospheric, composition of, 306, 306t
  conditioning of, in nose, 299–300, *299*
  expired, 306t, 307
  humidification of, 306, 306t
  pressure of, 302
Air embolism, in decompression sickness, 339
  in submarine escape, 340
Air hunger, 328
Airplane. See *Aviation physiology*.
Airway, ciliary movement in, 18
  obstruction of, in atelectasis, 327
Airway resistance, 296
  in emphysema, 326
Akinesia, in Parkinson's disease, 406–407
Alactacid oxygen debt, 660, *661*
Alanine, respiratory quotient of, 554
Alarm response, 445
Albino persons, vision in, 455
Albumin, 111
  diffusion of, through capillary pores, 230, 230t
  fatty acid transport with, 532
  formation of, 539
  osmotic pressure of, 234
  radioactive, in blood volume measurement, 268
Alcohol, gastritis from, 516
Alcoholic headache, 383
Aldosterone, 565
  activity of, 586
  cellular, 587
  circulatory system effects of, 587
  deficiency of, 591
  in arterial pressure control, 150, *150–151*
  in cardiac failure, 174
  in heat acclimatization, 547, 667
  in hydrogen ion secretion, 587
  in potassium secretion, 261, 276–277, *276–277*, 586–587
  in protein synthesis, 567
  in sodium absorption, 260, 586–587
  in volume-loading hypertension, 152
  radioimmunoassay of, 568, *568*
  renal effects of, 586–587
  renin-angiotensin system and, 588
  saliva composition and, 499
  secretion of, regulation of, 587–588
  structure of, 585–586, *586*
Aldosteronism, 593
  alkalosis from, 286
  potassium concentration and, 277
Alimentary regulation, 555
Alimentary tract. See also *Gastrointestinal tract*.
  anatomy of, 486, *487*
  food ingestion in, 489–491, *490*
  functions of, 486
  innervation of, 487–488
  layers of, 486–487, *487*
  movements in, 488–489, *489*
    in colon, 494–495, *494–495*
    in small intestine, 493–494, *493–494*
    in stomach, 491–493, *491*
    smooth muscle in, 487
Alkaloids, bitter taste of, 478

Alkalosis, 279
  bicarbonate-to-chloride ratio and, *284*, 285
  buffer systems and, 280
  effects of, 286
  in aldosterone excess, 587
  metabolic, 285–286
  renal correction of, 283
  respiratory, 285
  synaptic transmission effect of, 355
Allergen, 212
Allergy, 212–213. See also *Asthma*.
  basophils and, 204
  eosinophils and, 204
All-or-nothing principle, 51
Alpha efferent fibers, 388
Alpha globulin, 111
Alpha receptors, 442, 442t
Alpha waves, 428–429, *428–429*
Altitude, high, acclimatization to, 334–335
  oxygen pressure at, 332–335
  red blood cell production at, 195
  respiratory control at, 323
Alveolar ventilation, 298–299
  carbon dioxide effects on, 321–323, *321*, *323*
  hydrogen ion concentration and, 281, *281*
  in exercise, 323–324, *323*
  oxygen pressure effects on, 322–323, *323*
Alveoli, air in, composition of, 306–307, 306t, *307*
  vapor pressure in, 305, 306t
  air renewal in, 306, *307*
  carbon dioxide pressure in, 312
  carbon dioxide transport through, 312, *312*
  collapse of, 127. See also *Atelectasis*.
  destruction of, in emphysema, 326, *326*
  dryness of, 242
  edema of, 242
  macrophages in, 202
  opening of, at birth, 650
  oxygen diffusion from, 305–306
  oxygen in, pulmonary blood flow and, 125
  oxygen pressure in, 306, *307*, 311
    vs. altitude, 332–333, 333t
  physiology of, 307–308, *308–310*, 310
  pressure in, 295
Amacrine cells, 463–464, *463*
Ameboid locomotion, of leucocytes, 201
Ameloblasts, 615
Amenorrhea, 637
Amino acid(s), absorption of, 252, 515
  as neurotransmitters, 350
  catabolism of, growth hormone and, 571
  cotransport of, with sodium, 40, 515
  deaminated, in glycogenesis, 524
    oxidation of, 540
  deamination of, 539–540
  energy extraction from, 15–17, *16*
  essential, 539
  in blood, 538
    fetal, 643
  in body fluids, 270t
  in DNA, 22, *23*
  in extracellular fluid, 277
  in feeding regulation, 555
  in gastric secretions, 502
  in glucagon secretion, 601
  in gluconeogenesis, 529
  in muscular activity, 661
  in partial proteins, 554
  in protein digestion, 512, *512*
  insulin secretion and, 600

Amino acid(s) (*Continued*)
  nonessential, 539
  plasma concentration of, 538–539
    insulin and, 599–600
  protein formation from, 539
  reabsorption of, 253
  reaction of, in peptide linkage, 25
  release of, from cells, 538–539
  storage of, 538–539
  structure of, 537–538, *537*
  transamination of, 539–540
  transfer of, to RNA, 23–24, *24*, 24t
  transport of, 538–539
    cortisol effects on, 588–589
    growth hormone and, 571
    insulin in, 599
Ammonia, urea formation from, 540
Ammonia buffer system, bicarbonate-to-
    chloride ratio and, *284*, 285
  hydrogen ion transport by, 284
Ammonium chloride, in alkalosis treat-
    ment, 286
Amnesia, 422–423, 428
Amnion, 642
Amniotic fluid, formation of, 645
  ingestion of, 649
Amorphosynthesis, 373
AMP, in energy release, 523
Amphetamines, in exercise, 667
Amplification, in signal divergence, 357,
    357
  of control systems, 6
Ampulla, in vestibular apparatus, 396
  of vas deferens, 619, 620
Amygdala, behavioral functions of, 435
  in feeding regulation, 554
  in smell, 482
Amygdaloid nucleus, 404
Amyl nitrite, in angina pectoris, 173
Amylase, pancreatic, 503
  in carbohydrate digestion, 511, *511*
  in newborn, 652
Amyloidosis, 289
Anaerobic glycolysis, *526*, 528–529
Anaerobic metabolism, *658*, 659
Anal sphincter, 495, *495*
Analgesic system, of CNS, 380–381, *380*
Anaphase, *28*, 29
Anaphylaxis, 166, 212–213
  slow-reacting substance of, 300
  in asthma, 328
Anastomosis, of coronary arteries, 171, *171*
Anchoring filaments, of lymphatic capillar-
    ics, 238, *238*
Androgens. See also *Testosterone.*
  exercise and, 667
  newborn and, 653
  secretion of, 624
Androsterone, 624
Anemia, aplastic, 199
  cardiac function in, *159*, 160
  circulation effects of, 199
  from hemorrhage, 199
  hemolytic, 199
  hypochromic, 198
  in erythroblastosis fetalis, 215
  megaloblastic, 199
  oxygen therapy in, 329
  pernicious, 196, 199, 516
  red blood cell production stimulation in,
    195
  sickle cell, 199
Anesthesia, respiratory depression in, 325
  spinal, arterial pressure effect of,
    134–135, *135*
  synaptic transmission effect of, 355

Angina pectoris, 172–173
Angiogenesis factor, 133
Angioplasty, coronary, 173
Angiotensin, as vasoconstrictor, 144–146,
    145
  as vasodilator, 136
  hypertension caused by, 152–154, *153*
  in aldosterone secretion, 588
  in arterial pressure control, 150, *150–151*
  in compensated shock, 164
  in Goldblatt's hypertension, 153–154, *154*
  in kidney function, during hypertension,
    263–264
Angiotensin I, 145, *145*
Angiotensin II, 144–145, *145*
Angiotensinase, 145, *145*
Angiotensinogen, 145
Angiotension, in kidney function, during
    hypotension, 263–264
Angular acceleration, 397
Angular gyrus, 418
Annulospiral ending, in muscle spindle, 388
Anovulation, 638
Anterior pituitary gland. See *Pituitary
    gland, anterior.*
Anterolateral system, 370, 375, *375*
  pain transmission in, 379
  sensations transmitted by, 369–370
  vs. dorsal column–lemniscal system,
    369–370
Anthracosis, 127
Antibody(ies), 111
  action of, 209–210, *210*
  formation of, 209–210, *209–210*
  in blood transfusion, 213–214, 213t–214t
  in hyperthyroidism, 582
  in newborn, 653
  in radioimmunoassay, 568
  in saliva, 500
  nature of, 209, *209*
  sensitizing, 212
  specificity of, 208–209, 209
Anticoagulants, 220
  intravascular, 223–224
Anticodons, 23–24, *24*
Antidiuretic hormone, 565
  as vasoconstrictor, 144
  as vasodilator, 136
  fluid volume regulation by, 262
  formation of, 573–574
  function of, 574
  in compensated shock, 164
  in urine concentration, 258–259, *258*
  in urine dilution, 257, *257*
  inappropriate secretion of, 274
  sodium control by, 273–275, *274–275*
Antigen-antibody complex, in glomerular
    membrane, 286–287
Antigens, 207
  in blood transfusion, 213
  lymphocyte activation by, 208–209
  Rh factor, 214–215
  T cell binding of, 210–211
Antigravity muscles, excitation of, 395
Antihemophilic factor, 222
Anti-inflammatory effect, of cortisol,
    589–590
Antipyretics, 551
Antithrombin III, 223
Antithrombin-heparin cofactor, 223
Antrum, in follicular growth, 631
  of stomach, 491–492, *491*
Anxiety, cardiac output in, *159*
Aorta, abnormality of, *180*, 181
  baroreceptors in, 142
  oxygen pressure in, 311

Aorta (*Continued*)
  pressure changes in, in cardiac cycle,
    82–83, *83*
  pressure in, *119*, 119, 124, *124*
    at birth, 651
Aortic area, heart sounds in, 177, *177.*
Aortic bodies, respiratory control by, 322,
    322
Aortic pressure curve, *83*, 85
Aortic regurgitation, 178–179
  pressure pulse in, 123, *123*
Aortic stenosis, 178–179, *178*
Aortic valve, function of, 84–85, *84*
Aortic-coronary bypass, 173
Aphasia, 423
Aplastic anemia, 199
Apneustic center, 320
Apoferritin, 198, *198*
Apotransferrin, 198, *198*
Appetite, 489, 554–555
  for salt, 275
Apraxia, motor, 403
Aqueduct of Sylvius, 434
Aqueous humor, 244, *244*
  refractive index of, 448–449, *448*
Arachnoidal villi, 243, *243*
Arginine, 540
Arousal reaction, 426
Arrest reaction, 435
Arrhythmias, cardiac. See *Cardiac
    arrhythmias.*
Arterial oxygen saturation, in blood flow
    control, 130–132, *131*
Arterial pressure, 119, *119*
  autonomic control of, 444
  bleeding volume and, 163, *163*
  blood volume effect on, 271
  capillary pressure effects of, 232, *232*
  cardiac output and, 141
  centrifugal force effects on, 335
  control of, by atrial reflex, 144
    by baroreceptor reflexes, 141–142,
      142–143
    by capillary fluid shift, 146
    by hormones, 144–146, *145*
    by renal–body fluid system, 147–150,
      148–150, 153, *153*
    by renin-angiotensin system, 150,
      150–151
    by vasoconstrictors, 136
    by vasodilators, 136–137
    by vasomotor center, 143
    cardiac output and, *157*, 158
    fluid volume regulation and, 262, *262*
    long-term, 147–150, *148–151*, 153,
      153
    overall system for, 141
  glomerular filtration effects of, 251
  high. See *Hypertension.*
  hydrostatic effects on, 121
  in acute cardiac stimulation, 160
  in blood flow control, 132, *133*
  in circulatory shock, 162
  in eclampsia, 645
  in exercise, 184–185, 665
  in newborn, 652
  in spinal shock, 393
  mean, 140, *140*
  measurement of, 140–141, *140*
  normal, 139–140, *140*
  peripheral resistance and, 141
  pulmonary, 125–126, *126*
  pulses in, 122–123, *122–123*
  recording of, 113, *113*
  regulation of, 5–6
  spinal anesthesia effect on, 134–135, *135*

Arterial pressure (*Continued*)
  urinary output effect of, 147–150, *148–149*
  vs. cardiac output, 86, *86*
Arterioles, anatomy of, 130, *130*
  blood volume in, *119*
  dilatation of, 136
  function of, 118, 120
  hepatic, 505
  in microcirculation, 228, *229*
  of kidney, 248–249, *249*
    glomerular filtration effects on, 251
  pressure in, 119, *119*
  terminal. See *Metarterioles.*
Arteriosclerosis, 536. See also *Atherosclerosis.*
  in diabetes, 602–603
  in hypothyroidism, 583
Arteriovenous anastomosis, in heat transfer, 548
  in skin, 189–190, *189*
Arteriovenous fistula (shunt), cardiac function in, *159*, 160
Artery(ies), as pressure reservoir, 119–120
  blood volume in, *119*
  coronary. See *Coronary arteries.*
  distensibility of, 116
  function of, 118, 119–120
  hypertension effects on, 155
  pressure-volume curves for, 116, *116*
  pulse pressure in, 122–123, *122–123*
Articulation, 301, 423
Artifacts, in recording action potential, *54*, 55
Arytenoid cartilage, 301, *301*
Ascites, in nephrotic syndrome, 289
  in portal obstruction, 188
  in thiamine deficiency, 558
Ascorbic acid, 557t, 560
  in newborn diet, 653
Aspirin, as antipyretic, 551
  gastritis from, 516
Aster, *28*, 29
Astereognosis, 372
Asthma, 213, 300
  respiratory insufficiency in, 327–328
Astigmatism, 451–452, *451–452*
Astronauts. See *Space physiology.*
Atelectasis, 127
  respiratory insufficiency in, 327
Atherosclerosis. See also *Arteriosclerosis.*
  hypertension and, 155
  ischemic heart disease and, 171
  lipid metabolism and, 536
Athetosis, 406
Athletes. See *Exercise; Sports physiology.*
Atmosphere, artificial, in spacecraft, 336
  in submarine, 340
ATP. See *Adenosine triphosphate.*
ATP synthetase, 16, *527*, 528
ATPase, in myosin head, 61
  in smooth muscle contraction, 75
Atresia, of follicle, 31
Atrial fibrillation, 95, *95*, 104, *104*
  in valvular lesions, 179
Atrial flutter, 95, *95*, 104, *104*
Atrial natriuretic factor, 271–272
Atrial paroxysmal tachycardia, 104, *104*
Atrial premature contractions, 103, *103*
Atrial pressure, heart rate control and, 144
  in cardiac cycle, 82, *83*
  vs. cardiac output, 87, *87*
Atrial syncytium, 81
Atrioventricular block, 94, 102–103, *103*

Atrioventricular bundle, 81, *90*, 91
  block of, 102–103, *103*
  impulse transmission through, 92
Atrioventricular node, anatomy of, 90–91, *90*
  impulse transmission through, *90*, 91–93, *92*
Atrioventricular valves, 84–85, *84*
  sounds of, 177, *177*
Atrium (heart), anatomy of, 82, *82*
  depolarization of, 83, *83*
  hypertrophy of, 179
  impulse transmission through, *90*, 91
  pressure in, 120, 124–125. See also *Central venous pressure.*
  refractory period of, 81
Atrium (respiratory), 307, *309*
Atrophy, gastric, 516
  muscular, 67
Atropine, in bronchiolar obstruction, 300
Attention, 428
  hippocampus and, 436
Attenuation reflex, 473
Auditory association area, 417, *417*, 477, *477*
Auditory cortex, 417, *476-477*, 477–478
Auditory pathway, 476–477, *476*
Auditory receptive aphasia, 423
Auerbach's plexus, 488
Auscultation, in blood pressure measurement, 140–141, *140*
  of heart sounds, 177, *l77*
Autoimmunity, 212
Automaticity, of body, 6
Autonomic nervous system, 345, *345.* See also *Parasympathetic nervous system; Sympathetic nervous system.*
  accommodation control by, 469–470, *469*
  anatomy of, 439–442, *440–441*
  blood flow control by, 133–135, *134–135*
  control of, by brain stem, 445–446, *446*
  coronary blood flow control by, 170–171
  gastrointestinal tract control by, 488
  heart control by, 93–94
  in homeostasis, 4
  psychosomatic disorders and, 435
  pupillary aperture control by, *469*, 470
  reflexes of, 439. See also *Gastrointestinal reflexes; Spinal cord reflexes.*
Autoregulation. See also *Feedback.*
  of arterial pressure, 149–150, *150*
  of blood flow, 132, *133*
    gastrointestinal, 188
    renal, *262*, 263
  of glomerular filtration, 262–263, *262*
Autosomal chromosomes, 641
Aversion, limbic system and, 433–435, *434*
Aviation physiology, acceleratory forces in, 335–336, *336*
  oxygen pressure in, 332–335, *333*, 333t
A-V node. See *Atrioventricular node.*
Axis, electrical, in ECG, 105
Axon, 53, *53*
  in smooth muscle, 75
Axon hillock, *350*, 352
Axon terminals, acetylcholine secretion by, 69–70, *70*
Axoneme, 18–19, 621
Axoplasm, 53, *53*
Azathioprine, 216

B blood group, 213–214, 213t–214t
B cells, 208
  activation of, 209, 211

B cells (*Continued*)
  immune tolerance and, 211–212
  specificity of, 208–209
Baby. See *Infant.*
Backward movement, brain stem control of, 398
Bacteria, in colon, 516
  phagocytosis of. See *Phagocytosis.*
  removal of, in liver, 187
Bacterial enteritis, 508
Bainbridge's reflex, 144
Balance. See *Equilibrium.*
Baldness, 624–625
Bands, in myofibrils, 57–58, *58*, *64*
Baroreceptor reflex, 141–142, *142–143*
  in cardiac failure, 173–174
  in compensated shock, 164
Baroreceptors, adaptation of, 143, *143*
  anatomy of, 141–142, *142*
  arterial pressure regulation by, 5–6
  buffer function of, 142–143, *143*
  in shock compensation, 163
  postural change and, 142
  pressure response of, 142
  reflexes initiated by, 142, *142*
  resetting of, 143
Barrel chest, in asthma, 328
Bartholin's glands, 637
Basal ganglia, functions of, 405–406
  motor functions of, 404–407, *404–405*
  physiological anatomy of, 404–405, *404–405*
Basal metabolic rate, 545
  in hyperthyroidism, 582
  in hypothyroidism, 583
Base. See also *Acid-base balance.*
  definition of, 280
Basilar fibers, 474
Basilar membrane, 473–476, *473–475*
Basophil erythroblast, 195, *195*
Basophil myelocyte, *200*
Basophils, 204
  heparin production by, 223–224
Behavior, body temperature regulation by, 550
  control of, 436–437
Behavior function(s), amygdala in, 435
  hippocampus in, 436
  hypothalamus in, 432–435, *433–434*
  limbic system in, 432–435, *433–434*
  psychosomatic effects and, 435
Belching, 519
Bends, 338–339
Beriberi, 558
  cardiac function in, *159*, 160
Beta globulin, 111
Beta oxidation, of fatty acid, 533, *534*
Beta receptors, 442, 442t
Beta waves, 428–429, *428–429*
Betz cells, giant, 400–401
Bicarbonate. See also *Carbon dioxide; Sodium bicarbonate.*
  concentration of, in urine, 255t
  in alkalosis, 283
  in body fluids, 268, 270t
  in saliva, 499, *499*
  loss of, in diarrhea, 285
  reabsorption of, 254, 282–283, *282*
  reaction of, with hydrogen ion, 283
  removal of, from extracellular fluid, 283
  secretion of, by pancreas, 503–504
    in colon, 516
    in large intestine, 508
Bicarbonate buffer system, 280
Bicarbonate-to-chloride ratio, 284–285, *284*

Bifocals, 450
Bile, secretion of, 505–507, *505–507*, 506t
Bile acids, in fat absorption, 515
Bile ducts, 505, *505–506*
　pain in, 382–383, *382*
Bile salts, 505–506, 506t
　in extracellular fluid, 268
　in fat emulsification, 511, *512*
　in micelle formation, 512
Bilirubin, 199
　excretion of, 505–506, 506t
　in extracellular fluid, 268
　in newborn, 652
Bipolar cells, retinal, 462–463, *463*
Birth, 645–647, *646*
Birth control, 638
Bitter taste, 479
Black-out, from acceleratory forces, 335
Bladder, 290–291, *290–291*
　anatomy of, 290, *290*
　emptying of, 291, *291*, 445
　filling of, 290–291, *291*
　innervation of, 290
　sphincters of, 290, *290*
Blastocyst, 641–642
Bleeding disorders, 224–225
Bleeding volume, shock and, 163, *163*
Blind spot, 467
Blindness, 417
　color, 459, *459–460*
　night, 456
　odor, 481
Blood, amino acids in, 538
　carbon dioxide transport in, 315–316, *316*
　cleansing of, by kidney. See *Urine, formation of.*
　　by liver, 187
　　by spleen, 189
　conductance of, 114–115, *115*
　loss of, ADH secretion in, 574
　nutrient exchange between interstitial fluid and, 229–230, *230*, 230t
　osmolality of, in vascular control, 137
　oxygen concentration of, at high altitude, 333, *333*, 333t
　oxygen transport in, 312–315, *312–313*, *315*
　oxygen uptake of, 311, *311*
　pH of, 279
　physical characteristics of, 110–111
　typing of, 214, 214t
　viscosity of, 110–111, *111*, 199
　　in shock, 166
Blood cells. See also *Leukocytes; Red blood cells.*
　antigens in, 213
Blood circulation. See also *Blood flow; Circulation; Circulatory system.*
Blood clot. See also *Blood coagulation; Thrombosis.*
　dissolution (lysis) of, 219, 224
　formation of, 219–221, *219*
　organization of, 219
　propagation of, 221
　retraction of, 220–221
Blood clotting factors, 221–223, 221t, *222–223*
　disorders in, 224–225
Blood coagulation. See also *Anticoagulants; Blood clot; Hemostasis.*
　disorders of, 224–225
　disseminated intravascular, 167, 225
　in newborn, 652
　mechanism of, 220–224, *220*, 221t, *222–223*
　prevention of, 223–224

Blood flow, 112–113, *112–113*. See also *Circulation.*
　cerebral, 185–187, *185*.
　　in shock, 163
　control of, 129–137
　　acute, 130–132, *131*, *133*
　　autoregulation of, 132, *133*, *262*, 263
　　by arteries and arterioles, 120
　　by autonomic nervous system, 133–135, *134–135*
　　by heart, 85–86, *86*
　　cerebral, 185–187, *185*.
　　humoral, 135–137
　　in exercise, 184–185, *184*
　　in gastrointestinal system, 188
　　in heart, 170–171
　　long-term, 130, 132–134, *133*
　　mechanisms of, 130, *130*
　　metabolic, 131–132
　　myogenic, 132
　　oxygen demand theory of, 131
　　smooth muscle and, 76
　　through liver, 187
　　through skin, 190
　　types of, 129
　　vasodilator theory of, 131
　coronary, 169–173, 171
　　control of, 170–171
　　in compensated shock, 164–165, *164–165*
　　in exercise, 184–185
　　in ischemic heart disease, 171–173
　　in shock, 163
　　normal, 170, *170*
　factors affecting, 111–115, *112–115*
　glomerular filtration and, 251–252
　in acute cardiac stimulation, 160
　in capillaries, 229
　in exercise, 126–127
　in heart, 83–85, *83–84*
　in heat transfer, 548
　in hyperthyroidism, 580
　in kidney, 249, 251, *262*, 263
　in liver, 187, *187*
　in lungs, 125–126, *126*
　　obstruction of, 127
　in muscle, 664–665, *665*
　in myocardial infarction, 172
　in organs, 129–130, 130t
　in placenta, 645
　in renal medulla, 259
　in skeletal muscle, 183–185, *184*
　in skin, 189–190, *189*
　in spleen, 188–189, *189*
　in sweating, 190
　in tissues, 129–130, 130t
　laminar, 113
　measurement of, 112–113, *112–113*
　resistance to, 111–112, *112*, *114–115*, 115
　streamlined, 113
　turbulent, 113
　　in valvular disease, 178
　vs. oxygen availability, 130–132, *131*
Blood gases, in exercise, 664
Blood glucose concentration, 529
　between meals, 595
　cortisol effect on, 588
　glucagon and, 600–601
　growth hormone and, 571
　in alternating carbohydrate-lipid metabolism, 600
　in diabetes, 601
　in feeding regulation, 555
　in fetus, 463
　in insulin lack, *598*
　in newborn, 652

Blood glucose concentration (*Continued*)
　insulin secretion control by, 599–600
　low, 572, 600
　regulation of, 601
Blood groups, antigenicity and, 213
　O-A-B, 213–214, 213t-214t
　Rh factor, 214–215
Blood plasma. See *Plasma.*
Blood platelets. See *Platelet(s).*
Blood poisoning, 166–167
Blood pressure, 113–114, *113–114*. See also *Arterial pressure; Venous pressure.*
　blood flow effects of, 111–115, *112–115*
　distribution of, 119, *119*
　high. See *Hypertension.*
　in pulmonary circulation, 124–125, *124*
　measurement of, 113–114, *113–114*, 140–141, *140*
　standard units of, 113–114, *113*
Blood reservoir, liver as, 187
　lungs as, 125
　skin as, 190
　spleen as, 188–189, *189*
　veins as, 122
Blood transfusion, agglutination in, 214
　antigenicity in, 213
　in irreversible shock, 165, *166*
　kidney shutdown after, 215–216
　reaction to, 213–215
　typing before, 214, 214t
Blood vessels. See also *Arterial; Artery(ies); Vascular; Vein(s).*
　autonomic control of, 444
　diameter of, effect on conductance, 115, *115*
　growth of, in high altitude acclimatization, 334–335
Blood volume, average, 267
　cardiac failure and, 125
　cardiac output and, 158, 160
　control of, by renal-body fluid system, 147–150, *148–150*, 153, *153*
　　in compensated shock, 164
　　in hypertension, 153, *153*
　　mechanism of, 271–272, *271*
　distribution of, 118–119, *119*
　extracellular fluid balance and, 272, *272*
　in hypertension, 151–152
　in weightlessness, 337
　maternal, 645
　measurement of, 267–268
　of lungs, 125
　sympathetic nerve control of, 133
Blue baby, *180*, 181
Blue weakness, 459
Blue-sensitive pigment, 457–459, *458–459*
Body fluids. See also *Blood; Extracellular fluid; Fluid(s); Interstitial fluid; Intracellular fluid..*
　compartments of, 267–268
　dissolved nitrogen in, 338
　in exercise, 667
　osmolality of, 257, *257*
　osmolarity of, 272–275, *273–275*
　osmotic equilibria in, 269–271, *270*, 270t
　pH of, 279
　total water, 266–267, *267*, 267t
　volume of, 147–150, *148–150*, 153, *153*
　　control of, 149–150, *150*
Body temperature, 545–546, *546*
　abnormalities of, 550–552, *551*
　cardiac effects of, 88
　high, 550–551, *551*
　in exercise, 666–667
　in newborn, 652–653, *652*
　in shock, 167

Body temperature (*Continued*)
  low, 551–552
  regulation of, 548–550, *548–549*
    by skin, 189–190
    skin circulation effects of, 190
Body water, loss of, 266–267, 267t
  total, 266–267, *267*, 267t
Body weight, growth hormone and, 570, *570*
  in obesity, 556
  in starvation, 556, *557*
  thyroid hormones in, 579–580
Bombesin, in enteric plexus, 488
Bone, absorption of, 609–612, *610*, 614–615
  in space, 336–337
  acromegalic changes in, 572–573, *573*
  blood flow in, 130t
  calcification of, 608–609
  calcium in, 608–609
  compact, 608
  deposition of, 609–610, *610*
  diseases of, 614–615
  estrogen effects on, 633
  fracture of, 610
  growth of, 571–572
    testosterone effect on, 625
    vitamin C deficiency and, 560
  organic matrix of, 608
  remodeling of, 610
  strength of, 608
  vitamin D effects on, 606–607, *606*, 612
Bone fluid, 611–612
Bone marrow, aplasia of, 199
  blood cleansing function of, 207
  destruction of, red blood cell production and, 95
  leukocyte formation in, 200–201, 203
Bone salts, 608–609
Bony labyrinth, 395
Borders, visual perception of, 466, *466*
Bouton. See *Presynaptic terminals*.
Bowel. See *Intestine*.
Bowman, glands of, 481, *481*
Bowman's capsule, 248, *249*
  in lipoid nephrosis, 289
  pressure in, 251
Bradykinin, as cause of pain, 378–379
  as vasodilator, 136
  in asthma, 328
  in gastrointestinal blood flow, 188
  in sweating, 190
Brain. See also *Cerebellum; Cerebral cortex*.
  analgesic system of, 380–381, *380*
  blood flow in, 130t
    in shock, 163
  damage to, in heat stroke, 551
    in shock, 167
  edema of, 186–187
    respiratory depression in, 324–325
  effect of sound on, 477
  excess fluid in, 244
  function of, at lower level, 346–347
    in communication, 423
  functions controlled by, 346–347
    behavior, 432–436, *433*
    blood flow, 134–135, *134–135*
    micturition, 291
    respiration, in exercise, 324
    vasomotor center, *134*, 135
  glucose metabolism in, 601
    insulin and, 597
  pain in, 383
  respiratory control by, in exercise, 324

Brain (*Continued*)
  reticular activating system of, 425–428, *426–427*
  sinuses of, negative pressure in, 121, *121*
  vasomotor center control by, *134*, 135
Brain death, 431
Brain stem, antigravity support and, 394–395, *394*
  autonomic nervous system control of, 445–446, *446*
  connections of, with basal ganglia, 405
  in feeding regulation, 554
  motor pathways to spinal cord from, 394, *394*
  pain transmission to, 379–380, *379*
  sterotyped movement control by, 398
  structure of, 394, *394*
  swallowing and, 490
Brain tumor, CSF pressure and, 244
Brain waves, 428, *428*
Braxton Hicks's contractions, 646, *646*
Breast, development of, effects of estrogens on, 633
  effects of progesterone on, 634
  in pregnancy, 647–648
Breast feeding, 647–649, *648*, 649t
Breathing. See also *Respiration*.
  at birth, 650–651, *650*, 653
  periodic, 325
Breathing capacity, maximum, 298
Broca's area, 402, *402*, 423
Bronchi, *299*, 300
Bronchioles, *299*, 300, 307
  contraction of, in asthma, 327–328
Brunner's glands, 507
Brush border, in absorption, 513, *513*
  of carbohydrates, 511, 515
  of fat, 512, 515
  of ions, 514
  of protein, 515
Brush pile, in interstitium, 231
Bubbles, nitrogen, in decompression sickness, 339
Buccal glands, 499
Buffalo torso, 592
Buffer function, of baroreceptors, 142–143, *143*
Buffer nerves, 142–143
Buffer systems, acid-base, 280–281
  ammonia, 284–285, *284*
  bicarbonate, 280
  blood glucose, 601
  for calcium, 613
  in mucus, 498
  oxygen-hemoglobin, *313*, 314
  phosphate, 281–282
    hydrogen ion transport by, 283–284
  protein, 282
Bulbourethral glands, 619, *620*
Bundle branch block, 106, *106*
Bundle branches, 90, 91–92
Bundle of His, block of, 102–103, *103*
Burns, hypovolemic shock in, 166
Bursa of Fabricius, 207–208

C cells, 613
Caffeine, in exercise, 667
  synaptic transmission effect of, 355
Caisson disease, 338–339
Calcarine fissure, 465, *466*
Calcification, of atheromatous plaques, 536
  of bone, 608–609
Calcitonin, 565, 613–614, .613

Calcium channels, in action potential (smooth muscle), 74
  in presynaptic terminals, 348
Calcium ion, absorption of, 252, 560, 605–606
  in small intestine, 514
  parathyroid hormone and, 611–612
  testosterone and, 625
  vitamin D in, 606–607, *606*
  as vasoconstrictor, 137
  cardiac effects of, 88
  concentration of, in urine, 255t
  exchangeable, 609
  excitatory pulse of, 65
  excretion of, 612
  in acetylcholine channels, 70
  in body fluids, 270t
  in bone, 608–609
  in cardiac muscle contraction, 81–82
  in clotting, 222
  in excitation-contraction coupling, of smooth muscle, 74–75
  in extracellular fluid, 277
  in hormone mediation, 5677
  in hypoparathyroidism, 614
  in interstitial fluid, 607
  in lactation, 649
  in neurotransmission, 70
  in newborn diet, 653
  in plasma, 607, *607*
  in skeletal muscle contraction, 61
  in synaptic transmission fatigue, 355
  in tooth development, 616
  loss of, in weightlessness, 337
  neurotransmitter release and, 348
  parathyroid hormone effects on, 611–613, *611*, *613*
  reabsorption of, 254
Calcium ion concentration, abnormalities of, 607–608, *607*
  calcitonin effects on, 613
  control of, 613
  in calcitonin secretion, 613–614, *613*
  in parathyroid hormone secretion, 612, *613*
Calcium pump, 39–40
  in skeletal muscle, 65
  in smooth muscle relaxation, 75
Calcium-binding protein, 606
Calcium-sodium channels, in repetitive discharge, 52
  in sinoatrial node, 91
  slow, in cardiac muscle, 81
Calibration, of electrocardiogram, 98, 100
Callus, bone, 610
Calmodulin, 75
  in hormone mediation, 567
Calorie(s), 544
  daily requirements of, 545, 545t
  in foods, 553
Calorimetry, 544, *544*
Calsequestrin, 65
Canal of Schlemm, 244–245, *244*
Canaliculi, bile, 505, *505*
  intracellular, 501, *501*
Cancer, 30
  of prostate gland, 627
Capacitance, vascular, 116
Capillary(ies), alveolar, 307, *309*, 310–311
  anatomy of, 130, *130*
  blood flow in, 229
  blood volume in, *119*
  carbon dioxide pressure in, 312, *312*
  damage to, pulmonary edema and, 243
  function of, 118, 120

Capillary(ies) (*Continued*)
  glomerular, 250–251, *250*
  lymphatic, 237–238, *238*
  of kidney tubules, 249, *249*
  of muscle, during exercise, 184
  oxygen diffusion from, 311–312, *311*
  permeability of, 136, 241
    in shock, 165
  structure of, 228–229, *229*
  true, 228, *229*
  wall of, 229,*229*
Capillary bed, high vs. low pressure in, 250
Capillary exchange, 235–236
  diffusion in, 3
Capillary fluid shift, 146
Capillary membrane, alveolar, 307–308,
    308, 310, *310*
  diffusion through, 37, *37*, 229–230, *231*,
    230t
  fluid movement through, 231–236,
    231–233
  pores in, 229, *229*
  pulmonary, 242, *242*
Capillary pressure, 119, *119*, 231, 235
  at arterial end, 235
  at venous end, 235
  edema and, 241
  functional, 232–233
  hydrostatic effects on, 121
  in brain edema, 186–187
  measurement of, 232–233, *232*
  pulmonary, 242
Carbaminohemoglobin, 316
Carbohydrate metabolism. See also *Insulin.*
  blood glucose in, 529
  cortisol effects on, 588
  energy release in, by glycolytic pathway,
    525–529, *526, 527*
    by phosphogluconate pathway, 529
  glucogenesis in, 529
  glucose phosphorylation in, 524
  glycogen storage in, 524–525, *524*
  growth hormone and, 570–571
  in Cushing's syndrome, 592–593
  insulin in, 595–597, *597*, 600
  monosaccharide transport in, 523–524
  oxygen use in, 316
  thyroid hormones in, 579–580
  triglyceride synthesis in, 534–535, *535*
  vitamin B₁ in, 558
Carbohydrates. See also *Glucose.*
  absorption of, 514–515
  calories in, 553
  digestion of, 510–511
  in athletic performance, 658, 661, *661*
  in cell, 11
  in dental caries, 617
  digestive enzymes for, 503
  formation of, 14–15, 529
  in cell membrane, 10
  metabolism of. See *Carbohydrate metab-
    olism.*
  utilization of, in starvation, 557, *557*
Carbon dioxide. See also *Bicarbonate.*
  as vasodilator, 131
  diffusing capacity of, 310
  diffusion of, 303
    in placenta, 463
    in respiratory membrane, 308, *310*
    through capillary membranes, 230
  dissociation curve of, 316, *316*
  expiration of, 281–282
  hemoglobin binding with, 316
  in alveolar air, 306–307, 306t
  in cerebral blood flow regulation,
    185–186, *185*

Carbon dioxide (*Continued*)
  in colon, 519
  in extracellular fluid, 5
  in hydrogen ion secretion regulation, 282
  in respiratory control, 320–322, *321*
  in respiratory exchange ratio, 316
  in respiratory quotient, 554
  in spacecraft, 336
  in vascular control, 137
  pH and, 280–282
  removal of, 4
  solubility coefficient of, 302
  toxicity of, at high pressure, 338
  transport of, 315–316, *316*
    pressure differences in, 305–306
    to capillaries, 312, *312*
    to lungs, 312, *312*
Carbon dioxide pressure, 305–306
  alveolar ventilation effects of, 321–323,
    321, 323
  at high altitude, 333
  in alveoli, 306t, 307, 312
  in arterial blood, 312, *312*
  in capillaries, 312, *312*
  in cells, 312
  in exercise, 323–324, *324*
  in interstitial fluid, 312
  in periodic breathing, 325
Carbon dioxide–alveolar ventilation curve,
    in respiratory depression, *321*, 324
Carbon monoxide, hemoglobin binding
    with, 315
  in SCUBA diving, 339
  poisoning from, in submarine, 340
    oxygen therapy in, 329
Carbonate, in bone, 608
Carbonic acid, 280. See also *Bicarbonate;
    Carbon dioxide.*
  in acidosis, 285
  transport of, 315–316, *316*
Carbonic anhydrase, 282, 316
Carboxypolypeptidase, 503
  in protein digestion, 512, *512*
Carcinogens, 30
Carcinoid tumor, 136
Carcinoma, 30
Cardiac. See also *Coronary; Heart.*
Cardiac arrest, 96
  in cold exposure, 551
Cardiac arrhythmias, 94–96, *94–96*
  electrocardiogram of, 102–105, *103–105*
Cardiac cycle, 82–85, *82–84*
  current flow during, 100–101, *100*
  electrocardiogram and, 83, *83*
Cardiac failure, 173–177
  acute effects of, 173–175, *173*
  blood shift in, 125
  cardiac reserve in, 176–177, *176*
  cardiogenic shock in, 176
  classification of, 176
  compensated, *173*, 175
  decompensated, 175
  edema caused by, 241
  in thiamine deficiency, 558
  pulmonary edema and, 242–243, *242*
  unilateral left, 175–176
Cardiac function, baroreceptor reflex and,
    142
  effect of ions on, 87–88
  regulation of, 85–88, *86–87*
    by vasomotor center, 135
Cardiac impulse, transmission of, *90*,
    91–93, *92*
Cardiac index, 156–157, *157*
Cardiac muscle, action potentials of, 81,
    81, 99, *99*
  as syncytium, 80–81, *81*

Cardiac muscle (*Continued*)
  blood flow control in, 131
  compression of, coronary blood flow and,
    170, *170*
  contraction of, 81–82
  excitation-contraction coupling in, 81–82
  ischemia of, 171–173, *171*
  physiologic anatomy of, 80–82, *81–82*
Cardiac output, 112
  age effect on, 156–157, *157*
  arterial pressure and, 141
  bleeding volume and, 163, *163*
  blood volume effect on, 271
  curves for, 87, *87*
  definition of, 156
  effect of centrifugal force on, 335
  effects of exercise on, 156–157, *157*
  effects of pulmonary circulation on, 126–
    127
  high, 160
  in aldosterone abnormality, 587
  in cardiac failure, 173–176, *173*
  in essential hypertension, 154
  in exercise, 184–185, 665–666, *665*
  in hypertension, 151–152, *151*
  in hyperthyroidism, 580
  in myocardial infarction, 172
  in newborn, 652
  in pregnancy, 645
  in septic shock, 167
  in vasoconstrictor hypertension, 152–153,
    153
  in weightlessness, 337
  low, 159–160, *159*. See also *Shock.*
  mean circulatory pressure and, 116–117
  measurement of, 160–162, *161*
  metabolic effect on, 156, *157*
  normal values for, 156
  regulation of, 85–86, *86*, 157–160, *157,
    159*
    blood volume and, 158
    heart in, 157, 159
    in exercise, 158–159
    mean systemic filling pressure and,
      158–159
    metabolism and, 157, 158–159
    peripheral tissues and, 157–158
    venous return and, 157–158
Cardiac reserve, 176–177, *176*
  in patent ductus arteriosus, 180
Cardiac tamponade, in myocardial infarc-
    tion, 172
Cardiac toxicity, in hyperkalemia, 587
Cardiogenic shock, 162
  in myocardial infarction, 172
Cardio-Green dye, in indicator dilution
    method, 161, *161*
Cardiovascular system. See also *Blood ves-
    sels; Heart.*
  in exercise, 664–666, *665–666*
  thiamine deficiency and, 558
  thyroid hormones and, 580
Caries, 617
  saliva and, 500
Carina, cough reflex at, 301–302
Carnitine, in fatty acid metabolism, 533
Carnosine, in body fluids, 270t
Carotenoid pigments, 558
Carotid artery, baroreceptors in, 142, *142*
Carotid bodies, respiratory control by, 322,
    322
Carotid sinus, 142, *142*
Carpopedal spasm, 607, *607*
Carrier proteins, 10, 33
  in active transport, 39–40
    secondary transport, 40

Carrier proteins (*Continued*)
  in facilitated diffusion, 36
  in hydrogen ion regulation, 282
  in monosaccharide transport, 523
Carrier-mediated diffusion, 36
Cartilage, growth of, 571–572
  in trachea, 300
Cascade, clotting, 221–223, 221t, 222–223
  in glucagon-induced glycogenesis, 600
  of complement system, 210, *210*
  of enzymes, 566–567, *567*
Cataracts, 452
Catheter, in coronary angioplasty, 173
Cathode ray oscilloscope, membrane potential recording with, 54–55, *54*
Caudate nucleus, 401, 404–406, *404–405*
Cecum, reflex from, 494
Celiac disease, 518
Celiac ganglion, 488
Cell membrane, 8–10, *8–10*
  active transport through, 33, *33*, 38–40, *39–40*, 579
  carbohydrates of, 10
  cholesterol in, 536
  diffusion through, 33–38, *33*, 34t, *37–38*
  glucose transport through, 596–597, *597*
  in platelets, 219
  lipid barrier of, 9, *10*, 32–33, *33*
  monosaccharide transport through, 523–524
  phospholipids in, 536
  potentials. See *Membrane potential(s)*.
  proteins of, 9–10, *10*
  replenishment of, 15
  transport proteins of, 33, *33*
Cell(s), ameboid locomotion of, 17–18, *17*
  carbohydrate formation in, 14, *15*
  carbon dioxide pressure in, 312
  carbon dioxide transport to, 312, *312*
  characteristics of, 2
  ciliary movement of, 18–19, *18*
  cytoplasm of, 9, 10–12, *11–12*
  destruction of, by killer cells, 210, *210*
  deterioration of, in shock, 165
  differentiation of, 26
  digestion in, 14, *14*
  energy production in, 15–17, *16*
  energy utilization by, 543–544, *543*
  enzymes of, thyroid hormones and, 579
  functional systems of, 13–19
  genetic control of. See *Genetic control.*
  hair, 395–396, *395–396*, 475–476, *475*
  ingestion by, 13–14, *13*
  life cycle of, 27–30, *28*
  lipids in, 8, 14, *15*
  nucleus of, 8, *8*, 12–13, *12*
  organelles of, 8–12, *9–12*
  osmotic equilibrium in, 270–271, *270*
  oxygen diffusion into, *311*, 312
  oxygen pressure in, *311*
    metabolism and, 314–315, *315*
  protein formation in, 14, *15*, 24–25, *24–25*
  proteins in, 8–9
  pseudopodium of, 17, *17*
  reproduction of, 27–30, *28*
  structure of, 8–12, *8–12*
Cementum, 615, 617, *615*
Central lacteal, 513, *513*
Central nervous system. See also *Brain; Spinal cord.*
  depression of, in acidosis, 286
  effects of thyroid hormone on, 580
  in blood flow control, 134–135, *134–135*
  ischemic response of, 143
    in compensated shock, 164

Central nervous system (*Continued*)
  neuronal pool in, 356
  niacin deficiency and, 558
  oxygen toxicity and, 338
  smell sensation transmission to, *481*, 482
  synapses in. See *Synapse(s).*
  taste signal transmission to, 480, *480*
  vestibular apparatus connection to, 396–397, *396*
Central venous pressure, 120
  in cardiac failure, 173, *173*
Centrifugal force, 335
Centrioles, 9, *28*, 29
Centrosome, *641*
Cerebellar nuclei, 409, *409*
Cerebellum, divisions of, 408–409, *408*
  input system of, 407–409, *408*
  motor functions of, 407–411, *408–410*
  neuronal circuits of, 409–410, *409*
  output signals from, 409, *409*
  predictive functions of, 411
  vestibular apparatus connection to, 396, *396*
  voluntary movement control by, 410–411, *410*
Cerebral activity, blood flow and, 186
Cerebral circulation, 185–187, *185*
  in exercise, 184–185
Cerebral cortex. See also *Motor cortex.*
  activation of, 427–428
  as neuronal pool, 356
  communications and, 423
  dorsal column pathway to, 371, *371*
  function of, 347
  functions controlled by, 416–419, *417*
    hearing, 477–478, *477*
    sensitivity, 375–376
    vasomotor center, 135
  intellectual functions of. See *Intellectual functions.*
  memory and, 346, 419–423, *421*
  neuron columns in, 372
  pain perception in, 380
  physiological anatomy of, 415–416, *416*
  somatic sensory area II of, 371, *371*
  somatic sensory cortex of, 371–373, *371–372*
  visual information to, 466–467
Cerebral hemorrhage, hypertension and, 155
Cerebral palsy, from hypoxia, 650
Cerebropontile tract, *408*
Cerebrospinal fluid (CSF), 243–244, *243*
Cerebrovascular disease, respiratory depression, 324
Cerebrum, reticular activating system stimulation by, 426
Cervix, in parturition, 646–647, *646*
Chain reaction, in fibrillation, 95
Chain-terminating sequence, in RNA synthesis, 23
Channels, protein. See *Protein channels.*
Cheilosis, 559
Chemical potential, in osmosis, 269
Chemical theory, of smell, 482
Chemical thermogenesis, 550
Chemiosmotic mechanism, 526–528, *527*
Chemoreceptor system, respiratory control by, 322–323, *322–323*
Chemoreceptors, 363–364, 364t
Chemosensitive pain receptors, 378
Chemotactic substance, 212
Chemotaxis, in ameboid locomotion, 18
  in complement system, 210, *210*
  of leukocytes, 201, *201*

Chest. See also *Thorax.*
  current flow during ECG of, 100–101, *100*
Chest leads, for ECG, 102, *102*
Chewing, 489
Cheyne-Stokes breathing, 325
Chief cells, 500–501, *501*, 610–611
Chills, with fever, 550–551, *551*
Chloride, absorption of, 252
  in colon, 516
  in small intestine, 514
  at neuronal somal membrane, 350–351, *350*
  concentration of, in urine, 255t
  cotransport of, in urine concentration, 258
  in body fluids, 268, 270t
  in hydrochloric acid secretion, 500–501, *501*
  in saliva, 499, *499*
  loss of, alkalosis from, 285–286
  Nernst potential of, 351
  osmosis and, 37–38, *38*
  reabsorption of, 254
  regulation of, 284–285, *284*
Chloride channels, at synapse, 349
  in neuronal inhibition, 352–353
Chloride pump, at neuronal somal membrane, 350–351, *350*
Chloride-to-bicarbonate ratio, 284–285, *284*
Chlorpromazine, in schizophrenia, 437
Cholecalciferol, 606, *606*
Cholecystokinin, in feeding regulation, 556
  in gallbladder emptying, 505, *506*
  in gastrointestinal blood flow, 188
  in pancreatic secretion regulation, 504, *504*
  insulin secretion and, 600
  stomach motility and, 493
  structure of, 502–503
Cholera, 518
Cholesterol, 535–536, *535–536*
  digestion of, 511
  in bile, 506, 506t
  in chylomicrons, 515
  in extracellular fluid, 268
  in insulin lack, 598
  in lipid bilayer, 9
  plasma level of, 532
  secretion of, 506–507
Cholesterol esterase, digestive enzymes for, 503
Choline acetyltransferase, 348
Cholinergic fibers, 441–442
Cholinergic mediators, 441
Cholinesterase, 348. See also *Acetylcholinesterase.*
  neurotransmitter inactivation by, 349
Chondroitin sulfate, 608
  formation of, 14–15
Choroid, pigment in, 455
Choroid plexus, 243, *243*
Chorion, 462
Chorionic gonadotropin. See *Human chorionic gonadotropin*
Chromatic abberation, in accomodation, 470
Chromatids, 29
Chromatin, 12, *12*
Chromosomes, 9, 12, 28–29, *28*
  autosomal, 641
  daughter, 29
  sex, 620, 641
Chylomicrons, 515, 531–532
Chyme, 491–492
  absorption from, 513–515, *514*

Chyme (*Continued*)
  feces formation from, 515–516
  in ileum, 494
  in small intestine, 493–494
  neutralization of, 503–504
Chymotrypsin, 503
  in protein digestion, 512, *512*
Chymotrypsinogen, 503
Cilia, in fallopian tubes, 641
  in respiratory system, 300
  in vestibular apparatus, *395*, 396
  movement of, 18–19, *18*
Ciliary body, 244, *244*
Ciliary ganglion, 469, *469*
Ciliary muscle, 449, *449*
  autonomic control of, 443
Ciliary nerves, 469, *469*
Ciliary process, 244, *244*
Cimetidine, in gastric secretion, 503
  in peptic ulcer, 517
Cingulate gyrus, 432, *433*, 436
Circular fibers, 449, *449*
Circulation. See also *Blood flow.*
  cerebral, 185–187, *185.*
    in exercise, 184–185
  collateral, in heart, 171, *171*
  components of, 118
  fetal, 649, 651, *651*
  in newborn, 651–652, *651*
  in skin, 189–190, *189*
  micro-, anatomy of, 130, *130*
  portal, 187, *187*
    blockage of, 188
  pressure distribution in, 119, *119*
  pulmonary. See *Pulmonary circulation.*
  renal, pressures in, 250, *250*
  splanchnic, 187–189, *187, 189*
  splenic, 188–189, *189*
  systemic, 110, *111*, 119–123, *119,
    121–123*
    blood shift to pulmonary, 125
  micro-, 130, *130*
Circulatory filling pressure, 116–117
Circulatory shock, 162–167
  in aldosterone deficiency, 586–587
  in heat stroke, 551
Circulatory system, effects of centrifugal
    force on, 335
  extracellular fluid transport by, 3, *3–4*
  intracellular, 12
Circumvallate papillae, 479, *480*
Circus movement, 94–96, *94*
  arrhythmias from, 104–105, *104–105*
  in ventricular fibrillation, 172
Cirrhosis, of liver, 188
Cisternae, 63, *64*, 65
  in smooth muscle, 75
Citrate, as anticoagulant, 222
Citric acid cycle, 525–526, *527*
  insulin in, 597
Citrulline, 540
Clasmatocytes, 202
Claustrum, 404
Climate, artificial, in spacecraft, 336
  in submarine, 340
Climbing fibers, 409, *409*
Clitoris, sensation in, 637
Clone, of lymphocytes, 208–209
Clot. See *Blood clot.*
Clotting, disseminated intravascular, 225
CNS. See *Central nervous system*
Coagulation. See *Blood coagulation.*
Coated pits, 13, *13*
Cobalamin, 557t, 559
Cocaine, exercise and, 667

Cochlea, organ of Corti in, *472–474, 473,
    475–476*
  resonance in, 474–475
  sound attenuation in, 473
  sound transmission in, 473–474, *474*
  structure of, 473–474, *474*
  vibration in, 475, *475*
Cochlear duct, 395, *395*
Cochlear nerve, *472*, 475, *475*
Cochlear nuclei, *476*, 477
Codons, 22–23, *22–23*, 24t
Cold, extreme, 551–552
  cortisol function in, 589
  in thyroid stimulating hormone (TSH)
    secretion, 581
Cold receptors, 384–385, *384*, 548
Colitis, ulcerative, mass movement in, 495
Collagen, 538
  digestion of, 512
  in bone, 608–609
  in teeth, 615–616
  vitamin C deficiency and, 560
Collagen fiber bundles, in interstitium, 231,
    231
Collapse, of lungs, 295
Collateral circulation, in heart, 171, *171*
Collecting duct, 248, *249*
  hydrogen ion secretion by, 282
  potassium secretion in, 261
  reabsorption in, 253
  solute transport through, 258
  water reabsorption in, 259
Collecting lymphatic, 239, *239*
Collecting tube, sodium reabsorption in,
    260
Collecting tubule, 248, *249*
  hydrogen ion secretion by, 282
  potassium secretion in, 261
  reabsorption in, 253
Colloid, of thyroid gland, 576
Colloid goiter, 582–583
Colloid osmotic pressure, 231, *231,
    234–235*
  in glomerular capsule, 251
  plasma, in nephrotic syndrome, 289
  protein regulation and, 240
Colon, absorption in, 494–495, *494,
    515–516*
  movements of, 494–495, *494–495*
  pain in, 382
  secretions of, 508
  storage in, 494, *494*
Colony-stimulating factor, 203
Color blindness, 459, *459–460*
Color vision, cones in, 457, 458
  ganglion cells and, 465
  mechanism of, 458–459, *459–460*
  visual cortex and, 466
Colors, opponent, 465
Colostrum, 648
Coma, 431
  diabetic, 602–603
  in acidosis, 286, 355
  in uremia, 287–288
  oxygen toxicity and, 338
Communication, brain function in, 423
Compensation, in cardiac failure, 173–175,
    173
  in shock, 163–164, *164*
Complement complex, 209
Complement system, 209–210, *210*
Complete atrioventricular block, 103, *103*
Compliance, of lungs, 296, *296*
  of thorax, 296
  vascular, 116

Compliance (*Continued*)
  vascular, 116
    delayed, 117
    pulse pressure and, 122
Compound gland, 499, *499*
Compressed air sickness, 338–339
Concave lens, 451, *451*
Concentration, diffusion potential and, 45
  effect of, on diffusion, 36–37, *37*
  mental, 419
  molar, effect on osmosis, 38
  molecular, 269
  of urinary substances, 254, 255t,
    257–259, *258*
Concussion, respiratory depression in, 325
Conductance, in action potential, 49–50, *49*
  of blood, 114–115, *115*
Conduction, decremental, 354
  electrotonic, 463
  in heat loss, 546, *546*
  in smooth muscle, 72
  saltatory, 53–54, *53*
  velocity of, in cardiac muscle, 81
    in nerve fibers, 54
    in skeletal muscle, 63
Conduction deafness, 478
Conduction system, of heart, 90–93, *90–92*
  abnormalities in. See *Cardiac arrhyth-
    mias.*
  control of, 93–94
Conduction velocity, of nerve fibers,
    367–368, *367*
Conductive membrane, 53, *53*
Cones, 453–455, *453–455*
  in color vision, 457–459, *458–459*
  neural aspects of, 462–463, *463*
  signal transmission to ganglion cells by,
    465
  spectral sensitivity of, 458–459, *459*
Congenital defects, of heart, 179–181, *180*
Congestion, pulmonary, in cardiac failure,
    175–176
  in patent ductus arteriosus, 181
  systemic, in cardiac failure, 176
Connecting enzyme, 145, *145*
Consciousness, definition of, 420
Consolidation, of memory, 422
Constipation, 518
  defecation reflex and, 495
  headache in, 383
Contraception, 638
Constrictor waves, 491–492
Contraction(s). See also *Spasm.*
  coordination of, 402–403, *402*
  damping function in, 389–390, *390*
  motor cortex stimulation and, 401–402,
    401–402
  of antigravity muscles, 395
  of bladder, 291
  of cardiac muscle, 81–82, See also *Car-
    diac cycle.*
  of gallbladder, 505, *506*
  of gastrointestinal muscle. See *Mass move-
    ment; Mixing movement; Peristalsis.*
  of intestinal muscle, 487–488
  of lungs, 294–295, *294*
  of muscle, 657–658
  of skeletal muscle. See under *Skeletal
    muscle.*
  of smooth muscle. See under *Smooth
    muscle.*
  of stomach, in hunger, 554
  premature, in heart, 94
  uterine, 645–647, *646*
    Braxton Hicks's, 646, *646*

Contrast, visual, 464–466, *464*, *466*
Control systems, examples of, 5–6
  gain of, 6
Convection, in heat loss, 546, *546*
Convergence, in accommodation, 470
  of signals, 357, *357*
Convex lens, 451, *451*
Convulsions, in epilepsy, 431
  neuronal circuit instability in, 360
Coordination, muscular, 402–403, *402*
Cornea, refractive index of, 448–449, *448*
Corona radiata, 631, 641, *641*
Coronary arteries, anatomy of, 169, *170*
  angioplasty on, 173
  blood flow in, 169–173
    control of, 170–171
    normal, 170, *170*
  bypass of, 173
  collateral circulation in, 171, *171*
  ischemic disease of, 171–173, *171*
Coronary blood flow. See *Blood flow, coronary.*
Coronary occlusion, acute, 171–172
  cardiac reserve in, *176*
  injury current in, 106–107, *106–107*
  recovery from, 107, *107*
Corpus callosum, 418
Corpus luteum, 631–632, *631*
  in pregnancy, 644
Corti, organ of, *472–474*, 473, *475–476*
  spiral ganglion of, 475, 477, *475–476*
Corticocerebellar pathway, 407, *408*
Corticofugal pathway, 376
Corticospinal tract, 387, *387*, 400–401, *401*, *403*, 404
Corticosteroids. See *Glucocorticoids; Mineralocorticoids.*
Corticosterone, activity of, 586
Corticotropin. See *Adrenocorticotropic hormone.*
Corticotropin-releasing factor (CRF), 590, *590*
Cortisol, 565
  activity of, 586
  anti-inflammatory effects of, 589–590
  excess of, 592–593, *592*
  in carbohydrate metabolism, 588
  in fat metabolism, 589
  in gluconeogenesis, 529
  in protein metabolism, 588–589
  in stress, 589
  secretion of, abnormalities of, 591–593, *591*
    control of, 590–591, *590–591*
  structure of, 585–586, *586*
Cortisone, activity of, 586
Cough reflex, 300–301
Countercurrent mechanism, 257–259, *258*
Countertransport, sodium ion–hydrogen ion, 282
Cramps, muscular, 393
Cranial nerves, parasympathetic fibers in, 440
Creatine, formation of, in energy releasee, 658, *658*
  in body fluids, 270t
Creatinine, concentration of, in urine, 255t
  in extracellular fluid, 268
  reabsorption of, 253
Cretinism, 583–584
CRF (corticotropin-releasinng factor), 590, *590*
Crisis, in fever, 551, *551*
Crista ampullaris, *395*, 396
Critical frequency, for light fusion, 458
  of muscle contraction, 66

Cross-bridges, myosin, 58, 60–63, *60*
  in smooth muscle, 73
Crossed extensor reflex, *391*, 392
Crown, of tooth, 615, *615*
Crypts of Lieberkühn, 497–498, 507–508, *507*
CSF (cerebrospinal fluid), 243–244, *243*
Cuboidal epithelioid cells, 576
Cuneate nucleus, 370
Cupula, in vestibular apparatus, 396
Current of injury, 106–107, *106–107*
  in ventricular fibrillation, 172
Cushing's syndrome, 592–593, *592*
Cutaneous. See *Skin.*
Cyanide poisoning, blood flow in, 130–131
  oxygen therapy in, 329
Cyanocobalamin, in red blood cell production, 196
Cyanosis, 328
Cyclic adenosine monophosphate (cAMP), glucagon and, 600
  in glycogenolysis, 524–525
  in hormone mediation, 566–567, *567*
  in smooth muscle contraction, 76
  in thyroid hormone secretion, 580
  in water reabsorption, 259
Cyclosporin A, 216
Cylindrical lens, 451–452
Cystometrogram, 290–291, *291*
Cytochrome oxidase, 527, *527*
Cytochromes, 527, *527*
Cytoplasm, 8, *8–9*, 10–12, *11–12*
Cytosine, in DNA, 21, *21–22*
  in RNA, *22*, 23
Cytosol, 10

D antigen, 214–215
Dale principle, 350
Damping function, of cerebellum, 410
  of stretch reflex, 389–390, *390*
Dark, adaptation to, 457–458
Dead space, expiration and, 307
  in emphysema, 326
  in respiratory system, 298
  physiological, in high ventilation-perfusion ratio, 311
Deafness, 417, 478
Deamination, 539–540
Deceleration, 336
Decerebrate animal, 395
Decerebrate rigidity, 406
Decibel unit, 476
Decidual cells, 642
Deciduous teeth, 616
Decompression sickness, 338–339
Decremental conduction, 354
Deep cerebellar nuclei, 409, *409*
Deep sea diving physiology, 337–339, 337t
Deep sensation, 368
Defecation, 495, *495*
Defibrillation, ventricular, 96, *96*
Deglutition, 489–491, *490*
Dehydration, hypovolemic shock from, 166
  in diabetes mellitus, 602–603
7-Dehydrocholesterol, 606
Delivery, 645–647, *646*
Delta waves, 428–429, *428–429*
Dendrites, anatomy of, 347–348, *347*
  in neuronal pool, 356, *356*
  neuronal excitation and, 354
Denervation, muscular atrophy and, 67–68
Dense bodies, in smooth muscle, 72–73, *73*
Dental. See also *Teeth.*

Dental caries, 617
  saliva and, 500
Dental lamina, 616
Dentate nucleus, 409, *409*
Dentinal tubules, 616
Dentine, 615–617, *615–616*
Dentition, 616, *616*
Deoxyadenylic acid, in DNA, 21, *21*
Deoxycytidylic acid, in DNA, 21, *21*
Deoxyguanylic acid, in DNA, 21, *21*
Deoxyribonuclease, 503
Deoxyribonucleic acid (DNA), 12. See also *Genes.*
  formation of, 21–22, *21–22*
  in red blood cell production, 197
  in RNA synthesis, 23
  insulin and, 599
  proofreading of, 28
  repair of, 28
  replication of, 28
Deoxyribose, in DNA, 21, *21–22*
Deoxythymidylic acid, in DNA, 21, *21*
Depolarization, atrial, 83, *83*
  in action potentials, 48, 50–51, *50*
  in bundle branch block, 106, *106*
  in fibrillation, 95–96, *95*
  in injured cardiac muscle, 106–107, *106–107*
  in ventricular hypertrophy, 105, *105*
  of smooth muscle, without action potential, 74
  plateau in, 51–52, *52*
  ventricular, mean electrical axis in, 105
Depolarization waves, 98–100, *99*
Deposition, of bone, 609–610, *610*, 614–615
  of minerals, in teeth, 616–617
Depression, chemical transmitters and, 436–437
Depth, of focus, 450, *450*
  of sea, vs. gas volume, 337t
    vs. pressure, 337, 337t
  perception of, 452–453, *453*
Dermatitis, in niacin deficiency, 558
  in riboflavin deficiency, 559
Desoxycorticosterone, activity of, 586
Desynchronized sleep (REM), 429–430, *429*
Detrusor muscle, 290, *290*
Dexamethasone, activity of, 586
α-Dextrinase, 511, *511*
Diabetes, adrenal, 588
Diabetes insipidus, 273, *274*
Diabetes mellitus, 601–603. See also *Insulin.*
  acidosis in, 285, 602
  arteriosclerosis in, 602–603
  coma in, 602–603
  diet in, 602
  juvenile, 601–602
  maturity-onset, 601–602
  newborn and, 653
  pathophysiology of, 602
  treatment of, 602–603
Diagonal stepping reflex, 393, *393*
Dialysis, kidney, 288–289, *288*, 289t
Diapedesis, 195, 201
Diaphragm, 294
Diarrhea, 508, 518
  acidosis from, 285
Diastole, 82–83, *83*, 122
  coronary blood flow in, 170, *170*
  heart sounds in, in valvular lesions, 178, *178*
    pressure at, measurement of, 140–141, *140*

Diastole (*Continued*)
  heart sounds in, normal, 139–140, *140*
  sounds of, 177
  ventricles in, 83–84
DIC (disseminated intravascular coagulation) 167, 225
Diet. See also *Food; Nutrition.*
  composition of, 553
  in athletic performance, 658, 661–662, *661*
  in diabetes, 602
  taste and, 480
Differentiation, of cells, 26
Diffuse junctions, in smooth muscle contraction, 75
Diffusing capacity, in emphysema, 326
  in respiratory membrane, 310
  in tuberculosis, 328
  of oxygen, in exercise, 663–664, *664*
Diffusion, carrier-mediated, 36
  definition of, 33, *33*
  facilitated, 36
    in glucose transport, 597
  in gastrointestinal absorption, 513–514
  in interstitium, 231
  in renal tubules, 253
  in vitreous humor, 244
  membrane potentials caused by, 45–46, *45*
  net rate of, 36–37, *37*
    in osmosis, 269
  of gases, in liquids, 303, *303*
    in respiratory system, 301–303, *303*
    in tissue, 303
  of neurotransmitter, in smooth muscle, 75
  of oxygen. See *Oxygen, diffusion of.*
  of water, through cell membrane, 34
    through selectively permeable membrane, 37–38, *38*
  resting potential and, 47, *47*
  simple, *33*, 34
  through capillary membrane, 3, 4, 37, *37*, 229–230, *230*, 230t
  through cell membrane, 13, 33–38, *33*, 34t, *37–38*
  through lipid bilayer, 34
  through placental membrane, 642–643
  through protein channels, 34
  vs. active transport, 33
Diffusion coefficient, in respiratory membrane, 308
Diffusion potential, 45–46, *45*
Digestion. See also *Gastrointestinal secretion.*
  blood flow and, 188
  during chewing, 489
  hydrolysis in, 510–511
  in cells, 14, *14*
  in newborn, 652
  intracellular, 11
  of carbohydrates, 511, *511*
  of fat, 511–512, *512*
  of phagocytized particles, 202
  of proteins, 512, *512*
Digestive vesicles, 14, *14*
  phagocytosis of, 202
Digitalis, in cardiac failure, 175
Dihydroepiandrosterone, 624
Dihydrotestosterone, 624–625, *624*
1,25-Dihydroxycholecalciferol, 606–607, *606*
Dilatation, venous, cardiac output and, 159–160
Dilution, of urine, 257, *257*

Dilution principle, of blood volume measurement, 267–268
Diopter, 448–449, *448*
Dipalmitoyl lecithin, in alveoli, 295
Direction, of sound, 478
Disaccharides, digestion of, 510–511
Discs, in rods and cones, 454–457, *456-457*
  intercalated, 81, *81*
Disseminated intravascular coagulation, 225
  in septic shock, 167
Distal tubule, 248, *249*
  hydrogen ion secretion by, 282
  macula densa in, 263, *264*
  potassium secretion in, 261
  reabsorption in, 253
  sodium reabsorption in, 260
Distance, determination of, by eye, 452–453, *453*
Distensibility, vascular, 115–117, *116*
Distention, peristalsis from, 489, 493
Distractibility, 419
Diuresis, in diabetes mellitus, 602
  pressure, 147–150, *148*, 153
  water, 273, *274*
Diuretics, in cardiac failure, 175
Divergence, of signals, 357, *357*
Diver's paralysis, 338–339
Diving physiology, 337–339, 337t
  SCUBA, 339, *339*
  submarines and, 339–340
DNA. See *Deoxyribonucleic acid.*
DNA ligase, 28
DNA polymerase, 28
Dominance, of brain hemisphere, 417–418
L-Dopa, in Parkinson's disease, 407
Dopamine, as neurotransmitter, 350
  formation of, in reticular activating system, 427, *427*
  loss of, in Parkinson's disease, 406–407
  schizophrenia and, 437
Doppler effect, 113
Doppler flowmeter, 113, *113*
Dorsal column nucleus, 370, *370*
Dorsal column pathway, 370–371, *370*
Dorsal column–lemniscal system, anatomy of, 370–371, *370–371*
  in position sense, 374, *374*
  nerve fiber orientation in, 371
  sensations transmitted by, 369
  somatic sensory area I, 372–373
  somatic sensory association area of, 373
  somatic sensory cortex of, 371–372, *371–372*
  transmission in, 373–374, *373–374*
  vs. anterolateral system, 369–370
Dorsal horn, pain inhibitory complex of, 380, *380*
Dorsal respiratory group, 318–319, *319*
Dorsolateral white column, 371
Dreams, 429
Drinking, thirst and, 274–275
  water diuresis and, 273, *274*
Drugs, affecting neuromuscular transmission, 71
  alkalosis from, 285
  in exercise, 667
  in myasthenia gravis, 71
  synaptic transmission effect of, 355
Duct(s), bile, 505, *505–506*
  collecting. See *Collecting duct.*
  hepatic, 505, *507*
  lymph, 237–238, *238*
  salivary, 499, *499*
Ductus arteriosus, 651–652, *651*
  patent, 122–123, *123*, *178*, 179–180, *180*

Duodenocolic reflex, 495
Duodenum, bile entering, 505, *506*
  stomach emptying control by, 492–493
  ulcer in, 516–518, *517*
Dwarfism, 572
Dye, T-1824, in blood volume measurement, 267–268
Dye concentration curve, in cardiac output measurement, 161–162, *161*
Dynamic response, of spindle receptor, 388
Dynamic stretch reflex, 389, *389*
Dynein, 19
Dynorphin, in analgesic system, 381
Dysbarism, 338–339
Dyslexia, 417–418, 423, 467
Dysmetria, 410–411
Dyspnea, 328

Eardrum, 472–473, *472*
ECG. See *Electrocardiogram.*
Eclampsia, 645
Ectopic focus, 94, 103
Ectopic pacemaker, 93
Ectoplasm, in ameboid locomotion, 17, *17*
Eddy currents, in blood flow, 113
Edema, 272
  free fluid vesicles and, 231
  in heart failure, 175
  in nephrotic syndrome, 289–290
  in thiamine deficiency, 558
  in uremia, 287
  mechanism of, 240–241, *241*
  nonpitting, 589
  of brain, 186–187
    respiratory depression in, 324–325
  pulmonary. See *Pulmonary edema.*
Edinger-Westphal nucleus, 469–470, *469*
EEG. See *Electroencephalogram.*
Effector organs, receptors of, 442, 442t
Effectors, 345, *345*
Efferent arterioles, blood flow through, 248–250
  glomerular filtration and, 251, 263–264, *264*
Efferent lymphatics, 202, *202*
Efficiency, of heart, 85
  of muscle contraction, 65
Einthoven's triangle, *101*
Ejaculation, 623
Ejaculatory duct, 619, *620*, 623
Ejection, from ventricle, 84
Ejection fraction, 84
Elaboration of thought, 419
Elastic recoil, of lungs, 294–295
Elastin, 538
Electric current, defibrillation from, 96, *96*
  fibrillation from, 95–96, *95*
  flow of, during cardiac cycle, 100–101, *100*
  during ECG, 100–101, *100*
Electrical axis, in ECG, 105
Electrical potential. See also *Membrane potential(s).*
  at neuronal somal membrane, 351
  in diffusion, 36–37, *37*
  in neuronal inhibition, 352–353, *352*
Electrical stimulation, in pain relief, 381
  muscular atrophy and, 68
  of action potential, 54
Electrocardiogram, calibration of, *98*, 100
  cardiac arrhythmias and, 102–105, *103–105*
  in cardiac cycle, 83, *83*

Electrocardiogram (*Continued*)
  leads for, 101–102, *101–102*
  normal, 98–101, *98–100*
  recording of, 100
Electrochemical gradient, 38–39
Electrodes, for ECG, 101–102, *101–102*
Electroencephalogram, 428–429, *428–429*
  in epilepsy, 431, *432*
  in sleep, 429, *429*
Electrogenic pump, *45*, 46
Electrolytes, absorption of, in colon, 516
  glandular secretion of, 498
  in bile, 506, 506t
  secretion of, in large intestine, 508
Electromagnetic flowmeter, 112–113, *112*
Electromagnetic receptors, 363–364, 364t
Electron transport chain, 526–528, *527*
Electrotonic conduction, 463
Embolus, 225
  air, in submarine escape, 340
  nitrogen, in decompression sickness, 339
  pulmonary, 127, 225
Embryo. See also *Fetal; Fetus.*
  nutrition of, 642
Emission, 622–623
Emmetropia, 450, *450*
Emotion, in TSH secretion, 581
Emphysema, 127, 308, 311, 325–327, *326*
  respiration control in, 323
  smoking and, 664
Emulsification, by bile salts, 506
  of fat, 511, *512*
Enamel, of tooth, 615–617, *615–616*
Encephalin, in analgesic system, 380–381,
    380
End-diastolic volume, 84
End-feet. See *Presynaptic terminals.*
End-plate, 69
End-plate potential, in myasthenia gravis,
    71
  in neurotransmission, 70–71
End-systolic volume, 84
Endemic colloid goiter, 582–583
Endocrine glands. See specific gland; *Hor-
    mones.*
  in homeostasis, 4
Endocytosis, 13–14, *13*
Endolymph, in vestibular apparatus, 396–
    397
Endometrial cycle, 634–635, *634*
Endometrium, estrogen effects on, 633
  ovum implantation in, 641–642, *642*
Endoplasm, in ameboid locomotion, 17, *17*
Endoplasmic matrix, 10, *11*
Endoplasmic reticulum, 9, 10–11, *11–12.*
    See also *Sarcoplasmic reticulum.*
  agranular, *9*, 11, *11*
  granular, *9*, 11, *11*
  in glandular secretions, 498, *498*
  lipid formation by, 14, *15*
  protein formation by, 14, *15*
  ribosome attachment to, 25
Endorphins, in analgesic system, 380–381,
    380
Endotoxins, in DIC, 225
  in shock, 165
Endurance, muscular, 657–658
  glycogen in, 660–661, *661*
  muscular energy systems for, 659
Energy, ATP in, 522–523, 542–543, *543*
  balance of, in obesity, 556
  cellular, mitochondria and, 11, 15–17,
    16–17
  consumption of, in peptide linkage, 25
  for cardiac contraction, 85

Energy (*Continued*)
  for gaseous diffusion, 302
  for muscular contraction, 62
  for muscular work, 658–663, *658, 660–
    662*
  for respiration, 296–297
  in action potential recharging, 51, *51*
  in active transport, 39–40
  in food, 553
  in smooth muscle contraction, 73
  release of, from glucose, 525–529, *526–
    527*
    from proteins, 539–540
    in lipid metabolism, 533–535, *534–535*
  requirements of, for daily activities, 544–
    545, 545t
  storage of, as fat, 534–535
Energy currency, ATP and, 523
  of cell, 16
Engram, memory, 422
  sensory, 411–412
Enkephalins, as neurotransmitters, 350
  in enteric plexus, 488
Enteric lipase, 511, *512*
Enteric nervous system, 487–488
Enteritis, 508, 518
Enterogastric reflex, 492–493, 503
Enterokinase, 503
Enzyme(s), activation of, 27
  cascade of, 566–567, *567*
  cellular, thyroid hormones and, 579
  connecting, 145, *145*
  digestive, in cell, 11
  in cell membrane, 10
  in complement system, 210, *210*
  in platelets, 219
  inhibition of, 27
  intestinal, 508
  oxidative, 16
  pancreatic, 503–504, *504*
  proteolytic, as cause of pain, 378–379
    in phagocytosis, 202
    in saliva, 500
  secretion of, 498, *498*
  structural, in genetic control, 20
Eosinophil chemotactic substance, 212
Eosinophil metamyelocyte, *200*
Eosinophil myelocyte, *200*
Eosinophilic chemotactic factor, in asthma,
    328
Eosinophils, 204
Epididymis, 619, *620*, 621
Epilepsy, 431–432, *432*
  acidosis and, 355
  neuronal circuit instability in, 360
Epinephrine, adrenergic receptor effects of,
    442
  as vasoconstrictor, 144
  as vasodilator, 136
  bronchiole effect of, 300
  in fat utilization, 535
  in glycogenolysis, 524–525, 601
  in muscle blood flow control, 184
  release of, 444
  removal of, 442
Epithelial cells, brush border of. See *Brush
    border.*
EPSP (excitatory postsynaptic potential),
    351–352, *352*
Equatorial plate, 29
Equilibrium, during running, 366–367
  for capillary exchange, 235–236
  maintenance of, 395–398, *395–396*
  osmotic, in body fluids, 269–271, *270*,
    270t

Equilibrium (*Continued*)
  water-gas, 302
Equilibrium point, in arterial pressure con-
    trol, 148–149, *148*
Erection, female, 637
  male, 622–623, *623*
Erythema, 589
Erythroblast, 195, *195*
Erythroblastosis fetalis, 215
Erythrocytes. See *Red blood cells.*
Erythropoiesis, 194–197, *195–196*
Erythropoietin, 195–196, *196*
Escape, ventricular, 93, 103
Esophageal sphincter, in vomiting, 519
  lower, 491
  upper, 490
Esophagus, in swallowing, 490–491
  pain in, 382, *382*
  reflux in, 491, 500
  secretion from, 500
Estradiol, chemistry of, 632, *633*
Estriol, chemistry of, 632, *633*
Estrogens, 565–566
  chemistry of, 632, *633*
  in athletic performance, 656–657
  in breast development, 647
  in contraception, 638
  in endometrial cycle, 634
  in lactation, 648, *648*
  in pregnancy, *643*, 644, 646
  in uterine contractibility, 646
  intracellular functions of, 634
  sexual characteristics and, 633–634
  synthesis of, 632, *633*
Estrone, chemistry of, 632, *633*
Eunuchism, female, 636–637
Evaporation, in heat loss, 546–547, *546*
  water loss in, 266, 267t
Excitability, in alkalosis, 286
Excitation, by autonomic nervous system,
    442–443, 443t
  by neurotransmitters, 349
  in reciprocal circuit, 357–358, *358*
  interference patterns of, 469
  of action potential, 54
  of antigravity muscles, 395
  of ganglion cells, 464
  of heart, 90–93, *90–92*
    control of, 93–94
  of neurons, 436
    at dendrites, 354
  of rods, 455–457, *456-457*
Excitation-contraction coupling, in cardiac
    muscle, 81–82
  in skeletal muscle, 63, *64*, 65
  in smooth muscle, 74–75
Excitatory postsynaptic potential, 351–352,
    352
Excitatory pulse, of calcium ions, 65
Excitatory receptors, 76, 348
Excitatory state, of neuron, 354–355, *355*
Excitatory transmitter, 349
Excretion, fluid volume and, *258*, 261–262
  in placenta, 463
  of excess solutes, 257–259, *258*
  of excess water, 257, *257*
  of potassium, 260–261
  of sodium, 260
  of urea, 259–260
Exercise. See also *Sports physiology.*
  blood flow during, 183–185, *184*
  body fluids in, 667
  body heat in, 666–667
  cardiac effects of, 87, *87*
  cardiac output in, 156–159, *157*

Exercise (*Continued*)
 cardiac reserve and, 176, *176*
 cerebral blood flow in, 186
 coronary blood flow in, 170
 gastrointestinal blood flow in, 188
 glucose metabolism in, in muscle, 596–597, *597*
 in anemia, 199
 in patent ductus arteriosus, 181
 in weightlessness, 337
 lymphatic pump in, 239
 metabolic rate and, 544–545
 muscular hypertophy and, 67
 obesity and, 556
 oxygen debt in, 660, *660*
 oxygen transport rate in, 314
 oxygen uptake during, 311
 oxygen-diffusing capacity in, 310
 oxygen-hemoglobin buffering in, 314
 pulmonary circulation in, 126–127
 respiration in, 663–664, *663–664*
 respiratory control in, 320, 324–325, *324–325*
 salt in, 667
 smoking and, 664
 utilization coefficient, 313–314
 valvular lesions and, 179
 water loss from, 267
Exocytosis, 14–15
 in neurotransmitter release, 348
Exophthalmos, 582, *582*
Expansion, of lungs, 294–296, *294*
 surfactant and, 295
Expiration, air composition and, 306t, 307
 difficulty in, in asthma, 328
 neuronal control of, 319–320
 of carbon dioxide, 281–282
Expiratory reserve volume, 297–298
Extensor reflex, crossed, *391*, 392
Exteroceptive sensation, 368
Extracellular fluid, 267, *267*
 aldosterone effects on, 586–587
 bicarbonate increase in, 283–284, *284*
 bicarbonate removal from, 283
 calcium in, 277, 605–608, *606–607*
  bone and, 608–610, *609–610*
 carbon dioxide in, 5, 268, *268*
 components of, 3, 32, *32*, 268, *268*
  in renal failure, 287, *287*, 289t
 ions in, 277
 nutrients in, *3*, 4
 osmolarity of, 269–270, 270t, 272–275, *273–275*
 osmotic equilibrium in, 269–271, *270*, 271t
 oxygen in, 5
 phosphate in, 277, 607
 potassium control in, 276–277, *276–277*
 sodium concentration of, 272–275, *273–275*
 transport of, 3
 volume of, 272, *272*
  control of, 149–150, *150*
  in cardiac failure, 175–176
  vs. blood volume, 272, *272*
Extrafusal fibers, 388, *388*
Extraocular muscles, 467, *467*
 in hyperthyroidism, 582, *582*
Extrapyramidal tract, 401, *403*, 404
 lesions of, 403
Extrasystole, 103–104, *103*
Extrinsic pathway, clotting, 221–222, *222*
Eye. See also *Lens; Retina; Vision.*
 accommodation in, 449–450, *449–450*
 as camera, 448–449, *448*

Eye (*Continued*)
 autonomic control and, 443, 469–470, *469*
 cataracts of, 452
 depth perception in, 452–453, *453*
 disorders of, headache in, 383
 fixation of, 468–469, *468*
 fluid in, 244–245, *244*
 movements of, 402–403, 467–469, *467–469*
 optics of, 448–453
 pupillary aperture of, 450, *450*
 refractive errors in, 450–452, *450–452*
 visual acuity of, 452

F-actin, 61, *61*
Fabricius, bursa of, 207–208
Facilitated diffusion, 36, 597
Facilitation, in memory, 346
 in neuronal pool, 356, *356*, 358, *358*
 of neurons, 354
 presynaptic, in memory, 421
Facilitator terminal, in memory, 421–422, *421*
Factors, blood clotting, 221–223, 221t, *222–223*
 disorders in, 224–225
FAD (flavin adenine dinucleotide), 559
Fainting, in Stokes-Adams syndrome, 103
Fallopian tubes, ciliary movement in, 18
 ovum in, 641
 physiological anatomy of, 629, *630*
 progesterone effects on, 634
Fallot, tetralogy of, *180*, 181
Far-sightedness, 450–451
Fasciculus, medial longitudinal, 467
Fast channels, sodium, 52
Fast twitch, muscular, 662–663
Fastigial nucleus, 409, *409*
Fastigioreticular tract, 408
Fat. See also *Lipid(s); Triglycerides.*
 absorption of, 515
  in newborn, 652–653
 as insulation, 547–548
 body, in male vs. female, 656–657
 calories in, 553
 carbohydrate formation from, 529
 deposition of, 533–535
  estrogen in, 633–634
 digestion of, 503, 511–512, *512*
 formation of, insulin in, 597
 gallbladder emptying and, 505, *506*
 gallstones and, 507
 in extracellular fluid, 268
 in feces, 518
 metabolism of. See *Lipid metabolism.*
 metabolites of, in feeding regulation, 555
 mobilization of, in Cushing's syndrome, 592
 respiratory quotient of, 554
 stomach emptying and, 492–493
 storage of, 533–535
  in obesity, 556
  insulin in, 597
 utilization of, in starvation, 557, *557*
Fat cells, 533
Fatigue, in epilepsy, 431–432
 muscular, 67, 660
 of flexor reflex, 391
 of synaptic transmission, 355, 361
Fatty acids, absorption of, 515
 energy extraction from, 15–17, *16*
 formation of, from amino acids, 540
  from liver glucose, 596

Fatty acids (*Continued*)
 in fat digestion, 511–512, *512*
 in muscular activity, 661
 metabolism of, 533–534, *534–535*
 mobilization of, cortisol effects on, 589
 release of, in insulin lack, 598, *598*
 transport of, 532–533
 triglyceride formation from, 534, *535*
Feces, composition of, 516
 formation of, 515–516
 mixing of, 494–495
 mucus in, 508
 propulsive movement of, 495
 water loss in, 266, 267t
Feedback. See also *Autoregulation.*
 arterial pressure and, 150, *150–151*
 in accommodation, 469
 in ADH-thirst mechanism, 275
 in body temperature regulation, 548–550, *548–549*
 in calcium-calcitonin system, 613–614, *613*
 in control systems, 5–6
 in cortisol-ACTH system, 590–591, *590*
 in gastric secretion, 503
 in growth hormone–protein synthesis, 572
 in hypothalamic-pituitary-ovarian system, 635–636
 in labor initiation, 646, *646*
 in motor control, 404
 in neuronal pool, 359–360, *360*
 in osmoreceptor-ADH system, 273–274, *274*
 in pyloric pump, 492–493
 in respiratory center, 281–282
 in sleep-wakefulness cycle, 430–431
 in tendon reflex, 391
 in testosterone secretion, 626
 in thyroid hormone–TSH system, 581
 in vitamin D synthesis, 606–607, *606*
 motor control by, 411–413
 operon and, 26–27, *26*
 tubuloglomerular, 263
Feeding. See *Food.*
Feeding center, 554
Female athlete, 656–657
Female reproductive functions. See *Reproductive functions, female.*
Femoral vein, thrombosis of, 225
Fenestrae, 250
Ferritin, 197–198, *198*
Fertility, female, 637–638
 pineal gland in, 627
 sperm count and, 622
Fertilization, of ovum, 622, 638, 641
Fetal hemoglobin, 463
Fetus, blood constituents in, 643
 erythroblastosis fetalis in, 215
 gonadotropin effects on, 625, 644
 growth of, 649–650
 nutrition of, 642–643, 645
 testosterone in, 624, 644
Fever, 550–551, *551*
FFA (free fatty acid), 532
Fibrillation, 94–96, *95*
 atrial, 95, *95*, 104, *104*
  in valvular lesions, 179
 ventricular, 95–96, *95*, 104–105, *105*
  in myocardial infarction, 172
Fibrin, formation of, 220–221
 in platelet plug formation, 219
Fibrinogen, 111
 fibrin conversion from, 220–221
 formation of, 539

Fibrinogen (*Continued*)
  in semen, 621–622
  osmotic pressure of, 234
Fibrinolysin, 224
  in menstruation, *634*, 635
Fibrin-stabilizing factor, 219–220
Fibrous protein, 538
Fick method, 160–161, *161*
Field, of vision, 467, *467*
Fight or flight reaction, 445
Filaments, actin. See *Actin filaments*.
  anchoring, of lymphatic capillaries, 238, *238*
  myosin. See *Myosin filaments*.
Filling pressure, circulatory, 116–117
  systemic, cardiac output regulation and, 158–159
    in cardiac failure, 174
    in hemorrhagic shock, 162
Filtration, glomerular, 250–251, *250*
  dynamics of, 251–252
  in capillary, 235–236
Filtration coefficient, 236
  renal, 251
Filtration pressure, in capillary, 235
  renal, 251
Firing rate, of neuron, 354–355, *355*
Fistula, arteriovenous, cardiac function in, 160
Fixation, of eyes, 468–469, *468*
Flagellum, 18
Flatus, 516, 519
Flavin adenine dinucleotide, 559
Flavin mononucleotide, 559
Flavoprotein, 527
Flexing movement, brain stem control of, 398
Flexor reflex, 391–392, *391*
Flicking eye movement, 468, *469*
Flowmeter, 112–113, *112–113*
Fludrocortisone, 592
Fluid(s). See also *Body fluids*.
  in interstitium, 231
Fluid balance, in newborn, 652
Fluid intake. See also *Drinking*.
  average, 266
  blood volume and, 271, *271*
Fluid retention, edema caused by, 241
  in cardiac failure, 174
  in Goldblatt's hypertension, 153–154, *154*
Fluid volume, balance of, 269–271, *270*, 271t
  control of, 272, *272*
  distribution of, 231–236, *231–233*
  excretion of, 261–262, *262*
  regulation of, 261–262, *262*
Fluorine, in caries, 617
Flush, in fever, 551, *551*
Flutter, 94–95, *95*
  atrial, 95, *95*, 104, *104*
FMN (flavin mononucleotide), 559
Focusing, of eye, 449–450, *449*
  with corrective lens, 451–452, *451*
Foliate papillae, 479
Folic acid, 557t, 559
  in red blood cell production, 196–197
Follicle-stimulating hormone (FSH), 565
  in male sexual function, 625–626
  in ovarian cycle, 630–631, *630–631*, 635–636
Follicles, of thyroid gland, 576, *577*
  ovarian, 630–631, *631*, 636
  primordial, 629–630, *631*, 636
Follicular fluid, 631

Food. See also *Diet; Digestion; Metabolism; Nutrition*.
  energy in, 553
  in stomach, 491–492
  ingestion of, 489–491, *490*
  intake of, abnormality in, 556–557
    regulation of, 554–556
Foramen of Luschka, 243, *243*
Foramen of Magendie, 243, *243*
Foramen ovale, 651
Force, muscular, 657
Fovea, image fixation on, 468, *469*
  in accommodation, 470
  neural components of, 462–463, *463*
  visual acuity and, 452, 454, *454*
Fracture, of bone, 610
Frank-Starling law, 85–86, *86*, 157
  in exercise, 185
Free fatty acid, 532–533
Free fluid, in interstitium, 231
Free fluid vesicles, 231
Frequency, of sound, 476–477
Friction, in blood vessels, 543
Frontal cortex, in smell, 482
Fructose, glucose conversion from, 524
  in carbohydrate digestion, 511, *511*
  in semen, 621
  transport of, through cell membrane, 523
FSH. See *Follicle-stimulating hormone*.
Functional residual capacity, 298, 306, *307*
  in asthma, 306
Functional syncytium, in smooth muscle, 72
Fundus, of stomach, 491–492, *491*
Fungiform papillae, 479
Fusiform cells, in cerebral cortex, 415, *416*
Fusion, of light, 458, 465, 469

G-actin, 61
G cells, 502
G (gravity) force, 335–336
Gain, of control systems, 6
Galactose, glucose conversion from, 524
  in carbohydrate digestion, 511, *511*
  transport of, through cell membrane, 523
Gallbladder, bile storage in, 505, *506*
  pain in, 382–383, *382*
Galloping reflex, 393
Gallstones, bile storage in, 506–507, *507*
Gamma efferent coactivation, 390
Gamma efferent fibers, 388, 390
Gamma globulin, 111
  formation of, 539
Gamma motor nerve fibers, 388
Gamma-aminobutyric acid, as neurotransmitter, 350
Ganglion cells, retinal, 462, 464–466, *464*
Gangrene, hyperbaric oxygen therapy in, 340
  septic shock from, 167
Gap junction, in intestinal muscle, 487
  in smooth muscle, 72
Gas exchange, principles of, 301–303, *303*
  ventilation-perfusion ratio and, 310–311
Gas gangrene, hyperbaric oxygen therapy in, 340
Gases, diffusion of, through respiratory membrane, 307–308, *308–310*, 310
  in gastrointestinal tract, 516, 519
  pressures of, 302
  volume of, vs. sea depth, 337
Gastric. See also *Stomach*.
Gastric acid, in peptic ulcer, 517

Gastric atony, 517–518
Gastric atrophy, 516
Gastric glands, 491–492, 500–501, *501*
Gastric inhibitory peptide, 493
  insulin secretion and, 600
Gastric juice, neutralization of, 517
Gastric lipase, 511
Gastric mucosa, pernicious anemia and, 196
Gastric secretion, 445, 500–503, *501*
Gastrin, in gastrointestinal blood flow, 188
  in ileal emptying, 494
  in stomach emptying, 492
  insulin secretion and, 600
  secretion of, 500, 502–503
  structure of, 502–503
Gastrin cells, 502
Gastritis, 516
Gastrocolic reflex, 495
Gastroenteric reflex, 493
Gastroileal reflex, 494
Gastrointestinal absorption, anatomical basis of, 512–513, *513–514*
  in large intestine, 515–516
  in small intestine, 513–514, *514*
  mechanisms of, 513
Gastrointestinal blood flow, control of, 188
Gastrointestinal hormones, insulin secretion and, 600
Gastrointestinal reflexes, cecal, 494
  chewing, 489
  defecation, 495, *495*
  duodenocolic, 495
  enterogastric, 492–493, 503
  gastrocolic, 495
  gastroenteric, 493
  gastroileal, 494
  peristaltic, 493
  swallowing, 490
Gastrointestinal secretion, by large intestine, 508
  by small intestine, 507–508, *507*
  daily volume of, 499t
  esophageal, 500
  gastric, 500–503, *501*
  glands for, 497–498, *501–507*
  in liver, 505–507, *506–507*, 506t
  mechanism of, 498, *498*
  of bile, 505–507, *506–507*, 506t
  of electrolytes, 498, 508
  of mucus, 498–499
  of saliva, 499–500, *499–500*, 499t
  pancreatic, 503–504, *504*
  pH of, 499t
Gastrointestinal tract. See also *Alimentary tract*; specific parts, e.g., *Colon; Stomach*.
  autonomic control of, 443–444
  digestion in. See *Digestion*.
  disorders of, 516–519, *517*
  fetal, 649
  filling of, 555–556
  gas in, 516, 519
  motility of, food ingestion in, 489–491, *490*
    in colon, 494–495, *494–495*
    in small intestine, 493–494, *493–494*
    in stomach, 491–493, *491*
    principles of, 486–489, *487*
    types of, 488–489, *489*
  nutrients from, 4
  parasympathetic tone in, 444–445
  submucosa of, protective function of, 207
  thiamine deficiency and, 558
  thyroid hormone effects on, 580

Gating, of acetylcholine channels, 70
  of potassium channels, 49, *49*
  of protein channels, 34–36, *35*
  of sodium channels, 48–49, *49*
Gel, in interstitium, 231
General interpretative area, 417–419, *417*
Genes, 12. See also *Deoxyribonucleic acid (DNA)*.
  mutation of, 28, 30
  regulatory, 27
  steroid hormone action on, 567
  structural, 26, *26*
  structure of, 20–22, *20–23*
Genetic code, 22, *22–23*
Genetic control, 20–30
  genes in, 20–22, *20–23*
  genetic code in, 22, *22–23*
  in cancer, 30
  of cell differentiation, 26
  of cell reproduction, 27–30, *28*
  of cellular biochemical activity, 25–27, *26*
  of enzyme activity, 27
  RNA in, 22–24, *22–24*
Geniculocalcarine tract, 465
Germinal epithelium, tumors of, 627
GHRH (growth hormone-releasing hormone), 570, 572
Giantism, 572
Gigantocellular nucleus, 426–427, *427*
Gland(s), Bowman's, 481, *481*
  Brunner's, 507
  buccal, 499
  compound, 499, *499*
  gastric, 500–501, *501*
  mucous, 497, 500
  of gastrointestinal secretion, 497–498, *498, 501, 507*
  oxyntic, 500–501, *501*
  parotid, 499
  pyloric, 500, 503
  salivary, 499, *499*
  sublingual, 499
  submandibular, 499
  sweat, 547, *547*
Glaucoma, 245
Global aphasia, 423
Globulin(s), 111
  formation of, 539
  osmotic pressure of, 234
Globus pallidus, 401, 404, *404–405*, 406
Glomerular filtration, 250–251, *250*
  dynamics of, 251–252
  measurement of, 255
  rate of, 251
    in essential hypertension, 154
    in fluid volume regulation, 261–262
    urea excretion and, 260
Glomerular pressure, 251–252
Glomerulonephritis, 212, 286–287, 289
  cortisol in, 590
Glomerulotubular balance, 261–262, *262*
Glomerulus, 248, *481*, 482
Glossopharyngeal nerves, 142, *142*
  respiratory control by, 322, *322*
Glucagon, 565
  functions of, 600–601
  in glycogenolysis, 524–525
  secretion of, 601
Glucocorticoids, activity of, 586
  deficiency of, 591–592
  functions of, 588–591, *590–591*
  in fat utilization, 535
  in gluconeogenesis, 529
  in lipoid nephrosis, 289
  in transplantation, 216

Glucokinase, 524
  insulin effect on, 596
Gluconeogenesis, 529, 540
  cortisol effect on, 588
  glucagon in, 600–601
  in newborn, 652
  in starvation, 557
  insulin and, 596, 599
Glucose, absorption of, 252
  autonomic control of, 444
  concentration of, in urine, 255t
  diffusion of, through capillary pores, 230, 230t
  energy release from, 15–17, *16*, 525–529, *526–527*
  fatty acid formation from, 596
  formation of, by glycogenolysis, 524–525
    from amino acids, 540
  in blood. See *Blood glucose concentration*.
  in body fluids, 270t
  in carbohydrate digestion, 511, *511*
  in extracellular fluid, 268
  in muscular activity, 661–662
  metabolism of. See also *Carbohydrate metabolism*.
    growth hormone and, 571
    insulin in, 595–597, *597*
  phosphorylation of, 524
  polymer of. See *Glycogen*.
  reabsorption of, 253
  respiratory quotient of, 554
  sodium cotransport of, 40, 515
  transport of, insulin in, 523–524
    into fat cells, 598
    through cell membrane, 523–524, 596–597, *597*
  utilization of, cortisol effect on, 588
Glucose phosphatase, 596
Glucose phosphate, 596
Glucose-6-phosphate, formation of, 524
  in glycogenesis, 524, *524*
Glucostatic theory, of hunger, 555
Glutamate, as neurotransmitter, 350
Glutamic acid, in DNA, 22, *23*
Gluten enteropathy, 518
Glycerol, in gluconeogenesis, 529
  in glycogenesis, 524
  triglyceride formation from, 534, *535*
α-Glycerophosphate, 598
  in triglyceride formation, 534, *535*
Glycine, as neurotransmitter, 350
Glycocalyx, 10
Glycogen, breakdown of, 525–529, *526–527*
  formation of, 524, *524*
    insulin in, 595
  in cell, *9*
  in muscle, 596, 660–661, *661*
  release of, 596
  storage of, 524–525, *524*
    growth hormone and, 571
    in muscle, 596
Glycogenesis, 524, *524*
Glycogen–lactic acid system, *658*, 659–660, 662
Glycogenolysis, 524–525, *524*
  glucagon in, 600
Glycolipids, in cell membrane, 10
Glycolysis, 525–529, *526–527*
  anaerobic, *526*, 528–529
  control of, 528
  in exercise, *658*, 659
Glycoproteins, formation of, 14
  in cell membrane, 9–10
  in platelets, 219

Gnostic area, 417–419, *417*
GnRH (gonadotropin-releasing hormone), 635–636
Goblet cells, 497–498
Goiter, endemic, 582–583
  nontoxic, 583
  toxic, 579–582, *582*
Goitrogenic substance, 583
Goldblatt's hypertension, 153–154, *154*
Golgi apparatus, *9*, 11, *11*
  synthetic functions of, 14–15
Golgi tendon apparatus, 364, *364*, 374
Golgi tendon organs, 388–390, *390–391, 390*
Gonadotropin-releasing hormone (GnRH), 635–636
Gonadotropins, 566. See also *Follicle-stimulating hormone; Luteinizing hormone*.
  depression of, 636
  in male sexual function, 625–626
  in ovarian cycle, 630–631, *630–631*
Gracile nucleus, 370
Graft, rejection of, 216
Granular cell layer, in cerebral cortex, 409, *409, 415, 416*
Granulocyte-releasing factor, 203
Granulocytes, *200*, 201
  life span of, 201
Granulosa cells, 629, 631
  tumors of, 637
Graves' disease, 579–582, *582*
Gravity, 335. See also *Equilibrium*.
  body support against, 394–395, *394*
  lack of, 336–337
Green-sensitive pigment, 457–459, *458–459*
Ground substance, 608
Growth, estrogen in, 633, 657
  folic acid in, 559
  insulin in, 599, *599*
  of bone, vitamin C deficiency and, 560
  of cell, regulation of, 29–30
  of fetus, 649–650
  thyroid hormones in, 579
Growth factor, in cell regulation, 30
  in platelets, 219
Growth hormone, 565, 570
  in bone growth, 571–572
  in cartilage growth, 571–572
  in fat utilization, 535
  insulin and, 599, *599*
  metabolic effects of, 570–571
  secretion of, 572
    abnormalities of, 572–573, *573*
  weight gain and, 570, *570*
Growth hormone-releasing hormone (GHRH), 570, 572
Guanidine bases, in uremia, 287
Guanine, in DNA, 21, *21–22*
  in RNA, 22, 23
Guanosine triphosphate, in protein formation, 539
Gut. See *Colon; Intestine; Small intestine*.
Gynecomastia, 627

H band, in myofibrils, *58*
Habituation, 421–422, 434–435
Hair, distribution of, testosterone in, 624
  tactile, 364, *364*
Hair cells, 395–396, *395–396*
  in auditory mechanism, 475–476, *475*
Hair receptors, adaptation of, 365–366, *366*
Hair end-organ, 368
Hallucinations, hippocampus and, 436

Haloperidol, in schizophrenia, 437
Hand, movements of, coordination of, 403
Hangover, headache in, 383
Haustrations, 494
Haversian canal, 610, *610*
Hay fever, 213
Head, rotation of, 397
Headache, 383
  in hypoxia, 334
Healing, cortisol effect on, 590
  vitamin C deficiency and, 560
Hearing. See also *Sound.*
  central auditory mechanisms of, 476–477, *476*
  cerebral cortex function in, 477–478, *477*
  cochlea in, 472–475, *472–475*
  directional discrimination in, 478
  frequency range of, 476
  loss of, 417, 478
  loudness determination in, 476
  organ of Corti in, *473–475*, 475–476
  pitch determination in, 476
  sensitivity of, 473
  tympanic membrane in, 472–473, *472*
Heart. See also *Cardiac; Coronary.*
  abnormal rhythms of, 94–96, *94–96.* See also *Cardiac arrhythmias.*
  anatomy of, 123–124, *124*
  anemia effect on, 199
  autonomic control of, 444
  blood flow in, 130t
    in shock, 163
  blood volume in, *119*
  conduction system of, 90–93, *90–92*
    control of, 93–94
  congenital defects, *178*, 179–181, *180*
  depolarization of, plateau in, 51–52, *52*
  deterioration of, in cardiac failure, 176
    in shock, 164–165, *164–165*
  efficiency of, 85
  electrocardiogram of. See *Electrocardiogram.*
  excitation of, 90–93, *90–92*
    control of, 93–94
  exercise effect on, 159
  Frank-Starling law of, 85–86, *86*, 157
    in exercise, 185
  hypereffective, 87, *87*
  hypertension effects on, 155
  hypertrophy of, 87, *87*
    in exercise, 665
  hypoeffective, 87, *87*
  in cardiac output regulation, 157, 159
  in high altitude native, 335
  murmur of, in patent ductus arteriosus, *178*, 181
  nerves of, 86–87, *86*
  pain in, 172–173
    from viscera, 382, *382*
  rhythmicity of, 90–94, *90–92*
  stimulation of, 93–94
  structure of, 82, *82*
  valves of, function of, 84–85, *84*
    lesions of, *176*, 177–179, *178*
    sounds of, 177
Heart attack. See *Cardiac failure; Myocardial infarction.*
Heart block, 94, 102–103, *103*
  bundle branch, 106, *106*
  incomplete, 102–103, *103*
Heart disease, athletic performance in, 666
  ischemic, 171–173, *171.* See also *Coronary occlusion; Myocardial infarction.*
Heart rate, atrial reflex control of, 144
  control of, 86–87, *86*

Heart rate (*Continued*)
  control of, by sinoatrial node, 91, *91*
  fetal, 649
  in exercise, 665–666, *666*
Heart sounds, 85. See also *Phonocardiogram.*
  auscultation of, 177, *177*
  normal, 177
  of valvular lesions, 177–178, *178*
Heart strength, control of, 86–87, *86*
Heartbeat, dropped, 102–103, *103*
  restoration of, 96, *96*
Heartburn, 382
Heat. See also *Body temperature.*
  acclimatization to, 547, 667
  as cause of pain, 378–379
  body. See *Body temperature.*
  conduction of, to skin, 189
  conservation of, 549–550
  excessive, cortisol function in, 589
  loss of, 546–550, *546–549*
    in newborn, 652, *652*
  production of, 543–544, 546–550, *546–549*
    by nerve fibers, 51, *51*
    in skeletal muscle, 65
  sensation of, 384–385, *384*
  transfer of, from body core, 548
Heat stroke, 551, 666–667
Helicotrema, 474–475
Helium, in deep sea diving, 339
Helper cells, B cell activation by, 209
  function of, 210
Hematocrit, 110–111, *111*
Hemodynamics, 110
Hemoglobin, carbon dioxide with, 316
  carbon monoxide with, 315
  destruction of, 199
  fetal, 463
  formation of, 197, *197*
  in high altitude acclimatization, 334
  oxygen binding with, 312–314, *312–313*
  oxygen buffering function of, 5, 313, 314
  oxygen saturation of, at high altitude, 333, *333*, 333t
  oxygen transport by, 194
Hemoglobin S, 199
Hemoglobin-oxygen dissociation curve, 313–314, *313*
Hemolysis, 214
  in transfusion reaction, 214
Hemolytic anemia, 199
Hemolytic jaundice, 506
Hemophilia, 224–225
Hemorrhage, anemia from, 199
  cerebral, hypertension and, 155
  renin-angiotensin system and, 145–146, *145*
  shock caused by, 162–165, *163–165*
Hemosiderin, 197–198, *198*
Hemostasis, 218–219, *219.* See also *Blood coagulation.*
Henderson-Hasselbalch equation, 280
Henle, loop of. See *Loop of Henle.*
Henry's law, 302
Heparin, formation of, in basophils, 204
  in allergy, 212
  intravascular, 223–224
Hepatic. See also *Liver.*
Hepatic arterioles, 505
Hepatic cellular plates, 505, *505*
Hepatic duct, 505, *507*
Hepatic sinuses, 187, *187*
Hepatic sinusoids, 505, *505*
Hepatic vein, 187, *187*

Heredity, baldness and, 625
  in atherosclerosis, 536
  in athletic performance, 662–663
  in diabetes, 601
  in obesity, 556–557
Hering's nerves, 142, *142*
  respiratory control by, 322
Hering-Breuer inflation reflex, 319
Hermaphroditism, 653
Hexokinase, 524
Hexose monophosphate, in body fluids, 270t
High altitude. See *Altitude, high.*
High density lipoproteins, 532–533
High energy bonds, 522–523, 543, 658
High-pressure operations, physiology of, 337–339, 337t
Hilus, 202
Hippocampal gyrus, 432, *433*, 436
Hippocampus, functions of, 436
  memory consolidation by, 422–423
His, bundle of, block at, 102–103, *103*
Histamine, as cause of pain, 378–379
  as vasodilator, 131, 136
  bronchiolar effect of, 300
  in allergy, 212–213
  in anaphylaxis, 166
  in asthma, 328
  in gastric secretion, 503
Histiocytes, tissue, 202
Histones, 29
Hives, 213
Holistic theory, of thought, 419–420
Homeostasis, 3–5
Homunculi, *408*
Horizontal cells, retinal, 463–464, *463*
Hormone receptors, 566, *567*
Hormone-sensitive lipase, insulin effects on, 598
Hormone-sensitive triglyceride lipase, 532, 535
Hormones. See also specific gland; specific hormone.
  action mechanisms of, 566–567, *567*
  arterial pressure control by, 144–146, *145*
  blood flow regulation by, 135–137
  general, 564
  in fat utilization, 535
  in homeostasis, 4
  in newborn, 653
  in pancreatic secretion regulation, 504, *504*
  local, 564
  measurement of, 567–568
  nature of, 564–566, *565*
  sex. See *Sex hormones.*
  smooth muscle effects of, 76
  stomach emptying and, 492–493
Human chorionic gonadotropin, 566
  in infertility, 638
  in male sexual function, 625
  in pregnancy, 643–644, *643*
Human chorionic somatomammotropin, in pregnancy, 644, 648
Human somatomammotropin, 566
Humidification, of air, 299–300, *299*, 306, 306t
Humoral regulation, of blood flow, 135–137
Humors, of eye, 244–245, *244*
Hunger, 489, 554
Hunger center, 554
Hyaline membrane disease, 295, 327, 650–651

Hyaluronic acid, 608
  formation of, 14–15
Hyaluronidase, in sperm, 622
Hydrocephalus, 244
Hydrochloric acid, lack of, 516
  pepsin activation by, 501
  secretion of, 500–501, *501*
Hydrocortisone. See *Cortisol.*
Hydrogen, in colon, 519
  oxidation of, in metabolism, 526–527, *527*
Hydrogen bonding, in DNA, 21
Hydrogen ion, as vasodilator, 131
  bicarbonate reabsorption and, 282–283, *282*
  countertransport with sodium ion, 282
  in cerebral blood flow regulation, 185–186, *185*
  in vascular control, 137
  reaction of, with bicarbonate, 283
  secretion of, 252, 254, 282–284, *282, 284*
    aldosterone and, 587
  transport of, by ammonia buffer, 284, *284*
    by phosphate buffer, 283–284
Hydrogen ion concentration. See also *Acid; pH.*
  balance of, 279–280
  in taste, 479
  renal regulation of, 282–285, *282, 284*
  respiratory control by, 281–282, *281,* 320–322, *321*
Hydrogen peroxide, in iodide oxidation, 577
Hydrogen sulfide, in feces, 516
Hydrolysis, in digestion, 510–511
  of carbohydrates, 511, *511*
  of fat, 512, *512*
Hydrostatic pressure, blood pressure effects of, 120–121, *121*
  in lungs, 125–126
Hydroxyapatite, 608–609
  in tooth, 615–617
β-Hydroxybutyric acid, formation of, 534
  in insulin lack, 599
Hyperadrenalism, 592–593, *592*
Hyperbaric oxygen therapy, 340
Hypercalcemia, 88, 608
Hypercapnia, in emphysema, 327
Hypereffective heart, 87, *87*
Hyperemia, 132
Hyperglycemia. See also *Diabetes mellitus.*
  caused by glucagon, 600–601
Hyperglycemic factor, 600–601
Hyperinsulinism, in obesity, 557
Hyperkalemia, effect on heart, 88
  in Addison's disease, 277
  in aldosterone deficiency, 587
Hypermetropia, 450–451
Hyperopia, 450–451
Hyperosmolality, of medullary interstitial fluid, 258–259, *258*
Hyperparathyroidism, 614
Hyperpnea, in exercise, 324
Hyperpolarization, 52, *52*
  in neuronal inhibition, 352
  in retina, 456–457, *457*
  in sinoatrial node, 91
Hyperpyrexia, 551
Hypertension, 151–155
  cardiac output in, *159*
  causes of, 151
  effects of, 155
  essential, 154–155
  Goldblatt's, 153–154, *154*

Hypertension (*Continued*)
  in toxemia of pregnancy, 154
  pulmonary, in emphysema, 326–327
  spontaneous (hereditary), 154
  vasoconstrictor, 153–154, *153–154*
  ventricular hypertrophy in, 105, *105*
  volume-loading, 151–154, *151, 153–154*
Hyperthyroidism, 579–582, *582*
  cardiac function in, *159*, 160
Hypertonicity, 271
Hypertrophy, muscular, 67
  of atrium, 179
  of heart, 87, *87*
    in exercise, 665
  of muscle, 622
  of ventricle, 105, *105, 180*, 181
Hypoadrenalism, 591–592
Hypocalcemia, 607–608, *607*
  effect on heart, 88
Hypochromic anemia, 198
Hypoeffective heart, 87, *87*
Hypogastric nerves, in labor pain, 647
Hypoglycemia, 600
  growth hormone and, 572
Hypoglycemic shock, 597
Hypogonadism, 636–637
Hypokalemia, in aldosterone excess, 587
Hypoparathyroidism, 614
Hypophysis. See *Pituitary gland.*
Hypotension, kidney function and, 263–264
Hypothalamic-hypophysial portal system, 569–570, *569*, 635–636
Hypothalamic-inhibitory hormone, 570
Hypothalamic-releasing hormones, 569–570, *569*
Hypothalamus, anatomy of, 432, *433*
  behavioral functions of, 433–435, *434*
  in ACTH secretion regulation, 590–591, *590*
  in body temperature regulation, 548–550, *549, 552*
  in feeding regulation, 554
  in fluid volume control, 273–274, *273–274*
  in gonadotropin secretion, 626, 635–636
  in growth hormone secretion, 572
  in MSH secretion, 591
  in prolactin secretion, 648
  in sleep induction, 430
  in smell, 482
  in temperature control, 190
  in thyroid hormone secretion, 581
  in vasomotor control, 135
  output signals from, 432–434, *433–434*
  pituitary control by, 569
  posterior pituitary gland and, 573–574, *573*
  rage pattern in, 435
Hypothyroidism, 579–584, *583*
Hypotonicity, 271
Hypoventilation, hypoxia in, 328–329
Hypovolemia, shock caused by, 162–166, *163–165*
Hypoxia, at high altitude, 334
  erythropoietin formation and, 195–196, *196*
  in emphysema, 327
  in newborn, 650
  oxygen therapy in, 328–329
  synaptic transmission effect of, 355

I (isotropic) bands, 57, *58, 64*
Ileocecal sphincter, 494, *494*
Ileocecal valve, 494, *494*

Immune response, in blood transfusion, 213, 215
  Rh factor, 215
Immune system, cancer cell destruction by, 30
Immune tolerance, 211–212
Immunity, 206–212
  absence of, 207
  acquired, 207
  cell-mediated, 207, *208,* 210–211
  humoral, 207, *208,* 209–210
  in newborn, 653
  innate, 206
  vaccination and, 212
Immunoglobulin E antibodies, 212
Immunoglobulin M antibodies, 214
Immunoglobulins, 209, *209*
Immunosuppression, in transplantation, 216
Impedance matching, of ossicular system, 473
Inactivation gate, 48–49, *49*
Incisura, 85
Incomplete heart block, 102–103, *103*
Incus, 472, *472*
Indicator dilution method, 161–162, *161*
Indifferent electrode, for ECG, 102
Indirect calorimetry, 544, *544*
Inducer, genetic regulation by, 26
Infant, newborn, 650–653, *650–652*
Infarction, myocardial. See *Myocardial infarction.*
Infection, cortisol function in, 589
  generalized, septic shock from, 167
  resistance to. See *Leukocytes.*
Inferior colliculus, *476,* 477
Infertility, 638
Infinite gain principle, in arterial pressure control, 149
Inflammation, cortisol function in, 589–590
  leukocyte response to, 202–203
Information processing, in nervous system, 345–346
Ingestion, 489–491, *490*
  by cell, 13–14, *13*
Inhibin, 626, 635–636
Inhibition, by autonomic nervous system, 442–443, 443t
  by neurotransmitters, 349
  in reciprocal circuit, 357–358, *358*
  in retina, 463
  in vision, 464–465, *464*
  lateral, 374, *374*
    spatial patterns and, 358–359, *359*
  of muscle tone, 405–406
  of neuron, 352–353, *352*
  of neuronal pools, 356–358, *357–358*
  of smooth muscle, 76
  presynaptic, 353
    in memory, 421
  reciprocal, 392
  surround, 374, *374*
Inhibitor substance, genetic regulation by, 26
Inhibitory circuit, 357–358, *358*
  spatial patterns and, 358–359, *359*
Inhibitory postsynaptic potential, 352–353, *352*
Inhibitory receptors, 76, 348
Inhibitory transmitter, 349
Inhibitory zone, 356–357
Injury current, 106–107, *106–107*
  in ventricular fibrillation, 172
Innervation, reciprocal, 392
Insensible water loss, 266–267, 267t
Insomnia, 431

Inspiration, neuronal control of, 319
  neuronal reverberation in, 360
Inspiratory capacity, 297
Inspiratory reserve volume, 297–298
Insulation, body, 547–548
Insulin, 565
  excess of, in obesity, 557
  in carbohydrate metabolism, 595–597,
    597, 600
  in diabetes treatment, 602–603
  in fat metabolism, 535, 597–598, 598
  in glucose transport, 523–524
  in protein metabolism, 599–600, 599
  lack of, 597, 598–600, 598
  long-acting, 602
  secretion of, control of, 599–600
  short-acting, 602
  structure of, 595
Insulin antagonist, 603
Insulin clearance, 255
Insulin shock, in newborn, 653
Integrative function, of nervous system, 346
Intellectual functions. See also Memory;
    Thought.
  communication and, 423
  prefrontal area and, 419
  Wernicke's area and, 417–419, 417
Intention tremor, 410
Intercellular cleft, 229, 229
Interleukin 1, 209
Interleukin 2, 211
Internal environment, 3
Interneurons, 403–404, 403
Internodal pathways, in heart, 90–91, 90,
    92
Interphase, in cell reproduction, 27–28
Interpositus nucleus, 409
Interpretative function, of cerebral cortex,
    417–419, 417
Interstitial cell tumor, 627
Interstitial cells of Leydig, 623–624, 623,
    626
Interstitial fluid, 32, 230–231, 231. See also
    Lymph.
  calcium in, 607, 607
  carbon dioxide pressure in, 312
  carbon dioxide transport from, 312, 312
  constituents of, 268, 268
  entering lymphatic capillaries, 238, 238
  fluid movement between plasma and,
    231–236, 231–233
  medullary, hyperosmolality of, 258–259,
    258
  nutrient exchange between blood and,
    229–230, 230, 230t
  osmolarity of, 269–270, 270t
  oxygen diffusion from, 312
  oxygen diffusion into, 311–312, 311
  pH of, 279
  protein regulation in, 239–240
  pulmonary, 241–243, 242
Interstitial fluid colloid osmotic pressure,
    232, 234–235
Interstitial fluid pressure, 231, 231, 240
  edema and, 240–241, 241
  free, 241, 241
  in lung, 242
  lymph flow and, 239
  measurement of, 233–234, 233
Interstitial nucleus, 398
Interstitial space, dry state of, 240
Interstitium, 230–231, 231
Intestinal lipase, 508
Intestinal veins, vasoconstriction of, 188

Intestine. See Colon; Gastrointestinal;
    Small Intestine.
  absorption in, 512–513, 513–514
    of calcium, 606, 613
  blood flow through, 187–188
  emptying of, 445
  layers of, 486, 487
  obstruction of, shock in, 166
Intra-alveolar pressure, 295
Intracellular fluid, 267, 267
  components of, 3, 32, 32, 268, 268
  osmolality of, 269–270, 270t
  osmotic equilibrium in, 269–271, 270,
    271t
Intracellular vesicles, formation of, 15, 15
  function of, 15
Intrafusal fibers, 387–388, 388, 390
Intralaminar nucleus, 375
Intraocular fluid, 244–245, 244
Intrinsic factor, 516
  pernicious anemia and, 196
  secretion of, 500
Intrinsic pathway, clotting, 221–222, 222
Inulin, reabsorption of, 253
Involuntary fixation, mechanism of eye, 468
Iodide, oxidation of, 577
Iodide pump, 577, 577
Iodinase, 577, 577
Iodine, in thyroid hormone synthesis,
    576–577, 577–578
Iodine uptake test, in hyperthyroidism, 582
Iodopsin, 454–455
Ion channels, at synapse, 349
  effector receptors and, 442
Ionophore component, at synapse, 349
Ions. See also specific ion, e.g., Potassium
    ion; Sodium ion; Sulfate.
  absorption of, in small intestine, 514, 514
  active transport of, 39
  hydrated, transport of, 34, 34t
  osmotic effect of, 269
IPSP (inhibitory postsynaptic potential),
    352–353, 352
Iridocorneal angle, 244–245, 244
Iron, absorption of, in small intestine, 514
  in newborn diet, 653
  in pregnancy, 645
  loss of, 198
  metabolism of, 197–198, 198
Iron sulfide protein, 527
Ischemia, as cause of pain, 377, 382
  in migraine headache, 383
  cerebral, arterial pressure and, 143
    in compensated shock, 164
  in cardiac muscle, 171–173, 171
  of ventricles, in hypertension, 155
  toxin release in, in shock, 165
Ishihara's test chart, 459, 460
Islets of Langerhans, 565, 595, 596
  in newborn, 653
Isogravimetric method, for capillary pres-
    sure measurement, 232, 232
Isomaltase, 508
Isometric contraction, of muscle, 65–66, 66
  of ventricle, 84
Isometric relaxation, of ventricle, 84
Isosmotic absorption, 513–514
Isotonic muscle contraction, 65–66
Isotonicity, 271
Isovolumetric method, for capillary pres-
    sure measurement, 232
Isovolumic contraction, of ventricle, 84
Isovolumic relaxation, of ventricle, 84
Itching, 383–384

Jaundice, 506
  in erythroblastosis fetalis, 215
Jerk, muscle, 390
Joint proprioceptors, in respiratory control,
    324
Joint receptors, 374, 374
  adaptation of, 366, 366
  in equilibrium maintenance, 397–398
Junctional feet, 65
Junctional fibers, 92, 92
Juxtaglomerular cells, 144
  erythropoietin formation in, 195–196
Juxtaglomerular complex, 263, 264
Juxtamedullary nephron, 258

Kallidin, 136
  in gastrointestinal blood flow, 188
Kallikrein, 136
  in sweating, 190
Keratin, 538
Kernicterus, in erythroblastosis fetalis, 215
Ketogenesis, 540
α-Ketoglutaric acid, 540
Ketone bodies, in insulin lack, 599
Ketosis, in diabetes mellitus, 602
  in insulin lack, 598–599
  in starvation, 557
Kidney. See also Glomerular; Renal.
  acid-base balance and, 280, 282–285,
    282, 284
  aldosterone effects on, 586–587
  angiotensin effects on, 150
  blood flow in, 129, 130t, 249
  blood volume control by, 271–272, 271
  calcium regulation by, 277
  circulatory pressures in, 250–251, 250
  damage to, hypertension and, 155
  dialysis of, 288–289, 288, 289t
  diluting mechanism of, 257, 257
  edema and, 241
  erythropoietin formation in, 195–196
  failure of, 286–289, 287–288, 289t
    in transfusion, 215–216
  fetal, 649–650
  fluid retention and, in cardiac failure,
    174–175
  function of. See also Urine, formation of.
    in cardiac failure, 174–175
    in essential hypertension, 154–155
    in myocardial infarction, 172
    in shock, 167
  in homeostasis, 4
  in newborn, 652
  pain in, 382
  parathyroid hormone effects on, 611–612
  phosphate regulation by, 277
  physiologic anatomy of, 248–249,
    248–249
  plasma clearance in, 254–255
  potassium regulation by, 276–277,
    276–277
  protein loss by, 289–290
  removal of, hypertension and, 153–154,
    154
  renin-angiotensin system and, 145, 145
  sodium regulation by, 272–275, 273–275
  sympathetic stimulation of, 262
  tubules of. See also Collecting tubule;
    Distal tubule; Proximal tubule.
    absorption in, 249, 252–254, 252, 255t
    anatomy of, 248, 248
    secretion in, 249, 252–254, 252, 255t
  vitamin D synthesis in, 606, 606

Killer cells, 210, *210*
Kinesthesia, 374
Kinetochore, 29
Kinins, as vasodilator, 136
  in gastrointestinal blood flow, 188
Kinocilium, 396
Knee jerk, 390
Knob, synaptic. See *Presynaptic terminals.*
Knowing area, 417–419, *417*
Korotkoff's sounds, 140–141
Krause's corpuscles, 364, *364*
Krebs cycle, 525–526, *527*
Kupffer's cell, 187, 202
Kwashiorkor, 554

Labeled line principle, 365
Labor, 645–647, *646*
Labyrinth, in vestibular apparatus, 395
Lactase, 508, 511, *511*
Lactate, in body fluids, 270t
  in extracellular fluid, 277
Lactation, 647–649, *648*, 649t
  oxytocin effect on, 574
Lactic acid, as vasodilator, 131
  formation of, anaerobic, *526*, 528–529
  in cerebral blood flow regulation, 186
  in extracellular fluid, 268
  in glycogenesis, 524
  in muscular fatigue, 660
  removal of, 660
Lactic acid oxygen debt, 660, *661*
Lactic acid–glycogen system, *658*, 659–660, 662
Lactic dehydrogenase, 528
Lactose, breakdown of, 26
Langerhans, islets of, 565, 595, *596*
  in newborn, 653
Language, 418–419
Large intestine. See *Colon.*
Laryngeal spasm, in hypoparathyroidism, 614–615
Larynx, cough reflex at, 301–302
  in swallowing, 490
  in vocalization, 301, *301*
Last ditch stand arterial pressure control, 143
Latency, of thyroid hormones, 578, *578*
Lateral geniculate body, *463*, 465
Lateral inhibition, 374, *374*
  in vision, 464–465, *464*
Lateral olfactory area, 482
LATS (long-acting thyroid stimulator), 582
Leads, for ECG, 101–102, *101–102*
Leakage, of ions through nerve membrane, 47, *47*
  of sodium ion, in sinoatrial node, 91
Learning, 434–435
  hippocampus and, 436
  of skilled movements, 412–413
Lecithin, in bile, 506, 506t
Leg, venous valves in, 121–122, *121*
Lemniscal system. See *Dorsal column–lemniscal system.*
Lengthening reaction, 391
Lens, corrective, concave, 451, *451*
  convex, 451, *451*
  cylindrical, 451–452
  spherical, 451
  of eye, 448–449, *448*
    accommodation by, 449–450, *449*
    astigmatism, 451–452, *451*
    cataracts of, 452

Lens (*Continued*)
  of eye, focal autonomic control of, 443
    focal depth of, 450, *450*
    image formation by, 449
    refractive errors and, 450–451
    refractive index of, 448–449, *448*
Leprosy, hyperbaric oxygen therapy in, 340
Let-down, in milk secretion, 648
Leukemia, 204
Leukocytes, 199–204
  ameboid locomotion of, 17, 201
  characteristic of, 200, *200*
  genesis of, 200–201, *200*
  life span of, 201
Leukocytosis, 203
  inducing factor, 203
Leydig, interstitial cells of, 623–624, *623*, 626
LH. See *Luteinizing hormone.*
LHRH (luteinizing hormone–releasing hormone), 635–636
Lieberkühn, crypts of, 497–498, 507–508, *507*
Ligaments, of lens, 449, *449*
Ligand gating, of protein channels, 35, *35*
Ligand-activated gate, acetylcholine in, 70
Light, adaptation to, 457–458
  fusion of, 458, 465, 469
  intensity of, amacrine cells and, 464
    changes in, 465
  receptor potential and, 457
  rhodopsin decomposition by, 456, *456*
  sensitivity to, in retina, 463
  white, perception of, 459
Limb leads, for ECG, 101–102, *101–102*
Limbic cortex, 432, *433*, 436
Limbic system. See also *Amygdala; Hippocampus; Hypothalamus.*
  anatomy of, 432, *433*
  behavioral functions of, 433–434, *434*
  in smell, 482
Linear acceleration, 335–336, *336*, 397
Lines, visual perception of, 466, *466*
Lingual nerve, *480*
Liniments, action of, 381
Lipase, 511–512, *512*
  hormone-sensitive triglyceride, 532, 535
  intestinal, 508
  lipoprotein, 532
  tissue, 533
Lipid(s). See also *Cholesterol; Fat; Phospholipids; Triglycerides.*
  formation of, 14, *15*
  in cells, 8
  transport of, 531–532
  types of, 531
Lipid bilayer (lipid barrier), diffusion through, 34, 34t
  of cell membrane, 9, *10*, 32–33, *33*
Lipid metabolism, chylomicrons in, 531–532
  cortisol effects on, 589
  energy from, 533–535, *534–535*
  fat deposition in, 533
  fat mobilization in, 535
  fatty acid transport in, 532–533
  growth hormone and, 570–571
  in atherosclerosis, 536
  insulin in, 597–599, *598*
  liver function in, 533
  oxygen use in, 316
  thyroid hormones in, 579–580
Lipid-insoluble substances, diffusion of, 34
  through capillary membranes, 230

Lipid-soluble substances, diffusion of, 34, 229–230
Lipoid nephrosis, 289
β-Lipoprotein, 515
Lipoprotein lipase, 532
Lipoproteins, 532–533. See also *Cholesterol; Phospholipids.*
  in atherosclerosis, 536
  in insulin lack, 598
  in plasma, 268
Liver. See also *Hepatic.*
  anatomy of, 505, *505*
  as blood reservoir, 187
  bile secretion of, 505–507, *505–507*, 506t
  blood flow in, 129, 130t, 187
  blood pressure in, 188
  blood-cleansing function of, 187
  cirrhosis of, 188
  deterioration of, in shock, 165
  disorders of, clotting factors and, 224
  fat deposits in, 533
  glucose storage in, 595
  glycogen release from, 596
  glycogen storage in, 524–525, *524*
  in lipid metabolism, 533–534
  in newborn, 652
  lipoprotein formation in, 532
  mast cells in, 224
  nutrients from, 4
  pain in, 382
  proteins in, cortisol effects on, 589
  urea formation in, 540
  vitamin D conversion in, 606
Load reflex, 389–390
Lochia, 647
Locomotion, ameboid, 17–18, *17*
  reflexes of, 392–393, *393*
Locus ceruleus, 350, 427, *427*
  REM sleep and, 430
Long-acting thyroid stimulator (LATS), 582
Longitudinal tubules, 63, *64*, 65
Loop of Henle, 248, *249*
  hydrogen ion secretion by, 282
  in urine concentration, *258*, 258–259
  in urine dilution, 257, *257*
  potassium excretion in, 260–261
  reabsorption in, 253
  of sodium, 260
Loudness, determination of, 476
Low density lipoproteins, 532
  in atherosclerosis, 536
LRH (luteinizing hormone–releasing hormone), 570, 626
Lubrication, by mucus, 498–499
  in sexual act, 623, 637
Luminosity, perception of, 466
Lumirhodopsin, 456, *456*
Lung(s). See also *Pulmonary.*
  blood flow in, 125–126, *126*
    in patent ductus arteriosus, 180, *180*
    obstruction of, 127
  blood volume of, 125
  capacity of, 297–298, *297*
  carbon dioxide removal in, 4, 312, *312*
  carbon dioxide transport to, 312, *312*
  collapse of, 127, 295, 327
  compliance of, 296, *296*
  contraction of, 294–295, *294*
  expansion of, 294–296, *294*
    at birth, 650–651, *650*
    surfactant and, 295
  gas pressures in, 305–306
  hydrostatic pressure in, 125–126
  mast cells in, 224

Lung(s) (*Continued*)
  oxygen transport from, 314
  recoil of, 294–295
  sclerosis of, 127
Lupus erythematosus, 212
Luschka, foramina of, 243, *243*
Lutein cells, 632
Luteinization, 631–632
Luteinizing hormone (LH), 565
  in male sexual function, 625–626
  in ovarian cycle, 631–632, 635–636
Luteinizing hormone–releasing hormone
  (LRH), 570
  in male sexual function, 626
Luteotropic hormone–releasing hormone
  (LHRH), 635–636
Lymph, chylomicrons in, 515
  flow of, 239
    from lung, 242
  formation of, 238–239
Lymph channels, 237, *238*
Lymph nodes, 207
  macrophages in, 202, *202*
Lymph vessel, collecting, 239, *239*
Lymphatic capillaries, 237–238
Lymphatic obstruction, edema and, 241
Lymphatic system, 237–240, *238–239*
Lymphoblasts, 209
Lymphocytes, 200. See also *B cells; T cells.*
  clone of, 208–209
  entrapment of, in lymphoid tissue, 208
  release of, 210
  types of, 207
Lymphoid tissue, in immunity, 207–208
  lymphocyte entrapment in, 208
  lymphocyte release from, 210
Lymphokines, 209, 211
Lysis, of antigens, 210, *210*
Lysoferrin, 14
Lysosomal enzymes, in basophils, 204
Lysosomal membrane, effect of cortisol on,
  590
Lysosomes, *9*, 11
  digestion by, 14, *14*
  formation of, 15
Lysozyme, 14
Lytic complex, 210

Machinery murmur, *178*, 181
Macrophage migration inhibition factor,
  211
Macrophages, activation of, 211
  ameboid locomotion of, 17
  antigen liberation by, 209
  in lymph nodes, 202, *202*
  inflammation response by, 202–203
  phagocytosis by, 201–202
  properties of, 201–202
  tissue, 201–203, *202*
Macula, retinal, 454, *454*, 465, *466*
  vestibular, 395–396, *395*
Macula densa, 263, *264*
Magendie, foramen of, 243, *243*
Magnesium ion, absorption of, in small intestine, 514
  as vasodilator, 137
  concentration of, in urine, 255t
  in body fluids, 268, 270t
  in bone, 608
  reabsorption of, 254
Malabsorption, from small intestine, 518
Male, reproductive functions in. See *Reproductive functions, male.*

Male athlete, 656–657
Malleus, 472–473, *472*
Malocclusion, 617
Maltase, 508, 511, *511*
Maltose, digestion of, 511, *511*
Manic-depressive psychosis, chemical trans-
  mitters and, 436–437
Mannitol, in brain edema, 325
  reabsorption of, 253
Manometer, in blood pressure measure-
  ment, 113–114, *113*
Mark time, 393, *393*
Masculinization, in newborn female, 653
Mass movement, in colon, 495
Mast cells, 204
  heparin production by, 223–224
Mastication, 489
Mathematical thought, 418–419
Maturation, in red blood cell production,
  196–197
  of follicles, 631
  of ovum, 640
  of sperm, 621
Mean arterial pressure, 140, *140*
Mean circulatory filling pressure, 116–117
Mean electrical axis, of ventricles, 105
Mean systemic filling pressure, cardiac out-
  put regulation and, 158–159
  in cardiac failure, 174
  in hemorrhagic shock, 162
Meat, digestion of, 512
Mechanoreceptive sensation, 368
  detection of, 368–369
  transmission of, in anterolateral system,
    369–370, 374–375, *375*
    in dorsal column–lemniscal system,
      369–374, *370-374*
    in peripheral nerve fibers, 369
Mechanoreceptors, 363–364, *364*, 364t
Mechanosensitive pain receptors, 378
Meconium, 649
Medial geniculate nucleus, *476*, 477
Medial lemniscus, 370–371, *371*
Medial longitudinal fasciculus, 467, *467*
Medial olfactory area, 482
Median eminence, 570
Mediator, hormone, 566–567, *567*
Medulla, adrenal, function of, 440, 444
  brain, 394, *394*
Medullary sinus, 202, *202*
Megakaryocytes, 200, *200*
  platelet formation from, 219
Megaloblastic anemia, 199. See also *Perni-
  cious anemia.*
Megaloblasts, in red blood cell production,
  196
Meissner's corpuscles, 364, *364*, 368–369
Meissner's plexus, *487*, 488–489, 493
Melanin, 591
  in retina, 455
Melanocyte-stimulating hormone (MSH),
  secretion of, 591
Melanocytes, 591
Melatonin, in fertility, 627
Membrane, capillary. See *Capillary membrane.*
  conductive, 53, *53*
  glomerular, 250–251, *250*
  lysosome, 11
  nuclear, 8, *8–9*, 12
  of cell. See *Cell membrane.*
  of mitochondrion, 12, *12*
  osteolytic, 611–612
  periodontal, 615
  permeability of, 36

Membrane (*Continued*)
  respiratory, gas diffusion through,
    307–308, *308–310*, 310
  selectively permeable, 37–38, *38*, 269
Membrane channels. See *Protein channels.*
Membrane potential(s), 44–45. See also
  Action potential(s).
  from diffusion, 45–46, *45*
  in active transport, 45–46, *46*
  in neuronal inhibition, 352–353, *352*
  in retina, 457, *457*
  in smooth muscle, 73
  measurement of, 46, *46*
  physics of, 44–46, *45–46*
  recording of, 54–55, *54*
  resting. See *Resting potential(s).*
Membrane transport, by ATP, 16, *17*
Membranous labyrinth, 395, *395*
Memory, 346
  codification of, 422
  consolidation of, 422, 436
  loss of, 422–423
  mechanisms of, 420–422, *421*
  physiological basis of, 420–423
  primary, 420–422
  reward-punishment in, 434–435
  searching of, 422, 427–428
  secondary, 420–422
  sensory, 420
  storage of, 419
  types of, 420
  Wernicke's area and, 418
Memory engram, 422
Menarche, 630
Meningitis, headache in, 383
Menopause, 636
Menstrual cycle, 630–632, *630–631*,
  635–636
Menstruation, 634–635, *634*
  irregularity of, 637
  prevention of, 643–664
Mental function, at high nitrogen pressure,
  337–338
  in hypoxia, 334
  in shock, 167
Mercury manometer, in blood pressure
  measurement, 113–114, *113*
Meridional fibers, 449, *449*
Merkel's disk, 364, 368
Meromysin, 58
Mesencephalon, 394, *394*
  wakefulness and, 425–426, *426*
Mesenchymal tissue, 462
Mesenteric ganglia, 488
Mesenteric veins, vasoconstriction of, 188
Mesolimbic dopaminergic system, 437
Messenger RNA, 22–23, *23*, 24t, 25, *25*
  aldosterone effects on, 587
  insulin and, 599
Metabolator, 544, *544*
Metabolic acidosis, 285
Metabolic alkalosis, 285
Metabolic rate, basal, 545
  in hyperthyroidism, 582
  in hypothyroidism, 583
  in exercise, 544–545, 545t
  in newborn, 652, *652*
  measurement of, 544, *544*
  sympathetic stimulation and, 545
  thyroid hormones and, 545, 578–579
Metabolism, anaerobic, *658*, 659
  ATP in, 522–523
  autonomic control of, 444
  blood flow control and, 131–132
  cardiac output effect of, 156, *157*

Metabolism (*Continued*)
  growth hormone and, 570–571
  human chorionic somatomammotropin
      and, 644
  in action potential recharging, 51, *51*
  in hypovolemic shock, 167
  in leukemia, 204
  in newborn, 652
  in tooth development, 616
  insulin in. See *Insulin.*
  monosaccharide transport in, 523–524
  muscular, in exercise, 658–663, *658,*
      660–663
  of carbohydrates. See *Carbohydrate me-*
      tabolism.
  of fat. See *Lipid metabolism.*
  of iron, 197–198, *198*
  of proteins. See *Protein(s), metabolism*
      of.
  of testosterone, 624, *624*
  oxygen use in, 314–316, *315*
  respiratory quotient in, 554
Metaphase, *28,* 29
Metarhodopsin, 456, *456*
Metarterioles, anatomy of, 130, *130*
  in microcirculation, 228–229, *229*
Methane, in colon, 519
Methyl mercaptan, 482
Micelles, absorption of, 515
  in fat digestion, 512
Microcirculation, anatomy of, 130, *130*
Microglia, 202
Microphages, ameboid locomotion of, 17
Microtubules, *9,* 12
  in mitosis, 29
Microvilli, intestinal, 513, *513*
Micturition, 290–291, *290–291*
Migraine headache, 383
Milieu intérieur, 3
Milk, production of, 647–649, *648,* 649t
Milk teeth, 616
Milliosmole, 269
Mineralocorticoids, activity of, 586
  deficiency of, 591–592
  functions of, 586–588
Minerals, in bone. See *Bone.*
Minute respiratory volume, 298
Miosis, 470
Mitochondria, *9,* 11–12, *12*
  ATP formation in, 16, 526
  energy production in, 15–16, *16*
  fatty acid metabolism in, 533
  in sarcoplasm, 58–59, *59*
  in synaptic transmission, 348, *348*
  thyroid hormones and, 579
Mitosis, 27, *28,* 29
Mitotic apparatus, *28,* 29
Mitral area, for heart sounds, 177, *177*
Mitral cells, 481, *482*
Mitral stenosis, 178–179, *178*
Mitral valve, function of, 84, *84*
Mixing movement, 488
  in colon, 494–495
  in small intestine, 493, *493*
Mixing waves, 491–492
Modiolus, 474
Molar concentration, in osmosis, 38
Molecular concentration, 269
Molecular size, capillary membranes diffu-
      sion and, 230, 230t
Molecular weight, in diffusion, 36
Monoamine oxidase inhibitors, in depres-
      sion, 437
Monocytes, 200, *200*
  inflammation response by, 203

Monocytes (*Continued*)
  life span of, 201
  properties of, 201–202
Monoglycerides, absorption of, 515
  in fat digestion, 511–512, *512*
Monosaccharides. See also *Fructose; Galac-*
      tose; Glucose.
  absorption of, 514–515
  digestion of, 510–511, *511*
Moon face, 592, *592*
Morphine receptors, in analgesic system,
      381
Mossy fibers, 409, *409*
Motility. See *Gastrointestinal tract, motility*
      of.
Motion. See *Movement(s).*
Motor activity, voluntary, 390
Motor aphasia, 423
Motor apraxia, 403
Motor aspects, of communication, 423
Motor association area, 402–403, *402*
Motor axis, of nervous system, 345, *345*
Motor cortex, anatomy of, 400–403,
      401–402
  primary, 401–403, *401–402*
  vasomotor center control by, 135
Motor functions, 386. See also *Move-*
      ment(s).
  basal ganglia control of, 404–407,
      404–405
  cerebellar, 407–411, *408–410*
  cortical control of, 400–403, *401–402*
  of brain stem, antigravity support and,
      394–395, *394*
  in stereotyped movement, 398
  vestibular sensation, 395–398, *395–396*
  of nervous system, 345
  of spinal cord. See *Spinal cord reflexes.*
  sensory feedback, 411–413
  voluntary, initiation of, 413
Motor neurons, 347–348, *347–348,* 387, *387*
  spinal, 403–404, *403*
Motor unit, 66
Mountain climbing. See *Altitude, high.*
Movement receptors, 366–367
Movement(s). See also *Motor; Reflex(es).*
  axial, 406
  coordination of, 402–403, *402*
  girdle, 406
  gross intentional, 406
  of cell, 17–19, *17–18*
  of eye, 402–403, 467–468, *467–469*
  of gastrointestinal muscles. See *Gastroin-*
      testinal tract, motility of.
  of hand, 403
  of sperm, 621–622, 641, *641*
  rapid, establishment of, 412–413
  rotational, 403
  sensation of, in joint, 374, *374*
  sequential, 411
  skilled, establishment of, 412–413
  stereotyped, 398
  voluntary, 402–403, *402*
      cerebellar control of, 410–411, *410*
MSH (melanocyte-stimulating hormone),
      secretion of, 591
Mucosa, gastrointestinal, blood flow in, 188
  intestinal, anatomy of, 486, *487*
  of respiratory system, 300
Mucous cells, gastrointestinal, 497
Mucous glands, gastrointestinal, 497, 500
Mucous neck cells, 500, *501*
Mucus, in sexual act, 623, 637
  peptic ulcer and, 517
  properties of, 498–499

Mucus (*Continued*)
  secretion of, in large intestine, 508
  in small intestine, 507
  in stomach, 500–502
Multiple motor unit summation, 66
Multiple tracts, in signal divergence, 357,
      357
Murmur, heart, in patent ductus arteriosus,
      178, 181
  in valvular lesions, *178*
Muscarinic receptors, 442
Muscle(s), action of. See *Motor.*
  blood flow in, 129–130, 130t, 664–665,
      665
  cardiac. See *Cardiac muscle.*
  contraction of, ATP role in, 17, *17*
  development of, testosterone effects on,
      625
  effects of athletic training on, 662, *662*
  endurance of, 657–658
  glucose metabolism in, 596–597, *597*
  glycogen in, 660–661, *661*
  glycogen storage in, 524–525, *524,* 596
  hypertrophy of, 622
  in breathing, 295
  length of, comparison of, 388–389
  lengthening reaction of, 391
  metabolism in, in exercise, 658–663, *658,*
      660–663
  of eye movement, 467, *467*
  power of, 657
  recovery of, after exercise, 659–661,
      660–661
  size of, 657
  skeletal. See *Skeletal muscle.*
  smooth. See *Smooth muscle.*
  spasm of, 71, 403
      from reflex, 393
  strength of, 657, 662, *662*
  tendon on, 390–391, *390*
  vasodilatation of, cardiac output regula-
      tion and, 158–159
  weakness of, in shock, 167
Muscle action potential, 63
Muscle fiber(s), anatomy of, 57–59, *58–59*
  cardiac, 80, *81*
  extrafusal, 388, *388*
  fast twitch, 66, *66,* 622–663
  in smooth muscle, 71–72, *72*
  intrafusal, 387–388, *388,* 390
  slow twitch, 66, *66,* 622–663
Muscle impulse, 51
Muscle pump, 121–122
Muscle receptors, 387–390, *388–390*
Muscle spindle, 364, *364*
  adaptation of, 366, *366*
  continuous discharge of, 388–389
  in voluntary motor activity, 390
  innervation of, 387–388, *388*
  muscle length comparison by, 388–389
  receptor function of, 388–389, *388*
  signal averaging by, 389, *390*
  stretch reflex and, 389–390, *389–390*
  structure of, 388, *388*
Muscle tone, inhibition of, 405–406
  maintenance of, 403
Muscle twitch, 65–66, *66,* 662–663
Muscularis mucosae, anatomy of, 486, *487*
Musculoskeletal system, in homeostasis, 4
Mutation, in cancer, 30
  of genes, 28
Myasthenia gravis, 71
Mydriasis, 470
Myelin, degeneration of, 558
Myelin sheath, 52–53, *53*

Myeloblasts, 200
Myelocytes, *200*
Myenteric plexus, 488–489, 493
Myocardial infarction, 171–172, 176
    cardiac failure in, 173–175
    cardiac output in, *159*
    injury current in, 106–107, *106–107*
    recovery from, *173*, 174–175
Myoepithelial cells, 648
Myofibrils, 57–59, *58–59*
Myogenic mechanism, of blood flow control, 132, *133*
Myoglobin, iron in, 197
Myopia, 451
Myosin, in ameboid locomotion, 17
    in mitosis, 29
    in platelets, 219
Myosin cross-bridges, 58, 60–63, *60*
    in smooth muscle, 73
Myosin filaments, anatomy of, 57–58, *58–59*
    in cardiac muscle, 80, *81*
    in skeletal muscle contraction, 60–63, *60, 62*
    in smooth muscle, 72–73, *73*
    molecular characteristics of, 60–61, *60*
Myosin head, in skeletal muscle, 60–61
Myotactic reflex, 389–390, *389*
Myxedema, 583, *583*

Na-K ATPase, 579
NAD (nicotinamide adenine dinucleotide), 526–529, *527*, 558–559
NADH (nicotinamide adenine dinucleotide phosphate), 558–559
Narcosis, nitrogen, 337–338
Nasal field of vision, 467
Nasal structures, irritation of, headache in, 383
Natriuresis, pressure, 147–150, *148*, 153
Natriuretic factor, atrial, 271–272
Near-sightedness, 451
Neck, joint receptors of, 397–398
    muscles of, in breathing, 295
Necrosis, tubular, in shock, 167
NEFA (nonesterified fatty acid), 532
Negative feedback, in control systems, 5–6
    operon and, 26–27, *26*
Negative stretch reflex, 389
Neocerebellum, 408–409
Neonatal infant, 650–653, *650–652*
Neostriatum, 404–406, *405*
Nephritis, glomerular, 286–287
    pyelo-, 287
Nephron, anatomy of, 248–249, *248–249*
    function of, 249, *249*
    juxtamedullary, 258
Nephrosis, lipoid, 289
Nephrotic syndrome, 289–290
Nernst equation, 37, 45
Nernst potential, 45–46
    at neuronal somal membrane, 351
Nerve(s), blood flow control by, 133–135, *134–135*
    cardiac, 86–87, *86*
    controlling eye movement, 467–468, *467–468*
Nerve deafness, 478
Nerve endings, as pain receptors, 378
    in muscle spindle, 388
    somatic, 364, *364*
Nerve fiber(s), action potentials in. See *Action potential(s).*

Nerve fiber(s) (*Continued*)
    classification of, 367–368, *367*
    conduction velocity of, 367–368, *367*
    excitation of, 54
    heat production by, 51, *51*
    in cerebral cortex, 415, *416*
    in motor unit, 66
    membrane potentials and, 45–46, *45–46*
    motor, 388
    muscle fiber excitation by, 63
    myelinated, 52–53, *53*
    of spinal cord, sensory signal transmission in, 370, *370*
    orientation of, in dorsal column–lemniscal system, 371
    recharging of, 51, *51*
    resting potential of, 46–48, *47*
    type A, in pain transmission, 378–380, *379*
    type C, 378–380, *379*
    unmyelinated, 52–53, *53*
Nerve impulses, 51
    transduction of, sensory stimuli into, 365–367, *365–366*
Nerve trunk, signal transmission in, 52–53, *53*
Nervi erigentes, 440–441
Nervous system. See also *Autonomic nervous system; Central nervous system.*
    excitability of, in alkalosis, 286
    fetal, 649
    in homeostasis, 4
    information processing by, 345–346
    levels of, 346–347
    motor division of, 345, *345*
    sensory division of, 345, *345*
    thiamine deficiency and, 558
Neuritis, in thiamine deficiency, 558
Neurohypophysis, 573–574, *573*
Neuromuscular junction, acetylcholine and, 69–70
    anatomy of, 69, *70*
    drugs affecting, 71
    in skeletal muscle, 69–71, *70*
    in smooth muscle, 75–76, *75*
Neuromuscular transmission, 69–71, *70*
Neuron(s), axon hillock of, *350*, 352
    differences in, 348
    excitation of, 350–355, *350, 352, 355*
        in epilepsy, 431–432
    facilitation of, 354
    in cerebral cortex, 372
    in respiratory control, 318–320, *319*
        hydrogen ion stimulus by, 320–322, *321*
    inhibition of, 352–353, *352*
    motor, 387, *387*
    of brain stem, 394
    of reticular activating system, 426–427, *427*
    organization of, for signal relay, 356, *356*
    parasympathetic, 441
    postganglionic, in gastrointestinal tract, 488
    postsynaptic, 347, *348*, 349
    presynaptic, 347
    re-excitation of, 354
    resting, 351, *352*
    short circuiting of, 353
    sympathetic, 440, *440*
    synaptic functions of. See *Synapse(s).*
    threshold for excitation of, 352
    transmitter release by, 350
Neuronal circuits, after-discharge, 359–360, *359–360*

Neuronal circuits (*Continued*)
    facilitated, 422
    in dorsal column–lemniscal system, 373, *373*
    in motor control, 404–405, *405*
    of cerebellum, 409–410, *409*
    of stretch reflex, 389, *389*
    signal prolongation in, 359–360, *359–360*
    stability of, 360–361
Neuronal pools, 355–356, *356*
    inhibition of, 356–358, *357–358*
    signal prolongation by, 359–360, *359–360*
    signal transmission through, 356–358, *356–358*
    spatial pattern transmission through, 358–359, *358–359*
Neurotensin, in enteric plexus, 488
Neurotransmitters, 347, 349–350, 359t
    action of, duration of, 349
        on postsynaptic neuron, *348*, 349
    diffusion of, in smooth muscle, 75
    excitatory postsynaptic potential and, 351–352, *352*
    exhaustion of, 355
    function of, 348
    in behavior control, 436–437
    in sleep, 430–431
    in smooth muscle depolarization, 74
    re-uptake of, 349
    release by, 348
    synthesis of, 348–349
Neutral fat. See *Triglycerides.*
Neutralization. See also *Acid-base balance.*
    of antigens, 210
    of chyme, 503–504
    of gastric juice, 517
Neutrophil chemotactic substance, 212
Neutrophil metamyelocyte, *200*
Neutrophil myelocyte, *200*
Neutrophilia, 203
Neutrophils, 200
    chemotaxis and, 201, *201*
    inflammation response by, 202–203
    phagocytosis by, 201–202
    properties of, 201–202
Newborn infant, 650–653, *650–652*
    body temperature regulation in, 550
Niacin, in thiamine deficiency, 557t, 558–559
Nicotinamide adenine dinucleotide (NAD), 526–529, *527*, 558–559
Nicotinamide adenine dinucleotide phosphate (NADP), 558–559
Nicotine, exercise and, 664
Nicotinic acid, in thiamine deficiency, 557t, 558–559
Nicotinic receptors, 442
Night blindness, 456
Nightmares, 429
Nitrate, in extracellular fluid, 277
    reabsorption of, 254
Nitrogen, diffusion of, 303
    in deep sea diving, 337–339
    partial pressure of, 302
    solubility coefficient of, 302
Nitrogen narcosis, 337–338
Nitroglycerin, in angina pectoris, 173
Nociceptive reflex, 391–392, *391*
Nocireceptors, 363–364, 364t
Nocturnal emission, 622
Node of Ranvier, 53, *53*
    action potential at, 365, *365*
Nonesterified fatty acid, 532
Norepinephrine, action of, at synapse, 349
    adrenergic receptor effects of, 442

Norepinephrine (*Continued*)
  as neurotransmitter, 350
  as vasoconstrictor, 144
  as vasodilator, 136
  bronchiolar effects of, 300
  cardiac effects of, 93–94
  in action potential, 54
  in behavior control, 436–437
  in blood flow control, 135
    coronary, 170
    muscular, 184
    cutaneous, 190
  in fat utilization, 535
  in gastrointestinal tract control, 488
  release of, 444
  removal of, 441–442
  secretion of, in smooth muscle, 75–76
Nose, function of, 299–300. See also *Nasal.*
Nuclear envelope, 12–13
Nuclear membrane, 8, *8–9*, 12
Nuclear pores, 12–13, *12*
Nuclei, 8, *8*, 12–13, *12*
  cerebellar, 409, *409*
  in reticular formation, 394, *394*
  of brain stem, 398
  of reticular activating system, 426–427, *428*
  salivatory, 500, *500*
Nucleolus, 8, *9*, *12*, 13
  ribosome formation in, 24
Nucleoplasm, 8, 12, *12*
Nucleotides, in DNA, 21–22, *21–22*
  in RNA, *22*, 23
Nucleus parabrachialis, 319
Nucleus precommissuralis, 398
Nursing, 647–649, *648*, 649t
Nutrient demand theory, for blood flow control, 131
Nutrients. See also *Carbohydrates; Fat; Protein(s).*
  energy extraction from, 15–17, *16–17*
  exchange of, between interstitial fluid and blood, 229–230, *230*, 230t
  in extracellular fluid, 3, 4
  in muscular activity, 661–662, *661*
  reabsorption of, 253
Nutrition. See also *Diet; Food.*
  in pregnancy, 645
  of embryo, 642
  of fetus, 642–643, 645
  of newborn, 653
  regulation of, 555

O blood group, 213–214, 213t–214t
O-A-B blood groups, 213–214, 213t–214t
Obesity, 556–557
  in diabetes, 602
Obligatory degradation, of proteins, 540
Obstruction, edema and, 241
  in respiratory system, 300
  of intestines, shock in, 166
  of pylorus, 518
  of veins, cardiac output regulation and, 160
Obstructive jaundice, 506
Occipital cortex, eye movement control in, 468
Occlusion, coronary. See *Coronary occlusion.*
Oddi, sphincter of, 505, *506–507*
Odontoblasts, 615–616
Odor. See *Smell.*
Odor blindness, 481

Ohm's law, 112
Olfactory area, of brain, 482
Olfactory bulb, *481*, 482
Olfactory cells, 480–482, *481*
Olfactory hairs, 481, *481*
Olfactory membrane, 480–481, *481*
Oncogenes, 30
One-kidney hypertension, 153–154, *154*
One-sided sensation, 373
One-way conduction, through synapse, 347
On-off response, visual, 465
Operon, 26–27, *26*
Opiates, in analgesic system, 381
Opponent colors, 465
Opsonization, 210, *210*
Optic chiasm, 462, *463*
Optic disc, 467, *467*
Optic nerve, 462–463, *463*
  signals transmitted through, 464–465, *464*
Optic radiation, 462, *463*
Optic tract, 462, *463*
Optics, of eye, 448–453
Oral contraceptives, 638
Oral hygiene, saliva in, 500
Orbitofrontal area, 432, *433*, 436
  in smell, 482
Organ of Corti, *472–474*, 473, 475–476
Organelles, 8–12, *9–12*
Organic matrix, of bone, 608–610
Organification, of thyroglobulin, 577, *578*
Organs, transplantation of, 216
Orgasm, female, 637–638
  male, 623
Ornithine, 540
Orthochromatic erythroblast, 195, *195*
Oscillatory circuit, in after-discharge, 359–360, *360*
Oscilloscope, membrane potential recording with, 54–55, *54*
Osmolality, 38
  of blood, in vascular control, 137
  of body fluids, 257, *257*
Osmolarity, definition of, 269
  of body fluids, 269–270, 270t
Osmole, 38, 269
Osmoreceptors, 273–274, *274*
Osmosis, 269–271, *270*, 271t. See also *Osmotic.*
  across selectively permeable membrane, 37–38, *38*
  chemiosmosis, 526–528, *527*
  of water, in kidney tubule, 252–253
    in small intestine, 514, *514*
Osmosodium receptor, 273–274, *274*
Osmotic equilibria, in body fluids, 269–271, *270*, 270t
Osmotic pressure, 38, *38*, 269–271, *270*
  colloid, 231, *231*, 234–235
    in glomerular capsule, 251
    protein regulation and, 240
  in intestinal absorption, 514
  total, 234
Ossicular system, 472–473, *472*
Osteoblasts, 609–611, *609*, 614
Osteoclasts, 609–612, *609*, 614–615
Osteocytes, 609, 611
Osteoid, 609
Osteolysis, 611–612
Osteolytic membrane, 611–612
Osteomalacia, 615
Osteon, 610, *610*
Osteoporosis, in Cushing's syndrome, 593
Osteoprogenitor cells, 610, 612
Ostium, of fallopian tubes, 641
Otolith, 395–396, *395*

Ovarian cycle, 630–632, *630–631*, 635–636
  feedback effects in, 635–636
  fertile period in, 638
  irregularity of, 635–636
Ovary, abnormalities in secretion from, 636–637
  hormones of, 565–566. See also *Estrogens; Progestins;* and *Sex hormones, female.*
  physiological anatomy of, 629, *630*
Overheating, of body, 548
Overshoot potential, 81
Ovulation, 631, 636, 638
  endometrium during, 634, *634*
Ovum, fertilization of, 622, 638, 641, *641*
  implantation of, 641–642, *642*
  maturation of, 640
  transport of, 641
Oxalate, as anticoagulant, 222
Oxaloacetic acid, 526, *526*
Oxidation, beta, of fatty acid, 533, *534*
  in citric acid cycle, 525–527, *527*
  of amino acids, deaminated, 540
  of glucose, 525–529, *526–527*
  of hydrogen, in metabolism, 526–527, *527*
  of iodide, 577
Oxidative enzymes, 16
Oxidative phosphorylation, 526–528, *527*
Oxygen, alveolar, pulmonary blood flow and, 125
  at high altitude, 323
  consumption of, in exercise, 665, *665*
  deficiency of. See *Hypoxia.*
  diffusing capacity of, 310
    in exercise, 663–664, *664*
  diffusion of, 303, *303*
    in placenta, 642–643
    in respiratory membrane, 308, *310*
    through capillary membranes, 230
  hemoglobin binding with, 197, 312–314, *312–313*
  in alveolar air, 306–307, 306t
  in blood flow control, 130–132, *131*
    cerebral, 186
    muscular, 184
  in extracellular fluid, 5
  in respiratory exchange ratio, 316
  in spacecraft, 336
  metabolic use of, 314–315, *315*
  partial pressure of, 302
  respiratory control by, 320, 322–323, *322–323*
  solubility coefficient of, 302
  toxicity of, at high pressure, 338
  transport of, by hemoglobin, 194, 312–314, *312–313*
    dissolved, 315
    pressure differences in, 305–306
    rate of, 314
    to tissue, 311–312, *311*, 314
  uptake of, by pulmonary blood, 311, *311*
    in exercise, 663–664, *663-664*
  vasomotion and, 229
Oxygen buffer function, of hemoglobin, *313*, 314
Oxygen debt, 660, *660*
Oxygen demand, coronary blood flow and, 170
Oxygen demand theory, in blood flow control, 131
Oxygen Fick method, 160–161, *161*
Oxygen pressure, 305
  alveolar ventilation and, 322–323, *323*
  at high altitude, 332–335

Oxygen pressure (*Continued*)
  hemoglobin binding and, 313, *313*
  in alveoli, 306, *307*, 311
  in aorta, 311
  in cells, 311, *312*
    metabolism and, 314–315, *315*
  in exercise, 323–324, *324*, 664
  in interstitial fluid, 311, *311*
  in placenta, 462–643
  in respiratory control, 322, *322*
  in venous blood, 311
  vs. altitude, 332–334, *333*, 333t
Oxygen therapy, hyperbaric, 340
  in hypoxia, 328–329
Oxygenation, tissue, in red blood cell production, 195–196, *196*
Oxygen-helium mixture, in deep diving,
  339
Oxygen-hemoglobin, dissociation curve of,
  313–314, *313*
Oxyphil cells, 610, 611, *611*
Oxytocin, 565
  formation of, 574
  function of, 574
  in milk secretion, 648
  in sexual act, 637–638
  in uterine contractibility, 646

P wave, 83, *83*, 98, *98*
Pacemaker, ectopic, 93
  sinoatrial node as, 93
Pacemaker waves, in smooth muscle action
  potential, 74, *74*
Pacini's corpuscles, 364, *364*
  adaptation of, 365, *366*
  in position sensing, 374
  receptor potential of, 365, *365*
  stimulus strength detection by, 366–367
  vibration detection by, 369
Paget's disease, cardiac output in, *159*
Pain, ACTH secretion effects of, 590
  acute (fast onset), 377, 379–380, *379*
  hypovolemic shock from, 166
  in coronary disease, 172–173
  in head. See *Headache.*
  in hunger, 554
  inhibition of, 380–381, *380*
  itching and, 383–384
  labor, 647
  limbic system and, 433
  localization of, 380, 382
  measurement of, 378, *378*
  neuronal reverberation in, 360
  perception of, 365
  purpose of, 377
  referred, 381–383, *382*
  slow (chronic), 377–378, *379*, 380
  thermal, 384–385, *384*
  tickling and, 383–384
  transmission of, 379–380, *379*
  types of, 377–378
  visceral, 381–382, *382*
Pain control system, 380–381, *380*
Pain receptors, stimulation of, 378–379
Pain reflex, 391–392, *391*
Pain threshold, 378, *378*
Palate, in swallowing, 490
  taste buds on, 479
Palatopharyngeal folds, in swallowing, 490
Pancreas, physiological anatomy of, 595,
  596
  secretions of, 503–504, *504*, 595

Pancreatic amylase, 503
  in carbohydrate digestion, 511, *511*
  in newborn, 652
Pancreatic hormones, 565
Pancreatic lipase, 503
Pantothenic acid, 557t, 559
Papillae, on tongue, 479, *480*
Papillary muscle, 84
Para-aminohippuric acid clearance, 255
Paradoxical sleep (REM), 429–430, *429*
Parafollicular cells, 613
Parallax, moving, 453
Parallel circuit, in after-discharge, 359, *359*
Paralysis, diver's, 338–339
  in hypokalemia, 587
  in thiamine deficiency, 558
Paralysis agitans, 406–407
Parasites, eosinophils and, 204
Parasympathetic mediators, 441
Parasympathetic nervous system, accommodation and, 443, 449
  adrenergic fibers of, 441–442
  anatomy of, 440–441, *441*
  cholinergic fibers of, 441–442
  excitatory effects of, 442–443, 443t
  in arterial pressure, 444
  in bladder emptying, 445
  in blood flow control, 133–134, *134*
  in bowel emptying, 445
  in bronchiolar control, 300
  in coronary blood flow control, 170–171
  in defecation control, 495, *495*
  in gastric secretion, 445, 502
  in gastrointestinal function, 443–444, 488
  in heart control, 86–87, *86*, 93, 444
  in lens focusing, 443, 449
  in mucus secretion, 508
  in pupillary aperture control, 469, 470
  in salivary secretion, 445, 500, *500*
  in sexual act, female, 637
    male, 622–623, *623*
  inhibitory effects of, 442–443, 443t
  micturition and, 290
  organ effects of, 442–443, 443t
  pancreatic secretions and, 504, *504*
  psychosomatic disorders and, 435
  receptors of, 442, 442t
  reflexes and, 445
  vascular effects of, 444
Parasympathetic tone, 444–445
Parathyroid gland, hormones of, 566
  physiological anatomy of, 610–611, *611*
Parathyroid hormone, 566
  calcium control and, 277, 606–607, *606*,
    611–613, *611, 613*
  chemistry of, 611, *611*
  in hypoparathyroidism, 614
  in vitamin D synthesis, 606–607, *606*
  phosphate absorption and, 610–611, *611*
  secretion of, 612, *613*
Paraventricular nuclei, 573, *573*
Parietal opercular–insular area, of brain,
  480, *480*
Parietal (oxyntic) cells, 500–501, *501*
Parkinson's disease, 406–407
  schizophrenia in, 437
Parotid gland, 499
Paroxysmal tachycardia, 104–105, *104–105*
Pars intermedia, 591
Partial proteins, 554
Passive theory, of sleep, 430
Passive transport. See *Diffusion.*
Patent ductus arteriosus, 122–123, *123*,
  178, 179–180, *180*
Pco₂. See *Carbon dioxide pressure.*

Pellegra, 559
Pelvic nerves, 290
  gastrointestinal tract control by, 488
  mucus secretion and, 508
Pelvis, renal, 248
Pentagastrin, 503, 517
Pepsin, 501
  in protein digestion, 512, *512*
  lack of, 516
Pepsinogen, secretion of, 500–501
Peptic cells, 500–501, *501*
Peptic ulcer, 516–518, *517*
  pain in, 382–383
Peptidase, 508
  in protein digestion, 512, *512*
Peptide chain, 537–538
Peptide linkage, 25, 537–538
Peptides, as neurotransmitters, 350
  in antibodies, 209, *209*
  in gastrointestinal blood flow, 188
Peptone, 504
  in protein digestion, 512, *512*
Periaqueductal gray area, 380, *380*
Perimetry, 467, *467*
Periodic breathing, 325
Periodontal membrane, 615
Peripheral chemoreceptor system, respira-
  tory control by, 322–323, *322-323*
Peripheral nerves, pain transmission by,
  379
Peripheral resistance, total, 114
  arterial pressure and, 141
  cardiac output and, 160
  in essential hypertension, 154
  in hypertension, 151–152, *151*
  in vasoconstrictor hypertension, 152–
    153, *153*
Peripheral resistance unit (PRU), 114
Peripheral tissue, cardiac output regulation
  and, 157–158, *157*
Peristalsis, 488–489, *489*
  autonomic control of, 443–444
  in colon, 495
  in esophagus, 490–491
  in gallbladder emptying, 505
  in small intestine, 493–494
  in stomach, 491–492
Peristaltic rush, 493
Peritonitis, muscular spasm in, 393
  septic shock from, 167
Permeability, of capillaries, 136, 241
  in shock, 165
  of capillary pores, 230, 230t
  of glomerular membrane, 250–251, *250*
  of hepatic sinuses, 187
  of lipid bilayer, 34, 34t
  of lymphatic capillaries, 237–238
  of membrane, 36
  of protein channels, 34–35, *35*
Permeable membrane, 36, 269
Pernicious anemia, 196, 199, 516
Peroxidase, 577, *577*
Peroxisomes, formation of, 15
pH. See also *Hydrogen ion concentration.*
  formula for, 279
  in exercise, 323–324, *324*
  of body fluids, 279
  of chyme, 492
  of gastrointestinal secretions, 499t
  of urine, 284
Phagocytosis, 13–14, 200–202
  in complement system, 210
  in spleen, 189
  of hemoglobin, 199
Phagosome vesicle, 202

Pharynx, in swallowing, 489–490
Phasic receptors, 366–367
Phenols, in uremia, 287
Phonation, 301, *301*
Phonocardiogram, 177–178, *178.*
  in cardiac cycle, 83, *83*
Phosphagen system, 658–660, *658*, 662
Phosphatase, in glycogenolysis, 525
Phosphate, absorption of, 252, 605–606
    in small intestine, 514
    parathyroid hormone and, 611–612,
      611
  buffer system for, 280–281
    hydrogen transport by, 283–284
  concentration of, in urine, 255t
  excretion of, 612
  formation of, in energy release, 658, *658*
  high energy bond of, 16, 522–523, 543,
    658
  in ATP, 16
  in body fluids, 268, 270t
  in extracellular fluid, 277, 607
  in lactation, 649
  in tooth development, 616
  in uremia, 287
  precipitation of, in bone, 608–610
  reabsorption of, 254
Phosphocreatine, 543
  energy release from, 658–659, *658*
  in body fluids, 270t
Phosphogluconate pathway, 529
Phospholipase, 503
Phospholipids, 535–536, *535*
  digestion of, 511
  in chylomicrons, 515
  in extracellular fluid, 268
  in insulin lack, 598
  in lipid bilayer, 9
  in platelets, 219, 222
  plasma level of, 532
Phosphoric acid, in DNA, 21, *21–22*
Phosphorylase, in glycogenolysis, 524–525
  insulin inhibition by, 596
Phosphorylation, in glycogenolysis, 524–525
  of glucose, 524
  oxidative, 526–528, *527*
Photopsin, 457
Photoreceptor. See *Cones; Rods.*
Physical theory, of smell, 481–482
Piezoelectric effect, on bone, 610
PIF (prolactin inhibitory factor), 570, 648
Pigment. See also *Melanin.*
  carotenoid, 558
  in cones, 457–459, *458–459*
  in retina, 455
Piloerection, 549
Pinocytic channel, 229, *229*
Pinocytic vesicles, 229, *229*
Pinocytosis, 13, *13*
Pinpoint stimulus test, 373, *374*
Pitch, 476–477
Pituicytes, 573
Pituitary factor, unidentified, 588
Pituitary gland, 568–569, *569*
  anterior, hormones of, 570. See also *Ad-*
    renocorticotropic hormone.
  posterior, 573–574, *573*
Pituitary hormones, 565, 568–569
  in ovarian cycle, 635–636
Pituitary stalk, 573
Place principle, 476
Placenta, anatomy of, 642, *642*
  blood flow through, 645
  delivery of, 647
  diffusion in, 642–643

Placenta (*Continued*)
  estrogen secretion by, *643*, 644
  fetal circulation and, 651, *651*
  hormones of, 566
  progesterone secretion by, *643*, 644
Planning, of sequential movement, 411
Plaque, dental, 617
Plasma, 111
  amino acids in, 538–539
  calcium in, 605–608, *606–607*
  constituents of, 268, *268*, 289t
  flow of, interstitial fluid and, 231–236,
    231–233
    through kidney, 255
  in ascites, 188
  lipid concentrations in, 532
  loss of, hypovolemic shock from, 166
  osmolarity of, 269–270, 270t
  potassium in, 261
  urea in, 260
Plasma cells, 200
  antibody formation by, 209
Plasma clearance, 254–255
Plasma colloid osmotic pressure, 232, 234
Plasma proteins, concentration of, 234
  cortisol effects on, 589
  edema and, 241
  formation of, 539
  in glomerular filtrate, 251
  in newborn, 652
  loss of, in nephrotic syndrome, 289–290
  pressure caused by, 231, *231*, 234–235
  types, 111
  use of, 539
Plasmablasts, 209
Plasmin, 224
Plasminogen, 224
Plateau, in action potential, 51–52, *52*
  in cardiac muscle, 81, *81*
  in smooth muscle, 73–74, *74*
Platelet(s), 219
  in blood clot, 221
Platelet activating factors, in allergy, 212
Platelet plug, 218–219
Pleasure, limbic system and, 433–434, *434*
Pleura, pressure in, 295
Pluripotent hemopoietic stem cells, 207
Pneumonia, respiration control in, 323
  respiratory insufficiency in, 327
Pneumotaxic center, 318–319
PO2. See *Oxygen pressure.*
Poiseuille's law, 115
Polarization, in action potentials, 48
Polychromatophil erythroblast, 195, *195*
Polymorphonuclear basophils, 200, *200*
Polymorphonuclear eosinophils, 200, *200*
Polymorphonuclear neutrophils, 200, *200*
Polypeptide chains, 209, *209*
Polypeptides, in protein digestion, 512, *512*
Polysaccharides, digestion of, 510–511
Pons, 394, *394*
Pontile nuclei, 407, *408*
Pontocerebellar tract, 407, *408*
Pores, in capillary membrane, 229, *229*
    diffusion through, 230, 230t
  in glomerular membrane, 250–251, *250*
  in protein channels, 35–36, *35*
  nuclear, 12–13, *12*
Portal circulation, 187, *187*
  blockage of, 188
Portal venous pressure, 188
Portal venules, 505, *505*
Position sense, 374, *374*
Positive support reaction, 392
Postcentral gyrus, 371–372, *371*

Posterior pituitary gland, 573–574, *573*
Postganglionic fibers, parasympathetic, 441
  sympathetic, 440
Postsynaptic membrane, excitation of, 351–
    352, *352*
  inhibition at, 352–353, *352*
Postsynaptic neuron, 347, *348*, 349
Postsynaptic potentials, excitatory, 351–
    352, *352*
  inhibitory, 352–353, *352*
  summation of, 353–354
Post-tetanic potentiation theory, of mem-
    ory, 420–421
Postural change, baroreceptors and, 142
Posture, reflexes of, 392–393
Potassium channels, 35, *35*
  at synapse, 349
  in neuronal inhibition, 352–353
  in sinoatrial node, 90
Potassium chloride, in hydrochloric acid se-
    cretion, 500–501, *501*
Potassium ion. See also *Sodium-potassium*
    pump.
  absorption of, 252
    in small intestine, 514
  active transport of, 39, *39*, 579
  as cause of pain, 378–379
  as vasoconstrictor, 137
  as vasodilator, 131, 137
  cardiac effects of, 88
  concentration of, in urine, 255t
  conductance of, 49–50, *49*
  control of, in extracellular fluid, 276–277,
    276–277
  diffusion of, 35, *35*
  diffusion potential of, 47, *47*
  excretion of, 260–261
  in acetylcholine channels, 70
  in aldosterone secretion, 587–588
  in body fluids, 32, *32*, 268, 270t
  in bone, 608
  in saliva, 499, *499*
  in uremia, 287
  in ventricular fibrillation, 172
  leakage of, through nerve membrane, 47,
    47
  loss of, in exercise, 667
  membrane potentials and, 45–46, *45*
  Nernst potential of, 351
  reabsorption of, 254
  secretion of, 252, 254, 261, 276–277,
    276–277, 586–587
Potassium pump, at neuronal somal mem-
    brane, 350–351, *350*
Power, muscular, 657
  energy systems for, 659
Power failure syndrome. See *Cardiogenic*
    shock.
Power stroke, in muscle contraction, 62,
    62
P-Q interval, 100
Precapillary sphincter, 130, *130*, 228–229,
    229
  in blood flow control, 131
Precipitation, of antigens, 209
  of salts, in bone, 608–610, *609*
Precordial leads, for ECG, 102, *102*
Predictive function, of cerebellum, 411
  of prefrontal area, 419
Prednisone, activity of, 586
Pre-eclampsia, 645
Preferential channels, 130, *130*, 228, *229*
Prefrontal area, functions of, 419
Preganglionic fibers, parasympathetic, 441
  sympathetic, 440

Pregnancy, breast development in, 647–648
cardiac output in, *159*
hormones in, 643–644, *643*
maternal responses in, 644–645
nutrition in, 645
parathyroid glands in, 612
placenta in. See *Placenta.*
toxemia of, hypertension in, 154
Prelumirhodopsin, 456, *456*
Premature contractions, in heart, 94, 103–104, *103*
Premature infant, 653
Premature ventricular contractions, 103–104, *103*
Premotor cortex, 402–403, *402*
Preoptic receptors, 548
Prepyriform area, in smell, 482
Presbyopia, 449–450
Pressoreceptors. See *Baroreceptors.*
Pressure, barometric, vs. altitude, 332, 333t
blood. See *Blood pressure.*
capillary. See *Capillary pressure.*
cerebrospinal fluid, 243–244
diffusion and, 37, *37*
gaseous, 303, *303*
filtration, 251
in capillary, 235
glomerular, 251–252
hydrostatic, blood pressure effects of, 120–121, *121*
in lungs, 125–126
in bladder, 290–291, *291*
in pulmonary circulation, 124–125, *124*
in renal circulation, 250–251, *250*
interstitial fluid. See *Interstitial fluid pressure.*
intraocular, 244–245, *244*
lung recoil, 295
mean circulatory filling, 116–117
mean systemic filling, cardiac output regulation and, 158–159
negative, in brain sinuses, 121, *121*
of gases, across respiratory membrane, 308, 310
in air, 306–307, 306t
in alveoli, 306–307, 306t
in diffusion, 303, *303*
in lungs vs. tissue, 305–306
in respiratory system, 302
on cochlear fluid, 473
osmotic, 38, *38*, 269–271, *270*
in intestinal absorption, 514
total, 234
reabsorption, in capillary, 235
respiratory, 295
sensation of, 368–369
systemic filling, in cardiac failure, 174
in hemorrhagic shock, 162
vs. sea depth, 337, 337t
Pressure curve, aortic, *83*, 85
Pressure diuresis, 147–150, *148*, 153
Pressure natriuresis, 147–150, *148*, 153
Pressure pulse, arterial, 122–123, *122–123*
Pressure-volume curves. See *Volume-pressure curves.*
Pressurized operations, physiology of, 337–339, 337t
Prestitial nucleus, 398
Presynaptic facilitation, in memory, 421
Presynaptic inhibition, 353
in memory, 421
Presynaptic membrane, in memory, 421–422
Presynaptic neuron, 347

Presynaptic terminals, 348, *348*
excitatory, 356, *356*
in memory, 421–422
PRF (prolactin-releasing factor), 648
Primary auditory cortex, 477, *477*
Primary ending, in muscle spindle, 388
Primary follicle, 631, *631*
Primary memory, 420–422
Primary motor cortex, 400–403, *401–402*
Primary olfactory cortex, 482
Primary sensory area, of cerebral cortex, 416–417
Primary visual cortex, 465–467, *466*
Primordial follicle, 629–630, *631, 636*
Procarboxypolypeptidase, 503
Procoagulants, 220
Proerythroblast, 194–196, *195*
Progesterone, 565–556
functions of, 634
in breast development, 648
in endometrial cycle, 634–635
in lactation, 648, *648*
in pregnancy, *643*, 644
in uterine contractibility, 646
Progestins, chemistry of, 632, *633*
in contraception, 638
synthesis of, 632, *633*
Prognostication, 419
Prolactin, 565, 648, *648*
Prolactin inhibitory factor (PIF), 570, 648
Prolactin-releasing factor, (PRF), 648
Proliferative phase, of endometrial cycle, 634, *634*
Proline, in DNA, 22, *23*
Prolyl hydroxylase, 560
Prometaphase, 28, *29*
Promoter, in biochemical synthesis, 26, *26*
in RNA synthesis, 23
Promyelocyte, 200
Pronucleus, 641, *641*
Prophase, 28, *29*
Proprioceptive sensation, 368
Proprioceptors, in respiratory control, 324
in sensory engram, 411–412
neck, 397–398
Propulsive movement, in gastrointestinal tract. See *Peristalsis.*
Propylthiouracil, in hyperthyroidism, 582
Prostaglandins, as cause of pain, 378–379
as vasodilators, 136–137
in platelets, 219
in semen, 621
Prostate duct, 619
Prostate gland, abnormalities of, 626–627
anatomy of, 619, *620*
function of, 621
in sexual act, 623
Protein(s), absorption of, 515
activation of, 26, *26*
amino acid storage as, 538–539
amino acid transport to, 40
body, 536–538, *537*
buffer system for, 281
calories in, 553
carbohydrate formation from, 529
carrier. See *Carrier proteins.*
catabolism of, growth hormone and, 571
in Cushing's syndrome, 593
insulin and, 599
channel. See *Protein channels.*
dietary requirements of, 553
digestion of, 503, 512, *512*
digestive, in cell, 11
fibrous, 538

Protein(s) (*Continued*)
formation of, 14, *15.* See also *Ribonucleic acid.*
ATP role in, 16–17, *17*
in ribosomes, 24–25, *24–25*
in aldosterone secretion, 587
in body fluids, 268, *268*, 270t
in cell membrane, 9–10, *10*
in cells, 8–9
in interstitial fluid, 234–235
regulation of, 239–240
in lymph, 238–239
from lung, 242
in plasma. See *Plasma proteins.*
insulin and, 599
integral, 9–10, *10*
intracellular, 538
lipo-. See *Lipoproteins.*
metabolism of, 538–540
cortisol effects on, 588–589
insulin in, 599, *599*
obligatory loss of, 540
partial, 554
peripheral, 9–10, *10*
phagocytosis and, 13
reabsorption of, 253
receptor, at synapse, 348, 349
in smooth muscle contraction, 76
regulatory, 27
repressor, 26
sparing of, 540
structural, in genetic control, 20
surface receptor, 208–209
synthesis of, 539
growth hormone and, 570–571
hormonal effect on, 567
testosterone effect on, 625
thyroid hormones and, 579
transport, 33
utilization of, in starvation, 557, *557*
Protein channels, diffusion through, 34–36, *35*
ion leakage through, 47, *47*
net diffusion rate of, 36–37, *37*
Proteinase, in sperm, 622
Proteoglycan filaments, in interstitium, 231, *231*
Proteoglycans, in bone, 608
in cell membrane, 10
Proteolytic enzymes, as cause of pain, 378–379
in phagocytosis, 202
in saliva, 500
Proteose, 504
in protein digestion, 512, *512*
Prothrombin, thrombin conversion from, 220, *220*
Prothrombin activator, 220, *220*
formation of, 221–223, 221t
Protoplasm, 8
Protoporphyrin, 197, *197*
Proximal tubule, 248, *249*
hydrogen ion secretion by, 282
potassium excretion in, 260–261
reabsorption in, 253
sodium reabsorption in, 260
PRU (peripheral resistance unit), 114
Pseudopodium, 17–18, *17*
Psychogenic obesity, 556
Psychosis, chemical transmitters and, 436–437
Psychosomatic disorders, 435
Pteroylglutamic acid, 559
in red blood cell production, 196–197

Ptyalin, 511, *511*
Puberty, female, 630, 636
  male, 626
Pudendal nerve, 290, *290*
Pulmonary. See also *Lung(s).*
Pulmonary arteries, 124
  in patent ductus arteriosus, 180
  pressure in, 85, 24, *124*
  stenosis of, *180*, 181
Pulmonary capacity, 297–298, *297*
Pulmonary capillaries, pressure in, 124, *124*
Pulmonary circulation, 110, *111*, 123–127, *124*, *126*
  anatomy of, 123–124, *124*
  blood flow of, 125–126, *126*
  blood shift to systemic circulation, 125
  blood volume in, 125
  exercise effects on, 126–127
  pathological conditions affecting, 127
  pressures in, 124–125, *124*
Pulmonary congestion, in patent ductus arteriosus, 181
Pulmonary disease, cardiac output in, *159*
Pulmonary edema, death from, 243
  in cardiac failure, 175–176
  in myocardial infarction, 172
  in valvular lesions, 179
  mechanism of, 242–243, *242*
Pulmonary embolism, 127, 225
Pulmonary emphysema. See *Emphysema.*
Pulmonary hypertension, in emphysema, 326–327
Pulmonary interstitial fluid, 241–243, *242*
Pulmonary membrane. See *Respiratory membrane.*
Pulmonary resistance, total, 114
Pulmonary valve, function of, 84–85, *84*
Pulmonary veins, pressure in, 124–125
Pulmonary ventilation. See also *Alveolar ventilation; Respiration.*
  at high altitude, 334–335
  capacity of, 297–298, *297*
  in exercise, 663–664, *663*
  mechanics of, 294–297, *295-296*
  minute respiratory volume and, 298–299
  respiratory passageways in, 299–301, *299*
  volume of, 297, *297*
Pulmonary volume, 297, *297*
Pulmonary wedge pressure, 125
Pulmonic area, for heart sounds, 177, *177.*
Pulp, of tooth, 615–616, *615*
Pulse, radial, 123
  weak, 123
Pulse deficit, 123
Pulse pressure, 122–123, *122–123*
Pulsus paradoxus, 123
Pump. See also *Calcium pump; Sodium-potassium pump.*
  atrium as, 82–83
  electrogenic, *45*, 46
  hydrogen ion, 527–528
  iodide, 577, *577*
  lymphatic, 239–240
  osteocytic, 611
  potassium, 350–351, *350*
  pyloric, 492
  sodium, 350–351, *350*
  venous, 121–122
  ventricle as, 82–84, *83*
Punishment, limbic system and, 433–435, *434*
Pupillary aperture (opening), 450, *450*
  autonomic control of, 443, *469*, 470
Pupillary light reflex, *469*, 470

Purines, in DNA, 21, *21–22*
Purkinje cells, 409, *409*
Purkinje fibers, *90*, 92–93
  resting potential of, 81
Purkinje system, *90*, 91–92
Purpura, thrombocytopenic, 225
Pus, formation of, 203
Putamen, 401, 404–406, *404–405*
PVC (premature ventricular contractions), 103–104, *103*
Pyelonephritis, 287
Pyloric glands, 500, 503
Pyloric pump, 492
Pylorus, 491
  in emptying of stomach, 492
  obstruction of, 518
  sphincter of, 491
Pyramidal cells, 400
  in cerebral cortex, 415, *416*
Pyramidal tract, 400–401, *401*
Pyriform area, 432, *433*, 436
  in smell, 482
Pyrimidines, in DNA, 21, *21–22*
Pyrogens, 550
Pyridoxine, 557t, 559
Pyruvic acid, acetyl coenzyme A formation from, 525
  formation of, 525, *526*
  in anaerobic glycolysis, *526*, 528–529
  in cerebral blood flow regulation, 186
  in glycogenesis, 524

Q wave, 83, *83*
QRS complex, 83, *83*, 98, *98*
  action potential and, 99–100, *99*
Q-T interval, 100

R wave, 83, *83*, 98, *98*
Radial pulse, 123
Radiation, cancer and, 30
  in heat loss, 546, *546*
  in nuclear submarine, 340
  in space, 336
Radioactive iodine uptake, in hyperthyroidism, 582
Radioactive substances, in bone, 608
Radioimmunoassay, 567–568, *568*
Ragc, 435
Raising movement, brain stem control of, 398
Ramp signal, inspiratory, 319
Ranvier, node of, 53, *53*
  action potential at, 365, *365*
Raphe magnus nucleus, 380, *380*
Raphe nuclei, 405, 427, *427*
  as cause of sleep, 430
Rapid eye movement (REM) sleep, 428–429, *428*
Rapture of the depths, 337–338
Rate receptors, 366–367
Reabsorption, fluid volume regulation by, 262
  in capillary, 235
  in kidney tubules, 249, 252–254, *252*, 255t
  of bicarbonate, 282–283, *282*
  of fluid, 261–262
  of water, 259
Reabsorption pressure, in capillary, 235

Reading, 418–419
  saccadic movement in, 468–469
Reagins, 212
Receptor(s), acetylcholine, 442, 442t
  adrenergic, 442, 442t
  alpha, 442, 442t
  antigen, 210–211
  baro-. See *Baroreceptors.*
  beta, 442, 442t
  chemo-. See *Chemoreceptors.*
  cold, 384–385, *384*
  excitatory, 348
  head, 556
  hormone, 566, *567*
  inhibitory, 348
  joint, 366, *366*, 374, *374*, 397–398
  morphine, in analgesic system, 381
  movement, 366–367
  muscle, 387–390, *388–390*
  olfactory, 481–482
  osmosodium, 273–274, *274*
  pain, 378–379
  phasic, 366–367
  photo-. See *Cones; Rods.*
  position, 374, *374*
  rate, 366–367
  sensory. See *Sensory receptors.*
  stretch, 271–272
    in bladder, 291
    in inspiration control, 319
  swallowing, 490
  synaptic sensitivity of, 361
  temperature, 548
  thermal, 384–385
  tonic, 366–367
  volume, 271–272
  warmth, 384–385, *384*
Receptor potentials, 365, *365*, 456–457, *457*
  of hair cell, 476
Receptor proteins, at synapse, *348*, 349
  in aldosterone action, 587
  in smooth muscle contraction, 76
Receptor sites, for sodium-potassium pump, 39
Reciprocal inhibition, 392, 357–358, *358*
Reciprocal innervation, 392
Recording, of electrocardiogram, 100
Red blood cells, 194–199. See also *Hemoglobin.*
  deficiency of. See *Anemia.*
  destruction of, 198–199
  fetal, 649
  function of, 194
  genesis of, 194–197, *195–196*
  in weightlessness, 337
  iron metabolism and, 197–198, *198*
  maturation of, 196–197
  testosterone effect on, 625
  typing of, 214, 214t
Red nucleus, 398
Red-sensitive pigment, 457–459, *458-459*
Re-entrant pathway, 94
Referred pain, 381–383, *382*
Reflex(es), autonomic, 439
  Bainbridge, 144
  baroreceptor, 141–143, *142–143*
    in compensated shock, 164
  cecal, 494
  chewing, 489
  clinical use of, 390
  cord. See *Spinal cord reflexes.*
  cough, 300–301
  crossed extensor, *391*, 392
  defecation, 495, *495*

Reflex(es) (*Continued*)
  diagonal stepping, 393, *393*
  duodenocolic, 495
  enterogastric, 492–493, 503
  flexor, 391–392, *391*
  galloping, 393
  gastrocolic, 495
  gastroenteric, 493
  gastroileal, 494
  Hering-Breuer, 319
  in cardiac failure, 173–174
  in spinal shock, 393
  in swallowing, 490
  load, 389–390
  mark time, 393, *393*
  micturition, 290–291, *290–291*
  neck, in equilibrium maintenance, 398
  nociceptive, 391–392, *391*
  of locomotion, 392–393, *393*
  pain, 391–392, *391*
  peristaltic. See *Peristalsis*.
  positive support, 392
  postural, 392–393
  pupillary, *469*, 470
  scratch, 384
  spinal. See *Spinal cord reflexes*.
  spinal cord control of, 346
  stepping, 392–393
  stretch, 389–390, *389*
  sympathetic, in shock compensation, 163
  tendon, 390–391, *390*
  withdrawal, 391–392, *391*
Reflux, esophageal, 491, 500
Refraction, errors of, 450–451, *450–452*
Refractive index, of eye components, 448–449, *448*
Refractory period, circus movement and, 94–96, *94*
  in cardiac muscle, 81
Regulatory gene, 27
Regulatory mechanisms, 4–5. See also *Homeostasis*.
Regulatory protein, 27
Regulatory T cell, 211
Regulon, 27
Regurgitation, aortic, 178–179, *178*
  pressure pulse in, 123, *123*
  of heart valves, 178
Rehearsal, in memory transference, 422
Reinforcement, 434–435
Reissner's membrane, 473–474, *474*
REM sleep, 428–429, *428*
Remodeling, of bone, 610
Renal. See also *Kidney*.
Renal–body fluid system, in arterial pressure control, 147–150, *148–150*, 153, *153*
Renal fraction, 249
Renal function curve, 148–149, *148–149*
Renal output curve, 148–149, *148–149*
  in renin-angiotensin system, 150, *150*
Renin, 136
  as vasoconstrictor, 144–146, *145*
  in aldosterone secretion, 588
  in arterial pressure control, 150, *150–151*
  in cardiac failure, 174
  in Goldblatt's hypertension, 153–154, *154*
  in kidney function, during hypotension, 263–264
  secreted by tumor, in hypertension, 152–153
Repetitive discharge, in excitable tissues, 52, *52*
Repolarization, in action potential, 48, 51
  ventricular, 83, *83*, 99–100, *99*

Repolarization waves, 98–100, *99*
Repressor operator, 26, *26*
Repressor protein, 26
Reproduction, in homeostasis, 5
  of cell, 27–30, *28*
Reproductive functions, female, endometrial cycle in, 634–635, *634*
    fertility in, 638
    hormones in, 630, 643–644, *643*. See also *Estrogens; Progestins*.
    in pregnancy, 643–645, *643*
    lactation in, 647–649, *648*, 649t
    ovarian cycle in, 630–632, *630–631*, 635–636
    ovum maturation in, 640–642, *641–642*
    parturition in, 645–647, *646*
    physiological anatomy of, 629, *630*
    placenta in, 642–643, *642*
    sexual act in, 637–638
  male, abnormalities in, 626–627
    hormones in, 623–625, *623–624*
    physiologic anatomy of, 619, *620*
    sexual act in, 622–623, *623*
    spermatogenesis in, 619–622, *620*
Reservoir. See *Blood reservoir*.
Residual body, 14, *14*
Residual volume, 297–298
  in asthma, 328
Resistance, muscular, 662, *662*
  to blood flow. See *Vascular resistance*.
Resolution, 623, 637
Resonance, in cochlea, 474–475
  of voice, 301
Respiration. See also *Breathing; Pulmonary ventilation*.
  energy for, 296–297
  in exercise, 663–664, *663–664*
  pulsus paradoxus and, 123
  rate of, 298
    in acidosis, 286
    in high altitude acclimatization, 334–335
    in hypoxia, 334
  regulation of. See also *Respiratory center*.
    abnormalities in, 324–325
    by peripheral chemoreceptor system, 322–323, *322–323*
    chemical, 320–322, *321*
    during exercise, 323–324, *324–325*
    thyroid hormone effects on, 580
Respiratory acidosis, 285
  in deep sea diver, 338
Respiratory alkalosis, 285
Respiratory center, 318–320, *319*
  carbon dioxide excitation of, 5
  chemosensitive area of, 320–322, *321*
  depression of, 324–325
  high altitude adaptation of, 323
  hydrogen ion and, 281, *281*
Respiratory distress syndrome, in infant, 295, 327, 650–651
Respiratory exchange ratio, 316
Respiratory insufficiency. See also *Dyspnea*.
  in asthma, 327–328
  in atelectasis, 327
  in emphysema. See *Emphysema*.
  in hypoxia. See *Hypoxia*.
  in pneumonia, 327
  in tuberculosis, 328
Respiratory membrane, gas diffusion through, 307–308, *308–310*, 310
  inflammation of, in pneumonia, 327
  tuberculosis effects on, 328
Respiratory pressure, 295

Respiratory quotient, 554
Respiratory reserve, in patent ductus arteriosus, 180–181
Respiratory system, acid-base balance and, 280–282, *281*
  fetal, 649
  in newborn, 653
  nutrients from, 4
  water loss from, 266–267, 267t
Respiratory unit, 307
Resting expiratory level, 298
Resting potentials, in skeletal muscle, 63
  in cardiac muscle, 81
  in smooth muscle, 73
  of nerves, 46–48, *47*
  of neuronal soma, 350–351, *350*
  of sinoatrial node, 91
Resting stage, in action potentials, 48
Resuscitation, cardiac, 96, *96*
Reticular activating system, 425–428, *426–427*
  in epilepsy, 431–432
Reticular formation, 394–395, *394*
  control of stereotyped movements by, 398
Reticular nuclei, of brain stem, 401
Reticular system, in pain, 380
Reticulocyte, 195, *195*
Reticuloendothelial cells, of spleen, 189
Reticuloendothelial system, 202, *202*
Reticulospinal tract, 394, *394*, 401, *403*, 404
Reticulum, endoplasmic. See *Endoplasmic reticulum*.
Retina. See also *Cones; Rods*.
  amacrine cells of, 463–464, *463*
  bipolar cells of, 462–464, *463–464*
  blind spot in, 467, *467*
  depth of focus and, 450
  ganglion cells of, 464–466, *464*
  glucose metabolism in, 601
  horizontal cells of, 463–464, *463*
  image formation on, 449
  image size on, 452
  light adaptation of, 457–458
  light fusion by, 458
  neural organization of, 462–463, *463*
  pigment in, 455
  structure of, 453–455, *453–455*
Retinal, 456, *456*, 458
Retinal isomerase, 456, *456*
Retinene, 456, *456*, 458
Retinol, 456, *456*, 458, 557t, 558
Reverberatory circuit, in after-discharge, 359–360, *360*
  in crossed extensor reflex, 392
  in flexor reflex, 392
  in memory, 420
Reward, limbic system and, 433–435, *434*
Rh blood types, 214–215
Rheumatic fever, 212
  cortisol in, 590
  heart valve lesions from, 177–179, *178*
Rheumatoid arthritis, cortisol in, 590
Rhodopsin, 454–455
  in light adaptation, 457–458
  photochemistry of, 455–457, *456–457*
Rhythm method, of contraception, 638
Rhythmic contraction, of intestinal muscle, 487–488
Rhythmic stepping reflex, 392–393
Rhythmicity, of excitable tissues, 52, *52*
  of heart, 90–94, *90–92*
    abnormal, 94–96, *94–96*. See also *Cardiac arrhythmias*.
  of inspiration, 319

Rhythmicity (*Continued*)
    of signals, 360
    of sleep-wakefulness cycle, 430–431
Rib cage, in breathing, 294–295, *294*
Riboflavin, 557t, 559
Ribonuclease, 503
Ribonucleic acid (RNA), growth hormone
        and, 571
    in nucleolus, 13
    in transcription, 22–24, *22–24*, 24t
    in translation, 24–25, *24–25*
    insulin and, 599
    messenger, *22–23*, 23, 24t, 25, *25*
    ribosomal, 23–24
    synthesis of, 22–23, *22*
    thyroid hormones and, 579
    transfer, 23–24, *24–25*
    types of, *22–24*, 23–24, 24t
Ribose, in ATP, 16
    in RNA, 23
Ribosomal RNA, 23–24
Ribosomes, attachment of, endoplasmic
        reticulum and, 11, 25
    formation of, 13, 24
    growth hormone and, 571
    in glandular secretions, 498, *498*
    protein formation in, 24–25, *24–25*
    structure of, *25*
Rickets, 612, 614–615
Right atrial pressure. See *Central venous
        pressure*.
Rigidity, in Parkinson's disease, 406–407
RNA. See *Ribonucleic acid*.
RNA polymerase, *22*, 23
Rod receptor potential, 456–457, *457*
Rods, 453–455, *453–455*
    excitation of, 455–457, *456–457*
    neural aspects of, 462–463, *463*
Root, of tooth, 615, *615*
Rotation, brain stem control of, 398
    of head, 403
Rubrospinal tract, 401, *403*, 404
Ruffini's end organs, 364, *364*, 368–369,
        374
Running, energy expenditure in, 545t
    equilibrium in, 366–367, 397

S wave, 83, *83*, 98, *98*
S-A node. See *Sinoatrial node*.
Saccadic movement, 468–469
Saccharides, formation of, 14–15
Saccharin, 478
Saccule, 395, *395*, 397
Sacral parasympathetic nerves, 440–441,
        441
Sacral reflex, in spinal shock, 393
Sagittal sinus, negative pressure in, 121,
        121
Saliva, secretion of, 445, 499–500, *499–500*,
        499t
Salivary glands, 499, *499*
Salivatory nuclei, 500, *500*
Salt. See also *Sodium ion*.
    conservation of, 263–264
    craving for, 275
    excretion of, 147–150, *148*, 153
        in essential hypertension, 154
    intake of, arterial pressure and, 150,
        150–151
        in exercise, 667
        in hypertension, 151–152, *151*
        vs. output, 148–149, *148*, *149*
    retention of, in hypertension, 151–152

Saltatory conduction, 53–54, *53*
Salty taste, 479
Sarcolemma, 57, *58*
Sarcomere, anatomy of, 58, *58*
    length vs. tension of, 62–63, *62*
Sarcoplasm, 58–59
Sarcoplasmic reticulum, 59, *59*
    calcium release by, 63, *64*, 65
    in muscle action potential, 63, *64*
    in smooth muscle, 75
Sarcotubules, *64*
Satiety, 554
Satisfaction, limbic system and, 433–435,
        434
Scala media, 473–474, *473–474*
Scala tympani, *472–473*, 474
Scala vestibuli, *472–474*, 473–474
Schistosomiasis, eosinophils and, 204
Schizophrenia, 437
Schwann cells, 53, *53*
Sclerosis, of lungs, 127
Scotopsin, 456, *456*
Scratching, 384
SCUBA diving physiology, 339, *339*
Scurvy, 560
Second messenger, in hormone mediation,
        566–567, *567*
    in smooth muscle contraction, 76
    in thyroid hormone secretion, 580
Secondary ending, in muscle spindle, 388
Secondary memory, 420–422
Secondary sensory areas, 417, *417*
Secondary visual area, 466–467
Secretagogues, 502
Secretin, in gastrointestinal blood flow, 188
    in pancreatic secretion regulation, 504,
        504
    insulin secretion and, 600
    stomach motility and, 493
    structure of, 502–503
Secretion, gastrointestinal. See *Gastrointes-
        tinal secretion*.
    in kidney tubules, 249, 252–254, *252*,
        255t
    of ACTH, 590–591, *590*
    of aldosterone, 587–588
    of glucagon, 601
    of hydrogen ions, 282–284, *282*, *284*
    of insulin, 599–600
    of ions, aldosterone and, 586–587
    of parathyroid hormone, 612, *613*
    of potassium, 276–277, *276–277*
    of sweat, 547, *547*
    of testosterone, 623–624, *623*, 626
Secretory phase, of endometrial cycle, 634–
        635, *634*
Secretory vesicles, 11–12
    formation of, 15
    in glandular secretions, 498
Segmentation contraction, 493, *493*
Seizures. See *Epilepsy*.
Self-contained underwater breathing appa-
        ratus, 339, *339*
Self-excitation, of sinoatrial node, 91
Semen, 621–622
Semicircular canals, 395–397, *395*
Semilunar valves, function of, 84
    sounds of, 177
Seminal vesicle, 619, *620*, 621
Seminiferous tubules, 619–621, *620*
Sensation, auditory. See *Hearing*.
    deep, 368
        exteroceptive, 368
        itching, 383–384
        mechanoreceptive. See *Mechanoreceptive
            sensation*.

Sensation (*Continued*)
    modalities of, 365
    of smell, 480–482, *481*
    of taste, 478–480, *479–480*
    proprioceptive, 368
    sexual, female, 637
        male, 622–623
    tactile, 368–369
    thalamus function in, 375
    thermal, 384–385, *384*
    tickling, 383–384
    vestibular, 395–398, *395–396*
    visceral, 368
    visual. See *Vision*.
Senses, somatic, 368
Sensitivity, sensory, control of, 375–376
Sensory aphasia, 423
Sensory areas, of cerebral cortex, 416–417
Sensory aspects, of communication, 423
Sensory association area, of cerebral cor-
        tex, 416–417, *417*
Sensory engram, 411–412
Sensory feedback control, of motor func-
        tions, 411–413
Sensory information, processing of, 345–346
Sensory memory, 420
Sensory nerves, in skin, 358–359, *358*
Sensory receptors, 345, *345*, 363–376
    adaptation of, 365–366, *366*
    differential sensitivity of, 364–365
    joint, 366–367, *366*
    movement, 366–367
    phasic, 366–367
    position sense, 374, *374*
    potentials at. See *Receptor potentials*.
    predictive function of, 366–367
    rate, 366–367
    tactile, 368–369
    tonic, 366
    types of, 363–364, *364*, 364t
Sensory sensitivity, control of, 375–376
Sensory signals, separation of, in spinal
        cord, 371
    to cerebellum, 407, *408*
    to reticular activating system, 426
    transmission of, in anterolateral system,
        369–370, 374–375, *375*
        in dorsal column–lemniscal system,
            369–374, *370–374*
        in peripheral nerve, 369
        in spinal cord, 370, *370*
Sensory stimuli, detection of. See *Sensory
        receptors*.
    strength of, psychic interpretaton of, 367
        receptor adaptation and, 366
    transduction of, into nerve impulses,
        365–367, *365–366*
Sensory terminal, in memory, 421–422, *421*
Septic shock, 166–167
Serine, in DNA, 22, *23*
Serosa, 486, *487*
Serotonin, as cause of pain, 378–379
    as cause of sleep, 430
    as neurotransmitter, 350
    as vasodilator, 136
    in analgesic system, 380–381, *380*
    in behavior control, 436–437
    in enteric plexus, 488
Sertoli cells, *620*, 621, 626
Serum, from blood clot, 220–221
Servomechanism, in cerebellum, 411–412
Sex, in atherosclerosis, 536
Sex chromosomes, 620, 641
Sex hormones, exercise and, 667
    female, 630. See also under *Reproductive
        functions, female*.

Sex hormones (*Continued*)
   female, abnormalities in secretion of, 636–637
      in ovarian cycle, 630–632, 635–636
      in pregnancy, 643–644, *643*
   in athletic performance, 656–657, 667
   in contraception, 638
   male, 623–626, *623–624*
Sexual act, 622–623, *623*, 637–638
Sexual activity, from amygdala stimulation, 435
Sexual characteristics, estrogens in, 632–634
   testosterone in, 624
Sexual drive, 622, 637
Sexual functions. See *Reproductive functions.*
Sexual organs, female, 629, *629*
   estrogen effects on, 632–633
   male, 619, *620*
Sexual sensation, female, 637
   male, 622–623
Shivering, 549
   in heat stroke, 551
Shock, anaphylactic, 166
   cardiac output in, *159*
   cardiogenic, 162
      in myocardial infarction, 172
   circulatory, 162–167
      in adrenocortical hormone deficiency, 586–587
      in heat stroke, 551
   compensated, 163–163, *164*
   effects of, 167
   hemorrhagic, 162–165, *163–165*
   hypoglycemic, 597
   hypovolemic, 166
   insulin, in newborn, 653
   irreversible, 165–166
   nonprogressive, 163–164, *163*
   progressive, 163–165, *163–164*
   septic, 166–167
   spinal, 393
Short-circuiting, of neurons, 353
Shunt, in emphysema, 326
   in low ventilation-perfusion ratio, 310–311
   left-to-right (patent ductus arteriosus), 122–123, *123*, *178*, 179–180, *180*
   right-to-left (tetralogy of Fallot), *180*, 181
Sickle cell anemia, 199
Signal(s), averaging of, 389, *390*
   convergence of, 357, *357*
   definition of, 356
   divergence of, 357, *357*
   in reciprocal circuit, 357–358, *358*
   pain, transmission of, 379–380, *379*
   prolongation of, 359–360, *359–360*
   relaying of, 356–358, *356–358*
   rhythmic, 360
   sensory. See *Sensory signals.*
   spatial patterns and, 358–359, *358–359*
   thermal, transmission of, 385
   transmitted by optic nerve, 464–465, *464*
Silicosis, 127
Sinoatrial node, anatomy of, 90–91, *90*
   atrial premature contractions and, 103
   function of, 82, 90–91, *91*
   pacemaker function of, 93
Sinuses, cranial, negative pressure in, 121, *121*
   nasal, irritation of, headache in, 383
Skeletal muscle, after denervation, 67–68
   anatomy of, 57–59, *58–59*

Skeletal muscle (*Continued*)
   atrophy of, 67–68
   blood flow through, 183–185, *184*
   contraction of, 60–67, 183–184, *184*
      in single twitch, 65–66, *66*
      initiation of, 63, *64*, 65
      isometric vs. isotonic, 65–66, *66*
      maximal strength of, 67
      mechanics of, 66–67
      molecular mechanism of, 60–63, *60–62*
      speed of, 66, *66*
   control of, 357–358, *357*
   excitation of, by acetylcholine, 70–71
   fatigue of, 67
   hypertrophy of, 67
   impulse transmission to, 69–71, *70*
Skilled motor activity, 412
Skin, as reservoir, 190
   blood flow in, 130t, 189–190, *189*
   estrogen effects on, 634
   heat loss from, 546–548, *546–547*
   heat transfer to, 548
   sensory information from, spatial patterns in, 358–359, *358–359*
   temperature receptors in, 548
   testosterone effects on, 625
   thermal sensation and, 384–385, *384*
   vasoconstriction in, 549
   water loss from, 266–267, 267t
Skull, veins in, pressure in, 121
Sleep, 429–431, *429*
   EEG in, 429, *429*
   energy expenditure in, 545t
   induction of, 430
   physiological effects of, 431
   REM, 429–430
   slow wave, 429
   theories of, 430
   thyroid hormones and, 580
   vs. wakefulness, 430–431
Sleep spindles, 429
Sliding filament mechanism, 60, *60*
Slit-pores, in capillary membrane, 229, *229*
   in glomerular membrane, 250–251, *250*
Slow channels, in cardiac muscle, 81
   sodium, 52
Slow twitch, muscular, 662–663
Slow waves, in sleep, 428
   in smooth muscle action potential, 74, *74*
Small intestine, absorption in, 513–515, *514*
   malabsorption from, 518
   movements of, 493–494, *493–494*
   secretions of, 507–508, *507*
Smell, 480–482, *481*
   in learning, 436
Smoking, exercise and, 664
   peptic ulcer and, 517
Smooth muscle, action potential in, 73–74, *74*
   contraction of, 71–77, *72–75*
      energy requirements of, 73
      excitation-contraction coupling in, 74–75
      hormone effects on, 76
      maximum strength of, 73
      mechanical characteristics of, 76–77
      without action potential, 74, 76
   fiber size in, 71
   in bronchioles, 300
   intestinal, 487
   membrane potential in, 73
   neuromuscular junction in, 75–76, *75*
   relaxation of, 73
   tone of, 76–77

Smooth muscle (*Continued*)
   types of, 71–72, *72*
   visceral, 71–72, *72*, 74–75, *74–75*
Sodium bicarbonate, alkalosis from, 285
   in acidosis treatment, 286
Sodium channels, 35–36, *35*
   at synapse, 349
   fast, 52
   in action potential propagation, 50–51
   in neuronal inhibition, 352–353
   slow, 52
   voltage-gated, 48–49, *49*
Sodium chloride, in sweat, 547
Sodium ion, absorption of, 252, *252*, 586–587
   in colon, 516
   in small intestine, 514, *514*
   active transport of, 39, *39*, 257–258, *258*, 579
   as vasodilator, 137
   concentration of, in urine, 255t
   conductance of, 49–50, *49*
   control of, in extracellular fluid, 272–275, *273–275*
   cotransport of, with glucose, 515
   countertransport of, 282
   diffusion of, 35, *35*
   diffusion potential of, 47, *47*
   excretion of, 260, 271–272
      excessive, 274
   in acetylcholine channels, 70
   in aldosterone secretion, 588
   in body fluids, 32, *32*, 268, 270t
   in bone, 608
   in rod hyperpolarization, 457, *457*
   in saliva, 499, *499*
   leakage of, in sinoatrial node, 91
      through nerve membrane, 47, *47*
   membrane potentials and, 45–46, *45*
   Nernst potential of, 351
   osmosis and, 37–38, *38*
   reabsorption of, 254, 260
Sodium ion concentration, at neuronal somal membrane, 350–351, *350*
Sodium-potassium leak channels, 47, *47*
Sodium-potassium pump, 39, *39*
   in membrane potential, *45*, 46
   in resting potential, 46–47, *47*
   nerve fiber recharging by, 51, *51*
Sodium pump, at neuronal somal membrane, 350–351, *350*
Solubility coefficients, of gases, 302
Solutes. See specific solute, e.g., *Potassium ion; Sodium ion.*
Soma, 347–348, *347–348*
   resting potential of, 350–351, *350*
Somatic sensations, 368. See also *Mechanoreceptive sensation; Pain; Thermal sensation.*
Somatic senses, classification of, 368
Somatic sensory area, 345, *345*
Somatic sensory area I, 371–373, *371–372*
Somatic sensory area II, 371, *371*
Somatic sensory association area, 373
Somatic sensory cortex, 371–373, *371*, 400–401, *401*, 416, *416*
Somatomammotropin, human, 566
   in pregnancy, 644, 648
Somatomedins, 571–572
Somatostatin, in enteric plexus, 488
Somatotropic hormone. See *Growth hormone.*
Somatotropin. See *Growth hormone.*
Sound. See also *Hearing.*

Sound (*Continued*)
attenuation of, 473
conduction of, to cochlea, 472–473, *472*
direction of, 478
frequency of, 476–477
loudness of, 476
of heart. See *Heart sounds.*
patterns of, 477–478
pitch of, 476
transmission of, in cochlea, 473–474, *474*
Sour taste, 479
Space physiology, acceleratory forces in, 335–336, *336*
artificial climate in, 336
oxygen pressure in, 332–335, *333*, 333t
radiation hazards in, 336
weightlessness in, 336–337
Spasm, carpopedal, 607, *607*
laryngeal, in hypoparathyroidism, 614–615
muscular, 71, 403
from reflex, 393
vascular, 218
Spatial localization, in cerebellum, 408, *408*
Spatial orientation, in auditory system, 477
of nerve fibers, in dorsal column–lemniscal system, 371
Spatial patterns, perception of, 374, *374*
transmission of, 358–359, *358–359*
Spatial perception, in cerebral cortex, 417
Spatial summation, 66
of postsynaptic potentials, 353
of thermal sensations, 385
Speech, 301, *301*, 423
coordination of, 402, *402*
Sperm, 619–621, *620*
fertilization by, 641, *641*
flagellum of, 18
Spermatid, 620–621, *620*
Spermatocyte, 620, *620*, 626
Spermatogenesis, 619–621, *620*
feedback control of, 626
gonadotropin in, 625–626
Spermatogonia, 620, *620*, 625–626
Spermatozoon, 620, *620*
Spermiation, 621, 626
Spherical lens, 451
Sphincter. See specific structure, e.g., *Anal sphincter; Esophageal sphincter.*
Sphincter of Oddi, 505, *506–507*
Sphingomyelin, 53
Spike action potential, in smooth muscle, 73, *74*
Spike and dome pattern, in epilepsy, 432, *432*
Spinal cord, analgesic system of, 380–381, *380*
brain stem pathways to, 394, *394*
functions controlled by, 346
sensory signal transmitted by, 370, *370*
sexual sensation and, 622, *637*
transection of, 393
body temperature control by, 550
Spinal cord reflexes, activation of, 404
causing muscle spasm, 393
crossed extensor, *391*, 392
flexor, 391–392, *391*
muscle receptors in, 387–390, *388–390*
of locomotion, 392–393, *393*
organization for, 386–387, *387*
postural, 392–393
tendon, 390–391, *390*
Spinal motor neurons, stimulation of, 403–404, *403*

Spinal nerves, 133
Spinal shock, 393
Spindle, 29
Spinocerebellar tract, 408, *408*
Spinocervical pathway, 370–371, *370*
Spino-olivary pathway, 408, *408*
Spinoreticular pathway, 408, *408*
Spinothalamic tract, 375, *375*
Spiral ganglion of Corti, *472*, 475, 477, *475–476*
Spirometry, 297, *297*
Splanchnic circulation, 187–189, *187, 189*
Spleen, as reservoir, 188–189, *189*
blood cleansing function of, 189, 207
circulation in, 188–189, *189*
red blood cell destruction in, 198–199
Sports physiology, 656–667. See also *Exercise.*
body fluids in, 667
body heat in, 666–667
cardiovascular system in, 664–666, *665–666*
drugs and, 667
male vs. female athletes, 656–657
muscular metabolism in, 658–663, *658, 660, 663*
muscular strength in, 657–658
respiration in, 663–664, *663–664*
salt in, 667
Sprue, 518
Stapedius muscle, 473
Stapes, 472–475, *472, 474*
Starch, digestion of, 511, *511*
Starling equilibrium, 235–236
Starvation, 557, *557*
growth hormone and, 572
protein degradation in, 540
Static position sense, 374, *374*
Static pressure, 116–117
Static response, of spindle receptor, 388
Static stretch reflex, 389
Statoconia, 395–396, *395*
Steatorrhea, 518
causing osteomalacia, 615
Stenosis, aortic, 178–179, *178*
mitral, 178–179, *178*
of heart valves, 178, *178*
of pulmonary artery, *180*, 181
Stepping reflex, 392–393
Stercobilin, 516
Stereo sound perception, 478
Stereocilia, 396
Stereopsis, 453, *453*
Stereotyped movement, 398
Sterility, female, 638
Steroid hormones, in protein synthesis, 567
Stethoscope, heart sounds and, 177, *177*
Stigma, 631
Stilling test chart, 459
Stimulation, of action potential, 54
of reticular activating system, 426
Stimulatory field, 356
Stimulus, excitatory, 356, *356*
of pain receptors, 378–379
sensory. See *Sensory stimuli.*
subthreshold, 356, *356*
Stokes-Adams syndrome, 103
Stomach. See also *Gastric.*
emptying of, 492–493
in hunger, 554
mixing in, 491–492
motor functions of, 491–493
pain in, 382–383, *382*
storage in, 491

Storage iron, 198
Strength, muscular, 657, 662, *662*
Streptococcal infection, nephritis and, 286–287
Stress. See also *Sports physiology.*
ACTH secretion effects of, 590–591, *590*
Addisonian crisis in, 592
cortisol function in, 589
in peptic ulcer, 517
on bone, 610
Stress-relaxation, in compensated shock, 164
of blood vessels, 117
Stress response, 445
Stretch, in labor initiation, 646, *646*
Stretch receptors, 271–272
in bladder, 291
in inspiration control, 319
Stretch reflex, 389–390, *389*
Stroke, heat, 551
muscular spasm in, 403
Stroke volume, 84
in aortic lesions, 179
in exercise, 665–666, *666*
pulse pressure and, 122–123
Structural genes, 26, *26*
Strychnine, synaptic transmission effect of, 355
S-T segment shift, 106
Subconscious activity, of brain, 346–347
Sublingual glands, 499
Submandibular glands, 499
Submarines, health problems related to, 339–340
Submucosa, intestinal, anatomy of, 486, *487*
Submucosal plexus, 488
Subneural cleft, 69, *70*
Substance P, as neurotransmitter, 350
in enteric plexus, 488
Substantia gelatinosa, 379
Substantia nigra, 401, 404–406, *405*, 427, *427*
Subthalamic nucleus, 401
Subthreshold stimulus, 356
Succinyl CoA, in hemoglobin formation, 197
Sucrase, 508
Sucrose, digestion of, 511, *511*
reabsorption of, 253
Sugar, digestion of, 511, *511*
Sulfate, concentration of, in urine, 255t
in body fluids, 268, 270t
in extracellular fluid, 277
in uremia, 287
reabsorption of, 254
Summation, in neuronal pools, 357
of postsynaptic potential, 353–354
of thermal sensations, 385
Superior colliculi, 462, *463*
Superior olivary nucleus, sound direction and, 478
Superoxide, in oxygen toxicity, 338
Suppressor T cells, function of, 210, 212
Supraoptic nuclei, 573, *573*
Surface receptor proteins, 208–209
Surface tension, in lungs, 295
Surfactant, in alveoli, 295, 327
in respiratory distress syndrome, 650–651
in respiratory membrane, *310*
Surround inhibition, 374, *374*
Sustentacular cells, 481, *481*, 620, 621
Swallowing, 489–491, *490*
Sweating, 547, *547*
abolition of, 549

Sweating (*Continued*)
  control of, 190
  in exercise, 667
  in fever crisis, 551, *551*
  increased blood flow in, 190
  water loss from, 266–267, 267t
Sweet taste, 479
Sylvius, aqueduct of, 434
Sympathetic chain, 439–440, *440*
Sympathetic mediators, 441
Sympathetic nervous system, adrenal medulla and, 444
  adrenergic fibers in, 441–442
  alarm response in, 445
  anatomy of, 133, *134*, 439–440, *440*
  bronchiolar effect of, 300
  cholinergic fibers of, 441–442
  excitatory effects of, 442–443, 443t
  in arterial pressure control, 144–146, *145*, 444
  in blood flow control, 115, *115*, 133–135, *134–135*
    cerebral, 186
    coronary, 170–171
    cutaneous, 190
    gastrointestinal, 188
    muscular, 184–185
  in cardiac failure, 173–175, *173*
  in cardiac output regulation, 157, 160
  in ejaculation, 623
  in fluid volume regulation, 262
  in gastrointestinal function, 443–444, 488
  in heart control, 86–87, *86*, 93–94, 444
  in heat production, 550
  in psychosomatic disorders, 435
  in pupillary opening, 443
  in shock compensation, 163
  in sweating, 547, *547*
  in ventricular fibrillation, 172
  inhibitory effects of, 442–443, 443t
  mass discharges in, 445
  metabolic rate and, 545
  micturition and, 290, *290*
  organ effects of, 442–443, 443t
  receptors of, 442, 442t
  reflexes and, 445
  segmental distribution of, to organs, 440
  vascular effects of, 116, *116*, 444
Sympathetic tone, 444–445
Sympathetic vasoconstrictor fibers, 134
Sympathomimetic drugs, 442
Synapse(s), chemical, 347
  definition of, 347
  in information processing, 346
  memory and, 420–422, *421*
  physiological anatomy of, 347–350, *347–348*, 349t
  sensitivity of, 361
Synaptic after-discharge, 359, *359*
Synaptic body, of photoreceptor, 454–455, *454*
  of retina, 463
Synaptic cleft, 69, 348, *348*
Synaptic delay, 359
Synaptic gutter, 69, *70*
Synaptic knob. See *Presynaptic terminals.*
Synaptic receptors, sensitivity of, 361
Synaptic transmission, acidosis effects on, 355
  alkalosis effects on, 355
  dendrite function in, 354
  firing rate in, 354–355, *355*
  neuronal excitation in, 350–353, *350, 352*
  neuronal inhibition in, 352–353, *352*

Synaptic transmission (*Continued*)
  postsynaptic potential summation in, 353–354
Synaptic trough, 69, *70*
Synaptic vesicle, 348, *348*
Syncytium, cardiac muscle as, 80–81, *81*
  intestinal muscle as, 487
  drug effects on, 355
  fatigue of, 355, 361
  hypoxia effects on, 355
Syphilis, 127
Systemic circulation, 119–123, *119, 121–123*
  blood shift to pulmonary circulation, 125
Systemic filling pressure, cardiac output regulation and, 158–159
  in cardiac failure, 174
  in hemorrhagic shock, 162
Systole, 82–83, *83*, 122
  coronary blood flow in, 170, *170*
  heart sounds in, in valvular lesions, 178, *178*
  pressure at, measurement of, 140–141, *140*
    normal, 139–140, *140*
  sounds of, 177
  ventricle in, *83*, 84

T cell markers, 208–209
T cells, 207
  antigen binding of, 210–211
  B cell activation by, 209
  cytotoxic, 210–211
  helper, 210
  immune tolerance and, 211–212
  killer, 210, *210*
  regulatory, 211
  release of, 210
  specificity of, 208–209
  suppressor, 210, 212
T tubules, 63, *64*, 65
  in cardiac muscle, 81–82
T wave, 83, *83*, 98–99, *98*
  action potential and, 99–100, *99*
Tachycardia, paroxysmal, 104–105, *104–105*
Tactile hairs, 364, *364*
Tactile sensations, 368–369
Target tissue, 565
Taste, 478–480, *479–480*
  salivary secretion and, 500
Taste bud, 478–480, *479*
Tectorial membrane, 475, *475*
Tectospinal tract, 401, *403*, 404
Teeth, abnormalities of, 617
  forces on, in chewing, 489
  formation of, 616, *616*
  functions of, 615–616, *615*
  mineral exchange in, 616–617
Telophase, 28, *29*
Temperament, sex hormone effects on, 657
Temperature. See also *Body temperature.*
  diffusion effects of, 36
  perception of, 384
Temperature receptors, 548
Temporal field of vision, 467
Temporal summation, of muscle contraction, 66–67, *67*
  of postsynaptic potentials, 353–354
Tendon reflex, 390–391, *390*
Tendons, pulling of, 67
Teniae coli, 494
Tension, muscle, 390–391, *390*
Tensor tympani muscle, 473

Teratoma, 627
Terminal cisternae, 63, *64*, 65
Terminal knob, 348, *348*
Terminal(s), facilitator, 421–422, *421*
  presynaptic, 348, *348*
    excitatory, 356, *356*
    in memory, 421–422
    sensory, 421–422, *421*
Tertiary association area, 417–419, *417*
Testis, anatomy of, *620*
  descent of, 624, 644
  gonatotropin effects on, 625
  hormones of, 566
  interstitial cells of, 623–624, *623*
  tumors of, 627
Testosterone, 566
  action of, 625
  chemistry of, 624, *624*
  fetal testes and, 664
  functions of, 624–625
  in athletic performance, 656
  in spermatogenesis, 625–626
  metabolism of, 624, *624*
  secretion of, 623–624, *623*, 626
Tetanic simulation, in memory, 420–421
Tetanization, 66–67, *67*
Tetany, from hypocalcemia, 607–608, *607*
  in alkalosis, 286
  in hypoparathyroidism, 614
  in rickets, 614–615
Tetralogy of Fallot, *180*, 181
Thalamocortical system, 415–416, 427–428
Thalamus, cerebral cortex and, 415–416, *416*
  in smell, 482
  in somatic sensation, 370–371, *370–371*, 375
  motor control by, 404
  nuclei of, 405
  pain perception in, 380
  pain transmission to, 379–380, *379*
  wakefulness and, 425
Theca cells, 631
Theobromine, synaptic transmission effect of, 355
Theophylline, synaptic transmission effect of, 355
Thermal sensation, 384–385, *384*
Thermal signals, transmission of, 385
Thermogenesis, chemical, 550
Thermoreceptors, 363–364, 364t
Thermosensitive pain receptors, 378
Thermostat, hypothalamic, 548, *549*
Theta waves, 428–429, *428–429*
Thiamine, 557t, 558
  deficiency of, cardiac function in, 160
Thiamine pyrophosphate, 558
Thinking. See *Intellectual functions; Thought.*
Thiocyanate, in saliva, 500
Thirst, 274–275, *275*
Thirst center, 274, *274*
Thoracic duct, 237, *238*
Thorax. See also *Chest.*
  compliance of, 296
  expansibility of, 296
Thought, 419–423
Threshold, for action potential initiation, 50
  for excitation, of neuron, 352, 354–355
  for smell, 482
  for taste, 479
Threshold stimulus, 356, *356*
Threshold voltage, of sinoatrial node, 91, *91*

Thrombin, fibrin formation and, 220
  formation of, 220, *220*
Thrombocytopenia, 225
Thromboembolism, 225
Thromboplastin, release of, 221
Thrombosis, in atherosclerosis, 536
Thromboxane A, in platelets, 219
Thrombus, 225
  in coronary occlusion, 171
Thymine, in DNA, 21, *21–22*
Thymus gland, immune tolerance and, 211–212
  lymphocyte processing by, 207–208
Thyroglobulin, 576–578, *577*
Thyroid cartilage, 301, *301*
Thyroid cells, 577, *577*
Thyroid gland, anatomy of, 576, *577*
  blood flow in, 129, 130t
  diseases of, 581–584, *582–583*
  enlargement of. See *Goiter.*
Thyroid hormones, 565. See also *Thyroxine.*
  action of, 578, *578*
  formation of, 576–578, *577–578*
  functions of, 578–580
  growth and, 579
  in fat utilization, 535
  in protein synthesis, 567
  metabolic rate and, 545
  secretion of, 576–578, *577–578*
    regulation of, 580–581, *580*
Thyroid-stimulating hormone (TSH), 565, 570, 580–581, *580*
  in hypothyroidism, 582
Thyroid-stimulating hormone–releasing hormone, 570
Thyroiditis, 583
Thyrotoxicosis, 579–582, *582*
Thyrotropin, 580–581, *580*
  in heat production, 550
Thyrotropin-releasing hormone (TRH), 550, 581
Thyroxine, 565
  formation of, 576–577, *577–578*
  in gluconeogenesis, 529
  in heat production, 550
  metabolic rate and, 545
  release of, 578
  transport of, 578, *578*
Thyroxine-binding globulin, 578
Tickling, 383–384
Tidal volume, 297–298
Time calibration, of electrocardiogram, *98,* 100
Tissue, destruction of, as cause of pain, 377–379
  oxygen transport to, 311–312, *312*
  oxygenation of, in red blood cell production, 195–196, *196*
  transplantation of, 216
  vascularity of, changes in, 133
Tissue gel, in interstitium, 231
Tissue macrophages, 201–203, *202*
Tissue resistance, 296
Titration, of hydrogen ion with bicarbonate, 283
Tolerance, immune, 211–212
Tone, muscular, inhibition of, 405–406
  maintenance of, 403
  smooth, 76–77
Tongue, taste buds on, 479–480, *480*
Tonic contraction, of intestinal muscle, 487–488
  of smooth muscle, 76–77

Tonic receptors, 366–367
Tonotopic maps, 477
Tonsillar pillars, in swallowing, 490
Tooth. See *Teeth.*
Touch, disorders in, 373
  perception of, 365
  sensation of, 368–369
Toxemia, hypertension in, 154
Toxic goiter, 579–582, *582*
Trachea, *299,* 300
  closure of, in swallowing, 490
Tractus solitarius, 142, 318–319
  in swallowing, 490
Tranquilizers, reward-punishment and, 435
Transamination, 539–540
  pyridoxine in, 559
Transcription, insulin in, 599
  operon control of, 27
  RNA and, 22–24, *22–24,* 24t
  thyroid hormones and, 579
Transducers, in blood pressure measurement, 114, *114*
Transfer RNA, 23–24, *24–25*
Transferrin, 197–198, *198*
Transfusion. See *Blood transfusion.*
Translation, insulin in, 599
  RNA and, 24–25, *24–25*
  thyroid hormones and, 579
Transmission, neuromuscular, 69–71, *70*
  of mechanoreceptive sensation, in anterolateral system, 369–370, 374–375, *375*
    in dorsal column–lemniscal system, 369–374, *370–374*
    in peripheral nerve fibers, 369
  of pain, 379–380, *379*
    from viscera, 382
  of thermal signals, 385
Transmitter substance. See also *Neurotransmitters.*
  in action potential, 54
Transmitters. See *Neurotransmitters.*
Transplantation, 216
Transport, active. See *Active transport.*
Transport proteins, 33
Transport vesicles, 11, 14–15
Transverse tubules, 63, *64,* 65
  in cardiac muscle, 81–82
Trauma, cortisol function in, 589
  hypovolemic shock from, 166
Tremor, action, 410
  in hyperthyroidism, 580
  in Parkinson's disease, 406–407
  intention, 410
TRH (thyrotropin-releasing hormone), 550, 581
Tricarboxylic acid cycle, 525–526, *527*
Tricuspid area, for heart sounds, 177, *177*
Tricuspid valve, function of, 84
Tricyclic antidepressants, 437
Triglycerides. See also *Fat; Lipid(s).*
  digestion of, 511–512, *512*
  formation of, 515
  hydrolysis of, 532
  plasma level of, 532
  structure of, 531
  synthesis of, from carbohydrates, 534–535, *535*
    from proteins, 535
Trigone, 290, *291*
Triiodothyronine, 565
  formation of, 576–577, *577–578*
  release of, 578
  transport of, 578, *578*

Triolein, respiratory quotient of, 554
Tripping mechanism, in thirst, 275
Tristearin, 531
Trophoblastic cells, 641–642, *642*
Tropomyosin, 61, *61*
  in smooth muscle, 72
Troponin, 61, *61*
Trypsin, 503
  in protein digestion, 512, *512*
Trypsinogen, 503
TSH (thyroid-stimulating hormone), 565, 570, 580–581, *580*
  in hypothyroidism, 582
Tuberculosis, 127
  respiratory insufficiency in, 328
Tubular glands, gastrointestinal, 498, *501*
Tubular necrosis, in shock, 167
Tubules, dentinal, 616
  longitudinal, 63, *64,* 65
  micro-, *9,* 12
    in mitosis, 29
  of kidney, absorption in, 249, 252–254, *252,* 255t
    anatomy of, 248, *248*
    secretion in, 249, 252–254, *252,* 255t
    renal, potassium excretion in, 260–261
      sodium reabsorption in, 260
      urine concentration in, 257–259, *258*
      urine dilution in, 257, *257*
  sarco-, *64*
  transverse, 63, *64,* 65
    in cardiac muscle, 81–82
Tubuloglomerular feedback, 263
Tunneling operations, physiology of, 337–339, 337t
Turning movement, brain stem control of, 398
Twitch, muscular, 65–66, *66,* 662–663
Two-point discrimination test, 373, *374*
Tympanic membrane, 472–473, *472*
Typing, 412
  of blood, 214, 214t
  of tissue, 216
Tyrosine, in thyroglobulin synthesis, 577
  oxidation of, 577, *578*

Ubiquinone, 527
Ulcer, peptic, 516–518, *517*
Ulcerative colitis, mass movement in, 495
Ultrasonic Doppler flowmeter, 113, *113*
Umbilical artery, 642, *642*
Umbilical cord, anatomy of, *642*
Umbilical vein, 642, *642*
Uncus, 432, *433,* 436
  in smell, 482
Unidentified pituitary factor, 588
Uracil, in RNA, 23
Urate, absorption of, 252–254
  in extracellular fluid, 277
Urea, concentration of, in urine, 255t
  excretion of, 259–260
    conserving water and salt in, 263–264
    through placenta, 463
  formation of, 540
  in body fluids, 270t
  in extracellular fluid, 268
  reabsorption of, 253
Uremia, 287–288
  acidosis from, 285
  dialysis in, 288–289, *288,* 289t
Ureter, 290, *290*
  pain in, 382

Urethra, male, 619, *620*, 623
Urethral glands, 619, *620*
Uric acid, concentration of, in urine, 255t
  in extracellular fluid, 268
  in uremia, 287
Uridine diphosphate glucose, 524, *524*
Urinary output, after drinking, 273, *274*
  fluid volume regulation and, 261–262,
    262
  in cardiac failure, 174
  in renal–body fluid system, 147–150,
    148–149
  in renin-angiotensin system, 150, *150*
Urinary system, 248, *248*
  physiological anatomy of, 248–249, *248–
    249*
Urination, 290–291, *290–291*
Urine, formation of, 248–255
  autoregulation of, 262–263, *262*, *264*
  concentrated, 257–259, *258*
  dilute, 257, *257*. See also *Diabetes
    insipidus*.
    during hypotension, 263–264
    fluid volume control in, 261–262
    glomerular filtration and, 250–252, *250*
    plasma clearance and, 254–255
    potassium in, 260–261
    renal blood flow and, 249
    renal pressures and, 250, *250*
    sodium in, 260
    tubular activity in, 252–254, *252*, 255t
    urea in, 259–260
  in diabetes mellitus, 602
  pH of, 284
  substances in, 254, 255t
  transport of, through ureter, 290
  water loss in, 266, 267t
Urobilin, 516
Urogenital diaphragm, 290, *290*
Urticaria, 213
Uterine milk, 641
Uterus, contractions of, 645–647, *646*
  involution of, 647
  ovum implantation in, 641–642, *642*
  ovum transport to, 641
  oxytocin effect on, 574
  pain in, 383
  physiological anatomy of, 629, *630*
  progesterone effects on, 634
Utilization coefficient, 313–314
Utricle, 395, *395*, 397

Vaccination, 212
Vagina, estrogen effects on, 633
  physiological anatomy of, 629, *630*
Vagotomy, in peptic ulcer, 517–518
Vagus nerves, in cardiac function, 93, 133,
    134
  in gastric secretion, 502–503
  in gastrointestinal tract control, 488
  in respiratory control, 322, *322*
  in swallowing, 490–491
  parasympathetic fibers in, 440
  section of, 517–518
Valves, in lymphatic system, 238–239, *238–
    239*
  of heart, function of, 84–85, *84*
  venous, 121–122, *121*
Valvulae conniventes, intestinal, 512–513,
    513
Van Allen radiation belt, 336
Vapor pressure, of water, 302–303

Varicose veins, 122
Vas deferens, 619, *620*, 621
Vasa recta, 249, *249*
  in urine concentration, 258–259, *258*
Vascular. See also *Blood vessels*.
Vascular compliance, 116–117
  pulse pressure and, 122
Vascular distensibility, 115–117, *116*
Vascular fragility, vitamin C deficiency and,
    560
Vascular resistance, 111–112, *112*, 114–115,
    114–115
  at birth, 651
  units of, 114
Vascular spasm, 218
Vascularity, changes in, 133
Vasoactive intestinal polypeptide, 488
Vasoconstriction, 444–445
  in blood flow control, 134–135, *134–135*
  in gastrointestinal system, 188
  in skin, 190, 549
Vasoconstrictor tone, 134, *135*
Vasoconstrictors, 136
  arterial pressure control by, 144–146, *145*
  hypertension caused by, 152–154, *153*
  in diminished alveolar oxygen, 125
  in glomerular filtration, 263–264
  in muscular blood flow control, 184–185
Vasodilatation, 444–445
  baroreceptor reflex and, 142
  in brain oxygen deficiency, 186
  in coronary arteries, 170
  in gastrointestinal system, 188
  in skin, 190
  muscular, cardiac output regulation and,
    158–159
  smooth muscle relaxation in, 76
  thyroid hormones and, 580
Vasodilator feedback, in glomerular filtra-
    tion, 263–264
Vasodilator theory, in blood flow control,
    131
Vasodilators, 136–137
  in angina pectoris, 172–173
  in muscle, 183
Vasomotion, 229
Vasomotor center, arterial pressure regula-
    tion by, 5
  CNS ischemia and, 143
  control of, *134*, 135
  failure of, in shock, 165
  in blood flow control, 134–135, *134–135*
Vasomotor tone, 134, *135*
Vasopressin. See *Antidiuretic hormone*.
Vein(s), as blood reservoir, 122
  blood volume in, *119*
  collapse of, in standing position, 121, *121*
  dilatation of, baroreceptor reflex and,
    142
  distensibility of, 116
  function of, 118, 120–122, *121*
  lymph entering, 237, *238*
  obstruction of, cardiac output regulation
    and, 160
  pressure in. See *Venous pressure*.
  pressure-volume curves for, 116, *116*
  sympathetic stimulation of, 185
  valves of, 121–122, *121*
  varicose, 122
Velocity, of conduction, in cardiac muscle,
    81
  in nerve fibers, 54
  in skeletal muscle, 63
  of muscle contraction, 66, *66*

Venae cavae, pressure in, *119*
Venous plexus, subcutaneous, 189, *189*
Venous pressure, 119–122, *119*, *121*
  capillary pressure effects on, 232, *232*
  cardiac output regulation and, 158
  central, 120, 173, *173*
  centrifugal force effects on, 335
  in pulmonary circulation, 124–125
  portal, 188
Venous pump, 121–122
Venous return, cardiac output and, 85–86,
    157–160
  in circulatory shock, 162
  in exercise, 185
Venous system, in myocardial infarction,
    172
Ventilation. See *Alveolar ventilation; Pul-
    monary ventilation*.
Ventilation-perfusion ratio, 310–311
  in atelectasis, 327
  in emphysema, 326
  in pneumonia, 327
  in tuberculosis, 328
Ventral respiratory group, 318–320
Ventricle(s), anatomy of, 82, *82*, 123–124,
    124
  dilation of, in ventricular fibrillation, 172
  dropped beats in, 102–103, *103*
  emptying of, *83*, 84
  failure of, in aortic lesions, 179
  filling of, 83–84, *83*
  hypertrophy of, 105, *105*, *180*, 181
  ischemia of, in hypertension, 155
  mean electrical axis of, 105
  pressure in, 124, *124*
    in cardiac cycle, 82, *83*
  refractory period of, 81
  relaxation of, 84
  repolarization of, 83, *83*, 99–100, *99*
Ventricular contractions, premature, 103–
    104, *103*
Ventricular defibrillation, 96, *96*
Ventricular escape, 93, 103
Ventricular fibrillation, 95–96, *95*, 104–105,
    104
  in myocardial infarction, 172
Ventricular function curve, 86, *86*
Ventricular output curve, 86, *86*
Ventricular paroxysmal tachycardia, 104,
    104
Ventricular septum, defect of, *180*, 181
Ventricular syncytium, 81
Ventrobasal complex, 371, *371*, 375, *375*
  pain transmission to, 379–380, *379*
Ventromedial nuclei, in feeding regulation,
    554
Venules, anatomy of, 130, *130*
  function of, 118
  in microcirculation, 228–229, *229*
  pressure in, 119, *119*
Vermis, of cerebellum, 408, *408*
Vesicular follicle, 631, *631*
Vestibular apparatus, 395–397, *395–396*
  predictive function of, 366–367
Vestibular macula, 395–396, *395*
Vestibular membrane, 473–474, *474*
Vestibular nerve, 396–397, *396*
Vestibular nucleus, 394–395, *394*, 396
Vestibular sensation, 395–398, *395–396*
Vestibulocerebellar tract, 408
Vestibulospinal tract, 394, *394*, 401, *403*,
    404
Vibration, detection of, 369
  in cochlea, 474, 475

Vibration (*Continued*)
  of vocal cords, 301
  sensation of, 368–369
Villi, arachnoidal, 243, *243*
  intestinal, 512–513, *513–514*
  placental, 462, *642*
VIP (vasoactive intestinal polypeptide), 488
Viruses, neutralization of, 210–211
Visceral nucleus, 469
Visceral pain, 381–383, *382*
Visceral sensation, 368
Viscosity, of blood, in anemia, 199
Vision. See also *Eye.*
  color, cones in, 457, 458
    ganglion cells and, 465
      mechanism of, 458–459, *459-460*
      visual cortex and, 466
    contrast in, 464–466, *464, 466*
    fields of, 467, *467*
    fusion of, 458, 465
    in equilibrium maintenance, 398
    lateral geniculate body in, 465
    light adaptation in, 457–458, *458*
    pathway of, 462, *463*
    photochemistry of, 455–458, *456-458*
    retinal function in, 462–465, *463-464*
Visual acuity, 452
  fovea and, 454, *454*
Visual association area, 466–467
  of cerebral cortex, 416–417, *417*
Visual cortex, 416–418, 462, *463*
  image fusion and, 469
  primary, 465–467, *466*
Visual purple. See *Rhodopsin.*
Visual receptive aphasia, 423
Vital capacity, 298
  in tuberculosis, 328
Vitamin A, 557t, 558
  in light adaptation, 458
  in retina, 455
  in rhodopsin formation, 456, *456*
Vitamin B$_1$, 557t, 558
Vitamin B$_2$, 559
Vitamin B$_6$, 557t, 559
Vitamin B$_{12}$, 557t, 559
  in pernicious anemia, 516
  in red blood cell production, 196
Vitamin C, 557t, 560
  in newborn diet, 653
Vitamin D, 560
  deficiency of, 614–615
  in bone absorption-deposition, 612
  in calcium absorption, *606*, 606–607
  in hypoparathyroidism, 614
  in rickets, 615
Vitamin D$_3$, 606, *606*
Vitamin E, 560
Vitamin K, 560
  deficiency of, 224

Vitamins, formed in colon, 516
  in pregnancy, 645
  in red blood cell production, 196–197
  reabsorption of, 253
  requirements of, 557–558, 557t
Vitreous body, 244
Vitreous humor, 244, *244*
  refractive index of, 448–449, *448*
Vocal cords, 301, *301*
  coordination of, 402, *402*
  in swallowing, 490
Vocalization, 301, *301*, 423
Voice, testosterone effect on, 625
Voltage calibration, of electrocardiogram, *98*, 100
Voltage-gating, 48–49, *49*
  in presynaptic terminals, 348
  in sinoatrial node, 91
  of protein channels, 35, *35*
Volume-loading hypertension, 151–154, *151, 153–154*
Volume-pressure curves, in cardiac cycle, 82–83, *83*
  in edema, 240–241, *241*
  of arterial system, 116, *116*
  of lungs, in newborn, 650, *650*
  of venous system, 116, *116*
Volume receptors, 271–272
Voluntary fixation, mechanism of eye, 468
Voluntary motor activity, control of, 401–403, *401–402*
  initiation of, 390, 413
Vomiting, 519
  alkalosis from, 285–286

Wakefulness, cerebral cortex and, 347
  electroencephalogram in, 429, *429*
  in hypothalamic lesions, 430
  neuronal reverberation in, 360
  reticular activating system in, 425–428, *426–427*
  vs. sleep, 430–431
Walk-along theory of contraction, 61–62, *62*
Walking, energy expenditure in, 545t
  reflexes in, 392–393, *393*
  spinal cord control of, 346
Warmth receptors, 548
Water. See also *Body water.*
  absorption of, 252–253
    in colon, 516
    in small intestine, 513–514
  conservation of, 257–259, *258*, 263–264
  diffusion of, through capillary membranes, 230
    through cell membrane, 34
    through permeable membrane, 37–38, *38*

Water (*Continued*)
  evaporation of, in heat loss, 546–547, *546*
  excretion of, 257, *257*. See also *Diuresis.*
    in essential hypertension, 154
  formation of, in metabolism, 526–527, *527*
  gases in, partial pressures of, 302
  intake vs. output, 148–149, *148, 149*
  osmosis of, 270–271, *270*
    in small intestine, 514, *514*
  reabsorption of, 259
  retention of, in hypertension, 151–152
  secretion of, glandular, 498
    in large intestine, 508
  vapor pressure of, 302–303
    at high altitude, *333*, 333t
Water diuresis, 273, *274*
Wave summation, of muscle contraction, 66–67, *67*
Waves, brain, 428–429, *428–429*
  in electrocardiogram, 83, *83*, 98, *98*
  in small intestine, 493–494
  in stomach wall, 491–492
  micturition, 291
Weber-Fechner principle, 367
Wedge pressure, 125
Weight. See *Body weight.*
Weightlessness, in space, 336–337
Wernicke's aphasia, 423
Wernicke's area, 417–419, *417*
White blood cells. See *Leukocytes.*
White light, perception of, 459
Windows, of ear, *472, 474, 474*
Withdrawal reflex, 391–392, *391*
Word blindness, 417–418, 423, 467
Word deafness, 423
Words, formation of, 402, *402*
Work, of breathing, 296
Work output, in exercise, 665, *665*
Wound healing, cortisol effect on, 590
  vitamin C deficiency and, 560
Writing, 412

X chromosomes, 620, 641

Y chromosomes, 620, 641
Young-Helmholtz theory, 458–459

Z disc, in myofibrils, 58, *58*, 61
Zona glomerulosa cells, 593
Zona pellucida, 641